Williams'
Basic Nutrition
and Diet Therapy

EDITION
16

Williams' Basic Nutrition and Diet Therapy

Staci Nix, MS, RDN

Assistant Professor (Lecturer)
Department of Nutrition and Integrative Physiology
Adjunct Faculty, College of Nursing and School of Medicine
University of Utah
Salt Lake City, Utah

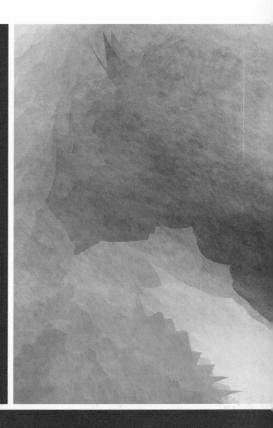

ELSEVIER

Elsevier
3251 Riverport Lane
St. Louis, Missouri 63043

Notice

International Standard Book Number: 978-0-323-65376-3

Senior Content Strategist: Sandy Clark
Senior Content Development Manager: Lisa P. Newton
Publishing Services Manager: Julie Eddy
Senior Project Managers: Richard Barber and Rachel E. McMullen
Design Direction: Renee Duenow

Printed in India

Last digit is the print number: 9   8   7   6   5   4   3   2

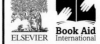

Working together
to grow libraries in
developing countries

www.elsevier.com • www.bookaid.org

Contributors

Theresa Dvorak, MS, RDN, CSSD, ATC
Assistant Professor (Lecturer)
Department of Nutrition and Integrative Physiology
University of Utah
Salt Lake City, Utah

Dana Gershenoff, MS, RDN, CDCES
Program Manager, Diabetes Professional Services
International Diabetes Center
Minneapolis, Minnesota

Melody Kienholz, BS, RDN, CSR
Renal Dietitian
Intermountain Medical Center Dialysis
Murray, Utah

Hailey Morris, MS, RDN
Graduate Student
University of Utah
Salt Lake city, Utah

Stacie Wing-Gaia, PhD, RDN, CSSD
Assistant Professor
Department of Exercise and Nutrition Sciences
Weber State University
Ogden, Utah

Kary Woodruff, PhD, RDN, CSSD
Assistant Professor (Lecturer)
Director of Clinical Experiences, Coordinated Master's
    Program
Department of Nutrition and Integrative Physiology
University of Utah
Salt Lake City, Utah

Jean Zancanella, MS, RDN
Associate Director, Coordinated Master's Program
Department of Nutrition and Integrative Physiology
University of Utah
Salt Lake City, Utah

ATC, Certified Athletic Trainer; *CDCES,* Certified Diabetes Care and Educator Specialist; *CSR,* Board Certification as a Specialist in Renal Nutrition; *CSSD,* Board Certified Specialist in Sports Dietetics; *RDN,* Registered Dietitian Nutritionist.

Reviewers

Kim Clevenger, EdD, MSN, RN, BC
Associate Professor of Nursing
Nursing
Morehead State University
Morehead, Kentucky

Kimberley Kelly, DNP, MSN, BSN, RN
School Director & VN Program Director The Vocational
  Nursing Institute Inc.
President of The Vocational Nursing Institute Inc.
CEO Compliance Review Services Inc.
Nursing Education Administration
The Vocational Nursing Institute, Inc.
Houston, Texas

Sandra A. Ranck, MSN, RN
Auburn Career Center
Concord Township, Ohio

Elizabeth A. Summers, MSN, CNE, RN
Coordinator of Practical Nursing Program
Cass Career Center
Harrisonville, Missouri

Preface

The field of nutrition is a dynamic human endeavor that is continuously expanding and evolving. Three main factors continue to change the face of nutrition. First, the science of nutrition continues to grow rapidly with exciting research. Discoveries in any field of science challenges some traditional ideas and lends to the development of new ones. Instead of focusing on nutrition in the treatment of disease, scientist and practitioners are expanding the search for disease prevention and life enhancement through optimized nutrition and healthy lifestyles. Thus was the spirit as scientists established the current Dietary Reference Intakes. Second, the rapidly increasing diversity of the United States population enriches our food patterns and presents a variety of health care opportunities and needs. Third, the public is increasingly aware of, and concerned about, health promotion and the role of nutrition. Clients and patients seek more self-directed involvement in their health care, and an integral part of that care is adequate and balanced nutrition.

This new edition continues to reflect upon the evolving face of nutrition science and evidence-based guidelines. Its guiding principle is our own commitment, along with that of our publisher, to the integrity of the material. Our goal is to produce a new book for today's needs, with updated content reflecting the most recently available scientific literature, and to meet the expectations and changing needs of students, faculty, and basic health care practitioners.

AUDIENCE

We have designed this text for students in nursing programs and for diet technicians or aides. It is also appropriate for programs in various allied health care professions.

CONCEPTUAL APPROACH

The purpose of this text is to introduce the foundational scientific principles of nutrition and their applications in person-centered care. As in previous editions, we make every attempt to explain new concepts carefully as we introduce them. In addition, our personal concerns are ever present, as follows: (1) that this introduction to the science and practice we love will continue to lead students and readers to enjoy learning about nutrition and stimulate further reading in areas of personal interest; (2) that caretakers will be alert to nutrition news and questions raised by their increasingly diverse clients and patients; and (3) that contact and communication with professionals in the field of nutrition will help build a strong team approach to clinical nutrition problems in all patient care.

ORGANIZATION

In keeping with the previous format, we have updated content to reflect current best practices and evidence-based guidelines.

In **Part 1,** *Introduction to Basic Principles of Nutrition Science,* Chapter 1 focuses on the directions of health care and health promotion, risk reduction for disease prevention, and community health care delivery systems, with emphasis on team-based care and the active role of clients in self-care. Descriptions and illustrations accompany the *Healthy People 2030,* the *Dietary Guidelines for Americans 2020-2025,* and the MyPlate guidelines. We have incorporated the Dietary Reference Intakes (DRIs) throughout chapter discussions in Part 1 as well as throughout the rest of the text. Current research updates all of the macronutrient, micronutrient, and energy chapters in the remainder of Part 1.

In **Part 2,** *Nutrition throughout the Life Cycle,* Chapters 10, 11, and 12 reflect current material on human growth and development needs in different parts of the life cycle. We reinforce the current guidelines for appropriate weight gain to meet the metabolic demands of pregnancy and lactation. Chapter 11 emphasizes the nutrient needs to support growth and the establishment of healthy eating habits throughout infancy, childhood, and adolescence. Chapter 12 focuses on sustaining a healthy lifestyle to reduce disease risks and support health maintenance for an aging adult population. In all cases, statistics represent the most recent publications available at the time of print.

In **Part 3,** *Community Nutrition and Health Care,* we have coordinated a strong focus on community nutrition with an emphasis on weight management and physical fitness as they pertain to health care benefits and risk reduction. We discuss the Nutrition Labeling and Education Act in terms of its current regulations and label format as well as its effects on food marketing. Chapter 13 covers and illustrates the complex issues of malnutrition and the cycle of despair. Highlights of food-borne diseases reinforce concerns about food safety in a changing marketplace. Chapter 14 highlights information on America's multiethnic cultural food patterns and various religious dietary practices. A seasoned educator in the cultural aspects of food made meaningful contributions and updates to this chapter. New information on the topics of obesity and genetics, along with the use of alternative weight-loss methods, is included in Chapter 15 by a certified specialist in weight management. A certified sports dietitian updated Chapter 16 and it discusses aspects of athletics, the proliferation of sports drinks, and the performance benefits of a well-hydrated and nourished athlete.

In **Part 4,** *Clinical Nutrition,* we have updated the chapters to reflect current medical nutrition therapy and approaches to nutrition education and management. As with previous editions, Drug-Nutrient Interaction boxes in this section address specific concerns with nutrition and medication interactions. Specific topics include developments in nutrition support, gastrointestinal disease, heart disease, diabetes mellitus, renal disease, surgery, cancer, and HIV. A certified diabetes care and educator specialist joined the team to update the content for Chapter 20 on nutrition for individuals with diabetes mellitus. Likewise, a certified renal dietitian provided updates to Chapter 21 on nutrition intervention for diseases of the kidneys. And an expert in medical nutrition therapy contributed updates to Chapter 22 on nutrition support.

CONTENT AND FEATURES

- **Book format and design.** The chapter format and use of color continue to enhance the book's appeal. Chapter concepts and overview, illustrations, tables, boxes, definitions, headings, and subheadings make the content easier to read and follow.
- **Learning supplements.** We have developed educational aids to assist both students and instructors in the teaching and learning process. Please see the *Ancillaries* section on the next page for more detailed information.
- **Illustrations.** Color illustrations, including artwork, graphs, charts, and photographs, help students and practitioners better understand the concepts and clinical practices presented.
- **Content threads.** This book shares an equivalent reading level and a number of features with other Elsevier books intended for students in demanding and fast-paced nursing curricula. Common features include; Key Concepts; Key Terms; Critical Thinking Questions; Chapter Challenge Questions; References; Further Reading and Resources; Glossary; and Cultural Considerations, For Further Focus, Drug-Nutrient Interactions, and Clinical Applications boxes. These common threads help promote and hone the skills these students must master. (See the Content Threads page after this preface for more detailed information on these learning features.)

LEARNING AIDS

This edition is especially significant because of its use of many learning aids throughout the text.

- **Part openers.** To provide the "big picture" of the book's overall focus on nutrition and health, we have introduced the four main sections as successive developing parts of that unifying theme.
- **Chapter openers.** To draw students immediately into the topic for study, each chapter opens with a short list of the basic concepts involved and a brief chapter overview leading into the topic to "set the stage."
- **Chapter headings.** Throughout each chapter, we have organized the material using special font or color to indicate the major headings and subheadings, providing easy reading and understanding of the key ideas. We have highlighted the main concepts and terms with bold type and italics.
- **Special boxes.** The inclusion of For Further Focus, Cultural Considerations, Drug-Nutrient Interactions, and Clinical Applications boxes leads students a step further on a given topic or presents a case study for analysis. These boxes enhance understanding of concepts through further exploration or application.
- **Case studies.** We have provided case studies to focus students' attention on related patient care problems within the **Next-Generation NCLEX® Examination-Style Unfolding Case Study** boxes. Questions for case analysis accompany each case. Students can use these examples for similar patient care needs in their own clinical assignments.
- **Diet therapy guides.** In clinical chapters, medical nutrition therapy guides provide practical help in patient care and education.
- **Definitions of terms.** We have presented the key terms important to students' understanding and application of the material in patient care in two ways. We have identified them in the body of the text and have listed them in a glossary at the back of the book for quick reference.
- **Summaries.** A brief summary in bulleted format reviews chapter highlights and helps students see how the chapter contributes to the book's "big picture." Students then can return to any part of the material for repeated study and clarification of details as needed.
- **Chapter Review Questions.** We have provided self-test questions in multiple-choice format at the end of each chapter to allow students to test their basic knowledge of the chapter's contents. In addition, each chapter includes Next-Generation NCLEX® Examination-style Case Study scenarios and questions.
- **References.** References throughout the text provide resources used in each chapter for students who may want to probe a particular topic of interest.
- **Further Reading and Resources.** To encourage further reading of useful materials, expand students' knowledge of key concepts, and help students apply material in practical ways for patient care and education, we have provided a brief list of annotated resources—including books, journals, and websites—at the end of the book.

ANCILLARIES

TEACHING AND LEARNING RESOURCES FOR THE INSTRUCTORS

Instructor Resources on Evolve: available at www.evolve.elsevier.com/Williams/basic/—provides a wealth of material to help you make your nutrition instruction a success. In addition to all of the Student Resources, we have provided the following for faculty:

- **TEACH Lesson Plans:** Modifiable lesson plans, based on the textbook chapter, provide a complete road map to link all parts of the educational package together. Instructors can modify or combine these lesson plans to meet particular scheduling and teaching needs.
- **Exam View Test Bank:** Contains approximately 700 multiple-choice and alternate-format questions for the NCLEX Examination. We have coded each question for correct answer, rationale, page reference, Nursing Process Step, NCLEX Client Needs Category, and Cognitive Level.
- **Image Collection:** Instructors may use these images in a unique presentation or as visual aids.
- **PowerPoint Presentations** with incorporated **Audience Response Questions** and unfolding **Case Study** to accompany each chapter.

FOR STUDENTS

- **Evolve Resources**
  - **Answers to Textbook Case Studies**—Students may find answers to detailed case studies in specific chapters of the textbook.
  - **Case Studies** engage students with the opportunity to apply the knowledge they have learned in real-life situations.
  - **Infant and Child Growth Charts, United States** are available to practice plotting and interpreting growth and development of children and adolescents.
  - **Self-Test Questions:** More than 350 self-assessment questions that provide students with practice questions and immediate feedback to help them prepare for exams.

- **Nutrition Resource Center website:** This informative website is available at http://nutrition.elsevier.com to provide the reader access to information about all Elsevier nutrition texts in one convenient location.

ACKNOWLEDGMENTS

Throughout this process, various staff members from Elsevier have kindly provided guidance and assistance, and I am grateful to them all. I would especially like to acknowledge the professionalism, fortitude, and diligence of Sandy Clark, Senior Content Strategist; Lisa P. Newton, Senior Content Development Manager; Richard Barber and Rachel McMullen, Senior Project Managers; and Renee Duenow, Design Director. Your vision for this text is the true power behind the print.

I would like to acknowledge the hard work and dedication of Sue Rodwell Williams, who began this series of nutrition texts designed for health care professionals and Elsevier's Nursing Marketing Department for supporting this book through its many editions. Their ability to bridge the gap between a product and the end point—students who will hopefully learn from and enjoy this text—is integral to the success of this project. The contributions from content experts covering pregnancy, lactation, childhood nutrition, cultural aspects of food, weight management, sports nutrition, nutrition support, diabetes, and renal nutrition lend an element of expertise to those chapters that will increase the value of the text overall. In addition, I am grateful to the reviewers who have provided constructive feedback on this edition. Your involvement provides the strength and thoroughness that authors cannot accomplish alone.

Finally, I want to thank my husband, family, and friends who have compassionately dealt with "the book" and me. Your abundant support sustains me.

Staci Nix

Contents

Food, Nutrition, and Health

Key Concepts

- Optimal personal and community nutrition are major components of health promotion and disease prevention.
- Nutrients in food are essential to our health and well-being.
- Food and nutrient guides help us to plan a balanced diet that is in accordance with our individual needs and goals.

We live in a world of rapidly changing elements, including our environment, food supply, population, and scientific knowledge. Within different environments, our bodies, emotional responses, needs, and health goals determine our individual nutrient needs. The study of food, nutrition, and health care focuses on **health promotion** from the individual level through the community level. Although we may define health and disease in a variety of ways, the primary basis for promoting health and preventing disease begins with a balanced diet and the nutrition it provides. The study of nutrition is of primary importance in the following two ways: it is fundamental for our own health, and it is essential for the health and well-being of our patients and clients.

HEALTH PROMOTION

BASIC DEFINITIONS

Nutrition and Dietetics

Nutrition is the food people eat and how their bodies use it. **Nutrition science** is the body of scientific knowledge that governs nutrient requirements for all aspects of life such as growth, activity, reproduction, and tissue maintenance. **Dietetics** is the health profession responsible for applying nutrition science to promote human health and treat disease. The nutrition authority on the health care team is the **registered dietitian nutritionist (RDN)** (also referred to as a *clinical nutrition specialist, a registered dietitian,* or a *public health nutritionist*). This health care professional carries the major responsibility of nutrition care for patients and clients.

Health and Wellness

High-quality nutrition supports good health throughout life, beginning with prenatal life and continuing through the end of life during advanced years. In its simplest terms, the word **health** is defined as the absence of disease. However, life experience shows that the definition of health is much more complex. It must include extensive attention to the roots of health for the meeting of basic needs (e.g.,

physical, mental, psychologic, and social well-being). This approach recognizes the individual as a whole and relates health to both internal and external environments. The concept of *wellness* broadens this approach one step further. Wellness seeks the full development of potential for all people within their given environments. It implies a balance between activities and goals, work and leisure, lifestyle choices and health risks, and personal needs versus others' expectations. The term *wellness* implies a positive dynamic state that motivates a person to seek a higher level of functioning, in which nutrition plays a chief role.

National Health Goals

The wellness movement continues to be a fundamental response to the burden of illness, disease treatment, and the rising costs of medical care on the health care system. Holistic health promotion focuses on personal choice when it comes to helping individuals and families

---

health promotion the active engagement in behaviors or programs that advance positive well-being.

nutrition the sum of the processes involved with the intake of nutrients as well as assimilating and using them to maintain body tissue and provide energy; a foundation for life and health.

nutrition science the body of science, developed through controlled research, that relates to the processes involved in nutrition internationally, clinically, and in the community.

dietetics the management of the diet and the use of food; the science concerned with nutrition planning and the preparation of foods.

registered dietitian nutritionist (RDN) a professional dietitian accredited with an academic degree from an undergraduate or graduate study program who has passed required registration examinations administered by the Commission on Dietetic Registration (CDR). The RDN and RD (registered dietitian) credentials are legally protected titles that may be used only by authorized practitioners. The term *nutritionist* alone is not a legally protected or licensed title in most states. See www.eatright.org for more details.

health a state of optimal physical, mental, and social well-being; relative freedom from disease or disability.

establish and sustain healthy lifestyles. The U.S. national health goals reflect this wellness philosophy in the *Healthy People* series published by the U.S. Department of Health and Human Services. The *Healthy People 2030* framework encompasses broad overarching goals and topic-specific objectives with the ultimate vision of a "society in which all people can achieve their full potential for health and well-being across the lifespan" (Figure 1.1).[1]

A major theme throughout the report is the access to and encouragement of healthy food choices, weight control, and education about modifiable nutrition-related risk factors for disease. The *Healthy People 2030* topics, objectives, interventions, resources, and national data are available on their website (www.healthypeople. gov). Some of the goals in the *Nutrition and Healthy Eating* category include the following:

- Promoting healthier food access
- Improving the presence of nutrition in the health care and worksite settings
- Improving the overall healthy weight status of the nation's population
- Reducing food insecurity
- Improving quality of food and nutrient consumption
- Reducing iron deficiency

The Leading Health Indicators are a small subset of the *Healthy People* objectives identified as high-priority issues affecting the overall health of the nation. Several indicators fall within the Nutrition and Healthy Eating category. The most recent course review did not find significant improvements in these nutrition-related Leading Health Indicators. In a nutshell, rising obesity and low vegetable consumption remain national health concerns in all age groups.[2] The Advisory Committee for *Healthy People 2030* are exploring creative means to foster collaboration among agencies at the national, state, local, and tribal levels, including public, private, and nonprofit sectors to achieve a healthier nation.[3]

Traditional and Preventive Approaches to Health

The preventive health care approach identifies existing risk factors and encourages positive lifestyle changes to reduce those risks *before* disease development. Alternatively, the traditional health care approach attempts treatment *after* symptoms of illness or disease exist (see the Drug-Nutrient Interaction box, "Introduction to Drug-Nutrient Interactions"). The traditional health care approach has much less value for lifelong positive health. Major chronic conditions (e.g., heart disease, cancer, diabetes) often develop long before overt symptoms arise.

🔗 Drug-Nutrient Interactions
SARA HARCOURT

Part of the traditional approach to medicine is "curing" the condition or disease. This often includes medications, surgery, or other interventions to alleviate symptoms or to treat the condition. For the purpose of the Drug-Nutrient Interaction boxes in this text, we will focus on the potential for interactions with nutrients in the diet and medications.

It is important to follow drug regimens strictly. Consuming some medications inappropriately can have potentially dangerous side effects, such as heart arrhythmias, hypertension, dizziness, and tingling in the hands and feet. Furthermore, some medications may interact with nutrients in food or dietary supplements, thereby creating a drug-nutrient interaction. The presence of food in the stomach may increase or decrease drug absorption, thus potentially enhancing or diminishing the effects of the intended medication. Consuming dietary supplements that contain vitamins and minerals at the same time as certain medications can pose potential risk. Knowing when a nutrient may influence the function of a drug and how to work with a client's diet is essential to the development of a complete medical plan.

In the following chapters of this book, look for the Drug-Nutrient Interaction boxes to learn about some of the more common interactions that may be encountered in the health care setting.

Healthy People 2030

Mission
To promote, strengthen, and evaluate the nation's efforts to improve the health and well-being of all people.

Overarching Goals
- Attain healthy, thriving lives and well-being free of preventable disease, disability, injury, and premature death.
- Eliminate health disparities, achieve health equity, and attain health literacy to improve the health and well-being of all.
- Create social, physical, and economic environments that promote attaining the full potential for health and well-being for all.
- Promote healthy development, healthy behaviors, and well-being across all life stages.
- Engage leadership, key constituents, and the public across multiple sectors to take action and design policies that improve the health and well-being of all.

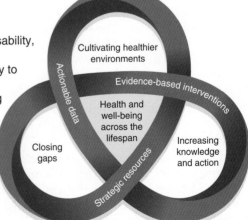

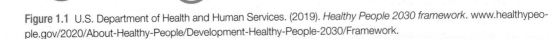

Figure 1.1 U.S. Department of Health and Human Services. (2019). *Healthy People 2030 framework*. www.healthypeople.gov/2020/About-Healthy-People/Development-Healthy-People-2030/Framework.

IMPORTANCE OF A BALANCED DIET

Signs of Good Nutrition

Health care professionals use a variety of markers to assess nutritional well-being. Physical appearance (e.g., health of eyes and hair), anthropometric measurements (e.g., weight, body composition), and biochemical markers (e.g., blood lipid levels, iron status) are a few of the objective indicators used to evaluate nutrition status. Well-nourished individuals are more able to recover from injury or illness and resist infectious diseases as compared with undernourished people. This is particularly important with our current trends of population growth and ever-increasing life expectancy. The national vital statistics report of 2019 stated that life expectancy in the United States is 76.1 years for men and 81.1 years for women, a slight decline over the previous 2 years.[4]

Food and Health

Food is a necessity of life. Our life situation and food choices (or limitations) will determine whether our bodies receive all of the components of proper nutrition. Nutrients may be categorized in many different ways, such as **essential** and **nonessential nutrients**; **energy-yielding** and **non–energy-yielding nutrients**; water-soluble and fat-soluble nutrients. For now, we will briefly discuss the six essential nutrients in human nutrition, which are the following:

Carbohydrates	Vitamins
Proteins	Minerals
Fats	Water

The core practitioners of the health care team (e.g., physician, dietitian, nurse) are aware of the important part that food plays in maintaining good health and recovering from illness. Therefore, assessing a client's nutrition status and identifying his or her nutrient needs are primary activities in the development of a personalized health care plan.

FUNCTIONS OF NUTRIENTS

To sustain life, the nutrients in foods must perform the following three basic functions within the body: provide energy, build tissue, and regulate metabolic processes.

Metabolism refers to the sum of all body processes that accomplish the basic life-sustaining tasks. Close relationships exist among all nutrients and their metabolic products. This is the fundamental principle of *nutrient interaction,* which involves two concepts. First, the individual nutrients have many specific metabolic functions, including primary and supporting roles. Second, no nutrient ever works alone; the following chapters clearly demonstrate this principle of nutrient interaction. Although scientists may separate nutrients for study purposes, remember that they do not exist that way in the human body nor in the food that we eat. They always interact as a dynamic whole to produce and maintain the body.

ENERGY SOURCES

We measure human energy in units called **kilocalories** (abbreviated as *kcalories* or *kcal*). Of the six essential nutrients, there are three energy-yielding nutrients. These include carbohydrates, fat, and protein. Alcohol is the only other energy-yielding substance in the diet. Because alcohol has no essential function in the body, it is not a *nutrient,* but it does provide 7 kcal per gram when consumed.

Carbohydrates

Dietary carbohydrates (e.g., starches, sugars) are the body's primary and preferred source of fuel for energy. Carbohydrates also maintain the body's reserve store of quick energy as **glycogen** (see Chapter 2). Each gram of carbohydrate consumed yields 4 kcal of body energy. In a well-balanced diet, carbohydrates from all sources should provide approximately 45% to 65% of the total kilocalories.

Fats

Dietary fats from both animal and plant sources provide the body's secondary or storage form of energy. This form is more concentrated, yielding 9 kcal for each gram consumed. In a well-balanced diet, fats should provide about 20% to 35% of the total kilocalories. Approximately two-thirds of this amount should be from plant sources, which provide monounsaturated and polyunsaturated fats, and no more than 10% of kilocalories should come from saturated fat (see Chapter 3).

---

essential nutrient a nourishing substance that a person must obtain from food because the body cannot make it for itself in sufficient quantity to meet physiologic needs.

nonessential nutrient a substance (e.g., saturated fat) that can be manufactured in the body by means of other nutrients. Thus, it is not essential to consume this nutrient regularly in the diet.

energy-yielding nutrient an essential nourishing substance that breaks down to yield energy within the body, including carbohydrate, fat, and protein.

non–energy-yielding nutrient a nourishing substance that does not break down to yield energy within the body, including vitamins, minerals, and water.

metabolism the sum of all chemical changes that take place in the body by which it maintains itself and produces energy for its functioning; products of the various reactions are called *metabolites.*

kilocalorie the general term *calorie* refers to a unit of heat measure, and it is used alone to designate the small calorie; the calorie that is used in nutrition science and the study of metabolism is the large Calorie, or kilocalorie, which avoids the use of large numbers in calculations; a kilocalorie, which is composed of 1000 calories, is the measure of heat that is necessary to raise the temperature of 1000 g (1 L) of water by 1° C.

glycogen a polysaccharide; the main storage form of carbohydrate in the body, which is stored primarily in the liver and muscle tissue.

Proteins

Ideally, the body will not use protein for energy. Rather, the body preserves protein for other critical functions, such as structure, enzyme and hormone production, fluid balance, and so on. However, if necessary energy from carbohydrates and fat is insufficient, the body may draw from dietary or tissue protein to obtain required energy. When used for energy, protein yields 4 kcal/g. In a well-balanced diet, protein should provide approximately 10% to 35% of the total kilocalories (see Chapter 4).

Thus, the recommended intake of each energy-yielding nutrient, as a percent of total kilocalories, is as follows:

- Carbohydrate: 45% to 65%
- Fat: 20% to 35%
- Protein: 10% to 35%

Figure 1.2 illustrates the acceptable ranges of caloric intake for each macronutrient as part of the whole diet. Because individual needs vary, there are no exact recommendations for any macronutrient. If the diet is on the lower end of kilocalories from one of the macronutrients, then a necessary increase in percentage of total kilocalories will come from one or both of the other macronutrients.

TISSUE BUILDING

Proteins

The primary function of protein is tissue building. **Amino acids** are the building blocks of protein that are necessary for constructing and repairing body tissues (e.g., organs, muscles, cells, blood proteins). Tissue building is a constant process that ensures the growth and maintenance of a strong body structure as well as the creation of vital substances for cellular functions.

Other Nutrients

Several other nutrients contribute to the building and maintenance of tissues. The following sections provide some examples.

Vitamins and minerals. Vitamins and minerals are essential nutrients that help to regulate many body processes. An example of the use of a vitamin in tissue building is that of vitamin C in developing collagen. Collagen is the protein found in fibrous tissues such as cartilage, bone

matrix, skin, and tendons. Two major minerals, calcium and phosphorus, participate in building and maintaining bone tissue. Another example is the mineral iron, which contributes to building the oxygen-carrier protein hemoglobin in red blood cells. Chapters 7 and 8 cover several other vitamins and minerals in detail with regard to their functions, which include tissue building.

Fatty acids. Fatty acids, the building blocks of lipids, help form the **phospholipids** that are necessary in all cell membranes. In addition, fatty acids facilitate the transport of fat-soluble nutrients throughout the body in the form of **lipoproteins**.

REGULATION AND CONTROL

The multiple chemical processes in the body that are necessary for providing energy and building tissue are carefully regulated and controlled to maintain a constant dynamic balance among all body parts and processes. Several of these regulatory functions involve essential nutrients. The following are a few examples.

Vitamins

Many vitamins function as coenzyme factors, which are components of cell enzymes, in the governing of chemical reactions during metabolism. This is true for most of the B-complex vitamins. In other words, the body must have an adequate supply of the B vitamins to yield energy (in the form of adenosine triphosphate [ATP]) from the metabolism of the energy-yielding nutrients (see Chapter 7).

Minerals

Many minerals also serve as coenzyme factors with enzymes in cell metabolism. For example, cobalt, which is a central constituent of vitamin B_{12} (cobalamin), functions with this vitamin in the synthesis of heme for hemoglobin formation.

Water and Fiber

Water and fiber also function as regulatory agents. In fact, water is the fundamental agent for life, providing the essential base for all metabolic processes. The adult body is approximately 50% to 70% water. Dietary fiber helps to regulate the passage of food material through the gastrointestinal tract, and it influences the absorption of nutrients.

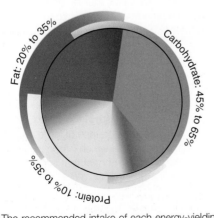

Figure 1.2 The recommended intake of each energy-yielding nutrient as a percentage of total energy intake.

amino acids the nitrogen-bearing compounds that form the structural units of protein; after digestion, amino acids are available for the synthesis of required proteins.

phospholipids class of lipids that are structural to the lipid bilayer of cell membranes. Composed of a glycerol backbone with two fatty acids and a phosphate group.

lipoprotein chemical complexes of fat and protein that serve as the major carriers of lipids in the plasma; they vary in density according to the size of the fat and protein load being carried (i.e., the lower the protein density, the higher the fat load); the combination package with water-soluble protein makes possible the transport of non–water-soluble fatty substances in the water-based blood circulation.

STATES OF NUTRITION

OPTIMAL NUTRITION

Receiving and using adequate nutrients through a varied and balanced diet facilitates the opportunity for achieving optimal nutrition. Balancing the intake of each essential nutrient covers the variations in health and disease and provides reserve supplies without unnecessary excesses.

MALNUTRITION

Malnutrition is a condition resulting from improper or insufficient diet. Both *undernutrition* and *overnutrition* are forms of malnutrition. Dietary surveys have shown that the average American diet is suboptimal. Intakes of fruits, vegetables, and dairy foods or dairy substitutes are lower than the recommended intake levels.[2] Meanwhile, the average consumption of undesirable components such as saturated fat, added sugar, alcohol, and sodium is considerably higher than recommended.[5] That does not necessarily mean that all of these individuals are malnourished. Nevertheless, it does indicate poor or limited dietary choices and suboptimal nutrient intake. Some people can maintain health on somewhat less than the optimal amounts of various nutrients in a state of borderline nutrition. However, on average, someone who is persistently receiving inadequate essential nutrients has a greater risk for physical illness and compromised immunity as compared with someone who is receiving optimal nutrition. This is particularly important for the very young and those of advanced age.[6] Such nutritionally deficient people are limited with regard to their physical work capacity, immune system function, and cognitive ability. They lack the nutrient reserves to meet added physiologic or metabolic demands from injury or illness or to sustain fetal development during pregnancy or proper growth during childhood.[7] This state may result from many situations including poor eating habits, a continuously stressful environment with little or no available food, or a disease state.

Undernutrition

Undernutrition, a subcategory of malnutrition, occurs when a person experiences depleted nutrient reserves and nutrient and energy intakes are not sufficient to meet daily needs or added metabolic stress. Many undernourished people live in conditions of poverty or illness. Such conditions influence the health of all involved but especially that of the most vulnerable populations: pregnant women, infants, children, and elderly adults. In the United States, one of the wealthiest countries in the world, widespread hunger and undernutrition still exist, which indicates that food security problems involve urban development issues, economic policies, and more general poverty-related issues (see the Cultural Considerations box, "Food Insecurity").

🌐 Cultural Considerations

Food Insecurity

Food insecurity is defined as the limited or uncertain availability of nutritious and adequate food. Fifteen million American households (i.e., 11.8% of all U.S. households) experience food insecurity annually. Homes with children report a significantly higher rate of food insecurity as compared with homes without children (15.7% and 10%, respectively).[1] *Hunger* is a chronic issue (i.e., persisting 8 months or more per year) within households that report food insecurity. There is widespread hunger and malnutrition among individuals living at or below the poverty level (defined as a household annual income of $24,858 for a family of four). The prevalence of food insecurity is disproportionally high in households that are headed by single mothers and in African-American and Hispanic households.[1]

Feeding America, which is the nation's largest organization of emergency food providers, "secures and provides food to families struggling with hunger, educates the public about the issue of hunger, and advocates for policies that protect people from going hungry."[2] The most recent *Hunger in America* report noted that 12 million children in the United States receive emergency food services annually. In addition, approximately 5% of *Feeding America* clients have completed some college or a 2-year college degree, and 5.7% have completed a 4-year college degree or higher level of education. College campuses are not immune to food insecurity or hunger: 10% of *Feeding America* clients are adults that are currently enrolled in higher education at part-time or full-time student status.[2]

Malnourished children are at an increased risk for stunted growth and episodes of infection and disease, which often have lasting effects on their intellectual development. Such problems may manifest as physical, psychologic, and sociofamilial disturbances in all age groups, with a significant negative impact on health status (including mental health), the quality of life, and the risk of chronic disease.[3] College students experiencing food insecurity report higher rates of depression and poorer academic performance than their food-secure counterparts.[4,5]

In addition to services offered by *Feeding America*, a variety of federal and nonfederal programs are available to address hunger issues in all cultural and age groups, such as the Supplemental Nutrition Assistance Program (SNAP), the Special Supplemental Nutrition Program for Women, Infants, and Children (WIC), and the National School Lunch Program (NSLP). The U.S. Department of Agriculture's Food and Nutrition Service provides detailed information about such programs on its website: www.fns.usda.gov.

REFERENCES
1. Coleman-Jensen, A., et al. (2018). *Household food security in the United States in 2017* (ERR-256). U.S. Department of Agriculture and Economic Research Service.
2. Weinfield, N., et al. (2014). *Hunger in America 2014 national report.* Chicago: Feeding America.
3. Chung, H. K., et al. (2016). Household food insecurity is associated with adverse mental health indicators and lower quality of life among Koreans: Results from the Korea National Health and Nutrition Examination Survey 2012-2013. *Nutrients, 8*(12).
4. Payne-Sturges, D. C., et al. (2018). Student hunger on campus: Food insecurity among college students and implications for academic institutions. *American Journal of Health Promotion, 32*(2), 349–354.
5. Wattick, R. A., Hagedorn, R. L., & Olfert, M. D. (2018). Relationship between diet and mental health in a young adult Appalachian college population. *Nutrients, 10*(8).

Undernutrition sometimes occurs in hospitalized patients as well. For example, acute trauma or chronic illness places added stress on the body, and the daily nutrient and energy intake may be insufficient to meet the needs of these individuals. This is common despite the supply of nutritionally balanced meals and nutrition support provided by the health care team at the hospital. Think about patients you have seen in a hospital: were they eager to eat? People are hospitalized because their health is in a state of serious distress. Illness and pain are often the cause for anorexia and decreased appetite. Thus, malnutrition, length of hospital stays, and adverse clinical outcomes are dependent upon and worsened by one another.[8-10]

Overnutrition

Some people are in a state of overnutrition, or excess nutrient and/or energy intake over time. Overnutrition is a form of malnutrition, especially when excess caloric intake produces harmful body weight (i.e., morbid obesity; see Chapter 15). Vitamin or mineral toxicities, another form of overnutrition, can also occur in people persistently using excessive dietary supplements (see Chapters 7 and 8).

NUTRIENT AND FOOD GUIDES FOR HEALTH PROMOTION

NUTRIENT STANDARDS

Most of the developed countries of the world have established nutrient standard recommendations. These standards serve as a reference for intake levels of the essential nutrients to meet the known nutrition needs of most healthy population groups. Although these standards are similar in many countries, they vary according to the philosophies of the scientists and practitioners with regard to the purpose and use of such standards. In the United States, we refer to these standards as the **Dietary Reference Intakes (DRIs)**.

U.S. Standards: Dietary Reference Intakes

Since 1941, the **Recommended Dietary Allowances (RDAs)** have been the authoritative source for setting standards for the minimum amounts of nutrients necessary to protect almost all people against the risk for nutrient deficiency. First published during World War II, the U.S. RDA standards serve as a guide for planning and obtaining food supplies for national defense and for providing population standards as a goal for good nutrition. The National Academy of Sciences revises and updates these standards as needed to reflect increasing scientific knowledge.

Public awareness and research attention have shifted from the original goal of *preventing deficiency disease* to reflect an increasing emphasis on nutrient requirements for *maintaining optimal health*. After World War II, nutrient deficiencies were a major concern to the health of the nation. However, that is not true today for the majority of the population. With food fortification and enrichment, few overt nutrient deficiencies exist in an otherwise balanced diet. This change of emphasis resulted in the DRIs project. This project examined essential nutrient quantities needed to produce optimal health. For example, the original goal was to find out how much vitamin C was necessary to prevent the disease scurvy. The current DRIs represent an ideal amount of each nutrient that will maximize the health benefits of each nutrient (i.e., the optimal amount of vitamin C one should consume to receive all of the health benefits of that nutrient). For some nutrients, this shift in focus made a notable difference in the recommendations; for others, the ideal intakes did not change.

The creation of the DRIs involved distinguished U.S. and Canadian scientists, who were divided into six functional panels (Box 1.1). They have examined thousands of nutrition studies addressing the health benefits of nutrients and the hazards of consuming too much of a nutrient. The working group of nutrition scientists responsible for these standards forms the Food and Nutrition Board of the Institute of Medicine. Publication of the original DRI recommendations took several years and a series of six volumes.[11-16] They will be updated as science or public policy indicates (such as the 2019 updates for sodium and potassium DRIs).[17]

The DRIs include recommendations for each sex and age group as well as recommendations for pregnancy and lactation (see Appendix B). For the first time, tolerable upper intake levels (ULs) identified the upper limits of safe nutrient intake. The DRIs encompass the following four interconnected categories of nutrient recommendations (Figure 1.3):

1. *Estimated Average Requirement (EAR).* The EAR is exactly what it sounds like: it is the mean, or average, dietary requirement of a nutrient in a specific population group.
2. *Recommended Dietary Allowance.* RDAs are established only when enough scientific evidence exists about a specific nutrient. It is set two standard deviations above the EAR to meet the needs of almost all (i.e., 97.5%) healthy individuals of a specific population group. Individuals should use the RDA as a guide to achieve optimal nutrient intake.
3. *Adequate Intake (AI).* The AI serves as the guide when insufficient scientific evidence is available to establish the RDA. Goals for individual intake may use both the RDA and the AI.

Box 1.1   **Dietary Reference Intake Panels of the Institute of Medicine of the National Academy of Sciences**

1. Calcium, vitamin D, phosphorus, magnesium, and fluoride
2. Folate and other B vitamins
3. Antioxidants
4. Macronutrients
5. Trace elements
6. Electrolytes and water

4. *Tolerable Upper Intake Level (UL).* This indicator is not a recommended intake. Rather, it sets the maximal intake that is unlikely to pose adverse health risks in almost all healthy individuals. For most nutrients, the UL refers to the daily intake from food, fortified food, and nutrient supplements combined.

Other Standards

Historically, Canadian and European standards have been similar to the U.S. standards. In less-developed countries, where factors such as the quality of available food must be considered, individuals refer to standards such as those set by the Food and Agriculture Organization and World Health Organization. Nonetheless, all standards provide a guideline to help health care providers who work with a variety of population groups to promote good health and prevent disease through sound nutrition.

FOOD GUIDES AND RECOMMENDATIONS

To interpret and apply nutrient standards, health care providers need practical food guides to use for nutrition education and food planning with individuals and families. Such tools include the U.S. Department of Agriculture's **MyPlate** system and the *Dietary Guidelines for Americans, 2020-2025.*

MyPlate

The MyPlate food guidance system (Figure 1.4) provides the public with a free nutrition education tool. The goal of this food guide is to promote variety, proportionality, moderation, gradual improvements, and physical activity.[18] Participants are encouraged to personalize their own plans via the public website www.choosemyplate.gov by creating a profile and entering their age, sex, weight, height, and activity level. The system will create a plan with individualized calorie levels and specific recommendations for serving amounts from each food group. In addition, the ChooseMyPlate site provides participants with worksheets, resources, and a variety of education tools for all age groups such as the following:
- Tip sheets on many nutrition topics
- Serving size information
- Healthy eating on a budget
- Recipes and menus
- Food safety and food waste information

Dietary Guidelines for Americans

The *Dietary Guidelines for Americans, 2020-2025* were established because of growing public concern that began in the 1960s and the subsequent Senate investigations studying hunger and nutrition in the United States. These guidelines address chronic health problems in an aging population and a changing food environment. A panel of experts updates the guidelines every 5 years. This publication encompasses a comprehensive evaluation of the scientific evidence regarding diet and health in a report jointly issued by the U.S. Department of Agriculture and the U.S. Department of Health and Human Services.[19]

Figure 1.5 shows the recommendations of the *Dietary Guidelines for Americans, 2020–2025.* The current guidelines continue to serve as a useful overall guide for promoting dietary and lifestyle choices that reduce the risk for chronic disease. No guidelines can guarantee health or well-being in an entire population because people differ widely with regard to their food

---

Dietary Reference Intakes (DRIs) reference values for the nutrient intake needs of healthy individuals for each sex and age group.

Recommended Dietary Allowances (RDAs) the average daily dietary intake level that is sufficient to meet the nutrient requirement of nearly all healthy individuals in a specified demographic group.

MyPlate a visual pattern of the basic five food groups—grains, vegetables, fruits, dairy, and protein—arranged on a plate to indicate proportionate amounts of daily food choices.

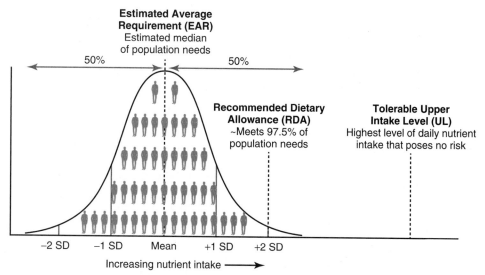

Figure 1.3 Bell curve representation of how the Estimated Average Requirement (EAR), Recommended Dietary Allowance (RDA), and Tolerable Upper Intake Level (UL) relate to one another within the DRI standards. Note that the RDA meets the needs of almost all healthy individuals. *SD,* standard deviation.

10 tips

*Nutrition
Education Series*

choose MyPlate

10 **tips** to a great plate

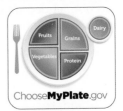

ChooseMyPlate.gov

Making food choices for a healthy lifestyle can be as simple as using these 10 Tips.
Use the ideas in this list to *balance your calories*, to choose foods to *eat more often*, and to cut back on foods to *eat less often*.

1 balance calories
Find out how many calories YOU need for a day as a first step in managing your weight. Go to www.ChooseMyPlate.gov to find your calorie level. Being physically active also helps you balance calories.

2 enjoy your food, but eat less
Take the time to fully enjoy your food as you eat it. Eating too fast or when your attention is elsewhere may lead to eating too many calories. Pay attention to hunger and fullness cues before, during, and after meals. Use them to recognize when to eat and when you've had enough.

3 avoid oversized portions
Use a smaller plate, bowl, and glass. Portion out foods before you eat. When eating out, choose a smaller size option, share a dish, or take home part of your meal.

4 foods to eat more often
Eat more vegetables, fruits, whole grains, and fat-free or 1% milk and dairy products. These foods have the nutrients you need for health—including potassium, calcium, vitamin D, and fiber. Make them the basis for meals and snacks.

5 make half your plate fruits and vegetables
Choose red, orange, and dark-green vegetables like tomatoes, sweet potatoes, and broccoli, along with other vegetables for your meals. Add fruit to meals as part of main or side dishes or as dessert.

6 switch to fat-free or low-fat (1%) milk
They have the same amount of calcium and other essential nutrients as whole milk, but fewer calories and less saturated fat.

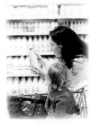

7 make half your grains whole grains
To eat more whole grains, substitute a whole-grain product for a refined product—such as eating whole-wheat bread instead of white bread or brown rice instead of white rice.

8 foods to eat less often
Cut back on foods high in solid fats, added sugars, and salt. They include cakes, cookies, ice cream, candies, sweetened drinks, pizza, and fatty meats like ribs, sausages, bacon, and hot dogs. Use these foods as occasional treats, not everyday foods.

9 compare sodium in foods
Use the Nutrition Facts label to choose lower sodium versions of foods like soup, bread, and frozen meals. Select canned foods labeled "low sodium," "reduced sodium," or "no salt added."

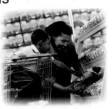

10 drink water instead of sugary drinks
Cut calories by drinking water or unsweetened beverages. Soda, energy drinks, and sports drinks are a major source of added sugar, and calories, in American diets.

USDA Center for Nutrition Policy and Promotion

Go to **www.ChooseMyPlate.gov** for more information.

DG TipSheet No. 1
June 2011
USDA is an equal opportunity provider and employer.

Figure 1.4 MyPlate food guidance system recommendations. (From the Center for Nutrition Policy and Promotion. [n.d.]. *Choose MyPlate mini-poster*. U.S. Department of Agriculture. Retrieved September 16, 2018, from www.choosemyplate.gov.)

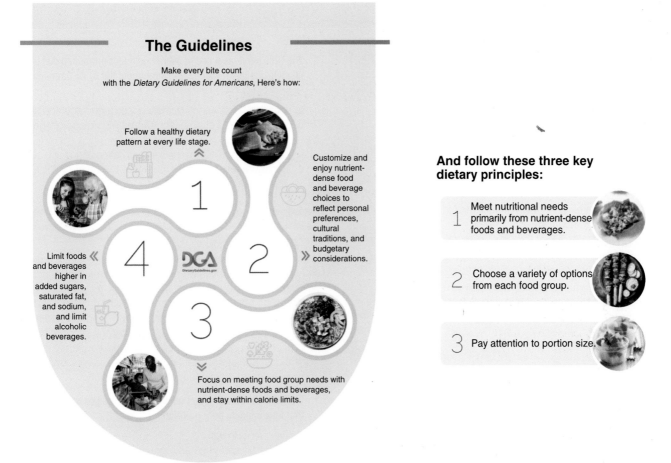

Figure 1.5 Summary of the *Dietary Guidelines for Americans, 2020-2025*. (From the U.S. Department of Agriculture and U.S. Department of Health and Human Services. [2020, December]. *Dietary guidelines for Americans, 2020-2025* [9th ed.]. www.dietaryguidelines.gov.)

needs and preferences. The goal is to help evaluate food habits and move toward general improvements.

The current DRIs, MyPlate guidelines, and *Dietary Guidelines for Americans, 2020-2025* are in accord with one another and supported by scientific literature. They reflect sound, although broad, guidelines for a healthy diet.

Other Recommendations

Organizations such as the American Cancer Society, the American Heart Association, and the American Diabetes Association also have their own independent dietary guidelines. In most cases, the *Dietary Guidelines for Americans, 2020-2025* serve as the model for advice set by various disease-specific organizations. This may seem a bit repetitive, but the difference is the added emphasis on the prevention of specific chronic diseases, such as heart disease, cancer, and diabetes.

INDIVIDUAL NEEDS

Person-Centered Care

Regardless of the type of food guide or recommendations used, health care professionals must remember that food patterns vary with individual needs, tastes, habits, living situations, economic status, and energy demands. Cookie-cutter meal plans without regard to the individual's preferences are not useful. Eating and appreciating food is one of the basic enjoyments of life. Thus, implementing dietary changes for oneself or for a client must recognize this concept. Use the food guides to identify healthy food groups to choose from and then use a person-centered approach to more specifically select suitable foods within those food groups to meet the client's needs.

Changing Food Environment

Our food environment has been rapidly changing in recent decades. American food habits appear to have deteriorated in some ways, with a heightened reliance on fast, processed, and prepackaged foods. However, Americans do recognize the relationship between food and overall health. More than ever, Americans are being selective about what they eat. Regardless of how much the food environment changes, the one thing that never goes out of style is the invention of food fads and popular diets. Health care professionals can address such concerns with a person-centered approach and ensure that the general dietary needs are satisfied in accordance with the DRIs. Following a fad diet is a personal preference. If health care professionals dismiss such preferences in favor of a cookie-cutter meal plan, they are more likely to garner resistance from the client instead of making any potential improvements.

Putting It All Together

Summary

- Good food and key nutrients are essential to life and health.
- In our changing world, an emphasis on health promotion and disease prevention by reducing health risks has become a primary health goal.
- The importance of a balanced diet for meeting this goal via the functioning of its nutrients is fundamental. Functions of nutrients include providing energy, building tissue, and regulating metabolic processes.
- Malnutrition exists in the United States in both overnutrition and undernutrition states.
- Food guides that help with the planning of an individualized healthy diet include the DRIs, MyPlate, and *Dietary Guidelines for Americans, 2020-2025*.
- A person-centered approach is best when developing individual dietary recommendations that consider personal factors.

Chapter Review Questions

See answers in Appendix A.

1. *Healthy People 2030* focuses on the ultimate vision of _____.

   a. a society in which all people can achieve their full potential for health and well-being
   b. a society in which there is zero tolerance for disease
   c. a society in which local plant sources supply all food in the United States
   d. a society consuming a primarily plant-based diet

2. Nutrient interactions involve the following two concepts: _____.

   a. nutrients have specific metabolic functions and work together to maintain the body
   b. nutrients have specific metabolic functions and work independently to maintain the body
   c. nutrients generally have independent functions in a healthy body but interact to promote healing during illness
   d. specific nutrients have similar metabolic functions and may be substituted for one another

3. The most important and unique role of dietary protein is to _____.

   a. provide energy
   b. build tissue
   c. provide essential fatty acids
   d. function as a coenzyme

4. Forms of malnutrition include _____.

   a. overnutrition only
   b. undernutrition only
   c. conditions associated with poverty only
   d. overnutrition and undernutrition

5. The DRIs serve as a useful overall guide for promoting dietary and lifestyle choices for all people throughout life by recommending _____.

   a. ideal intakes for each nutrient according to age and sex
   b. minimum intakes of each nutrient regardless of age and sex
   c. optimal intakes of each nutrient regardless of age and sex
   d. minimum intakes of each nutrient to prevent deficiency diseases

Next-Generation NCLEX® Examination-style Case Study

See answers in Appendix A.

A 45-year-old female (Ht.: 5'4" Wt.:135 lbs.) loves to run and lift weights, but she injured her foot 3 months ago. Since she has not been able to exercise, she has focused on eating mostly fruits and vegetables to avoid gaining weight. She reports avoiding grains such as bread, rice, and pasta. Her appetite has declined after getting a cold for the second time this month, so she eats small amounts of food frequently throughout the day. She states that her energy level is very low and that she has felt fatigued since the time of her injury.

1. From the list below, select all of the client's signs and symptoms that may indicate poor nutrition.

   a. Frequent illness
   b. High fruit and vegetable consumption
   c. Prolonged injury
   d. Fatigue
   e. Eliminating a food group from the diet
   f. Small frequent meals throughout the day

2. Choose the *most likely* options for the information missing from the statements below by selecting from the list of options provided.
   By eliminating most grains from her food intake, her diet may not provide adequate ___1___. This could cause her to feel fatigued, as these nutrients have a role in ___2___.

OPTION 1	OPTION 2
B vitamins	providing calories
vitamin C	bone development
phosphorous	collagen synthesis
calcium	eye function
vitamin A	energy metabolism

3. From the list below, select all of the Dietary Reference Intake categories that would be appropriate to identify the client's individual nutrient needs.

   a. Estimated Average Requirement
   b. Dietary Guidelines for Americans
   c. Recommended Daily Allowance
   d. Adequate Intake
   e. MyPlate
   f. Tolerable Upper Intake Level
   g. Daily Values

4. From the list below, select all the resources that would be beneficial for her health care provider to use to demonstrate healthy eating patterns.

    a. MyPlate
    b. Dietary Guidelines for Americans
    c. Healthy People Initiative
    d. Dietary Reference Intakes
    e. Estimated Average Requirements

5. Using the Acceptable Macronutrient Distribution ranges, identify the grams of each nutrient that the client needs based on a 2000-calorie diet. Place an X in the box that corresponds to the correct macronutrient recommendation for each of the corresponding columns.

OPTIONS	CARBOHYDRATES	PROTEIN	FAT
45 – 78 g			
225 – 325 g			
50 – 175 g			
900 – 1300 g			
200 – 700 g			
400 – 700 g			

6. At a follow-up visit, the client reports the changes listed below in her dietary habits. Place an X under "effective" for all changes that demonstrate a good understanding of the MyPlate recommendations. Place an X under "ineffective" for all changes that are not effective in meeting her MyPlate recommendations.

DIETARY CHANGES	EFFECTIVE	INEFFECTIVE
Makes ½ of her grains whole grains		
Fills ¼ of her plate with fruits and vegetables		
Drinks whole milk		
Replaced sweet tea with water		
Eats meals on a bigger plate		
Eats at the table to limit distractions		
Chooses canned vegetables with sodium		

Additional Learning Resources

Please refer to this text's Evolve website for answers to the Case Study questions:

http://evolve.elsevier.com/Williams/basic/

References and **Further Reading and Resources** in the back of the book provide additional resources for enhancing knowledge.

2

Carbohydrates

Key Concepts

- Carbohydrate foods are practical energy sources because of their wide availability, relatively low cost, and exceptional storage capabilities.
- Carbohydrates vary from simple to complex in composition, thus providing quick and extended energy for the body.

- Dietary fiber, which is an indigestible carbohydrate, performs several key functions to promote overall health within the gastrointestinal tract.

As discussed in Chapter 1, key nutrients in food sustain life and promote health. The unique functions of each nutrient provide the body with three essential elements for life: (1) energy to do work; (2) building materials to maintain form and functions; and (3) control agents to regulate these processes efficiently. These three basic functions of nutrients are closely related, and it is important to remember that no nutrient ever works alone.

This chapter looks specifically at the body's primary fuel source: carbohydrates. Carbohydrates are plentiful in the food supply, and they are an important contribution to a well-balanced diet. After learning about and critically evaluating the true function of carbohydrates within the body, you should be able to better interpret the incongruity between health care professionals and fad diet enthusiasts regarding the use, abuse, and misunderstanding of this macronutrient.

NATURE OF CARBOHYDRATES

RELATION TO ENERGY

Basic Fuel Source

Energy is required for organisms to live. All energy systems must have a basic fuel supply. In the Earth's energy system, vast energy resources from the sun enable plants, through photosynthesis, to transform solar energy into starch (a complex carbohydrate), which is the stored fuel form in plants. The human body can rapidly break down plant sources of carbohydrates through digestion and metabolism to yield our major source of energy, the simple carbohydrate glucose.

Throughout this text, we will use the term *energy* interchangeably with the terms *calorie, kilocalorie,* and *kcal* (see the definition of *kilocalorie* in Chapter 1). Our bodies need energy to survive. Both involuntary (e.g., heart and lung function) and voluntary actions (e.g., walking, talking) require energy, and that energy is derived from the fuel within the food that we eat.

> **photosynthesis** the process by which plants that contain chlorophyll are able to manufacture carbohydrates by combining carbon dioxide and water; sunlight is used as energy, and chlorophyll is a catalyst.

Energy System

A successful energy system, whether a living organism or a machine, must be able to do the following three things to reap energy from a fuel source:

1. Change the crude fuel to a refined fuel that the machine is designed to use.
2. Transport the refined fuel to the places that need it.
3. Burn the refined fuel in the special equipment set up at these places.

The body does these three things more efficiently than any manmade machine. It digests food containing complex carbohydrates such as starch (a crude fuel) to liberate simple carbohydrates such as glucose (a refined fuel). The body then absorbs and, through blood circulation, carries the refined fuel to cells that need it. Our cells metabolize glucose in their specific and intricate equipment. Ultimately, the process of cellular metabolism liberates energy in the form of adenosine triphosphate (ATP). We classify carbohydrates as quick-energy foods because the human body can rapidly digest the starches and sugars that we eat to yield energy.

Dietary Importance

Practical reasons also exist for the large quantities of carbohydrates found in diets all over the world. First, carbohydrates are widely available and easily grown (e.g., grains, legumes, vegetables, fruits). In some areas, carbohydrate foods make up almost the entire diet. Second, carbohydrates are relatively low in cost as compared with many other food items. Third, carbohydrate foods are easily stored. Modern processing and packaging can extend the shelf life of carbohydrate products, allowing for long-term storage without spoilage (e.g., rice, corn, wheat).

Whole and enriched grains are important contributors to the overall diet quality and intake of several key nutrients (e.g., fiber, folate, iron).[1,2] In addition, diets high in whole grains are associated with a reduced risk of certain chronic diseases.[3] Thus, one of the *Healthy People 2030* objectives is to increase the consumption of whole grains in the diets of all individuals over the age of 2 years.[4] Likewise, the *Dietary Guidelines for Americans, 2020-2025* encourage people to make at least half of all grains consumed whole grains.[5] Nevertheless, current dietary trends in the United States are such that about 44% of the carbohydrates consumed are in the form of sugar rather than complex carbohydrates.[6]

CLASSES OF CARBOHYDRATES

A carbohydrate is composed of carbon (C), hydrogen (H), and oxygen (O). Its abbreviated name, *CHO,* is the combination of the chemical symbols of its three components. The term **saccharide** denotes a carbohydrate class name, and it comes from the Latin word *saccharum,* which means "sugar." The number of saccharide units within the structure of a carbohydrate determines its classification: *mono*saccharides have one unit; *di*saccharides have two units; and *poly*saccharides have many units. Monosaccharides and disaccharides are small, simple structures of only one and two saccharide units, respectively; thus, we refer to them as **simple carbohydrates.** Polysaccharides are large, complex compounds of many saccharide units in long chains; thus, we refer to them as **complex carbohydrates.** For example, starch, which is the most significant polysaccharide in human nutrition, is composed of many coiled and branching chains in a tree-like structure. Each of the multiple branching chains is composed of 24 to 30 units of glucose. During digestion, a gradual release of each glucose unit supplies a steady source of energy over time. Table 2.1 summarizes these classes of carbohydrates and demonstrates their basic structure.

Monosaccharides

The three single saccharides are glucose, fructose, and galactose. Monosaccharides, which are the building blocks for all carbohydrates, require no digestion. They are quickly absorbed from the intestine into the bloodstream and transported to the liver. Depending on the immediate energy demands, the body will either use the monosaccharides for energy or store them as **glycogen** for later use.

Glucose. The basic single sugar in human metabolism is glucose, which is the form of sugar circulating in the blood. It is the primary fuel for cells. We do not usually encounter glucose, a moderately sweet sugar, as such in the diet, except in corn syrup or some processed food items. The body's supply of glucose mainly comes from the digestion of starch. The predominantly occurring form of natural glucose is *dextrose.*

Fructose. Fruit and honey are two of the food sources with the highest concentration of fructose. People sometimes misclassify honey as a sugar substitute; but because it *is* a sugar, we cannot consider it a substitute.

Table 2.1   Summary of Carbohydrate Classes

CHEMICAL CLASS NAME	CLASS MEMBERS	SOURCES
Monosaccharides (simple carbohydrates)	Glucose (dextrose)	Corn syrup (commonly used in processed foods)
	Fructose	Fruits, honey
	Galactose	Lactose (milk, milk products)
Disaccharides (simple carbohydrates)	Sucrose	Table sugar (sugar cane, sugar beets)
	Lactose	Milk, milk products
	Maltose	Molasses
		Starch digestion, intermediate
		Sweetener in food products
Polysaccharides (complex carbohydrates)	Starch	Grains and grain products (cereal, bread, crackers, baked goods)
		Rice, corn, bulgur
		Legumes
		Potatoes and other vegetables
	Glycogen	Storage form of carbohydrate in animal tissue (not a dietary source)

The amount of fructose found in fruits depends on the degree of ripeness. As a fruit ripens, some of its stored starch turns to sugar. Fructose is the sweetest of the simple sugars.

High-fructose corn syrups, which are manufactured by changing the glucose in cornstarch into fructose, are heavily used in processed food products, canned and frozen fruits, and soft drinks. These syrups are inexpensive sweeteners and significantly contribute to the high sugar intake in the United States. The per-capita consumption of high-fructose corn syrup increased dramatically in the late 1970s and early 1980s to a height of 11 teaspoons (tsp) per person per day in 1999.[7] Although reports from the most recent years show a decline in high-fructose corn syrup intake, the overall intake of caloric sweeteners as a whole remains excessively high. Figure 2.1 demonstrates the total added sugar in the American diet and how much comes from high-fructose corn syrup. Note that high-fructose corn syrup is only one of the sweeteners regularly used in the typical American diet.

---

saccharide the chemical name for sugar molecules; may occur as single molecules in monosaccharides (glucose, fructose, galactose), two molecules in disaccharides (sucrose, lactose, maltose), or multiple molecules in polysaccharides (starch, dietary fiber, glycogen).

simple carbohydrates sugars with a simple structure of one or two single-sugar (saccharide) units; a monosaccharide is composed of one sugar unit, and a disaccharide is composed of two sugar units.

complex carbohydrates large complex molecules of carbohydrates composed of many sugar units (polysaccharides); the complex forms of dietary carbohydrates are starch and dietary fiber.

glycogen a complex carbohydrate found in animal tissue that is composed of many glucose units linked together.

Galactose. Galactose does not usually exist as a free monosaccharide in the diet; rather, it is a product of lactose (milk sugar) digestion.

Disaccharides

Disaccharides are simple double sugars that are composed of two single-sugar units linked together. The three disaccharides that are important in human nutrition are sucrose, lactose, and maltose.

$$\text{Sucrose} = \text{Glucose} + \text{Fructose}$$

$$\text{Lactose} = \text{Glucose} + \text{Galactose}$$

$$\text{Maltose} = \text{Glucose} + \text{Glucose}$$

Sucrose. What we know as common table sugar is sucrose. Its two single-sugar units are glucose and fructose. Manufacturers harvest sucrose from sugar cane or sugar beets, and we use it in the form of granulated, powdered, or brown sugar. Molasses, which is a by-product of sugar production, is also a form of sucrose. When people speak of sugar in the diet, they usually mean sucrose.

Lactose. Mammary glands form the disaccharide in milk, called lactose. Its two single-sugar units are glucose and galactose. Lactose is the only common sugar that plants do not produce. It is less soluble and less sweet than sucrose. Cow's milk contains approximately 4.8% lactose, and human milk contains approximately 7% lactose. Because lactose promotes the absorption of calcium, the presence of both nutrients in milk is advantageous for absorption.

Maltose. We do not find maltose as such in food form (naturally). It is an intermediate product of starch digestion. Glucose units make up the entirety of starch. Therefore, during the chemical breakdown of starch in

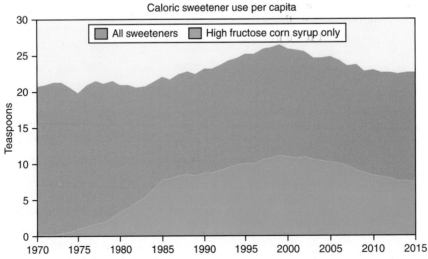

Figure 2.1 Daily intake of all caloric sweeteners and high-fructose corn syrup in the United States per person. (Data from U.S. Department of Agriculture and Economic Research Service. [2019]. *Caloric sweeteners: Per capita availability adjusted for loss.* www.ers.usda.gov/data-products/food-availability-per-capita-data-system/.)

the gastrointestinal tract, we release many disaccharide units of maltose. Food manufacturers use synthetically derived maltose in various processed foods.

Polysaccharides

Polysaccharides are complex carbohydrates that are composed of many sugar units. The important polysaccharides in human nutrition include starch, glycogen, and dietary fiber.

Starch. Starches are the most significant polysaccharides in the diet. We find polysaccharides in grains, legumes, and other vegetables and in some fruits in small amounts. Starches are more complex in structure than simple sugars, so they break down more slowly and supply energy over a longer period. Cooking starch improves its flavor and also softens and ruptures the starch cells, thereby making digestion easier and faster. Starch mixtures thicken when cooked, because the portion that encases the starch granules has a gel-like quality that thickens the starch mixture in the same way that pectin causes jelly to set.

The Dietary Reference Intakes (DRIs; see Chapter 1) recommend that 45% to 65% of total kilocalories consumed come from carbohydrates, with a greater portion of that intake coming from complex carbohydrates.[8] For countries in which starch is the staple food, carbohydrates make up an even higher proportion of the diet. The major food sources of starch (Figure 2.2) include grains in the form of cereal, pasta, crackers, bread, and other baked goods; legumes in the form of beans and peas; potatoes, rice, corn, and bulgur; and other vegetables, especially of the root variety.

We use the term *whole grain* to refer to food products such as flours, breads, or cereals derived from grains that retain the three key elements of a grain: the outer bran layers, the inner germ, and the endosperm and thus the nutrients found within (e.g., fiber, protein, vitamins, and minerals) (Figure 2.3). *Refined* grains are grains that have had one or more of the fundamental parts of the whole grain removed during the milling process. *Enriched* grains are grains that have first been

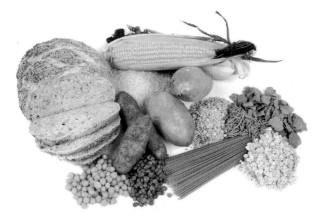

Figure 2.2 Complex carbohydrate foods. (Copyright iStock Photo; Credit: robynmac.)

refined and then enriched with a select few of the nutrients that were lost during the refining process. See the For Further Focus box, "Enriched and Fortified Foods," for more details on enriched and fortified foods.

For Further Focus

Enriched and Fortified Foods

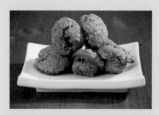

Significant portions of nutrients are lost when whole grains are refined. To make up for some of these losses, manufacturers enrich the grains with a few vitamins and minerals that were lost during the refining process. Some of these key nutrients are added back at levels higher than what would normally be found in whole grains (e.g., folate), but most are not added back at all.

NUTRIENTS LOST DURING THE REFINING PROCESS

Nutrients typically not added back	Nutrients added back to enriched grains
Protein	Riboflavin
Fiber	Niacin
Vitamin B_6	Thiamin
Choline	Folate
Vitamin B_{12}	Iron
Vitamin A	
Vitamin E	
Vitamin K	
Calcium	
Magnesium	
Phosphorus	
Potassium	
Zinc	
Copper	
Manganese	
Selenium	

As you can see, enriching refined grains does help to restore the nutritive value for a few nutrients, but it leaves the product generally inferior to its original whole-grain state.

Fortified foods are foods that have nutrients added to them that would not naturally occur in that food regardless of how it was processed (e.g., calcium-fortified orange juice). Many enriched grains, such as ready-to-eat breakfast cereals, are also fortified with additional vitamins and minerals that would not have been found in the whole grain (e.g., vitamin C).

Glycogen. Glycogen is a significant carbohydrate found in the body, as opposed to a polysaccharide consumed in the diet. The liver and muscles contain glycogen, where it is in constant metabolic use (i.e., broken down to form glucose for immediate energy needs and synthesized for storage) and is crucial to the body's metabolism and energy balance. The small stores of tissue glycogen help to sustain normal blood glucose levels during short-term fasting periods

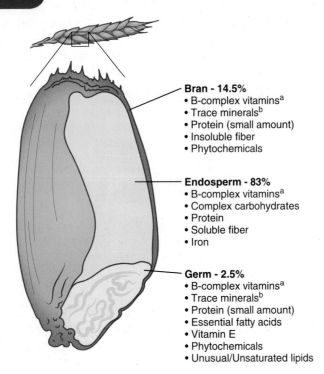

Bran - 14.5%
• B-complex vitamins[a]
• Trace minerals[b]
• Protein (small amount)
• Insoluble fiber
• Phytochemicals

Endosperm - 83%
• B-complex vitamins[a]
• Complex carbohydrates
• Protein
• Soluble fiber
• Iron

Germ - 2.5%
• B-complex vitamins[a]
• Trace minerals[b]
• Protein (small amount)
• Essential fatty acids
• Vitamin E
• Phytochemicals
• Unusual/Unsaturated lipids

[a]thiamin, niacin, riboflavin, pantothenic acid
[b]iron, zinc, iodine, copper, manganese, selenium

Figure 2.3 Kernel of wheat showing bran layers, endosperm, and germ. (Courtesy Eileen Draper.)

(e.g., sleep), and they provide immediate fuel for muscle action. These reserves also protect cells from depressed metabolic function and injury. Chapter 20 covers the process of blood glucose regulation with regard to glycogen breakdown in detail.

Dietary fiber

Humans lack the necessary **enzymes** to digest dietary fiber; therefore, these polysaccharides do not have a direct energy value like other carbohydrates. However, their indigestibility makes them an important dietary asset. High-fiber foods, such as whole grains, vegetables, fruit, and legumes, provide bulk to the diet, increase satiety, and are naturally nutrient-dense foods. Individuals who regularly consume diets high in plant-based fiber-rich foods are at reduced risk for several chronic diseases.[3,9-11]

We refer to dietary fiber as either soluble or insoluble (Table 2.2). Cellulose, lignin, and most hemicelluloses are not soluble in water. The rest of the dietary fibers (i.e., most pectins, β-glucans, gums, mucilages) are water soluble. Recommendations for fiber consumption may relate to the water-solubility distinction and the particular function of the fiber. For example, certain types of soluble fiber are capable of binding bile acids in the gastrointestinal tract and ultimately improving blood lipid levels.[12,13] Alternatively, large particles in nonfermentable insoluble fiber are helpful for the prevention of constipation by increasing the water and mucus secretions in the large intestine.[14] However, you will notice from Table 2.2 that many of these functions overlap the soluble/insoluble categories and many

high-fiber foods contain both types of fiber. It is more important to include a variety of high-fiber foods in the diet than to be overly concerned with the specific form of fiber found in your grains, fruits, and vegetables. In the section that follows, we will cover a few key points for the three most common forms of dietary fiber.

Cellulose. Cellulose is the chief component of cell walls in plants and is the most abundant dietary fiber. It is notable in human nutrition for adding important bulk to fecal matter. This bulk helps to move the food mass along, it stimulates normal muscle action in the intestine, and it forms soft feces for the elimination of waste products. The main sources of cellulose are the stems and leaves of vegetables and the coverings of seeds and grains. Within the same area of the plant, phosphorus is stored in the form of phytic acid; this compound is undigested in humans because of the lack of a necessary enzyme (phytase). Phytic acid is a strong **chelator** of important minerals (see the Drug-Nutrient Interaction box, "Phytic Acid and Mineral Absorption").

Drug-Nutrient Interaction

Phytic Acid and Mineral Absorption

Some naturally occurring compounds found in food can bind minerals, thereby making them unavailable for absorption. Phytic acid is one such compound. Legumes, wheat bran, and seeds contain phytic acid. The same foods are also a good source of iron; however, because of the phytic acid interference, as little as 2% of the available iron may be absorbed and used by the body.

A diet that consists of high-fiber foods containing phytic acid coupled with a low intake of iron-rich foods (e.g., meat, poultry) may intensify iron deficiency. This can especially be a problem in the developing world where grains and legumes are a staple in the diet. Iron-deficiency anemia is one of the most serious health problems in the world today with a disproportionate burden placed on developing countries.[1]

Although iron-deficiency anemia is not nearly as common in the United States as in developing countries, it is a concern among pregnant and premenopausal women. If the anemia is severe enough, a physician may prescribe an iron supplement. The consumption of foods that contain high amounts of phytic acid along with the supplement would inhibit iron absorption just as it would if the iron were part of the food.

Phytic acid binds to other minerals that have a similar charge as iron, including calcium, magnesium, and zinc. Calcium supplements are often prescribed for those who may be losing bone mass (e.g., postmenopausal women) or for those who do not get enough calcium in the diet (e.g., teens, the elderly). Calcium supplements taken along with food sources of phytic acid may not be available for absorption. When recommending that clients take an iron or calcium supplement, also advise them to take the supplement with foods that do not contain phytate to maximize the bioavailability of the minerals and minimize the drug-nutrient interaction.

REFERENCE
1. Kassebaum, N. J. (2016). The global burden of anemia. *Hematol Oncol Clin North Am, 30*(2), 247–308.

| Table 2.2 | Summary of Dietary Fiber Classes |

DIETARY FIBER CLASS	SOURCE	FUNCTION
Insoluble Fiber		
Cellulose	Main cell wall constituent of plants (stalks and leaves of vegetables; outer coverings of seeds, such as are found in whole grains)	Holds water; reduces elevated colonic intraluminal pressure
Hemicellulose	Cell wall plant material (bran, whole grains)	Holds water and increases stool bulk; reduces elevated colonic pressure; binds bile acids, thus decreasing serum cholesterol level
Lignin	Woody part of plants (broccoli stems; fruits with edible seeds, such as strawberries and flaxseeds)	Antioxidant; binds bile acids, thus decreasing serum cholesterol level; binds minerals
Soluble Fiber		
Algal polysaccharides	Algae, seaweeds	Used as thickener in food products
β-Glucans	Oats and barley bran	Binds bile acids, thus decreasing serum cholesterol level
Gums	Oats, legumes, guar, barley	Decreases gastric emptying; slows digestion, gut transit time, and glucose absorption
Mucilages	Psyllium husk, flaxseed	Holds water
Pectins	Intercellular plant material (fruit)	Binds bile acids, thus decreasing serum cholesterol level; binds minerals

Lignin. Lignin, which is the only noncarbohydrate type of dietary fiber, is a large compound that forms the woody part of certain plants. It binds the cellulose fibers in plants, thereby giving added strength and stiffness to plant cell walls. Flax and sesame seeds are particularly good dietary sources of lignin. The unique antioxidant properties of this dietary fiber lend it to additional health benefits as a protector against oxidative stress.[15]

Noncellulose polysaccharides. Hemicellulose, pectins, gums, mucilages, and algal substances are noncellulose polysaccharides. They absorb water and swell to a larger bulk, thus slowing the emptying of the food mass from the stomach (aiding satiety), binding bile acids in the intestine, and preventing spastic colon pressure by providing bulk for normal muscle action. Noncellulose polysaccharides also provide fermentable material for the **gut microbiota.**

---

enzymes the proteins produced in the body that digest or change nutrients in specific chemical reactions without being changed themselves during the process; digestive enzymes in gastrointestinal secretions act on food substances to break them down into simpler compounds. (An enzyme usually is named after the substance [i.e., substrate] on which it acts, with the common word ending of -ase; for example, sucrase is the specific enzyme for sucrose, which it breaks down into glucose and fructose.)

chelator a ligand that binds to a metal to form a metal complex.

gut microbiota microorganisms found in the gastrointestinal tract.

Dietary Intake. In general, the food groups that provide needed dietary fiber include whole grains, legumes, vegetables, and fruits with as much of their skin remaining as possible. Table 2.3 provides the grams of carbohydrate and dietary fiber per serving of commonly used foods. Whole grains provide a special natural "package" of the complex carbohydrate starch and the fiber in its coating. In addition, whole grains contain an abundance of vitamins and minerals.

Many health organizations recommend an increase in the consumption of complex carbohydrates in general and dietary fiber in particular.[5,8,9] Risk factors for certain chronic diseases of adulthood (e.g., hypertension, diabetes, obesity) appear to be lower in individuals who regularly consume diets high in fiber-rich foods.[10,12,16-18] The protective role of fiber in overall health continues to be an active area of research.

The Food and Nutrition Board of the Institute of Medicine has always indicated that we should not try to achieve desirable fiber intake exclusively by adding concentrated fiber supplements to the diet. Instead, the recommendations are to eat a high-fiber diet that is rich in whole foods. The recommended daily intake of fiber for women and men aged 19 to 50 years old is 25 and 38 g/day, respectively.[8] This intake requires the consistent daily intake of whole grains, legumes, vegetables, fruits, seeds, and nuts. Unfortunately, the average American falls disconcertingly short of the recommended servings of these food groups on a daily basis. In fact, only 13% of adults (≥18 years of age) in the United States consume the recommended servings of fruit per day, less than 9% of adults meet the daily serving recommendations for

Table 2.3 **Carbohydrate Content, Dietary Fiber, and Caloric Value for Selected Foods**

FOOD SOURCE	SERVING SIZE	CARBOHYDRATE (G)	DIETARY FIBER (G)	TOTAL KILOCALORIES
Concentrated Sweets				
Sugar				
Granulated	1 tsp	4.2	0	16
Powdered	1 tsp	2.49	0	10
Maple	1 tsp	2.73	0	11
Honey	1 Tbsp	17.3	0	64
Syrup				
High-fructose corn	1 Tbsp	14.44	0	53
Maple	1 Tbsp	13.42	0	52
Jam and preserves	1 Tbsp	13.77	0.2	56
Carbonated beverage, cola	12 oz	35.18	0	136
Candy				
Skittles	1 package (1.8 oz)	46.42	0	205
Starburst fruit chews	1 package (2.07 oz)	48.72	0	241
Twizzlers	4 pieces from an 8-oz package	35.88	0	158
Baked Goods				
Brownie	1 square (1 oz)	18.12	0.6	115
Butter cookie	1 medium (1 oz)	19.53	0.2	132
Doughnut, glazed	1 medium (3-inch diameter)	22.86	0.7	192
Fruit				
Apple, raw with skin	1 medium (3-inch diameter)	25.13	4.4	95
Apricots, dried, no sugar added	½ cup	27.69	3.2	106
Banana	1 medium (7½ to 7⅞ inches long)	26.95	3.1	105
Cherries, sweet, raw	15 cherries	19.69	2.6	77
Orange	1 medium (2⅞-inch diameter)	17.56	3.1	69
Pineapple	1 slice (3½-inch diameter × ¾-inch thick)	11.02	1.2	42
Strawberries	10 medium (1¼-inch diameter)	9.22	2.4	38
Vegetables				
Asparagus, cooked	½ cup	3.7	1.8	20
Beans, kidney, cooked	½ cup	20.18	5.7	112
Broccoli, cooked	½ cup	5.6	2.6	27
Carrots, raw	½ cup chopped, raw	6.13	1.8	26
Corn, sweet, yellow, cooked	½ cup, cut	15.63	1.8	72
Green beans (snap beans, cooked)	½ cup	4.92	2	22
Lettuce, green leaf, raw	1 cup shredded	1	0.5	5
Potato, with skin, baked	1 medium (2¼ to 3¼ inches in diameter)	36.59	3.8	161
Potato, sweet, baked	1 medium (2-inch diameter, 5 inches long)	23.61	3.8	103
Squash, summer	½ cup cooked slices	3.41	1	17
Tomatoes, red, raw	½ medium (2¾ -inch diameter)	2.39	0.7	11
Dairy Products				
Milk				
Skim	1 cup	12.15	0	83
2%	1 cup	13.5	0	138

Table 2.3	Carbohydrate Content, Dietary Fiber, and Caloric Value for Selected Foods—cont'd			
FOOD SOURCE	**SERVING SIZE**	**CARBOHYDRATE (G)**	**DIETARY FIBER (G)**	**TOTAL KILOCALORIES**
Whole	1 cup	11.03	0	146
Cheese				
Cheddar	½ cup, shredded	0.72	0	228
Cottage, 2% milk fat	½ cup	4.14	0	97
Grain Products				
Bread				
Wheat	1 slice	14.34	1.2	78
White	1 slice	12.6	0.7	66
Rye	1 slice	15.46	1.9	83
Cereal (Dry)				
Corn flakes	1 cup	22.20	0.3	101
Rice, puffed	1 cup	12.57	0.2	56
Wheat, shredded	1 cup	39.89	6.1	172
Cereal (Cooked)				
Grits, corn, cooked with water	1 cup	37.93	2.1	182
Oatmeal, cooked with water	1 cup	28.08	4.0	166
Wheat, cooked with water	1 cup	33.15	3.9	150
Crackers, saltines	5	11.03	0.4	62
Pasta, cooked	1 cup	39.07	6.7	176
Rice				
Brown	½ cup, cooked	22.39	1.8	108
White	½ cup, cooked	26.59	0.3	121

Data from the Nutrient Data Laboratory. (n.d.). *USDA National Nutrient Database for Standard Reference.* U.S. Department of Agriculture, Agricultural Research Service. Retrieved September 22, 2018, from ndb.nal.usda.gov/.

vegetables, and less than 8% of adults consume the recommended servings per day of whole grains.[19,20] In other words, the average American diet is very low in foods that provide necessary fiber. Subsequently, the mean fiber intake for adults in the United States is 17.3 g per day.[6] These averages are remarkably lower than the recommended fiber intake and may contribute to health problems.

Health professionals can assist members of the public with evaluating their fiber intake by educating and encouraging the use of nutrition facts labels. Food labels list the total dietary fiber found in each serving of food. Manufacturers may also voluntarily list the specific type of fiber (i.e., soluble or insoluble) on the nutrition facts label.

As with many things in nutrition, too much of a good thing also can be problematic. Sudden increases in fiber intake can result in uncomfortable gas, bloating, and constipation. Fiber intake should be gradually increased (along with water intake) to an appropriate amount for the individual. In addition, excessive amounts of dietary fiber can trap (by chelation) small amounts of minerals and prevent their absorption in the gastrointestinal tract. This function of fiber is beneficial when trapping or binding bile acids, but it may compromise nutrition status if fiber intake greatly exceeds the recommendations to the point of reducing mineral absorption. See the Case Study box, "Carbohydrates and Fiber."

Other Sweeteners

Sugar alcohols and alternative sweeteners often replace the use of regular sugar. *Nutritive* sweeteners contribute to the total calorie intake (e.g., sugar alcohols). *Nonnutritive sweeteners* or *alternative sweeteners* are sugar substitutes that do not have a notable caloric value.

Nutritive sweeteners. The sugar alcohols sorbitol, mannitol, and xylitol are the alcohol forms of sucrose, mannose, and xylose, respectively. Sugar alcohols provide 2 to 3 kcal/g as compared with other carbohydrates, which provide 4 kcal/g. The most well-known sugar alcohol is sorbitol, which is widely used as a sucrose substitute in various foods, candies, chewing gum, and beverages. Both glucose and sugar alcohols are absorbed in the small intestine. However, sugar alcohols are absorbed more slowly and do not increase the blood sugar level as rapidly as glucose. Therefore, food manufacturers may use sugar alcohols in products that are intended for individuals who cannot tolerate a high blood sugar level (e.g., those with diabetes). Another

NEXT-GENERATION NCLEX® EXAMINATION-STYLE UNFOLDING CASE STUDY
Carbohydrates and Fiber

See answers in Appendix A.

A 38-year-old male with a history of obesity, diabetes, and high total cholesterol (240 mg/dl) has uncontrolled blood glucose levels (120 mg/dl). He has come to see the registered dietitian nutritionist (RDN) for diet recommendations. The RDN collected and analyzed a 1-day diet history. The analysis indicated that he consumed a total of 1850 calories, 260 g of carbohydrate, and 19 g of fiber.

1. Highlight or circle the foods listed below that are *most likely* to raise the client's blood glucose.

   Breakfast: sweetened cheerios (2 c.), skim milk (1 ¼ c.), banana (1 medium), black coffee (8 oz)

   Lunch: turkey sandwich (2 pieces of white bread, 3 oz turkey, tomato, lettuce); pretzels (1 c.); carrots (1/2 c.); sweet tea (16 oz)

   Dinner: chicken breast (4 oz), mashed potatoes with butter (3/4 c.), green beans (1/2 c.), dinner Roll, soda (12 oz)

2. Choose the *most likely* options for the information missing from the statements below by selecting from the list of options provided.

   According to dietary guidelines, the client is _____ the total percent of calories from carbohydrate and needs to _____ the total grams of fiber in his diet to meet recommendations.

OPTIONS	
within	decrease
above	below
increase	

After analyzing the client's diet, the nurse identifies changes that can promote glucose control and reduction of cholesterol.

3. Choose the *most likely* options for the information missing from the statements below by selecting from the list of options provided.

   After analyzing the client's diet, the nurse identifies high intake of _____ carbohydrates containing _____ sugars most likely contribute to high blood glucose levels.

OPTIONS	
refined	slow digesting
simple	unprocessed
complex	natural

4. Use an X to identify foods in the client's diet that are indicated appropriate, contraindicated, and irrelevant given the background provided.

FOOD ITEM	INDICATED	CONTRAINDICATED	IRRELEVANT
Dinner roll			
Chicken breast			
Soda			
Cheerios			
Pretzels			
Skim milk			
Mashed potatoes with butter			
Banana			
Black Coffee			

The client is in the clinic for a follow up visit. A month ago, he received diet education regarding choosing complex carbohydrates and increasing fiber intake to 50 grams per day. His assessment shows that his blood glucose is now within normal limits (90 mg/dl) and his total cholesterol levels have improved (200 mg/dl). However, the client mentions that while he has lost some weight and felt more energized, he has also been experiencing stomach discomfort, bloating, gas, and has irregular bowel movements.

5. Choose the *most likely* options for the information missing from the statements below by selecting from the list of options provided.

   Upon hearing these symptoms, the nurse educates the client that large amounts of ____1____ may be causing gastrointestinal discomfort, but it also may have contributed to his ____2____ levels due to its ability to form gels and absorb ____3____.

OPTION 1	OPTION 2	OPTION 3
iron	cholesterol	fat
fiber	iron	enzymes
carbohydrate	glucose	bile salts

6. For each assessment, use an X to indicate whether the interventions were effective (helped to meet expected outcomes), ineffective (did not help to meet expected outcomes), or unrelated (not related to the expected outcomes).

ASSESSMENT FINDING	EFFECTIVE	INEFFECTIVE	UNRELATED
Blood glucose 87 mg/dl			
Total cholesterol 195 mg/dl			
Client reports reduced bowel movements			
Client describes stomach pains throughout the day			
Client walks one mile daily			
Client's clothes have been fitting him better			
Client reports less acne on his skin			

advantage of using a sugar alcohol to replace sugar is a lowered risk of dental caries, because oral bacteria cannot use the alcohol for fuel. The downside of using excessive amounts of sugar alcohols in food products is that the slowed digestion may result in osmotic diarrhea.

Nonnutritive sweeteners. Manufacturers produce nonnutritive sweeteners for use as an alternative or artificial sweetener in food products. Because nonnutritive sweeteners do not provide kilocalories, they provide the sweet taste without contributing to an individual's total energy intake. People typically associate these sweeteners with "diet foods." The artificial sweeteners that are approved for use in the United States are acesulfame-K, advantame, aspartame, luo han guo (monk fruit extract), neotame, saccharin, stevia, and sucralose.[21] Nonnutritive sweeteners are much sweeter than sucrose; therefore, the same sweet taste comes from only extremely small quantities of the product. Table 2.4 provides a summary of nutritive and nonnutritive sweeteners and their relative sweetness value as compared with table sugar.

FUNCTIONS OF CARBOHYDRATES

BASIC FUEL SUPPLY

The main function of carbohydrates is to provide fuel for the body. Carbohydrates burn in the body at the rate of 4 kcal/g; thus, the fuel factor of carbohydrates is 4. The cellular metabolism throughout the body requires a readily available source of energy, which carbohydrates provide. Fat also serves as a source of fuel, but the body requires only a relatively small amount of dietary fat to supply the essential fatty acids (see Chapter 3).

RESERVE FUEL SUPPLY

The total amount of carbohydrate in the body, including stored glycogen and blood sugar, is small. Healthy, well-nourished adults store approximately 100 g of glycogen in the liver, which is about 8% of the liver mass weight. On average, 300 to 400 g of glycogen can be stored in the skeletal muscle, accounting for 1% to 2% of the muscle mass weight. Without refueling, the total amount of available glucose in the muscle provides enough energy for 1 to 2 hours of aerobic activity at 66% maximum capacity. Therefore, we must eat carbohydrate foods regularly throughout the day to maintain euglycemia, prevent tissue protein catabolism, and satisfy energy demands.

Glycogen in the liver primarily maintains blood glucose levels and protects cells from depressed metabolic function. Constant carbohydrate availability is essential for proper functioning of the central nervous system. The brain has no stored supply of glucose; therefore, it is dependent on a minute-to-minute supply of glucose from the blood. Sustained and profound shock from low blood sugar may cause brain damage and can result in coma or death.

sugar alcohols nutritive sweeteners that provide 2 to 3 kcal/g; examples include sorbitol, mannitol, and xylitol; these are produced in food-industry laboratories for use as sweeteners in candies, chewing gum, beverages, and other foods.

sorbitol a sugar alcohol that is often used as a nutritive sugar substitute; it is named for where it was discovered in nature, in ripe berries of the *Sorbus aucuparia* tree; it also occurs naturally in small quantities in various other berries, cherries, plums, and pears.

euglycemia normal blood glucose level.

Table 2.4   Sweetness of Sugars and Artificial Sweeteners

SUBSTANCE	SWEETNESS VALUE RELATIVE TO SUCROSE
Nutritive Sweeteners	
D-Tagatose	75 to 92
Glucose	74
Erythritol	60 to 80
Isomalt	45 to 65
Isomaltulose	50
Lactitol	30 to 40
Maltitol	90
Mannitol	50 to 70
Sorbitol	50 to 70
Sucrose	100
Trehalose	45
Xylitol	100
Nonnutritive Sweeteners (Approved for Use in the U.S.)[a] and Associated Brand Names	
Acesulfame-K Sweet One, Sunett	200
Advantame	20,000
Aspartame NutraSweet, Equal, Sugar Twin	200
Luohan guo extract (*Siraitia grosvenorii*) Nectresse, Monk Fruit in the Raw, PureLo	100 to 250
Neotame Newtame	7000 to 13000
Saccharin Sweet and Low Sweet Twin, Sweet'N Low Necta Sweet	200 to 700
Stevia (*Stevia rebaudiana*) Truvia, PureVia, Enliten	200 to 400
Sucralose Splenda	600

[a]Some artificial sweeteners provide a small amount of calories. Example: 1 packet of Splenda provides 3 kcal, and 1 packet of Equal provides 4 kcal. Because the relative sweetness compared to sucrose is so great, very little of the artificial sweeteners is necessary to achieve the same level of sweetness as sugar and thus the kilocalories provided are minimal.
Modified from Fitch, C., et al. (2012). Position of the Academy of Nutrition and Dietetics: Use of nutritive and nonnutritive sweeteners. *J Acad Nutr Diet, 112*(5), 739–758; and U.S. Food and Drug Administration. (2018). *Additional information about high-intensity sweeteners permitted for use in food in the United States.* Retrieved September 30, 2018, from www.fda.gov/Food/IngredientsPackagingLabeling/FoodAdditivesIngredients/ucm397725.htm.

METABOLIC REGULATOR

Carbohydrates help to regulate protein and fat metabolism. If dietary carbohydrate is sufficient to meet energy needs, the body will not sacrifice protein for fuel. This protein-sparing action of carbohydrate protects protein for its major roles in tissue growth and maintenance. The other macronutrients cannot serve as a substitute for these crucial functions. Likewise, with sufficient carbohydrate for energy, we do not need fat to supply large amounts of energy. This is significant, because a rapid breakdown of fat may result in the production of ketones, which are products of incomplete fat oxidation in the cells. Ketones are strong acids. The conditions of acidosis or ketosis upset the normal acid-base balance of the body and could result in cellular damage in severe cases. This *antiketogenic effect* is one protective action of carbohydrates.

FOOD SOURCES OF CARBOHYDRATES

STARCHES

Starch is the most important carbohydrate in a balanced diet. Nutrient-dense starches such as rice, wheat, corn, legumes, and potatoes provide important sources of fiber and other essential nutrients (see Table 2.3).

SUGARS

It is too simplistic to declare that we should avoid all sources of "sugar" in a healthy diet. After all, the form of carbohydrate provided in fruit is a disaccharide (a simple sugar). The difference between this type of sugar and the "added sugar" in candy is that fruit also provides fiber, water, vitamins, and minerals. The problem with excess added sugar in the diet (e.g., sweets, desserts, candy, soda drinks) is the large quantities of "empty calories" consumed, often to the exclusion of other important foods that are sources of essential nutrients. As with most things, moderation is the key.

See the For Further Focus box, "Carbohydrate Complications," for a brief discussion of two controversial topics in mass-media coverage of nutrition: the glycemic index and "net carbs."

DIGESTION OF CARBOHYDRATES

MOUTH

The digestion of carbohydrates begins in the mouth and progresses through the successive parts of the gastrointestinal tract. Two types of actions accomplish it: (1) muscle actions that mechanically break the food mass into smaller particles and (2) chemical processes in which specific enzymes break

---

 For Further Focus

Carbohydrate Complications

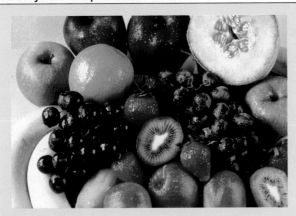

GLYCEMIC INDEX
The glycemic index (GI), which was developed by researchers at the University of Toronto in the early 1980s, was thought to be an ideal tool for controlling blood glucose levels, specifically for individuals with diabetes. However, the use of this tool has been controversial.

How It Works
The GI ranks foods according to how fast blood glucose levels rise after consuming a specific amount (50 g) as compared with a reference food such as white bread or pure glucose. Foods that produce a higher peak in blood sugar within 2 hours of eating them earn a higher GI ranking. Thus, low-GI foods do not produce high blood glucose spikes and are favorable. In addition, low-GI foods are generally high in fiber.

Complications of Use
The primary reason why this tool is controversial is its high variability. The GI of a food can vary significantly in the following ways:
- From person to person
- With the quantity of food eaten
- From one time of day to another
- When a food is eaten alone versus when it is eaten with other foods
- Depending on the ripeness, variety, cooking method used, degree of processing, and site of origin

In addition, the GI of a food does not indicate the nutritious quality of the food. For example, ice cream has a lower GI value than pineapple.

Potential Benefits of Consistent Use
One recently published meta-analysis concluded that individuals with type 2 diabetes who were consuming a low-GI diet had improved long-term blood glucose control (as measured by glycosylated hemoglobin A1c).[1] Other studies evaluating the long-term benefits of a low-GI diet on risks for developing type 2 diabetes and cardiovascular risk factors have not been consistent. A healthy diet focusing on nutrient-dense foods such as fruits, vegetables, and whole grains naturally has a lower GI than the standard American fare. Health professionals generally agree that it is appropriate to consider low-GI diets in the context of an otherwise healthy diet as an additional complementary step in improving the overall diet quality for some individuals.[2]

For Further Focus—cont'd

Carbohydrate Complications

NET CARBS

Food manufacturers invented a category of carbohydrates called "net carbs" as a marketing tactic to capitalize on the low-carbohydrate diet craze. The U.S. Food and Drug Administration regulates all information provided in the nutrition facts label, including total carbohydrates, dietary fiber, and sugars, and it does not acknowledge or approve of the "net carb" category.

Development of this concept occurred during the height of carbohydrate-phobic diets. Food manufacturers reasoned that they could simply subtract these carbohydrates from the total carbohydrates in a food serving because dietary fiber and sugar alcohols have lower GI values. For example, a food may have 30 g of total carbohydrates with 18 g of sugar alcohols and 3 g of fiber, thereby leaving 9 g of "net carbs." Manufacturers also refer to these as "impact carbs" or "active carbs."

Problems With the "Net Carb" Theory

- Sugar alcohols do have calories and can raise blood sugar levels.
- We do not know the safety of excessive use of sugar alcohols in foods, but this type of labeling encourages manufacturers to increase the use of products such as sorbitol to lower their "net carb" claim.
- Excess intake of sugar alcohols can cause diarrhea.
- The idea of zero "net carbs" does not explain the fact that the food still has calories.

The bottom line is that there are no successful shortcuts to an overall healthy diet. Diets that avoid high-carbohydrate containing foods, such as fruits, vegetables, grains, and legumes are missing significant sources of essential nutrients and fiber that other food groups do not provide. For weight management, no substitute exists for the formula of "calories in must equal calories out." Total calories count more than the quantity—or lack thereof—of "net carbs."

REFERENCES

1. Ojo, O., et al. (2018). The effect of dietary glycaemic index on glycaemia in patients with type 2 diabetes: A systematic review and meta-analysis of randomized controlled trials. *Nutrients*, *10*(3).
2. Augustin, L. S., et al. (2015). Glycemic index, glycemic load and glycemic response: An international scientific consensus summit from the International Carbohydrate Quality Consortium (ICQC). *Nutr Metab Cardiovasc Dis*, *25*(3), 795–815.

down the nutrients into still smaller usable metabolic products. *Mastication*, or the chewing of food, breaks food into fine particles and mixes it with saliva. During this process, the parotid glands, which lie under each ear at the back of the jaw, secrete the enzyme salivary amylase (also called *ptyalin*). Salivary amylase acts on starch to begin its breakdown into **dextrins** and disaccharides (primarily maltose). Monosaccharides do not require further digestion for absorption.

STOMACH

Wavelike contractions of the stomach muscles continue the mechanical digestive process. This action, called *peristalsis*, further mixes food particles with gastric secretions. There are no carbohydrate-specific enzymes released in the stomach. Gastric secretions include hydrochloric acid, which inhibits the action of salivary amylase swallowed from the mouth. However, before the food completely mixes with the acidic gastric secretions, more than 20% to 30% of the starch may have cleaved into units of maltose. Muscle action continues to mix the food mass and then moves it to the lower part of the stomach. Here the food mass is a thick and creamy chyme, ready for its controlled emptying through the pyloric valve and into the duodenum, which is the first portion of the small intestine.

SMALL INTESTINE

Peristalsis continues to help with digestion in the small intestine by mixing and moving chyme along the length of the organ. Carbohydrate-specific enzymes from the pancreas and the intestine complete the chemical digestion of carbohydrate in the small intestine.

Pancreatic Secretions

Secretions from the pancreas enter the duodenum through the common bile duct. These secretions contain the starch-splitting enzyme *pancreatic amylase* for the continued breakdown of starch into disaccharides and monosaccharides.

Intestinal Secretions

Enzymes from the **brush border** (i.e., microvilli) of the intestinal tract contain three disaccharidases: *sucrase, lactase,* and *maltase*. These enzymes act on their respective disaccharides to render the monosaccharides—glucose, galactose, and fructose—ready for absorption directly into the **portal** blood circulation.

Lactose intolerance, which is the inability to break lactose down into its monosaccharide units, results from insufficient lactase activity. Symptoms include bloating, gas, abdominal pain, and diarrhea. A

---

dextrins intermediate starch breakdown products.

brush border the cells that are located on the microvilli within the lining of the intestinal tract; the microvilli are tiny hair-like projections that protrude from the mucosal cells that help to increase surface area for the digestion and absorption of nutrients.

portal an entrance or gateway; for example, the portal blood circulation designates the entry of blood vessels from the intestines into the liver; it carries nutrients for liver metabolism, and it then drains into the body's main systemic circulation to deliver metabolic products to body cells.

congenital deficiency of lactase during infancy is rare. The decreased production of lactase after infancy affects approximately 65% of people worldwide, with a much higher prevalence in certain countries and ethnic groups (see the Cultural Considerations box, "Ethnicity and Lactose Intolerance").[22]

Figure 2.4 provides a summary of the major aspects of carbohydrate digestion through the successive parts of the gastrointestinal tract. Chapter 5 covers the overall process of the absorption and metabolism of all energy-yielding nutrients (i.e., carbohydrate, fat, and protein).

RECOMMENDATIONS FOR DIETARY CARBOHYDRATE

DIETARY REFERENCE INTAKES

The Dietary Reference Intakes (DRIs) include acceptable macronutrient intake ranges for each of the energy-yielding nutrients as a portion of the total kilocalories, or energy needs. The DRIs recommend that 45% to 65% of total caloric intake come from carbohydrate foods.[8] This translates to 225 to 325 g of carbohydrates for a 2000 kcal/day diet. As noted earlier, the recommended fiber intake is 25 g/day for women and 38 g/day for

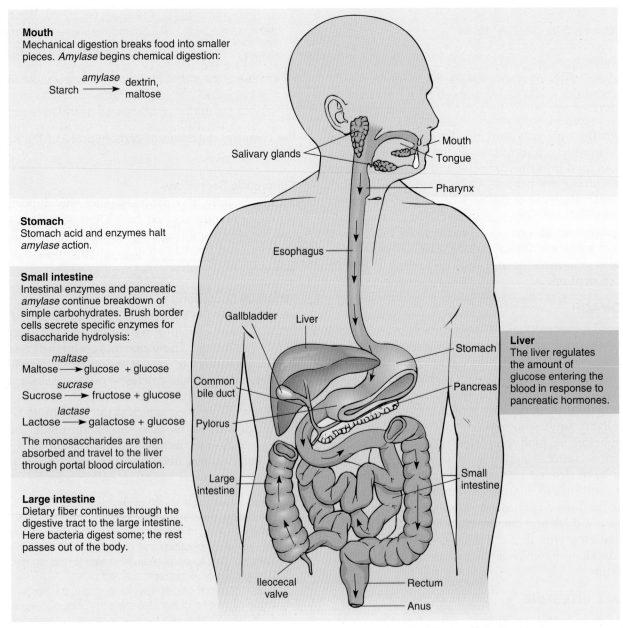

Mouth
Mechanical digestion breaks food into smaller pieces. *Amylase* begins chemical digestion:

$$Starch \xrightarrow{amylase} dextrin, maltose$$

Stomach
Stomach acid and enzymes halt *amylase* action.

Small intestine
Intestinal enzymes and pancreatic *amylase* continue breakdown of simple carbohydrates. Brush border cells secrete specific enzymes for disaccharide hydrolysis:

$$Maltose \xrightarrow{maltase} glucose + glucose$$
$$Sucrose \xrightarrow{sucrase} fructose + glucose$$
$$Lactose \xrightarrow{lactase} galactose + glucose$$

The monosaccharides are then absorbed and travel to the liver through portal blood circulation.

Large intestine
Dietary fiber continues through the digestive tract to the large intestine. Here bacteria digest some; the rest passes out of the body.

Liver
The liver regulates the amount of glucose entering the blood in response to pancreatic hormones.

Mouth
Tongue
Salivary glands
Pharynx
Esophagus
Gallbladder
Liver
Stomach
Common bile duct
Pancreas
Pylorus
Large intestine
Small intestine
Ileocecal valve
Rectum
Anus

Figure 2.4 Summary of carbohydrate digestion. Note: Enzymes are in *italics*. (Courtesy Rolin Graphics.)

Cultural Considerations

Ethnicity and Lactose Intolerance

Lactose intolerance or malabsorption results when the enzyme that is necessary for lactose digestion (lactase) is absent or deficient from the brush border cells of the small intestine. This condition, known as *hypolactasia*, usually does not present side effects until less than 50% of the enzyme is active.[1] If the disaccharide lactose cannot be hydrolyzed into its respective monosaccharides (i.e., glucose and galactose), then the unabsorbed sugar attracts excess fluid into the gut. Normal bacteria found in the colon can partially metabolize the lactose entering the large intestine, thereby producing large amounts of gas and discomfort.

It is difficult to estimate the overall prevalence of lactose intolerance in the United States. However, it is possible to determine the racial and ethnic groups with a higher incidence. African Americans, Asian Americans, Hispanic Americans, and Native Americans have higher rates of lactose intolerance as compared with Americans of Northern European descent.[2]

Individuals with lactose intolerance can usually tolerate some low-lactose milk products, such as hard cheese. Lactose intolerance is not an allergy, and most affected individuals can handle varying levels of lactose in their diet. Individuals can determine their tolerance by gradually introducing small amounts of lactose-containing foods into the diet, while noting any side effects. Most individuals can tolerate up to 12 g of lactose before symptoms arise.[1] The strong genetic link to lactose intolerance indicates that a drastic change to dietary lactose tolerance will probably not occur over a lifetime. However, many individuals do experience slight fluctuations in tolerance.

REFERENCES

1. Deng, Y., et al. (2015). Lactose intolerance in adults: Biological mechanism and dietary management. *Nutrients, 7*(9), 8020–8035.
2. Suchy, F. J., et al. (2010). National Institutes of Health Consensus Development Conference: Lactose intolerance and health. *Ann Intern Med, 152*(12), 792–796.

men aged 19 to 50 years old. The DRIs are slightly lower for adults over the age of 50 (21 g/day for women and 30 g/day for men).[8] We can achieve these recommendations by choosing carbohydrate foods such as whole grains, legumes, vegetables, and fruits. In addition, the DRIs recommend limiting added sugar to no more than 25% of the total calories consumed. See the Clinical Applications box, "What Is Your Dietary Reference Intake for Carbohydrates?" to calculate your personal carbohydrate recommendation.

DIETARY GUIDELINES FOR AMERICANS

The *Dietary Guidelines for Americans* are evidence-based guidelines for the promotion of health (see Figure 1.5). The guidelines advise individuals to do the following with regard to carbohydrate-rich foods[5]:

- Consume at least half of all grains as whole grains.
- Increase vegetable and whole fruit intake. Eat a variety of vegetables from all subgroups—dark green; red and orange; beans, peas, and lentils; starchy; and other vegetables.
- Choose more nutrient-dense foods and less foods and beverages with added sugar.
- Reduce the intake of calories from added sugars to less than 10% of total calories in the diet starting at age 2. Avoid foods and beverages with added sugars for those younger than age 2.

MYPLATE

The MyPlate food guidance system provides recommendations that are specific to age, sex, height, weight, and physical activity when reported as part of the MyPlate plan (see Chapter 1, Figure 1.4).[23] This is a free resource about dietary sources of and serving recommendations for carbohydrates, including the consumption of fiber, whole grains, fruits, vegetables, and added sugars.

Clinical Applications

What Is Your Dietary Reference Intake for Carbohydrates?

Using the current Dietary Reference Intakes (DRIs), calculate the amount of calories and grams of carbohydrates recommended for your daily consumption. This requires you to know how many total calories you consume on a daily basis.

Step 1: Keep track of everything you eat for 1 day. You can use the USDA's FoodData Central (found at: fdc.nal. usda.gov), to look up each item you eat and calculate your daily food intake. This is your *total energy intake*. (Chapter 6 discusses the evaluation of total energy intake relative to body weight and activity needs.)

Total energy intake = _____ kcal

Step 2: Multiply your total energy intake by 45% (0.45) and 65% (0.65) to get the recommended number of *kilocalories from carbohydrates (CHO)*.

_____ total kcal × 0.45 = _____ kcal
_____ total kcal × 0.65 = _____ kcal

Example:
2200 total kcal × 0.45 = 990 kcal
2200 total kcal × 0.65 = 1430
Thus, the recommended range of total kilocalories from CHO for this example is 990 to 1430 kcal/day.

Step 3: Determine how many *grams of CHO* you need based on these recommendations.

Each gram of CHO has 4 kcal; therefore, divide your recommended range of kilocalories from CHO (as determined in step 2) by 4.

_____ kcal/day from CHO ÷ 4 = _____ g of CHO/day

Example:
990 to 1430 kcal/day from CHO ÷ 4 = 247.5 to 357.5 g of CHO/day.

Continued

Clinical Applications—cont'd

What Is Your Dietary Reference Intake for Carbohydrates?

Thus, after rounding to the nearest whole number, the recommended range of total grams of CHO for this example is 248 to 358 g of CHO/day.

Step 4: What is the maximum amount of total kilocalorie consumption that can come from *added sugars,* according to the DRIs? Manufacturers add sugars to food and beverages during production. The majority of added sugars in American diets come from candy, soft drinks, fruit drinks, pastries, and other sweets.

Multiply your total energy intake by 25% (0.25) to get the maximum number of *kilocalories from added sugars.*

_____ total kcal × 0.25 = _____ kcal

Example:

2200 total kcal × 0.25 = 550 kcal

Thus, the maximum amount of total kilocalories from added sugar for this example is 550 kcal/day.

Step 5: Determine the number of grams of added sugar by dividing the maximum kcal/day of added sugar by 4.

_____ kcal/day from added sugar ÷ 4 = _____ g of added sugar/day

Example:

550 kcal/day from added sugar ÷ 4 = 137.5 g of added sugar/day

Therefore, the 137.5 g of added sugar is the recommended *limit* per day for this example.

NOTE: There is no dietary need for added sugar in the diet. This is only a reference for a *maximum* consumption. The *Dietary Guidelines for Americans* further recommends limiting added sugar to 10% of total kilocalories in the diet.

Putting It All Together

Summary

- The primary source of energy for most of the world's population is carbohydrate-rich plant-based foods. For the most part, these food products can be stored easily and are relatively low in cost.

- Two basic types of carbohydrates supply energy: simple and complex. Simple carbohydrates are single- and double-sugar units (i.e., monosaccharides and disaccharides, respectively). Because simple carbohydrates are easy to digest and absorb, they provide quick energy. Complex carbohydrates (i.e., polysaccharides) are composed of many sugar units linked together. They break down more slowly and thus provide sustained energy over a longer period.

- Dietary fiber is a complex carbohydrate that is not digestible by humans. It mainly occurs as the structural parts of plants, and it provides important bulk in the diet, affects nutrient absorption, and benefits health.

- Carbohydrate digestion starts briefly in the mouth with the initial action of salivary amylase to begin digesting starch into smaller units. No enzyme for starch digestion is present in the stomach, but muscle action continues to mix the food mass and move it to the small intestine, where pancreatic amylase continues the chemical digestion. Final starch and disaccharide digestion occurs in the small intestine with the action of sucrase, lactase, and maltase to produce single-sugar units of glucose, fructose, and galactose. These monosaccharides are then absorbed into the portal blood circulation to the liver.

Chapter Review Questions

See answers in Appendix A.

1. John is trying to increase dietary fiber in his diet. A good food choice to recommend is _____.
   a. whole-grain toast with apple slices
   b. toaster pastry with blueberry filling
   c. hot dog on white bun
   d. milkshake with low-fat potato chips

2. A client asks the nurse for examples of refined grains. The nurse may give the following examples of refined grains: _____.
   a. popcorn and steel-cut oats
   b. carrots and celery
   c. chocolate chip cookies and saltine crackers
   d. parmesan cheese and cantaloupe

3. Jeremy's primary care physician recently diagnosed him with lactose intolerance. He comes into the clinic with complaints of gas and bloating. A review of the foods eaten reveals the most likely cause to be _____.
   a. roasted chicken with parsley
   b. chocolate ice cream
   c. baked potato with butter
   d. dried fruit mix

4. Anna requires 2100 calories per day. An appropriate amount of carbohydrate calories per day for her would be _____.
   a. 210–525 calories
   b. 420–735 calories
   c. 765–1105 calories
   d. 945–1365 calories

5. Which of the following food items would most likely provide the quickest source of energy?
   a. Oat bran muffin
   b. Orange juice
   c. Pretzels
   d. 2% milk

Next-Generation NCLEX® Examination-style Case Study

See answers in Appendix A.

A 20-year-old college soccer player (Ht.: 5'8" Wt.:140 lbs.) complains of fatigue and lack of energy throughout the day. She struggles to finish workouts and her coaches are becoming disappointed in her performance. She is trying to reduce her body fat as much as possible. She provided the following 24-hour recall:

Breakfast: eggs (2) with cheese, spinach (¼ c.), and whole milk (8 oz.)

Lunch: chicken breast (6 oz.) with broccoli (½ c.) drizzled with cheese

Snack: carrots (½ c.) with ranch dressing and string cheese

Dinner: salmon (8 oz.), cauliflower rice (¾ c.), and asparagus (½ c.)

1. From the list below, identify nutrition concerns regarding the client's diet.

   a. Lack of carbohydrate-rich foods
   b. Lack of protein-rich foods
   c. Lack of fat-rich foods
   d. Lack of fruits
   e. Lack of grains
   f. Excessive carbohydrates

2. Choose the *most likely* options for the information missing from the statements below by selecting from the list of options provided.

   The client may not be maintaining ___1___. Failing to refuel ___2___ stores can cause fatigue and ___3___ catabolism.

OPTION 1	OPTION 2	OPTION 3
hyperglycemia	fat	muscle
euglycemia	glycogen	bone
hypoglycemia	protein	mineral

3. Select the correct amount of carbohydrates in grams using the Acceptable Macronutrient Distribution Range based on the client's calorie needs of 2400 kcals/day.

   a. 160-223 g/day
   b. 125-173 g/day
   c. 280-360 g/day
   d. 480-390 g/day
   e. 270-390 g/day

4. From the list below, identify appropriate meal choices containing complex carbohydrates that would be best for the client to consume before her workouts.

   a. Eggs with bacon and milk
   b. Cheese and egg omelet
   c. Oatmeal with strawberries, milk, and a hardboiled egg
   d. Cinnamon roll with icing
   e. Toast with peanut butter, banana slices, and milk

5. For each assessment, use an X to indicate whether the interventions were effective (helped to meet expected outcomes), ineffective (did not help to meet expected outcomes), or unrelated (not related to the expected outcomes).

ASSESSMENT FINDING	EFFECTIVE	INEFFECTIVE
Feels energized throughout the day		
Completes her workouts with less unplanned breaks		
Fears foods such as pasta and rice		
Feels satisfied after meals		
Has irregular bowel movements		
Consumes 200 g of carbohydrate/day		

Additional Learning Resources

Please refer to this text's Evolve website for answers to the Case Study questions:
http://evolve.elsevier.com/Williams/basic/
References and **Further Reading and Resources** in the back of the book provide additional resources for enhancing knowledge.

Key Concepts

- Dietary fat is essential to the body as an energy fuel and a structural material.
- Foods from animal and plant sources supply distinct forms of fat that affect health in different ways.
- Excess dietary fat, especially in an otherwise unbalanced diet, is a risk factor for poor health.

General awareness regarding health concerns and the risk of chronic disease from poor food selections has influenced dietary choices for decades. More knowledge of "heart-healthy" fats is helpful for the public to identify beneficial sources of dietary fat and to create a well-rounded diet.

This chapter examines the various aspects of fat as an essential nutrient, a concentrated storage form of energy, and a savory food component. In addition, we will review the types of fat and the health implications when dietary fat intake or body fat goes unchecked.

THE NATURE OF FATS

DIETARY IMPORTANCE

Fats are a concentrated fuel source for the human energy system. A large amount of energy can be stored in a relatively small space within adipose tissue as compared with carbohydrates that are stored as glycogen. As such, fats supplement carbohydrates (the primary fuel) as an additional energy source. In food, fats occur in the form of either solid fat or liquid oil. Fats are not soluble in water, and they have a greasy texture.

STRUCTURE AND CLASSES OF FATS

The name of the chemical group of fat and fat-related compounds is **lipids,** which comes from the Greek word *lipos,* meaning "fat." Several fat-related compounds (e.g., **glycolipid**) and health conditions of the body (e.g., **hyperlipidemia**) contain the word *lipid.*

All lipids are composed of the same basic chemical elements as carbohydrates: carbon, hydrogen, and oxygen. The majority of dietary fats are **glycerides,** which are composed of **fatty acids** attached to a glycerol backbone. Most natural fats, whether in animal or plant sources, have three fatty acids attached to their glycerol base, thus the chemical name of **triglyceride** (Figure 3.1).

Fatty acids are classified as short-, medium-, or long-chain. The chains contain carbon atoms with a methyl group (CH_3) on one end (also known as the *omega end*) and an acid carboxyl group (COOH) on the

other end. Short-chain fatty acids have 2 to 4 carbons, medium-chain fatty acids have 6 to 10 carbons, and long-chain fatty acids have more than 12 carbons. Additional significant characteristics, such as saturation or essentiality, classify fatty acids as well. Other types of fat in the body include combination molecules such as lipoproteins and phospholipids. The following sections briefly describe each of the lipid types.

Saturated Fat

When a substance is described as **saturated,** it contains all of the material that it is capable of holding (Figure 3.2A). For example, a saturated sponge holds all of the water that it can contain. Similarly, fatty acids are saturated or unsaturated according to whether hydrogen ions fill each available spot on the carbon backbone. Thus, a saturated fatty acid is heavy and dense (i.e., solid at room temperature). If most of the fatty acids in a triglyceride are saturated, we call that fat a *saturated fat.* Most saturated fats are of animal origin. Figure 3.3 shows a variety of foods with saturated fat, including meat, dairy, and eggs.

lipids the chemical group name for organic substances of a fatty nature; the lipids include fats, oils, waxes, and other fat-related compounds such as cholesterol.

glycolipid a lipid with a carbohydrate attached.

hyperlipidemia high lipid levels in the blood.

glycerides the chemical group name for fats; fats are formed from a glycerol base with one, two, or three fatty acids attached to make monoglycerides, diglycerides, and triglycerides, respectively; glycerides are the principal constituents of adipose tissue, and they are found in animal and vegetable fats and oils.

fatty acids the major structural components of fats.

triglycerides the chemical name for fats in the body or in food; three fatty acids attached to a glycerol base.

saturated the state of being filled; the state of fatty acid components being filled in all their available carbon bonds with hydrogen, thus making the fat more solid at room temperature; such solid food fats are generally from animal sources.

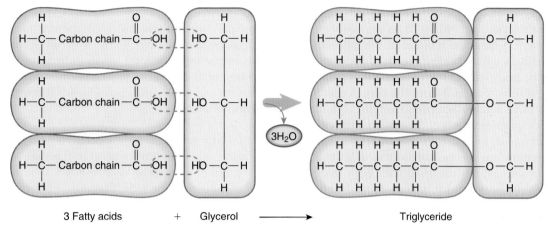

3 Fatty acids   +   Glycerol ⟶ Triglyceride

Figure 3.1 A triglyceride contains three fatty acids bound to a glycerol molecule.

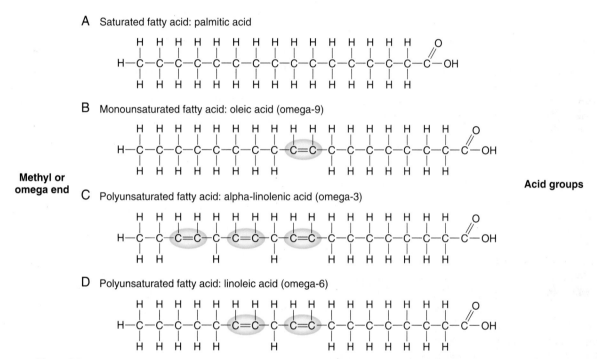

A Saturated fatty acid: palmitic acid

B Monounsaturated fatty acid: oleic acid (omega-9)

Methyl or omega end

Acid groups

C Polyunsaturated fatty acid: alpha-linolenic acid (omega-3)

D Polyunsaturated fatty acid: linoleic acid (omega-6)

Figure 3.2 Types of fatty acids. (A) Saturated palmitic acid. (B) Monounsaturated oleic acid (an omega-9 fatty acid). (C) Polyunsaturated alpha-linolenic acid (an omega-3 fatty acid). (D) Polyunsaturated linoleic acid (an omega-6 fatty acid). (Modified from Grodner, M., Escott-Stump, S., & Dorner, S. [2016]. *Nutritional foundations and clinical applications: A nursing approach* [6th ed.]. St. Louis: Mosby.)

Unsaturated Fat

A fatty acid that is not completely filled with all of the hydrogen that it can hold is unsaturated; as a result, it is less heavy and less dense (i.e., liquid at room temperature). If most of the fatty acids in a triglyceride are unsaturated, we call that fat an *unsaturated fat.* If the fatty acids have one unfilled spot (i.e., one double bond between the carbon atoms), the fat is called a *monounsaturated fat* (see Figure 3.2B). Examples of foods that contain monounsaturated fats include the vegetable oils: olive, canola (rapeseed), peanut; nuts such as macadamia, hazelnuts, almonds, and pecans; and avocados. If the fatty acids have two or more unfilled spots (i.e., more than one double bond between the carbon atoms), the fat is called a *polyunsaturated fat*

(see Figure 3.2C and D). Examples of foods that contain polyunsaturated fats are the vegetable oils: safflower, sunflower, corn, and soybean. Fats from plant and fish sources are mostly unsaturated (Figure 3.4). However, notable exceptions are the tropical oils (palm and coconut oils), which are predominantly saturated fats despite originating from a plant.

The location of the first double bond from the omega end (i.e., the methyl group end) on an unsaturated fatty acid determines another form of classification. For example, when the first double bond is on the third carbon from the methyl end, we call it an *omega-3 fatty acid* (see Figure 3.2C). When the first double bond starts on the sixth carbon from the methyl end, we call it an *omega-6 fatty acid* (see Figure 3.2D).

Essential fatty acids. We apply the term *essential* or *non-essential* to a nutrient according to its necessity in the diet. A nutrient is essential if either of the following is true: (1) its absence will create a specific deficiency disease or (2) the body cannot manufacture it in sufficient amounts and must obtain it from the diet. A diet with 10% or less of its total kilocalories from fat is unlikely to supply adequate amounts of the essential fatty acids. The only fatty acids known to be essential for complete human nutrition are the polyunsaturated fatty acids linoleic acid and alpha-linolenic acid. Both essential fatty acids serve important functions related to tissue strength, cholesterol metabolism, muscle tone, blood clotting, and heart action. As with all essential nutrients, essential fatty acids must come from the foods we eat. With an adequate dietary supply of the essential fatty acids, the body is capable of manufacturing saturated, monounsaturated, and other polyunsaturated fatty acids, as well as cholesterol. Therefore, no Dietary Reference Intake (DRI) exists for fat compounds other than the two essential fatty acids.[1]

The terms *omega-3 fatty acid* and *alpha-linolenic acid* are not interchangeable terms (despite the frequent erroneous use). This is also a point of confusion for *omega-6 fatty acid* and *linoleic acid*. There are several omega-3 and omega-6 fatty acids, of which alpha-linolenic and linoleic are two examples. Other examples of omega-3 fatty acids are eicosapentaenoic acid and docosahexaenoic acid. Thus, it is not accurate to use the vague term *omega-3* when indicating the particular essential fatty acid *alpha-linolenic acid*. The same is true for omega-6 and linoleic acid: the terms are not synonymous.

Trans-fatty acids. Naturally occurring unsaturated fatty acid molecules have a bend in the chain of atoms at the point of the carbon double bond. We call this form *cis*, meaning "same side," because both of the hydrogen atoms around the carbon double bond are on the same side of the bond. When manufacturers partially hydrogenate vegetable oils to produce a more solid, shelf-stable fat, the normal bend changes so that the hydrogen atoms on either side of the carbon double bond move to opposite sides. We call this form *trans*, meaning "opposite side," and it is most commonly the result of *hydrogenation*. Figure 3.5 shows the *cis* form and the *trans* form of a fatty acid; note the location of the hydrogen atoms relative to the double bond in each configuration.

Commercially hydrogenated fats in margarine, snack items, fast food, and many other food products used to be high in trans fat. Trans fats are unnecessary in human nutrition and pose a great number of negative health consequences related to all-cause mortality and cardiovascular disease (CVD).[2-4] In fact, the evidence was so convincing that the U.S. Food and Drug Administration (FDA) ruled that partially hydrogenated oils (the primary source of trans fats in human food) are no longer recognized as a safe product in the food supply and issued a deadline of June 2018 for the removal of such fats from the food supply.[5] Some food companies were allowed an extension on this ruling (up to 2 years) to accommodate foods previously released into the food supply, but additional food manufacturing may not use products containing trans fats.

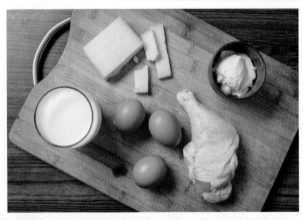

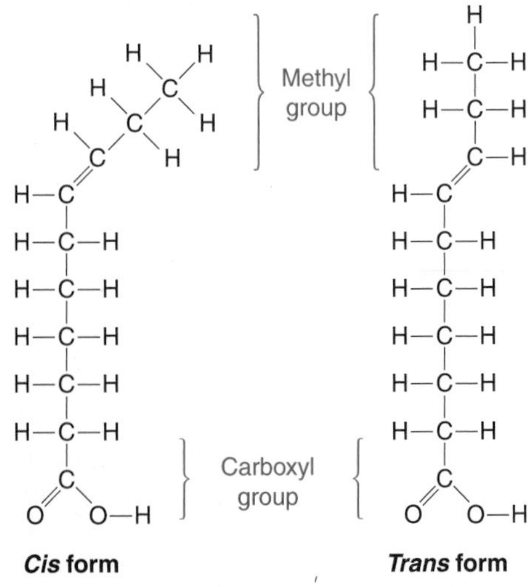

Figure 3.3 Dietary sources of saturated fats. (Copyright iStock Photo; Credit: dutourdumonde.)

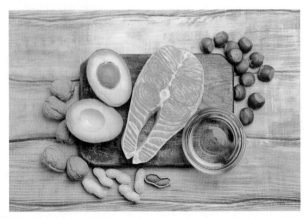

Figure 3.4 Dietary sources of unsaturated fats. (Copyright iStock Photo; Credit: JulijaDmitrijeva.)

Figure 3.5 *Cis* and *trans*-fatty acid configuration.

The dietary recommendations by the *Healthy People* initiative, the Institute of Medicine, and the *Dietary Guidelines for Americans* are to avoid trans fat in the diet as much as possible.[1,6-8]

Lipoproteins

Lipoproteins, which are the major vehicles for lipid transport in the bloodstream, are combinations of triglycerides, protein (apoprotein), phospholipids, cholesterol, and other fat-soluble substances (e.g., fat-soluble vitamins). Because fat is insoluble in water and because blood is predominantly water, fat cannot freely travel in the bloodstream; it needs a water-soluble carrier. The body solves this problem by wrapping small particles of fat in a covering of protein, which is **hydrophilic**. The blood then transports these packages of fat to and from the cells throughout the body to supply needed nutrients. A lipoprotein's relative load of fat and protein determines its density. The higher the protein load, the higher the lipoprotein's density. The lower the protein load, the lower the lipoprotein's density (Figure 3.6). Low-density lipoproteins (LDLs) carry fat and cholesterol to cells. High-density lipoproteins (HDLs) carry free cholesterol from body tissues back to the liver for metabolism. Circulating levels of lipoproteins are indicative of lipid disorder risks and the underlying blood vessel disease atherosclerosis. Chapter 19 covers these relationships in detail.

Phospholipids

Phospholipids are triglyceride derivatives in which a phosphate group replaces one fatty acid. The result is a molecule that is partially **hydrophobic** and partially hydrophilic because of the phosphate group. We call this an *amphiphilic molecule,* in which the hydrophilic heads face outward to the aqueous environment and the hydrophobic heads bind fats and oils and face each other. Phospholipids are major constituents in cell membranes and allow for membrane fluidity.

Lecithin. Lecithin, which is a major phospholipid produced by the liver, is a key building block of cell membranes as a component of the lipid bilayer. The amphiphilic quality of lecithin makes it ideal for transporting fats and cholesterol throughout the body. Most foods made from animal products provide dietary lecithin because all cell membranes contain it. Liver and egg are particularly rich sources.

Eicosanoids. Eicosanoids are signaling hormones that exert local control over multiple functions in the body (e.g., the inflammatory response, blood clotting, blood pressure regulation). They also serve as messengers for the central nervous system. Eicosanoids are synthesized from fatty acids released from phospholipids and are divided into four classes: (1) prostaglandins; (2) prostacyclins; (3) thromboxanes; and (4) leukotrienes.

Sterols

Sterols are a subgroup of steroids, and they are amphipathic in nature. *Phytosterols* are plant-made sterols and *zoosterols* are animal-made sterols. Sterols play a variety of important roles, including membrane fluidity and cellular signaling. Cholesterol is the most significant zoosterol.

---

linoleic acid an essential fatty acid that consists of 18 carbon atoms and 2 double bonds. The first double bond is located at the sixth carbon from the omega end, making it an omega-6 fatty acid. Found in vegetable oils.

alpha-linolenic acid an essential fatty acid with 18 carbon atoms and 3 double bonds. The first double bond is located at the third carbon from the omega end, making it an omega-3 fatty acid. Found in soybean, canola, and flaxseed oil.

cholesterol a fat-related compound called a sterol that is synthesized only in animal tissues; a normal constituent of bile and a principal constituent of gallstones; in the body, cholesterol is primarily synthesized in the liver; in the diet, cholesterol is found in animal food sources.

hydrophilic water loving.

hydrophobic water fearing.

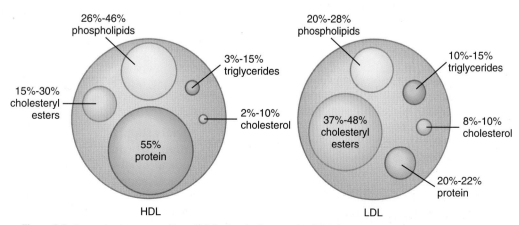

Figure 3.6 Approximate composition of high-density lipoproteins (HDLs) and low-density lipoproteins (LDLs).

Cholesterol. Cholesterol is vital to cell membranes; it is a precursor for some hormones, and it plays other important roles in human metabolism. It occurs naturally in foods of animal origin. The main food sources of cholesterol in the diet of U.S. adults are meat, eggs, baked goods, and milk.[9] To ensure that it always has the relatively small amount of cholesterol necessary for sustaining life, the human body synthesizes endogenous cholesterol in many body tissues, particularly in the liver as well as in small amounts in the adrenal cortex, the skin, the intestines, the testes, and the ovaries. Consequently, no biologic requirement for dietary cholesterol exists, and there is not a DRI for cholesterol consumption. The *Dietary Guidelines for Americans, 2020-2025* agree with the DRI recommendations to consume a diet low in cholesterol by choosing lean sources of meat that are also low in saturated fat.[1,8] Dietary cholesterol intake is only one of several influential factors in determining one's serum cholesterol levels (a risk factor for CVD). However, even small increases in LDL cholesterol fractions can increase the risk for CVD over time.[10-12] Thus, consuming a balanced diet with adequate fiber and that is also low in dietary cholesterol, saturated fats, and trans fats reduces the overall risk for CVD as it relates to serum cholesterol levels.

FUNCTIONS OF FAT

FAT IN FOOD
Energy
In addition to carbohydrates, fats serve as a fuel source for cellular energy. The body can efficiently convert excess caloric intake from any macronutrient into stored fat for later use. Fat is a much more concentrated form of fuel, yielding 9 kcal/g when burned by the body as compared with carbohydrate's yield of 4 kcal/g.

Essential Nutrients
Dietary fat supplies the body with the essential fatty acids (linoleic and alpha-linolenic acid). As long as we consume adequate amounts of the essential fatty acids, our bodies are capable of endogenously producing other fats and cholesterol as needed. In addition, foods high in fat are frequently a good source of fat-soluble vitamins (see Chapter 7), and dietary fat aids in the absorption of those vitamins.

Flavor and Satisfaction
Fat in the diet adds flavor to foods and contributes to a feeling of satiety after a meal. The slower rate of digestion of fats (as compared with that of carbohydrates and protein) causes some of these effects. This satiety also results from the fuller texture and body that fat gives to food and the slower emptying time of the stomach that it necessitates. The absence of satiation while an individual is consuming a low-fat or fat-free diet may contribute to dissatisfaction with such weight-loss attempts that remove too much dietary fat.

Fat Substitutes
Several fat substitutes, which are compounds that are not absorbed and thus contribute little or no kilocalories, are available to improve flavor and physical texture to low-fat/fat-free foods and to help reduce total dietary fat intake. The U.S. FDA considers fat substitutes that are currently on the market safe. However, the risks and benefits of long-term use of fat substitutes are not well established. There are many different types of fat substitutes. Two of the more common examples are Simplesse (CP Kelco, Atlanta, GA), which is made by reshaping the protein of milk whey or egg whites, and Olean (Olestra, Procter & Gamble, Cincinnati, OH), which is an indigestible form of sucrose.

FAT IN THE BODY
Adipose Tissue
Adipose tissue, located throughout the body, is the main storage site for fat. A web-like padding of fat tissue supports and protects vital organs, and a layer of fat directly under the skin is important for the regulation of body temperature.

Cell Membrane Structure
Fat forms the fatty center of cell membranes, thereby creating the selectively permeable lipid bilayer. Embedded within this layer are proteins that allow for the transport of various nutrients in and out of the cells. In addition, the protective myelin sheath that surrounds neurons is largely composed of fat.

FOOD SOURCES OF FAT
FATTY ACID COMPOSITION
People commonly classify foods as being a source of one type of fat or another. In reality, most foods contain a combination of different types of fats. For example, we generally think of olive oil as a "heart-healthy" monounsaturated fat. Although it is a significant source of monounsaturated fat (74% of the fatty acids), olive oil is also composed of 15% saturated fatty acids and 11% polyunsaturated fatty acids. Another prime example is beef fat. It is true that beef fat is mostly saturated fat (52% of the fatty acids are saturated), but a hefty 44% of fatty acids are monounsaturated and 4% are polyunsaturated.[13] Very few things in nutrition are all or nothing. Keep this in mind as you read the following section, where we categorize fats according to the predominant, but not exclusive, source of fat.

Animal Fats
The chief dietary supply of saturated fat and cholesterol comes from animal sources, the most concentrated of which include meat fats (e.g., bacon, sausage), dairy fats (e.g., cream, ice cream, butter, cheese), and egg yolks.

Adipose fat stored in the cells of adipose (fatty) tissue.

The exceptions to this rule are the tropical oils: coconut and palm oil. These tropical oils are plant-based fats but are composed predominantly of saturated fatty acids (e.g., 91% of the fat in coconut oil is saturated).[13] The American diet has traditionally featured meats and other foods of animal origin. The U.S. Department of Agriculture reports that animal products in particular (e.g., meat, poultry, fish, eggs, dairy products) contribute 38% of the total fat to U.S. diets as well as 54% of the saturated fat and almost all of the cholesterol (95%).[14] Some animal fats also contain small amounts of unsaturated fats. For example, a 6-oz serving of sockeye salmon provides 3.2 g of monounsaturated fat and 2.3 g of polyunsaturated fat, in addition to 1.6 g of saturated fat.[13]

Although animal products do supply saturated fat and cholesterol to the diet, not all types of animal-derived foods are created equal. Two important dietary factors that are associated with a higher risk of chronic disease such as heart disease, stroke, and type 2 diabetes are a high intake of processed meat and a low intake of omega-3 fats from seafood.[15-17] Diets that derive the majority of their protein and fat from lean poultry or fish do not share the same high-risk profiles.[18] Thus, one dietary recommendation to help reduce the overall risk of chronic disease is to choose lean, unprocessed meat and seafood products in place of their high saturated fat or processed counterparts.[8,19,20]

Plant Fats

Plant foods supply mostly monounsaturated and polyunsaturated fats, including the essential fatty acids. Vegetable oils (e.g., safflower, corn, cottonseed, soybean, peanut, olive; see Figure 3.4) are particularly good sources of unsaturated fats. However, as indicated previously, the exceptions are coconut and palm oils; these plants provide mostly saturated fats, and commercially processed food items use these fats frequently.

PHYSICAL CHARACTERISTICS OF FOOD FAT

For practical purposes, we can categorize food fats as either visible or invisible fats.

Visible Fat

The obvious fats are easy to see and include butter, margarine, separate cream, salad oils and dressings, lard, shortening, fatty meats (e.g., bacon, sausage, salt pork), and the visible fat of any meat. Visible fats are easier to control in the diet than those that are less apparent.

Invisible Fat

Some dietary fats are less visible, so individuals who want to control dietary fat must be aware of these food sources. Invisible fats include cheese, the cream portion of homogenized milk, nuts, seeds, olives, avocados, and lean meat. Invisible fats are those that you cannot cut out of the food. Even when all of the visible fat has been removed from meat (e.g., the skin on poultry and the obvious fat on the lean portions), approximately 25% of the total fat surrounding the muscle fibers remains.

Table 3.1 provides a list of commonly eaten foods and their fat content according to type of fat.

FOOD LABEL INFORMATION

The FDA food-labeling regulations for nutrition facts panel content provide the following mandatory and voluntary (italicized in following list) information relating to dietary fat in food products (Figure 3.7):
- Total fat
- Saturated fat
- Trans fat
- *Polyunsaturated fat*
- *Monounsaturated fat*
- Cholesterol

Table 3.1	Fat in Food Servings					
FOOD	SERVING SIZE	TOTAL FAT (G)	SATURATED FAT (G)	MONO-UNSATURATED FAT (G)	POLY-UNSATURATED FAT (G)	TRANS FATS (G)
Fats						
Butter	1 Tbsp	11.5	7.2	3.3	0.4	0.5
Cream cheese	1 Tbsp	3.4	2	0.9	0.2	0.1
Margarine	1 Tbsp	11	2	3	3	3
Mayonnaise	1 Tbsp	12	1.5	2.5	7	0
Salad dressing, Italian	2 Tbsp	6.2	0.9	1.7	3.2	Trace
Bread and Grains						
Bagel, wheat	1 (98 g)	1.5	0	0.3	0.9	0
Muffin, blueberry	1 medium (113 g)	18.2	3.2	5.5	9.2	0.2
Pasta, cooked	½ cup	0.6	0.1	0.08	0.2	0
Rice, white, cooked	½ cup	0.2	0.06	0.07	0.06	0

Continued

Table 3.1 **Fat in Food Servings—cont'd**

FOOD	SERVING SIZE	TOTAL FAT (G)	SATURATED FAT (G)	MONO-UNSATURATED FAT (G)	POLY-UNSATURATED FAT (G)	TRANS FATS (G)
Dairy						
Cheese, cheddar	2 oz	18.9	10.7	5.3	0.5	0.6
Cheese, feta	2 oz	12.2	7.5	2.6	0.3	0
Ice cream, vanilla	½ cup	7.3	4.5	2	0.3	0
Milk, low-fat	1 cup	2.4	1.5	0.7	0.1	0
Milk, skim	1 cup	0.4	0.3	0.1	0	0
Milk, whole	1 cup	8	4.6	2	0.5	0
Yogurt, frozen, vanilla	½ cup	4	2.5	1.2	0.2	Trace
Yogurt, plain, whole milk	6 oz	5.5	3.6	1.5	0.2	
Eggs, Fish, Meat, and Nuts						
Beef, ground, cooked	3 oz	12.4	4.8	5.4	0.4	0
Beef, rib eye steak, lean only	3 oz	9	3.6	4.1	0.5	0.4
Bologna, beef and pork	3 oz	24.6	9.3	10.5	1.1	0
Chicken, breast meat and skin, cooked	3 oz	6.6	1.9	2.6	1.4	0
Duck, meat and skin, cooked	3 oz	24	8.2	11	3.1	0
Egg	1 large	6.7	2	2.7	1.5	0.4
Nuts, almonds	1 oz	14	1	9	3.5	Trace
Nuts, walnuts	1 oz	18.5	1.7	2.5	13.4	0
Tuna, yellowfin, cooked	3 oz	0.5	0.17	0.1	0.15	Trace
Other						
Danish pastry, cheese	1 medium (71 g)	15.5	4.8	8	1.8	0
French fries	1 medium serving (117 g)	17.2	2.7	7	6.3	0.1

Fruit and Vegetables contain only trace amounts of any type of fat.

Agricultural Research Service. (2018). *USDA Food Composition Databases*. U.S. Department of Agriculture. Retrieved May 15, 2019, from ndb.nal.usda.gov.

The FDA has approved a series of health claims that link one or more dietary components to the reduced risk of specific diseases.[21] Approved health claims that involve dietary fat include the following:

- A diet that is low in total fat may reduce the risk of some cancers.
- Diets that are low in saturated fat and cholesterol may reduce the risk of coronary heart disease.

See the label claim information published by the FDA (search "health claims" at www.fda.gov) for more information about approved health claims. This website provides updates regarding approved health claims, pending claims, and the appropriate use of the claims on food products. Chapter 13 covers food labels and health claims further.

DIGESTION OF FATS

As with other macronutrients (i.e., carbohydrates and proteins), fats are broken down into their basic building blocks, fatty acids, through the process of mechanical and chemical digestion (summarized in Figure 3.8).

MOUTH

When an individual eats fat-containing food, some initial fat breakdown may begin in the mouth by the action of *lingual lipase*, an enzyme that the Ebner gland at the back of the tongue secretes. Lingual lipase is only important for digestion during infancy. For adults, the primary digestive action that occurs in the mouth is mechanical. Foods are broken into smaller particles through chewing and moistening for passage into the stomach.

STOMACH

Little if any chemical digestion of fat occurs in the stomach. General muscle action continues to mix the fat with the stomach contents. However, no significant amounts of fat enzymes are present in the

Nutrition Facts

8 servings per container
Serving size   2/3 cup (55g)

Amount per serving
Calories   230

	% Daily Value*
Total Fat 8g	**10%**
Saturated Fat 1g	**5%**
Trans Fat 0g	
Cholesterol 0mg	**0%**
Sodium 160mg	**7%**
Total Carbohydrate 37g	**13%**
Dietary Fiber 4g	**14%**
Total Sugars 12g	
Includes 10g Added Sugars	**20%**
Protein 3g	
Vitamin D 2mcg	10%
Calcium 260mg	20%
Iron 8mg	45%
Potassium 235mg	6%

* The % Daily Value (DV) tells you how much a nutrient in a serving of food contributes to a daily diet. 2,000 calories a day is used for general nutrition advice.

Figure 3.7 Example of nutrition facts panel. (From the U.S. Food and Drug Administration. [2018]. *Changes to the Nutrition Facts label*. U.S. Department of Health and Human Services. Retrieved October 10, 2018, from www.fda.gov/Food/GuidanceRegulation/GuidanceDocumentsRegulatoryInformation/LabelingNutrition/ucm385663.htm.)

gastric secretions except *gastric lipase* (tributyrinase), which acts on emulsified butterfat. The primary gastric enzymes act on protein in the food mix. Meanwhile, mechanical movements prepare fat for its major, enzyme-specific breakdown in the small intestine.

SMALL INTESTINE

Fat digestion largely occurs in the small intestine, where the major enzymes that are necessary for the chemical changes are present. These digestive agents come from three major sources: an emulsification agent from the gallbladder and two specific enzymes from the pancreas and the small intestine.

Bile

The liver first produces **bile** in large dilute amounts. It is then stored and concentrated in the gallbladder so that it is ready for use during fat digestion as needed. The fat that comes into the duodenum, which is the first section of the small intestine, stimulates the secretion of *cholecystokinin*, a hormone that the glands in the intestinal walls release. In turn, cholecystokinin causes the gallbladder to contract, relax its opening, and subsequently secrete bile into the intestine by way of the common bile duct. Bile is not an enzyme that acts in the chemical digestive process; rather, it functions as an **emulsifier.** This emulsification process accomplishes the following two important tasks: (1) it separates the fat into small particles, thereby greatly increasing the total surface area available for enzymatic action and (2) it lowers the surface tension of the finely dispersed and suspended fat particles, thus allowing the enzymes to penetrate more easily. The bile also provides an alkaline medium that is necessary for the action of *pancreatic lipase*, which is the chief lipid enzyme.

Pancreatic and Intestinal Enzymes

Pancreatic juice flowing into the small intestine contains one enzyme for triglycerides and another for cholesterol. First, pancreatic lipase breaks off one fatty acid at a time from the glycerol base of triglycerides. One free fatty acid plus a diglyceride and then another fatty acid plus a monoglyceride are liberated in turn (Figure 3.9). Each succeeding step of this breakdown occurs with increasing difficulty. In fact, the separation of the final fatty acid from the remaining monoglyceride is such a slow process that less than one-third of the total fat present reaches complete breakdown. The final products of fat digestion to be absorbed are fatty acids, monoglycerides, and glycerol.

The enzyme *cholesterol esterase* acts on cholesterol esters (not free cholesterol) to form a combination of free cholesterol and fatty acids in preparation for absorption into the lacteals (lymph vessels) and finally into the bloodstream (see Chapter 5). The small intestine secretes an enzyme in the intestinal juice called *lecithinase*, which breaks down lecithin for absorption. Some small amounts of remaining fat may pass into the large intestine for fecal elimination.

Figure 3.8 summarizes fat digestion in the successive parts of the gastrointestinal tract.

Absorption

Fat absorption into the gastrointestinal cells and bloodstream is more complex than the absorption of other macronutrients. Triglycerides are not soluble in water and thus cannot directly enter the bloodstream, which is mostly water. Within the small intestine, bile salts surround the monoglycerides and fatty acids to form **micelles.** Found in the middle of the packaged micelle are the non–water-soluble fat particles (e.g., fatty acids, monoglycerides), whereas the hydrophilic parts face outward. This structure allows the products of lipid digestion to travel to the brush border membrane. Once there, fats are absorbed into the epithelial cells of the intestine. *Enterohepatic circulation* is the process by which bile is absorbed and transported by the portal vein to the liver for reuse. Some medications used to lower blood cholesterol levels work by removing bile acid from this recycling process (see the Drug-Nutrient Interaction box, "Questran and Bile").

Mouth
Mechanical digestion breaks food into smaller pieces. Chemical digestion begins to a small degree with the secretion of *lingual lipase.*

Stomach
Peristalsis continues to mechanically mix fats with water and acid. *Gastric lipase* hydrolyzes butterfat.

Small intestine
Bile, stored in the gallbladder, enters the small intestine from the common bile duct to emulsify fat. The combined actions of chemical and mechanical digestion expose the greatest possible fat surface area to *pancreatic lipase:*

Emulsified triglycerides

pancreatic ↓ *lipase*

Fatty acids, monoglycerides, glycerol

Monoglycerides, fatty acids, and bile form micelles for absorption.

Mucosal cell
Re-formed triglycerides combine with cholesterol, phospholipids, and proteins to form chylomicrons, ready for absorption into the lymphatic system.

Large intestine
Some fats are partially digested; the rest pass through unchanged, exiting in feces.

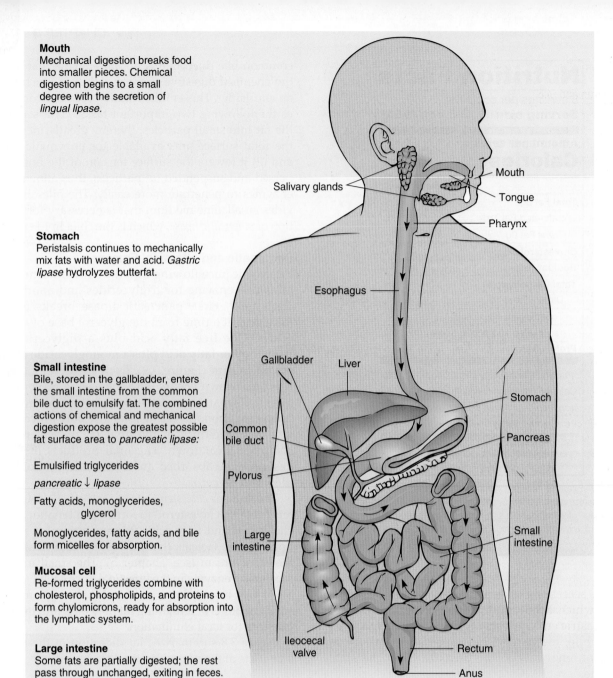

Figure 3.8 Summary of lipid digestion. Note: Enzymes are in *italics*. (Courtesy Rolin Graphics.)

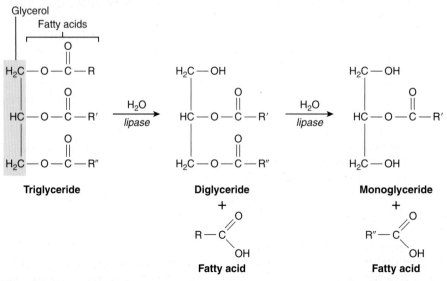

Figure 3.9 Enzymatic digestion of triglycerides into diglycerides, monoglycerides, and free fatty acids.

Questran and Bile

The liver produces bile and it is composed primarily of bile acids, salts, cholesterol, and phospholipids. The liver takes cholesterol out of circulation and uses it each time it manufactures bile. However, the gallbladder releases bile into the small intestine, where it emulsifies fat. After completing its task, the body reabsorbs bile along with the fat and fat-soluble nutrients for efficient recycling by the body. Thus, we need very little dietary cholesterol to produce bile.

Questran (cholestyramine) is an antihyperlipidemic that works by taking bile out of the recycling loop by binding it in the gastrointestinal tract and preventing its reabsorption. The bile is then excreted in the feces. Because the body depends on bile for the digestion of dietary fat, the liver will have to make more bile and will use circulating blood cholesterol to produce replacement bile. As such, Questran can lower blood cholesterol levels in individuals at risk for cardiovascular disease by forcing cholesterol out of the circulation to manufacture bile. Soluble fiber acts in much the same way to lower circulating cholesterol levels (see Chapter 2).

Bile acid sequestrants decrease the absorption of bile in addition to other fat-soluble nutrients such as vitamins A, D, E, and K. Individuals taking bile acid sequestrants on a long-term basis should be aware of good dietary sources of fat-soluble vitamins to ensure adequate intake and avoid potential nutrient deficiencies.

Monoglycerides and fatty acids that make it into the intestinal cells via micelle transport reconstruct to form triglycerides again. A new carrier called a **chylomicron** will package the triglycerides, along with cholesterol, phospholipids, and proteins (Figure 3.10). This lipoprotein particle formed within the intestinal cell allows the products of fat digestion to enter the circulation. Chylomicrons first enter the lacteals, then the lymphatic circulatory system, and then eventually the bloodstream. Figure 3.11 provides a summary of fat absorption through the process of micelle production and the formation of chylomicrons.

bile an emulsifying agent produced by the liver and transported to the gallbladder for concentration and storage; it is released into the duodenum in response to the hormone cholecystokinin to facilitate enzymatic fat digestion by acting as an emulsifier.

emulsifier an agent that breaks down large fat globules into smaller, uniformly distributed particles; the action is accomplished chiefly in the intestine by bile acids, which lower the surface tension of the fat particles, thereby breaking the fat into many smaller droplets and facilitating contact with the fat-digesting enzymes.

micelles packages of free fatty acids, monoglycerides, and bile salts; the hydrophobic fat particles are found in the middle of the package, whereas the hydrophilic part faces outward and allows for the absorption of fat into intestinal mucosal cells.

chylomicron a lipoprotein formed in the intestinal cell that is composed of triglycerides, cholesterol, phospholipids, and protein; chylomicrons allow for the absorption of fat into the lymphatic circulatory system before entering the blood circulation.

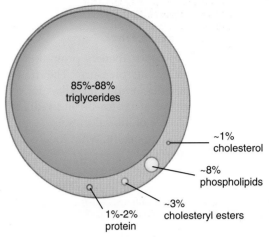

Figure 3.10 Approximate composition of a chylomicron.

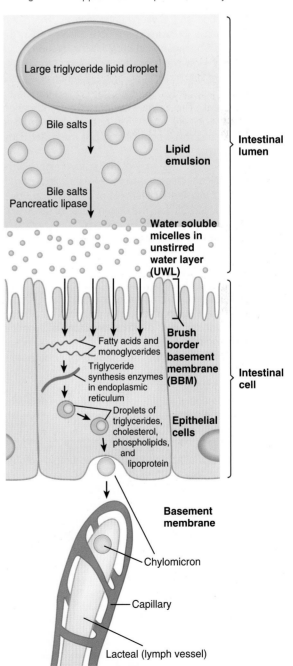

Figure 3.11 Summary of fat absorption. (From Mahan, L. K., & Escott-Stump, S. [2008]. *Krause's food & nutrition therapy* [12th ed.]. St. Louis: Saunders.)

RECOMMENDATIONS FOR DIETARY FAT

DIETARY FAT AND HEALTH

Fat in food enhances flavor, thereby providing a sense of satisfaction and eating pleasure. The traditional American diet provides ample fat kilocalories. The current average intake of fat for all individuals over the age of 2 years is 36% of kilocalories.[22]

If fat is vital to human health, what then is the concern about fat in the diet?

🌐 Cultural Considerations

Ethnic Differences in Lipid Metabolism

Dietary patterns and habits form at an early age because of family influence and environmental factors. The dietary fat intake of some individuals is much different from that of others in part because of cultural norms, customs, and food availability. However, since the unveiling of the human genome, we are learning that biologic differences also exist that may affect the ways in which our bodies handle the nutrients we eat. The prevalence of, and complications resulting from, obesity have long been known to differ among ethnic and racial populations, but the exact cause remains uncertain.

Women are often the subjects of study in obesity research. A significant difference in race exists with regard to the incidence of women 20 years old or older who are overweight in the United States. The current rates of overweight and obesity are[1]:

- 80.6% of black or African-American women
- 78.8% of Hispanic or Latina women
- 84.5% of Mexican women
- 64.6% of white women

Researchers have found that Caucasian and African-American obese women differ significantly in their adipose tissue activity and ability to effectively store triglycerides as subcutaneous fat.[2] Such biologic differences in lipid metabolism and adipose tissue activity may contribute to metabolic disorders. African-American women demonstrate impaired triglyceride storage activity in adipose tissue, which is associated with insulin resistance and other obesity-related disorders.[3] This may help explain why the risks associated with excess body fat may be worse for some than others.

These types of differences continue to unfold with ongoing genetic studies. Differences such as these will also guide individuals in their dietary and lifestyle choices with regard to how their bodies will respond to specific nutrients and long-term energy balance. The path from fat in our food to fat on our bodies continues to provide many questions for inspection and evaluation.

REFERENCES

1. National Center for Health Statistics. (2018). *Health, United States, 2017: With special feature on mortality*. Hyattsville, MD.
2. White, U. A., et al. (2018). Racial differences in in vivo adipose lipid kinetics in humans. *Journal of Lipid Research*, 59(9), 1738–1744.
3. Allister, C. A., et al. (2015). In vivo 2H2O administration reveals impaired triglyceride storage in adipose tissue of insulin-resistant humans. *Journal of Lipid Research*, 56(2), 435–439.

Health Problems

Research continues to indicate that health problems from excess dietary fat are specific to certain types of fat. We must consider the whole diet before making any conclusions about the health of a diet. In addition, not all individuals metabolize and process fat the same. See the Cultural Considerations box, "Ethnic Differences in Lipid Metabolism," for more details on this topic.

Amount of fat. Too many kilocalories in the diet, regardless of the source—fat, carbohydrates, or protein—will exceed the requirement of immediate energy needs. The surplus is stored as body fat. Excess body fat, particularly in the abdominal region, is associated with higher rates of all-cause mortality and risk factors for chronic diseases such as diabetes, hypertension, and heart disease.[23-25] How much fat is in your own daily diet? See the Clinical Applications box entitled "How Much Fat Are You Eating?" to assess your fat intake.

👁 Clinical Applications

How Much Fat Are You Eating?

Keep an accurate record of everything that you eat and drink for 1 day. Be sure to include all fat or other nutrient seasonings used with your foods (e.g., salad dressing, sauce, mayonnaise). If you want a more representative picture, use the USDA FoodData Central (fdc.nal.usda.gov), or another program to which you have access, to look up each food consumed and evaluate your average intake over a 3- to 7-day period.

Step 1: Calculate the total kilocalories and grams for each of the energy-yielding nutrients (i.e., carbohydrates, fat, and protein) in everything that you eat. Multiply the total grams of each energy nutrient by its respective fuel factor:

Fat: _____ g × 9 (kcal/g) = _____ kcal

Protein: _____ g × 4 (kcal/g) = _____ kcal

Carbohydrate: _____ g × 4 (kcal/g) = _____ kcal

Step 2: Add the kilocalories from each macronutrient to determine the total kilocalories consumed.

Step 3: Calculate the percentage of each energy-yielding nutrient in your total diet:

Example: (Fat kcal ÷ Total kcal) × 100 = % Fat kcal in diet

Step 4: Compare the amount of fat in your diet with the DRI recommendations (20% to 35% fat).

Type of fat. As discussed earlier, the type of dietary fat matters. Historically, we have accepted that an excess of cholesterol and saturated fat in the diet, which comes predominantly from animal food sources, is a specific risk factor for atherosclerosis, the underlying blood vessel disease that contributes to heart disease (see Chapter 19). However, if we replace saturated and trans fats in the diet with omega-6 polyunsaturated fatty acids or carbohydrates, there are little to no health benefits.[26-28] On the other hand, if saturated and trans fats are replaced with omega-3 polyunsaturated fats or a combination of both omega-3 and omega-6 polyunsaturated fats, there is a favorable result to lipid profiles and may be protective against some forms of heart and circulatory disease.[3,27,29-31] The American Heart Association concluded in its recent Presidential Advisory Report that diets favoring fat intake from unsaturated fats, such as the Mediterranean diet, lower the risk of cardiovascular disease and all-cause mortality by reducing LDL cholesterol and blood triglycerides.[31]

Trans-fatty acids. Observed effects of diets that are high in trans-fatty acids include an increase in LDL cholesterol levels, a reduction in the protective HDL cholesterol levels, an increase in the atherogenic index and endothelial dysfunction, and an increased production of atherosclerotic inflammatory cytokines.[2,4,32] As noted earlier, the FDA recently removed trans-fatty acids from the list of generally recognized as safe (GRAS) food additives.[5] Thus, the use of partially hydrogenated oils (the primary source of trans-fatty acids in the food supply) is no longer allowed in any food product, thereby drastically reducing the consumption of trans fats in the United States.

Essential fatty acid deficiency. Fat-free diets may lead to essential fatty acid deficiency with clinical manifestations. Omega-3 fatty acids are especially necessary for normal function of the brain, the central nervous system, and the cell membranes. Inadequate essential fatty acid intake is linked to many health problems, such as hair loss, dermatitis, impaired wound healing, compromised immunity and brain function, and growth retardation in children.

Health Promotion

The ongoing movement in American health care is toward health promotion and disease prevention through the reduction of risk factors related to chronic disease. Heart disease continues to be a leading cause of death, and there are many efforts aimed at reducing the various risk factors that lead to this disease. Poor diets contribute to these risk factors, which include obesity, diabetes, elevated levels of blood triglycerides, and hypertension. In the past, health care providers saw such risk factors only in adults. However, physicians are increasingly diagnosing children and adolescents with the same conditions. The Centers for Disease Control and Prevention reported that 21% of all youth between the ages of 6 and 19 years have abnormal lipid levels. Of those individuals, youth with a body mass index (BMI) in the obese category have a significantly higher prevalence (43.3%) of cardiovascular health risk than normal-weight children (13.8%).[33] Healthier eating habits are especially important for children in high-risk families (e.g., families with identified lipid disorders and heart disease at young ages).

Additional lifestyle risk factors for chronic disease include smoking, excessive stress, and physical inactivity, especially among middle-aged and older individuals. Maintaining an ideal body weight requires diligence in keeping the body's total daily caloric intake in balance with the total daily energy use. Chapter 15 covers in detail low-fat diets, fad diets, and other issues that affect weight management.

DIETARY REFERENCE INTAKES

The current DRIs recommend that 20% to 35% of the total kilocalories in the diet come from fat, that less than 10% of the kilocalories come from saturated fats, and that dietary cholesterol be limited to a maximum of 300 mg/day. No DRI or Tolerable Upper Intake Level is set for trans-fatty acids. The National Academy of Sciences recommends limiting trans-fat intake to as low as possible while maintaining a nutritionally adequate diet.[1] Fat is an essential part of the diet; therefore, diets that are completely devoid of fat are equally unhealthy and can result in a deficiency of essential fatty acids.

Vegetable oils are the primary source of our essential fatty acids, both of which are polyunsaturated fats. The DRI for linoleic acid is 17 g/day for men and 12 g/day for women. Seed oils (e.g., flax, canola, and soybean) and dark green leafy vegetables are the best source of alpha-linolenic acid. People usually consume much less alpha-linolenic acid than linoleic acid. The recommendation for alpha-linolenic acid intake is 1.6 and 1.1 g/day for men and women, respectively.[1]

Dietary Guidelines for Americans

In line with the current national health goal of health promotion through disease prevention by reducing identified risks of chronic disease, the *Dietary Guidelines for Americans, 2020-2025* recommend the following with regard to dietary fat intake:[8]

- For individuals over the age of 2 years, consume less than 10% of calories from saturated fatty acids. Replace saturated fats in the diet with unsaturated fats, particularly polyunsaturated fats.
- The guidelines agree with the DRI recommendations to limit trans fat and dietary cholesterol consumption to be as low as possible without compromising the nutritional adequacy of the diet.
- Choose fat-free or low-fat milk and milk products.
- Choose protein foods that are lean and nutrient dense (e.g., lean meats, poultry, and eggs; seafood; beans, peas, and lentils; and nuts, seeds, and soy products).
- Use oils to replace solid fats where possible (e.g., vegetable oils and oils in food, such as seafood and nuts).

MyPlate

The MyPlate food guidance system provides recommendations for designing a diet that reflects the DRI and *Dietary Guidelines for Americans* recommendations for fat intake within a well-balanced diet. After an individual plan is determined on the basis of age, sex, height, weight, and physical activity level, other helpful tips and resources are available through the free website www.choosemyplate.gov, such as information about how to choose lean protein sources, where to find essential fatty acids, tips for eating out, and sample menus.[6]

Putting It All Together

Summary

- Fat is an essential nutrient that serves important body needs as a backup storage fuel (secondary to carbohydrate) for energy. Fat also supplies important tissue needs as a structural material for cell membranes, a protective padding for vital organs, an insulation source to maintain body temperature, and a covering material for nerve fibers.
- Food fats have different forms and health implications. Saturated fat and cholesterol come from primarily animal food sources. Plant food sources are the richest source of unsaturated fats and may reduce health risks when used in place of trans fats in a well-balanced diet.
- When we eat various foods that contain triglycerides and cholesterol, several specific digestive agents, including bile and pancreatic lipase, prepare and break down fats. Within the endothelial cell, chylomicrons incorporate fatty acids and monoglycerides and transport them through the lymphatic system into the bloodstream.
- Replacing saturated in the diet with unsaturated fats is ideal for health promotion and disease prevention.

Chapter Review Questions

See answers in Appendix A.

1. Margaret has been reading information from the Internet regarding the health benefits of coconut oil in the diet. What type of fat does coconut oil primarily contain?

   a. Saturated
   b. Monounsaturated
   c. Polyunsaturated
   d. Trans fat

2. Elevated levels of blood lipids are referred to as _____.

   a. hyperglycemia
   b. hyperlipidemia
   c. hypertension
   d. hypernatremia

3. Mary's doctor advises her to follow a low saturated fat diet to help reduce the risk of heart disease. Which of the following foods would you most likely recommend as part of this meal plan?

   a. Beef curry made with ghee and whole coconut milk
   b. Skinless chicken and vegetables sautéed with olive oil
   c. Baked potato topped with chili, butter, and sour cream
   d. Turkey sausage and egg biscuit

4. Jeremy consumed 1800 calories of which 50 grams were from fat. What percentage of the total calories come from fat?

   a. 11%
   b. 25%
   c. 30%
   d. 42%

5. Bile from the gallbladder serves as a (an) _____ rather than an enzyme in the chemical digestive process.

   a. alkali
   b. acid
   c. emulsifier
   d. catalyst

Next-Generation NCLEX® Examination-style Case Study

See answers in Appendix A.
A 50-year-old male (Ht.: 5'10" Wt.: 200 lbs.) has a history of high cholesterol. His diet history shows frequent consumption of red meat, cheese, and fast food, with very little fruits or vegetables. The family physician placed him on Questran, an antihyperlipidemic. A couple of months later he noticed that his skin felt very dry and his vision was blurry.

1. From the list below, select the diet factors that may contribute to the client's high cholesterol.

   a. High intake of omega-3 fatty acids from red meat
   b. High intake of saturated fats from foods such as meat and dairy
   c. Low intake of omega-3 fatty acids from foods such as fish
   d. Low intake of unsaturated fats from foods like coconut and palm oil
   e. High intake of saturated fats from foods like olive oil and nuts
   f. Low intake of unsaturated fats from foods like olive oil and nuts

2. Choose the *most likely* options for the information missing from the statements below by selecting from the list of options provided.

   The client has a high intake of ___1___ fat, which can raise cholesterol levels. These fats are generally ___2___ at room temperature.

OPTION 1	OPTION 2
unsaturated	solid
polyunsaturated	volatile
saturated	liquid
essential	gelatinous

3. Choose the *most likely* options for the information missing from the statements below by selecting from the list of options provided.

   The client's symptoms of dry skin and blurred vision may be a result of his diet and medication. Questran binds to _____1_____ and inhibits reabsorption in the colon. This increases the use of _____2_____ circulating in the bloodstream (to create more bile in the liver) but can also reduce absorption of _____3_____.

OPTION 1	OPTION 2	OPTION 3
cholesterol	fat soluble vitamins	chyme
chyme	cholesterol	bile
bile	chyme	cholesterol
fat soluble vitamins	bile	fat-soluble vitamins

4. From the list below, identify topics that may be important to discuss with the client to improve his conditions.

   a. Identifying different types of fats and their impact on the body
   b. Foods containing vitamins A, D, E, and K
   c. How to follow the ketogenic diet
   d. Importance of avoiding all types of fats
   e. Dietary guidelines regarding dietary fat
   f. MyPlate guidelines and meal planning

5. The registered dietitian found that the client's energy needs are ~2250 kcals/day. Use the DRI's to find the client's recommended range of grams from total fat and maximum number of grams from saturated fat. Place an X in the box that corresponds to the correct macronutrient recommendation for each of the corresponding columns.

OPTIONS	FAT	SATURATED FAT
450–788		
25		
32		
50–88		
38		
225		

6. Evaluate the client's new attempt to follow the *Dietary Guidelines for Americans, 2020-2025* to determine if the education was effective or ineffective. Place an X under "effective" for all changes that demonstrate a good understanding of the recommendations. Place an X under "ineffective" for all changes that are not effective.

DIETARY CHANGES	EFFECTIVE	INEFFECTIVE
Consumes 35% kcals from saturated fat		
Chooses fat-free milk and dairy		
Chooses lean cuts of chicken over red meats		
Uses butter instead of olive oil		
Increases fruit and vegetable intake		
Consumes foods from all food groups		

Additional Learning Resources

Please refer to this text's Evolve website for answers to the Case Study questions:
http://evolve.elsevier.com/Williams/basic/
References and **Further Reading and Resources** in the back of the book provide additional resources for enhancing knowledge.

Proteins

Key Concepts

- Dietary protein provides the amino acids that are necessary for building and maintaining body tissue.
- The composition of amino acids making up a single protein determines the quality of that protein and its ability to meet the body's needs.
- As with all essential nutrients, consuming adequate dietary protein is essential to life and health.

A myriad of proteins in the body make life possible. Each specific protein has a unique structure that allows it to perform a designated task. Amino acids are the building blocks of all proteins. People obtain amino acids from a variety of foods. This chapter looks at the nature of proteins, both in food and in human bodies. It explains why protein balance is essential to life and health, and it discusses how a nutritious diet can maintain that balance.

THE NATURE OF PROTEIN

FUNCTIONS OF AMINO ACIDS

Building Blocks

All proteins, whether in our bodies or in the food we eat, are composed of amino acids. Peptide bonds join amino acids together (Figure 4.1) in chain sequences that are unique to each individual protein. A *dipeptide* contains two amino acids joined together. When three amino acids bond together, we call that a *tripeptide*. *Polypeptides* are chains of up to 100 amino acids linked together. A single *protein* may contain hundreds of amino acids bound together. When we eat protein-rich foods, the digestive process deconstructs the protein into single amino acids by breaking the peptide bonds. The type of protein found in food is distinct to each dietary source. For example, dairy foods contain the protein casein; egg whites contain albumin, and wheat products contain gluten. If provided an adequate supply of dietary protein, the body will reassemble all needed proteins from the individual amino acids after digestion and absorption.

To maintain its solvency, each protein chain adopts a folded form, which can fold and unfold in accordance with metabolic needs. Because proteins are relatively large, complex molecules, they are occasionally subject to mutations or malformations in structure. For example, protein-folding mistakes are involved in Alzheimer disease, cystic fibrosis, and other hereditary diseases.

Dietary Importance

The word *amino* refers to compounds that contain nitrogen. Like carbohydrates and fats, proteins have a basic structure of carbon, hydrogen, and oxygen. However, unlike carbohydrates and fats, protein is approximately 16% nitrogen. As such, protein is the primary source of nitrogen in the diet. In addition, some proteins contain small but valuable amounts of the minerals sulfur, phosphorus, iron, and iodine. Our diet must supply all nine essential amino acids to the body. These amino acids are also known as *indispensable*.

CLASSES OF AMINO ACIDS

There are 20 amino acids vital to life and health. These amino acids fit into one of the following classifications according to whether the body can make them: indispensable, dispensable, or conditionally indispensable in the diet (Box 4.1).[1] Formerly, we referred to these classifications as *essential, nonessential,* or *conditionally essential*, respectively. Some people still refer to them as such.

Indispensable Amino Acids

The human body cannot manufacture nine of the amino acids in sufficient quantity or at all. We refer to these amino acids as indispensable. As the word *indispensable* implies, we cannot exclude these amino acids from the diet without compromising health. Under normal circumstances, the body synthesizes the remaining 11 amino acids to meet continuous metabolic demands throughout the life cycle.

Dispensable Amino Acids

The word *dispensable* can be confusing; all amino acids have essential tissue-building and metabolic functions in the body. However, the term refers to five amino acids that the body can synthesize from other amino acids, if the necessary building blocks and enzymes are

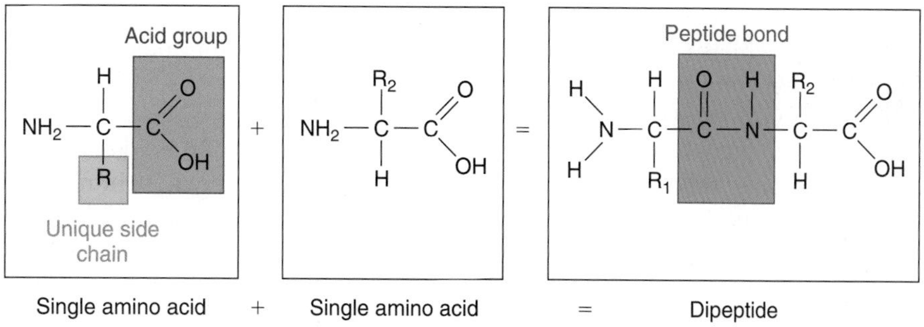

Figure 4.1 Amino acid structure. (Modified from Mahan, L. K., & Escott-Stump, S. [2008]. *Krause's food & nutrition therapy* [12th ed.]. Philadelphia: Saunders.)

| Box **4.1** | Indispensable, Dispensable, and Conditionally Indispensable Amino Acids |

INDISPENSABLE	DISPENSABLE	CONDITIONALLY INDISPENSABLE
Histidine	Alanine	Arginine
Isoleucine	Aspartic acid	Cysteine
Leucine	Asparagine	Glutamine
Lysine	Glutamic acid	Glycine
Methionine	Serine	Proline
Phenylalanine		Tyrosine
Threonine		
Tryptophan		
Valine		

available. These amino acids are needed by the body for a healthy life, but they are dispensable (i.e., not necessary) in the diet.

Conditionally Indispensable Amino Acids

We classify the remaining six amino acids as *conditionally indispensable*. Normally, the body can synthesize these amino acids (along with the dispensable amino acids). However, under certain physiologic conditions, we must consume these amino acids in the diet. Arginine, cysteine, glutamine, glycine, proline, and tyrosine are indispensable when endogenous sources cannot meet the metabolic demands (i.e., we do not have enough precursors to make them ourselves). For example, the human body can make cysteine from the essential amino acid methionine. However, when the diet is deficient in methionine and there are inadequate precursors to synthesize cysteine, the diet must provide cysteine. Thus, cysteine is an indispensable amino acid during that time. Severe physiologic stress, illness, and genetic disorders also may render an amino acid conditionally indispensable.

Phenylketonuria (PKU) is a genetic disorder in which the affected individual lacks the enzyme needed to convert phenylalanine to tyrosine. Therefore, tyrosine becomes an indispensable amino acid for individuals with PKU. In addition, because the conversion of phenylalanine cannot take place, phenylalanine levels in the blood may rise to toxic levels. Individuals with

PKU must follow a specific phenylketonuria diet that avoids certain foods (see the Drug-Nutrient Interaction box, "Aspartame and Phenylketonuria").

Drug-Nutrient Interaction

Aspartame and Phenylketonuria

SARA HARCOURT

Aspartame is a non-nutritive sweetener (i.e., it does not provide any nutrients or calories) that is composed of two amino acids: aspartic acid and phenylalanine. Synthetically made, aspartame's structure more closely resembles a protein than a carbohydrate. However, by adding a methanol group, the end product tastes sweet. Food manufacturers use it in foods and beverages as a high-potency sweetener, and it is approximately 200 times sweeter than sucrose (table sugar). Therefore, we need only a little bit to sweeten a food to the same degree as with sugar.

Phenylketonuria (PKU) is a disease in which an individual lacks the enzyme *phenylalanine hydroxylase*. Without this enzyme, the body cannot metabolize phenylalanine and thus it accumulates in the blood. High levels in the blood are toxic to brain tissue, and this can result in mental degradation and possibly death. Individuals with PKU must follow a strict diet with careful intake of phenylalanine that supports growth but that does not exceed tolerance. Those with PKU should avoid all foods that contain aspartame because of its concentrated phenylalanine content.

Foods that contain phenylalanine, such as aspartame (e.g., *NutraSweet* and *Equal*) have warnings on their packages for individuals with PKU.

Following is a list of common foods that contain aspartame:
- Chewing gum
- Diet sodas
- Frozen desserts
- Gelatins
- Puddings
- Reduced calorie condiments
- Sugar-free candies and cookies
- Yogurt

BALANCE

In terms of nutrition, *balance* refers to the relative intake and output of substances in the body to maintain the equilibrium obligatory for health in various circumstances throughout the life span. Life-sustaining protein and the nitrogen that it supplies are part of this balance.

Protein Balance

Catabolism is the process by which the body breaks down tissue proteins into their amino acid building blocks. Our body will then resynthesize other proteins, as needed, through the process of **anabolism**. To maintain nitrogen balance, a process called **deamination** will remove the part of the amino acid that contains nitrogen, convert it into ammonia, and then excrete it as urea in the urine. Depending on the need, the body will use that non-nitrogen carbon backbone to build a carbohydrate, a fat, or another amino acid. The rate of this protein and nitrogen turnover varies in different tissues in accordance with the degree of metabolic activity and the available supply of amino acids.

Tissue turnover is a continuous process of reshaping, building, and adjusting to maintain overall protein equilibrium within the body. With this finely balanced system, healthy individuals have a small dynamic pool of amino acids from tissue protein and dietary protein that is available to meet metabolic needs (Figure 4.2).

Nitrogen Balance

A person's nitrogen balance indicates how well the body is maintaining its tissue. The intake and use of dietary protein are measured by the amount of nitrogen supplied by food protein and the amount of nitrogen excreted in the urine. For example, 1 g of urinary nitrogen results from the digestion and metabolism of 6.25 g of protein. Thus, if we excrete 1 g of nitrogen in the urine for every 6.25 g of protein consumed, then the body is in nitrogen balance. This balance is the normal pattern in adult health. However, at different times of life or in states of malnutrition or illness, the balance may shift to be either positive or negative.

Positive nitrogen balance. A positive nitrogen balance exists when the body holds on to more nitrogen than it excretes, thus storing more nitrogen in the form of protein (by building tissue) than it is losing (by breaking down tissue). This situation occurs normally during periods of rapid growth, such as infancy, childhood, adolescence, pregnancy, and lactation. A positive nitrogen balance also occurs in individuals recovering from illness or malnutrition. In such cases, we use protein to meet increased needs for tissue building and its associated metabolic activity.

Negative nitrogen balance. A negative nitrogen balance occurs when the body excretes more nitrogen than it keeps. This happens when the body has an inadequate dietary supply of protein and/or total energy. In this case, it is necessary for the body to catabolize body tissue containing protein to meet other critical functions. Ongoing malnutrition, illness, and starvation are examples of periods when negative nitrogen balance may occur.

Kwashiorkor is a classic protein deficiency disease characterized by negative nitrogen balance in individuals suffering from dietary protein insufficiency. This condition may occur even when kilocalories from carbohydrates and fat are adequate. The failure to maintain the nitrogen balance may not become apparent for some time, but it eventually causes the loss of muscle tissue, the impairment of body organs and functions, and an increased susceptibility to infection. Extended periods of negative nitrogen balance in children may cause growth retardation, morbidity, and (eventually) mortality.

FUNCTIONS OF PROTEIN

PRIMARY TISSUE BUILDING

Protein is the fundamental structural material of every cell in the body. In fact, the largest dry-weight portion of the body is protein. Body protein (e.g., the lean mass

> **catabolism** the metabolic process of breaking down large substances to yield smaller building blocks.
> **anabolism** the metabolic process of building large substances from smaller parts; the opposite of catabolism.
> **deamination** the removal of the nitrogen-containing part (amino group) from an amino acid.

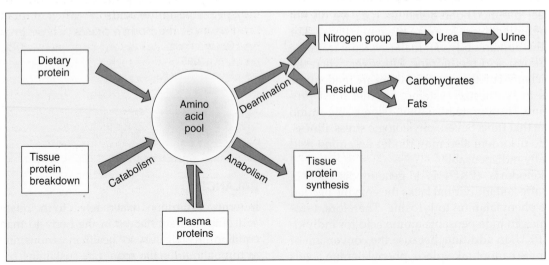

Figure 4.2 The balance between protein compartments and the amino acid pool.

of muscles) accounts for approximately three fourths of the dry matter in most tissues, excluding bone and adipose tissue. Protein makes up the bulk of the muscles, internal organs, brain, nerves, skin, hair, and nails; it is a vital part of regulatory substances such as enzymes, hormones, and blood plasma. There is an ever-constant need for tissue repair and replacement. The primary functions of protein are to repair worn-out, wasted, or damaged tissue and to build new tissue.

ADDITIONAL BODY FUNCTIONS

In addition to its basic tissue-building function, protein has other critical body functions related to energy, water balance, metabolism, and the body's defense system. Box 4.2 lists the major functions of protein.

Water and pH Balance

There are three compartments of fluids within the body: intravascular, intracellular, and interstitial (see Chapter 9). Cell membranes, which are not freely permeable to protein, separate the body compartments. Because protein attracts water, plasma proteins such as albumin help to control water balance throughout the body by exerting osmotic pressure. This pressure maintains the normal circulation of tissue fluids within the appropriate compartments.

The normal pH of blood is between 7.35 and 7.45. However, constant metabolic functions throughout the body release acidic and alkaline substances, thereby affecting the overall acidity and alkalinity of blood. The unique structure of proteins—a combination of a carboxyl acid group and a base group—allows them to act as buffering agents by releasing or taking up excess acid within the body. If blood reaches a pH in either extreme (i.e., too acidic or too alkaline), plasma proteins denature, which can result in death.

Metabolism and Transportation

Various metabolic functions in the body that use enzymes, transport agents, and hormones are dependent upon protein. Digestive and cell enzymes are proteins that control metabolic processes. Enzymes that are required for the digestion of carbohydrates (amylase), fats (lipase), and proteins (proteases) are proteins in structure. Protein also acts as a vehicle to carry nutrients throughout the body. For example, lipoproteins are protein-dependent transport carriers of fat within the water-soluble environment of blood. Other examples are hemoglobin, which is the vital oxygen carrier in the red blood cells, and transferrin, which is the iron transport protein in blood. Peptide hormones (e.g., insulin, glucagon) are also proteins that play a major function in the metabolism of glucose (discussed further in Chapter 20).

---

osmotic pressure the pressure that is produced as a result of osmosis across a semipermeable membrane.

Box **4.2** Functions of Protein
• Structural tissue building • Water balance through osmotic pressure (e.g., albumin) • Buffer agent to help maintain pH balance • Digestion and metabolism through enzymatic action (e.g., amylase, lipase, proteases) • Cell signaling (hormones) and transport (e.g., hemoglobin and transferrin) • Immunity (antibodies) • Source of energy (4 kcal/g)

Immune System

Several aspects of the immune system depend on adequate protein availability. For example, special white blood cells (i.e., lymphocytes) and antibodies are part of the body's immune system that helps defend against disease and infection. Consequently, compromised immune function is a classic symptom of protein deficiency.

Energy System

As described in previous chapters, carbohydrates are the primary fuel source for the body's energy system. Dietary and stored fat are efficient supplemental sources of fuel. In times of need, protein may furnish additional fuel to sustain body heat and energy, but this is a less efficient backup source for use only when the supply of carbohydrate and fat is insufficient. The available fuel factor of protein is 4 kcal/g.

FOOD SOURCES OF PROTEIN

TYPES OF DIETARY PROTEIN

Most foods contain a mixture of different proteins that complement one another. Animal and plant foods provide a wide variety of many nutrients, including protein. We classify dietary proteins as complete or incomplete, depending on their amino acid composition.

Complete Proteins

Complete proteins are proteins that contain all nine indispensable amino acids in sufficient quantity and ratio to meet the body's needs. These proteins are primarily of animal origin (e.g., egg, milk, cheese, meat, poultry, fish; Figure 4.3A). However, there are a couple of exceptions to this rule. For example, gelatin is an incomplete protein of animal origin, and soy is a complete protein of plant origin. Gelatin is a relatively insignificant protein because it lacks the three essential amino acids tryptophan, valine, and isoleucine, and it has only small amounts of leucine. Soybeans and food products made from soy (e.g., tofu, soymilk) are the only plant-based sources of complete proteins (Figure 4.3B). This is one reason why it is easy for vegans/vegetarians to maintain a healthy protein balance in their diet without consuming animal products.

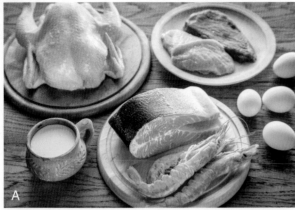

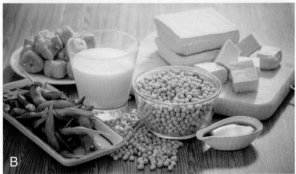

Figure 4.3 (A) Sources of complete protein from animal foods. (B) Sources of complete protein from soybeans. (Copyright iStock Photos; A, Credit: AlexPro9500; B, Credit: naito8)

Incomplete Proteins

Incomplete proteins are proteins that are deficient in one or more of the nine indispensable amino acids. These proteins are generally of plant origin (e.g., grains, legumes, nuts, seeds), but they are found in foods that make valuable contributions to the overall sum of dietary protein. As mentioned above, the exception is soy protein, which is a complete protein of plant origin.

VEGETARIAN DIETS

Vegetarian diets contain predominately, if not exclusively, plant-based foods. Approximately 3.3% of the U.S. adult population (about 8 million adults) consistently follow a vegetarian diet.[3] Several reasons lead people to choose a vegetarian diet, including taste preference, environmental and animal cruelty concerns, health incentives, religious adherence, and aversion to the consumption of animal products. Alternatively, a diet that is void of animal products is not always a choice. In some areas in the world, vegetarianism is a result of the lack of resources and availability of animal products.

Types of Vegetarian Diets

Vegetarian diets differ according to the beliefs or needs of the individuals who are following such food patterns. In general, the following four basic types describe most vegetarians:

1. *Lacto-vegetarians:* These vegetarians accept only dairy products from animal sources to supplement their basic diet of plant foods. The use of milk and milk products (e.g., cheese) with a varied mixed diet of whole or enriched grains, legumes, nuts, seeds, fruits, and vegetables in sufficient quantities to meet energy needs provides a balanced diet.
2. *Ovo-vegetarians:* The only animal foods included in the ovo-vegetarian diet are eggs. Because eggs are an excellent source of complete proteins, individuals regularly consuming eggs do not have to be overly concerned with complementary proteins (discussed in the next section).
3. *Lacto-ovo-vegetarians:* These vegetarians follow a food pattern that allows for the consumption of dairy products and eggs (Figure 4.4). Their diet excludes flesh from meat, poultry, pork, fish, and seafood.
4. *Vegans:* Vegans consume no foods originating from or containing animal products. Their food pattern consists entirely of plant foods (e.g., whole or enriched grains, legumes, nuts, seeds, fruits, vegetables). The use of soybeans, soymilk, soy bean curd (tofu), and processed soy protein products enhances the nutrition value of the diet. A well-planned diet with sufficient food intake ensures adequate nutrition.

A vegetarian diet (including the vegan option) can meet the current recommendations for all essential nutrients, including protein.[2] In addition, vegetarian diets are appropriate throughout all stages of life, including pregnancy, infancy, childhood, adolescence, and older age as well as for those with an athletic lifestyle.[2]

Complementary Proteins

Consuming a mixture of plant-based proteins provides adequate amounts of amino acids, particularly when the person expands the basic use of various grains to include soy and other dried legumes (e.g., beans and peas). Because most plant proteins lack one or more of the indispensable amino acids, vegetarians should choose a variety of plant foods to ensure that the various plants will provide all amino acids. This is the art of combining plant protein foods so that they complement one another and supply all indispensable amino acids (see the Cultural Considerations box, "Indispensable Amino Acids and Their Complementary Food Proteins").

A balanced vegetarian eating pattern throughout the day, together with the body's small reserve of amino acids, ensures an overall amino acid balance. The underlying requirement for vegetarians—as for all people—is to eat a sufficient amount of varied foods to meet the normal nutrient and energy needs.[2]

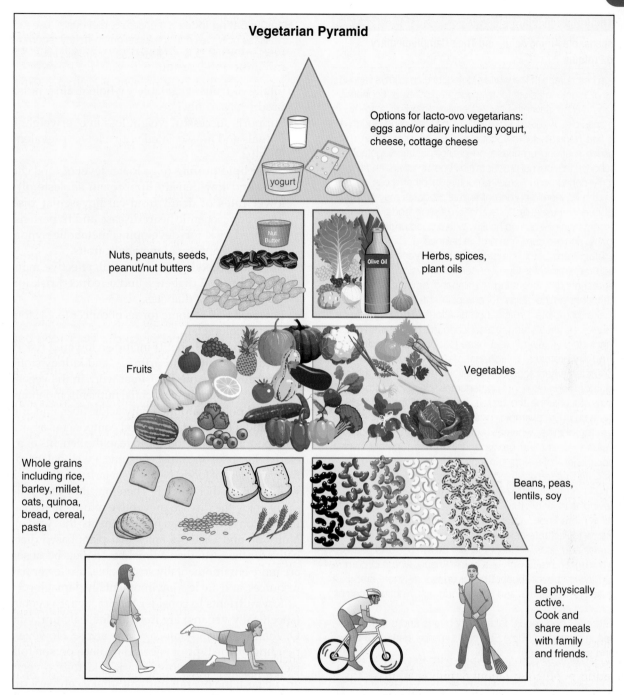

Figure 4.4 Lacto-ovo-vegetarian diet pyramid.

Cultural Considerations

Indispensable Amino Acids and Their Complementary Food Proteins

A large percentage of the worldwide population follows various forms of vegetarian diets for religious, traditional, or economic reasons. Many Seventh-Day Adventists follow a lacto-ovo-vegetarian diet, whereas individuals of the Hindu and Buddhist faiths are generally lacto-vegetarian. The Mediterranean diet has such a strong emphasis on grains, pastas, vegetables, and cheese that animal products (i.e., beef, chicken, and pork) are only consumed in small amounts. In other areas of the world, the economic burden of animal products may be cost prohibitive for the regular consumption of such foods. Any form of a vegetarian diet can be healthy with a good understanding of how to achieve complete protein balance.

Protein from both animal and plant sources can satisfy protein requirements. One concern often voiced related to a vegetarian diet is getting a balanced amount of the indispensable amino acids to complement each other and to make complete protein combinations. However, such concerns are usually unnecessary because vegetarian diets that include a variety of plant-based foods provide sufficient high-quality protein to match that of omnivorous diets.

Complementary food combinations are made by mixing families of foods (e.g., grains, legumes, dairy for lacto-vegetarians) to balance the dietary intake of all indispensable amino acids. For example, grains are low in threonine and high in methionine, whereas legumes are just the opposite. Therefore, consuming grains and legumes together overcomes the lack of a single amino acid from either group. Experts note that former mindful combination of complementary plant proteins within every given meal is unnecessary; achieving a balance throughout the day with a variety of foods is more important.[1] Following are sample food combinations to illustrate complementary protein combinations:

- *Grains and peas, beans, or lentils:* brown rice and beans; whole-grain bread with pea or lentil soup; wheat or corn tortilla with beans; peanut butter on whole-wheat bread; Indian dishes of rice and dal (a legume); Chinese dishes of tofu and rice
- *Legumes and seeds:* falafel; soy beans and pumpkin or sesame seeds; Middle Eastern hummus (garbanzo beans and sesame seeds) or tahini
- *Grains and dairy (for lacto-vegetarians):* whole-wheat pasta and cheese; yogurt and a multigrain muffin; cereal and milk; a cheese sandwich made with whole-grain bread
  See the Further Reading and Resources section at the back of your text for evidence-based resources on vegetarian diets.

REFERENCE

1. Melina, V., Craig, W., & Levin, S. (2016). Position of the Academy of Nutrition and Dietetics: Vegetarian Diets. *J Acad Nutr Diet*, 2016. 116(12): p. 1970–1980.

Health Benefits and Risk

Some of the most notable benefits of vegetarianism include the following:[2,4-17]

- Better quality diet for nutrient intake as indicated by the **Healthy Eating Index** (e.g., lower levels of dietary saturated fat and cholesterol consumption; higher

Healthy Eating Index a measure of diet quality used to assess how well a food plan aligns with key recommendations of the *Dietary Guidelines for Americans*.

intake of fruits, vegetables, whole grains, nuts, soy products, and fiber).
- Supports successful weight loss in overweight individuals and is associated with a lower prevalence of obesity.
- Better lipid profiles (e.g., lower level of total cholesterol and low-density lipoprotein cholesterol) and lower rates of death from cardiovascular disease, including ischemic heart disease and hypertension.
- Reduced risk for developing metabolic syndrome with lower abnormal metabolic traits.
- Improved blood glucose control, effective management of type 2 diabetes, and a reduced risk for developing type 2 diabetes.
- Lowered risk of some forms of cancer (e.g., stomach cancer, colorectal).
- Other possible benefits include a lowered risk of diverticulitis, cataracts, arthritis, and kidney stones.

The preventive mechanism at work in the vegetarian diet is the rich supply of essential nutrients, monounsaturated and polyunsaturated fatty acids, fiber, and antioxidants and a lower intake of food components associated with poor health outcomes. To reap the benefits of a vegetarian lifestyle, one must consume a well-balanced diet from a variety of foods. Not all vegetarians follow an ideal well-balanced diet, though. Therefore, they do not necessarily enjoy the disease-preventive returns noted earlier. In addition to the human health benefits, the Academy of Nutrition and Dietetics notes that plant-based diets are better for the earth than animal-based diets because they are more environmentally sustainable, use fewer natural resources, and are less environmentally damaging.[2]

Key nutrients to consider for practicing vegetarians (specifically vegans) are iron, iodine, calcium, vitamin D, vitamin B_{12}, and omega-3 fatty acids.[2] However, depending on the type of vegetarian diet a person follows (semi-vegetarian, lacto-vegetarian, lacto-ovo-vegetarian, vegan), the overall nutrient intake can vary drastically and may not be different from omnivorous diets for any specific nutrient. In addition, some research shows that these same nutrients of concern (specifically calcium and vitamin D) are more of a concern in individuals who are omnivores but are at risk because of income level, overweight status, or race as opposed to vegetarian status.[18] Table 4.1 outlines the reasons for concern and effective ways to overcome these barriers.

DIGESTION OF PROTEIN

MOUTH

After consuming a food that contains protein, the body must break down the protein into the necessary ready-to-use building blocks (i.e., amino acids). The successive parts of the gastrointestinal tract complete this task

Table 4.1 **Nutrient Considerations for Vegetarians**[a]

NUTRIENT	CONCERN	SOLUTION
Alpha-linolenic acid (and other omega-3 fatty acids)	Few plant foods are good sources of alpha-linolenic acid	Regularly include sources of alpha-linolenic acid in the diet, such as seeds (flax, chia, hemp), walnuts, canola oil, soy products, and foods fortified with docosahexaenoic acid (DHA), or take DHA supplements that are derived from microalgae
Calcium	Oxalates, phytate, and fiber reduce the absorption of calcium found in spinach, beet greens, and Swiss chard	Regularly consume plant foods that are high in calcium and low in oxalates, such as Chinese cabbage, broccoli, Napa cabbage, collards, kale, okra, and turnip greens in addition to calcium-fortified foods such as orange juice, plant-based milks, and tofu
Iodine	Plant-based diets are low in iodine unless iodized salt is used	Consume sea vegetables or use iodized salt on occasion
Iron	Plant foods contain non-heme iron, which is less bioavailable than the heme iron found in animal foods and which is sensitive to inhibitors such as phytate and polyphenolytics	Consume high-iron plant foods with dietary sources of vitamin C and citric acid, which enhance iron absorption
Protein	Plant protein quality varies; not sure how to obtain all essential amino acids	Consume a variety of plant foods throughout the day, including soy products
Vitamin B_{12}	Vitamin B_{12} is not found in plant foods	Choose foods that are fortified with B_{12}, such as soy milk, breakfast cereal, nutritional yeast; or use a vegetarian friendly dietary supplement
Vitamin D	Other than endogenously produced vitamin D from sunlight exposure, the primary source of this vitamin is fortified cow's milk	Choose foods that are fortified with vitamin D, such as soymilk, rice milk, orange juice, and breakfast cereal. If the regular consumption of fortified foods and sun exposure do not meet needs, consider a vegetarian-friendly dietary supplement
Zinc	Plant foods high in phytates bind zinc and prevent absorption	Regularly consume foods such as nuts, soy products, zinc-fortified cereals, and soaked and sprouted beans, grains, and seeds

[a]Not all nutrients in this table are of specific nutrient deficiency concern for vegetarians. These are common nutrients that vegetarians frequently have questions about and the solution to any real or perceived concerns.
Source: Melina V., Craig, W., & Levin, S. (2016). Position of the Academy of Nutrition and Dietetics: Vegetarian diets. *J Acad Nutr Diet*, 116(12), 1970–1980.

through mechanical and chemical digestion. The mechanical breaking down of protein begins with chewing in the mouth. The food particles are mixed with saliva and passed on to the stomach as a semisolid mass.

STOMACH

Because proteins are such large and complex structures, a sequence of enzymes is necessary for digestion and for the liberation of individual amino acids, which is the primary form needed for absorption. Unlike the enzymes that digest carbohydrates and fats, we store all enzymes involved in protein digestion (i.e., proteases) as inactive **proenzymes** called **zymogens**. The body will activate zymogens according to need. The proteases cannot be stored in an active form because the cells and organs that produce and store them (which are made of structural proteins) would also be subject to digestion upon exposure.

The chemical digestion of protein begins in the stomach. In fact, the stomach's chief digestive function is to carry out the first stage of the enzymatic breakdown of protein. The following three agents in the gastric secretions help with this task.

Hydrochloric Acid

Hydrochloric acid begins the unfolding and denaturing of the complex protein chains. This unfolding makes the individual peptide bonds (see Figure 4.1) more available for enzymatic action. Hydrochloric acid also provides the acid medium that is necessary to activate the gastric enzyme specific to proteins.

Pepsin

A single layer of chief cells in the stomach wall produce the inactive proenzyme called *pepsinogen*. Next, the hydrochloric acid within the gastric juices changes pepsinogen to the active enzyme **pepsin**. Pepsin begins splitting the bonds between the protein's long chain of amino acids, which changes the large protein into short chains of polypeptides. If the protein stayed in the stomach longer, pepsin would continue this breakdown until only the individual amino acids remained. However, with the normal gastric emptying time, pepsin only completes the first stage of breakdown.

Rennin

The gastric enzyme **rennin** is present only during infancy and childhood, and it is especially important for the infant's digestion of milk. Rennin and calcium act on the casein of milk to produce a curd. By coagulating milk into a more solid curd, rennin prevents the food from passing too rapidly from the infant's stomach to the small intestine.

proenzyme an inactive precursor (i.e., a forerunner substance from which another substance is made) that is converted to the active enzyme by the action of an acid, another enzyme, or other means.

zymogen an inactive enzyme precursor.

pepsin the main gastric enzyme specific to proteins; it begins breaking large protein molecules into shorter-chain polypeptides; gastric hydrochloric acid is necessary for its activation.

rennin the milk-curdling enzyme of the gastric juice of human infants and young animals (e.g., calves); rennin should not be confused with renin, which is an important enzyme produced by the kidneys that plays a vital role in the activation of angiotensinogen to angiotensin I.

SMALL INTESTINE

Although protein digestion begins in the acidic medium of the stomach, the alkaline medium of the small intestine completes the process. Enzymes from the secretions of both the pancreas and the intestine take part in this process.

Pancreatic Secretions

The following three enzymes produced by the pancreas continue breaking down proteins until they are small enough for absorption:

1. **Trypsin:** When food contacts the intestinal cells in the duodenum (the first section of the small intestine), the cells release the enzyme **enterokinase**. Enterokinase then activates the zymogen *trypsinogen* (released from the pancreas) into trypsin. Trypsin works on proteins and large polypeptide fragments that arrive from the stomach. This enzymatic action breaks long protein chains into small polypeptides and dipeptides.

2. **Chymotrypsin:** Trypsin that is already present in the gut will activate the zymogen *chymotrypsinogen* (released from the pancreas) into chymotrypsin. The active enzyme then continues the protein splitting process similar to trypsin.

3. **Carboxypeptidase:** This enzyme attacks the acid (i.e., carboxyl) end of the peptide chains, thereby producing small peptides and some free amino acids. Trypsin also serves as the activator of this zymogen by activating *procarboxypeptidase* (released from the pancreas) into carboxypeptidase.

Figure 4.5 summarizes the activation sequence for these proteases.

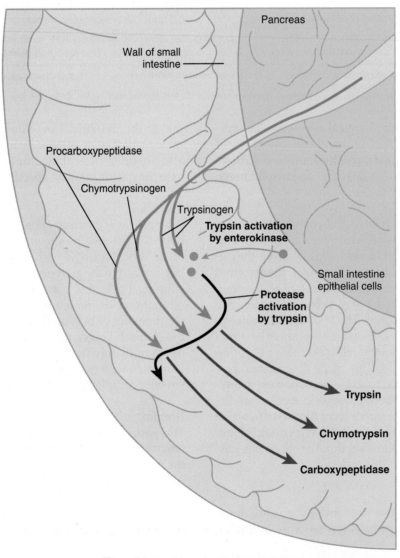

Figure 4.5 Summary of protease activation.

Intestinal Secretions

Glands in the intestinal wall produce the following two protein-splitting enzymes to complete the breakdown of protein (mostly in the form of di-, tri-, and polypeptides at this point) and liberate the remaining amino acids:

1. **Aminopeptidase:** This enzyme attacks the nitrogen-containing (i.e., amino) end of the peptide chain and releases amino acids one at a time, thereby generating peptides and free amino acids.
2. **Dipeptidase:** This is the final enzyme in the protein-splitting system. Dipeptidase completes the job by breaking the remaining dipeptide bond to release two individual amino acids.

This finely coordinated system of protein-splitting enzymes breaks down the large, complex proteins into progressively smaller peptide chains and frees each individual amino acid. This is a tremendous overall task. The amino acids are now ready to be absorbed directly into the portal blood circulation for use in the building of body tissues. Figure 4.6 summarizes this remarkable system of protein digestion.

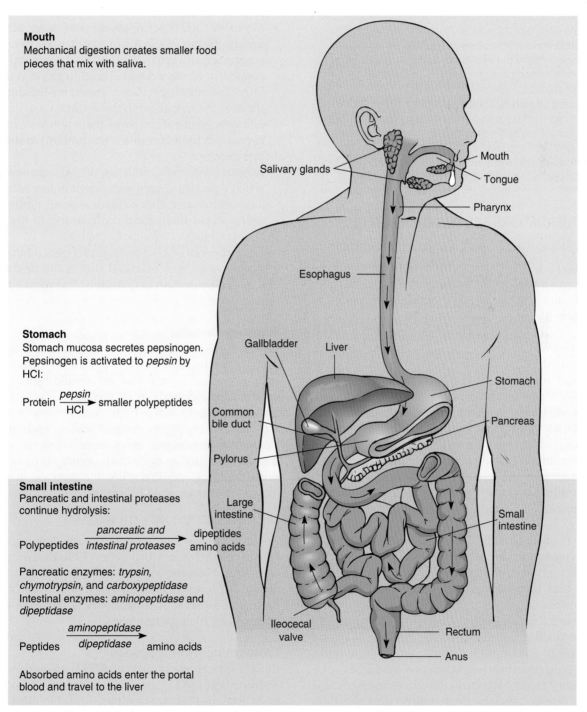

Mouth
Mechanical digestion creates smaller food pieces that mix with saliva.

Stomach
Stomach mucosa secretes pepsinogen. Pepsinogen is activated to *pepsin* by HCl:

$$\text{Protein} \xrightarrow[\text{HCl}]{pepsin} \text{smaller polypeptides}$$

Small intestine
Pancreatic and intestinal proteases continue hydrolysis:

$$\text{Polypeptides} \xrightarrow{\substack{\textit{pancreatic and} \\ \textit{intestinal proteases}}} \substack{\text{dipeptides} \\ \text{amino acids}}$$

Pancreatic enzymes: *trypsin*, *chymotrypsin*, and *carboxypeptidase*
Intestinal enzymes: *aminopeptidase* and *dipeptidase*

$$\text{Peptides} \xrightarrow[\textit{dipeptidase}]{\textit{aminopeptidase}} \text{amino acids}$$

Absorbed amino acids enter the portal blood and travel to the liver

Figure 4.6 Summary of protein digestion. Note: Active enzymes are in *italics.* (Courtesy Rolin Graphics.)

trypsin a protein-splitting enzyme secreted as the inactive proenzyme trypsinogen by the pancreas and that is activated by enterokinase (or the presence of active trypsin); works in the small intestine to reduce proteins to shorter-chain polypeptides and dipeptides.

enterokinase an enzyme produced and secreted in the duodenum in response to food entering the small intestine; it activates trypsinogen to its active form of trypsin.

chymotrypsin a protein-splitting enzyme secreted as the inactive zymogen chymotrypsinogen by the pancreas; after it has been activated by trypsin, it acts in the small intestine to continue breaking down proteins into shorter-chain polypeptides and dipeptides.

carboxypeptidase a specific protein-splitting enzyme secreted as the inactive zymogen procarboxypeptidase by the pancreas; after it has been activated by trypsin, it acts in the small intestine to break off the acid (i.e., carboxyl) end of the peptide chain, thereby producing smaller-chained peptides and free amino acids.

aminopeptidase a specific protein-splitting enzyme secreted by glands in the walls of the small intestine that breaks off the nitrogen-containing amino end (i.e., NH_2) of the peptide chain, thereby producing smaller-chained peptides and free amino acids.

dipeptidase the final enzyme in the protein-splitting system that releases free amino acids from dipeptide bonds.

RECOMMENDATIONS FOR DIETARY PROTEIN

INFLUENTIAL FACTORS OF PROTEIN NEEDS

The following three factors influence the body's requirement for protein: (1) tissue growth; (2) the quality of the dietary protein; and (3) the additional needs that result from illness or disease.

Tissue Growth

During rapid growth periods of the human life cycle, more protein per unit of body weight is necessary to build new tissue and to maintain existing tissue. Human growth is most rapid during fetal growth throughout gestation, during infant growth the first year of life, and during adolescent growth. Childhood is a sustained time of continued growth, but this occurs at a somewhat slower rate than the three previously mentioned periods. For adults, protein requirements level off to meet tissue-maintenance needs, but individual needs vary.

Dietary Protein Quality

The bioavailability of a protein and its composition of amino acids significantly influence its dietary quality and relative value in human nutrition.[19,20] For example, incomplete protein sources (i.e., plant foods) have a lower quality score than complete protein sources (i.e., animal products and soy) because of the lack of one or more indispensable amino acids. However, as noted earlier, when one consumes complementary incomplete protein sources together, this strategy overcomes any single amino acid shortfall. There are several methods available to assess the comparative protein quality of various foods and estimate the protein requirements to meet human needs. Each method has strengths and limitations. The following list provides examples of methods used to rate protein quality and/or used to estimate protein needs.[21-23]

- *Protein efficiency ratio* (PER) *rating*: Based on the weight gain of a growing test animal in relation to its intake of a specific protein source.
- *Protein digestibility-corrected amino acid score* (PDCAAS): Rates the protein source according to the amount of indispensable amino acids contained (i.e., amino acid score) and the digestibility of the whole protein.
- *Digestible indispensable amino acid score* (DIAAS): Similar to the PDCAAS in that it rates the protein source according to the amino acid score and the digestibility of the protein. The difference is that the DIAAS method specifically measures the digestibility of each amino acid in the ileum.
- *Nitrogen balance*: Compares the amount of nitrogen consumed (which comes from protein) to the nitrogen excreted.
- *Indicator amino acid oxidation* (IAAO): Assumes that when a protein source is deficient in any indispensable amino acid that oxidation of all amino acids will prevent them from contributing to the amino acid pool for protein use in the body.

Regardless of one's personal preference for protein foods, a varied and balanced diet is the best way to obtain quality protein in quantities that meet a healthy person's needs.

Illness or Disease

Illness or disease, especially when fever and catabolic tissue breakdown accompany it, raises the body's need for protein and kilocalories for rebuilding tissue and meeting the demands of an increased metabolic rate. Traumatic injury often requires extensive tissue rebuilding. After surgery, wound healing and the restoration of losses require extra protein. Extensive tissue destruction, such as that which occurs with burns and pressure sores, requires a notable increase in protein intake for a successful healing and grafting process.

DIETARY DEFICIENCY OR EXCESS

As with any nutrient, moderation and balance are the keys to health. Too much or too little dietary protein can be problematic for overall body function. In addition, sufficient overall energy intake from carbohydrate and fat sources is necessary to conserve protein for its many biologic functions.

Protein-Energy Malnutrition

Protein-energy malnutrition (PEM) or severe acute malnutrition (SAM) may occur in a variety of situations. The most severe cases are found in areas where all foods—not just protein-rich foods—are in short supply. Children are at the highest risk for experiencing malnutrition because of their high needs during rapid growth and development. However, PEM can affect anyone at any point throughout the life cycle, particularly during the advanced years of life. Individuals who are 65 years old or older and who need homecare services, those living in rural areas, and especially women are at increased risk for suffering from PEM worldwide despite the social or economic development of their home country.[24] An overall energy deficiency often accompanies PEM as well. However, individuals with high protein needs during infection or disease (e.g., acquired immunodeficiency syndrome, cancer, liver failure) sometimes experience PEM despite seemingly adequate total dietary intake. As previously mentioned, protein has many critical functions in the body. Thus, the consequences of a dietary deficiency relate directly to these functions. Without the amino acid building blocks, the body cannot synthesize needed structural (i.e., muscle) or functional proteins (i.e., enzymes, antibodies, and hormones).

Two severe forms of PEM are kwashiorkor and marasmus. Characteristics of the two forms of PEM are different. Kwashiorkor, which is the more frequently fatal of the two forms, may result from an acute deficiency of protein, whereas marasmus results from a more chronic deficiency of many nutrients, of which protein is one. The result with either form is stunted growth, a weakened immune system, and poor development.

Kwashiorkor. Kwashiorkor is more common among children between the ages of 18 and 24 months, who have been breastfed all their lives and are then rapidly weaned, often because of the arrival of a younger sibling. Switching the child from the nutrient-balanced breast milk to a dilute diet of mostly carbohydrates and small amounts of incomplete protein triggers the condition (e.g., a grain-based diet). The children may receive adequate total kilocalories, but they lack enough high-quality bioavailable protein sources. The term *kwashiorkor* is a Ghanaian word that refers to the disease that takes over the first child when the second child is born.

Characteristics of kwashiorkor include generalized edema and fatty liver resulting from inadequate protein availability to maintain fluid balance and to transport fat away from the liver (Figure 4.7). However, the exact etiology of kwashiorkor clinical manifestations is not well defined. Research suggests that there may be factors beyond recent weaning and poor quality protein intake involved in the development of the distinctive edema, such as oxidative stress, infection, and traumatic emotional/environmental events.[25]

Marasmus. Individuals with marasmus have an emaciated appearance with little or no body fat. This is a chronic form of energy and protein deficiency; in other words, it is a result of starvation. Stunted growth and development are more severe with this form of malnutrition. Marasmus can affect individuals of all ages with inadequate food sources.

Excess Dietary Intake

The body has a finite need for protein. When a person has met their dietary protein needs, the body deaminates extra protein so that it can store the carbon backbone as fat or use it as energy. Eating excess protein does not build muscle; only exercising with enough protein to support growth can do that. One of the associated problems with diets that are heavily laden with excess animal protein is that protein foods of animal origin are generally also high in saturated fat and cholesterol (see Chapter 3). In addition, if a person fills up on high-protein foods, little room is left for fruits, vegetables, and other whole grains, which are packed with essential vitamins, minerals, and fiber.

Although most protein and amino acid supplements are not harmful in small doses, they are unnecessary in a balanced diet. However, taking excessive single amino acid dietary supplements can be harmful if it is to the exclusion of other essential amino acids, thereby creating an overall imbalance. A growing body of research indicates that high dietary intakes and circulating levels of branched chain amino acids are associated with an increased risk for insulin resistance and other cardiometabolic diseases.[26-28]

DIETARY GUIDES

Dietary Reference Intakes

The Recommended Dietary Allowances (RDAs) continue to be the principal dietary guide for protein consumption, and they are part of the Dietary Reference Intake standards. The RDAs are set to meet the nutrient

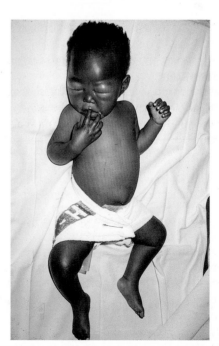

Figure 4.7 Kwashiorkor. The infant shows generalized edema, which is seen in the form of puffiness of the face, arms, and legs. (Reprinted from Kumar, V., Abbas, A. K., Fausto, N., et al. [2007]. *Robbins basic pathology* [8th ed.]. Philadelphia: Saunders.)

requirements of most healthy people. Thus, severe physical stress (e.g., illness, disease, surgery) can increase a person's requirement for protein beyond the standard RDA.

Similar to carbohydrate and fat recommendations, the National Academy of Sciences set the DRIs for proteins as a percentage of the total kilocalorie ingestion. Most children and adults are able to meet their protein needs when 10% to 35% of their total calories come from protein.[1] The RDA standards relate to the age, sex, and weight of the average person, and they reflect the analysis of available nitrogen-balance studies. Another method for estimating protein needs is relative to ideal body weight. Using this method, the RDA for both men and women is set at 0.8 g of high-quality protein per kilogram of desirable body weight per day (i.e., 0.8 g/kg/d; see the Clinical Applications box, "Calculating Dietary Reference Intake for Protein" and the For Further Focus box, "Dietary Protein Intake versus Recommendations").[1] Dietary recommendations are higher for infants and for pregnant and breastfeeding women to meet the metabolic needs of growth (see Appendix B).

Dietary Guidelines for Americans

As previously stated, the standard American diet provides adequate protein, the majority of which generally comes from animal products. There are potential health risks associated with a diet in which excess animal products take the place of other nutrient-dense fruits, vegetables, and whole grains in the meal plan. The key is to create dietary habits that allow for a variety of all food groups, without an excess in any area.

The *Dietary Guidelines for Americans, 2020–2025* recommend the following with regard to protein-rich foods:[29]

- Choose a variety of protein foods, including seafood, lean meat and poultry, eggs, beans and peas, soy products, and unsalted nuts and seeds.
- Consume at least 8 oz per week of seafood from a variety of sources that are lower in methylmercury.
- Replace protein foods that are high in sodium and saturated fat with more nutrient-dense options.

Table 4.2 provides a comparison of protein-rich food portions.

MyPlate

As with the other macronutrient recommendations from the MyPlate guidelines, Americans are encouraged to consume a variety of foods to meet all of their nutrient needs (see Figure 1.4).[30] The MyPlate website (www.choosemyplate.gov) includes tips for choosing lean sources of meat, poultry, and fish as well as vegetable protein sources such as beans, nuts, and seeds. Individuals can obtain a personalized MyPlate plan by entering their age, sex, height, weight, and physical activity level. Sample menus for omnivores and eating tips for vegetarian lifestyles are also available.

Clinical Applications

Calculating Dietary Reference Intake for Protein

There are two ways to calculate a person's dietary recommendation for protein. Let's work through an example for both calculations.

DIETARY REFERENCE INTAKES OF ACCEPTABLE MACRONUTRIENT DISTRIBUTION RANGE:[1]

To calculate the protein needs of an individual who is consuming 2200 kcal/day based on the Dietary Reference Intake recommendation of 10% to 35% of total kilocalories, complete the following calculations:

Example: 2200 kcal × 0.10 = 220 kcal/day *and* 2200 kcal × 0.35 = 770 kcal/day

thus giving a range of 220 to 770 kcal/day from protein. Now let's convert protein kcals to grams of protein by dividing kcals by the fuel factor of 4.

Example: 220 kcal ÷ 4 kcal/g = 55 g *and* 770 kcal ÷ 4 kcal/g = 192.5 g

thus giving a recommended range of 55 g to 192.5 g of protein per day to satisfy the acceptable macronutrient distribution range for protein.

RECOMMENDED DIETARY ALLOWANCE RELATIVE TO IDEAL BODY WEIGHT:[1]

To calculate the protein needs of a woman who is 5 feet, 4 inches tall with an ideal body weight of 120 lb (see Chapter 15 for ideal body weight calculations) based on the Recommended Dietary Allowance of 0.8 g of protein/kg of body weight per day, perform the following calculations:

Example: First, convert weight in pounds to weight in kg (2.2 lb = 1 kg):

120 lb ÷ 2.2 lb/kg = 54.5 kg

Next, multiply weight in kg by the RDA of 0.8 g/kg/d:

Example: 54.5 kg × 0.8 g/kg = 43.6 g of protein per day

Therefore, a woman who measures 5 feet, 4 inches tall and who is consuming 2200 kcal/day with a minimum of 10% of her calories coming from high-quality protein will obtain more than her Recommended Dietary Allowance for protein of 43.6 g per day.

Now, calculate your own dietary needs for protein based on both your total kcal intake and your body weight. Does your usual food intake meet your protein needs?

REFERENCE

1. Food and Nutrition Board and Institute of Medicine. (2002). *Dietary reference intakes for energy, carbohydrate, fiber, fat, fatty acids, cholesterol, protein, and amino acids*. Washington, DC: National Academies Press.

Dietary Protein Intake versus Recommendations

The U.S. Department of Agriculture's "What We Eat in America" report noted that the average daily protein intake of men and women 20 years and older is 97 g and 69 g per day, respectively; and that Americans over the age of 2 years consume an average of 16% of total kcals from protein, which is well within the DRI of 10% to 35% of kilocalories.[1]

New methods of assessing protein quality (e.g., DIAAS and PDCAAS discussed in the *Dietary Protein Quality* section) challenge the current RDA recommendation of 0.8 g/kg/d. Based on these methods, some researchers conclude that protein intake requirements could be slightly higher at 0.91 g/kg/day to better meet body needs.[2]

Nevertheless, the average person most likely meets their dietary protein requirements when consuming the usual American fare. For example, let us consider the needs of a 150-lb man consuming a typical 2440-kcal diet. Based on the national average, we can assume that roughly 16% of his kilocalories are coming from protein, which equals ~ 98 g of protein per day:

$$2440 \text{ kcal} \times 16\% \text{ protein} = 390 \text{ kcal} \div 4 \text{ kcal/g} = 98 \text{ g protein}$$

Meanwhile, the same 150-lb (68-kg) man would only require approximately 62 g of protein to meet his needs even at the higher recommendation of 0.91 g/kg/d. Thus, we can conclude that additional consumption of protein through supplements is unnecessary for the majority of the American population. Even if a person needed extra protein because of metabolic stress or high growth rates, they would most likely meet those needs by consuming the standard American fare.

REFERENCES

1. Agricultural Research Service. (2018). Nutrient intakes from food and beverages: Mean amounts consumed per individual, by gender and age. In *What we eat in America* (NHANES, 2015–2016). U.S. Department of Agriculture.
2. Food and Agriculture Organization of the United Nations. (2013). Dietary protein quality evaluation in human nutrition. Report of an FAO Expert Consultation. *FAO Food and Nutrition Paper, 92*, 1–66.

Table 4.2 Foods That Are High in Protein[a]

FOOD	SERVING SIZE	PROTEIN (g)
Goose, meat only, roasted	3 oz	29
Veal, loin, lean only, braised	3 oz	28.5
Chicken, breast, meat only, roasted	3 oz	26.4
Beef, top round, trimmed of fat, grilled	3 oz	25.6
Turkey, breast, meat only, roasted	3 oz	25.6
Pork, sirloin, boneless, roasted	3 oz	25.2
Tuna, fresh, yellowfin, cooked with dry heat	3 oz	24.8
Liver, chicken, pan fried	3 oz	21.9
Beef, ground, 70% lean, 30% fat, pan browned	3 oz	21.7
Salmon, Atlantic, cooked with dry heat	3 oz	21.6
Lamb, shoulder, trimmed to ¼ inch of fat, broiled	3 oz	20.8
Duck, meat only, roasted	3 oz	20
Tuna, canned in water, drained	3 oz	20
Halibut, fresh, cooked with dry heat	3 oz	19.2
Scallops, steamed	3 oz	17.5
Haddock, cooked with dry heat	3 oz	17
Tofu, fried	3 oz	16
Ham, sliced, 11% fat	3 oz	14.1
Soy burger, cooked	3 oz	13.3
Oysters, cooked with moist heat	3 oz	9.7
Cottage cheese, 2% milk fat	3 oz	8.9
Milk, 1% fat	1 cup	8.2
Lentils, boiled	3 oz	7.7
Chickpeas (garbanzo beans), cooked	3 oz	7.5
Peanut butter, smooth	2 Tbsp	7.1
Soy milk	1 cup	7
Cheese, cheddar	1 oz	6.8
Egg, whole, hard-boiled	1 large	6.3
Cheese, blue	1 oz	6
Yogurt, plain, skim milk	3 oz	4.9
Kidney beans, boiled	3 oz	4.1

[a]Listed in decreasing order of protein per serving.
Data from Agricultural Research Service. (n.d.). *USDA Food Composition Database*. U.S. Department of Agriculture. Retrieved May 17, 2019, from ndb.nal.usda.gov/ndb/

Putting It All Together

Summary

- Protein provides the human body with amino acids, which are its primary tissue-building units. Of the 20 common amino acids, 9 are indispensable in the diet, because the body cannot manufacture them.
- Complete proteins contain all of the indispensable amino acids. Complete protein food sources are mostly of animal origin. Plant protein foods mostly provide incomplete proteins lacking in one or more of the indispensable amino acids. The exception is soy protein, which is of plant origin and provides a good source of complete proteins.
- A constant turnover of tissue protein occurs between tissue anabolism and tissue catabolism. Adequate dietary protein and a reserve pool of amino acids help to maintain this overall protein balance. Nitrogen balance is a measure of overall protein balance.
- A mixed diet including a variety of foods, together with sufficient non-protein kilocalories from carbohydrates and fats, supplies the body with a balance of protein and other nutrients.
- Vegan diets contain only plant proteins. Other vegetarian diets may include dairy products, eggs, and sometimes fish. All vegetarian lifestyles can provide balanced nutrition with planning and variety.
- After we eat protein-containing foods, a powerful digestive team of six protein-splitting enzymes breaks peptide bonds to liberate individual amino acids for absorption.
- Growth needs and the nature of the diet in terms of protein quality and energy intake determine a person's protein requirements. Clinical influences on protein needs include fever, disease, surgery, and other trauma to body tissues.

Chapter Review Questions

See answers in Appendix A.

1. Amino acids are unique as compared to carbohydrates and fats because of the presence of _____ in their structure.

   a. carbon
   b. hydrogen
   c. phosphorus
   d. nitrogen

2. Which of the following foods contain complete proteins?

   a. Corn
   b. Eggs
   c. Whole-grain bread
   d. Peanuts

3. The zymogens procarboxypeptidase and chymotrypsinogen are activated by the enzyme _____ in the small intestine.

   a. pepsin
   b. aminopeptidase
   c. trypsin
   d. dipeptidase

4. Protein requirements would most likely be the highest for which of the following individuals (based on the information provided)?

   a. 16-year-old active teenager
   b. 26-year-old sedentary lawyer
   c. 47-year-old female pilot
   d. 72-year-old grandfather

5. Based on the RDA acceptable macronutrient range for protein, how many grams of protein should be included in the diet of an individual consuming 2100 kcal per day?

   a. 40 g to 58 g
   b. 53 g to 184 g
   c. 105 g to 195 g
   d. 208 g to 320 g

Next-Generation NCLEX® Examination-style Case Study

See answers in Appendix A.

A 9-year-old boy is small for his age. His parents are concerned about his growth. They are vegan and have raised him on a vegan diet for his entire life. They also mention that their son is a particularly picky eater. He refuses to eat foods such as nuts, dried beans, and soy. A 24-hour diet recall is collected.

Breakfast: 1 piece of toast with jelly, 8 oz. orange juice
Lunch: 1 cup of whole-wheat pasta with tomato sauce
Snack: 1 apple
Dinner: 1 cup white rice with ½ cup of carrots

1. From the list below, identify all nutrition concerns related to the client's history.

   a. Food aversion combined with a vegan diet
   b. Consuming inadequate amounts of dispensable amino acids
   c. Consuming inadequate calories
   d. Consuming inadequate protein
   e. Diet providing adequate amounts of amino acids for muscle growth
   f. Consuming inadequate amounts of indispensable amino acids

2. Choose the *most likely* options for the information missing from the statements below by selecting from the list of options provided.

   From this client's diet recall, it does not appear that they are combining an appropriate array of different ____1____ to ensure his intake of complementary proteins. This practice is important because most vegan-friendly foods on their own are deficient in one or more of the nine ____2____ amino acids.

OPTION 1	OPTION 2
whole-grains	dispensable
animal-based foods	nonessential
plant-based foods	indispensable
dairy-based foods	conditionally indispensable

3. Choose the *most likely* options for the information missing from the statements below by selecting from the list of options provided.

The client may be in a state of _____ since he is not getting all of the needed amino acids. He can combine different plant foods with different amino acid profiles to help achieve a _____ nitrogen balance and encourage growth.

OPTIONS	
metabolism	positive
anabolism	negative
catabolism	neutral
insufficient	

4. From the list below, select all the dietary interventions that are appropriate for the client in order to facilitate growth.

a. Increase total calories to increase amino acids
b. Increase plant-based protein foods to increase protein and amino acid intake
c. Consume dairy products containing all amino acids
d. Use protein supplements such as whey protein
e. Eat more soy products

5. From the list below, select all the diet combinations with complementary amino acids that are appropriate for the client consuming a vegan diet.

a. Whole wheat pasta with cheese
b. Beans and rice
c. Peanut butter on whole wheat bread
d. Yogurt with a whole wheat muffin
e. Tofu and rice
f. Whole wheat toast with grape jelly

Additional Learning Resources

Please refer to this text's Evolve website for answers to the Case Study questions:
http://evolve.elsevier.com/Williams/basic/
References and **Further Reading and Resources** in the back of the book provide additional resources for enhancing knowledge.

Digestion, Absorption, and Metabolism

Key Concepts

- Through a coordinated system of mechanical and chemical digestive processes, our gastrointestinal tract breaks food down into smaller substances, liberating nutrients for biologic use.
- Distinct organ structures and functions accomplish these tasks through the successive parts of the gastrointestinal system.

- Absorption, transport, and metabolism allow for the distribution, use, and storage of nutrients throughout the body.

As described in previous chapters, nutrients that the body requires do not come ready to use; rather, they are packaged as foods in a variety of forms. Therefore, whole food must be broken down into smaller substances for absorption and metabolism to meet the body's needs. The preceding chapters cover the digestion of the macronutrients: carbohydrates, fat, and protein.

This chapter views the overall process of food digestion and nutrient absorption as one continuous whole that involves a series of successive events. In addition, we review the metabolism and the unique body structures and functions that make this process possible.

DIGESTION

BASIC PRINCIPLES

Body cells cannot use food in the form in which we eat it. We must first liberate individual nutrients from one another for absorption and cellular use to sustain life. This process involves many steps, including digestion, absorption, transport, and metabolism.

Figure 5.1 shows the different parts of the gastrointestinal (GI) tract and accessory organs. The individual parts of the GI system work systematically together as a whole to complete the process of digestion and metabolism. Food components travel through this system until they ultimately are absorbed and delivered to the cells or excreted as waste.

> **digestion** the process by which food is broken down in the gastrointestinal tract to release nutrients in forms that the body can absorb.
>
> **absorption** the process by which nutrients are taken into the cells that line the gastrointestinal tract.
>
> **transport** the movement of nutrients through the circulatory system from one area of the body to another.
>
> **metabolism** the sum of the vast number of chemical changes in the cell that ultimately produce the materials that are essential for energy, tissue building, and metabolic controls.

MECHANICAL AND CHEMICAL DIGESTION

Food goes through a series of mechanical and chemical changes within the GI tract to allow for nutrient absorption. Together, these actions encompass the overall process of digestion.

Chapters 2, 3, and 4 cover the mechanical and chemical actions that occur during the digestion of the macronutrients. Of the micronutrients, most vitamins and minerals require little to no digestion. There are some exceptions (e.g., vitamins A and B_{12}, biotin) that require digestion, or hydrolysis, before absorption can take place. Water does not require digestion, and it is easily absorbed into the general circulation. This chapter explores those actions as a whole and interdependent process. Chapters 7, 8, and 9 cover vitamins, minerals, and water in detail.

Mechanical Digestion: Gastrointestinal Motility

Beginning in the mouth, the muscles and nerves in the walls of the GI tract coordinate their actions to provide the necessary motility for digestion to ensue. This automatic response to the presence of food enables the system to break up the food mass swallowed in each bite and move it along the digestive pathway.

Muscles. Layers of smooth muscle in the GI wall interact to provide two general types of movement: (1) muscle tone or tonic contraction, which ensures the continuous passage of the food mass and valve control along the way, and (2) periodic muscle contraction and relaxation, which are rhythmic waves that mix the food mass and move it forward. *Peristalsis* is the alternating muscular contractions and relaxations that force the contents forward in the GI tract. The term comes from the Greek words *peri*, meaning "around," and *stalsis*, meaning "contraction."

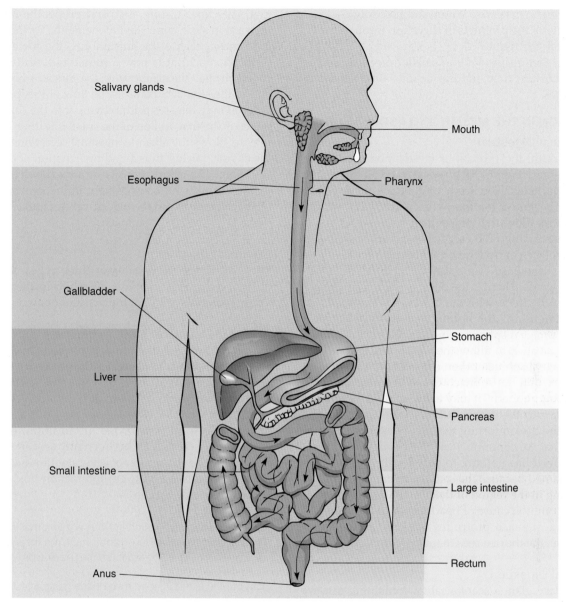

Figure 5.1 The gastrointestinal system. Through the successive parts of the system, multiple activities of digestion liberate food nutrients for cellular use. (Courtesy Rolin Graphics.)

Nerves. Nerves regulate muscular action along the GI tract. The *intramural nerve plexus* is a complex network of nerves in the GI wall that extends from the esophagus to the anus. These nerves do three things: (1) control muscle tone in the wall; (2) regulate the rate and intensity of the alternating muscle contractions; and (3) coordinate all of the various movements. When all is well, these finely tuned movements flow together like those of a great symphony, without conscious awareness. However, when all is not well, we recognize the discord as pain. Chapter 18 addresses such problems and diseases of the GI tract.

Chemical Digestion: Gastrointestinal Secretions

A number of secretions work together to make chemical digestion possible. Secretory cells in the intestinal tract and the nearby accessory organs produce each of the constituents for precise jobs in chemical digestion. The secretory action of these cells or glands responds to stimulus from the presence of food, nerve impulses, or hormonal stimuli. The major types of secretions are the following:

1. *Hydrochloric acid and buffer ions:* We need hydrochloric acid and buffer ions to produce the correct pH (i.e., the degree of acidity or alkalinity) that is necessary for enzymatic activity.
2. *Enzymes:* Digestive enzymes are proteins produced in the body. Their specific design allows them to break down large macronutrients (e.g., triglycerides) into smaller building blocks (e.g., glycerol and fatty acids).
3. *Mucus:* Mucus lubricates and protects the mucosal tissues that line the GI tract and helps to moisten the food mass.

4. *Water and electrolytes:* Water and electrolytes assist in carrying the products of digestion through the GI tract into the tissues.

5. *Bile:* Bile emulsifies fat into smaller pieces to expose more surface area for the actions of fat-splitting enzymes.

DIGESTION IN THE MOUTH AND ESOPHAGUS

Mechanical Digestion

In the mouth, the process of mastication (i.e., biting and chewing) begins to physically break food into smaller particles. The teeth and oral structures are particularly suited for this work. After chewing the food, we swallow the mixed mass of food particles, and it passes down the esophagus, largely as a result of nerve reflex–controlled autonomic peristaltic waves. Muscles at the base of the tongue facilitate the swallowing process. Then, if the body is in the upright position, gravity helps with the movement of food down the esophagus. At the entrance to the stomach, the gastroesophageal sphincter muscle relaxes, much like a one-way valve, to allow the food to enter. The gastroesophageal sphincter then constricts again to retain the food within the stomach cavity. If the sphincter is not working properly, it may allow acid-mixed food to seep back into the esophagus from the stomach. The result is the discomforting feeling of gastroesophageal reflux (what we commonly call "heartburn").

Heartburn has nothing to do with the heart, but it was so named because the sensations are perceived as originating in the region of the heart. A hiatal hernia is another common cause of heartburn; this occurs when part of the stomach protrudes upward into the chest cavity (i.e., the thorax; see Chapter 18).

Chemical Digestion

The salivary glands secrete saliva containing **salivary amylase** (also called *ptyalin*). *Amylase* is the general name for any starch-splitting enzyme. Small glands at the back of the tongue (i.e., von Ebner's glands) secrete lingual lipase. Lipase is the general name for any fat-splitting enzyme. However, in this case, food does not remain in the mouth long enough for much chemical action to occur. During infancy, lingual lipase is a more relevant enzyme for the digestion of milk fat. The salivary glands also secrete a mucous material that lubricates and binds food particles to facilitate the swallowing of each food bolus (i.e., lump of food material). Mucous glands also line the esophagus, and their secretions help to move the food mass toward the stomach.

DIGESTION IN THE STOMACH

Mechanical Digestion

Under sphincter muscle control from the esophagus, which joins the stomach at the cardiac notch, the food enters the fundus (i.e., the upper portion of the stomach) in individual bolus lumps. Within the stomach, muscles gradually knead, store, mix, and propel the food mass forward in slow, controlled movements. By the time the food mass reaches the antrum (i.e., the lower portion of the stomach), it is now a semiliquid, acid-food mix called **chyme.** The *pyloric valve*, a sphincter muscle at the end of the stomach, controls the flow at this point. This valve slowly releases acidic chyme into the duodenum, which is the first section of the small intestine. The slow release allows the alkaline intestinal secretions to buffer the chyme quickly, thus avoiding irritation of the mucosal lining. The caloric density of a meal, which mainly results from its fat composition, influences the rate of stomach emptying at the pyloric valve. Figure 5.2 shows the major parts of the stomach.

Chemical Digestion

The gastric secretions contain three types of materials that help with chemical digestion in the stomach. These materials are acid, mucus, and enzymes.

Acid. The hormone **gastrin** stimulates parietal cells within the lining of the stomach to secrete hydrochloric acid. Hydrochloric acid creates the necessary degree of acidity for gastric enzymes to work, and it activates the first protease, pepsinogen, in the stomach. As you will recall from Chapter 4, *protease* is the general name for any protein-splitting enzyme. In addition, the acidic environment created by hydrochloric acid in the stomach aids in the absorption of several vitamins and minerals (see the Drug-Nutrient Interaction box, "Acidity for Nutrient Absorption").

---

salivary amylase a starch-splitting enzyme that is secreted by the salivary glands in the mouth and that is commonly called ptyalin (from the Greek word *ptyalon*, meaning "spittle").

chyme the semifluid food mass in the gastrointestinal tract that is present after gastric digestion.

gastrin a hormone that helps with gastric motility, stimulates the secretion of gastric acid by the parietal cells of the stomach, and stimulates the chief cells to secrete pepsinogen.

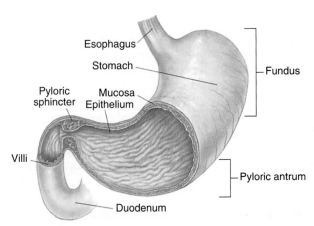

Figure 5.2 Stomach. (Reprinted from Raven, P. H., & Johnson, G. B. [1992]. *Biology* [3rd ed.]. New York: McGraw-Hill.)

Drug-Nutrient Interaction

Acidity for Nutrient Absorption

The body controls the pH of the gastrointestinal tract contents by secreting acidic or alkaline buffering agents. The release of hydrochloric acid in the stomach lowers the pH and makes stomach content very acidic; and bicarbonate, secreted from the pancreas into the small intestines, neutralizes the pH. Hormones and a feedback system that is constantly fine-tuning the environment of the gastrointestinal tract for optimal performance control the release of hydrochloric acid and bicarbonate.

Hydrochloric acid in the stomach has many functions. The acid kills microorganisms, activates pepsinogen, and begins the digestive process of proteins. In addition, the downstream absorption of several vitamins and minerals depends on the exposure to an acidic environment in the stomach. Specifically, the interaction with hydrochloric acid increases the bioavailability of vitamin B_{12}, calcium, iron, and magnesium further along the GI tract. Therefore, situations that cause a decrease in hydrochloric acid secretion in the stomach can reduce the bioavailability of these vitamins and minerals, increase the bacterial load,[1] and potentially alter the digestive process of protein.

Proton pump inhibitors (PPIs) are a class of drugs that reduce the release of acid in the stomach. Over-the-counter and prescription-grade acid suppressors are some of the most commonly used medications in the United States, and people frequently use them for extended periods. Although we do not yet understand the extent of micronutrient deficiency resulting from the chronic use of PPIs, the clinical implications could be significant. This is a particularly important consideration for individuals at risk for malnutrition. The American Gastroenterological Association's advice for best practices is to ensure clients on long-term PPI therapy are adequately meeting their recommended dietary allowance (RDA) for these micronutrients to avoid complications.[1]

REFERENCE
1. Freedberg, D. E., Kim, L. S., & Yang, Y. X. (2017). The risks and benefits of long-term use of proton pump inhibitors: Expert review and best practice advice from the American Gastroenterological Association. *Gastroenterology*, *152*(4), 706–715.

Mucus. Mucus protects the stomach lining from the erosive effect of hydrochloric acid. Mucus also helps to bind, mix, and move the food mass along the GI tract.

Enzymes. Chief cells in the stomach secrete the zymogen pepsinogen. Hydrochloric acid activates pepsinogen to become the protein-splitting enzyme pepsin. Other cells produce small amounts of a gastric lipase called *tributyrinase*, which works on tributyrin (i.e., butterfat); however, this is a relatively minor activity in the stomach.

Various sensations, emotions, hormones, and foods stimulate the nerve impulses that trigger these secretions. The concept of the stomach "mirroring the person within" is not without merit. For example, anger and hostility increase secretions, whereas fear and depression decrease secretions and inhibit blood flow and motility.

DIGESTION IN THE SMALL INTESTINE

Up to this point, the digestion of food has largely been mechanical, and it has resulted in the delivery of a semifluid mixture of fine food particles and watery secretions to the small intestine. Thus, the major task of chemical digestion and the absorption that follows occur in the small intestine. The intricately developed structural parts, synchronized movements, and array of enzymes of the small intestine allow for the final steps of mechanical and chemical digestion.

Mechanical Digestion

Under the control of nerve impulses, the muscular walls of the small intestine stretch from the food mass and hormonal stimuli, and the intestinal muscles produce several types of movement that aid digestion, as follows:

- *Peristaltic waves* slowly push the food mass forward, sometimes with long, sweeping waves over the entire length of the intestine.
- *Pendular movements* from small, local muscles sweep back and forth, thereby stirring the chyme at the mucosal surface.
- *Segmentation rings* from the alternating contraction and relaxation of circular muscles progressively chop the food mass into successive soft lumps and then mix them with GI secretions.
- *Longitudinal rotation* by long muscles that run the length of the intestine rolls the slowly moving food mass in a spiral motion to mix it and expose new surfaces for absorption.
- *Surface villi motions* stir and mix the chyme at the intestinal wall, thereby exposing additional nutrients for absorption.

Chemical Digestion

The small intestine, together with the GI accessory organs (i.e., the pancreas, liver, and gallbladder), supply many secretory materials to accomplish the major chore of chemical digestion. The pancreas and intestines secrete enzymes that are specific for the digestion of each macronutrient.

Pancreatic enzymes.
1. *Carbohydrate:* **Pancreatic amylase** converts starch into disaccharides such as maltose and sucrose.
2. *Protein:* Trypsin and chymotrypsin split large protein molecules into smaller and smaller peptide fragments and finally into single amino acids. Carboxypeptidase removes end amino acids from peptide chains.

3. *Fat:* **Pancreatic lipase** converts triglycerides into monoglycerides and free fatty acids.

Intestinal enzymes.

1. *Carbohydrate:* Disaccharidases (i.e., maltase, lactase, and sucrase) split their respective disaccharides (i.e., maltose, lactose, and sucrose) into monosaccharides (i.e., glucose, galactose, and fructose).
2. *Protein:* The intestinal enzyme enterokinase activates trypsinogen (released from the pancreas) to become the protein-splitting enzyme trypsin. Aminopeptidase removes end amino acids from polypeptides. Dipeptidase splits dipeptides into their two remaining amino acids.

Mucus. The intestinal glands secrete large quantities of mucus. Mucus protects the mucosal lining from the irritation and erosion that would result from exposure to the highly acidic gastric contents entering the duodenum and from the activated proteases further downstream.

Bile. Bile is an emulsifying agent and an important part of fat digestion and absorption. The liver produces bile and the gallbladder stores it so that it is readily available when fat enters the intestine.

Hormones. An alkaline environment in the small intestine, with a pH greater than 8, is necessary for the activity of the pancreatic enzymes. Thus, acidic stomach content entering the small intestine triggers the release of the hormone **secretin**. In response, the pancreas secretes bicarbonate to neutralize the chyme. In addition, secretin, which the mucosal glands in the first part of the intestine produce, controls the emission of pancreatic enzymes and slows gastric contractions.

When fat is present, the intestinal mucosal glands secrete the hormone **cholecystokinin** (CCK). CCK prompts the release of pancreatic juices and bile from the gallbladder to emulsify fat. The presence of glucose and fat in the duodenum actives **gastric inhibitory peptide** (GIP) secretion from the enterocytes of the small intestine. GIP stimulates insulin secretion from the pancreas in preparation for glucose absorption and inhibits gastric secretions and motility. The benefits of slowing down GI contractions and motility are that the long process of fat digestion has time to occur and the physical distention of the small intestine increases satiety throughout this process.

Figure 5.3 shows the arrangement of the accessory organs to the duodenum, which is the first section of the small intestine. These organs make up the biliary system. We sometimes refer to the liver as the "metabolic capital" of the body, because it performs numerous functions for the metabolism of all converging nutrients (Box 5.1). Chapter 18 reviews the liver's many metabolic functions in detail.

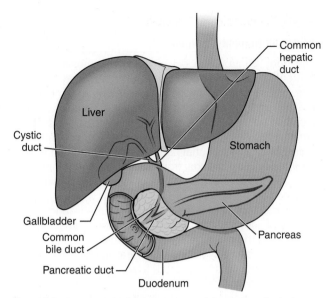

Figure 5.3 Organs of the biliary system and the pancreatic ducts.

pancreatic amylase a major starch-splitting enzyme that is secreted by the pancreas and that acts in the small intestine.

pancreatic lipase a major fat-splitting enzyme produced by the pancreas and secreted into the small intestine to digest fat.

secretin a hormone that stimulates gastric and pancreatic secretions. Secretin stimulates the secretion of pepsinogen from the chief cells of the stomach. In response to a low pH in the duodenum, secretin stimulates the pancreatic release of bicarbonate to increase the pH to an alkaline environment.

cholecystokinin (CCK) a hormone secreted from the mucosal epithelium of the small intestine in response to the presence of fat and certain amino acids in chyme. CCK inhibits gastric motility, increases the release of pancreatic enzymes, and stimulates the gallbladder to secrete bile into the small intestine.

gastric inhibitory peptide (GIP) a hormone secreted from the enterocytes of the duodenum and jejunum in response to the presence of glucose and fat. GIP stimulates insulin secretion from the pancreas and inhibits gastric motility.

Figure 5.4 illustrates the various nerve and hormone controls that influence digestion. Although each of the macronutrient chapters provide small individual summaries of digestion, Figure 5.5 presents a general summary of the entire digestive process so that you can view the overall process as one continuous and integrated whole.

ABSORPTION AND TRANSPORT

When digestion is complete, we have simplified whole food into molecules small enough for absorption. The process reduces carbohydrates to the monosaccharides glucose, fructose, and galactose. We have freed fatty acids and monoglycerides from triglycerides and individual amino acids from complex proteins. In addition, vitamins and minerals are liberated. With a water base for solution and transport, in addition to the

Box 5.1   Functions of the Liver

MAJOR FUNCTIONS
- Bile production
- Synthesis of proteins and blood clotting factors
- Metabolism of hormones and medications
- Regulation of blood glucose levels
- Urea cycle: converts excess ammonia into urea to remove the waste products of normal metabolism

SPECIFIC METABOLIC FUNCTIONS REGARDING THE MACRONUTRIENTS
- Lipolysis: breaking down lipids into fatty acids and glycerol
- Lipogenesis: building up lipids from fatty acids and glycerol

- Glycolysis: breaking down glucose into pyruvate to enter the Krebs cycle
- Gluconeogenesis: converting noncarbohydrate substances into glucose
- Glycogenolysis: breaking down glycogen into individual glucose units
- Glycogenesis: combining units of glucose to store as glycogen
- Protein degradation: breaking down proteins into single amino acids
- Protein synthesis: building complete proteins from individual amino acids

This is not an exhaustive list of all functions performed by the liver.

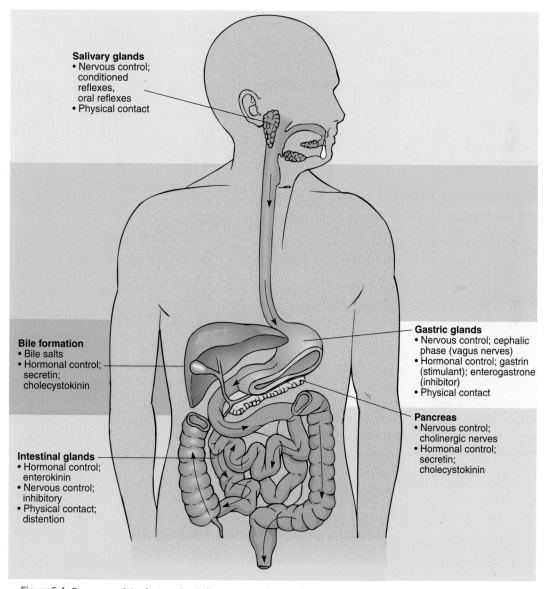

Figure 5.4 Summary of the factors that influence secretions in the gastrointestinal tract. (Courtesy Rolin Graphics.)

necessary electrolytes, the whole fluid, food-derived mass is now primed for absorption. For many nutrients, especially certain vitamins and minerals, the point of absorption becomes the vital gatekeeper that determines how much of a given nutrient is available for cellular use. Although the GI tract is efficient, we do not absorb 100% of all nutrients consumed because

of varying degrees of bioavailability. A nutrient's bioavailability depends on the following: (1) the amount of nutrient present in the GI tract; (2) the competition among nutrients for common absorptive sites; and (3) the form in which the nutrient is present (see the Clinical Applications box, "Micronutrient Bioavailability and Competitive Absorption"). The dietary intake

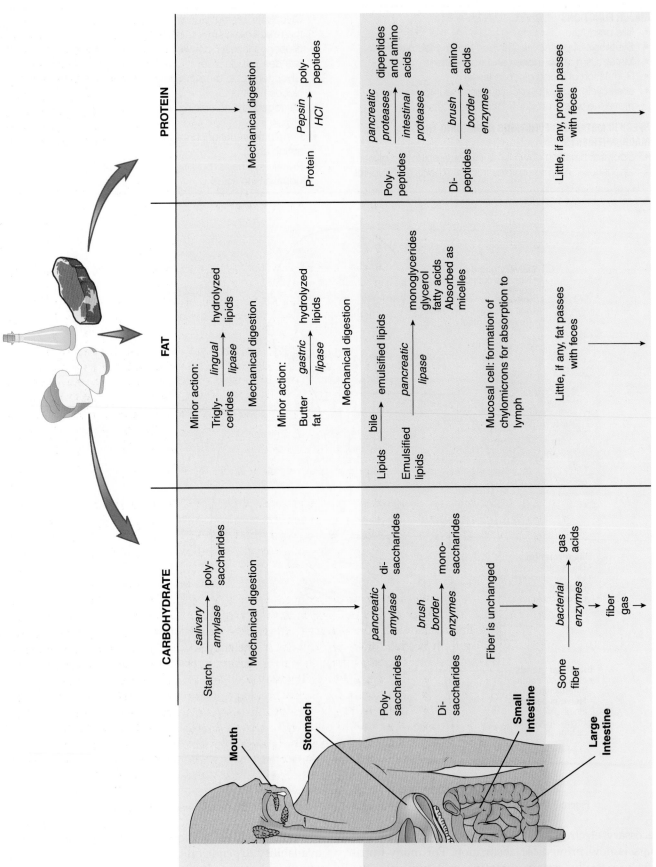

Figure 5.5 Summary of the digestive processes. Note: Enzymes are in *italics*. (Courtesy Rolin Graphics.)

recommendations (i.e., the DRIs) for all macronutrients and micronutrients take into account this varying degree of bioavailability.

ABSORPTION IN THE SMALL INTESTINE

Absorbing Structures

Three important structures of the intestinal wall surface (Figure 5.6) are particularly adapted to ensure the

maximal absorption of essential nutrients in the digestive process:

- *Mucosal folds:* Like the hills and valleys of a mountain range, the surface of the small intestine piles into many folds. It is easy to see mucosal folds when examining the intestinal tissue.
- *Villi:* Closer examination under a regular light microscope reveals small, finger-like projections that

---

Clinical Applications

Micronutrient Bioavailability and Competitive Absorption

Iron and zinc deficiency are two of the most common micronutrient deficiencies worldwide (along with vitamin A and iodine).[1,2] Subsequently, we often use food fortification or enrichment and dietary supplements containing these nutrients as a means for improving intake. However, just because we consume the added micronutrients, it does not mean that we can absorb or use them within the body. Many factors regulate nutrient bioavailability, including the presence of other nutrients and natural compounds within the food.

Iron and zinc enrichment in grain products has several factors working against the absorption of either nutrient. For example, the phytic acid found in grain products decreases the bioavailability of iron, zinc, and calcium by binding to the minerals and preventing absorption.[3] In addition, divalent cations compete for absorption throughout the gastrointestinal tract. For example, iron, copper, and zinc compete for binding to transporter molecules during absorption. Thus, a high level of any one divalent metal will reduce the bioavailability of the other divalent minerals.

Does this mean that it is a waste of time to include such products in the diet? No, not at all. Reduced bioavailability is not the same as blocked absorption. Reduced bioavailability only means that a smaller percent of the nutrient consumed is actually absorbed. Fortunately, the body is extremely efficient and does not depend on 100% absorption of all nutrients consumed. If you are working with a client who is taking a dietary supplement to correct for a nutrient deficiency, it is prudent to check for factors inhibiting or enhancing the bioavailability of that particular nutrient. That way, you can help clients make ideal choices about when to take their supplements, what foods to take them with or avoid, and what foods to consume to help stabilize the supply of the nutrients of concern.

REFERENCES

1. Peng, W., & Berry, E. M. (2018). Global nutrition 1990-2015: A shrinking, hungry, and expanding fat world. *PLoS One, 13*(3), e0194821.
2. World Health Organization. (2018). *Malnutrition.* Retrieved May 17, 2019, from www.who.int/news-room/fact-sheets/detail/malnutrition.
3. Moretti, D., et al. (2014). Bioavailability of iron, zinc, folic acid, and vitamin A from fortified maize. *Annals of the New York Academy of Sciences, 1312,* 54–65.

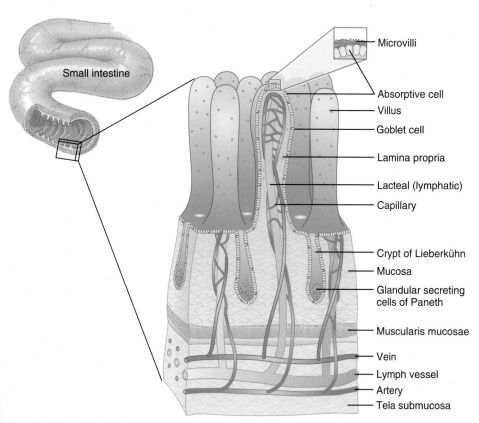

Figure 5.6 The intestinal wall. A diagram of the villi of the human intestine that shows its structure and the blood and lymph vessels. (Reprinted from Mahan, L. K., & Escott-Stump, S. [2008]. *Krause's food & nutrition therapy* [12th ed.]. Philadelphia: Saunders.)

cover the folds of the mucosal lining. These little **villi** further increase the exposed surface area. Each villus has an ample supply of blood vessels to receive protein, carbohydrate, and water-soluble micronutrients. Each villus also has a lymph vessel to receive fat-soluble nutrients. We call this lymph vessel a *lacteal*, because the fatty chyme is creamy at this point and looks like milk.

- *Microvilli:* Even closer examination with an electron microscope reveals a covering of smaller projections on the surface of each tiny villus. We call the covering of **microvilli** on each villus the *brush border,* because it looks like bristles on a brush.

These three unique structures of the inner intestinal wall—folds, villi, and microvilli—combine to make the inner surface nearly 600 times greater than the area of the outer surface of the intestine. In the absence of muscular contractions, the length of the small intestine

---

mucosal folds the large, visible folds of the mucous lining of the small intestine that increase the absorbing surface area.

villi small protrusions from the surface of a membrane; finger-like projections that cover the mucosal surfaces of the small intestine and that further increase the absorbing surface area.

microvilli extremely small, hair-like projections that cover all of the villi on the surface of the small intestine and that greatly increase the total absorbing surface area.

---

is approximately 6 m (20 ft) for the average adult. This remarkable organ is well adapted to deliver nutrients from digested food into the circulation for use within the body's cells. Far from being the lowly "gut," the small intestine is one of the most highly developed, exquisitely fashioned, and specialized tissues in the body.

Absorption Processes

A number of absorbing processes complete the task of moving vital nutrients across the inner intestinal wall and into the body circulation. These processes include diffusion, energy-driven active transport, and pinocytosis (Figures 5.7 and 5.8):

- *Simple diffusion* is the force by which particles move outward in all directions from an area of greater concentration to an area of lesser concentration. Small materials that do not need the help of a protein channel to move across the mucosal cell membranes use this method.
- *Facilitated diffusion* is similar to simple diffusion, but it makes use of a protein channel for the carrier-assisted movement of larger items across the mucosal cell membrane.
- *Active transport* is the force by which particles move against their concentration gradient. Active transport mechanisms usually require some sort of carrier to help transport the particles across the membrane. For example, glucose enters absorbing cells through an

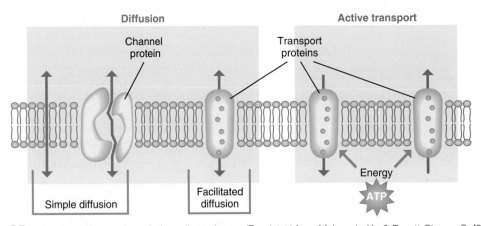

Figure 5.7 Transport pathways through the cell membrane. (Reprinted from Mahan, L. K., & Escott-Stump, S. [2012]. *Krause's food & nutrition therapy* [13th ed.]. Philadelphia: Saunders.)

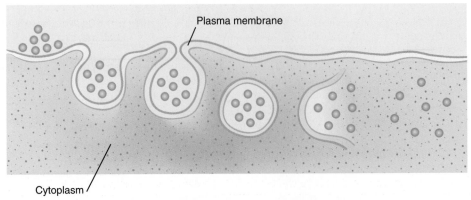

Figure 5.8 Pinocytosis; the engulfing of a large molecule by the cell.

active transport mechanism that involves sodium as a partner.

- *Pinocytosis* is the penetration of larger materials by attaching to the thick cell membrane before the cell engulfs it (see Figure 5.8).

ABSORPTION IN THE LARGE INTESTINE

Water

The main absorptive task that remains for the large intestine is to absorb water. Most of the water that enters the large intestine is absorbed in the first half of the colon. Only a small amount (approximately 100 mL) remains to form the feces for elimination.

Dietary Fiber

Humans do not digest dietary fiber because we lack the specific enzymes that are capable of breaking the beta bonds between the molecules found in fiber. However, fiber contributes important bulk to food mass and helps to form feces. The formation and passage of intestinal gas is a normal process of healthy digestion, but it can be problematic for some individuals (see the Clinical Applications box, "The Sometimes Embarrassing Effects of Digestion").

Figure 5.9 shows the approximate location of absorption of each nutrient as well as the route through which it is absorbed (i.e., lymph or blood) throughout the GI tract.

TRANSPORT

After freeing and absorbing individual nutrients from whole food, the circulatory systems must transport them to various cells throughout the body. This transportation requires the work of both the vascular and the lymphatic systems.

Vascular System

The vascular system is composed of veins and arteries, and it is responsible for supplying the entire body with nutrients, oxygen, and many other vital substances that are necessary for life via the blood. In addition, the vascular system transports waste (e.g., carbon dioxide, nitrogen) to the lungs and kidneys for removal.

🔹 Clinical Applications

The Sometimes Embarrassing Effects of Digestion

After eating certain foods, some people complain of the discomfort or embarrassment of gas. Gas is a normal by-product of digestion, but when it becomes painful or apparent to others, it may become a physical and social dilemma.

Typical adults will release between 0.5 and 1.75 L of gas daily. The majority of the gas in the GI tract originates from swallowing air. The rest is a by-product of bacteria in the colon. We release gas via the mouth as belching or the anus as flatus. Sometimes extra gas collects in the stomach or intestine, thereby creating an embarrassing—although usually harmless—situation.

STOMACH GAS

Trapped air bubbles may accumulate in the stomach. This occurs when a person eats too fast, drinks through a straw, or otherwise takes in extra air while eating. Burping releases some gas, but the following tips may help to avoid uncomfortable situations:

- Avoid carbonated beverages.
- Chew with the mouth closed.
- Do not gulp, drink from a can or through a straw, or eat while overly nervous.

INTESTINAL GAS

Intestinal gas forms in the colon, where bacteria attack fermentable residues and cause them to decompose and produce gas. Carbohydrates release hydrogen, carbon dioxide, and methane—in varying degrees dependent upon the types and amounts of bacteria in the gut. All three products are odorless (although sometimes noisy) gases. Protein produces hydrogen sulfide and volatile compounds such as indole and skatole, which add a distinctive aroma to the expelled air. Changing the diet to include less fermentable residue foods can improve symptoms.[1] However, problem foods are specific to individuals and may depend on the type and quantity of bacteria in their gut.

The following suggestions may help to control flatulence:

- Cut down on simple carbohydrates (e.g., sugars). Especially observe milk's effect, because lactose intolerance may be the culprit. Substitute cultured forms, such as yogurt or milk treated with a lactase product such as Lactaid (McNeil Nutritionals, Fort Washington, PA).
- Use a prior leaching process before cooking dry beans to remove indigestible saccharides such as raffinose and stachyose. Although humans cannot digest these substances, they provide a feast for bacteria in the intestines. This simple procedure eliminates a major portion of these gas-forming saccharides. First, put washed, dry beans into a large pot; add 4 cups of water for each pound of beans (approximately 2 cups); and boil the beans uncovered for 2 min. Remove the pot from the heat, cover it, and let it stand for 1 hour. Finally, drain and rinse the beans, add 8 cups of fresh water, bring the water to a boil, reduce the heat, and simmer the beans in a covered pot for 1 to 2 hours or until beans are tender. Season as desired.
- Eliminate known food offenders. These vary from person to person, but some of the most common offenders are beans (if they are not prepared for cooking as described), onions, cabbage, and high-fiber wheat and bran products.

Once achieving relief, slowly add more complex carbohydrates and high-fiber foods back into the diet. After tolerating small amounts, try moderate increases. If no relief occurs, a medical provider can help rule out or treat an overactive gastrointestinal tract.

REFERENCE

1. Azpiroz, F., et al. (2014). Effect of a low-flatulogenic diet in patients with flatulence and functional digestive symptoms. *Neurogastroenterology and Motility, 26*(6), 779–785.

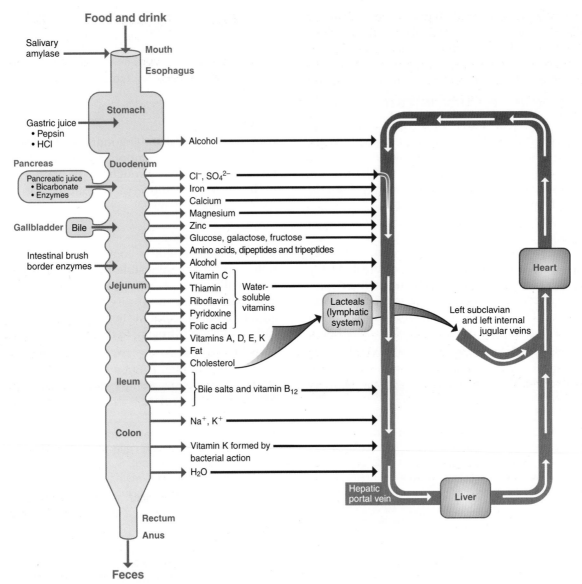

Figure 5.9 Sites of secretion and absorption in the gastrointestinal tract. (Modified from Mahan, L. K., & Escott-Stump, S. [2008]. *Krause's food & nutrition therapy* [12th ed.]. Philadelphia: Saunders.)

Most of the products of digestion are water-soluble nutrients, which can therefore be absorbed into the vascular system (i.e., the blood circulatory system) directly from the intestinal cells. The nutrients travel first to the liver for immediate use by the **hepatocytes** before dispersing to other cells throughout the body. *Portal circulation* is the portion of circulation from the intestines to the liver.

Lymphatic System

The lymphatic system provides an alternative route for fat-soluble nutrient absorption because fats are not water soluble. These fat molecules first pass into the lacteals in the villi, then flow into the larger lymph vessels of the body, and eventually enter the bloodstream through the thoracic duct.

hepatocytes cells of the liver.

METABOLISM

At this point, the digestive processes have broken down the individual macronutrients in food into their respective building blocks (i.e., monosaccharides, amino acids, and fatty acids), and we have absorbed them into the bloodstream or the lymphatic system. Now the body can convert the macronutrients into needed energy or store it for later use.

In addition, the micronutrients (i.e., vitamins and minerals) are free for absorption. Once absorbed, the micronutrients disperse throughout the body for their many critical functions.

CATABOLISM AND ANABOLISM

Metabolism is the sum of the chemical reactions that occur within a living cell to maintain life. The mitochondrion of the cell is the work center in which all metabolic reactions take place. The two types of metabolism are catabolism and anabolism. Catabolism is the breaking down of large substances into smaller units. For example, breaking down stored glycogen into its smaller building blocks (i.e., glucose) is a catabolic reaction. Anabolism is the opposite; it is the process by which cells build large substances from smaller particles, such as building a complex protein from single amino acids.

The Krebs cycle (also known as the *citric acid cycle* and the *tricarboxylic acid* [*TCA*] *cycle*) is the hub of energy production that occurs in the mitochondria of the cell. It is not so much that we *produce* energy here. Rather, the mitochondria convert energy into a form that the body can use. The combined processes of metabolism (i.e., catabolic and anabolic reactions) ensure that the body has much needed energy in the form of adenosine triphosphate (ATP). Figure 5.10 is a simplified illustration of macronutrient breakdown and shows how macronutrients enter the final step of energy production to ultimately supply cells with ATP.

The rate of ATP production fluctuates, and it speeds up or slows down depending on energy needs at a given time. Energy needs are minimal during sleep, but they increase dramatically during strenuous physical activity. Chapter 6 covers energy supply and demand further.

ENERGY DENSITY

Because carbohydrates have 4 kcal/g and fat has 9 kcal/g, the metabolism of glucose yields less energy (i.e., ATP) than the metabolism of fat, gram for gram. However, the body prefers to use glucose as its primary source of energy. We can use protein as a source of energy as well, but this is an inefficient use of protein, and it results in extra nitrogen waste. The body only breaks down protein for energy when glucose and fatty acids are unavailable.

STORING EXTRA ENERGY

If the amount of food consumed yields more energy than is needed to maintain voluntary and involuntary actions, the remaining energy is stored for later use in the body. The human body is a highly efficient organism. Energy or kilocalories in excess of needs are not wasted. Excess glucose can easily be stored as glycogen in the liver and muscles for quick energy when required. Glycogenesis is the anabolic process of converting extra glucose into glycogen.

Once the glycogen reserves are full, additional excess energy from carbohydrates, fat, or protein is stored as fat in adipose tissue. Lipogenesis is the building up of triglycerides for storage in the adipose tissue of the body. Both glycogen and stored fat are available for use when energy demands require it. Chapter 6 discusses energy balance and the factors that influence it further.

Excess protein intake is not "stored as muscle." The body uses amino acids to build functional and structural proteins as needed, and the liver maintains some free amino acids to meet rapid needs of the body. However, protein intake beyond the body's requirements is broken down further. During this process, we remove the nitrogen unit

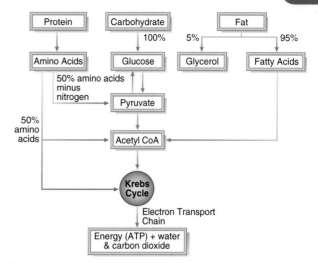

Figure 5.10 Catabolic pathways. (Modified from Peckenpaugh, N. J. [2007]. *Nutrition essentials and diet therapy* [10th ed.]. Philadelphia: Saunders.)

and convert the remaining carbon chain into glucose or fat for storage. Gluconeogenesis is the conversion of noncarbohydrate sources (e.g., amino acids) to glucose.

Although alcohol is not a nutrient, it does provide 7 kcal/g. Therefore, alcohol intake adds to the overall supply of energy (see the For Further Focus box, "What About Alcohol?").

ERRORS IN DIGESTION AND METABOLISM

THE GENETIC DEFECT

Certain food intolerances stem from underlying genetic disease. For genetic diseases involving metabolism, the necessary enzyme controlling the cell's use of an essential nutrient is missing, thereby preventing normal nutrient metabolism. Although there are many inherited metabolic disorders, we will only focus on a select few within this text. Three examples of genetic defects are phenylketonuria (PKU), galactosemia, and glycogen storage diseases.

Phenylketonuria

Phenylalanine hydroxylase is the enzyme that is responsible for metabolizing the essential amino acid phenylalanine. PKU is a rare autosomal recessive genetic disorder resulting from a lack of phenylalanine hydroxylase. Without this enzyme available for phenylalanine metabolism, phenylalanine will build up to toxic levels in the body. Although the disease is not curable, it is treatable through diet. If left untreated, PKU causes severe irreversible brain damage and central nervous system damage. Other possible symptoms and side effects include irritability, hyperactivity, developmental problems, convulsive seizures, and psychiatric disorders.

PKU affects approximately 1 in every 10,000 to 15,000 live births in the United States.[1] Screening tests began during the 1960s, and they are now mandatory at birth in all areas of the United States. A simple blood test can identify affected infants, and thus treatment can start immediately. With proper treatment, children with PKU

For Further Focus

What About Alcohol?

DOES ALCOHOL PROVIDE ENERGY?
Yes. Alcohol contributes to the overall energy intake in the form of calories. Alcohol yields 7 kcal/g. This is more than both carbohydrates and protein, which yield 4 kcal/g each.

IS ALCOHOL A NUTRIENT?
No. Unlike carbohydrates, fats, proteins, vitamins, minerals, and water, alcohol performs no essential function in the body. Alcohol is not stored in the body, but if consumed in large quantities, the by-products of metabolism may accumulate to toxic amounts.

HOW IS ALCOHOL DIGESTED?
About 85% to 95% of alcohol is absorbed without any chemical digestion. Alcohol is one of the few substances that can be absorbed directly into the circulation from the stomach. The presence of food in the stomach slows the rate of alcohol absorption into the blood. What is not absorbed in the stomach is absorbed in the small intestine and sent directly to the liver for detoxification and metabolism.

HOW IS ALCOHOL METABOLIZED?
Alcohol metabolism takes precedence over the metabolism of nutrients in the body because it is a toxin. The primary by-product of alcohol metabolism is acetaldehyde, which is the culprit for the destruction of healthy tissue that is associated with alcoholism. After detoxifying the alcohol, the liver uses the remaining by-products to produce fatty acids. The process of lipogenesis combines fatty acids with glycerol to form triglycerides, which are stored in the liver. A single drinking binge can result in an accumulation of fat in the liver. Repeated episodes over time can lead to fatty liver disease, which is the first stage of alcoholic liver disease.

Alcohol metabolism is a priority for the liver. Blood alcohol concentrations peak at approximately 30 to 45 minutes after one drink, which is defined as 12 oz of beer, 5 oz of wine, or 1.5 oz of 80-proof distilled spirits. The liver can only work at a designated speed to metabolize and rid the body of alcohol, regardless of the quantity consumed. When consumption exceeds the rate of metabolism, alcohol and its metabolites begin to accumulate in the blood and circulate throughout the body.

Several factors influence an individual's ability to metabolize alcohol, including sex, age, food intake, body weight and composition, genetics, and medications.

MORE INFORMATION
To find out more about alcohol and its dangers, benefits, and associated diseases, refer to the following websites:
- Mayo Clinic: *site search for alcohol*: www.mayoclinic.org
- Alcoholics Anonymous: www.aa.org
- National Institute on Alcohol Abuse and Alcoholism: www.niaaa.nih.gov

---

can grow normally and have healthy lives. The treatment is a low-phenylalanine diet for life consisting of a supplemental nutrition formula designed specifically for individuals with PKU and low-protein food products (see also the Drug-Nutrient Interaction box, "Aspartame and Phenylketonuria," in Chapter 4). Unfortunately, the prescribed diet is somewhat unpalatable, and lifelong adherence is low.[2] Successful management requires intensive family counseling by a metabolic team. Research into cell-directed therapy and more permanent treatment guidelines is ongoing.[3-7]

Galactosemia
Galactosemia is a genetic disease caused by a missing enzyme that alters normal carbohydrate metabolism. Galactosemia is an autosomal recessive disorder (similar to PKU) and it affects approximately 1 in every 30,000 to 60,000 live births.[8] The missing enzyme, galactose-1-phosphate uridyltransferase, is one that converts galactose to glucose. Because galactose comes from the breakdown of lactose (milk sugar), affected individuals must eliminate all sources of lactose from the diet. When it is not treated, galactosemia causes fatal brain and liver damage. Newborn screening programs, which are required in all states, identify affected infants. If treatment begins immediately, they may recover some complications and avoid life-threatening damage.

Treatment is a strict galactose-free diet, with special formulas for infants and lactose-free food guides. Individuals with galactosemia must follow the diet for life. Despite rigorous treatment, patients generally experience complications at some point in life such as cognitive disability, speech problems, neurologic and/or movement disorders, and ovarian dysfunction for women.[9] Currently, globally accepted treatment protocols that are successful in avoiding all complications do not exist. However, despite known gaps in knowledge surrounding successful treatment, experts recently proposed universal guidelines for diagnosis, treatment, and follow-up for the first time.[10] These guidelines are beyond the scope of this text but you may refer to reference number 10 in this chapter for full details (see references in the back of the book).

Glycogen Storage Diseases
Glycogen storage diseases (GSDs) are a group of rare genetic defects that inhibit the normal metabolic pathways of glycogen. This disease occurs in 1 of every 100,000 live births in the United States.[11] Twelve distinct forms of GSD result from the absence of the required enzymes that are necessary for the synthesis or breakdown of glycogen. The enzyme that is missing distinguishes the exact form of GSD and the tissue affected. The liver is the primary site of glycogen metabolism; therefore, hepatic forms of GSD (e.g., von Gierke disease or type I glycogenosis) affect the glucose availability of the whole body. Myopathic forms of GSD inhibit normal glycogen metabolism in the striated muscles and are less severe than hepatic forms. An example of a myopathic form is McArdle disease (i.e., type V glycogenosis).

The focus of dietary treatment for individuals with GSD is to avoid hypoglycemia through a balanced carbohydrate diet. Because they are not able to use stored glycogen for blood glucose balance during periods of fasting (e.g., overnight, between meals), a constant and steady intake of available glucose is imperative for cell function throughout the body.

OTHER INTOLERANCES OR ALLERGIES

Other problems with digestion and metabolism are the result of food intolerances or allergies. An example of an error in digestion is lactose intolerance, which results from the inability to digest lactose.

Lactose Intolerance

A deficiency of any one of the disaccharidases (i.e., lactase, sucrase, or maltase) in the small intestine may produce a wide range of GI problems and abdominal pain because the body cannot digest the specific sugar involved (see Chapter 2). Lactose intolerance is the most common, and it manifests as varying degrees of intolerance. With this condition, there is insufficient lactase to break down the milk sugar lactose; thus, lactose accumulates in the intestine, causing abdominal cramping and diarrhea. Individuals with lactose intolerance carefully avoid milk and all dairy products containing lactose to remain symptom free. Alternatively, they may consume milk treated with a commercial lactase product or lactose-free milk substitute products (e.g., soy, almond, rice milk).

Allergies

Allergies are inappropriate immune responses to substances that are not otherwise harmful. Food allergies are not necessarily problems with digestion or metabolism but can affect the gastrointestinal tract and its normal function. One example is celiac disease. Celiac disease is an allergy to the proteins known as gluten. The response is a cellular destruction of the GI tract lining. As a result, digestion of all nutrients is negatively affected. Chapter 18 covers issues involving GI disorders and allergies in more detail.

Putting It All Together

Summary

- The multiple metabolic tasks that sustain life require that cells receive key nutrients after the digestion, absorption, and transport of food.
- Mechanical digestion consists of spontaneous muscular activity that is responsible for the initial mechanical breakdown by mastication and the movement of the food mass along the GI tract by motions such as peristalsis.
- Chemical digestion involves enzymatic action that breaks food down into progressively smaller components and then releases its nutrients for absorption.
- Absorption involves the passage of nutrients from the intestines into the mucosal lining of the intestinal wall. It primarily occurs in the small intestine as a result of the work of highly efficient intestinal wall structures.
- The lymphatic and blood circulation transport absorbed nutrients throughout the body.
- Metabolism is the sum of the body processes that change food energy from the macronutrients into various forms of body energy. Metabolism is a balance of both anabolic and catabolic reactions.
- Genetic diseases of metabolism result from missing enzymes that control the metabolism of specific nutrients. Treatment diets in each case limit or eliminate the offending nutrient involved or provide the nutrient that cannot be derived endogenously.

Chapter Review Questions

See answers in Appendix A.

1. If you chew a piece of bread in the mouth for a long time, it begins to taste sweet because of the action of the enzyme _____.

   a. pepsin
   b. mucus
   c. amylase
   d. lipase

2. _____ is an example of mechanical digestion.

   a. Mastication
   b. Amylase secretion
   c. Active transport
   d. Simple diffusion

3. A 45-year-old female is considering eating 2.5 times the recommended protein for her body to build more lean muscle. Which of the following would be an appropriate response?

   a. Encourage her to proceed because the extra protein will build more muscle.
   b. Explain to her that excess protein intake is broken down and used for energy if needed or stored as fat.
   c. Explain that the extra protein intake will build muscle as long as she increases calorie intake as well.
   d. Encourage her to eat more fruit and vegetables rather than protein, to build muscle mass.

4. Upon admission to the hospital from hypothermia and starvation, a 23-year-old would most likely be in a state of _____.

   a. catabolism
   b. anabolism
   c. glycogenesis
   d. lipogenesis

5. A woman who has a large surgical resection of the small intestine would most likely have difficulty with _____.

   a. storing bile
   b. secreting pepsin
   c. digesting food
   d. producing chyme

Next-Generation NCLEX® Examination-style Case Study

See answers in Appendix A.

A 12-year-old female is experiencing frequent abdominal cramps, bloating, gas, and diarrhea. She feels tired and reports suffering recurrent headaches. She notices her stomach pains shortly after eating foods such as cereal and milk, bean and cheese burritos, and ice cream. She skips meals often because she is worried that it will make her feel ill.

1. Based on information provided, the nurse anticipates that the client has_____.

   a. phenylketonuria
   b. galactosemia
   c. lactose intolerance
   d. glycogen storage disease
   e. grohn's disease

2. Choose the *most likely* options for the information missing from the statements below by selecting from the list of options provided.

   The client is not producing adequate amounts of the intestinal enzyme ____1____, allowing ____2____ to move into the ____3____ instead of undergoing digestion and absorption.

OPTION 1	OPTION 2	OPTION 3
galactase	sucrose	ileum
lipase	glucose	colon
maltose	lactose	duodenum
lactase	maltase	jejunum

3. From the list below, select all of the appropriate dietary interventions to alleviate the client's symptoms.

   a. Avoid dairy products
   b. Consume lactose-free products
   c. Consume products with added lactase
   d. Only eat animal-based foods until symptoms subside
   e. Consume fat-free dairy products
   f. Experiment with low-lactose containing foods to identify a threshold
   g. Avoid all products containing gluten

4. You are educating the client on appropriate food choices. Place an X under "effective" for all changes that would help eliminate the client's symptoms. Place an X under "ineffective" for all changes that would not be effective.

FOODS	EFFECTIVE	INEFFECTIVE
Lactaid milk		
Almond milk		
Eggs		
Cheese		
Cow's milk		
Yogurt		
Soy milk		

Additional Learning Resources

Please refer to this text's Evolve website for answers to the Case Study questions:
http://evolve.elsevier.com/Williams/basic/
References and **Further Reading and Resources** in the back of the book provide additional resources for enhancing knowledge.

Energy Balance

Key Concepts

- The body uses energy released from chemical bonds within food in various forms.
- The body uses most of its energy supply to meet basal metabolic needs.
- A balance between the intake of food energy and the output of body work maintains life and health.
- States of energy imbalance may manifest as a body weight that is underweight or overweight.

Through the process of metabolism, our bodies continually convert energy from the food that we eat into the form of cellular energy that we use for work and activity. According to intake and output demands, either we use fuel or we store it. This chapter looks at the big picture of energy balance among all of the energy-yielding nutrients and demonstrates how we measure, cycle, and use energy to meet the body's metabolic demands.

HUMAN ENERGY SYSTEM

ENERGY NEEDS

Both voluntary and involuntary actions require energy. Thus, the maintenance of life and health depends upon a constant supply of energy.

Involuntary Body Work

The greatest use of energy in the body is the result of involuntary work, which includes all of the activities that happen without conscious effort. These activities consist of such vital processes as circulation, respiration, digestion, and absorption as well as many other internal activities that maintain life. Involuntary body functions require energy in various forms, such as chemical energy (in many metabolic products), electrical energy (in brain and nerve activities), mechanical energy (in muscle contraction), and thermal (i.e., heat) energy to maintain body temperature.

Voluntary Work and Exercise

Voluntary work includes all of the actions related to a person's conscious activities of daily living and physical activity. Although it may seem like we burn more calories performing these intentional actions throughout the day, that usually is not the case.

MEASUREMENT OF ENERGY

In common usage, we refer to the energy found in food and the energy expended in physical actions as a calorie. However, in human nutrition, we use the term *kilocalorie* (i.e., 1000 calories) to designate the large calorie unit that nutrition scientists use to avoid dealing with too many zeros. A kilocalorie (abbreviated as *kcalorie* or *kcal*) is the amount of heat that is necessary to raise 1 kg of water 1° C. When referring to body or food energy, we will always refer to the kilocalorie in this text. Most people do not realize that there is a difference between a calorie and a kilocalorie. People often use the terms interchangeably in common language, but they should never be confused in the scientific literature.

The international unit of measure for energy is the joule (J). To convert kilocalories (kcal) into kilojoules (kJ), multiply the number of kilocalories by 4.184 (e.g., 200 kcal × 4.184 = 836.8 kJ). Nutrition facts labels on food products in most of the world express energy in units of kilojoules instead of kilocalories.

FOOD AS FUEL FOR ENERGY

We use energy in the form of adenosine triphosphate (ATP) for voluntary and involuntary body functions. ATP is a metabolic end product of the energy-yielding foods consumed (see Figure 5.10). The body must have an adequate supply of fuel to balance energy demands for healthy weight maintenance. As explained earlier in this book, the only three energy-yielding nutrients are the macronutrients carbohydrate, fat, and protein. Carbohydrates and fat are the body's primary fuel sources. The body uses protein for energy only when other fuel sources are not available.

Fuel Factors

Metabolism of each energy-yielding substance provides the body with a specific quantity of ATP units. We refer to

---

calorie a measure of heat; the energy necessary to do work is measured as the amount of heat produced by the body's work; the energy value of a food is expressed as the number of kilocalories that a specified portion of the food will yield when it is oxidized in the body.

this quantity as their respective fuel factor or energy density (see Chapter 5). Note that we have used the term *substance* instead of energy-yielding *nutrients*. That is because ethanol (i.e., beverage alcohol from fermented grains and fruits) also supplies energy but is not a nutrient. The fuel factors are as follows: carbohydrate, 4 kcal/g; fat, 9 kcal/g; protein, 4 kcal/g; and alcohol, 7 kcal/g.

Energy and Nutrient Density

The term *density* refers to the degree of concentrated material in a given substance. More material in a smaller volume of a given substance increases the density. Thus, the concept of *energy density* refers to a high concentration of energy (i.e., kilocalories) in a small amount of food. Of the three energy-yielding nutrients, foods that are high in fat have the highest energy density. Similarly, we can evaluate foods in terms of their *nutrient density*. A food with a high nutrient density means that it has a relatively high concentration of vitamins and minerals in a smaller volume of a given food. Some foods are both energy and nutrient dense, which means that they provide a lot of both kilocalories and micronutrients. *Empty calorie* foods are the direct opposite of a nutrient-dense food.

Examples of foods that would fit into each category are the following:

- Energy dense: butter, oil, French fries, fried meats (e.g., fried chicken), ice cream
- Nutrient dense: vegetables, fruits, legumes, whole grains, lean protein (e.g., non-fatty fish, white meat or lean chicken), and low-fat dairy/dairy-substitute products
- Energy and nutrient dense: avocados, cheese, seeds (e.g., sunflower seeds), nuts, nut butters (e.g., peanut butter, almond butter)
- Empty calories: sugar-sweetened beverages (e.g., soda), pastries, donuts, cakes

Food guides such as MyPlate and the *Dietary Guidelines for Americans* (see Figures 1.4 and 1.5) recommend foods that are nutrient dense as opposed to only energy dense.[1,2]

ENERGY BALANCE

Similar to matter, we can neither create nor destroy energy. When we say that energy is "produced," what we really mean is that it is transformed (i.e., changed in form and cycled through a system). Consider the human energy system as part of the total energy system on Earth. In this sense, two energy systems support life—one within the body and the much larger one surrounding us—as follows:

1. *External energy cycle:* In the environment, the ultimate source of energy is the sun and its vast nuclear reactions. With the use of water and carbon dioxide as raw materials, plants transform the sun's radiation into stored energy (mainly carbohydrate with some fat and protein). The food chain continues as animals eat plants and the products of other animals (e.g., meat, milk, eggs).

2. *Internal energy cycle:* When people eat plant and animal foods, the stored energy of the food in its complex form (e.g., polysaccharides, triglycerides) is broken down into simple fuels (e.g., glucose and fatty acids) available to meet the energy needs on a cellular level. Voluntary and involuntary actions of the body require energy in many forms, such as chemical, electrical, mechanical, and thermal energy. As this internal energy cycle continues, water is excreted, carbon dioxide is exhaled, and heat is radiated, thereby returning these end products to the external environment. The overall energy cycle continually repeats itself to sustain life.

ENERGY INTAKE

The total overall energy balance within the body depends on the energy intake in relation to the energy output. The sources of energy for all bodily functions are the energy-yielding substances acquired through food and caloric drinks. We use stored energy in the body tissues (e.g., adipose tissue) to supplement this dietary supply.

Estimating Dietary Energy Intake

One can estimate personal energy intake by recording a day's actual food consumption and calculating its energy value. There are several methods available to accomplish this, such as using food labels to gather nutrient information of foods consumed throughout the day, using various databases to look up the energy value of foods eaten, or by using online or mobile apps that allow the user to enter portions of food consumed to calculate total daily intake. One such freely available online database that allows users to search for individual foods is the United States Department of Agriculture's (USDA) FoodData Central (fdc.nal.usda.gov). This database provides an extensive list of nutrients found in approximately 275,000 foods. You can search by food item, food group, or brand name. Some of the online and smartphone mobile apps allow users to enter their personal (e.g., sex, age, activity level) and **anthropometric** data so that it can compare their recorded energy intake to their estimated energy output through physical activity and **basal energy expenditure** (BEE). The accuracy of any method employed depends on the precision of the food consumption and physical activity recorded and entered by the user.[3-5]

Stored Energy

Throughout times of fasting, such as during sleep, or the extreme stress of starvation, the body draws from its stored energy.

Glycogen. In a well-nourished person, there is a 12- to 48-hour reserve of glycogen in the liver and muscles.

The body will quickly deplete this supply if we do not replenish it through daily carbohydrate intake. Glycogen stores maintain normal blood glucose levels during periods of sleep. However, the first meal of the day, breakfast (which is so named because it "breaks the fast"), has a significant function for restoring those supplies and meeting subsequent energy needs.

Adipose tissue. Although the amount of fat storage in the body is larger than that of glycogen storage, the supply varies among persons. Unlike glycogen stores, there is a relatively unlimited amount of energy that one can store as fat. In addition, fat provides more kilocalories per gram than any other fuel source, thus making it an efficient storage form.

Muscle mass. We can elicit energy from protein used to build muscle mass. However, this lean tissue serves important structural functions, and it is preferably not sacrificed for energy use. Only during longer periods of fasting or starvation does the body turn to this tissue for energy.

ENERGY OUTPUT

The necessary activities to sustain life—normal body functions, the regulation of body temperature, and the processes of tissue growth and repair—use energy from food and body reserves. *Metabolism* is the sum of the total chemical changes that occur during all of these activities (see Chapter 5). The following three demands for energy determine the body's total energy requirements: (1) basal energy expenditure; (2) physical activity; and (3) the thermic effect of food.

Basal Energy Expenditure

The term *basal energy expenditure* (BEE) or basal metabolic rate (BMR) refers to the sum of all internal activities of the body while at total rest; we express it in kilocalories per day. For example, if an individual's BEE were 1500 kcal, that would represent the amount of energy that this particular person would need to consume, on average, over a 24-hour period to maintain his or her current weight while at complete rest. On occasion, people use the terms *BEE* and resting energy expenditure (REE) interchangeably. However, a technical difference exists between BEE and REE. We must measure BEE when an individual is at absolute digestive, physical, mental, thermal, and emotional rest. It is rather difficult to maintain the stringent conditions required to measure a true BEE; therefore, it is more common to measure a person's REE. The REE is up to 10% higher than a true BEE measurement, but one can minimize the differences through compliance to best practices protocol when measuring REE.[6-8]

The majority (60% to 75%) of the average person's total energy expenditure (TEE) is used to meet basal energy demands alone. In addition, a few small but highly active organs use the majority of that energy.[9,10] The

anthropometric the physical measurements of the human body that are used for health assessment, including height, weight, body composition.

basal energy expenditure (BEE) the amount of energy (in kcal) needed by the body for the maintenance of life when a person is at complete digestive, physical, mental, thermal, and emotional rest (i.e., 10 to 12 hours after eating and 12 to 18 hours after physical activity); measured immediately upon waking. Also referred to as basal metabolic rate (BMR).

thermic effect of food an increase in energy expenditure caused by the activities of digestion, absorption, transport, and metabolism of ingested food; a meal that consists of a usual mixture of carbohydrates, protein, and fat increases the energy expenditure equivalent to approximately 10% of the food's energy content (e.g., a 300-kcal piece of pizza would elicit an energy expenditure of 30 kcal to digest the food).

resting energy expenditure (REE) the amount of energy (in kcal) needed by the body for the maintenance of life at rest over a 24-hour period; this is often used interchangeably with the term *basal energy expenditure*, but in actuality it is slightly higher because the protocol for measurement does not put the person at complete rest. Also referred to as resting metabolic rate (RMR).

combined weight of the brain, heart, liver, and kidneys equals only 5% to 7% of an adult's total body weight. Nevertheless, these highly active organs account for approximately 80% of the body's REE. Thus, the size and function of highly metabolically active organs and tissues account for the majority of individual variability for REE and total energy needs.[11,12] There are many methods available for predicting a person's REE based on body size and the size of the organs with high metabolic activity. The evolution of these formulas has been ongoing for more than a century.

Measuring basal energy expenditure or resting energy expenditure. Direct calorimetry is a method of measuring energy use that involves specially engineered metabolic chambers in which subjects relax while their energy expenditure, in the form of heat production, is directly measured. There are few such facilities available; thus, clinicians rarely use this method for measuring energy expenditure.

Alternatively, dietitians sometimes measure BEE or REE in clinical practice (e.g., hospital patients with altered metabolism, athletes, subjects in research laboratories) with the use of indirect calorimetry. This method measures the amount of energy that a person uses while at rest. A portable metabolic cart allows the person to breathe into an attached mouthpiece or ventilated hood system while lying down, and the normal exchange of oxygen and carbon dioxide is measured (Figure 6.1). The technician can calculate the metabolic rate with a high degree of accuracy from the rate of gas exchange.[13]

Several handheld devices developed over the past couple of decades are intended to provide an alternative, portable, fast, and less expensive method for measuring REE via indirect calorimetry (e.g., MedGem and BodyGem [Microlife USA, Clearwater, FL]) (Figure 6.2).[14] The test subject holds the device while breathing exclusively into the mouthpiece. Some of the available handheld devices measure only oxygen consumption to calculate a client's REE, whereas other devices measure both oxygen and carbon dioxide exchange similarly to the metabolic cart.[15] The usefulness and reliability of such devices remain unclear for some populations.[16-20]

Predicting basal energy expenditure or resting energy expenditure. A rudimentary formula for calculating basal energy needs is to multiply 0.9 kcal/kg body weight for women and 1 kcal/kg body weight for men by the number of hours in a day. Thus, examples of how we can estimate the daily basal metabolic needs (in kilocalories) for men and women are as follows:

For a 154-lb man:

$$1 \text{ kcal} \times \text{kg body weight} \times 24 \text{ hours}$$
(1) Convert pounds to kilograms: 154 lb ÷ 2.2 = 70 kg
(2) 1 kcal × 70 kg × 24 hr = 1680 kcal/day

For a 121-lb woman:

$$0.9 \text{ kcal} \times \text{kg body weight} \times 24 \text{ hours}$$
(1) convert pounds to kilograms: 121 lb ÷ 2.2 = 55 kg
(2) 0.9 kcal × 55 kg × 24 hr = 1188 kcal/day

Obviously, this simple equation does not take into account personal distinctions such as age, height, activity level, fitness, or any other factor that would alter energy needs. This formula is useful in determining the energy needs of groups of people to get an overall estimate. For example, if we have a group of people going on a backpacking trip and need to determine how much food to take, we could start with this formula. Using the average weight of the group members for the formula, plus additional kilocalories added for activity, we could estimate how many

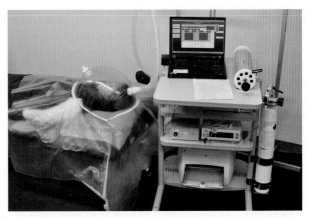

Figure 6.1 Measuring resting metabolic rate with a metabolic cart. (Courtesy Susie Parker-Simmons, United States Olympic Committee.)

kilocalories should be available per person per day. By multiplying that number by the number of people in the group and the number of days for the trip, we could have an approximate estimate of the number of kilocalories the group would need to transport. It is not precise enough to use in a clinical setting or for specific individual needs.

The Mifflin-St. Jeor equations, the Harris-Benedict equations, and the equations that were used for the 2002 Dietary Reference Intake (DRI) values provide an alternate method of estimating the REE or BEE that is more specific to the individual (Box 6.1). Of these equations, the Mifflin-St. Jeor equation is the most commonly used REE measurement for healthy people.[21] However, predictive formulas are not reliable for some clients because of disease state, age (at either end of the spectrum), or obesity status. Therefore, indirect calorimetry measurements are the only accurate methods for reliably calculating energy needs for some clients.[8,22-25]

Factors that influence basal energy expenditure. Practitioners should keep in mind that several factors influence the BEE when interpreting test results. In addition to the influence from organs of the body with high metabolic activity, other major factors that

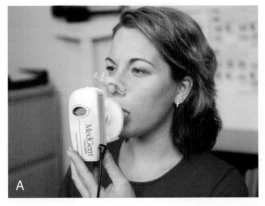
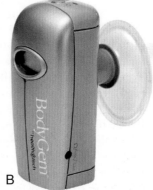

Figure 6.2 (A) MedGem and (B) BodyGem devices, which are used to determine the resting metabolic rate. (Courtesy Microlife USA, Clearwater, FL.)

Box 6.1 Equations for Estimating Resting Energy Needs

MIFFLIN-ST. JEOR[1]
Men

TEE (kcal/day) = (10 × Weight [kg] + 6.25 × Height [cm] − 5 × Age [yr] + 5) × PA[a]

Women

TEE (kcal/day) = (10 × Weight [kg] + 6.25 × Height [cm] − 5 × Age [yr] − 161) × PA[a]

HARRIS-BENEDICT[2]
Men

TEE (kcal/day) = (66.47 + 5 × Height [cm] + 13.75 × Weight [kg] − 6.755 × Age) × PA[a]

Women

TEE (kcal/day) = (655.1 + 1.85 × Height [cm] + 9.56 × Weight [kg] − 4.676 × Age) × PA[a]

1.200 = Sedentary (little or no exercise; desk job)

1.375 = Lightly active (light exercise/sports 1 to 3 days/wk)

1.550 = Moderately active (moderate exercise/sports 3 to 5 days/wk)

1.725 = Heavy exercise (hard exercise/sports 6 to 7 days/wk)

2002 Dietary Reference Intake Energy Calculation[b,3]

EER = TEE + Energy deposition

Children 0 to 36 Months Old

0 to 3 months: (89 × Weight [kg] − 100) + 175 kcal

4 to 6 months: (89 × Weight [kg] − 100) + 56 kcal

7 to 12 months: (89 × Weight [kg] − 100) + 22 kcal

13 to 36 months: (89 × Weight [kg] − 100) + 20 kcal

Boys 3 to 8 Years Old

EER = 88.5 − (61.9 × Age [yr]) + PA × (26.7 × Weight [kg] + 903 × Height [m]) + 20 kcal

Boys 9 to 18 Years Old

EER = 88.5 − (61.9 × Age [yr]) + PA × (26.7 × Weight [kg] + 903 × Height [m]) + 25 kcal

PA COEFFICIENT USED FOR BOYS 3 TO 18 YEARS OLD

1.00 if PAL is estimated to be ≥1.0 but <1.4 (sedentary)

1.13 if PAL is estimated to be ≥1.4 but <1.6 (low active)

1.26 if PAL is estimated to be ≥1.6 but <1.9 (active)

1.42 if PAL is estimated to be ≥1.9 but <2.5 (very active)

Girls 3 to 8 Years Old

EER = 135.3 − (30.8 × Age [yr]) + PA × (10.0 × Weight [kg] + 934 × Height [m]) + 20 kcal

Girls 9 to 18 Years Old

EER = 135.3 − (30.8 × Age [yr]) + PA × (10.0 × Weight [kg] + 934 × Height [m]) + 25 kcal

PA COEFFICIENT USED FOR GIRLS 3 TO 18 YEARS OLD

1.00 if PAL is estimated to be ≥1.0 but <1.4 (sedentary)

1.16 if PAL is estimated to be ≥1.4 but <1.6 (low active)

1.31 if PAL is estimated to be ≥1.6 but <1.9 (active)

1.56 if PAL is estimated to be ≥1.9 but <2.5 (very active)

Men 19 Years Old and Older

EER = 662 − (9.53 × Age [yr]) + PA × (15.91 × Weight [kg] + 539.6 × Height [m])

PA COEFFICIENT FOR MEN 19 YEARS AND OLDER

1.00 if PAL is estimated to be ≥1.0 but <1.4 (sedentary)

1.11 if PAL is estimated to be ≥1.4 but <1.6 (low active)

1.25 if PAL is estimated to be ≥1.6 but <1.9 (active)

1.48 if PAL is estimated to be ≥1.9 but <2.5 (very active)

Women 19 Years Old and Older

EER = 354 − (6.91 × Age [yr]) + PA × (9.36 × Weight [kg] + 726 × Height [m])

PA COEFFICIENT FOR WOMEN 19 YEARS AND OLDER

1.00 if PAL is estimated to be ≥1.0 but <1.4 (sedentary)

1.12 if PAL is estimated to be ≥1.4 but <1.6 (low active)

1.27 if PAL is estimated to be ≥1.6 but <1.9 (active)

1.45 if PAL is estimated to be ≥1.9 but <2.5 (very active)

REFERENCES
1. Mifflin, M. D., et al. (1990). A new predictive equation for resting energy expenditure in healthy individuals. *Am J Clin Nutr*, 51(2), 241–247.
2. Roza, A. M., & Shizgal, H. M. (1984). The Harris Benedict equation reevaluated: Resting energy requirements and the body cell mass. *Am J Clin Nutr*, 40(1), 168–182.
3. Food and Nutrition Board and Institute of Medicine. (2002). *Dietary reference intakes for energy, carbohydrate, fiber, fat, fatty acids, cholesterol, protein, and amino acids.* Washington, DC: National Academies Press.

EER, Estimated energy requirement; *PA*, physical activity; *PAL*, physical activity level; *TEE*, total energy expenditure.

[a]The PA coefficients for men and woman noted above are applicable to both the Mifflin-St. Jeor and the Harris-Benedict equations.

[b]Each age-specific and sex-specific equation for the 2002 Dietary Reference Intake Energy Calculations has a specific set of PA coefficients. Make sure to use the PA coefficients associated with the specific equation used.

affect BEE are body composition, growth periods, body temperature, hormonal status, and disease state as follows:

- *Body composition:* Lean body mass includes muscles, bones, connective tissue such as ligaments and tendons, and internal organs. One of the largest contributors to overall metabolic rate is the relative percent of metabolically active lean body mass.[26] The more lean body mass a person has, the higher the person's BEE. This is because lean tissues have a significantly greater metabolic activity than adipose tissue. Other factors (e.g., sex, age, height) primarily influence the metabolic rate proportionally as they relate to the lean body mass and overall body size. For example, males usually have more lean body mass than females, younger people usually have more lean body mass than elderly individuals, and taller people generally have more lean body mass than short people.

- *Growth periods:* BEE rises considerably during pregnancy, which is a period of rapid growth for both the pregnant woman and fetus. However, this value is highly variable among women, and it is correlated with total weight gain and prepregnancy fat stores.

BEE increases above prepregnancy rates with the progression of pregnancy; average increases with each trimester are 4.5%, 10.8%, and 24%, respectively.[27] During rapid growth periods in childhood and adolescence, human growth hormone stimulates cell regeneration and raises BEE to support anabolism. As growth and the rate of cellular regeneration slow with age, so does BEE.

- *Body temperature:* Changes in body temperature significantly alter the body's total energy expenditure. A fever will increase the BEE as the immune system works to fight infection. In states of starvation and malnutrition, the process of **adaptive thermogenesis** results in lowered heat production to conserve energy and thus BEE decreases. In cold weather, especially in freezing temperatures, BEE rises in response to the generation of more body heat to maintain normal core temperature.

- *Hormonal status:* The presence or absence of hormones also influences a person's energy expenditure. For example, epinephrine and growth hormone increase the metabolic rate to varying degrees relative to duration of hormone secretion.

  Thyroid hormone plays a significant role in regulating metabolism. Thyroid function tests can measure the activity of the thyroid gland, serum **thyroxine** levels, thyroid-stimulating hormone levels, serum protein-bound iodine levels, and radioactive iodine uptake levels. Such tests are not associated with a kilocalorie amount in terms of total energy needs. However, the tests may gauge a person's overall metabolic function. Individuals with an underactive thyroid gland may develop hypothyroidism, which manifests as a decreased metabolic rate. Oral medications such as levothyroxine can successfully treat hypothyroidism (see the Drug-Nutrient Interaction box, "Absorption of Levothyroxine," for more information about hypothyroid medication interactions). Conversely, hyperthyroidism occurs when the thyroid gland is overactive (see the Cultural Considerations box, "Hypermetabolism and Hypometabolism: What Are They and Who Is at Risk?").

- *Disease state:* Depending on the disease and presence of inflammation, the BEE may be increased or decreased. The best method for obtaining accurate estimates of BEE in such individuals is to use direct or indirect calorimetry measurements.[8]

---

adaptive thermogenesis an adjustment to heat production in response to changing environmental influences (e.g., external temperature, diet).

thyroxine (T$_4$) an iodine-dependent thyroid prohormone; the active hormone form is T3; it is a major controller of basal metabolic rate.

🔵 Drug-Nutrient Interaction

Absorption of Levothyroxine

Health care providers may prescribe the synthetic hormone levothyroxine (Synthroid) to treat hypothyroidism. It is absorbed primarily in the jejunum and ileum of the small intestine. Taking levothyroxine on an empty stomach maximizes absorption, which suggests the importance of gastric acid. The presence of food delays or prevents the drug's absorption. Thus, patients should take the medication at least 1 hour before or 2 hours after a meal. A consistent medication and eating schedule is imperative for normalization of the thyroid hormones through levothyroxine treatment.

Many nutrition factors affect the absorption of the drug. Medications, dietary supplements, and foods that interfere with levothyroxine absorption include the following:[1,2]

- Medications: antacids, beta-blockers, bile acid sequestrants, ciprofloxacin, orlistat, phosphate binders, proton pump inhibitors, raloxifene, simethicone, tricyclic antidepressants
- Dietary supplements: calcium and iron supplements, chromium picolinate
- Foods or nutrients: milk, soy, papaya, fiber, coffee, grapefruit juice

Gastrointestinal disorders (e.g., celiac disease, lactose intolerance, *Helicobacter pylori* infection, bowel resection, inflammatory bowel disease, hypochlorhydria, chronic gastritis, motility disorders) and disorders of the accessory organs involved in digestion (e.g., pancreatic insufficiency, liver cirrhosis) all affect the absorptive ability of the digestive system and consequently interfere with the absorption of levothyroxine.[1,2]

Celiac disease is an autoimmune disorder that affects about 1% of the general population. Individuals with celiac disease are more likely to have additional autoimmune disorders such as Hashimoto thyroiditis, an autoimmune thyroid disorder.[3] It is important to note that when a person has celiac disease or another malabsorption disorder (e.g., lactose intolerance), levothyroxine absorption will not improve sufficiently with higher doses of the drug until dietary restrictions for the disorder are followed.

REFERENCES

1. Virili, C., et al. (2019). Gastrointestinal malabsorption of thyroxine. *Endocr Rev, 40*(1), 118–136.
2. Skelin, M., et al. (2017). Factors affecting gastrointestinal absorption of levothyroxine: A review. *Clin Ther, 39*(2), 378–403.
3. Bibbo, S., et al. (2017). Chronic autoimmune disorders are increased in coeliac disease: A case-control study. *Medicine (Baltimore), 96*(47), e8562.

Physical Activity

Physical activity involved in work, recreation, and activities of daily living also influence the individual variations in energy output (see Chapter 16). In addition to increasing energy expenditure and reducing the risk of chronic diseases, exercise has positive effects on health-related quality of life throughout the life span.[28-31] Table 6.1 provides a list of various activities and the amount of kilocalories used per pound of body weight per hour. Although mental work or study does

Hypermetabolism and Hypometabolism: What Are They and Who Is at Risk?

Hypermetabolism and hypometabolism are conditions in which the metabolic rate is either significantly higher (hyper) or lower (hypo) than expected. Because the thyroid gland is responsible for producing the hormone thyroxine, a significant controller of the metabolic rate, such conditions usually result from malfunctions of the thyroid gland. Clinically, we refer to hypermetabolism and hypometabolism involving the thyroid gland as *hyperthyroidism* and *hypothyroidism*, respectively.

An individual with hyperthyroidism has a significantly higher metabolic rate and higher energy needs than expected. Neither the person's lean tissue mass, age, nor sex explains such high energy needs. This individual likely has an overactive thyroid gland, which means that he or she produces too much thyroxine. As a result, the normal energy intake recommendations do not meet this client's needs. For example, a woman who is 25 years old, 5 feet and 5 inches tall, and weighs 125 lb normally needs approximately 2200 kcal/day to maintain her weight if she engages in a moderate level of activity. However, the same woman with hyperthyroidism may need 1.5 to 2.5 times as many kilocalories per day to maintain her current weight.

Conversely, individuals with hypothyroidism do not produce enough thyroxine for their body size and therefore require less energy than expected to maintain their current body weight. The Dietary Reference Intakes for energy for an individual with hypothyroidism are too high and would likely result in weight gain. However, effective medications are available for hypothyroidism. Typically, both hyperthyroidism and hypothyroidism present during young adulthood.

Congenital hypothyroidism (CH), which occurs in 1 out of every 2000 to 4000 live births in the United States, is a type of hypothyroidism that is present at birth and that can result in mental disability and slowed growth if it is not treated.[1] Newborn screening for CH began during the 1970s and is now standard. The risk of CH is linked to gestational age, birth weight, sex, and ethnicity. Infants who weigh less than 4.5 lb or more than 10 lb at birth have a significantly higher risk of developing CH. Females of any weight are significantly more likely to have CH than males. The incidence rate of CH in the United States is twice as high in Hispanic newborns and 44% higher in Asian and Native Hawaiian or other Pacific Islander newborns as compared with Caucasian newborns; it is 30% lower in African-American newborns as compared with Caucasian newborns.[2]

Improved methods and frequency of testing have drastically increased the number of diagnosed and treated cases of CH in the United States. The close monitoring of basal metabolism and total energy expenditure is an important aspect of the treatment. Modifications to medications and energy intake, as needed, help control weight and prevent long-term complications.

REFERENCES
1. National Institutes of Health. (2018). *Congenital hypothyroidism.* Genetics Home Reference. https://ghr.nlm.nih.gov/condition/congenital-hypothyroidism#resources
2. Hinton, C. F., et al. (2010). Trends in incidence rates of congenital hypothyroidism related to select demographic factors: Data from the United States, California, Massachusetts, New York, and Texas. *Pediatrics, 125*(Suppl. 2), S37–S47.

not require additional kilocalories, muscle tension, restlessness, and agitated movements may slightly increase energy needs for some individuals.

The energy expenditure that we use for physical activity goes beyond the BEE. It is difficult to keep track of all energy that we use explicitly for physical activity to calculate the total energy requirement. Instead, we can estimate the energy that we use for physical activity by categorizing our physical activity (PA) level in accordance with standard values. This PA factor is then multiplied by the estimated or measured BEE. The PA factor (or *PA coefficient*) is dependent on lifestyle and the formula used to estimate BEE. For example, an individual who works at a desk job and who has little or no leisure activity would have a PA factor of approximately 1.2 according to the Mifflin-St. Jeor equation. To estimate the total energy expenditure for this individual, you would multiply the person's BEE by a PA factor of 1.2 (see Box 6.1).

Thermic Effect of Food

After eating, a person requires extra energy for the physical process of digestion, absorption, and transportation of nutrients to the cells. We refer to this overall stimulating effect as the *thermic effect of food*. Approximately 5% to 10% of the body's total energy needs for metabolism relate to the digestion and storage of nutrients from food. Another way to think about it is to assume that 5% to 10% of the calories in a food consumed will be used during the digestion of that food.

Total Energy Expenditure

A person's TEE includes the energy needs for BEE, his or her physical activities, and the thermic effects of food (Figure 6.3). Total energy requirements vary considerably between individuals. To maintain energy balance, food energy intake must match body energy output as an average over time. An energy imbalance in which energy intake consistently exceeds energy output eventually leads to weight gain (see the Case Study box, "Weight Loss and Hypothyroidism"). To correct the imbalance, one could decrease food kilocalorie intake and/or increase energy output through physical activity. Extreme and unhealthy weight loss may occur when food energy intake does not meet body energy requirements for extended periods. Treatment may be complex and will depend on the cause of the weight loss, whether intentional or unintentional (see Chapter 15).

The Clinical Applications box entitled "Evaluate Your Daily Energy Requirements" provides a

Table 6.1	Energy Expenditure per Pound per Hour During Various Activities
ACTIVITY	**kcal/lb/h[a]**
Aerobics, moderate	2.95
Bicycling	
Light: 10 to 11.9 mph	2.72
Moderate: 12 to 13.9 mph	3.63
Fast: 14 to 15.9 mph	4.54
Mountain biking	3.85
Daily Activities	
Cleaning	1.36
Cooking	0.91
Driving a car	0.91
Eating, sitting	0.68
Gardening, general	1.81
Office work	0.82
Reading, writing while sitting	0.70
Sleeping	0.41
Shoveling snow	2.72
Running	
5 mph (12 min/mile)	3.63
7 mph (8.5 min/mile)	5.22
9 mph (6.5 min/mile)	6.80
10 mph (6 min/mile)	7.26
Sports	
Boxing, in ring	5.44
Field hockey	3.63
Golf	2.04
Rollerblading	4.42
Skiing, cross country, moderate	3.63
Skiing, downhill, moderate	2.72
Soccer	3.85
Swimming, moderate	3.14
Tennis, doubles	2.27
Tennis, singles	3.63
Ultimate Frisbee	3.63
Volleyball	1.81
Walking	
Moderate: ≈3 mph (20 min/mile), level	1.50
Moderate: ≈3 mph (20 min/mile), uphill	2.73
Brisk: ≈3.5 mph (17.14 min/mile), level	1.72
Fast: ≈4.5 mph (13.33 min/mile), level	2.86
Weight Training	
Light or moderate	1.36
Heavy or vigorous	2.72

[a]Multiply the activity factor by the weight in pounds by the fraction of hour spent performing the activity: Example: A 150-lb person plays soccer for 45 minutes. Therefore, the equation would be as follows: 3.85 (i.e., the factor from the table) × 150 (lb) × 0.75 (h) = 433.13 calories burned. Energy expenditure depends on the physical fitness of the individual and the continuity of exercise.
Modified from Nieman, D. C. (2003). *Exercise testing and prescription: A health-related approach* (5th ed.). New York: McGraw-Hill.

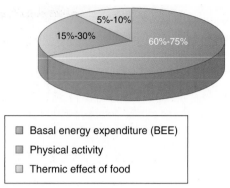

5%-10%
15%-30%
60%-75%

◼ Basal energy expenditure (BEE)
◼ Physical activity
◻ Thermic effect of food

Figure 6.3 The contributions of basal energy expenditure, physical activity, and the thermic effect of food to total energy expenditure.

step-by-step example for evaluating your energy needs. You may also wish to record your food and activities for a day and to calculate your energy intake (i.e., kilocalories in) and output (i.e., kilocalories out). Because it is difficult to keep track of what you are doing for 24 hours of the day, the estimate from this method is often different from the equations for estimating REE (i.e., Mifflin-St. Jeor, Harris Benedict).

RECOMMENDATIONS FOR DIETARY ENERGY INTAKE

GENERAL LIFE CYCLE
Growth Periods
During periods of rapid growth, extra energy per unit of body weight is necessary to build new tissue. Compare the kcal/lb estimates from birth to age 18 in Table 6.2. Note that the kcal/lb needs reflect the rapid growth occurring during infancy and adolescence, with continuous but slower growth taking place between these periods. The rapid growth of the fetus and

Table 6.2	Approximate Caloric Allowances from Birth to the Age of 18 Years
AGE (yr)	**kcal/lb**
Infants	
Birth to 0.5	33.4
0.6 to 1.0	35.6
Children	
1 to 2	36.2
Boys	
3 to 8	32
9 to 13	26.3
14 to 18	24
Girls	
3 to 8	29.7
9 to 13	23.8
14 to 18	19.3

Data from the Food and Nutrition Board and Institute of Medicine. (2002). *Dietary reference intakes for energy, carbohydrate, fiber, fat, fatty acids, cholesterol, protein, and amino acids*. Washington, DC: National Academies Press.

NEXT-GENERATION NCLEX® EXAMINATION-STYLE UNFOLDING CASE STUDY
Weight Loss and Hypothyroidism

See answers in Appendix A.

A 32-year-old female (Ht.: 5'4", Wt.: 160 lbs., BMI: 27 kg/m²) comes into the office with a history of hypothyroidism. She has been experimenting with intermittent fasting, but wakes up feeling very low-energy. She also has not been successful in losing any weight. She is looking for diet advice to help her lose weight. The registered dietitian nutritionist (RDN) collected and analyzed a 1-day diet record and found that her daily calorie consumption is approximately 1,800.

1. **Highlight or circle the foods from the client's diet that are nutrient-dense.**

   Breakfast: Cinnamon Roll, Apple Juice, Yogurt
   Lunch: Grilled Chicken Wrap (w/lettuce, tomato, spinach), Potato Chips, Sweet Tea, Almonds
   Dinner: Chicken Fried Steak, Baked Potato, Butter (with potato), Asparagus, Cookies

2. **Choose the *most likely* options for the information missing from the statements below by selecting from the list of options provided.**

   The client is most likely feeling low-energy due to the ____1____ of ____2____ stores throughout the night after long periods of fasting for 12-48 hours. These stores are responsible for maintaining ____3____ levels during sleep.

OPTION 1	OPTION 2	OPTION 3
depletion	fat	blood glucose
repletion	protein	energy
activation	glycogen	triglyceride

Using the Mifflin-St. Jeor equation, you determine that her total energy expenditure is ~1900 kcals. This is above her usual intake, yet she still struggles to lose weight. You know that there are many factors that may lower basal energy expenditure.

3. **From the list below, select all factors that could potentially lower the client's basal energy expenditure below normal.**

   a. Low lean body mass
   b. Pregnancy
   c. Fasting
   d. Hypothyroidism
   e. Hyperthyroidism
   f. Female sex
   g. Hormone imbalance
   h. Sedentary lifestyle

4. **Choose the *most likely* options for the information missing from the statements below by selecting from the list of options provided.**

   You determined that the client's hypothyroidism leads to ____1____ production of ____2____, which slows metabolism. This would require the client have a ____3____ calorie deficit to facilitate weight loss.

OPTION 1	OPTION 2	OPTION 3
increased	levothyroxine	larger
appropriate	thyroxine	smaller
reduced	thyroid stimulating hormone	gradual

The client returns to the office for a follow-up appointment one month later. She has started swimming (3.85 kcals/hr) for 1 hr/day on 6 days/week and mentioned that she made other lifestyle changes as well. She is happy with her weight loss and would like to maintain her current body weight. However, she is not sure how many calories she is expending with all of these lifestyle changes.

5. **Choose the *most likely* options for the information missing from the statements below by selecting from the list of options provided.**

   Considering this client's new exercise regimen, the nurse found the client's BEE (kcal/kg/hr) and TEE (kcal/day) to be ____1____ and ____2____ respectively.

OPTION 1	OPTION 2
1570 kcals/day	2187 kcals/day
2200 kcals/day	1570 kcals/day
1700 kcals/day	1700 kcals/day

6. **Select all of the lifestyle factors the client may have implemented that would most likely be effective in facilitating weight loss.**

   a. Choosing nutrient-dense foods
   b. Increasing daily physical activity
   c. Increasing fruit and vegetable consumption
   d. Choosing calorie dense foods
   e. Increasing exercise
   f. Reduce large amounts of calories by fasting
   g. Reducing calories gradually and moderately
   h. Consume variety of foods from each food group
   i. Eliminate food groups
   j. Consume more processed foods than whole foods

the placenta as well as other maternal tissues make increased energy intake during pregnancy and lactation highly important (see Chapter 10).

Adulthood

Energy needs decline with age, but the specific amount of decline is highly individual. Once we achieve full adult height, energy needs level off to meet requirements for tissue maintenance, tissue repair, and physical activity. Historical data indicated that the average decline in BEE was 1% to 2% per kg of fat-free mass per decade.[32] However, more recent data indicate that BEE is much more specific to each person, lifestyle, and disease state during the adult years and is more complex to predict. As the aging process continues, the relative size of the organs with high metabolic activity (e.g., brain, liver, kidneys, heart, gut) gradually declines. Because these organs are major drivers of the metabolic energy needs of the adult, the BEE declines relative to the decline in organ size.[33] Adults who sustain highly active lifestyles and conserve skeletal muscle mass are likely

Clinical Applications

Evaluate Your Daily Energy Requirements

Your estimated energy requirement (in kcal) per day is the sum of your body's three uses of energy, which are as follows: basal energy expenditure (also known as basal metabolic rate), thermic effect of food, and physical activity. Let us work through a couple of estimated energy requirement calculations together. Then you can plug in your own values to evaluate your daily energy balance. For our examples, we will use the Estimated Energy Requirement (EER) formula from the 2002 Dietary Reference Intakes. Other formulas are also available in Box 6.1.

EER FORMULA FOR THE 2002 DIETARY REFERENCE INTAKES FOR MEN AND WOMEN OVER 19 YEARS OF AGE:

Men 19 years old and older = 662 − (9.53 × Age [yr]) + Physical activity (PA) × (15.91 × Weight [kg] + 539.6 × Height [m])

Women 19 years old and older = 354 − (6.91 × Age [yr]) + PA × (9.36 × Weight [kg] + 726 × Height [m])

PHYSICAL ACTIVITY

Abbreviated as PA, PA coefficient, or PAL (physical activity level) in the formula. The PA level is the ratio of the total energy expenditure to the basal energy expenditure.

LIFESTYLE	PA FACTOR FOR MEN	PA FACTOR FOR WOMEN
Sedentary: Mostly resting with little or no planned strenuous activity and only performing those tasks that are required for independent living	1.0	1.0
Low Active: In addition to the activities of a sedentary lifestyle, the added equivalent of a 1.5- to 3-mile walk at a speed of 3 to 4 mph for the average-weight person[a]	1.11	1.12
Active: In addition to the activities identified for a sedentary lifestyle, an average of 60 min of daily moderate-intensity physical activity (e.g., walking at 3 to 4 mph for 3 to 6 miles/day) or shorter periods of more vigorous exertion (e.g., jogging for 30 min at 5.5 mph)	1.25	1.27
Very Active: In addition to the activities of a sedentary lifestyle, an activity level equivalent to walking at 3 to 4 mph for 12 to 22 miles/day (approximately 5 to 7 hours per day) or shorter periods of more vigorous exertion (e.g., running 7 mph for approximately 2.5 hours/day)	1.48	1.45

[a]For example, a man who weighs 70 kg and is 1.77 m tall and a woman who weighs 57 kg and is 1.63 m tall, based on the reference body weights for adults.

Let Us Work Through Our First Example

We have a 22-year-old woman who weighs 130 lb. She is 5 feet and 5 inches tall and is maintaining a regular physical exercise program. She is currently consuming approximately 2300 kcal/day. First, we will need to convert all of her measurements into metric terms:

Conversions: 1 pound = 2.2 kg; 39.37 in = 1 m

Thus, our client is 130 lb ÷ 2.2 = 59 kg; 5 ft 5 in = 65 inches ÷ 39.37 = 1.651 m.

Now, we will insert her numbers into the formula provided for women using an active PA coefficient of 1.27 for women:

EER = 354 − (6.91 × 22 yr old) + 1.27 [PA] × (9.36 × 59 kg + 726 × 1.651 m)

EER = 354 − 152 + 1.27 × (552.24 + 1198.63)

EER = 2426 kcal/day

Conclusion: According to our calculations and her reported kcal intake of 2300 kcal/day, our client is likely to lose weight over time. Her energy intake is approximately 126 kcal/day less than her energy output. Because 1 lb of body fat equals approximately 3500 kcal, she could lose about 1 lb every 28 days with her current eating and exercise routine.

Let Us Work One More Example Together

We have a 41-year-old man who weighs 195 lb (88.64 kg). He is 6 feet (1.829 m) tall and eats an average of 3100 kcal/day while maintaining a low active lifestyle (PA = 1.11). Work through the calculations on your own to make sure you are getting the order of operations correct. Check your work against the numbers below.

EER = 662 − (9.53 × 41 yr old) + 1.11 [PA] × (15.91 × 88.64 kg + 539.6 × 1.829 m)

EER = 662 − 390.73 + 1.11 × (1410.26 + 986.93)

EER = 2932 kcal/day

Conclusion: This man will likely gain weight with his current exercise and meal plan, because he is consuming approximately 168 kcal more than he is expending. Approximately how many pounds will he gain per month?

Now, calculate your own daily energy requirements and estimate your energy balance status. Are you in energy balance?

If you would like to use Table 6.1 to estimate your specific energy use according to your actual activities for a full day, follow the steps below:

1. Estimate the time that you spent on a given activity by adding the total minutes that you spent on that activity throughout the day and then converting those minutes to hours (or decimal fractions of hours) for the day (e.g., total minutes of an activity ÷ 60 minutes/h = hours of that activity).
2. Multiply the total time for a given type of activity by your weight (in lb) and by the average kilocalories per hour for that activity (e.g., total time [h] × wt [lb] × kcal/h = total kcal/day for that activity).
3. Finally, add together kilocalories used for all activities during the 24-hour period to get the day's total energy expenditure (e.g., total kcal/day of all activities = total energy expenditure for 1 day from activities).

to experience a less dramatic decline in energy needs than their counterparts with a less active lifestyle and resultant loss of lean muscle mass. Meanwhile, adults suffering morbidity have a higher BEE than their peers of the same sex, age, and body composition do, demonstrating that disease plays a role in the overall metabolic demands on the body.[34-36]

A notable decline in the metabolic rate occurs around 40 to 50 years of age.[11] Some of these changes relate directly to the increase in fat mass and loss of fat-free mass that accompanies menopause in women.[37,38] Therefore, to maintain energy balance, food choices should reflect a decline in caloric density and place greater emphasis on increased nutrient density, particularly after the fourth or fifth decade of life.

DIETARY REFERENCE INTAKES

To determine recommendations for energy intake, the Food and Nutrition Board of the Institute of Medicine considered the average energy intake of individuals who were healthy, free living, and maintaining a healthy body weight as determined by **body mass index** measurements (see inside back cover of text for body mass index chart).[6] Table 6.3 gives the mean total energy expenditure throughout the lifecycle. Note the average height, weight, body mass index, and physical activity level within each age and sex group. The DRIs for vitamins and minerals are set at two standard deviations *above the mean* to meet the needs of 97.5% of the population. However, experts set the DRIs for energy *at the mean* for the

Table 6.3 Median Height, Weight, and Recommended Energy Intake

AGE (yr)	MEAN WEIGHT (kg [lb])	MEAN HEIGHT (m [in])	MEAN BODY MASS INDEX (kg/m²)	BASAL ENERGY EXPENDITURE (kcal/day)	MEAN PHYSICAL ACTIVITY LEVEL	MEAN TOTAL ENERGY EXPENDITURE (kcal/day)
Infants						
Birth to 0.5	6.9 (15)	0.64 (25)	16.9	—	—	501
0.6 to 1.0	9 (20)	0.72 (28)	17.2	—	—	713
Children						
1 to 2	11 (24)	0.82 (32)	16.2	—	—	869
Males						
3 to 8	20.4 (45)	1.15 (45)	15.4	1035	1.39	1441
9 to 13	35.8 (79)	1.44 (57)	17.2	1320	1.56	2079
14 to 18	58.8 (130)	1.70 (67)	20.4	1729	1.80	3116
19 to 30	71 (156)	1.80 (71)	22.0	1769	1.74	3081
31 to 50	71.4 (157)	1.78 (70)	22.6	1675	1.81	3021
51 to 70	70 (154)	1.74 (69)	23.0	1524	1.63	2469
71+	68.9 (152)	1.74 (69)	22.8	1480	1.52	2238
Females						
3 to 8	22.9 (50)	1.20 (47)	15.6	1004	1.48	1487
9 to 13	36.4 (80)	1.44 (57)	17.4	1186	1.60	1907
14 to 18	54.1 (119)	1.63 (64)	20.4	1361	1.69	2302
19 to 30	59.3 (131)	1.66 (65)	21.4	1361	1.80	2436
31 to 50	58.6 (129)	1.64 (65)	21.6	1322	1.83	2404
51 to 70	59.1 (130)	1.63 (63)	22.2	1226	1.70	2066
71+	54.8 (121)	1.58 (62)	21.8	1183	1.33	1564
Pregnant						
First trimester						+0
Second and third trimesters						+300/day
Lactating						
First 12 months						+500/day

Data from Food and Nutrition Board and Institute of Medicine. (2002). *Dietary reference intakes for energy, carbohydrate, fiber, fat, fatty acids, cholesterol, protein, and amino acids*. Washington, DC: National Academies Press.

population to avoid encouraging overconsumption of kilocalories.

DIETARY GUIDELINES FOR AMERICANS

The *Dietary Guidelines for Americans* address energy needs by making the following recommendations:[2]

- Choose a healthy eating pattern at an appropriate calorie level to help achieve and maintain a healthy body weight, support nutrient adequacy, and reduce the risk of chronic disease.
- To meet nutrient needs within calorie limits, choose a variety of nutrient-dense foods across and within all food groups in recommended amounts.
- Meet nutrition needs primarily through whole foods.
- Limit calories from added sugars and saturated fats.
- Meet the Physical Activity Guidelines for Americans.

> **body mass index** the body weight in kilograms divided by the square of the height in meters (kg/m^2); this measurement correlates with body fatness and the health risks associated with obesity.

MYPLATE

The MyPlate website (www.choosemyplate.gov) can help you to determine an individualized calorie level and corresponding serving sizes from each of the food groups to meet energy and nutrient density needs on the basis of age, sex, weight, height, and activity level.[1] The site also provides helpful information for maintaining a balance between food intake and energy output through physical activity.

Putting It All Together

Summary

- In the human energy system, food provides energy. In the United States, we measure energy in kilocalories. Energy from food cycles through the body's internal energy system in balance with the sun-powered external environment's energy system.
- Metabolism is the sum of the body processes that are involved in converting food into various forms of energy available for use within the cells. When food is not available, the body draws on its stored energy, which is in the forms of glycogen, fat, and muscle protein.
- The following elements make up almost all of a person's total energy expenditure: (1) basal energy expenditure, which makes up the largest portion of energy needs; (2) energy for physical activities; and (3) the thermic effect of food.
- Energy requirements vary throughout life and are altered in disease states.

Chapter Review Questions

See answers in Appendix A.

1. **Which of the following individuals most likely has the highest energy needs per pound of body weight?**

    a. 38-year-old male administrative assistant
    b. 72-year-old grandmother
    c. 22-year-old college student
    d. 7-month-old baby boy

2. **Which of the following helps maintain normal blood glucose levels during sleep hours?**

    a. Cholesterol stores
    b. Protein stores
    c. Glycogen stores
    d. Vitamin D stores

3. **A measure of a client's metabolic rate could be determined using**

    _____.

    a. glycogen levels
    b. indirect calorimetry
    c. physical activity records
    d. body temperature

4. **Jenny is trying to lose weight and has decreased her energy intake by 250 kcal per day. How long should it take her to lose 1 lb of body fat if all other factors remain stable?**

    a. Approximately 8 days
    b. Approximately 14 days
    c. Approximately 27 days
    d. Approximately 32 days

5. **Calculate the amount of kilocalories in 1 cup of milk that contains 4 g of fat, 10 g of protein, and 15 g of carbohydrate.**

    a. 90 kcal
    b. 120 kcal
    c. 136 kcal
    d. 145 kcal

Next-Generation NCLEX® Examination-style Case Study

See Answers in Appendix A.

A 70-year-old female (Ht.: 5'4" 210 lbs.) experiences pain in her joints and has trouble moving around the house. She gained a significant amount of weight during the decade after going through menopause. She reports not making any notable changes to her diet throughout this same period. She does not participate in physical activity and her muscles do not feel as strong as they used to. She is looking for help to lose weight.

1. **From the list below, select all the factors that influence the client's energy balance.**

    a. Menopause increases basal energy expenditure
    b. Menopause decreases basal energy expenditure
    c. Energy needs decrease with age
    d. Energy needs increase with age
    e. Reduced physical activity increases basal energy expenditure
    f. Reduced physical activity decreases basal energy expenditure
    g. Reduction in muscle mass
    h. Reduced energy needs required by organs

2. Choose the *most likely* options for the information missing from the statements below by selecting from the list of options provided.

The client is most likely consuming more energy than she is expending; this creates a(n) ____1____ energy balance, causing her to ____2____ weight.

OPTIONS	
negative	gain
positive	lose
neutral	maintain

3. Use an X to identify effective and ineffective interventions to help the client lose weight.

INTERVENTION	EFFECTIVE	INEFFECTIVE
Reduce physical activity		
Increase nutrient-dense foods		
Reduce calorie-dense food		
Skip meals		
Build muscle mass through regular physical activity		
Create a positive energy balance		
Create a negative energy balance		

4. Using the client's weight (kg), height (cm), and age (years), find her energy needs using the Mifflin St. Jeor equation. Use a physical activity factor of 1.0 for sedentary individuals.
Women: $(10 \times W + 6.25 \times Ht - 5 \times A - 161) \times PA$

   a. 2610 kcals/day
   b. 1755 kcals/day
   c. 1459 kcals/day
   d. 2200 kcals/day
   e. 2000 kcals/day
   f. 1200 kcals/day

Additional Learning Resources

Please refer to this text's Evolve website for answers to the Case Study questions:
http://evolve.elsevier.com/Williams/basic/
References and **Further Reading and Resources** in the back of the book provide additional resources for enhancing knowledge.

Vitamins

Key Concepts

- Vitamins are noncaloric, essential nutrients that are necessary for many metabolic tasks.
- Certain health problems result from inadequate or excessive vitamin intake.
- Vitamins occur in a variety of foods, along with energy-yielding macronutrients.

- The body uses vitamins to make the coenzymes that are required for some enzymes to function.
- Whole foods such as fruits, vegetables, nuts, and grains are also a source of valuable phytonutrients.
- The need for particular vitamin supplements depends on a person's vitamin and health status.

This chapter answers some of the questions about vitamins: What do they do? How much of each vitamin does the human body need? From what foods do they come? Do we need to take dietary supplements? The scientific study of nutrition, on which experts rely upon to establish the Dietary Reference Intake (DRI) guidelines, continues to expand the body of nutrition knowledge. Thus, the answers to these questions have evolved through years of research and discovery.

This chapter looks at the vitamins both as a group and as individual nutrients. It explores general and specific vitamin needs as well as reasonable and realistic dietary supplement use.

THE NATURE OF VITAMINS

Scientists discovered most of the vitamins that we know about today during the early 1900s while searching for cures of classic diseases that they thought were associated with dietary deficiencies. At first, scientists assigned letters of the alphabet to each vitamin in the order of its discovery; however, they eventually abandoned this practice in favor of more specific names related to a vitamin's chemical structure or body function. We use the letter designation and contemporary name in this text.

DEFINITION

Upon the discovery of each vitamin, the following two defining characteristics emerged:

1. It must be a vital organic substance that is not a macronutrient (i.e., carbohydrate, fat, or protein), and it must be necessary to perform a specific metabolic function or to prevent a deficiency disease.
2. The body cannot manufacture it in sufficient quantities to sustain life, so the diet must provide it.

Because the body needs vitamins only in small amounts, we call them *micro*nutrients. The total volume of vitamins that a healthy person normally requires each day would barely fill a teaspoon. Thus, the units of measure for vitamins—milligrams or micrograms—are exceedingly small and difficult to visualize (see the For Further Focus box, "Small Measures for Small Needs"). Nonetheless, all vitamins are essential to human life.

For Further Focus

Small Measures for Small Needs

Early during the age of scientific development, scientists realized that they needed an internationally understood common language of measures to exchange rapidly emerging scientific knowledge. Thus, the metric system was born. French scientists established this system in the mid-1800s and named it *Le Système International d'Unités*, which we abbreviate as *SI units*. The use of these more precise units is now widespread, especially because it is mandatory for all purposes in most countries. The U.S. Congress passed the official Metric Conversion Act in 1975, but the United States has been slower to apply the metric system to common use as compared with other countries. However, the use of this system in scientific work is explicit worldwide.

Let us compare the two metric measures that we use for vitamins in the United States. Below are the Recommended Dietary Allowances (RDAs) equated with common measures to demonstrate just how small our needs really are.

- A *milligram* (mg) is equal to one thousandth of a gram (28 g = 1 oz; 1 g is equal to approximately ¼ tsp). We measure RDAs in milligrams for thiamin, riboflavin, niacin, pyridoxine, pantothenic acid, choline, and vitamins C and E.
- A *microgram* (mcg or μg) is equal to one millionth of a gram. We measure RDAs in micrograms for vitamins A (retinol equivalents), B_{12}, D, and K and for folate and biotin.

It is surprising that the total amount of vitamins that we need each day would scarcely fill a teaspoon; however, that small amount makes the difference between life and death over time.

FUNCTIONS OF VITAMINS

Although each vitamin has its specific metabolic tasks, general functions of vitamins include the following: (1) components of coenzymes; (2) antioxidants; (3) hormones that affect gene expression; (4) components of cell membranes; and (5) components of the light-sensitive rhodopsin molecule in the eyes (e.g., vitamin A).

Metabolism: Enzymes and Coenzymes

Enzymes act as catalysts, and vitamin-dependent coenzymes are an integral part of some enzymatic processes. Thus, without adequate vitamins these enzymes cannot catalyze their metabolic reactions. For example, several of the B vitamins (i.e., thiamin, niacin, and riboflavin) are part of coenzymes. These coenzymes are, in turn, integral parts of enzymes that metabolize glucose, fatty acids, and amino acids to release energy for cellular use.

Tissue Structure and Protection

Some vitamins are involved in tissue or bone building. For example, vitamin C is vital to the synthesis of collagen, which is a structural protein in the skin, ligaments, and bones. In fact, the word *collagen* comes from a Greek word meaning "glue." Collagen is like glue in its capacity to add tensile strength to body structures. Vitamins (e.g., A, C, and E) also act as antioxidants to protect cell structures and to prevent damage caused by free radicals.

Prevention of Deficiency Diseases

When a vitamin deficiency becomes severe, the function of that vitamin becomes apparent because the body can no longer perform that vitamin's specific function. For example, insufficient dietary vitamin C causes the classic vitamin deficiency disease scurvy. Scurvy is a hemorrhagic disease that is characterized by bleeding in the joints and other tissues and by the breakdown of fragile capillaries under normal blood pressure; these are all symptoms that are directly related to vitamin C's role in producing collagen. Collagen is what makes capillary walls strong. Untreated scurvy leads to internal membrane disintegration and death.

VITAMIN METABOLISM

The way in which our bodies digest, absorb, and transport vitamins depends on the vitamin's solubility. Vitamins are traditionally classified as either fat soluble (vitamins A, D, E, and K) or water soluble (vitamin C and all of the B vitamins). Refer to Figure 5.9 for the general absorptive sites of vitamins throughout the small intestines.

Fat-Soluble Vitamins

Intestinal cells absorb fat-soluble vitamins along with dietary fat as a micelle and then incorporate all fat-soluble nutrients into chylomicrons. From the intestinal cells, chylomicrons enter the lymphatic circulation and then the blood (see Chapter 3 for details on fat absorption).

The body's ability to store each vitamin, and the capacity of the liver and kidneys to clear it, determines its potential for toxicity. Unlike water-soluble vitamins, the liver and adipose tissue can store fat-soluble vitamins for long periods. This storage capacity is beneficial during times of inadequate dietary intake because the body can use this reserve to meet bodily needs. Conversely, fat-soluble vitamin accumulation in storage sites of the body is the reason that excess intake can result in toxicity over time.

Water-Soluble Vitamins

Intestinal cells easily absorb water-soluble vitamins. From these cells, the vitamins move directly into the portal blood circulation. Because blood is mostly water, the transport of water-soluble vitamins does not require the assistance of carrier proteins.

With the exception of cobalamin (vitamin B_{12}) and pyridoxine (vitamin B_6), the body does not store water-soluble vitamins to any significant extent. Therefore, the body relies on the frequent intake of foods that are rich in water-soluble vitamins.

DIETARY REFERENCE INTAKES

The DRIs are recommendations for nutrient intake by healthy population groups. Refer to Chapter 1 for details on the four categories that make up the DRIs. This chapter's discussion of vitamins and the following chapters that discuss minerals, fluids, and electrolytes refer to the various DRI recommendations (especially the RDAs) whenever possible.

This chapter consists of the following sections: (1) Fat-Soluble Vitamins; (2) Water-Soluble Vitamins; (3) Plant Nutrients; and (4) Nutrient Supplementation.

SECTION 1: FAT-SOLUBLE VITAMINS

The fat-soluble vitamins are vitamins A, D, E, and K.

VITAMIN A (RETINOL)

FUNCTIONS

Vitamin A plays a role in vision, growth, tissue strength, and immunity.

Vision

Scientists gave vitamin A the chemical name retinol because of its major task in the retina of the eye. The aldehyde form, retinal, is part of a light-sensitive pigment in retinal cells called *rhodopsin* (also known as *visual purple*). Rhodopsin enables the eye to adjust to different amounts of available light. Vitamin A–related compounds (i.e., the carotenoids lutein and zeaxanthin) are abundant in the macular pigment of the retina, where their antioxidant properties protect the macula.[1,2]

antioxidant a molecule that prevents the oxidation of cellular structures by free radicals.

catalysts substances that increase the rate at which a specific chemical reaction proceeds but are not consumed during the reaction.

scurvy a hemorrhagic disease caused by a lack of vitamin C that is characterized by diffuse tissue bleeding, painful limbs and joints, thickened bones, and skin discoloration from bleeding; bones fracture easily, wounds do not heal, gums swell and tend to bleed, and the teeth loosen.

retinol the chemical name of vitamin A; the name is derived from the vitamin's visual functions related to the retina of the eye, which is the back inner lining of the eyeball, which catches the light refractions of the lens to form images interpreted by the optic nerve and the brain and which makes the necessary light–dark adaptations.

carotenoids organic pigments that are found in plants; known to have functions such as scavenging free radicals, reducing the risk of certain types of cancer, and helping to prevent age-related eye diseases; more than 600 carotenoids have been identified, with β-carotene being the most well known.

Growth

Retinoic acid and retinol are involved in skeletal and soft-tissue growth through their roles in protein synthesis and the stabilization of cell membranes. The constant need to replace old cells in the bone matrix, the gastrointestinal tract, and other areas requires adequate vitamin A intake.

Tissue Strength and Immunity

The other retinoids (i.e., retinoic acid and retinol) help to maintain healthy epithelial tissue, which is the protective tissue covering all body surfaces (i.e., the skin and the inner mucous membranes in the nose, throat, eyes, gastrointestinal tract, and genitourinary tract). These tissues are the primary barrier to infection. Vitamin A is also important as an antioxidant and in the production of immune cells that are responsible for fighting bacterial, parasitic, and viral attacks.

REQUIREMENTS

Vitamin A requirements reflect its two basic forms found in food and stored in the body. The summary table for fat-soluble vitamins (see Table 7.5) and the DRI tables in Appendix B list the established RDAs for vitamin A.

Food Forms and Units of Measure

Dietary vitamin A occurs in two forms:

1. Preformed vitamin A or retinol: The active vitamin A found in food products of animal origin.
2. Provitamin A or β-**carotene**: A pigment in yellow, orange, and deep green fruits or vegetables that the human body can convert to retinol. Carotenoids are a family of compounds that are similar in structure; β-carotene and lutein are the most common in foods. Box 7.1 lists some of the known carotenoids.

In the typical American diet, a significant amount of vitamin A is in the *pro*vitamin A form (i.e., β-carotene). We convert quantities of carotenoids and preformed vitamin A to retinol equivalents to have a common system for measurement. The body can make 1 mcg of retinol from the following quantities of vitamin A food sources: 12 mcg of dietary β-carotene, 2 mcg of supplemental β-carotene, or 24 mcg of either α-carotene or β-cryptoxanthin. An older measure that is sometimes used to quantify vitamin A is the International Unit (IU). One IU of vitamin A equals 0.3 mcg of retinol or 0.6 mcg of β-carotene.

Body Storage

The liver can store large amounts of retinol. In healthy individuals, the liver stores approximately 80% of the body's total vitamin A. Thus, the liver is particularly susceptible to toxicity when a person supplements with excessive vitamin A. Tissues such as adipose tissue, the eyes, lungs, skin, spleen, and testes store the remaining vitamin A in the body.

DEFICIENCY

Dietary vitamin A deficiency is the leading cause of preventable blindness in children worldwide and a significant risk factor for mortality resulting from measles and diarrhea.[3] In 1991, 39% of children in low- and middle-income countries were deficient in vitamin A. The current rate of worldwide vitamin A deficiency is slightly lower, at a rate of 29%, subsequent to massive efforts of vitamin A supplementation.[4]

Dietary vitamin A inadequacy disrupts the continuous regeneration of rhodopsin, which the human eye needs for vision. If left untreated, conjunctival and corneal changes lead to a progressive series of ocular diseases, known collectively as **xerophthalmia,** beginning with night blindness, slow adaptation to darkness, glare blindness, and **Bitot's spots**. Persistent vitamin A deficiency will eventually progress to corneal xerosis, ulceration, and **keratomalacia** (Figure 7.1).

As with all nutrients, vitamin A's deficiency symptoms relate directly to its functions. Therefore, a lack of dietary vitamin A may also compromise growth, reproduction, immune systems, and the epithelial tissue.

Box 7.1 **Carotenoids**

Carotenes: orange pigments that contain no oxygen
- α-Carotene
- β-Carotene
- γ-Carotene
- δ-Carotene
- Lycopene

Xanthophylls: yellow pigments that contain some oxygen
- α- and β-Cryptoxanthin
- Lutein
- Lycophyll
- Neoxanthin
- Violaxanthin
- Zeaxanthin

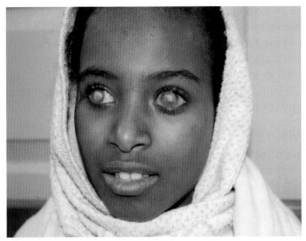

Figure 7.1 Corneal blindness from vitamin A deficiency. (Courtesy Lance Bellers. In Burton, M. J. [2009]. Prevention, treatment and rehabilitation. *Community Eye Health*, 22[71]:33–35.)

TOXICITY

Symptoms of *hypervitaminosis A* (excessive vitamin A intake) include bone pain, dry skin, fatigue, anorexia, and loss of hair. Vitamin A toxicity may cause liver injury with portal hypertension, which is elevated blood pressure in the portal vein, and ascites, which is fluid accumulation in the abdominal cavity. Because of the potential for toxicity, the DRI committee set the upper (intake) level (UL) of retinol for adults at 3000 mcg/day.[5] Toxicity symptoms usually result from the overconsumption of preformed vitamin A rather than of the carotenoids. Excessive vitamin A consumption during pregnancy is a known **teratogen**, which is the reason that acne treatment with medications containing high amounts of vitamin A (e.g., Accutane, Retin-A) is contraindicated during pregnancy.

The absorption of dietary carotenoids is dose dependent at high intake levels. However, the prolonged excessive intake of foods that are high in β-carotene causes a harmless orange tint to the skin. The orange tint disappears once the person discontinues the excessive intake. On the other hand, β-carotene supplements can reach concentrations in the body that promote oxidative damage, cell division, and the destruction of other forms of vitamin A.

---

carotene a group name for the red and yellow pigments (α-, β-, and γ-carotene) that are found in plant foods; β-carotene is most important to human nutrition because the body can convert it to vitamin A, thus making it a primary source of the vitamin.

xerophthalmia progressive ocular disease, frequently caused by vitamin A deficiency, beginning with severe dryness of the cornea and conjunctiva.

Bitot's spots white or gray conjunctival lesions developing on the cornea resulting from vitamin A deficiency.

keratomalacia drying and clouding of the cornea resulting from vitamin A deficiency.

teratogen a substance or factor resulting in birth defects or miscarriage of an embryo or fetus.

FOOD SOURCES AND STABILITY

Fish liver oils, liver, egg yolks, butter, and cream are sources of preformed natural vitamin A. Milk fat also contains preformed vitamin A. Because low-fat and fat-free dairy products do not contain milk fat, they also do not contain naturally occurring preformed vitamin A. However, food manufacturers of low-fat and fat-free milk fortify their products with vitamin A. Thus, all types of commercially prepared cow's milk are a good source of this vitamin. Some good sources of β-carotene are dark-green, leafy vegetables such as collard greens, kale, and spinach as well as dark-orange vegetables and fruits such as carrots, sweet potatoes or yams, pumpkins, melon, and apricots. Table 7.1 provides some comparative food sources of vitamin A.

β-Carotene and preformed vitamin A require emulsification by bile salts before they are absorbed into the intestine. Preformed vitamin A is efficiently absorbed at a rate of 75% to 100%. The absorption of β-carotene is significantly more variable with an absorption rate ranging from 3% to 65%.[6] The capriciousness of this range is attributable to factors such as dietary source, gastric content, nutrient status, drug-nutrient interactions, and genetic factors. Furthermore, even if the carotenoids are successfully absorbed, the body is only able to bioconvert roughly ½ of the carotenoids into

Table **7.1** Food Sources of Vitamin A		
ITEM	**QUANTITY**	**AMOUNT (MCG OF RETINOL EQUIVALENTS)**
Fruits and Vegetables		
Carrots, raw	½ cup	534
Collard greens, boiled	½ cup	361
Pumpkin, boiled	½ cup, mashed	353
Spinach, boiled	½ cup	472
Sweet potato, baked, in skin	1 medium (114 g)	1096
Meat, Poultry, Fish, Dry Beans, Eggs, and Nuts		
Beef liver, pan fried	3 oz	6582
Chicken liver, pan fried	3 oz	3652
Egg yolk, fresh, raw	2 large	130
Milk and Dairy Products		
Cream, heavy, whipping	½ cup	247
Milk, low-fat 1%, fortified	8 oz	142
Milk, skim, fortified	8 oz	149
Fats, Oils, and Sugars		
Fish oil, cod liver	1 Tbsp	4080

Data from the Nutrient Data Laboratory. (n.d.). *USDA Food Composition Databases*. U.S. Department of Agriculture, Agricultural Research Service. Retrieved January 24, 2019, from ndb.nal.usda.gov/ndb/.

active vitamin A. The body incorporates both forms into chylomicrons (along with fat) inside the intestinal cells. The chylomicrons then pass through the lymphatic system and into the bloodstream for circulation.

Heat and oxygen exposure reduce the stability of retinol. Quick cooking methods that use little water help to preserve vitamin A in food.

VITAMIN D (CALCIFEROL)

Vitamin D was mistakenly classified as a vitamin in 1922 by its discoverers when they cured rickets with fish oil, which is a natural source of vitamin D.[7] Today, we know that the compounds produced by animals (i.e., **cholecalciferol** or vitamin D_3) and the compounds produced by some organisms (i.e., **ergocalciferol** or vitamin D_2) are **prohormones** rather than true vitamins. Vitamins D_2 and D_3 are both physiologically relevant to human nutrition, and we collectively refer to them as *calciferol*.

Upon exposure to ultraviolet light, humans are able to convert the precursor 7-dehydrocholesterol, a compound that is in the epidermal layer of our skin, into cholecalciferol. Similarly, organisms such as invertebrates and fungi are capable of converting the precursor ergosterol into ergocalciferol after they receive ultraviolet irradiation.

The body must activate cholecalciferol and ergocalciferol in two successive hydroxylation reactions to yield the active and functional form of vitamin D, **calcitriol**. The first hydroxylation reaction occurs in the liver to produce calcidiol (also known as 25-hydroxycholecalciferol and 25-hydroxyvitamin D_3). The enzyme **1α-hydroxylase** then catalyzes the second hydroxylation reaction in the kidneys to produce calcitriol (also known as 1,25-dihydroxycholecalciferol and 1,25-dihydroxyvitamin D_3). Figure 7.2 illustrates the activation process of vitamin D in the body.

FUNCTIONS

The most commonly recognized functions of vitamin D are its role in bone mineralization and the homeostasis of calcium and phosphorus. However, vitamin D receptors are located on cells throughout the body. Other processes that vitamin D takes part in include immune function; neuromuscular function; and cell proliferation, differentiation, and apoptosis.

Calcium and Phosphorus Homeostasis

Maintaining calcium homeostasis in the blood is a critical function of vitamin D. Calcitriol acts physiologically with two other hormones—parathyroid hormone and the thyroid hormone calcitonin—to control calcium and phosphorus absorption and metabolism. Calcitriol stimulates the following: (1) the intestinal cell absorption of calcium and phosphorus; (2) the renal reabsorption of calcium and phosphorus; and (3) the osteoclastic **resorption** of calcium and phosphorus from trabecular bone. All of these mechanisms work together to maintain blood calcium and phosphorus homeostasis (see Figure 7.2).

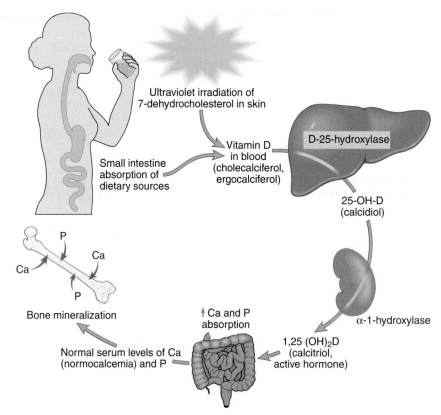

Figure 7.2 Vitamin D activation from skin synthesis and dietary sources. Normal vitamin D metabolism maintains blood calcium levels. (Modified from Kumar, V., Abbas, A., Fausto, N., & Mitchell, R. [2007]. *Robbins basic pathology* [8th ed.]. Philadelphia: Saunders.)

cholecalciferol the chemical name for vitamin D₃ in its inactive form; it is often shortened to *calciferol*.

ergocalciferol the chemical name for vitamin D₂ in its inactive form; it is produced by some organisms (not humans) upon ultraviolet irradiation from the precursor ergosterol.

prohormone a precursor substance that the body converts to a hormone; for example, a cholesterol compound in the skin is first irradiated by sunlight and then converted through successive enzyme actions in the liver and kidney into the active vitamin D hormone, which then regulates calcium absorption and bone development.

calcitriol the activated hormone form of vitamin D.

1α-hydroxylase the enzyme in the kidneys that catalyzes the hydroxylation reaction of 25-hydroxycholecalciferol (i.e., calcidiol) to calcitriol, which is the active form of vitamin D; 1α-hydroxylase activity is increased by parathyroid hormone when blood calcium levels are low.

resorption the destruction, loss, or dissolution of a tissue or a part of a tissue by biochemical activity (e.g., the loss of bone, the loss of tooth dentin).

Bone Mineralization

Osteoporosis involves a loss of bone density that leads to brittle bones and spontaneous fractures. Because calcitriol regulates the rate of calcium and phosphorus resorption from bone, doctors use it clinically to reduce the risk and progression of osteoporosis.[8]

REQUIREMENTS

Establishing requirements for vitamin D is difficult because the skin produces it and because the number of natural food sources is limited. Dietary vitamin D requirements vary according to individual exposure to sunlight, the latitude where people reside, and even the concentration of melanin in a person's skin.

In the northern hemisphere, particularly above approximately 40 degrees latitude, significantly less sunlight is present throughout the winter months. Because the amount of vitamin D produced in the skin is relative to the intensity of the sun exposure, there is less opportunity for endogenous vitamin D production during the winter at these latitudes. Similarly, melanin concentration in the skin affects individual variability of vitamin D production because melanin absorbs ultraviolet radiation in a way that is similar to that of sunscreen. Therefore, darker-skinned people synthesize less vitamin D than lighter-skinned people do even if they receive the same amount of sun exposure.

The current DRI for vitamin D is 600 IU/day for most adults (see Table 7.5 and Appendix B). However, national data show that adults in the United States only consume approximately 188 IU (4.7 mcg) of vitamin D from food and beverage daily.[9]

DEFICIENCY

A chronic calcitriol deficiency and/or low calcium intake during childhood causes **rickets**. Children with

rickets have soft long bones that bend under the child's weight (Figure 7.3). In addition to causing skeletal malformations, inadequate vitamin D intake prevents children from attaining their peak bone mass, thereby contributing to the development of osteoporosis or **osteomalacia** as adults. Many other chronic diseases have been associated with vitamin D deficiency, including muscle weakness, several types of cancer, coronary heart disease, hypertension, stroke, tuberculosis, obesity, type 2 diabetes, macular degeneration, neurologic disorders (e.g., Alzheimer and Parkinson disease), and several autoimmune diseases (e.g., type 1 diabetes, multiple sclerosis, rheumatoid arthritis).[10] However, it is still debatable whether vitamin D deficiency is a cause or result of such diseases, or if supplementation would alter the pathology of such diseases.[11]

There is not a universally accepted method for assessing vitamin D status nor an agreement on the vitamin D levels that constitute normal. The most recent publication by the Endocrine Society proposing global standards are as follows: (1) assess vitamin D status using 25-hydroxyvitamin D levels (>50 nmol/L = sufficiency, 30–50 nmol/L = insufficiency, and <30 nmol/L = vitamin D deficiency); (2) give infants 400 IU/d (10 mcg) of vitamin D from birth to 12 months of age, regardless of feeding method; and (3) all children and adults should meet their DRI for vitamin D through diet and/or supplementation (a minimum of 600 IU/d).[12] However, other data show that 600 IU/d of vitamin D is inadequate to keep the blood levels of 25-hydroxyvitamin D at the goal of more than 50 nmol/L and instead recommend 1040 IU (26 mcg) daily to meet the needs of 97.5% of the adult population.[13] As of the printing of this text, the DRI committee for

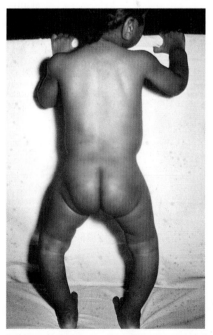

Figure 7.3 A child with rickets; note the bowlegs. (Reprinted from Kumar, V., Abbas, A., Fausto, N., & Mitchell, R. [2007]. *Robbins basic pathology* [8th ed.]. Philadelphia: Saunders.)

U.S. standard recommendations has not yet adopted these recommendations.

TOXICITY

Excessive dietary intake of vitamin D can be toxic, especially for infants and children. Symptoms of toxicity or hypervitaminosis D include fragile bones, kidney stones, and the calcification of the soft tissues (e.g., kidneys, heart, lungs). The prolonged intake of excessive cholecalciferol in dietary supplement form may produce elevated blood calcium concentrations (i.e., hypercalcemia) and calcium deposits in the kidney nephrons, which interfere with overall kidney function. The UL for vitamin D among people who are older than 9 years of age is 4000 IU/day (100 mcg).[14] The cutaneous production of vitamin D will not cause vitamin D toxicity. Most people will not exceed the UL of vitamin D through food intake alone. However, individuals who consume diets that are high in fatty fish and fortified milk in addition to taking dietary supplements that contain vitamin D may be at risk for toxicity.

FOOD SOURCES AND STABILITY

Fatty fish are one of the only good natural sources of vitamin D (Table 7.2). Therefore, a large portion of daily vitamin D intake comes from fortified foods. Because milk is a common food that also contains calcium and phosphorus, it is a practical food to fortify with vitamin D. The standard commercial practice is to add 400 IU per quart. Food manufacturers often fortify butter substitutes (e.g., margarine) and dairy

substitutes (e.g., soy or rice milk products) with vitamin D as well.

Vitamin D is relatively stable under most conditions that involve heat, aging, and storage.

VITAMIN E (TOCOPHEROL)

Early vitamin studies identified a nutrient that was necessary for animal reproduction.[15] This substance was named **tocopherol** from two Greek words: *tophos*, meaning "childbirth," and *phero*, meaning "to bring," with the *-ol* ending indicating its alcohol functional group. Scientists thought tocopherol was an antisterility vitamin. However, they soon realized that this effect was only present in rats and a few other animals and not in humans. Scientists have since discovered a number of related compounds. Tocopherol is the generic name for this entire group of homologous fat-soluble nutrients, which are designated as α-, β-, γ-, and δ-tocopherol or tocotrienol. Of these eight nutrients, α-tocopherol is the only one that is significant in human nutrition and thus used to calculate dietary needs.[16]

FUNCTIONS

The most vital function of α-tocopherol is its antioxidant action in tissues. In addition, vitamin E has other important roles such as immune function and cell signaling that drives gene expression. Scientists are still exploring the many metabolic pathways in which vitamin E is involved.[17]

Antioxidant Function

α-Tocopherol is the body's most abundant fat-soluble antioxidant. The polyunsaturated fatty acids (see Chapter 3) in the phospholipids of cell and organelle membranes are particularly susceptible to free radical oxidation. α-Tocopherol intercepts this oxidation process and protects the polyunsaturated fatty acids from damage.

Relation to Selenium Metabolism

Selenium is a trace mineral that, as part of the selenium-containing enzyme glutathione peroxidase, works with α-tocopherol as an antioxidant. Glutathione peroxidase is the second line of defense for preventing free radical

Table **7.2**	Food Sources of Vitamin D	
ITEM	**QUANTITY**	**AMOUNT (INTERNATIONAL UNITS)**
Meat, Poultry, Fish, Dry Beans, Eggs, and Nuts		
Salmon, sockeye, cooked	3 oz	570
Salmon, sockeye, canned, drained solids	3 oz	730
Tuna, light, canned in oil, drained solids	3 oz	229
Whitefish, mixed species, smoked	3 oz	435
Milk and Dairy Products		
Milk, low-fat 2%, fortified	1 cup (8 fl oz)	120
Soymilk, vitamin-D fortified	1 cup (8 fl oz)	119
Fats, Oils, and Sugars		
Fish oil, cod liver	1 Tbsp	1360

Data from the Nutrient Data Laboratory. (n.d.). *USDA Food Composition Databases*. U.S. Department of Agriculture, Agricultural Research Service. Retrieved January 24, 2019, from ndb.nal.usda.gov/ndb/.

rickets a disease of childhood that is characterized by the softening of the bones from an inadequate intake of vitamin D and insufficient exposure to sunlight; it is also associated with impaired calcium and phosphorus metabolism.

osteomalacia soft bones typically caused from a vitamin D or calcium deficiency.

tocopherol the chemical name for vitamin E, which was named by early investigators because their initial work with rats indicated a reproductive function; in people, vitamin E functions as a strong antioxidant that preserves structural tissues such as cell membranes.

damage to membranes. Glutathione peroxidase spares α-tocopherol from oxidation, thereby reducing the dietary requirement for α-tocopherol. Similarly, α-tocopherol spares glutathione peroxidase from oxidation, thus reducing the dietary requirement for selenium.

REQUIREMENTS

The summary table for fat-soluble vitamins (see Table 7.5) and the DRI tables in Appendix B list the requirements for α-tocopherol in milligrams per day.

DEFICIENCY

The fetus normally accrues α-tocopherol, along with body fat, during the final 1 to 2 months of gestation. Thus, premature infants who missed the period for fat and fat-soluble vitamin accumulation are particularly vulnerable to hemolytic anemia. Without adequate vitamin E for antioxidant protection, the red blood cell membrane phospholipids and proteins are susceptible to oxidation and destruction. Without supplemental vitamin E treatment, the continued loss of functioning red blood cells leads to hemolytic anemia.

A dietary deficiency of vitamin E is rare; the only cases occur in individuals who cannot absorb or metabolize fat. In such cases, the α-tocopherol deficiency disrupts the normal synthesis of myelin, which is the protective phospholipid-rich membrane that covers the nerve cells. The major nerves that are disturbed are the spinal cord fibers that affect physical activity and the retina of the eye, which affects vision.

TOXICITY

α-Tocopherol from food sources has no known toxic effects on people. Supplemental α-tocopherol intakes that exceed the UL of 1000 mg/day may interfere with vitamin K activity and blood clotting. Although the exact mechanism is unknown, this may be problematic for individuals who are deficient in vitamin K or for clients who are receiving anticoagulation therapy.[18]

FOOD SOURCES AND STABILITY

The richest sources of α-tocopherol are vegetable oils (e.g., wheat germ, soybean, safflower). Note that vegetable oils are also the richest sources of polyunsaturated fatty acids, which α-tocopherol protects. Other food sources of α-tocopherol include nuts, seeds, and fortified cereals. Table 7.3 provides a list of food sources of vitamin E.

α-Tocopherol is unstable to heat and alkalis.

VITAMIN K

In 1929 Henrik Dam, a biochemist at the University of Copenhagen, discovered a hemorrhagic disease in chicks that were eating a diet devoid of all lipids. Dam hypothesized that an unidentified lipid factor was missing in the chicks' feed. Dam called it *koagulations vitamin* or *vitamin K,* and we still use the assigned letter today.[19] Dam later succeeded in isolating the agent

Table 7.3	Food Sources of Vitamin E as α-Tocopherol	
ITEM	QUANTITY	AMOUNT (mg OF α-TOCOPHEROL)
Bread, Cereal, Rice, and Pasta		
Great Grains, Cranberry Almond Crunch, Post, ready-to-eat cereal	1 cup	3.6
Oatmeal Squares, Quaker, ready-to-eat cereal	1 cup	2.72
Fruits and Vegetables		
Apricots, dried	½ cup	2.81
Avocado, raw	½ cup	3.06
Spinach, cooked, boiled	½ cup	1.87
Turnip greens, cooked, boiled	½ cup	2.18
Nuts and Seeds		
Almonds, oil roasted	1 oz	7.36
Hazelnuts	1 oz	4.26
Sunflower seeds	1 oz	10.3
Fats, Oils, and Sugars		
Cottonseed oil	1 Tbsp	4.80
Safflower oil	1 Tbsp	4.64
Sunflower oil	1 Tbsp	5.59

Data from the Nutrient Data Laboratory. (n.d.). *USDA Food Composition Databases.* U.S. Department of Agriculture, Agricultural Research Service. Retrieved January 24, 2019, from ndb.nal.usda.gov/ndb/.

from alfalfa and identifying it, for which he received the Nobel Prize for physiology and medicine. As with many of the vitamins, several homologous forms of vitamin K make up the group. The major dietary form of vitamin K in plants is **phylloquinone**. Intestinal bacteria synthesize menaquinone, a secondary form of vitamin K. Menaquinone contributes approximately half of our daily supply of vitamin K. Menadione is a synthetic precursor of vitamin K, but the U.S. Food and Drug Administration banned it from dietary supplement use because of its toxic effects.

FUNCTIONS

Vitamin K has two well-established functions in the body: blood clotting and bone development.

Blood Clotting

The blood-clotting process is the earliest discovered and most well-known function of vitamin K. Vitamin K is essential for maintaining the normal blood concentrations of four blood-clotting factors. Prothrombin (i.e., clotting factor II) was the first identified and characterized of these vitamin–K-dependent blood factors. Prothrombin, which the liver synthesizes, converts to thrombin upon activation. Thrombin then initiates the conversion of fibrinogen to fibrin to form the blood clot (Figure 7.4).

phylloquinone a fat-soluble vitamin of the K group that is found primarily in green plants.

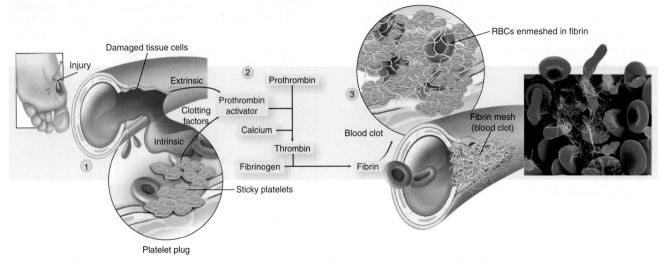

Figure 7.4 The blood-clotting mechanism. The complex clotting mechanism can be distilled into three steps: (1) the release of clotting factors from both injured tissue cells and sticky platelets at the injury site, which form a temporary platelet plug; (2) a series of chemical reactions that eventually result in the formation of thrombin; and (3) the formation of fibrin and the trapping of blood cells to form a clot. (Modified from Thibodeau, G. A., & Patton, K. T. [2012]. *Anatomy & physiology* [8th ed.]. St. Louis: Mosby.)

Phylloquinone is an antidote for the effects of excessive anticoagulant drug doses, and it may be used to control and prevent certain types of hemorrhages. Fat-soluble vitamins are more completely absorbed when bile is present. Thus, conditions that hinder the release of bile into the small intestine decrease the bioavailability of vitamin K and ultimately increase the length of time that is required for blood to form a clot. When a patient receives bile salts with vitamin K concentrate, the blood-clotting time returns to normal. See the Drug-Nutrient Interaction box entitled "Vitamin K Considerations With Anticoagulant and Antibiotic Medications" for additional information about special medication considerations related to vitamin K.

 Drug-Nutrient Interaction

Vitamin K Considerations With Anticoagulant and Antibiotic Medications

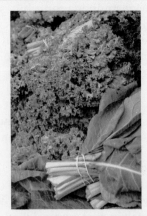

(Copyright iStock Photo; Credit: LindasPhotography.)

ANTICOAGULATION MEDICATIONS

Anticoagulation medications such as warfarin act to reduce the overall production of blood-clotting factors. Because the primary action of vitamin K is the manufacturing of these same blood-clotting proteins, the amount of vitamin K–rich foods that a person eats can affect the medication dose necessary for optimal coagulation control. Some individuals taking anticoagulation medications believe that they should completely avoid all foods that are rich in vitamin K. However, doing so would lead to an undesirable and unnecessary restriction of numerous nutrient-rich vegetables and the many vitamins and minerals found within these foods. Alternatively, clients should strive to eat a diet with a relatively consistent amount of vitamin-K–rich foods such as dark, leafy greens. A dietitian can educate clients about foods that are rich in vitamin K and help them to achieve a balance between their medication level and their desired vitamin K intake.

ANTIBIOTICS

Healthy bacteria in the gut synthesize one form of vitamin K, menaquinone. This source is significant for meeting overall vitamin K needs for most individuals. The long-term use of medications that destroy gastrointestinal bacteria, such as oral antibiotics, also eliminates this valuable source of vitamin K. Health care providers should advise clients to maintain their daily intake of food sources of vitamin K during and after treatment with antibiotics (see Table 7.4).

Bone Development

Several proteins involved in bone metabolism require vitamin K–dependent modifications to function. The most abundant noncollagenous protein in bone matrix, osteocalcin, is one of the vitamin K–dependent proteins. Vitamin K is involved in the modification of the glutamic acid residues of osteocalcin to form calcium-binding γ-carboxyglutamic acid residues. Like the blood-clotting proteins, osteocalcin binds calcium; unlike the blood-clotting proteins, it forms bone crystals.

REQUIREMENTS

Because intestinal bacteria synthesize menaquinone, a constant supply is normally available to support body needs. Currently not enough scientific evidence is available to establish an RDA; thus, AIs are the reference values instead. The summary table for fat-soluble vitamins (Table 7.5) and the DRI tables in Appendix B list the established AIs for vitamin K.

DEFICIENCY

Primary deficiency of vitamin K is not common. However, a deficiency (i.e., hypoprothrombinemia) may occur as a secondary result of another clinical condition. Individuals who have severe malabsorption disorders (e.g., Crohn's disease) or who receive chronic

Table 7.4 Food Sources of Vitamin K

VEGETABLES	QUANTITY	AMOUNT (mcg)
Beet greens, cooked, boiled	1 cup, chopped	697
Collard greens, cooked from frozen, drained	1 cup, chopped	1060
Mustard greens, cooked, drained	1 cup, chopped	830
Spinach, cooked, drained	1 cup, chopped	889
Swiss chard, cooked, drained	1 cup, chopped	573
Turnip greens, cooked from frozen, drained	1 cup, chopped	851

Data from the Nutrient Data Laboratory. (n.d.). *USDA Food Composition Databases.* U.S. Department of Agriculture, Agricultural Research Service. Retrieved January 24, 2019, from ndb.nal.usda.gov/ndb/.

Table 7.5 Summary of Fat-Soluble Vitamins

VITAMIN	FUNCTIONS	RECOMMENDED INTAKE (ADULTS)	DEFICIENCY	TOLERABLE UPPER INTAKE LEVEL (UL) AND TOXICITY	SOURCES
Vitamin A (retinol, retinal, and retinoic acid) Provitamin A (carotene)	Vision cycle: adaptation to light and dark; tissue growth, especially skin and mucous membranes; reproduction; immune function	Men, 900 mcg/d; women, 700 mcg/d	Night blindness; xerophthalmia; susceptibility to epithelial infection; impaired immunity, growth, and reproduction	UL: 3000 mcg/d Hair loss; skin irritation; bone pain, liver damage; birth defects	Retinol (animal foods): cod liver oil, liver, egg yolk, cream, butter, fortified dairy products Provitamin A (plant foods): dark green and deep orange vegetables (e.g., spinach, collard greens, pumpkin, sweet potatoes, carrots)
Vitamin D (cholecalciferol, ergocalciferol)	Maintain calcium and phosphorus homeostasis; calcification of bones and teeth; growth	Between the ages of 1 and 70 years, 600 IU/d; 70 years of age or older, 800 IU/day	Rickets and growth retardation in children; osteomalacia in adults	UL: 1000 to 4000 IU/d Calcification of soft tissue; kidney damage	Synthesized in the skin with exposure to sunlight, fortified milk products, fatty fish, fish oils
Vitamin E (α-tocopherol)	Antioxidant	Adults, 15 mg/day	Breakdown of red blood cells; anemia; nerve damage; retinopathy	UL: 1000 mg/d (from supplements) Inhibition of vitamin K activity in blood clotting	Vegetable oils, vegetable greens, wheat germ, nuts, seeds
Vitamin K (phylloquinone, menaquinone)	Normal blood clotting and bone development	Men, 120 mcg/d; women, 90 mcg/d	Bleeding tendencies; hemorrhagic disease; poor bone growth	UL: Not set Interference with anticoagulation drugs	Synthesis by intestinal bacteria, dark green leafy vegetables

treatment with antibiotics that kill intestinal bacteria are susceptible to vitamin K inadequacy.

Infants do not have adequate vitamin K stores at birth because vitamin K does not efficiently transfer through the placenta during gestation, and the intestinal tract of a newborn does not yet have vitamin K–producing gut flora. Consequently, infants routinely receive vitamin K injections at birth to prevent hemorrhaging.

TOXICITY

The DRI committee did not set a UL for vitamin K because toxicity is rare.

FOOD SOURCES AND STABILITY

Green, leafy vegetables such as spinach, collard greens, and kale are the best dietary sources of vitamin K, providing 100 to 1000 mcg of phylloquinone per cup of cooked food (Table 7.4).

Phylloquinone is fairly stable, although it is sensitive to light and irradiation. Therefore, manufacturers package clinical preparations in dark bottles.

Table 7.5 provides a summary of the fat-soluble vitamins.

SECTION 2: WATER-SOLUBLE VITAMINS

The water-soluble vitamins are vitamin C and all of the B vitamins.

VITAMIN C (ASCORBIC ACID)

FUNCTIONS

Vitamin C has several critical functions in the body. It acts as an antioxidant and as a cofactor of enzymes, and it plays a role in many metabolic and immunologic activities.

Connective Tissue

Ascorbic acid is necessary to build and maintain strong tissues through its involvement in collagen synthesis. Collagen is especially important in tissues of mesodermal origin, including connective tissues (e.g., ligaments, tendons, bone matrix, other binding lattices that hold together and give tensile strength to tissues) and other tissues that contain connective tissue (e.g., cartilage, tooth dentin, capillary walls).

Every time the amino acids proline or lysine are added during collagen synthesis, they are hydroxylated (i.e., OH is added) to form hydroxyproline and hydroxylysine by the ascorbic acid–dependent enzymes prolyl hydroxylase and lysyl hydroxylase, respectively. Iron is a cofactor for both enzymes, and ascorbic acid is required to maintain the iron atoms in these enzymes in their active ferrous (Fe^{2+}) form.

> **primary deficiency** deficiency of a nutrient resulting from inadequate dietary intake; different from secondary causes, in which the deficiency is due to malabsorption or other bioavailability hindrances.
>
> **ascorbic acid** the chemical name for vitamin C; the vitamin was named after its ability to cure scurvy.

Hydroxyproline and hydroxylysine form covalent bonds with other residues, which strengthen collagen's structure. When ascorbic acid is plentiful, collagen and the connective tissues in which it is integral quickly develop. Blood vessels are particularly dependent on ascorbic acid's role in collagen synthesis to help their walls resist stretching from the force of blood through them.

General Body Metabolism

The more metabolically active body tissues (e.g., adrenal glands, brain, kidney, liver, pancreas, thymus, spleen) contain the highest concentrations of ascorbic acid. When stimulated, the adrenal glands draw upon ascorbic acid. This use of ascorbic acid during adrenal stimulation suggests an increased need for ascorbic acid during stress. Other enzymes that require ascorbic acid perform very diverse functions, including the following: (1) the conversion of the neurotransmitter dopamine to the neurotransmitter norepinephrine; (2) the synthesis of carnitine, a mitochondrial fatty acid transporter that is involved in extracting energy from fatty acids; (3) the oxidation of phenylalanine and tyrosine; (4) the metabolism of tryptophan and folate; and (5) the maturation of some bioactive neural and endocrine peptides. Furthermore, ascorbic acid helps the body to absorb nonheme iron by keeping it in its bioactive reduced ferrous form (Fe^{2+}), thereby making it available for hemoglobin production and helping to prevent iron deficiency anemia.

Antioxidant Function

Similar to the function of vitamin E, ascorbic acid is an antioxidant that works to protect the body from damage caused by free radicals. Free radicals lead to oxidative stress, which is associated with increased risks of inflammatory diseases, Alzheimer's disease, cancer, and heart disease.

REQUIREMENTS

The summary table for water-soluble vitamins (see Table 7.13) and the DRI tables in Appendix B list the established requirements for vitamin C. Because cigarette smoke increases oxidative stress and free radicals in body tissues, the DRI committee recommends an additional 35 mg/day of vitamin C for smokers (see the Clinical Applications box, "Ascorbic Acid Needs in Smokers").

Clinical Applications

Ascorbic Acid Needs in Smokers

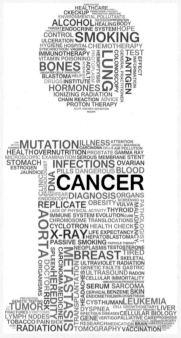

(Copyright iStock Photo; Credit:gguy44.)

Free radicals are reactive molecules that can disrupt the normal structure of DNA, proteins, carbohydrates, and fatty acids. Such damage increases the risk of cancer, cardiovascular disease, and a myriad of other health problems. Cigarette smoke is one environmental source of free radicals—for both the smoker and anyone inhaling secondhand smoke. Cigarette smoke causes deleterious effects to many major organ systems in the body.[1,2] The body fights free radicals with antioxidants such as vitamins A, E, and C and minerals such as selenium and zinc. Antioxidants help neutralize free radicals and work to protect the body on a cellular level.

As free radical production increases so does the need for antioxidants. Ascorbic acid is the specific antioxidant essential to the process of breaking down the toxic compounds found in cigarette smoke. Thus, cigarette smokers deplete their supply of ascorbic acid more rapidly than nonsmokers do. In addition to the general health recommendation of discontinuing the habit of smoking, it is recommended that cigarette smokers consume extra vitamin C to help fight the oxidative stress and cellular damage invoked by smoking.[3]

REFERENCES

1. Alberg, A. J., Shopland, D. R., & Cummings, K. M. (2014). The 2014 Surgeon General's Report: Commemorating the 50th anniversary of the 1964 report of the advisory committee to the U.S. surgeon general and updating the evidence on the health consequences of cigarette smoking. *American Journal of Epidemiology, 179*(4), 403–412.
2. Goel, R., et al. (2017). Variation in free radical yields from U.S. marketed cigarettes. *Chemical Research in Toxicology, 30*(4), 1038–1045.
3. Food and Nutrition Board and Institute of Medicine. (2000). *Dietary reference intakes for vitamin C, vitamin E, selenium, and carotenoids*. Washington, DC.

DEFICIENCY

Signs of ascorbic acid deficiency include tissue bleeding (e.g., easy bruising, pinpoint skin hemorrhages; Figure 7.5A), joint bleeding, susceptibility to bone fracture, poor wound healing, bleeding gums, and tooth loss (Figure 7.5B). Extreme deficiency results in the disease scurvy.

The name *ascorbic acid* comes from the Latin word *scorbutus*, meaning "scurvy," and the prefix *a-*, meaning "without"; thus, the term *ascorbic* means "without scurvy." In developed countries today, we do not see frank scurvy often, but we do see vitamin C deficiency in combination with other forms of overt malnutrition.

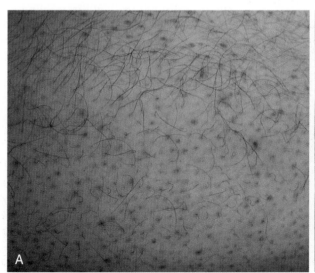
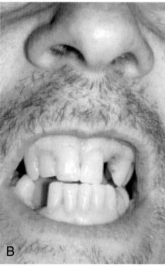

Figure 7.5 Scurvy observed on the skin and in the mouth. (A, From Al-Dabagh, A., et al. [2013]. A disease of the present: Scurvy in "well-nourished" patients. *J Am Acad Dermatol, 69*[5], e246–7. B, Courtesy Nicholas D. Magee, Royal Victoria Hospital. In Minerva. [2003]. *Br Med J, 326*[7379], 60.)

TOXICITY

The UL for ascorbic acid is 2000 mg/day. Although we can excrete most excessive intakes of water-soluble vitamins in the urine, the body clears levels of more than 2000 mg/day less efficiently. Excessive vitamin C may cause gastrointestinal disturbances (e.g., nausea, abdominal cramps) and osmotic diarrhea.

FOOD SOURCES AND STABILITY

The best food sources of ascorbic acid include citrus fruits, bell peppers, and kiwis. Additional good sources include berries, broccoli, tomato juice, and other green and yellow vegetables (Table 7.6).

Exposure to air and heat readily oxidizes ascorbic acid. Ascorbic acid is not stable in alkaline mediums; thus, adding baking soda to foods to preserve color destroys the ascorbic acid content. Acidic fruits and vegetables retain their ascorbic acid content better than nonacidic foods, and the vitamin is highly soluble in water. The more water added for cooking, the more ascorbic acid leaches out of the fruit or vegetable into the cooking water.

THIAMIN (VITAMIN B₁)

The name of the vitamin **thiamin** comes from the presence of the thiazole ring in its structure.

FUNCTIONS

Thiamin is a component of the coenzyme thiamin pyrophosphate, which is involved in several metabolic reactions that ultimately provide the body with energy in the form of adenosine triphosphate (ATP). Thiamin is especially necessary for the healthy function of systems that are in constant action and in need of energy, such as the gastrointestinal tract, the nervous system, and the cardiovascular system.

REQUIREMENTS

The dietary requirement for thiamin relates directly to its function in energy and carbohydrate metabolism. As the body's demand for ATP escalates, so does the use of, and necessity for, most of the B vitamins. Consequently, more thiamin intake is necessary during pregnancy, lactation, and other conditions or lifestyles that raise the total kilocalorie use above average. Diseases and conditions that accelerate glucose metabolism, such as fever, also increase the body's use of thiamin. The summary table for water-soluble vitamins (see Table 7.13) and the DRI tables in Appendix B list the established requirements for thiamin.

DEFICIENCY

Due to thiamin's involvement in the generation of ATP, a deficiency of the nutrient will have downstream effects on energy availability. The gastrointestinal tract relies on a steady supply of energy for muscular activity. Therefore, a lack of dietary thiamin may result in constipation, indigestion, and a poor appetite. The central nervous system also depends on constant energy. Without sufficient thiamin, alertness and reflexes decrease, and apathy, fatigue, and irritability may result. If the thiamin deficit continues, nerve irritation, pain, and prickly or numbing sensations may eventually progress to paralysis.

Beriberi is the chronic thiamin deficiency disease. This paralyzing disease was especially prevalent in countries that relied heavily on polished white rice as a food staple. The name describes the disease well; it is Singhalese for "I can't, I can't," because afflicted people are too ill to do much. In industrialized societies, thiamin deficiency is principally associated with chronic alcoholism and poor diet. Alcohol inhibits the intestinal absorption of thiamin. Alcohol-induced thiamin deficiency causes a debilitating brain disorder known as *Wernicke encephalopathy*, which affects mental alertness, short-term memory, and muscle coordination.

TOXICITY

The kidneys clear excess thiamin; therefore, there is no evidence of toxicity from oral intake, and no UL exists.

FOOD SOURCES AND STABILITY

Although thiamin is widespread in most plant and animal tissues, the amount is usually small. Thus, thiamin deficiency is a distinct possibility when food intake is markedly curtailed (e.g., with alcoholism or exceedingly inadequate diets). Good food sources of thiamin include yeast, pork, whole or **enriched** grains (e.g., flour, bread, cereals), and legumes (Table 7.7). Some raw fish contain a thiamin-degrading enzyme (i.e., thiaminase) and consequently are not good sources.

Table 7.6	Food Sources of Vitamin C	
ITEM	**QUANTITY**	**AMOUNT (mg)**
Vegetables		
Mustard spinach, raw	1 cup, chopped	195
Pepper, red, sweet, raw	½ cup, chopped	95
Pepper, yellow, sweet, raw	½ cup, chopped	137
Tomato, juice, canned	½ cup	85
Fruits		
Kiwi	½ cup, sliced	83
Lemon juice	8 fl oz	94
Orange juice	8 fl oz	124
Orange, navel	1 medium	83
Pineapple	1 cup pieces	93
Strawberries	1 cup	90

Data from the Nutrient Data Laboratory. (n.d.). *USDA Food Composition Databases*. U.S. Department of Argiculture, Agricultural Research Service. Retrieved January 24, 2019, from ndb.nal.usda.gov/ndb/.

Table 7.7   Food Sources of Thiamin

ITEM	QUANTITY	AMOUNT (mg)
Bread, Cereal, Rice, and Pasta		
Oat Blenders with honey and almond, Malt-O-Meal, ready-to-eat cereal	1 cup	0.84
Wheat Bran Flakes, Ralston, ready-to-eat cereal	1 cup	2.0
Whole Hearts oat cereal, Weet-abix, ready-to-eat cereal	1 cup	1.1
Meat, Poultry, Fish, Dry Beans, Eggs, Nuts, Seeds		
Beans, black, cooked	1 cup	0.42
Ham, sliced, regular (11% fat)	3 oz	0.53
Nuts, macadamia, raw	3 oz	1.0
Pork loin, lean, boneless, roasted	3 oz	0.48

Data from the Nutrient Data Laboratory. (n.d.). *USDA Food Composition Databases*. U.S. Department of Agriculture, Agricultural Research Service. Retrieved January 24, 2019, from ndb.nal.usda.gov/ndb/.

Neutral or alkaline environments destroy thiamin. As with other water-soluble vitamins, prepared foods retain more thiamin when we consume the cooking water along with the dish rather than discard it.

RIBOFLAVIN (VITAMIN B₂)

The name riboflavin comes from the vitamin's chemical nature. It is a yellow-green fluorescent pigment that contains ribose, which is a monosaccharide with five carbons.

FUNCTIONS

Riboflavin is active in its coenzyme forms: flavin adenine dinucleotide (FAD) and flavin mononucleotide (FMN). These two flavin coenzymes are required for macronutrient metabolism to produce ATP via the Krebs cycle and the electron transport chain (see Chapter 5). Flavoproteins are involved in a number of other metabolic reactions as well. Some examples of riboflavin-dependent reactions include converting the amino acid tryptophan to niacin (vitamin B₃), converting retinal to retinoic acid, and synthesizing the active form of folate.

REQUIREMENTS

Riboflavin needs relate specifically to total energy requirements for age, level of exercise, body size, metabolic rate, and rate of growth. As with thiamin, the expert committee set the RDA for riboflavin to correspond with the average energy use of each population group. Energy needs above the estimated average level means higher riboflavin needs as well. The summary table for water-soluble vitamins (see Table 7.13) and the DRI tables in Appendix B list the established requirements for riboflavin.

DEFICIENCY

Riboflavin deficiency particularly affects areas of the body with rapid cell regeneration. Symptoms include cracked lips and mouth corners; a swollen, red tongue; burning, itching, or tearing eyes caused by extra blood vessels in the cornea; and a scaly, greasy dermatitis in the skin folds. Riboflavin deficiency usually occurs in conjunction with other B vitamin and nutrient deficiencies (e.g., protein malnutrition) rather than alone. A rare riboflavin-specific deficiency has been given the general name *ariboflavinosis* (i.e., without riboflavin). Its symptoms are tissue inflammation and breakdown and poor wound healing; even minor injuries become easily aggravated and do not heal well.

TOXICITY

There have not been any reported adverse effects of riboflavin intake from food or supplements. Thus, there is no UL for riboflavin.

FOOD SOURCES AND STABILITY

One of the most frequently consumed natural food source of riboflavin is cow's milk. Each serving of milk contains about 0.5 mg of riboflavin. Other good sources include enriched grains, animal protein sources such as meats (especially beef liver), almonds, and soybeans. Table 7.8 provides a summary of riboflavin food sources.

Light destroys riboflavin; therefore, containers that prevent light penetration (e.g., opaque plastic or cardboard) will better preserve the vitamin in foods such as milk.

thiamin the chemical name of vitamin B₁; this vitamin was discovered in relation to the classic deficiency disease beriberi, and it is important in body metabolism as a coenzyme factor in many cell reactions related to energy metabolism.

beriberi a disease of the peripheral nerves that is caused by a deficiency of thiamin (vitamin B₁) and is characterized by pain (neuritis) and paralysis of legs and arms, cardiovascular changes, and edema.

enriched descriptive term for foods to which vitamins and minerals have been added back after a refining process that caused a loss of some nutrients; for example, iron may be lost during the refining process of a grain, so the final product will be enriched with additional iron.

riboflavin the chemical name for vitamin B₂; it has a role as a coenzyme factor in many cell reactions related to energy and protein metabolism.

niacin the chemical name for vitamin B₃; this vitamin was discovered in relation to the deficiency disease pellagra; it is important as a coenzyme factor in many cell reactions related to energy and protein metabolism.

Table 7.8 Food Sources of Riboflavin

ITEM	QUANTITY	AMOUNT (mg)
Bread, Cereal, Rice, and Pasta		
Corn Burst, Malt-O-Meal, ready-to-eat cereal	1 cup	0.85
Wheat Bran flakes, Ralston, ready-to-eat cereal	1 cup	3.1
Meat, Poultry, Fish, Dry Beans, Eggs, and Nuts		
Almonds, dry roasted	½ cup	0.83
Beef liver, braised	3 oz	2.9
Chicken liver, simmered	3 oz	1.7
Soybeans, raw	½ cup	0.81
Milk and Dairy Products		
Milk, skim or whole	8 fl oz	0.43
Soy milk	8 fl oz	0.5
Yogurt, plain, low fat	8 fl oz	0.53

Data from the Nutrient Data Laboratory. (n.d.). *USDA Food Composition Databases*. U.S. Department of Agriculture, Agricultural Research Service. Retrieved January 24, 2019, from ndb.nal.usda.gov/ndb/.

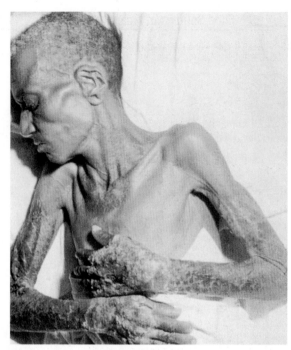

Figure 7.6 Pellagra, which results from a niacin deficiency. (Reprinted from McLaren, D. S. [1992]. *A colour atlas and text of diet-related disorders* [2nd ed.]. London: Mosby–Year Book.)

NIACIN (VITAMIN B₃)

FUNCTIONS

Niacin is part of two coenzymes. The role of one of the niacin-containing coenzymes (nicotinamide adenine dinucleotide, NAD) is the metabolism of the macronutrients. You should notice the theme among the B vitamin functions with regard to their role in macronutrient metabolism. The function of this niacin-containing coenzyme is similar to that of the coenzymes containing riboflavin and thiamin. The other niacin-containing coenzyme (nicotinamide adenine dinucleotide phosphate, NADP) is involved in DNA repair and steroid hormone synthesis.

REQUIREMENTS

Factors such as age, growth, pregnancy and lactation, illness, tissue trauma, body size, and physical activity—all of which affect energy needs—influence niacin requirements. Because the body can make some of its needed niacin from the essential amino acid tryptophan, the DRI committee states the total niacin requirements in terms of niacin equivalents (NEs) to account for both sources. Approximately 60 mg of tryptophan can yield 1 mg of niacin; thus, 60 mg of tryptophan equals 1 NE. The summary table for water-soluble vitamins (see Table 7.13) and the DRI tables in Appendix B list the established requirements for niacin.

DEFICIENCY

Symptoms of general niacin deficiency are weakness, poor appetite, indigestion, and various disorders of the skin and nervous system. Sunlight-exposed skin areas develop a dark, scaly dermatitis. Extended deficiency may result in central nervous system damage with resulting confusion, apathy, disorientation, and neuritis. The four Ds: *d*ermatitis, *d*iarrhea, *d*ementia, and *d*eath (Figure 7.6) characterize the niacin deficiency disease pellagra. When therapeutic doses of niacin are given, symptoms from pellagra improve. Pellagra was common in the United States and parts of Europe during the early 20th century in regions where corn (which is low in niacin) was the staple food. In the southern United States, more than 3 million cases of pellagra resulted in an estimated 100,000 deaths between 1900 and 1940.[20]

TOXICITY

Excessive niacin intake can produce adverse physical effects, unlike high intakes of thiamin and riboflavin. Although no evidence exists of adverse effects from consuming niacin that naturally occurs in food, evidence does exist for excessive niacin consumption and adverse effects from nonprescription vitamin supplements and niacin-containing prescription medications. The primary toxicity reaction is a reddened flush on the skin of the face, arms, and chest that is accompanied by burning, tingling, and itching. This reaction also occurs in many clients who therapeutically use niacin as a treatment for hypercholesterolemia (see the Clinical Applications box, "Niacin as a Treatment for High Cholesterol"). The UL is 35 mg/day.[21]

FOOD SOURCES AND STABILITY

Meat is a good source of niacin. Most dietary niacin in the United States comes from meat, poultry,

Clinical Applications

Niacin as a Treatment for High Cholesterol

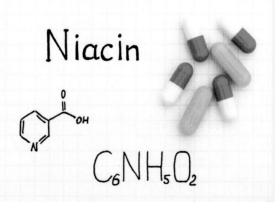

(Copyright iStock Photo; Credit:Ekaterina79.)

In addition to the many other important functions of niacin, high-dose niacin supplements can improve blood lipid profiles. Elevated blood levels of low-density lipoprotein (LDL) cholesterol and triglycerides increase the risk for cardiovascular disease. At doses of 1500 to 2000 mg/d, niacin decreases both LDL and triglyceride levels. In addition, pharmacologic doses of niacin improve high-density lipoprotein (HDL) cholesterol levels; this is the "good" cholesterol.[1] When health care providers use niacin in this way, it is functioning as a drug rather than as a vitamin. People should use niacin *only* as an adjunct therapy while under

medical supervision. Patients with cardiovascular disease that are undergoing treatment with statins, and whose LDL cholesterol is well controlled, do not benefit further from supplemental niacin; thus, guidelines do not recommend taking both.[1]

Appreciating the potential role of niacin at pharmacologic dosing requires an understanding of the possible side effects. The RDA for niacin in adult men and women is 16 mg/d and 14 mg/d, respectively. The UL for niacin is 35 mg/d.[2] Not surprisingly, a long-term dose of 2000 mg/d has substantial side effects. Adverse effects from pharmacologic dosing are the same as the toxicity effects: flushing of the skin, tingling sensation in the extremities, abdominal discomfort, nausea, peptic ulcer, and potential complications of hyperglycemia in individuals with diabetes. Some individuals may even experience liver damage if they continue supplementing unsupervised for months or years at a time. Physicians periodically check liver enzymes for clients on niacin supplementation or statin medications to monitor side effects of either medication.

REFERENCES

1. Jellinger, P. S., et al. (2017). American Association of Clinical Endocrinologists and American College of Endocrinology guidelines for management of dyslipidemia and prevention of cardiovascular disease. *Endocrine Practice, 23*(Suppl. 2), 1–87.
2. Food and Nutrition Board and Institute of Medicine. (1998). *Dietary reference intakes for thiamin, riboflavin, niacin, vitamin B6, folate, vitamin B12, pantothenic acid, biotin, and choline.* Washington, DC.

Table 7.9   Food Sources of Niacin

ITEM	QUANTITY	AMOUNT (mg OF NIACIN EQUIVALENTS)
Bread, Cereal, Rice, and Pasta		
Blueberry Mini Spooners, Malt-O-Meal, ready-to-eat cereal	1 cup	7.7
Cap'n Crunch's OOPS! All berries, Quaker, ready-to-eat cereal	1 cup	7.7
Crisp Rice, Ralston, ready-to-eat cereal	1 cup	9.6
Wheaties cereal, General Mills	1 cup	13.3
Meat, Poultry, Fish, Dry Beans, Eggs, and Nuts[a]		
Beef liver, braised	3 oz	14.9
Chicken, breast, boneless, roasted	3 oz	8.9
Chicken liver, pan-fried	3 oz	11.8
Fish, yellowtail, cooked, dry heat	3 oz	7.4
Peanuts, oil roasted	½ cup	11
Tuna, yellowfin, cooked, dry heat	3 oz	18.8

[a]The body can convert the amino acid tryptophan into niacin. Therefore, foods that are high in tryptophan also are significant sources of niacin.
Data from the Nutrient Data Laboratory. (n.d.). *USDA Food Composition Databases.* U.S. Department of Agriculture, Agricultural Research Service. Retrieved January 24, 2019, from ndb.nal.usda.gov/ndb/.

or fish (Table 7.9). Enriched and whole-grain breads, bread products, and ready-to-eat cereals have ample levels of niacin. Peanuts are another good source of niacin.

Niacin is stable in acidic mediums and in heat, but it is lost in cooking water unless the water is retained and consumed (e.g., in soup).

VITAMIN B₆

The name **pyridoxine** comes from the pyridine ring in the structure of this vitamin. The term *vitamin B₆* collectively refers to a group of six related compounds: pyridoxine, pyridoxal, pyridoxamine, and their respective activated phosphate forms. Two of the phosphorylated compounds are the coenzymes pyridoxal 5′-phosphate and pyridoxamine 5′-phosphate.

pellagra the deficiency disease caused by a lack of dietary niacin and an inadequate amount of protein that contains the amino acid tryptophan, which is a precursor of niacin; pellagra is characterized by skin lesions that are aggravated by sunlight as well as by gastrointestinal, mucosal, neurologic, and mental symptoms.

pyridoxine the chemical name of vitamin B₆; in its activated phosphate form (i.e., B_2PO_4), pyridoxine functions as an important coenzyme factor in many reactions in cell metabolism that are related to amino acids, glucose, and fatty acids.

FUNCTIONS

Pyridoxal 5'-phosphate, which is the metabolically active form of vitamin B_6, has an essential role in protein metabolism and in many cell reactions that involve amino acids. It is involved in neurotransmitter synthesis and, thus, in brain and central nervous system activity. Unlike most water-soluble vitamins, vitamin B_6 is stored in tissues throughout the body, particularly muscle. It participates in amino acid absorption, ATP production, the synthesis of the heme portion of hemoglobin, and niacin formation from tryptophan. Enzymes that make use of vitamin B_6 coenzymes are also involved in carbohydrate and fat metabolism.

REQUIREMENTS

Vitamin B_6 is involved in amino acid metabolism; therefore, needs vary directly in response to protein intake and utilization. The summary table for water-soluble vitamins (see Table 7.13) and the DRI tables in Appendix B list the established requirements for vitamin B_6.

DEFICIENCY

A vitamin B_6 deficiency is unlikely, because more of the vitamin is available in a typical diet than is required. A vitamin B_6 deficiency causes abnormal central nervous system function with hyperirritability, neuritis, and possible convulsions. Vitamin B_6 deficiency is one cause of microcytic hypochromic anemia, because it is required for heme synthesis (part of the red blood cell protein hemoglobin).

TOXICITY

High vitamin B_6 intake from food does not result in adverse effects, but large supplemental doses can cause uncoordinated movement and nerve damage. Symptoms improve upon discontinuation of the supplemental overdosing. Studies that linked vitamin B_6 to nerve damage led the DRI committee to set the UL for adults at 100 mg/day.[21]

FOOD SOURCES AND STABILITY

Vitamin B_6 is widespread in foods. Good sources include grains, enriched cereals, liver and kidney, and other meats (Table 7.10). Legumes contain limited amounts of vitamin B_6.

Vitamin B_6 is stable to heat but sensitive to light and alkalis.

FOLATE

Scientists first discovered folate in dark green, leafy vegetables; thus, earning the name *folate*, which originates from the Latin word *folium*, meaning "leaf." In nutrition, the term *folate* refers loosely to a large class of folic acid–derived molecules (i.e., pteroylglutamic acid) found in plants and animals. The most stable form of folate is folic acid, which is the form that manufacturers use in vitamin supplements and fortified food products. Foods rarely contain this form of folate (i.e.,

Table 7.10 Food Sources of Vitamin B_6 (Pyridoxine)

ITEM	QUANTITY	AMOUNT (mg)
Bread, Cereal, Rice, and Pasta		
All-Bran cereal, Kellogg's	½ cup	3.72
Complete Wheat Flakes cereal, Kellogg's	1 cup	2.67
Mueslix cereal, Kellogg's	⅔ cup	1.96
Total Whole Grain cereal, General Mills	1 cup	2.67
Fruits and Vegetables		
Banana	1 medium (118 g)	0.43
Potato, baked, with skin	1 medium (173 g)	0.54
Meat, Poultry, Fish, Dry Beans, Eggs, and Nuts		
Beef liver, fried	3 oz	0.87
Chicken, light meat, boneless, grilled	3 oz	0.98
Chickpeas (garbanzo beans), canned, solid and liquid	½ cup	0.57
Pistachios, raw	1 oz	0.48
Salmon, cooked, dry heat	3 oz	0.8
Tuna, yellowfin, cooked, dry heat	3 oz	0.88

Data from the Nutrient Data Laboratory. (n.d.). *USDA Food Composition Databases*. U.S. Department of Agriculture, Agricultural Research Service. Retrieved January 24, 2019, from ndb.nal.usda.gov/ndb/.

folic acid) naturally. We convert folate to, and use it as, the coenzyme tetrahydrofolic acid (TH_4) in the body.

FUNCTIONS

TH_4 participates in DNA synthesis (with the enzyme thymidylate synthetase) as well as cell division. TH_4 is involved in the synthesis of the amino acid glycine, which in turn is required for heme synthesis and thus hemoglobin synthesis.

TH_4 also participates in the reduction of blood homocysteine concentration and indirectly in gene expression (with the enzyme methionine synthase). **Hyperhomocysteinemia** is common in patients with cardiovascular disease. However, whether this contributes to or is merely an effect of cardiovascular disease is controversial because lowering homocysteine levels through folic acid supplementation does not subsequently alter the risk for cardiovascular events or all-cause mortality.[22]

REQUIREMENTS

We use dietary folate equivalencies (DFEs) to express the DRI for folate because the bioavailability of naturally occurring food folate differs from that of synthetic folic acid. One mcg of DFE equals 1 mcg of food folate, 0.5 mcg of folic acid taken on an empty stomach, or 0.6 mcg of folic acid taken with food. Because of the role of folate in cell division during embryogenesis, adequate preconception and pregnancy intakes reduce the occurrence of a neural tube defect. Thus, the DRIs include a special recommendation that all women who are capable of becoming pregnant take 400 mcg/day of synthetic folic acid from fortified foods or supplements in addition to natural folate found in a varied diet. The DRI recommendations (listed in the summary tables for water-soluble vitamins [see Table 7.13] and in Appendix B) are aimed at providing adequate safety allowances that include specific population groups that are at risk for deficiency, such as pregnant women, adolescents, and older adults.[21]

DEFICIENCY

Folate deficiency impairs DNA and RNA synthesis. Thus, a lack of dietary folate quickly affects rapidly dividing cells. When red blood cells cannot divide, the result is large and immature erythrocytes (i.e., megaloblastic macrocytic anemia). If left untreated, symptoms may progress to poor growth in children, weakness, depression, and neuropathy. Pregnant and lactating women are particularly susceptible to diminished blood folate concentrations and anemia because of their higher needs.

Neural tube defects (NTDs) such as **spina bifida** and **anencephaly** are some of the most common birth defects in the United States, occurring in approximately 7 in every 10,000 live births (Figure 7.7).[23] This defect occurs within the first 28 days after conception, often before a woman realizes that she is pregnant. Although the exact causes of NTDs are not known, adequate stores of folic acid before conception and during early gestation reduce the risk for NTD–affected pregnancies.[24,25]

TOXICITY

There are no known negative effects from the consumption of food sources of folate. However, some evidence shows that excessive folic acid can mask biochemical indicators of vitamin B_{12} deficiency. Prolonged B_{12} deficiency can result in permanent nerve damage; therefore, the DRI committee set the adult UL for supplemental folic acid at 1000 mcg/day.[21]

FOOD SOURCES AND STABILITY

Folate is widely distributed in foods (Table 7.11). Rich sources include green, leafy vegetables; orange juice; legumes; and chicken liver. Since January 1998, as part of an effort to reduce the occurrences of NTDs, the United States has required all manufacturers of certain grain products (e.g., enriched white

---

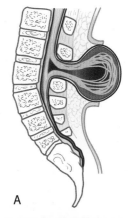

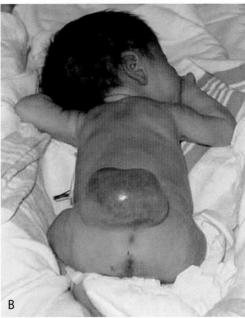

Figure 7.7 (A) Myelomeningocele. (B) Spina bifida in a child at birth with a cutaneous defect over the lumbar spine. (B, Courtesy Dr. Robert C. Dauser, Baylor College of Medicine, Houston, TX.)

---

flour; white rice; corn grits; cornmeal; noodles; fortified breakfast cereals, bread, rolls, and buns) to fortify with folic acid. The fortification of the general food supply has successfully reduced the prevalence of NTDs in the United States by approximately 28%. This translates to roughly an averted 1300 NTD-affected births annually because of folate fortification.[23] Although there are other non–folate-related causes for NTDs, supplemental folic acid does improve the folate status of women and improves pregnancy outcome.

The special DRI recommendation that women who are capable of becoming pregnant consume folic acid from supplements or fortified foods is one of only two current RDAs that specifically recommend consuming vitamin sources in addition to those available in a varied diet of natural foods.

Heat destroys folate. When submerging foods into cooking water, the folate easily leaches out into the water. Food processing, storage, and preparation can destroy as much as 50% to 90% of food folate.

---

hyperhomocysteinemia the presence of high levels of homocysteine in the blood; associated with cardiovascular disease.

spina bifida a congenital defect in the embryonic fetal closing of the neural tube to form a portion of the lower spine, which leaves the spine unclosed and the spinal cord open to various degrees of exposure and damage.

anencephaly the congenital absence of the brain that results from the incomplete closure of the upper end of the neural tube.

Table 7.11 Food Sources of Folate

ITEM	QUANTITY	AMOUNT (mcg OF DFE)
Bread, Cereal, Rice, and Pasta		
Grape-nuts, Post, ready-to-eat cereal	½ cup	200
Maple Brown Sugar LIFE Cereal, Quaker, ready-to-eat cereal	¾ cup	460
Toasted Multigrain Crisps, Quaker, ready-to-eat cereal	1 cup	420
Wheat Bran flakes, Ralston, ready-to-eat cereal	¾ cup	400
Fruits and Vegetables		
Asparagus, frozen, cooked	½ cup	122
Edamame, frozen, prepared	1 cup	482
Orange juice, fresh	1 cup, 8 oz	41
Spinach, cooked, boiled	½ cup	131
Meat, Poultry, Fish, Dry Beans, Eggs, and Nuts		
Chicken liver, simmered	3 oz	491
Garbanzo beans (chick-peas), cooked, boiled	½ cup	141
Lentils, cooked, boiled	½ cup	179
Turkey, liver, simmered	3 oz	587

Data from the Nutrient Data Laboratory. (n.d.). *USDA Food Composition Databases*. U.S. Department of Agriculture, Agricultural Research Service. Retrieved January 24, 2019, from ndb.nal.usda.gov/ndb/.

COBALAMIN (VITAMIN B$_{12}$)

Cobalamin earned its name from the single gray atom of the trace mineral cobalt at the center of its corrin ring. The term *vitamin B$_{12}$* originally referred to the synthetic pharmaceutical molecule cyanocobalamin. In nutrition, it has become a term for all cobalamin derivatives, including the two biologically active coenzyme derivatives methylcobalamin and deoxyadenosylcobalamin.

FUNCTIONS

Vitamin B$_{12}$ is essential for DNA synthesis and cell division. There are two cobalamin-dependent coenzymes with critical biologic activity.

Methylcobalamin is a coenzyme that is required for the catalytic activity of two of the same enzymes as tetrahydrofolic acid: methionine synthase and serine hydroxymethyltransferase. Thus, like tetrahydrofolic acid, methylcobalamin participates in the reduction of blood homocysteine concentration and indirectly in gene expression. Methylcobalamin is also involved in the production of the amino acid glycine, which in turn is required for heme synthesis and, therefore, hemoglobin synthesis.

Deoxyadenosylcobalamin is a coenzyme for the mitochondrial enzyme methylmalonyl-coenzyme A mutase, which is involved in the metabolism of fatty acids that have an odd number of carbon atoms.

REQUIREMENTS

The amount of dietary vitamin B$_{12}$ needed for normal human metabolism is small, consisting of only a few micrograms per day. A mixed diet that includes animal foods easily provides this much and more. The summary table for water-soluble vitamins (see Table 7.13) and the DRI tables in Appendix B list the established requirements for vitamin B$_{12}$. The DRIs include a special recommendation that both men and women who are 50 years old and older meet their RDA with vitamin B$_{12}$–fortified foods or supplements because of decreased absorption with age.[21]

DEFICIENCY

The vast majority of cobalamin deficiency cases are due to poor absorption from food as opposed to inadequate intake. A component of the gastric digestive secretions called *intrinsic factor* is necessary for the absorption of vitamin B$_{12}$ by intestinal cells (Figure 7.8). Gastrointestinal disorders that destroy the cells in the stomach (e.g., atrophic gastritis) disrupt the secretion of intrinsic factor and hydrochloric acid, both of which we need for vitamin B$_{12}$ absorption. Diseases affecting the small intestine such as Crohn's disease may prevent vitamin B$_{12}$ absorption in the ileum.

There are reported cases of primary vitamin B$_{12}$ deficiency from inadequate intake in vegans (see Chapter 4). Because foods made with animal products are the only natural sources of vitamin B$_{12}$, vegans must rely on dietary supplements or foods fortified with cobalamin to meet their dietary requirements. For example, fortified almond milk has approximately 3 mcg per 8

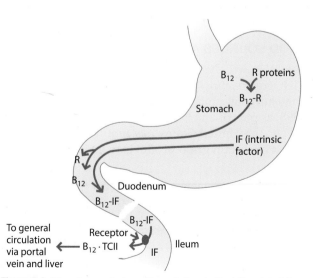

Figure 7.8 Digestion and absorption of vitamin B$_{12}$. (Reprinted from Mahan, L. K., & Escott-Stump, S. [2011]. *Krause's food & nutrition therapy* [13th ed.]. Philadelphia: Saunders.)

oz cup. A conscientious vegan choosing B_{12}-fortified vegan friendly foods should not have a problem with inadequate intake.

The general symptoms of vitamin B_{12} deficiency include nonspecific symptoms such as fatigue, anorexia, and nausea. In advanced cases, a multitude of conditions may develop, including hematologic (e.g., **pernicious anemia**), neurologic (e.g., peripheral neuropathy), and digestive (e.g., glossitis) manifestations. In such cases, the health care provider will most often administer the vitamin B_{12} via hypodermic injection to bypass the absorption defect.

TOXICITY

The DRI committee did not establish a UL for vitamin B_{12} because it does not appear to produce adverse effects in healthy individuals when intake from food or supplements exceeds bodily needs.

FOOD SOURCES AND STABILITY

Vitamin B_{12} is bound to protein in foods. All dietary vitamin B_{12} originates from bacteria that inhabit the gastrointestinal tracts of herbivorous animals. Thus, the only naturally occurring food sources are of animal origin or come from bacteria found on unwashed plants. Human intestinal bacteria also synthesize vitamin B_{12}, but it is not bioavailable. The richest dietary sources are beef liver, lean meat, clams, oysters, herring, and crab (Table 7.12).

Vitamin B_{12} is stable throughout ordinary cooking processes.

PANTOTHENIC ACID

The name **pantothenic acid** refers to this substance's widespread functions in the body and its widespread availability in foods of all types. The name comes from the Greek word *pantothen*, meaning "from every side." Pantothenic acid is present in all living things, and it is essential to all forms of life.

cobalamin the chemical name for vitamin B_{12}; this vitamin is found mainly in animal protein food sources; it is closely related to amino acid metabolism and the formation of the heme portion of hemoglobin; the absence of hydrochloric acid and intrinsic factor leads to pernicious anemia and degenerative effects on the nervous system.

pernicious anemia a form of megaloblastic anemia resulting from vitamin B_{12} deficiency. Frequently caused by destroyed gastric parietal cells that produce intrinsic factor; without intrinsic factor, vitamin B_{12} cannot be absorbed.

pantothenic acid a B-complex vitamin that is found widely distributed in nature and that occurs throughout the body tissues; it is an essential constituent of the body's main activating agent, coenzyme A.

FUNCTIONS

Pantothenic acid is part of coenzyme A (CoA), which is a carrier of acetyl moieties or larger acyl moieties. It is involved in cellular metabolism as well as protein acetylation and protein acylation.

Acetyl CoA is involved in energy extraction from the fuel molecules glucose, fatty acids, and amino acids. CoA also is involved in the biosynthesis of the following: (1) sphingolipids, which are found in neural tissue; (2) some amino acids; (3) isoprenoid derivatives (e.g., cholesterol, steroid hormones, vitamins A and D); (4) δ-aminolevulinic acid, which is the precursor of the porphyrin rings in hemoglobin, the cytochromes of the electron transport chain, and the corrin ring of vitamin B_{12}; (5) the neurotransmitter acetylcholine; and (6) melatonin, which is a sleep inducer that is derived from the neurotransmitter serotonin.

REQUIREMENTS

The usual intake range of pantothenic acid in the American diet is 4 to 7 mg/day. The summary table for water-soluble vitamins (Table 7.13) and the DRI tables in Appendix B list the AIs for pantothenic acid.

DEFICIENCY

Given its widespread natural occurrence, pantothenic acid deficiencies are unlikely. Individuals fed synthetic diets that contain virtually no pantothenic acid are the only known cases of deficiency.

TOXICITY

No observed adverse effects have been associated with pantothenic acid intake in people or animals. Therefore, the DRI committee has not established a UL for this vitamin.

FOOD SOURCES AND STABILITY

Pantothenic acid occurs as widely in foods as in body tissues. All animal and plant cells contain pantothenic acid, and it is especially abundant in animal tissues, whole-grain cereals, fortified cereals, and sunflower seeds. Milk, eggs, and some vegetables contain smaller amounts.

Pantothenic acid is stable to acid and heat, but it is sensitive to alkalis.

Table **7.12**	Food Sources of Vitamin B_{12} (Cobalamin)	
ITEM	**QUANTITY**	**AMOUNT (mcg)**
Meat, Poultry, Fish, Dry Beans, Eggs, and Nuts[a]		
Beef liver, pan-fried	3 oz	83
Clams, cooked, moist heat	3 oz	84
Mussels, cooked, moist heat	3 oz	20
Oysters, Pacific, cooked, moist heat	3 oz	25

[a]Food manufacturers fortify several vegan-friendly meat and dairy substitute products (e.g., soy milk, tofu) with vitamin B_{12}.
Data from the Nutrient Data Laboratory. (n.d.). *USDA Food Composition Databases*. U.S. Department of Agriculture, Agricultural Research Service. Retrieved January 24, 2019, from ndb.nal.usda.gov/ndb/.

Table 7.13   Summary of Vitamin C and the B-Complex Vitamins

VITAMIN	FUNCTIONS	RECOMMENDED INTAKE (ADULTS)	DEFICIENCY	TOLERABLE UPPER INTAKE LEVEL (UL) AND TOXICITY	SOURCES
Vitamin C (ascorbic acid)	Antioxidant; collagen synthesis; helps prepare iron for absorption and release to tissues for red blood cell formation; metabolism	Men, 90 mg; women, 75 mg; smokers: an additional 35 mg/d	Scurvy (deficiency disease); sore gums; hemorrhages, especially around bones and joints; anemia; tendency to bruise easily; impaired wound healing and tissue formation; weakened bones	UL: 2000 mg Diarrhea	Citrus fruits, kiwi, tomatoes, strawberries, peppers, pineapple
Thiamin (vitamin B_1)	Normal growth; coenzyme in carbohydrate metabolism; normal function of heart, nerves, and muscle	Men, 1.2 mg; women, 1.1 mg	Beriberi (deficiency disease); *gastrointestinal:* loss of appetite, gastric distress, deficient hydrochloric acid; *central nervous system:* fatigue, nerve damage, paralysis; *cardiovascular:* heart failure, edema of the legs	UL not set; toxicity unknown	Pork, whole grains, enriched cereals, legumes, yeast
Riboflavin (vitamin B_2)	Normal growth and energy; coenzyme in protein and energy metabolism	Men, 1.3 mg; women, 1.1 mg	Ariboflavinosis; wound aggravation; cracks at the corners of the mouth; a swollen red tongue; eye irritation; dermatitis	UL not set; toxicity unknown	Milk; meats, almonds, soybeans, enriched cereals
Niacin (vitamin B_3, nicotinamide, nicotinic acid)	Coenzyme in energy production; normal growth; skin health	Men, 16 mg of niacin equivalents; women: 14 mg of niacin equivalents	Pellagra (deficiency disease); weakness; loss of appetite; diarrhea; scaly dermatitis; neuritis; confusion	UL: 35 mg Skin flushing	Meat, poultry, fish, whole grains, enriched cereals
Vitamin B_6 (pyridoxine)	Coenzyme in amino acid metabolism: protein synthesis; heme formation; brain activity; carrier for amino acid absorption	Between the ages of 19 and 50 years, 1.3 mg; men 50 years of age or older, 1.7 mg; women 50 years of age or older, 1.5 mg	Anemia; hyperirritability; convulsions; neuritis	UL: 100 mg Nerve damage	Enriched cereals, legumes, meats, poultry, seafood
Folate (folic acid, folacin)	Coenzyme in DNA and RNA synthesis; amino acid metabolism; red blood cell maturation	400 mcg of dietary folate equivalents	Megaloblastic anemia (large immature red blood cells); poor growth; neural tube defects	UL: 1000 mcg Masks vitamin B_{12} deficiency	Fortified cereals, liver, asparagus, spinach, legumes, orange juice
Cobalamin (vitamin B_{12})	Coenzyme in synthesis of heme for hemoglobin; myelin sheath formation to protect nerves	2.4 mcg	Pernicious anemia; poor nerve function	UL not set; toxicity unknown	Liver; lean meats, seafood
Pantothenic acid	Formation of coenzyme A; fat, cholesterol, protein, and heme formation	Adequate intake, 5 mg	Unlikely because of widespread distribution in most foods	UL not set; toxicity unknown	Meats, eggs, milk, whole grains, enriched cereals, sunflower seeds, vegetables
Biotin	Coenzyme A partner; synthesis of fatty acids, amino acids, and purines	Adequate intake, 30 mcg	Natural deficiency unknown	UL not set; toxicity unknown	Liver, egg yolk, soy flour, nuts

BIOTIN

FUNCTIONS

Biotin is a coenzyme for five carboxylase enzymes. Carboxylase enzymes transfer carbon dioxide moieties from one molecule to another in the following biotin-dependent enzymes:

1. *α-Acetyl-CoA carboxylase:* Involved in fatty acid synthesis
2. *β-Acetyl-CoA carboxylase:* Involved in inhibiting fatty acid breakdown during the hours after starch, sucrose, or fructose is consumed
3. *Pyruvate carboxylase:* Involved in synthesizing glucose during fasting (gluconeogenesis) or during short bursts of energy (from lactic acid)
4. *Methylcrotonyl-CoA carboxylase:* Involved in the degradation of the amino acid leucine
5. *Propionyl-CoA carboxylase:* Involved in the breakdown of the three-carbon fatty acid propionic acid

REQUIREMENTS

The amount of biotin needed for metabolism is extremely small (i.e., measured in micrograms). The summary table for water-soluble vitamins (see Table 7.13) and the DRI tables in Appendix B list the AIs for biotin.

DEFICIENCY

There are no known natural biotin dietary deficiencies. A rare inborn error of metabolism called *biotinidase deficiency* can result in neurologic disturbances in untreated cases, but it is treatable with lifelong oral biotin supplementation.

Uncooked egg whites contain a protein called *avidin*. Avidin binds the micronutrient biotin. Consequently, consuming raw eggs inhibits biotin absorption.

TOXICITY

There are no known cases of toxicity or other adverse effects from the consumption of biotin by people or animals. No data currently support setting a UL for biotin.

FOOD SOURCES AND STABILITY

Biotin is widely distributed in natural foods, but it is not equally absorbed from all of them. For example, the biotin in corn and soy meal is completely bioavailable (i.e., able to be digested and absorbed by the body). However, almost none of the biotin in wheat is bioavailable. The best food sources of biotin are liver, cooked egg yolk, soy flour, cereals (except bound forms in wheat), meats, tomatoes, and yeast. The bacteria that normally inhabit the gut also synthesize biotin, which is available for intestinal cell absorption.

Biotin is a stable vitamin, but it is water soluble. Table 7.13 provides a summary of the water-soluble vitamins.

CHOLINE

Choline is a water-soluble nutrient that is associated with the B-complex vitamins. The Institute of Medicine established an AI of choline for the first time in the 1998 DRIs.[21]

FUNCTIONS

Choline is important for maintaining the structural integrity of cell membranes as a component of the phospholipid lecithin (i.e., phosphatidylcholine). Choline is also involved in lipid transport (i.e., lipoproteins), homocysteine reduction, and the neurotransmitter acetylcholine, which is involved in involuntary functions, voluntary movement, and long-term memory storage, among other things.

REQUIREMENTS

The DRI tables in Appendix B list the established AIs for choline.

DEFICIENCY

There are reported cases of fatty liver disease from choline deficiency in patients who are receiving long-term parenteral nutrition devoid of choline.[26] There remains speculation about a multitude of other potential adverse effects resulting from choline deficiency, such as birth defects, neural tube defects, neurologic disorders, and fatty liver disease.[27]

TOXICITY

Very high doses of supplemental choline have resulted in depressed blood pressure, fishy body odor, sweating, excessive salivation, and reduced growth rate. The UL for adults is 3.5 g/day.[21]

FOOD SOURCES AND STABILITY

A wide variety of foods naturally contains choline. Soybean products, eggs, liver, and other meat products are especially rich sources of choline.

Choline is a relatively stable nutrient. It is water soluble, as are all of the B-complex vitamins.

SECTION 3: PLANT NUTRIENTS

PHYTOCHEMICALS

In addition to the vitamins discussed so far in this chapter, there are other bioactive molecules found in plants called *phytochemicals* that have multifaceted health benefits. Phytochemicals are organic molecules. The term *phytochemical* comes from the Greek word *phyton,* meaning "plant." Scientists believe that fruits, vegetables, beans, nuts, and whole grains provide thousands of phytochemicals, many of which remain unidentified. People frequently use the terms phytochemical and *phytonutrient* interchangeably.

FUNCTION

Phytochemicals have a wide variety of functions, some of which include antioxidant and anti-inflammatory activity, hormonal actions, interactions with enzymes and DNA replication, and antibacterial effects. Diets that are high in phytochemicals from fruits and vegetables appear to protect against cardiovascular disease, cancer, obesity, and other chronic diseases.[28-31] The beneficial effects of phytochemicals are thought to result from the synergistic actions of multiple constituents as opposed to the actions of isolated compounds, which, in part, explains why taking a dietary supplement with only one of the known phytochemicals (e.g., carotene, lycopene) does not have the same advantageous effects as consuming many phytochemicals in whole food form.

RECOMMENDED INTAKE

There are no established DRIs for phytochemicals. Phytochemicals give fruits and vegetables their specific colors; thus, consuming a colorful variety of fruits, vegetables, whole grains, and nuts will provide a rich supply of phytochemicals. MyPlate guidelines recommend filling half of your plate with fruits and veggies each time you eat to consume 1.5 to 2 cups of fruit and 2 to 3 cups of vegetables daily.[32] They specifically recommend choosing a wide variety of vegetables and focusing on whole fruits to maximize nutrient density and quality (Figure 7.9). Unfortunately, only 12.2% of U.S. adults meet their fruit intake recommendations, and a mere 9.3% of adults meet their vegetable intake recommendations, on average.[33] Meanwhile, large-scale international meta-analysis studies show that people eating 7 to 10 servings of fruits and vegetables per day (the equivalent of 550–800 g/d) have the lowest risk

for all-cause mortality.[31] Considering how few Americans meet even the minimum recommendation for fruit and vegetable intake, it is safe to say that most of us could enhance our phytochemical profile, and improve our overall health, by increasing our fruit and veggie choices daily. See the Cultural Considerations box, "The American Diet," for more details.

FOOD SOURCES

Whole and unrefined foods such as vegetables, fruits, legumes, nuts, seeds, whole grains, and certain vegetable oils (e.g., olive oil) are rich sources of phytochemicals. Foods derived from animals and those that have been processed and refined are almost devoid of phytochemicals.

The following is a list of seven typical fruit and vegetable colors along with the phytochemical or phytochemical class that these plants usually contain. The specified phytochemical or phytochemical class is generally present in plant foods of other colors as well. However, color is one prominent indicator that a significant quantity of the identified phytochemical or phytochemical class is present in a food. Flavonoids are the exception that is worth noting. Although orange-yellow foods are a good source of flavonoids, other significant sources include purple grapes, black tea, olives, onions, celery, green tea, oregano, and whole wheat, none of which have an orange-yellow color.

- *Red* foods provide lycopene.
- *Yellow-green* foods provide zeaxanthin.
- *Red-purple* foods provide anthocyanin.
- *Orange* foods provide β-carotene.
- *Orange-yellow* foods provide flavonoids.
- *Green* foods provide glucosinolate.
- *White-green* foods provide allyl sulfides.

By consuming one fruit or vegetable from each of these seven color categories regularly, individuals get a variety of phytochemicals. Thousands of other phytochemicals are also widely distributed in fruits, vegetables, grains, soybeans, legumes, and nuts.

SECTION 4 NUTRIENT SUPPLEMENTATION

The Dietary Supplement Health and Education Act (DSHEA) of 1994 officially defined supplements as a product (other than tobacco) that has the following characteristics:

- It is intended to supplement the diet.
- It contains one or more dietary ingredients (including vitamins, minerals, herbs or other botanicals, amino acids, and other substances) or their constituents.
- It is intended to be taken by mouth as a pill, capsule, tablet, or liquid.
- It is labeled on the front panel as being a dietary supplement.

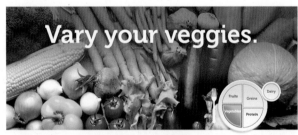

Find your healthy eating style. #MyPlateMyWins   ChooseMyPlate.gov

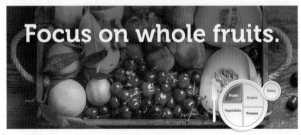

Find your healthy eating style. #MyPlateMyWins   ChooseMyPlate.gov

Figure 7.9 MyPlate recommendations for fruit and vegetable choices to reap the benefits of variety and whole food choices. (U.S. Department of Agriculture. [n.d.]. *What is MyPlate?* Retrieved January 5, 2019, from www.choosemyplate.gov/vary-your-veggies-0 and www.choosemyplate.gov/focus-fruits.)

The American Diet

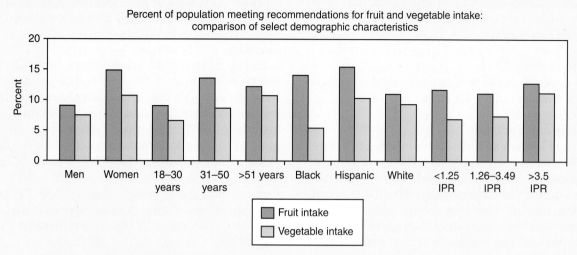

Percent of population meeting recommendations for fruit and vegetable intake: comparison of select demographic characteristics

IPR: Income to poverty ratio
Source: Lee-Kwan, S. H., et al. (2017). Disparities in state-specific adult fruit and vegetable consumption - United States, 2015. *MMWR Morb Mortal Wkly Rep, 66*(45), 1241–1247.

Individuals should be able to satisfy their vitamin, mineral, and phytochemical needs by consuming the recommended servings from each food group in accordance with the MyPlate guidelines. However, the typical "American diet" is far from what the MyPlate or *Dietary Guidelines for Americans* recommends. According to the Centers for Disease Control and Prevention (CDC), very few Americans consume the minimum servings of fruit and vegetable daily.[1] Although no group excels, there are some notable differences between select demographic characteristics in average fruit and vegetable intake.

How do you measure up? Can you say that your diet is better than the average American? What about your family and friends? Preventing nutrient deficiency is always preferable to disease treatment; hence, the old saying: "An apple a day keeps the doctor away."

The CDC provides recommendations for increasing access to, and intake of, fruits and vegetables in their 2018 State Indicator Report on Fruit and Vegetables.[2] See the www.cdc.gov website for more information on state-specific recommendations.

REFERENCES

1. Lee-Kwan, S. H., et al. (2017). Disparities in state-specific adult fruit and vegetable consumption - United States, 2015. *MMWR Morb Mortal Wkly Rep, 66*(45), 1241–1247.
2. Centers for Disease Control and Prevention. (2018). *State indicator report on fruits and vegetables*. Atlanta, GA: Centers for Disease Control and Prevention, U.S. Department of Health and Human Services.

The U.S. Food and Drug Administration regulates dietary supplements in the United States. The Office of Dietary Supplements (ods.od.nih.gov), which is housed within the National Institutes of Health, has the following mission: "to strengthen knowledge and understanding of dietary supplements by evaluating scientific information, stimulating and supporting research, disseminating research results, and educating the public to foster an enhanced quality of life and health for the U.S. population."[34]

The use of dietary supplements is common in the United States. About half of the population regularly take a dietary supplement.[35] The most commonly used supplement is the multivitamin or multimineral variety. It is the position of the Academy of Nutrition and Dietetics that micronutrient supplements are warranted only when individuals cannot meet their nutrient needs through diet alone.[36] Whole foods should provide adequate nutrients when people eat a healthy and varied diet in accordance with the MyPlate guidelines. However, because very few Americans currently eat in the ways that these guidelines recommend, inadequate nutrient consumption is possible.[33] Although dietary vitamin and mineral supplements may be beneficial for bridging this gap, it is also possible to exceed the UL for certain nutrients. Of interest is that the use of dietary supplements is most common among the healthiest people rather than among those who need supplementation the most.

RECOMMENDATIONS FOR NUTRIENT SUPPLEMENTATION

Health care professionals should be aware that people often fail to notify their health care providers about the use of dietary supplements. Drug-nutrient interactions are more common with dietary supplements than with whole foods; thus, it is important to ask clients specifically about their use of vitamin, mineral, macronutrient, or herbal supplements. Although dietary supplements may not be necessary for everyone, there are some instances in which supplemental forms of specific nutrients are recommended based on age, lifestyle, or disease state.

LIFE CYCLE NEEDS

Vitamin needs fluctuate with age and with situations that occur throughout the life cycle.

Pregnancy and Lactation

The DRI guidelines explicitly establish separate recommendations for women during pregnancy and lactation that take into account the increased nutrient demands that occur during this period. To reduce the risk of neural tube defects, the DRI committee recommends that pregnant women and women who are capable of becoming pregnant increase their intake of folic acid from fortified foods and/or dietary supplements in addition to the folate that is already present in their diets.[21] Women may find meeting the increased nutrient needs of pregnancy difficult by diet alone because of intolerances, food preferences, or other factors that can marginalize their diet. Supplements may then become a practical way of ensuring adequate intake to meet increased nutrient demands.

Infants, Children, and Adolescents

The American Academy of Pediatrics recommends that all breastfed infants receive 400 IU of supplemental vitamin D daily to help prevent rickets. Infants who are not breastfed, children, and adolescents who do not consume at least 1 quart/day of vitamin D–fortified milk or otherwise have an intake of 400 IU of vitamin D should also receive supplemental vitamin D daily.[12]

Older Adults

The aging process may increase the need for some vitamins because of decreased food intake and less efficient nutrient absorption, storage, and usage (see Chapter 12). The Institute of Medicine recommends that people who are 50 years of age or older take 2.4 mcg/day of vitamin B_{12} from fortified foods and/or dietary supplements.[21]

LIFESTYLE AND HEALTH STATUS

Personal lifestyle choices also influence individual needs for nutrient supplementation.

Restricted Diets

People who habitually follow fad diets may find meeting many of the nutrient intake standards difficult, particularly if their meals provide fewer than 1200 kcal/day. Very restrictive diets may cause multiple nutrient deficiencies. A wise weight-reduction program should meet all nutrient needs. As mentioned earlier, vegans need supplemental vitamin B_{12} in fortified foods or dietary supplements, because the only natural food sources of

this vitamin are of animal origin. Individuals following a vegan diet pattern should also ensure adequate intake of other key nutrients, such as calcium, vitamin D, and omega-3 fatty acids. If there is concern for dietary adequacy, a dietary supplement may be beneficial.[37]

Smoking

Smoking cigarettes adversely affects health in many ways, including reducing the body's vitamin C reserve. Research shows that smokers have significantly less serum vitamins C and E than nonsmokers.[38] The Institute of Medicine set the RDA of vitamin C at 35 mg/day higher for smokers to compensate for the oxidative stress that is induced by smoking.[16] The additional vitamin C does not necessarily need to come from a dietary supplement; however, if the person continues to smoke and does not consume additional vitamin C–rich foods, a dietary supplement may be advisable.

Alcohol

The chronic or abusive use of alcohol can interfere with the absorption of B-complex vitamins, especially thiamin, folate, and vitamin B_6. Multivitamin supplements that are rich in B vitamins may partially mitigate the effects. However, decreased alcohol use must accompany this nutrition therapy to rectify the alcohol-induced deficiency.

Disease

Evidence does not support the use of multivitamin and multimineral dietary supplements to prevent chronic disease. However, for individuals with certain diseases, dietary supplements may help combat particular nutrient deficiencies. In states of disease, malnutrition, malabsorption, debilitation, or hypermetabolic demand, each patient requires careful nutrition assessment. Nutrition support, including therapeutic supplementation as indicated, is part of the total medical treatment. A dietitian plans dietary and supplemental medical nutrition therapy to meet the client's clinical requirements.[36]

SUPPLEMENTATION PRINCIPLES

BASIC PRINCIPLES

The following basic principles may help to guide nutrient supplementation decisions:
- *Read the labels carefully.* The Nutrition Labeling and Education Act of 1990 standardized and defined label terminology on food products in an effort to ensure that health claims on food packaging are clear and truthful.
- *Vitamins, like drugs, can be harmful in large amounts.* The only time that larger vitamin doses may be helpful is when severe deficiency exists or when nutrient absorption or metabolism is inefficient. Individuals should consult a scientifically based supplement-savvy medical provider.

- *Professionally determined individual needs govern specific supplement usage.* Each person's need should be the basis for supplementing nutrients. This prevents excessive intake, and the expense of purchasing dietary supplements, which may have a cumulative effect over time.

- *All nutrients work together to promote good health.* Consuming large amounts of one vitamin may induce deficiencies of other vitamins or nutrients.

- *Food is the best source of nutrients.* Whole foods are the best "package deals" in nutrition. Foods provide wide varieties of nutrients in every bite as compared with the dozen or so provided by a dietary supplement. In addition, by itself, a vitamin can do nothing. It is catalytic, so it must have a substrate (i.e., carbohydrate, protein, fat, or their metabolites) on which to work. With the careful selection of a wide variety of foods and with good storage techniques, meal planning, and preparation techniques, most people can obtain ample amounts of essential nutrients from their diets.

- *Evaluate the information.* The Further Reading and Resources section at the back of this textbook provides a list of reliable organizations and resources related to dietary supplements.

MEGADOSES

At high pharmacologic concentrations, vitamins no longer operate strictly as nutritional agents. Nutrients and drugs can do the following: (1) participate in or improve physiologic conditions or illnesses; (2) prevent diseases; or (3) relieve symptoms. However, many people are unaware of the similarities between drugs and vitamins. Most people realize that too much of any drug can be harmful or even fatal and take care to avoid overdosing. However, too many people do not apply this same logic to nutrients and only realize the dangers of vitamin megadoses when they experience toxic side effects.

The liver can store large amounts of fat-soluble vitamins, especially vitamin A. Therefore, there is a great potential for toxicity from megadoses of fat-soluble vitamins, including liver, bone, and brain damage in extreme cases.[39-42] Megadoses of one vitamin can also produce toxic effects and lead to a secondary deficiency of another nutrient. In addition, hyperphysiologic levels of one vitamin may increase the need for other nutrients with which it works in the body, thereby effectively inducing a deficiency. Excess supplementation may alter the bioavailability of a vitamin that shares an absorptive site with another vitamin. By overloading these absorptive pathways, the nutrient in highest quantities may render the other vitamin unavailable for absorption.

Herbal products are also widely used as dietary supplements in the United States. Although the benefits and risks of herbal products are outside the scope of this textbook, there are references provided here that detail the danger for liver, heart, and kidney toxicity from specific herb and dietary supplements. Please see the list of references at the back of the textbook and note the five part series by AC Brown published between 2017 and 2018.[43-47]

FUNCTIONAL FOODS

The term *functional food* has no consistently recognized definition. Generally, "functional foods" include any foods or food ingredients that may provide a health benefit beyond its basic nutrient value. We also refer to such foods as *nutraceuticals* or *designer foods*. The position of the Academy of Nutrition and Dietetics is that such whole foods—having been fortified, enriched, or enhanced in some way—could be beneficial when regularly consumed as part of a varied diet.[48] The regulation of functional foods is complicated by the fact that the current governing body (the Food and Drug Administration) does not define or recognize functional foods. Box 7.2 gives examples of functional food categories.

Experts have not established recommendations for functional food intake because scientific evidence on which to base such recommendations is insufficient. However, over the past decade, there has been a focused research effort on determining the clinical efficacy of functional foods. If efficacy is clearly substantiated and reliable assessments for accurately quantifying active constituents in foods are in place, then expert committees will work to establish recommendations for intake. Until such recommendations are established, the daily intake of foods from all food groups—including functional foods—is the best way to meet macronutrient and micronutrient needs.

Box 7.2	Functional Food Categories and Selected Food Examples[a]

FUNCTIONAL FOOD CATEGORY	SELECTED FUNCTIONAL FOOD EXAMPLES
Conventional foods (whole foods)	Orange juice
Contain natural bioactive food compounds	Soy-based foods Yogurt
Modified foods	Calcium-fortified orange juice
Bioactive ingredients obtained by enrichment or fortification	Folate-enriched breads
Food ingredients that are synthesized	Indigestible carbohydrates

From Crowe, K. M., et al. (2013). Position of the Academy of Nutrition and Dietetics: Functional foods. *J Acad Nutr Diet, 113*(8), 1096–1103.
[a]Note: Medical foods and dietary supplements are not functional foods.

Putting It All Together

Summary

- Vitamins are organic, noncaloric food substances that are necessary in minute amounts for explicit metabolic tasks. A balanced diet usually supplies sufficient vitamins.
- The fat-soluble vitamins are A, D, E, and K. They mainly affect body structures (i.e., bones, rhodopsin, cell membrane phospholipids, and blood-clotting proteins).
- The water-soluble vitamins are vitamin C (ascorbic acid), the eight B-complex vitamins (i.e., thiamin, riboflavin, niacin, pyridoxine, folate, cobalamin, pantothenic acid, and biotin), and choline. Their major metabolic tasks relate to their roles in coenzyme factors, except for vitamin C, which is a biologic reducing agent that quenches free radicals and supports collagen synthesis.
- All water-soluble vitamins—especially vitamin C—are easily oxidized, so care must be taken to minimize the exposure of food surfaces to air or other oxidizers during storage and preparation. With few exceptions, all nutrients in foods are more bioavailable and beneficial to the body than nutrients in supplements.
- Whole and unrefined plant foods contain phytochemicals. A diet that is high in phytochemicals from a variety of sources is associated with a decreased risk for chronic disease.
- Vitamin supplementation is beneficial in some situations. Megadoses of water-soluble or fat-soluble vitamins can have detrimental effects.
- Functional foods are whole foods with added nutrients, such as vitamins, minerals, herbs, fiber, protein, or essential fatty acids that may have beneficial health effects.

Review Questions

See answers in Appendix A.

1. **Mary wants to increase her intake of foods rich in β-carotene. Which of the following foods would be the best source?**

   a. Whole-wheat bread
   b. Spinach
   c. Scrambled egg
   d. Wheat germ

2. **Based on the information provided, people who _____ would be more likely to experience a vitamin D deficiency.**

   a. have darker skin and live at higher latitudes
   b. have darker skin and live at lower latitudes
   c. have lighter skin and live at higher latitudes
   d. have lighter skin and live at lower latitudes

3. **The best food choice for a woman with a severe wound who needs adequate vitamin C to help promote healing would be _____.**

   a. stuffed green peppers
   b. whole-wheat toast with Swiss cheese
   c. a chocolate milkshake
   d. grilled chicken

4. **Dermatitis, diarrhea, dementia, and death characterize deficiency symptoms associated with _____.**

   a. beri-beri
   b. scurvy
   c. rickets
   d. pellagra

5. **Megaloblastic anemia is associated with _____ deficiency.**

   a. vitamin C
   b. selenium
   c. protein
   d. folate

Next-Generation NCLEX® Examination-style Case Study

See answers in Appendix A.

A 65-year-old female (Wt.: 155 lbs. Ht.: 5'10") has a history of deep vein thrombosis. She has felt unusually tired lately, so she came to the clinic. Her medical history reveals the following:

   She has had frequent nose bleeds for the last 2 weeks
   She is taking Warfarin (anticoagulant) as prescribed
   She had a urinary tract infection (3 weeks ago); client reported completing her antibiotics and feels better
   No change in weight since last visit
   Multiple bruises on arms and legs
   Client reports eating well with good appetite
   Client states that she tries to avoid as much vitamin K as possible to avoid interaction with Warfarin
   Blood pressure 122/83 mm/Hg

1. **From the list below, select all of the history and assessment findings that require follow-up.**

   a. She has had frequent nose bleeds for the last 3 weeks
   b. She is taking Warfarin as prescribed
   c. Weight has not changed since last visit (3 weeks ago)
   d. Multiple bruises appear on arms and legs
   e. Client is eating well and has good appetite
   f. Finished antibiotics for recent urinary tract infection (3 weeks ago)
   g. Client states that she tries to avoid as much vitamin K as possible to avoid interaction with Warfarin
   h. Blood pressure 122/83 mm/Hg

2. **Choose the *most likely* options for the information missing from the statements below by selecting from the list of options provided.**

   The client's anticoagulant medication ___1___ the function of vitamin K, which is to help ___2___ blood clots.

OPTION 1	OPTION 2
counteracts	prevent
enhances	form
facilitates	remove
provides	transfer

3. Choose the *most likely* options for the information missing from the statements below by selecting from the list of options provided.

The gut contains ____1____ that synthesize vitamin K. The client's recent use of antibiotics most likely ____2____ this source of vitamin K and may have ____3____ the function of Warfarin, causing the blood to be less viscous.

OPTION 1	OPTION 2	OPTION 3
tissue	eliminated	reduced
bacteria	created	enhanced
organs	transported	neutralized
villi	absorbed	inhibited

4. Place an X under "effective" to identify appropriate recommendations for this client. Place an X under "ineffective" to identify recommendations that would not be effective.

RECOMMENDATIONS	EFFECTIVE	INEFFECTIVE
Stop taking Warfarin		
Avoid taking antibiotics again in the future		
Consume consistent amounts of vitamin K daily		
Avoid as much vitamin K as possible		
Take vitamin and mineral supplements consistently		

5. From the list below, identify food sources of vitamin K to include in the client's daily meal plan.

a. Hamburger patty
b. Spinach
c. Collard Greens
d. Black beans
e. Kale
f. 1% fat cow's milk

6. Place an X under "effective" for all of the client's outcomes that indicate the intervention was effective. Place an X under "ineffective" for all outcomes that indicate the intervention was not effective.

OUTCOMES	EFFECTIVE	INEFFECTIVE
Client states that her blood clots a lot quicker		
She is not sure how much vitamin K she eats daily		
She continues to have bruising on arms and legs		
Her nose bleeds have discontinued		
She feels more energetic		
She can identify foods with vitamin K and includes them in her diet		

Additional Learning Resources

Please refer to this text's Evolve website for answers to the Case Study questions:
http://evolve.elsevier.com/Williams/basic/
References and **Further Reading and Resources** in the back of the book provide additional resources for enhancing knowledge.

8 Minerals

Key Concepts

- The human body requires a variety of minerals to perform its numerous metabolic tasks.
- A mixed diet of varied foods providing adequate energy intake is the best source of the minerals necessary for life.
- Of the total amount of minerals that a person consumes, only a relatively limited amount is bioavailable to the body.

Over the course of Earth's history, shifting oceans and plate tectonics have deposited minerals throughout its crust. These minerals move from rocks to soil to plants to animals and people. Not surprisingly, the mineral content of the human body is similar to that of the Earth's crust.

In nutrition, we focus on mineral elements: single atoms that are simple compared with vitamins, which are large, complex, organic compounds. Minerals perform a wide variety of metabolic tasks that are essential to human life. The amount of each mineral that we need ranges from relatively large for major minerals to exceedingly small for the trace minerals.

NATURE OF MINERALS IN HUMAN NUTRITION

Most living matter is composed of four elements: hydrogen, carbon, nitrogen, and oxygen, which are the building blocks of life. The minerals that are necessary to human nutrition are elements widely distributed in nature. Of the 118 elements on the periodic table, 25 are essential to human life. These 25 elements, in varying amounts, perform a variety of metabolic functions.

CLASSES OF MINERALS

Minerals occur in varying amounts in the body. For example, a relatively large amount (approximately 1.5%) of our total body weight is calcium, most of which is in the bones. A 150-lb adult has approximately 2.25 lb of calcium in the body. On the other hand, the total iron content of the human body is much smaller. The same adult weighing 150 lb has only approximately 0.11 oz of iron in his or her body. In both cases, the amount of each mineral is specific to its task.

The varying amounts of individual minerals in the body are the basis for classification into two main groups: major and trace minerals.

Major Minerals

The term *major* refers to the amount of a mineral in the body and not its relative importance to human nutrition. Major minerals have a recommended intake of more than 100 mg/day. The seven major minerals are calcium, phosphorus, sodium, potassium, magnesium, chloride, and sulfur. The food that we eat must provide all necessary minerals, because the body cannot manufacture any of them.

Trace Minerals

The remaining 18 elements make up the group of trace minerals. These minerals are no less important to human nutrition than the major minerals; however, smaller amounts of them are in the body. Trace minerals have a recommended intake of less than 100 mg/day. Box 8.1 provides a list of all of the minerals that are essential to human nutrition.

FUNCTIONS OF MINERALS

Minerals are involved in most of the body's metabolic processes. They are involved in building tissue as well as activating, regulating, transmitting, and controlling metabolism. For example, sodium and potassium are key players in water balance, calcium and phosphorus are required for osteoblasts to build bone, and iron is critical to the oxygen carrier hemoglobin. We cover the specific functions for each mineral within its respective section.

MINERAL METABOLISM

The point of intestinal absorption and the point of tissue uptake are usually the controlling factors in overall mineral metabolism.

Digestion

Minerals are absorbed and used in the body in their ionic forms, which means that they are carrying either a positive or a negative electrical charge. Unlike the macronutrients, minerals do not require a great deal of mechanical or chemical digestion before absorption occurs.

Box 8.1 Major Minerals and Trace Minerals in Human Nutrition

MAJOR MINERALS[a]	TRACE MINERALS
Calcium (Ca)	**Essential[b]**
Phosphorus (P)	Iron (Fe)
Sodium (Na)	Iodine (I)
Potassium (K)	Zinc (Zn)
Chloride (Cl)	Selenium (Se)
Magnesium (Mg)	Fluoride (F⁻)
Sulfur (S)	
Copper (Cu)	**Essentiality Unclear**
Manganese (Mn)	Silicon (Si)
Chromium (Cr)[c]	Tin (Sn)
Molybdenum (Mo)	Cadmium (Cd)
Cobalt (Co)	Arsenic (As)
Boron (B)	Aluminum (Al)
Vanadium (V)	
Nickel (Ni)	

[a]Required intake of more than 100 mg/day.
[b]Required intake of less than 100 mg/day.
[c]Essentiality is currently under review.

Absorption

The following general factors influence how much of a mineral is absorbed from the gastrointestinal tract.

- Food form: minerals from animal sources are usually more readily absorbed than those from plant sources
- Body need: more is absorbed if the body is deficient than if the body has sufficient quantities
- Tissue health: if disease disturbs the absorbing intestinal surface, its absorptive capacity is greatly diminished (e.g. celiac disease, bowel resection)

The absorptive method for each mineral depends on its physical properties. Some minerals require active transport for absorption, whereas others enter the intestinal cells by diffusion. Compounds found in foods may also affect the absorptive efficiency. For example, the presence of fiber, phytate, or oxalate—all of which are found in a variety of whole grains, fruits, and vegetables—can bind certain minerals in the gastrointestinal tract, thereby inhibiting or limiting their absorption.

Transport

Minerals enter the portal blood circulation and travel throughout the body bound to plasma proteins or mineral-specific transport proteins (e.g., iron is bound to the protein **transferrin** in circulation).

Tissue Uptake

Hormones control the uptake of some minerals into their target tissue. For example, **thyroid-stimulating hormone (TSH)** controls the uptake of iodine from the blood into the thyroid gland depending on the amount that the thyroid gland needs to make the hormone **thyroxine**. When the demand for thyroxine is elevated, TSH stimulates the thyroid gland to take up iodine and the kidneys to retain more iodine. When the thyroxine concentration is normal, the anterior pituitary gland releases less TSH, thereby resulting in less iodine uptake by the thyroid gland and more excretion of iodine into the urine by the kidneys.

Occurrence in the Body

There are several different forms of minerals found throughout the body tissues. The two basic forms in which minerals occur in the body are as free ions in body fluids (e.g., sodium in tissue fluids) and as covalently bound minerals that may bind with another mineral (e.g., calcium and phosphorus in **hydroxyapatite**) or with organic substances (e.g., iron that is bound to heme and globin to form the organic compound hemoglobin).

MAJOR MINERALS

CALCIUM

The intestinal absorption of dietary calcium depends on the food form and hormonal control. Calcium found in plant-based foods is sometimes bound to oxalate or phytate and thus not readily available. The interaction of the hormones vitamin D, parathyroid hormone, and calcitonin (from the thyroid gland) directly controls calcium's intestinal absorption and use, along with indirect control by the **estrogen hormones**.

Functions

Calcium has four key functions in the body.

Bone and tooth formation. The bones and teeth contain approximately 99% of the body's calcium. Removing hydroxyapatite from bone leaves a collagen matrix. If dietary calcium is insufficient during critical periods (e.g., the initial formation of the fetal skeleton, childhood growth, or the rapid growth of long bones during adolescence), then it could hinder the construction and density of healthy bones. Calcification of the teeth happens before they erupt from the gums; thus, insufficient dietary calcium later in life does not affect tooth structure as it does bone structure.

Blood clotting. Calcium is essential for the formation of fibrin, which is the protein matrix of a blood clot.

transferrin a protein that binds and transports iron through the blood.

thyroid-stimulating hormone (TSH) hormone released from the anterior pituitary gland that regulates the activity of the thyroid gland; also known as *thyrotropin*.

thyroxine (T$_4$) an iodine-dependent thyroid prohormone; the active hormone form is T$_3$; it is the major controller of basal metabolic rate.

hydroxyapatite (Ca$_{10}$[PO$_4$]$_6$[OH]$_2$) the major mineral component of normal bone and teeth; provides structure and rigidity to bone; primary storage site of calcium and phosphorus in the body.

estrogen hormones sex hormones produced primarily by the ovaries.

Muscle and nerve action. Calcium ions are required for muscle contraction and the release of neurotransmitters from neuron synapses.

Metabolic reactions. Calcium is necessary for many general metabolic functions in the body. Such functions include the intestinal absorption of vitamin B_{12}, the activation of the fat-splitting enzyme pancreatic lipase, and the secretion of insulin by the β cells of the pancreas. Calcium also interacts with the cell membrane proteins that govern the membrane's permeability to nutrients.

Requirements

A varied diet that provides enough calcium to meet the Dietary Reference Intake (DRI) should provide sufficient calcium nourishment for the body. The summary table for major minerals (see Table 8.3) and the DRI tables in Appendix B provide the DRIs for calcium.

Deficiency

Insufficient dietary calcium during the growth years increases the risk for various bone deformities. Rickets is one such bone disease caused by a chronic vitamin D deficiency and subsequent poor absorption of calcium. **Hypocalcemia** relative to blood phosphorus concentration results in muscle spasms and tetany. The most common calcium-related clinical issue today is **osteoporosis** (Figure 8.1). Historically, the medical community recognized osteoporotic bone fractures as a problem among postmenopausal women primarily. However, with the increase in life expectancy, osteoporotic bone fractures are progressively more common among elderly men as well.[1,2] In the United States, 16% of men and almost 30% of women over the age of 50 years meet the diagnostic criteria for osteoporosis, of which hip fractures are the most common complication (see the Cultural Considerations box, "Bone Health in Sex and Racial Groups").[3] With

---

🌐 Cultural Considerations

Bone Health in Sex and Racial Groups

Low bone mass is defined as a bone mineral density (BMD) of between 1 and 2.5 standard deviations below the mean of a matched reference group (see image below). Any of the following three criteria are diagnostic for osteoporosis in postmenopausal women and men over the age of 50: a BMD of ≥2.5 standard deviations below the mean of the reference group, a low trauma fracture, or a qualifying fracture risk assessment (FRAX) score.

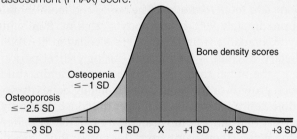

SD = Standard deviation
x = Population mean

Demonstration of what a standard deviation looks like on a normal bell curve.

Osteoporosis affects a significant number of older adults. Currently, 46% of men and 77% of women over the age of 80 years are living with osteoporosis in the United States.[1] An additional 47 million Americans are living with low bone mass, which is a significant risk factor for osteoporosis.[2]

Osteoporosis is often thought of as a "white woman's disease." Although it is true that women carry more than double the risk for osteoporosis, this debilitating bone disease is problematic for men and other racial groups as well. With regard to differences among racial groups, non-Hispanic black men and women have the highest BMD and therefore the lowest risk for osteoporosis compared with Hispanic, non-Hispanic white, and non-Hispanic Asian Americans.[2] Even though no racial group is free from osteoporosis, the exact reasons for these differences are unclear.

Many variables contribute to the development of either strong or fragile bones. Some variables include age, body weight, physical activity, hormonal influences, and dietary intakes of several vitamins and minerals (not just calcium) throughout life. Nutrition provides the materials needed for tissue deposition, maintenance, and repair. BMD and the collagen matrix formation determine overall bone strength. The structural protein collagen accounts for more than 20% of the dry weight of total bone mass and 90% of the organic bone matrix. Collagen degradation leads to osteoporosis. As such, the vitamins and minerals that are critical for a strong collagen and bone matrix also are integral to overall bone health. A balance of several nutrients is important for healthy bone building, including protein; calcium; phosphorus; copper; magnesium; manganese; potassium; zinc; and vitamins C, D, and K.

Osteoporosis is largely a preventable disease. It is also a costly disease. Coupled with the general trends of an aging population, this bone disease is a serious national concern. Because BMD reaches a peak mass by the average age of 30 years, the years prior are vital for establishing healthy bones. Maximizing peak bone mass ensures a greater reserve of bone mineral and collagen so that, as age-associated degradation ensues, effects are postponed or abated altogether. A healthy diet following the MyPlate guidelines should provide all of the essential nutrients to support the generation of strong bones.

For more information about osteoporosis, please see the National Institutes of Health website on Osteoporosis and Related Bone Diseases (search "osteoporosis" at www.niams.nih.gov).

See the National Osteoporosis Foundation for additional information on the FRAX score (search "FRAX score" at www.nof.org).

REFERENCES

1. Wright, N. C., et al. (2017). The impact of the new National Bone Health Alliance (NBHA) diagnostic criteria on the prevalence of osteoporosis in the USA. *Osteoporosis International, 28*(4), 1225–1232.
2. Looker, A. C., et al. (2017). Trends in osteoporosis and low bone mass in older US adults, 2005-2006 through 2013-2014. *Osteoporosis International, 28*(6), 1979–1988.

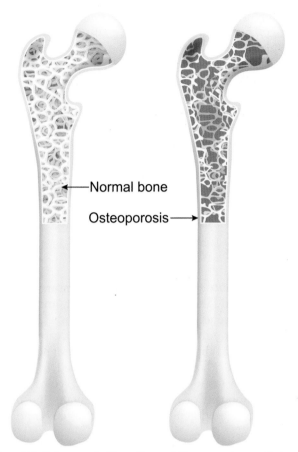

Normal bone

Osteoporosis

Figure 8.1 Osteoporosis. Normal bone *(left)* versus osteoporotic bone *(right)*. (Copyright iStock Photo.)

a global average cost exceeding $42,000 per fracture, the medical and societal burdens of osteoporotic hip fractures are a significant liability to the health care system worldwide.[4]

Osteoporosis is not a primary calcium deficiency disease as such; rather, it results from a combination of factors that create an overall loss of bone density. These factors include the following: (1) chronic calcium deficiency resulting from inadequate calcium intake or poor intestinal calcium absorption related to deviations in the amounts of hormones that control calcium absorption and metabolism; (2) inadequate weight-bearing physical activity, which stimulates muscle insertion into bones and significantly influences bone strength, shape, and mass; and (3) side effects of medications that cause bone loss over time. Although not all risk factors are easily modified (e.g., medications), some risk factors are effectively reduced with healthy lifestyle changes (e.g., a Mediterranean diet and regular physical activity).[5,6]

Bone is a dynamic tissue, with both new bone formation and bone resorption occurring constantly. This bone remodeling can affect up to 50% of total bone mass annually in young children and approximately 5% of bone mass in adults. Unfortunately, bone resorption often outpaces bone formation in postmenopausal women and in aging men. The dynamics involved in this process are multifactorial and not fully

understood. Increased calcium intake alone—whether from food sources or dietary supplement—does not prevent osteoporosis in susceptible adults or successfully treat diagnosed cases of osteoporosis. Therapies that reduce bone loss in osteoporosis include combinations of the various factors that are involved in the building of bones: adequate dietary calcium, the active hormonal form of vitamin D, estrogens, and weight-bearing physical activity. In addition, there are a variety of medications in use for the treatment and prevention of bone loss; however, the long-term compliance of such therapy is poor in the United States.[7,8]

The period of life during which bone density is reaching its peak is an especially important time to obtain adequate dietary calcium. However, food intake studies report that the average calcium intake of females from adolescence through adulthood is generally well below the DRIs. Teenage girls consume 857 mg/day of calcium on average, whereas the Recommended Daily Allowance (RDA) is 1300 mg/day.[9] Deficiencies during this critical period of bone development may have long-term negative outcomes with regard to overall bone strength and risk for osteoporosis.[10,11]

Toxicity

The toxicity of calcium from food sources is unlikely. However, a tolerable upper intake level (UL) for calcium has been set at 2000 to 3000 mg/day (depending on age) because of the negative effects of excessive calcium supplementation over time. **Hypercalcemia** is associated with the calcification of soft tissue and the decreased bioavailability of several essential nutrients (e.g., iron, magnesium, phosphorus, and zinc).

Food Sources

Milk and milk products are important dietary sources of readily available calcium. Milk that is used in cooking (e.g., in soups, sauces, or puddings) or in milk products such as yogurt, cheese, and ice cream is an excellent source of calcium. Calcium-fortified soy products, fruit juices, and other food products (e.g., cereals, cereal bars) are high in bioavailable calcium. In addition, several plants provide a natural source of calcium. Calcium in low-oxalate greens such as bok choy, collard greens, kale, and turnip greens is absorbed and can be an important source of calcium for vegetarians. Oxalic acid is a compound that is found in plants such as spinach, rhubarb, Swiss chard, beet greens, and certain other vegetables and nuts that forms an insoluble salt with calcium (calcium oxalate),

hypocalcemia a serum calcium level that is below normal.
osteoporosis an abnormal thinning of the bone that produces a porous, fragile, lattice-like bone tissue with enlarged spaces that are prone to fracture or deformity.
hypercalcemia a serum calcium level that is above normal.

thus interfering with the intestinal absorption of calcium. Phytate, which is another plant compound in grains such as wheat, can also bind with calcium and interfere with its intestinal absorption. Table 8.1 lists food sources of calcium.

In addition to food sources, calcium intake from supplements is widespread. Surveys show that 14% of adults in the United States take calcium supplements specifically, whereas 35% of the total population take a multivitamin and mineral supplement that contains calcium.[12] The bioavailability of supplemental calcium depends on the dose and the timing of meals relative to taking the supplement. Calcium is best absorbed in doses of 500 mg or less and when taken with food rather than on an empty stomach (see the For Further Focus box, "Calcium From Food or Supplements").

PHOSPHORUS

Functions

The phosphorus atom is most commonly bound to four oxygen atoms to form the phosphate molecule (PO_4^{3-}). Phosphorus functions in the following metabolic processes.

Bone and tooth formation. The calcification of bones and teeth depends on the deposition of hydroxyapatite by osteoblasts in bone's collagen matrix. The ratio of calcium to phosphorus in typical bone is approximately 1.5:1 by weight.

Energy metabolism. Phosphate is necessary for the controlled oxidation of carbohydrate, fat, and protein to release the energy in their covalent bonds (as a component of thiamin pyrophosphate), and it captures energy for use in the body as a component of adenosine triphosphate. Phosphate is also involved in protein construction (as a component of RNA), cell function (as a component of cell enzymes activated by phosphorylation), and genetic inheritance (as a component of DNA).

Acid-base balance. Phosphate is an important chemical buffer that helps maintain the pH homeostasis of body fluids.

Requirements

The typical American diet contains approximately 1350 mg of phosphorus daily, which meets the body's needs at all stages of life.[9] Refer to the DRI tables in Appendix B or the summary table for major minerals (see Table 8.3) for the DRIs of phosphorus.

Deficiency

Phosphate (the dietary form of phosphorus) is widely distributed in foods; thus, a deficiency is rare. The only evidence of deficiency has been among people who persistently consumed large amounts of antacids containing aluminum hydroxide.[13,14] The aluminum ion (Al^{3+}) binds with phosphate, thereby making the phosphate unavailable for intestinal absorption. **Hypophosphatemia**, characterized by weakness, loss of appetite, fatigue, and pain, results in bone loss over time.

Toxicity

Hyperphosphatemia from food intake is equally rare. However, if phosphorus intake is significantly higher than calcium intake for a long period, bone resorption may occur. The DRI guidelines list the UL for phosphorus at 4 g/day for people between the ages of 9 and 70 years.[15]

Table 8.1   Food Sources of Calcium

ITEM	QUANTITY	AMOUNT (mg)
Bread, Cereal, Rice, and Pasta		
Cream of Wheat cereal, prepared with water	1 cup	154
Multigrain bagel	1 bagel (81 g)	100
Tortilla, flour	1 (8 inch)	97
Vegetables[a]		
Beet greens, cooked	½ cup, chopped	82
Collards, cooked	½ cup, chopped	134
Rhubarb, cooked	½ cup, chopped	174
Fruits		
Orange juice, fortified with calcium	8 fl oz	350
Meat, Poultry, Fish, Dry Beans, Eggs, and Nuts		
Salmon, pink, canned, drained solids with bone	3 oz	241
Sardines, canned in oil, solids with bone	3 oz	325
Soybeans, green, raw	½ cup	252
Soybeans, green, boiled	½ cup	130
Tofu, raw, firm, prepared with calcium sulfate	½ cup	861
Milk and Dairy Products or Their Substitutes		
Cheese, parmesan, grated, reduced fat	1 oz	314
Milk, skim	8 fl oz	300
Soy milk, calcium fortified	8 fl oz	301
Tofu yogurt	8 fl oz	309
Yogurt, plain, skim milk	8 fl oz	452

[a]Low bioavailability.
Data from Agricultural Research Service. (2019). *USDA Food Composition Databases.* U.S. Department of Agriculture. Retrieved January 22, 2019, from ndb.nal.usda.gov.

For Further Focus

Calcium From Food or Supplements

Good health is not a simple matter, and our bodies are no simple machines. They require many nutrients to function properly, and the diet must provide these. One of the major minerals our bodies require is calcium. Data from the National Health and Nutrition Examination Study (NHANES) indicate that the average dietary intake of calcium by females falls well below the DRI. Unfortunately, this trend begins in the adolescent years. The graph below represents the average calcium intake for females by age group relative to their DRI. Note that at no point does the average calcium intake meet or exceed the established calcium needs.

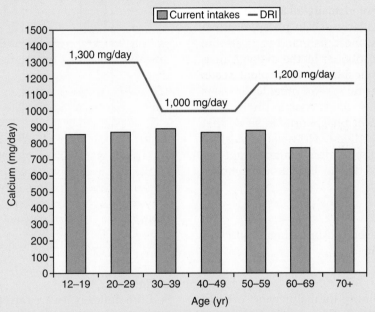

Data from Agricultural Research Service. (2018). Nutrient intakes from food and beverages: Mean amounts consumed per individual, by gender and age. In *What we eat in America* (NHANES 2015-2016). U.S. Department of Agriculture; and Food and Nutrition Board. (2011). *Dietary reference intakes for calcium and vitamin D*. Institute of Medicine. Washington, DC: National Academies Press.

Over the past decade, Americans' food choices have changed in ways that directly affect calcium-rich food consumption. For example, many Americans have replaced milk with soft drinks; they are eating out more often at restaurants (which typically contain less calcium than homemade meals); there is a trend for perpetual dieting (and dairy products are often one of the first foods to go); and there is a lack of risk acknowledgments regarding the importance of calcium-rich foods and health.

The best overall source of calcium is dairy products. The primary reason for this is that, unlike calcium supplements, calcium-rich foods supply the body with other beneficial nutrients as well, including protein; vitamins A, B_{12}, and D (if fortified); magnesium; potassium; riboflavin; niacin; and phosphorus. Some nondairy foods naturally contain calcium, including fish with bones (e.g., canned sardines), soybeans, collards, mustard greens, and rhubarb.[a] Most people find that meeting the DRI for calcium exclusively from nondairy foods can be challenging because the calcium concentration in nondairy foods is relatively low. For example, half a cup of chopped, cooked, collards has 134 mg of calcium, whereas 8 oz of skim milk contains 300 mg.[1] Furthermore, several vegetables contain phytates and oxalates that form insoluble complexes with calcium and thus decrease their bioavailability to the body. This makes the relative amount of calcium meaningfully less from vegetable sources.

The best way to improve one's overall diet is to consume a variety of foods that are high in calcium, preferably from dairy or fortified dairy substitute sources. However, calcium-fortified foods and supplements may be necessary for some people to meet their recommended intake of calcium. Calcium from supplements come in a variety of forms, including calcium carbonate, citrate, phosphate, lactate, and gluconate. The amount of calcium absorbed into the body from these sources varies considerably. Of the calcium supplements, calcium carbonate provides a bioavailable form of calcium that matches the bioavailability of calcium from milk.[2] Regardless of the source of your dietary calcium, take a moment to consider the overall value of your diet, and assess whether you should make improvements—particularly if you are still in the stage of life when bone density is accruing.

REFERENCES

1. Agricultural Research Service. (2019). *USDA Food Composition Databases*. U.S. Department of Agriculture. Retrieved January 15, 2019, from ndb.nal.usda.gov.
2. Greupner, T., Schneider, I., & Hahn, A. (2017). Calcium bioavailability from mineral waters with different mineralization in comparison to milk and a supplement. *Journal of the American College of Nutrition*, 36(5), 386–390.

[a]The bioavailability of calcium from some vegetables is very poor.

hypophosphatemia a serum phosphorus level that is below normal.
hyperphosphatemia a serum phosphorus level that is above normal.

Food Sources

Phosphorus is part of all living tissue found in animal and plant cells; therefore, phosphorus is sufficient in the natural food supply of virtually all animals. High-protein foods are particularly rich in phosphorus, so milk and milk products, meat, fish, and eggs are the primary sources of phosphorus in the average diet. The bioavailability of phosphorus from plant seeds (e.g., cereal grains, beans, nuts, peas, other legumes) is much lower, because these foods contain phytic acid, which is a storage form of phosphorus in seeds that humans cannot directly digest. However, a healthy flora of gut bacteria will provide a limited supply of phytase, the enzyme needed to liberate phosphorus from phytic acid.

SODIUM

Sodium is plentiful in the body. Approximately 0.2% of the adult body is sodium.

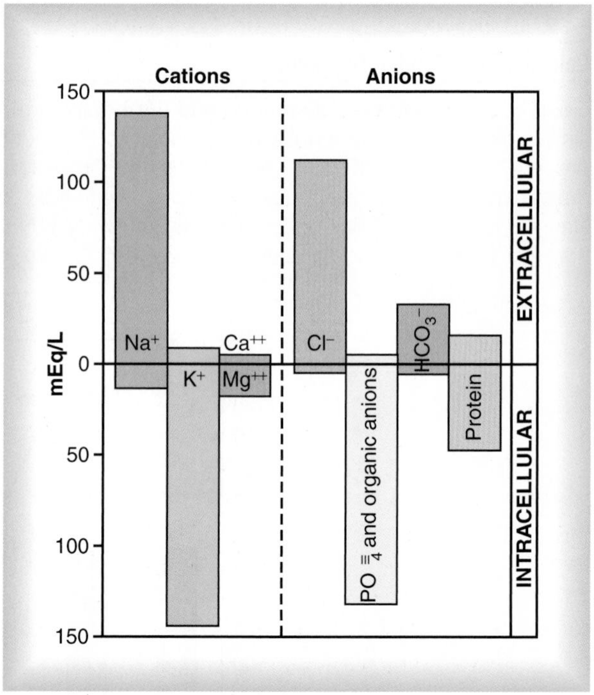

Figure 8.2 The ionic composition of the major body fluid compartments. (Reprinted from Guyton, A. C., & Hall, J. E. [2006]. *Textbook of medical physiology* [12th ed.]. Philadelphia: Saunders.)

Functions

The main function of sodium is the maintenance of body water balance (see Chapter 9). Sodium also has important tasks in muscle action and nutrient absorption.

Water balance. Ionized sodium concentration is the major influence on the volume of extracellular water (Figure 8.2). Variations in sodium concentration largely control the movement of water across biologic membranes by osmosis. Sodium is also an integral part of the digestive juices that are secreted into the gastrointestinal tract, most of which are reabsorbed by the intestinal cells.

Muscle action. Sodium and potassium ions are necessary for the normal response of stimulated neurons, the transmission of nerve impulses to muscles, and the contraction of muscle fibers.

Nutrient absorption. Sodium-dependent glucose transporters, which are a vital part of intestinal cells, allow for the passage of glucose and galactose from the intestinal lumen into the intestinal cells.

Requirements

The body is able to function on various amounts of dietary sodium through mechanisms designed to conserve or excrete the mineral as needed. Individual sodium needs vary greatly depending on growth stage, sweat loss, and medical conditions (e.g., diarrhea, vomiting). The summary table for major minerals (see Table 8.3) and the DRI tables in Appendix B provide the DRIs for sodium.

Deficiency

Sodium deficiencies are rare, because the body's need is low, and individual intake in the United States is typically high. An exception is during heavy sweating, such as by those who are engaged in heavy labor or strenuous physical exercise in a hot environment for an extended period (e.g., more than 2 hours). Commercial sports drinks, which replace sodium, glucose, and fluid, are useful to restore losses during such activities. Although sweat is relatively low in sodium, drinking too much plain water during lengthy strenuous exercise can further dilute blood sodium concentration and exacerbate **hyponatremia** complications. Hyponatremia can result in acid-base imbalances, muscle cramping, and worse, if left untreated.

Toxicity

The sodium content of the average American diet, which contains a high amount of processed foods, usually far exceeds the recommended intake range. Women consume an average of 3 g/day of sodium, and men consume an average of 4.1 g/day (approximately 2 to 3 times the recommended amount).[9] Excessive dietary sodium increases the blood pressure in salt-sensitive individuals, which is approximately 50% of people with hypertension.[16-18] However, for most people with healthy kidneys and adequate water intake, the kidneys excrete excess sodium in the urine. The acute excessive intake of sodium chloride (i.e., table salt) causes the accumulation of sodium in the blood (i.e., **hypernatremia**) and extracellular spaces. This sodium pulls water out of cells into the extracellular space by osmosis, thereby causing edema. Nevertheless, the DRI committee recently concluded that there is insufficient evidence at this time to establish a UL for sodium.[19]

Food Sources

Common table salt used in cooking, seasoning, preserving, and processing foods is the main dietary source of sodium. Sodium also occurs naturally in foods, and it is generally most prevalent in foods of animal origin. Natural food sources provide enough sodium to meet the body's needs. When people regularly consume food from manufacturers that add salt and other sodium compounds to processed foods as a preservative, sodium intake dramatically increases. For example, cured ham has approximately 30 times more sodium than raw pork. Natural, unprocessed food sources of sodium include animal products, such as milk, meat, and eggs, and vegetables, such as carrots, beets, leafy greens, and celery (see Appendix C for the sodium and potassium content of foods).

POTASSIUM

The adult body is approximately 0.4% potassium, which is approximately twice the amount of sodium.

Functions

Potassium is involved with sodium in the maintenance of the body water balance, and it has many other metabolic functions.

Water balance. Potassium is the major intracellular electrolyte. Its osmotic effect holds water inside the cells and counterbalances the osmotic effect of sodium, which draws water out of the cells and into the extracellular fluid compartments (see Figure 8.2).

Metabolic reactions. Potassium plays a role in energy production, the conversion of blood glucose into stored glycogen, and the synthesis of muscle protein.

Muscle action. Potassium ions also play a role in nerve impulse transmission to stimulate muscle action. Along with magnesium and sodium, potassium acts as a muscle relaxant that opposes the muscle contraction effect of calcium. The heart muscle is sensitive to potassium levels; therefore, there are systems in place to regulate blood potassium concentrations tightly.

Insulin release. Potassium is necessary for the release of insulin from pancreatic β cells in response to rising blood glucose concentrations.

Blood pressure. Sodium is one of the main dietary factors associated with hypertension. However, the sodium and potassium molar ratio may be more pertinent to hypertensive risk factors than the amount of dietary sodium alone. A potassium intake that is equal to the sodium intake may help to prevent the pathogenesis of hypertension; such is the basis for the Dietary Approaches to Stop Hypertension (DASH) diet (covered in Chapter 19). The National Heart, Lung, and Blood Institute provides a plethora of resources on the DASH diet (search "DASH diet" at www.nhlbi.nih.gov).

Requirements

The average American diet provides 2.6 g/day of potassium, which is adequate for women but is less than the established Adequate Intake (AI) of 3.4 g/day for men.[9] The *Dietary Guidelines for Americans, 2020–2025* encourage the consumption of potassium through an increased daily intake of fruit, vegetables, legumes, and low-fat dairy products.[20] The summary table for major minerals (see Table 8.3) and the DRI tables in Appendix B provide the DRIs for potassium.

Deficiency

Symptoms of potassium deficiency are well defined but seldom related to inadequate dietary intake. **Hypokalemia** is more likely to develop during clinical situations such as prolonged vomiting or diarrhea, severe malnutrition, or surgery. Hypokalemia is sometimes a concern while a person is using antihypertensive medications, particularly those that cause urinary potassium loss (known as "potassium-wasting" diuretics). Characteristic symptoms of potassium deficiency include heart muscle weakness with possible cardiac arrest, respiratory muscle weakness with breathing difficulties, poor intestinal muscle tone with resulting bloating, and overall muscle weakness.

Toxicity

As with sodium, the kidneys normally excrete excess potassium so that toxicity does not occur. However, if oral potassium intake is excessive or if intravenous potassium causes **hyperkalemia,** the heart muscle can weaken to the point at which it stops beating. There is not a UL for potassium from food sources.

Food Sources

Potassium is an essential part of all living cells; thus, it is abundant in natural foods. The richest dietary sources of potassium are unprocessed foods: fruits such as oranges and bananas, vegetables such as potatoes and leafy green vegetables, fish, whole grains,

---

hyponatremia a serum sodium level that is below normal.
hypernatremia a serum sodium level that is above normal.
hypokalemia a serum potassium level that is below normal.
hyperkalemia a serum potassium level that is above normal.

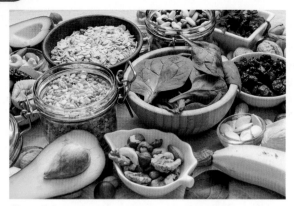

Figure 8.3 Foods rich in potassium. (Copyright iStock Photo.)

Table 8.2	Food Sources of Potassium	
ITEM	**QUANTITY**	**AMOUNT (MG)**
Bread, Cereal, Rice, and Pasta		
Raisin Bran Cereal, Malt-O-Meal	½ cup	161
Wheat germ, toasted cereal	½ cup	535
Vegetables		
Beet greens, boiled	½ cup	654
Potato, russet, baked, with skin	1 medium (173 g)	952
Sweet potato, baked in skin	1 medium (114 g)	542
Swiss chard, boiled	½ cup	480
Fruits		
Apricot, dried	¼ cup	550
Banana	1 medium (118 g)	422
Orange juice, fresh	8 fl oz	496
Prunes, dried, pitted	½ cup	637
Raisins, seeded	¼ cup	299
Meat, Poultry, Fish, Dry Beans, Eggs, and Nuts		
Beans, white, boiled	½ cup	502
Clams, cooked, moist heat	3 oz	534
Halibut, cooked, dry heat	3 oz	449
Soybean, green, raw	½ cup	794
Soybeans, roasted	½ cup	1264
Milk and Dairy Products		
Milk, skim	8 fl oz	382
Yogurt, plain, low fat	8 fl oz	352

Data from Agricultural Research Service. (2019). *USDA Food Composition Databases*. U.S. Department of Agriculture. Retrieved January 22, 2019, from ndb.nal.usda.gov.

legumes, seeds, and milk products (Figure 8.3). Those who eat the recommended number of servings of fruits and vegetables daily usually have an ideal potassium intake. Plant sources of potassium are highly water soluble; therefore, much of the potassium is lost when fruits and vegetables are boiled or blanched (unless one consumes the water as well). Table 8.2 lists food sources of potassium.

CHLORIDE

Chloride is the chemical form of chlorine in the body. Chloride accounts for approximately 0.2% of the body's weight, and it is widely distributed throughout tissues.

Functions

Chloride helps to maintain water and acid-base balances. The extracellular fluid compartments of the body hold the majority of the body's chloride content (see Figure 8.2). Its two significant functions involve digestion and respiration.

Digestion. Chloride (Cl^-) is one element of the hydrochloric acid (HCl) secreted in the gastric juices. The action of gastric enzymes requires that stomach fluids have a pH of approximately 1.0.

Respiration. Red blood cells (RBCs) transport carbon dioxide, which is a by-product of cellular metabolism, to the lungs, where they expel it during respiration. Within the RBCs, the enzyme carbonic anhydrase combines carbon dioxide (CO_2) with water (H_2O) to form carbonic acid (H_2CO_3). Carbonic acid then dissociates into a bicarbonate ion (HCO_3^-) and a proton (H^+). Bicarbonate ions move out of the RBCs and into the plasma, and chloride ions (Cl^-) move in the opposite direction, thereby maintaining the balance of negative charges on either side of the RBC membrane. The *chloride shift* is essentially an exchange of a bicarbonate ion with a chloride ion in the plasma.

Requirements

The summary table for major minerals (see Table 8.3) and the DRI tables in Appendix B provide the DRIs for chloride. The need for chloride gradually declines after the age of 50 years.

Deficiency

A dietary deficiency of chloride does not occur under normal circumstances. Because the normal intake and output of chloride from the body parallel that of sodium, conditions that lead to a sodium deficiency also can lead to a chloride deficiency. The primary reason for chloride deficiency is excessive loss of HCl through vomiting, which results in metabolic alkalosis from disturbances in the acid-base balance (see Chapter 9).

Toxicity

The only known dietary cause of chloride toxicity is severe dehydration, when the concentration of chloride is too great. The DRI committee has not set a UL for chloride.

Food Sources

Sodium chloride (i.e., ordinary table salt) provides the majority of dietary chloride consumption. The kidneys efficiently reabsorb chloride when dietary intake is low.

MAGNESIUM

Approximately 0.1% of the adult body weight is magnesium, and 60% of that magnesium is in the bones.

Functions

Magnesium has widespread metabolic functions, and it is in all body cells. About 99% of body magnesium is intracellular, with the remaining 1% found in the extracellular space.

General metabolism. Magnesium is a necessary cofactor for more than 300 enzymes that make use of nucleotide triphosphates (e.g., adenosine triphosphate) for activating or catalyzing reactions that produce energy, synthesize body compounds, or help to transport nutrients across cell membranes.

Protein synthesis. Magnesium is a cofactor for enzymes that activate amino acids for protein synthesis and that synthesize and maintain DNA. When cells replicate, they must produce new proteins, and this process requires magnesium.

Muscle action. Magnesium ions are involved in the conduction of nerve impulses that stimulate muscle contraction as part of magnesium adenosine triphosphate (MgATP). Pumps that require MgATP for energy drive calcium out of the myofibrillar spaces into the sarcoplasmic reticulum.

Basal energy expenditure. MgATP is involved in the secretion of thyroxine, thus helping the body to maintain a normal metabolic rate and to adapt to cold temperatures.

Requirements

The average American only consumes about 84% of the recommended intake for magnesium, with a median daily intake of 345 mg/day for men and 272 mg/day for women.[9] The summary table for major minerals (Table 8.3) and the DRI tables in Appendix B provide the DRIs for magnesium.

Deficiency

A primary deficiency of magnesium is rare among people who consume balanced diets. Clinical situations such as renal disorders, starvation, persistent vomiting, or diarrhea with a loss of magnesium-rich gastrointestinal fluids display symptoms of **hypomagnesemia**. Other causes of hypomagnesemia include genetic mutations that alter magnesium uptake or retention, chronic use of proton pump inhibitors, pancreatitis, uncontrolled diabetes mellitus, and chronic

hypomagnesemia a serum magnesium level that is below normal.

malnutrition with alcoholism.[21] In severe cases, hypomagnesemia can be life threatening. Other mineral deficiencies, such as hypocalcemia and hypokalemia, frequently accompany cases of hypomagnesemia. Deficiency symptoms relate to cardiovascular and neurologic instability such as muscle weakness, tetany, and cardiac arrhythmia, which can be fatal.[22]

Toxicity

Magnesium from food is unlikely to cause problems at high intake levels. Therefore, the DRI committee set a UL for magnesium intake from supplements and pharmaceutical preparations only. The UL from nonfood sources is 350 mg/day for people who are 9 years old and older; it is less for younger children.[15] Individuals consuming excessive magnesium from supplements or nonfood sources (e.g., medications) may experience nausea, vomiting, and diarrhea.

Food Sources

Unprocessed foods have the highest concentrations of magnesium. Major food sources of magnesium include nuts, soybeans, legumes, whole grains, oats, and cocoa. More than 80% of the magnesium in cereal grains is lost with the removal of the germ and outer layers. Significant amounts of magnesium may also be present in drinking water in regions that have hard water with a high mineral content.

SULFUR

Functions

As part of the amino acids cysteine and methionine, sulfur is an essential part of protein structure, and it is present in all body cells. It participates in widespread metabolic and structural functions, and it is a component of the vitamins thiamin and biotin.

Hair, skin, and nails. Disulfide bonds between cysteine residues in the protein keratin are essential to the structure of the hair, skin, and nails.

General metabolic functions. Sulfhydryl or thiol groups (i.e., covalently bonded sulfur and hydrogen atoms) form high-energy bonds that make various metabolic reactions energetically favorable.

Vitamin structure. Sulfur is a component of thiamin and biotin, which act as coenzymes in cell metabolism.

Collagen structure. The disulfide bonding of cysteine residues is necessary for collagen superhelix formation, and it is therefore important in the building of connective tissue.

| Table 8.3 | Summary of Major Minerals |

MINERAL	FUNCTIONS	RECOMMENDED INTAKE (ADULTS)	DEFICIENCY	TOLERABLE UPPER INTAKE LEVEL (UL) AND TOXICITY	SOURCES
Calcium (Ca)	Bone and teeth formation; blood clotting; muscle contraction and relaxation; nerve transmission	Between ages of 19 and 50 years, 1000 mg; between ages of 51 and 70 years, 1200 mg in women and 1000 mg in men; 70 years or older, 1000 mg	Tetany, rickets, osteoporosis	UL: 2500 mg Hypercalcemia; interferes with absorption of other nutrients	Dairy products, canned fish with bones, fortified foods (e.g., orange juice, cereal, soy products)
Phosphorus (P)	Bone and tooth formation; energy metabolism; DNA and RNA; acid-base balance	700 mg	Unlikely, but can cause bone loss, loss of appetite, and weakness	UL: 4 g Bone resorption (loss of calcium)	High-protein foods (e.g., meat, dairy, fish, eggs)
Sodium (Na)	Major extracellular fluid control; water and acid-base balance; muscle action; transmission of nerve impulse and resulting contraction; nutrient absorption	Adequate intake: 14 years or older, 1.5 g	Fluid shifts, acid-base imbalance, cramping	UL not set Hypertension in salt-sensitive people; edema	Table salt, processed foods (e.g., luncheon meats, salty snacks)
Potassium (K)	Major intracellular fluid control; acid-base balance; regulation of nerve impulse and muscle contraction; blood pressure regulation; metabolic reactions	Adequate intake: men, 3.4 g; women, 2.6 g	Irregular heartbeat, difficulty breathing, muscle weakness	UL not set Cardiac arrest	Fresh fruits and vegetables, dairy, legumes, whole grains
Chloride (Cl)	Acid-base balance (chloride shift); hydrochloric acid (digestion)	Adequate intake: between ages of 19 and 50 years, 2.3 g; between ages of 51 and 70 years, 2.0 g; 71 years or older, 1.8 g	Hypochloremic alkalosis with prolonged vomiting or diarrhea	UL not set Toxicity unlikely	Table salt, processed foods
Magnesium (Mg)	Coenzyme in metabolism, muscle and nerve action; helps with thyroid hormone secretion	Men, 400 to 420 mg; women, 310 to 320 mg	Tremor, spasm, ventricular arrhythmia	UL 350 mg (from supplements) Nausea; vomiting; diarrhea	Whole grains, nuts, seeds, legumes, spinach, cocoa
Sulfur (S)	Essential constituent of cell protein, hair, skin, nails, vitamin, and collagen structure; high-energy sulfur bonds in energy metabolism	Diets that are adequate in protein contain adequate sulfur	Unlikely	UL not set Toxicity unlikely	Meat, eggs, cheese, milk, nuts, legumes

Requirements

Dietary requirements for sulfur are not stated as such, because sulfur is supplied by protein foods that contain the amino acids methionine and cysteine.

Deficiency

Sulfur deficiency states only occur with general protein malnutrition and the deficient intake of the sulfur-containing amino acids.

Toxicity

Sulfur is unlikely to reach toxic concentrations in the body because of dietary intake; thus, there is no UL.

Food Sources

A diet that contains adequate protein contains adequate sulfur. Sulfur is only available to the body as part of the amino acids methionine and cysteine and in the vitamins thiamin and biotin. Thus, animal protein foods are the main dietary sources of sulfur. Sulfur is widely available in meat, eggs, milk, cheese, legumes, and nuts.

Table 8.3 provides a summary of the major minerals.

TRACE MINERALS

IRON

The human body contains approximately 3 to 4 g of iron. As with several other nutrients, iron is essential for life, but it can be toxic in excess. Thus, the body has exquisite systems for balancing iron intake and excretion and for efficiently transporting iron into and out of cells to maintain homeostasis. The transport protein transferrin binds and conveys iron throughout the body. Iron is stored with ferritin in the liver, the spleen, and other tissues (Figure 8.4).

Functions

Iron serves as the functional part of hemoglobin, and it plays a role in the body's general metabolism.

Hemoglobin synthesis. Approximately 70% of the body's iron is in RBC hemoglobin. Iron is a component of heme, which is the nonprotein part of hemoglobin. Hemoglobin delivers oxygen to the cells to participate in oxidation and metabolism processes. Iron also is part of myoglobin, a protein found in muscle cells, which is structurally and functionally analogous to hemoglobin in blood.

General metabolism. Iron is necessary for glucose metabolism, antibody production, drug detoxification by the liver, collagen and purine synthesis, and the conversion of β-carotene to active vitamin A.

Requirements

Iron needs vary throughout life, depending on growth and development. The summary table for trace minerals (see Table 8.7) and the DRI tables in Appendix B provide the DRIs for iron.

Women require extra iron to cover the losses that occur during menstruation. Throughout pregnancy, the RDA of iron for women increases from 18 mg/day to 27 mg/day. This increase often requires the addition of an iron supplement, because neither the typical American diet nor the iron stores of many women can meet the increased iron demands of pregnancy. The average iron intake of women in the United States is 12.1 mg/day, which is considerably less than the RDA.[9] The DRI committee estimated that vegetarians need 1.8 times more iron than omnivores owing to the lower bioavailability of iron from plant sources.[23] However, the current consensus is that the body adapts to low bioavailable iron sources and is able to maintain adequate iron status without iron supplementation.[24]

Deficiency

When a person has *anemia*, it means that they have a decreased number of circulating RBCs, decreased hemoglobin, or both. *Iron-deficiency anemia* is the most prevalent form of anemia worldwide and significantly contributes to the global burden of disease.[25] Almost 33% of the world's population is anemic, and adequate iron availability could ameliorate the majority of those cases (approximately 63%).[26] Other causes of anemia include micronutrient deficiencies other than iron, chronic infections, and genetic mutations that inhibit hemoglobin synthesis or survival. The percentage of packed RBCs (i.e., hematocrit), the RBC hemoglobin level, or the percentage of transferrin saturation, all of which correspond to the metabolism of iron (see Figure 8.4), are the most common diagnostic tools used to screen for iron-deficiency anemia.

Iron-deficiency anemia disproportionately burdens preschool-aged children and pregnant women, which happen to be the two populations with the most severe long-term detrimental complications from iron deficiency (Figure 8.5). The World Health Organization estimates that more than 800 million women and children suffer from iron-deficiency anemia worldwide, with the predominant onus in regions of low socioeconomic status.[27] Increased mortality and poor cognitive and functional outcomes result from iron-deficiency anemia in these populations.

Iron-deficiency anemia may have several causes, including the following: (1) inadequate dietary iron intake (i.e., primary deficiency); (2) excessive blood loss; (3) a lack of gastric hydrochloric acid, which liberates iron for intestinal absorption; (4) the presence of inhibitors of iron absorption (e.g., phytate, phosphate, tannin, oxalate); and (5) the manifestation of intestinal mucosal lesions that affect the absorptive surface area.

Toxicity

Iron toxicity from a single large dose (20 to 60 mg per kg of body weight) results in potentially lethal clinical manifestations.[28] In the United States, iron overdose from supplements is one of the leading causes of

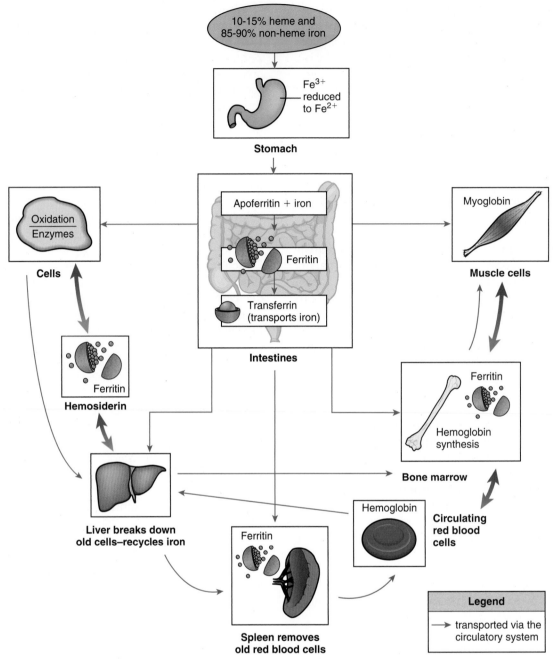

Figure 8.4 The absorption and metabolism of iron.

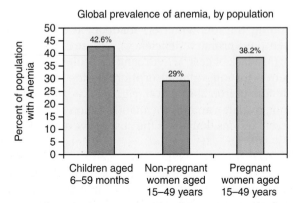

Figure 8.5 The global prevalence of anemia (as a percent of the population) for women and children. (Data from World Health Organization. [2015]. *The global prevalence of anaemia in 2011.* Geneva: World Health Organization.)

poisoning among young children who are less than 6 years old. Symptoms include nausea, vomiting, and diarrhea. If left untreated, iron toxicity causes free radical damage that overwhelms the body's ability to neutralize the oxidative stress by antioxidants. Symptoms may progress to gastrointestinal bleeding, shock, metabolic acidosis, and potentially fatal liver damage. The UL for iron is 40 mg/day for children (birth to 18 years) and 45 mg/day for adults.[23]

Hemochromatosis may result from five types of genetic mutations, but it is most commonly the result of a mutation in the hemochromatosis *(HFE)* gene. The congenital disease is an autosomal recessive disorder that leads to iron overload, even though iron intake is within the normal range. This disorder affects from 1 in 150 to 250 individuals of northern

European descent.[29] Afflicted individuals absorb excessive amounts of iron from food; over time, the iron accumulation causes widespread organ damage (usually presenting between the ages of 40 and 60 years). Treatment involves frequent bloodletting (i.e., therapeutic phlebotomy) of approximately 400 to 500 mL of whole blood to reestablish normal serum iron levels.[30] If treatment begins before pervasive damage occurs, individuals with hemochromatosis have a normal life expectancy.

Food Sources

The typical Western diet provides an average of 7 mg of iron per 1000 kcal of energy intake.[31] Iron is widely distributed in the U.S. food supply, primarily in meat, fortified cereals, and some vegetables (Figure 8.6). Liver and fortified cereal products are especially good sources. The body absorbs iron more easily when consumed along with vitamin C. Iron in food occurs in two forms: heme and nonheme. Heme iron is the most efficiently absorbed form of dietary iron, but it contributes the least to the total iron intake. Only 40% of the animal food sources and no plant-based foods provide heme iron (Table 8.4). Nonheme iron is less efficiently absorbed, because it is more tightly bound in foods, yet most of our food sources (i.e., 60% of the animal food sources and all the plant food sources) contain nonheme iron. Consuming food sources of vitamin C and moderate amounts of lean meats, fish, or poultry in the same meal enhances the absorption of nonheme iron. Enriched and fortified cereal products are a good source of nonheme iron. Table 8.5 lists food sources of iron.

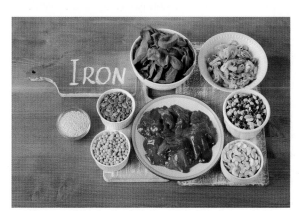

Figure 8.6 Food sources of dietary iron. (Copyright iStock Photo.)

Table **8.4** | **Characteristics of the Heme and Nonheme Portions of Dietary Iron**

	HEME	NONHEME
Food sources	None in plant sources; 40% of iron in animal sources	All iron in plant sources; 60% of iron in animal sources
Absorption rate	Rapid; transported and absorbed intact	Slow; tightly bound in organic molecules

ferritin the storage form of iron.
hemochromatosis genetic disease resulting in iron overload.
thyrotropin-releasing hormone (TRH) a hormone produced by the hypothalamus that stimulates the release of thyroid-stimulating hormone by the pituitary.

Table **8.5** | **Food Sources of Iron**

ITEM	QUANTITY	AMOUNT (mg)
Bread, Cereal, Rice, and Pasta		
Grape-Nuts, Post, ready-to-eat cereal	½ cup	16.24
Honey Bunches of Oats, Post, ready-to-eat cereal	1 cup	16.18
Oatmeal Squares, Quaker, ready-to-eat cereal	1 cup	16.52
Toasted Multigrain Crisp, ready-to-eat	1 cup	17.04
Fruits and Vegetables		
Seaweed, spirulina, dried	½ cup	15.96
Spinach, boiled, drained[a]	½ cup	3.21
Meat, Poultry, Fish, Dry Beans, Eggs, and Nuts		
Beef, plate steak, lean only, grilled	3 oz	5.46
Chicken, giblets, simmered	3 oz	5.47
Lamb, liver, pan-fried	3 oz	8.67
Nuts, coconut milk, canned	1 cup	7.46
Oysters, wild, cooked, moist heat	3 oz	7.83
Pork, liver, braised	3 oz	15.23
Soybeans, boiled	½ cup	4.42
Soybeans, mature seeds, raw	½ cup	15.70

[a]Low bioavailability.
Data from Agricultural Research Service. (2019). *USDA Food Composition Databases.* U.S. Department of Agriculture. Retrieved January 22, 2019, from ndb.nal.usda.gov.

IODINE

The average adult body contains only 15 to 20 mg of iodine.

Functions

Iodine's basic function is as a component of thyroxine (T_4), a hormone synthesized by the thyroid gland that helps to control the basal metabolic rate. The hypothalamus and the pituitary gland ultimately control T_4 synthesis. A sensitive system of feedback mechanisms helps maintain adequate T_4 levels in the body.

The hypothalamus excretes **thyrotropin-releasing hormone (TRH)**. TRH, in turn, stimulates the release of TSH from the anterior pituitary gland. TSH controls the thyroid gland uptake of iodine from the bloodstream and the release of triiodothyronine (T_3) and T_4 into the circulation (Figure 8.7). Blood T_4 concentration acts as a feedback mechanism to determine how much

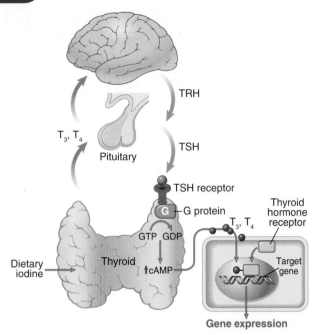

Figure 8.7 Uptake of iodine for triiodothyronine and thyroxine production. (Reprinted from Guyton, A. C., & Hall, J. E. [2006]. *Textbook of medical physiology* [12th ed.]. Philadelphia: Saunders.)

TRH the hypothalamus releases and how much TSH the pituitary gland releases. As blood T_4 concentration decreases, the hypothalamus and the pituitary gland are stimulated to release more TRH and TSH, respectively. *Serum protein-bound iodine* is the transport form of iodine in the blood.

Requirements

To maintain desirable tissue levels of iodine, the adult body's minimal requirement is 50 to 75 mcg/day; therefore, to provide an extra margin of safety, the RDA is 150 mcg/day for all people who are 14 years of age and older.[23] The summary table for trace minerals (see Table 8.7) and the DRI tables in Appendix B provide additional DRIs for iodine.

Deficiency

The World Health Organization maintains that iodine-deficiency disorders are the easiest and least expensive of all nutrient disorders to avert; however, they remain the number-one cause of preventable brain damage worldwide (see the Clinical Applications box, "Micronutrient Deficiencies and Vulnerable Populations").[32] Geographic regions with mountains or frequent flooding that deplete the soil of iodine are more susceptible to iodine-deficiency disorders. Access to iodized salt has reduced the global prevalence of iodine deficiency in the last few decades.[33] However, nearly 30% of the world's population still has insufficient access to iodine; these individuals are at high risk for the following deficiency diseases.[34]

Goiter. A **goiter** is an enlarged thyroid gland (Figure 8.8). When starved for iodine, the thyroid gland cannot

> **goiter** an enlarged thyroid gland that is usually caused by a lack of iodine to produce the thyroid hormone thyroxine.

produce a normal amount of T_4. Because of a low blood T_4 concentration, the pituitary gland continues to release more TSH. Large amounts of TSH overstimulate the nonproductive thyroid gland, thereby increasing its size greatly. An iodine-starved thyroid gland may weigh 0.45 to 0.67 kg (1 to 1.5 lb) or more. Although the thyroid is one of the larger endocrine glands, it normally weighs only 10 to 20 g in an adult.

Cretinism and congenital hypothyroidism. Cretinism is a congenital disorder resulting from insufficient thyroid hormone to the fetus during gestation. One reason for unavailable thyroid hormones is maternal iodine deficiency throughout pregnancy. Common characteristics of cretinism include physical deformity, dwarfism, mental retardation, and auditory disorders. During pregnancy, the mother's need for iodine takes precedence over the iodine needs of the developing fetus. Thus, the fetus suffers from iodine deficiency and continues to do so after birth. The physical and mental development of these children is severely impeded and irreversible.

Congenital hypothyroidism is a disorder resulting from insufficient thyroid hormone during gestation attributable to genetic defects in the metabolic pathways of the thyroid hormones. The severity of defects can vary greatly, but early treatment can help prevent further damage (see the Cultural Considerations box, "Hypermetabolism and Hypometabolism: What Are They and Who Is At Risk?," in Chapter 6).

Impaired mental and physical development. Studying the long-term effects of a single nutrient deficiency is difficult. When a person or a population is deficient in one nutrient, they are likely deficient in other nutrients as well. In addition, there are usually other contributing factors influencing the results of such studies (e.g., sociodemographic, ethnic, lifestyle factors). That said, studies indicate that children born to women with even mild iodine deficiency during pregnancy have a significant reduction in their intelligence quotient despite adequate dietary intake throughout childhood.[35] Long-term severe iodine deficiency during childhood and adolescence appears to delay growth and the onset of puberty, both of which the normalization of dietary iodine levels may correct.[36,37]

Hypothyroidism. Hypothyroidism occurs when a poorly functioning thyroid gland does not make enough T_4, thereby greatly reducing the basal metabolic rate. There are many causes of hypothyroidism, including both iodine deficiency and iodine toxicity.[38] Iodine deficiency is the most common cause of hypothyroidism worldwide. Symptoms include fatigue; depression; weight gain; thin, coarse hair; dry skin; poor cold tolerance; infertility;

⌂ Clinical Applications

Micronutrient Deficiencies and Vulnerable Populations

Micronutrient deficiencies, particularly those occurring during infancy, have the potential to compromise health throughout the entire life cycle. Severe conditions may manifest as an intergenerational cycle beginning with poor growth and intellectual impairments and culminating as morbidity and an increased risk for mortality. Preventing the onset of this cycle is a powerful tool for positively improving the global burden of disease.[1]

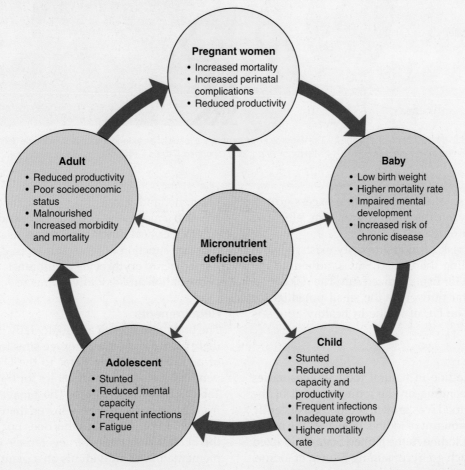

The populations most vulnerable to micronutrient deficiencies and overt malnutrition are pregnant women and children from birth to age 5. The micronutrients of greatest concern worldwide for these susceptible individuals are iron, iodine, zinc, folate, and vitamin A. Many foods enriched or fortified in developed nations include these very nutrients; examples include bread and grain products enriched with folate and iron, milk fortified with vitamin A, and salt fortified with iodine. In areas of the world without such food systems in place, the prevalence of micronutrient deficiencies, frequently occurring concurrently, are substantially higher with extensive cost to nations and far reaching consequences over generations.

The three recommended readings provided here are for further study, practical application, and clinical consideration for resource-poor countries.

- Yakoob, M. Y., & Lo, C. W. (2017). Nutrition (micronutrients) in child growth and development: A systematic review on current evidence, recommendations and opportunities for further research. *J Dev Behav Pediatr, 38*(8), 665–679.
- Bailey, R. L., West, K. P., Jr., & Black, R. E. (2015). The epidemiology of global micronutrient deficiencies. *Ann Nutr Metab, 66*(Suppl. 2), 22–33.
- Millward, D. J. (2017). Nutrition, infection and stunting: The roles of deficiencies of individual nutrients and foods, and of inflammation, as determinants of reduced linear growth of children. *Nutr Res Rev, 30*(1), 50–72.

REFERENCE
1. Bailey, R. L., West, K. P., Jr., & Black, R. E. (2015). The epidemiology of global micronutrient deficiencies. *Annals of Nutrition & Metabolism, 66*(Suppl. 2), 22–33.

and hoarse voice. In severe and rare cases, hypothyroidism can advance to myxedema coma and death.[39]

Toxicity

When trying to correct for long-term iodine deficiency, practitioners must be careful of over-supplementing. Excess iodine supplementation may lead to thyrotoxicosis or iodine-induced hyperthyroidism. Individuals with underlying thyroid dysfunction are more susceptible to iodine toxicity from chronic or acute doses than are individuals without existing thyroid dysfunction.

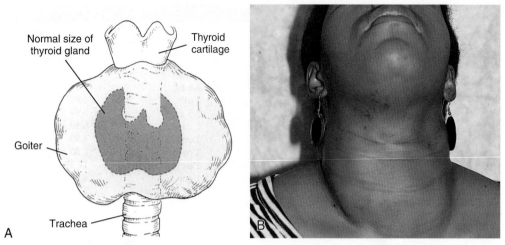

Figure 8.8 (A) Illustration of a goiter. (B) The extreme enlargement is a result of an extended duration of iodine deficiency. (B, Reprinted from Swartz, M. H. [2014]. *Textbook of physical diagnosis* [7th ed.]. Philadelphia: Saunders.)

Iodine toxicity may present as iodine-excess goiter, autoimmune thyroiditis, hypothyroidism, elevated TSH, and ocular damage.

Although the risk of iodine toxicity exists, several countries (including the United States) adhere to the recommendation for using iodized salt. The risk for iodine deficiency far outweighs the small potential for iodine toxicity. The UL of iodine in healthy adults is 1100 mcg/day.[23]

Food Sources

The amount of iodine in natural food sources varies considerably depending on the iodine content of the soil in which the food was grown. Seafood consistently provides a good amount of iodine. However, the major reliable source of iodine in the United States is iodized table salt, with each gram containing 77 mcg of iodine.

ZINC

Zinc is an essential trace mineral with wide clinical significance. The amount of zinc in the adult body is approximately 1.5 g to 4 g.

Functions

Zinc is required for the optimal function of 200 to 300 enzymes. DNA, RNA, and protein synthesis, as well as energy metabolism and food intake regulation, are among the many biochemical and physiologic functions in which zinc is critically involved. Zinc has three major roles in metalloenzymes, including (1) participation in catalytic functions, (2) maintenance of structural stability, and (3) involvement in regulatory functions. These metalloenzymes are active in all major metabolic pathways and are involved in the formation or hydrolysis of proteins, lipids, and carbohydrates. All aspects of the immune system are reliant on adequate zinc availability.[40] Reproduction, optimal activity of growth hormone, and successful synaptic neurotransmission are also among the activities dependent upon zinc. Another critical function of zinc is its role in the structure and function of biomembranes. Zinc functions as a stabilizer of erythrocyte membranes, thus decreasing peroxidation and oxidative damage.

Requirements

The body relies on an adequate daily intake of zinc, as there are no significant storage sites to access in times of poor consumption. Refer to the DRI tables in Appendix B or the summary tables for trace minerals (see Table 8.7) for zinc RDAs. The bioavailability of zinc from plant-based foods is lower than that of animal-based food products, but this does not appear to lower the overall zinc status of vegetarians or warrant supplementation of individuals on a plant-based diet.[24]

Deficiency

Adequate zinc intake is imperative for good health during periods of rapid tissue growth, such as pregnancy, childhood, and adolescence. Inadequate zinc intake, and overt zinc deficiency, is a considerable nutrition concern in developing countries.[41] Zinc deficiency contributes to a myriad of health issues such as inflammation and oxidative stress; dermal and epidermal tissue breakdown; fetal malformations and stunted growth; and diarrheal diseases, poor wound healing, and overall compromised immune function.[42,43] People with poor appetites, who subsist on marginal diets, or who have chronic wounds or illnesses with excessive tissue breakdown, are particularly vulnerable to zinc deficiency.

Acrodermatitis enteropathica (AE) is a rare autosomal recessive disorder causing severe zinc deficiency and death if it is not treated. Patients with this condition are not able to absorb sufficient zinc from the gut. Classic

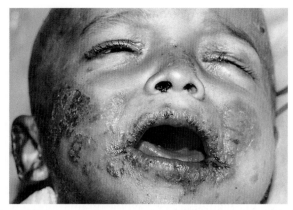

Figure 8.9 Skin lesions that are characteristic of severe zinc deficiency in a patient with acrodermatitis enteropathica. (From Kumar, V., Abbas, A. K., Fausto, N. [2005]. *Robbins and Cotran pathologic basis of disease* [7th ed.]. Philadelphia: Saunders.)

symptoms of acrodermatitis enteropathica begin with skin lesions and progress to severely compromised immune function (Figure 8.9). Oral zinc supplements at high doses are successful (if properly diagnosed soon after birth) in treating this inborn error of metabolism.

Toxicity

As with several other minerals, zinc toxicity from food sources alone is uncommon. Excessive intake by dietary supplements is generally self-limiting because of the side effects of nausea, vomiting, and abdominal

Table 8.6   Food Sources of Zinc

ITEM	QUANTITY	AMOUNT (mg)
Bread, Cereal, Rice, and Pasta		
Oat Blenders with almonds and honey, Malt-O-Meal, ready-to-eat cereal	¾ cup	5.36
Wheat Bran flakes, Ralston, enriched, ready-to-eat cereal	¾ cup	18.66
Meat, Poultry, Fish, Dry Beans, Eggs, and Nuts		
Beef, chuck, short ribs, lean only, braised	3 oz	10.44
Crab, Alaskan king, cooked, moist heat	3 oz	6.48
Lobster, northern, cooked, moist heat	3 oz	3.44
Oyster, eastern, farmed, cooked, dry heat	3 oz	38.38
Oysters, eastern, wild, cooked, moist heat	3 oz	66.81
Soybean, mature seeds, roasted	½ cup	2.70
Milk and Dairy Products		
Yogurt, plain, skim milk	8 fl oz	2.20

Data from Agricultural Research Service. (2019). *USDA Food Composition Databases*. U.S. Department of Agriculture. Retrieved January 22, 2019, from ndb.nal.usda.gov.

For Further Focus

Zinc Barriers

Most individuals eating a well-rounded diet that includes either meat products or zinc-fortified, vegetarian-friendly meat substitutes satisfy their bodies' need for zinc. The average daily adult zinc intake in the United States is 13.2 mg for men and 9.4 mg for women, both of which meet the sex-specific DRIs.[1] However, that intake level does not meet the DRI for pregnant or lactating women, which is 11 mg and 12 mg, respectively.[2] That said, *consuming* zinc and *absorbing* zinc are not the same thing.

Although the prevalence of zinc deficiency is lower in developed countries and in areas that habitually consume meat than in developing countries, there remains a risk of inadequate zinc status for some individuals. Susceptible individuals may unknowingly compromise their zinc health by choosing foods and supplements that reduce zinc's bioavailability. Here are some examples:

- Excessive dietary fiber or phytate-containing foods may hinder absorption and create a negative zinc balance.
- Vitamin and mineral supplements may contain iron-to-zinc ratios of greater than 3:1 and thus provide enough iron to inhibit zinc absorption.
- Animal foods, which are rich in readily available zinc, are consumed less by cholesterol-conscious individuals.
  Low levels of zinc can reduce the amount of carrier-proteins available to transport iron and vitamin A to their target tissues.

The following suggestions may help to increase dietary zinc bioavailability:

- Include some form of animal food (e.g., meat, poultry, seafood) or vegetarian-acceptable fortified food in the diet each day to ensure an adequate intake of zinc.
- Avoid the excessive use of alcohol.[3]
- Avoid "crash" diets, which are typically low in many micronutrients.
- If taking a dietary supplement of zinc, do so separately from iron supplements and do not exceed the DRI.

REFERENCES

1. Agricultural Research Service. (2018). Nutrient intakes from food and beverages: Mean amounts consumed per individual, by gender and age. In *What we eat in America* (NHANES 2015-2016). U.S. Department of Agriculture.
2. Food and Nutrition Board. (2001). *Dietary reference intakes for vitamin A, vitamin K, arsenic, boron, chromium, copper, iodine, iron, manganese, molybdenum, nickel, silicon, vanadium, and zinc.* Institute of Medicine. Washington, DC: National Academies Press.
3. Skalny, V., et al. (2018). Zinc deficiency as a mediator of toxic effects of alcohol abuse. *European Journal of Nutrition*, 57(7), 2313–2322.

pain. The UL for zinc of 40 mg/day was established based on the negative effects of excess zinc supplementation on copper metabolism.[23] Excessive zinc intake inhibits copper absorption, thereby resulting in a zinc-induced copper deficiency.

Food Sources

The greatest food source of zinc in the United States is meat, which supplies approximately 70% of the dietary zinc consumed. Seafood (particularly oysters) is another excellent source of zinc. Legumes and whole grains are reasonable sources of zinc, but the zinc in these foods is less available for intestinal absorption because of phytate binding (see the For Further Focus box, "Zinc Barriers," for additional information about inhibitors to zinc absorption). A balanced diet usually meets adult needs for zinc. Table 8.6 lists food sources of zinc.

SELENIUM

Functions

Selenium is present in all body tissues except adipose tissue. The highest concentrations of selenium are in the liver, kidneys, heart, and spleen. Selenium is an essential part of the enzyme *glutathione peroxidase*, which is an antioxidant that protects the lipids in cell membranes from oxidative damage. An abundance of selenium may spare vitamin E to an extent, because selenium and vitamin E protect against free radical damage. Selenium is also a component of many proteins in the body known as *selenoproteins*. One such selenoprotein is type 1 iodothyronine 5′-deiodinase, which is the enzyme required to convert T_4 to T_3.

Requirements

Refer to the summary table for trace minerals (see Table 8.7) and in the DRI tables in Appendix B for the DRIs of selenium.

Deficiency

Inadequate selenium negatively alters immune function and increases the opportunity for oxidative stress, specifically within the thyroid gland. Selenium intake varies worldwide along with soil selenium availability. Geographic areas with a poor soil content of selenium are more susceptible to selenium deficiency syndromes such as *Kashin-Bek disease* and *Keshan disease*. Kashin-Bek disease causes chronic arthritis and joint deformity. Keshan disease, which is named after the area in China where it was discovered, is a disease of the heart muscle that primarily affects young children and women of childbearing age. Left untreated, it can lead to heart failure resulting from cardiomyopathy (i.e., degeneration of the heart muscle).

Toxicity

The most common symptoms of selenium toxicity are hair loss, joint pain, nail discoloration, and gastrointestinal upset (i.e., nausea, vomiting, and diarrhea). Most known cases of dietary selenium toxicity are in isolated regions of the world where the soil has extremely high levels of selenium. The UL for selenium is 400 mcg/day for people who are 14 years old and older.[44]

Food Sources

Most selenium in food is highly available for intestinal absorption. The amount of selenium in food depends on the quantity of selenium in the soil used to graze animals and grow plants. However, diverse food distribution systems mitigate local differences in soil selenium concentrations. Pork, turkey, lamb, chicken, and organ meats (e.g., beef liver) are consistently good sources of selenium. Fish, whole grains, and other seeds are a decent source of selenium, but the quantity will vary. Brazil nuts are an exceptionally good source of selenium with 1342 mcg per ½ cup serving.[45] The average adult intake of selenium in the United States is 115.5 mcg/day.[9]

The following sections briefly review the remaining essential trace minerals.

FLUORIDE

Fluoride forms a strong bond with calcium; thus, it accumulates in calcified body tissues such as bones and teeth. Fluoride's main function in human nutrition is to prevent the development of dental caries. Fluoride strengthens the ability of teeth to withstand the erosive effect of bacterial acids. The use of fluoridated toothpaste (0.1% fluoride) and improved dental hygiene habits have greatly benefited dental health. Additionally, the fluoridation of the public water supply is responsible for an added decline in dental caries, and health care cost, during recent decades.[46]

The summary table for trace minerals (see Table 8.7) and the DRI tables in Appendix B provide the DRIs for fluoride. The DRI committee set the UL for fluoride at 10 mg/day for people who are 9 years old and older to avoid dental **fluorosis** (Figure 8.10).[15]

Crab, shrimp, raisins, grape juice, hot breakfast cereals (Cream of Wheat, grits, and oatmeal), and tea provide significant sources of fluoride. Cooking in fluoridated water raises the fluoride concentration in many foods. People who are using well water should periodically check the fluoride concentration of their water, because some well water contains markedly high natural sources of fluoride.

COPPER

We sometimes refer to copper as the "iron twin," because we metabolize them both in much the same way, and both are components of cell enzymes. Both of these minerals are also involved in energy production and hemoglobin synthesis. Primary deficiency of copper is rare.

---

fluorosis an excess intake of fluoride that causes the yellowing of teeth, white spots on the teeth, and the pitting or mottling of tooth enamel.

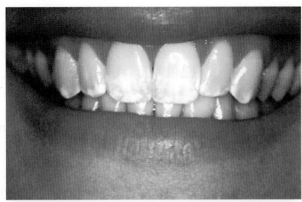

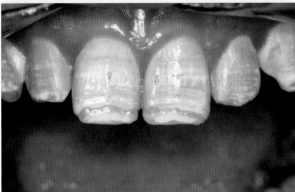

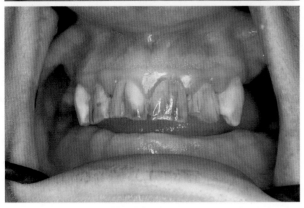

Figure 8.10 Fluorosis.

Copper is involved in two severe inborn errors of metabolism. The first is *Menkes disease*, which is a lethal X-linked genetic disease of copper metabolism. Treatment with subcutaneous copper administration, beginning within the first 30 days of life, decreases the progressive nature of the disease.[47] Otherwise, individuals with Menkes disease progress through neurodegeneration and connective tissue deterioration and do not survive past childhood. *Wilson disease* is a rare autosomal recessive genetic disorder that manifests as abnormally high deposits of copper in the body, particularly within the liver and brain. Without treatment, Wilson disease causes liver and nerve damage that ultimately leads to death. However, there are oral drug therapies for Wilson disease that dramatically improve prognosis and may stabilize or even reverse deleterious effects of the disease.[48] Provided that individuals are compliant with medications for life, they may experience a normal life span.

The summary table for trace minerals (see Table 8.7) and the DRI tables in Appendix B provide the DRIs for copper. The UL for copper is 10 mg/day to avoid gastrointestinal upset and liver damage.[23] Copper is widely distributed in natural foods. Organ meats (especially liver), veal, beef, lamb, oysters, and legumes are the richest food sources of copper.

MANGANESE

There are approximately 14 mg of manganese in an adult body weighing 150 lb. Manganese functions like many other trace minerals: as a component of cell enzymes. Manganese-dependent enzymes catalyze many important metabolic reactions. These metabolic reactions include metabolism of carbohydrates, amino acids, and cholesterol; formation of bone and cartilage; and wound healing through its role in manganese-activated glycosyltransferases. In some magnesium-dependent enzymes, manganese may serve as a substitute for magnesium, depending on the availability of these two minerals. The intestinal absorption and bodily retention of manganese are inversely associated with serum ferritin concentration.

There are no known manganese deficiencies among humans consuming an unrestricted diet. Long-term exposure to manganese dust causes *inhalation toxicity* in miners and other industrial workers. The excess manganese accumulates in the liver and the central nervous system, thereby producing severe neuromuscular symptoms that are similar to those of Parkinson disease. There is also a potential for manganese toxicity among clients who are receiving parenteral nutrition with standard trace element supplementation because the bioavailability of manganese is approximately 95% greater when administered parenterally than if it is absorbed enterally.[49] In addition, these clients may experience an impaired elimination pathway; thus, manganese accumulates and damages the brain. In addition, individuals with either iron-deficiency anemia or selenium deficiency are at higher risk for hypermanganesemia. The UL of manganese from dietary sources is 11 mg/day for healthy adults.[23]

The summary table for trace minerals (see Table 8.7) and the DRI tables in Appendix B provide the DRIs for manganese. The most commonly consumed food sources of manganese are of plant origin. Whole grains, cereal products, and soybeans are the richest food sources.

MOLYBDENUM

Molybdenum is better absorbed than many minerals, and inadequate dietary intake is unlikely. The amount of molybdenum in the body is exceedingly small. Molybdenum is the functional catalytic component in several cell enzymes involved in oxidation-reduction reactions. The summary table for trace minerals (see Table 8.7) and the DRI tables in Appendix B provide the DRIs for molybdenum. There is a UL for molybdenum of 2000 mcg/day for adults because of symptoms similar to gout at very high doses (>10 g/day).[23] The amounts of molybdenum in foods vary considerably depending on the soil in which they are grown.

Table 8.7   Summary of Selected Trace Elements

MINERAL	FUNCTIONS	RECOMMENDED INTAKE (ADULTS)	DEFICIENCY	TOLERABLE UPPER INTAKE LEVEL (UL) AND TOXICITY	SOURCES
Iron (Fe)	Hemoglobin and myoglobin formation; cellular oxidation of glucose; antibody production	Men, 8 mg; women between ages of 19 and 50 years, 18 mg; women who are 50 years old or older, 8 mg	Anemia, pale skin, impaired immune function	UL: 45 mg Nausea; vomiting; diarrhea; liver, kidney, heart, and central nervous system damage; hemochromatosis	Liver, meats, whole grains, enriched grains, dark green vegetables, soybeans
Iodine (I)	Synthesis of thyroxine, which regulates cell oxidation and basal metabolic rate	150 mcg	Goiter, cretinism, hypothyroidism, hyperthyroidism	UL: 1100 mcg Goiter	Iodized salt, seafood
Zinc (Zn)	Essential enzyme constituent; protein metabolism; storage of insulin; immune system; sexual maturation	Men, 11 mg; women, 8 mg	Compromised immunity, oxidative stress (inflammation), stunted growth, congenital malformations	UL: 40 mg Nausea; vomiting; abdominal pain; zinc-induced copper deficiency, altered lymphocyte response	Meat, seafood (especially oysters), enriched grains, soybeans
Selenium (Se)	Forms glutathione peroxidase; spares vitamin E as an antioxidant; protects lipids in cell membrane	55 mcg	Impaired immune function, Keshan disease, heart muscle failure	UL: 400 mcg Brittleness of hair and nails; gastrointestinal upset	Seafood, kidney, liver, meats, whole grains, Brazil nuts
Fluoride (F-)	Constituent of bone and teeth; helps prevent dental caries	Adequate Intake: men, 4 mg; women, 3 mg	Increased dental caries	UL: 10 mg Dental fluorosis	Fluoridated water, toothpaste
Copper (Cu)	Associated with iron in energy production, hemoglobin synthesis, iron absorption and transport, and nerve and immune function	900 mcg	Anemia, bone abnormalities; Menkes disease	UL: 10 mg Wilson disease, which results in liver and nerve conduction damage	Liver, seafood, whole grains, legumes, nuts
Manganese (Mn)	Activates reactions in urea synthesis, energy metabolism, lipoprotein clearance, and synthesis of fatty acids	Adequate Intake: men, 2.3 mg; women, 1.8 mg	Clinical deficiency present only with protein-energy malnutrition	UL: 11 mg Inhalation toxicity in miners, which results in neuromuscular disturbances	Cereals, whole grains, soybeans, legumes, nuts, tea, vegetables, fruits
Molybdenum (Mo)	Constituent of many enzymes	45 mcg	Unlikely	UL: 2 mg Toxicity unlikely	Organ meats, milk, whole grains, leafy vegetables, legumes
Chromium (Cr)	Potentially associated with glucose metabolism	Adequate Intake: men, 35 mcg; women, 25 mcg	Unlikely	UL not set Toxicity unlikely	Whole grains, cereal products, brewer's yeast

CHROMIUM

The European Food Safety Authority concluded that chromium is not an essential element in human nutrition in 2014.[50] The DRI committees in the United States and Canada have not reevaluated the data for chromium's essentiality since the last publication of the DRIs in 2001. Several researchers believe that it is time to remove chromium from the list of essential elements for human nutrition because there is no evidence of chromium deficiency and there are no high-quality studies illuminating essential functions of chromium.[51]

The DRI committee included chromium in the most recent recommendations but did not establish a UL.[23] The summary table for trace minerals (see Table 8.7) and the DRI tables in Appendix B provide the DRIs for chromium. The food content of chromium is difficult to establish and will vary according to soil mineral content where plants are cultivated or animals graze.

Table 8.7 provides a summary of selected trace elements.

OTHER ESSENTIAL TRACE MINERALS

RDAs and AIs were not set for the remaining trace minerals: aluminum, arsenic, boron, nickel, silicon, tin, and vanadium. At the time of the last DRI publication, not enough data were available to establish such recommendations.[23] Although the complete process of their metabolism is unclear, experts consider most of these minerals essential to the nutrition of specific animals and may be essential to human nutrition as well. Because these minerals occur in such small amounts, they are difficult to study, and dietary deficiency is highly unlikely.

The available research data regarding boron, nickel, and vanadium are sufficient to establish a tolerable UL level. The adult ULs for both boron and vanadium were set based on data gathered from animal studies: for boron, the UL is 20 mg/day; for vanadium, it is 1.8 mg/day. The adult UL for arsenic was set at 1 mg/day.[23]

MINERAL SUPPLEMENTATION

Dietary supplement use in the United States fluctuates along with socioeconomic status. Individuals with the most food security, highest socioeconomic status, and arguably the least likely to need supplemental nutrients are the *most likely* to use dietary supplements on a regular basis.[52] With very few exceptions, a well-rounded, healthy diet can meet the nutrient needs of most individuals.

The same principles discussed in Chapter 7 for vitamin supplementation apply to mineral supplementation. Special needs during growth periods and in clinical situations may merit specific mineral supplements. Before taking or recommending supplements, consider the potential nutrient-nutrient interactions and drug-nutrient interactions. Several dynamics can hinder mineral bioavailability (see the Drug-Nutrient Interaction box, "Mineral Depletion").

 Drug-Nutrient Interaction

Mineral Depletion

Medications interact with minerals through two major mechanisms: either by blocking absorption or by inducing renal excretion. The following are examples of drug-nutrient interactions that may alter whole-body mineral status:

- *Diuretics:* People who require the long-term use of diuretic drugs for the treatment of hypertension may need to pay special attention to certain minerals that are also lost. Along with excess water, excreted minerals include sodium, potassium, magnesium, and zinc. The intake of foods that are high in these minerals is generally enough to regain homeostasis. Some diuretics (e.g., spironolactone) are potassium sparing and thus extra potassium is not necessary.
- *Chelating agents:* Chelation therapy removes excess metal ions from the body. Penicillamine treats Wilson disease and rheumatoid arthritis and helps to prevent kidney stones. It attaches to zinc and copper, thereby blocking absorption and leading to the excretion and possible depletion of both minerals.
- *Antacids:* The acidic environment of the stomach is required for the absorption of many drugs and nutrients, including minerals. The chronic use of antacids alters the environment such that mineral deficiencies can occur. Phosphate deficiency is a concern for individuals who are chronically using over-the-counter antacids. In extreme cases, hypercalcemia may result, causing damage to soft tissues.

LIFE CYCLE NEEDS

Specific periods of rapid growth throughout the life cycle may warrant mineral supplementation.

Pregnancy and Lactation

Women require additional copper, iodine, iron, magnesium, manganese, molybdenum, selenium, and zinc to meet the demands of rapid fetal growth during pregnancy. DRIs remain elevated for several minerals throughout lactation to meet both mother and infant needs. Not all women will require dietary supplements to meet these increased needs, though. A healthy, balanced diet including a variety of foods from all food groups will meet most nutrient requirements. However, iron supplementation during pregnancy is common because it is challenging to meet the DRI recommendations for this mineral through dietary intake alone.

Adolescence

Rapid bone growth during adolescence requires increased calcium, phosphorus, and magnesium.[15,53] If an adolescent's diet is chronically lacking in the minerals critical for bone development at this vital stage, then the risk increases for osteoporosis in later adult years. Too little dietary calcium prevents the realization of maximum bone density and may lead to the resorption of calcium from bone to maintain an appropriate blood calcium concentration. With the rise in soft drink consumption coupled with the decline of calcium-containing drinks (i.e., milk or milk substitutes) consumed in the United States, there is reason for concern about poor bone growth during these important years.

Another consideration during the adolescent years is folate and iron for teenage girls. Depending on the adequacy of their diet, supplements containing iron and folate may benefit adolescent girls as they begin menstruating to support iron stores and maintain adequate folate status in the event of pregnancy.

Adulthood

Healthy adults who consume well-balanced and varied diets do not require mineral supplements. A well-rounded and varied diet in combination with adequate physical activity and exercise maintains optimal bone health in most adults. There is widespread use of calcium and vitamin D supplements in the hopes of improving bone health and reducing the risk of fracture in advanced years. However, at any adult age, vitamin D and calcium supplementation alone neither prevents nor successfully treats osteoporosis.

CLINICAL NEEDS

People with certain clinical problems or those at high risk for developing such problems may require mineral supplements. Because it is not possible to cover every disease state that alters mineral needs in this textbook, note that some clinical situations increase the body's use of certain minerals beyond what the average diet can supply. In those cases, clients can consult with a registered dietitian nutritionist on how to improve overall nutrient intake, which may necessitate dietary supplements.

Putting It All Together

Summary

- Minerals are elements that are widely distributed in foods. Minerals build body tissue; activate, regulate, and control metabolic processes; and transmit neurologic messages.
- The classification of minerals as a trace or major mineral depends on the relative amount found in the body. Major minerals are necessary in larger quantities than trace minerals, and they make up 60% to 80% of all of the inorganic material in the body. Trace minerals, which are necessary in quantities as small as a microgram, make up less than 1% of the body's inorganic material.
- RDAs have not been set for all minerals. However, AIs or ULs have been set for almost all essential minerals without RDAs.
- Mineral supplementation—along with vitamin supplementation—continues to be a hot topic of research. There are periods that occur throughout the life cycle and specific disease states that may warrant supplementation. However, in most situations, a balanced diet provides an adequate supply of all of the essential nutrients.

Chapter Review Questions

See answers in Appendix A.

1. It is particularly beneficial for growing adolescents to consume foods with highly bioavailable forms of calcium such as _____.

   a. yogurt
   b. baked beans
   c. orange slices
   d. chicken livers

2. Phosphorus functions in metabolic processes to maintain health by _____.

   a. assisting in the formation of fibrin to form clots
   b. controlling the uptake of iodine from the blood
   c. capturing energy in the form of adenosine triphosphate
   d. carrying oxygen to the cells for oxidation and metabolism

3. A woman taking a diuretic medication to manage her blood pressure complains of overall weakness, difficulty breathing, and a feeling of abdominal bloating. These symptoms may be characteristic of _____.

   a. sodium toxicity
   b. potassium deficiency
   c. excess potassium intake
   d. iron toxicity

4. The doctor told her client with high blood pressure to reduce his dietary sodium intake. Of the following options, which is a food choice that is likely to have the highest sodium content?

   a. Whole grain toast with blackberry jam
   b. Pork loin with cranberry sauce
   c. Homemade beef and bean burrito
   d. Olive and feta cheese salad with crackers

5. Hypothyroidism is characterized by _____.

   a. thin, coarse hair; weight gain; poor cold tolerance
   b. thin, coarse hair; general nervousness; weight loss
   c. acne-like skin lesions, weight loss, increased appetite
   d. weight gain, heat intolerance, dwarfism

Next-Generation NCLEX® Examination-style Case Study

See answers in Appendix A.

A 70-year-old female (Ht.: 5'8" Wt.: 130 lbs.) fractured her right talus, although she is unsure how it happened. She goes to a swimming class twice a week. She has a family history of hypertension. She has a history of hyperthyroidism but frequently forgets to take her medication. She does not have a large appetite and rarely drinks alcohol. Her primary care physician diagnosed her with osteoporosis. A dietary recall is collected.

Breakfast: piece of toast with peanut butter and banana
Lunch: saltine crackers (5), chicken noodle soup (1 c.), and
   hot tea (8 oz.)
Snack: applesauce (1/2 c.)
Dinner: pinto beans (1/2 c.), piece of cornbread, cooked
   spinach (1/4 c.), and hot tea (8 oz.)
Dessert: hard caramel candies (3)

1. From the list below, select all of the client's risk factors related to the client's diagnosis.

   a. BMI
   b. Age
   c. Hyperthyroidism
   d. Alcohol use
   e. Family history
   f. Exercise patterns
   g. Sex

2. From the list below, identify potential nutrient concerns from the client's dietary recall.

   a. Low in calories
   b. Low in fruits
   c. Low in vegetables
   d. Inadequate sources of calcium
   e. Excessive phosphorous
   f. Excessive iron

3. Choose the *most likely* options for the information missing from the statements below by selecting from the list of options provided.

   In addition to the client's diet, her poorly controlled hyperparathyroidism causes _____ from the bones to be _____, making them weak and brittle.

OPTIONS	
potassium	resorbed
calcium	calcified
iodine	oxidized

4. Place an X under "effective" to identify appropriate recommendations to improve this client's bone density. Place an X under "ineffective" to identify recommendations that would not be effective.

INTERVENTION	EFFECTIVE	INEFFECTIVE
Consume dairy products		
Consume fortified foods with calcium		
Consume plant products with minimal oxalate acid		
Consume plant products with oxalate acid		
Take a vitamin D supplement		
Increase low intensity exercise		
Participating in resistance exercise		
Consistently take thyroid medication		

5. From the list below, select all of the foods necessary for client education that provide a good source of calcium.

   a. Milk
   b. Eggs
   c. Cheese
   d. Sardines
   e. Bok Choy
   f. Spinach
   g. Calcium fortified soy products
   h. Chicken
   i. Calcium fortified orange juice

Additional Learning Resources

Please refer to this text's Evolve website for answers to the Case Study questions:

http://evolve.elsevier.com/Williams/basic/

References and **Further Reading and Resources** in the back of the book provide additional resources for enhancing knowledge.

Water and Electrolyte Balance

Key Concepts

- Water compartments inside and outside of the cells maintain a balanced distribution of total body water.
- The concentration of various solute particles in water determines the internal shifts and movement of fluid in the body.

- Water and electrolyte balance has many checks and balances beginning at the cellular level and involves organ and hormonal controls.
- A state of **dynamic equilibrium** among the body's water and acid-base balance system influences the entire body to sustain life.

Water is the most vital nutrient to human existence. Humans can survive far longer without food than without water. Only the continuous need for air is more demanding.

One of the most basic nutrition tasks is ensuring a balanced distribution of water to all body cells. Water is critical for the physiologic functions that are necessary to support life. This chapter briefly looks at the finely developed water and electrolyte balance systems in the body, examines how these systems work, and describes the various parts and processes that maintain them.

BODY WATER FUNCTIONS AND REQUIREMENTS

WATER: THE FUNDAMENTAL NUTRIENT

Basic Principles

Three basic principles are essential to an understanding of the balance and uses of water in the human body.

A unified whole. The human body forms one continuous body of water that is contained by a protective envelope of skin. Water moves to all parts of the body, and it is controlled by solvents within the water and membranes that separate the compartments. Virtually every space inside and outside of cells is filled with water-based body fluids. Within this environment, we are able to sustain all processes that are necessary for life.

Body water compartments. Within the framework of human physiology, the key word *compartment* refers to dynamic areas within the body. Discussions of body water may focus on *total body water* or water specific to distinct intracellular or extracellular compartments throughout the body that are separated by membranes. The body's dynamic mechanisms constantly shift water to places of greatest need and maintain equilibrium

among all parts. We cover the individual compartments later in this chapter.

Particles in the water solution. The concentration and distribution of particles in water (e.g., sodium, chloride, calcium, magnesium, phosphate, bicarbonate, protein) control the internal shifts and balances among the compartments of water throughout the body.

Homeostasis

W.B. Cannon, a physiologist, viewed the principles of **homeostasis** as "body wisdom."[1] Early in the 20th century he applied the term *homeostasis* to the body's capacity to maintain its life systems, despite what enters the system from the outside. The body has a great capacity to use numerous finely balanced homeostatic mechanisms to protect its vital water supply.

BODY WATER FUNCTIONS

Body water performs the following critical functions.

Solvent

Water provides the basic liquid solvent for all chemical reactions within the body. The **polarity** of water effectively ionizes and dissolves many substances.

dynamic equilibrium the process of maintaining balance (i.e., equilibrium) through constant change or motion by energy or action (i.e., dynamic).

homeostasis the state of relative dynamic equilibrium within the body's internal environment; a balance that is achieved through the operation of various interrelated physiologic mechanisms.

polarity the interaction between the positively charged end of one molecule and the negatively charged end of another (or the same) molecule.

Transport

Water circulates throughout the body in the form of blood and various other secretions and tissue fluids. In this circulating fluid, the many nutrients, secretions, metabolites (i.e., products formed from metabolism), and other materials can be carried anywhere in the body to meet the needs of all body cells.

Thermoregulation

Water is necessary to help maintain a stable body temperature. As the body temperature rises, we produce sweat that evaporates from the skin, thereby cooling the body.

Lubricant

Water also has a lubricating effect on moving parts of the body. For example, fluid within joints (i.e., synovial fluid) helps to provide smooth movement and prevents damage from constant friction.

BODY WATER REQUIREMENTS

The Dietary Reference Intake (DRI) for water reflects the median total water intake reported by participants in the Third National Health and Nutrition Examination Survey (NHANES). These recommendations include water from beverages and food and are the amounts required to meet the needs of healthy individuals who are relatively sedentary and living in temperate climates.[2] To meet adult fluid needs, the average sedentary woman should consume 2.7 L (91 oz) of total water per day. Because approximately 19% of total water intake comes from food, this leaves 74 oz (approximately 9.25 cups or 2.2 L) of fluids in the form of beverages per day, with the remaining portion provided by food. A sedentary man should aim for 3.7 L (125 oz) of total water per day. Assuming that approximately 0.7 L of water is obtained from food (19%), a man should drink 101 oz (approximately 12.6 cups or 3 L) of fluid in the form of beverages daily.[2] Table 9.1 lists the Adequate Intake (AI) values of fluid for all individuals.

The body's requirement for water varies in accordance with several aspects: environment, activity level, functional losses, metabolic needs, age, and other dietary influences. Modifications to these factors will subsequently alter the individual requirement for fluid intake.

Surrounding Environment

Both the external climate and internal heat produced from physical work can increase the body temperature. Whatever the cause, high body temperature results in water loss through sweat and requires fluid intake for replacement. On the opposite end of the spectrum, cold temperatures and altitude result in elevated respiratory water loss, hypoxia- or cold-induced diuresis, and increased energy expenditure, all of which raise water needs as well.[2]

Activity Level

Heavy work and physical activity increase the water requirement for two reasons: (1) more water is lost in sweat and respiration and (2) more water is necessary for the increased metabolic demands of physical activity.

Fluid intake needs during activity are highly variable and depend on body size, sweat rates, and type of activity. Thus, specific hydration plans should be determined on an individual basis. For the average person, fluid balance through normal dietary intake is sufficient to maintain homeostasis. Athletes may require more specificity to their fluid intake regimen before, during, and after exercise because of prolonged or intense training sessions. Current guidelines recommend that athletes drink between 5 and 10 mL/kg of body weight of fluid at least 2 hours before exercise to ensure euhydration and at least 20 to 24 oz of fluid for every pound of body weight that is lost during exercise.[3] See the For Further Focus box entitled "Hydrating with Water, Sports Drink, or Energy Drink" and Chapter 16 for more information on the fluid needs of athletes.

Table 9.1   Adequate Intake of Water (Liters Per Day)[a]

AGE	MALE			FEMALE		
	FROM FOOD	FROM BEVERAGES	TOTAL WATER	FROM FOOD	FROM BEVERAGES	TOTAL WATER
Birth to 6 months	0.0	0.7	0.7	0.0	0.7	0.7
7 to 12 months	0.2	0.6	0.8	0.2	0.6	0.8
1 to 3 years	0.4	0.9	1.3	0.4	0.9	1.3
4 to 8 years	0.5	1.2	1.7	0.5	1.2	1.7
9 to 13 years	0.6	1.8	2.4	0.5	1.6	2.1
14 to 18 years	0.7	2.6	3.3	0.5	1.8	2.3
>19 years	0.7	3.0	3.7	0.5	2.2	2.7
Pregnancy, 14 to 50 years				0.7	2.3	3.0
Lactation, 14 to 50 years				0.7	3.1	3.8

[a]1 L = 33.8 oz; 1 L = 1.06 qt; 1 cup = 8 oz.
Data from the Food and Nutrition Board. (2004). *Dietary Reference Intakes for water, potassium, sodium, chloride, and sulfate*. Institute of Medicine. Washington, DC: National Academies Press.

For Further Focus

Hydrating with Water, Sports Drink, or Energy Drink

Sports drinks began with a solution called *Gatorade*, a beverage that its developers named for their university's football team. They reasoned that, if they analyzed the sweat of their players, they could then replace the lost minerals and water in a drink that contained some flavoring, coloring, and sugars to make it acceptable; it would taste better and have more benefits than plain water. Although Gatorade proved beneficial for some athletes, most do not need it during general nonendurance exercise.

The ideal fluid to prevent dehydration depends on how demanding the exercise is and how long it lasts. For exercise bouts of less than 90 minutes, physically fit athletes can usually maintain hydration with plain water. However, endurance athletes need both water and fuel (i.e., carbohydrate), especially during hot weather, for exercise lasting more than 60 to 90 minutes. For athletes who lose substantial amounts of water and sodium through sweat, electrolyte replacement is also an important consideration. Although rare, hyponatremia can be fatal. The most common cause of hyponatremia among endurance athletes is excess sodium loss through sweat combined with fluid replacement by plain water. Water dilutes the plasma sodium even more, thereby exacerbating the condition. Thus, experts recommend sports drinks that contain electrolytes, particularly sodium, as well as carbohydrate for athletes participating in endurance or high-intensity exercise lasting over an hour. Because the personal sweat rate and electrolyte concentrations vary considerably, so do the actual amount of electrolytes needed by each athlete.[1]

Other products entering the sports-drink market add large amounts of vitamins and minerals to their solutions. These extra vitamins do not help an athlete's performance. Furthermore, a perspiring athlete could easily consume a megadose of vitamins after drinking four or five bottles of such products on a hot day.

Energy drinks and energy shots have become popular, especially among adolescent and young adult athletes. The potential performance benefit from these products primarily comes from the caffeine and/or carbohydrate content.[2] Because the safety and efficacy of many of the added ingredients, such as taurine, guarana, and gingko biloba, are not well established, and the actual amount of these ingredients contained in the product is typically unknown, athletes are encouraged to use a sports nutrition product with established research, such as traditional sports drinks, to satisfy hydration needs.

Although sports drinks may meet the needs of athletes who are competing in physically demanding endurance events, those who are participating in less demanding sports activities do not require them. Water is the best solution for regular needs, and it costs far less.

REFERENCES

1. McDermott, B. P., et al. (2017). National athletic trainers' association position statement: Fluid replacement for the physically active. *Journal of Athletic Training, 52*(9), 877–895.
2. Souza, D. B., et al. (2017). Acute effects of caffeine-containing energy drinks on physical performance: A systematic review and meta-analysis. *European Journal of Nutrition & Food Safety, 56*(1), 13–27.

Functional Losses

When any disease process interferes with the normal functioning of the body, water requirements are likely affected. For example, with gastrointestinal problems such as prolonged diarrhea, large amounts of water may be lost. Uncontrolled diabetes mellitus causes an excess loss of water through urine because of high blood glucose levels. In such cases, the replacement of lost water and electrolytes is vital to prevent dehydration.

Metabolic Needs

Metabolic processes require water. A general rule is that approximately 1000 mL of water is necessary for the metabolism of every 1000 kcal consumed. Inadequate fluid availability leads to metabolic and functional abnormalities on a cellular level.

Age

Age plays an important role in determining water needs. High fluid intake (via breast milk or breast milk substitute) is critical during infancy because an infant's body content of water is particularly high (approximately 70% to 75% of their total body weight) and because a relatively large amount of this body water is outside of the cells and thus is more easily lost. As body composition changes throughout the life span, so do relative water needs per kilogram of body weight.

Caffeine and Medications

Certain dietary constituents and medications can affect water requirements because of their natural **diuretic** effects. Although the intake of caffeine in high concentrations (≥300 mg) has a minor acute diuretic effect, the end result does not appear to be a loss in total body fluid.[4,5] The metabolism of caffeine varies among individuals; however, the routine intake of caffeine diminishes its influence over time.

Several medications contain diuretics specifically for reducing overall body fluid, as in the case of antihypertensive medications (e.g., furosemide [Lasix], bumetanide [Bumex], spironolactone [Aldactone]). Monitoring individuals who are taking medications that promote water loss for dehydration and electrolyte imbalance, particularly upon beginning the medication, is an important aspect of patient care (see the Drug-Nutrient Interaction box, "Drug Effects on Water and Electrolyte Balance").

DEHYDRATION

Dehydration is the excessive loss of total body water. The percentage of total body weight lost in fluid indicates the relative severity of dehydration. Symptoms are apparent after a 1% to 2% loss of normal weight.

diuretic any substance that induces urination and subsequent fluid loss.

Drug Effects on Water and Electrolyte Balance

Some medications can affect fluid and electrolyte balance. Drugs with anticholinergic properties, such as the antidepressant amitriptyline and the antipsychotic chlorpromazine, may result in a thickening of the saliva and dry mouth. Individuals who are using these medications may need to increase their fluid intake to help alleviate such side effects.

We categorize antidepressants relative to their activity in the brain. Selective serotonin reuptake inhibitors (SSRIs, such as Paxil, Zoloft, Prozac, Celexa), tricyclics, serotonin and norepinephrine reuptake inhibitors (SNRIs, such as Effexor, Cymbalta), and norepinephrine and dopamine reuptake inhibitors (NDRIs, such as Wellbutrin) have oral and gastrointestinal side effects that include taste changes, nausea, vomiting, and dry mouth. Clients can avoid some of the negative side effects by drinking 2 to 3 L of water per day and maintaining a consistent sodium intake.

The adrenal glands release corticosteroids. However, a number of medical conditions require additional exogenous corticosteroid administration. Some examples include inflammation, asthma, arthritis, severe allergies, and intestinal disorders. As a side effect, prescription corticosteroids (e.g., prednisone, methylprednisolone, and hydrocortisone) increase the excretion of several nutrients, including potassium. Clients on long-term corticosteroid treatments should be encouraged to increase their daily intake of fluids and of foods that are good sources of potassium to maintain an adequate body balance.

Loop diuretics (e.g., Lasix) and thiazide diuretics (e.g., hydrochlorothiazide) increase the urinary excretion of fluids, thereby lowering blood volume and treating hypertension. Minerals are lost in the urine along with fluid excretion. Anyone taking these medications should increase the amount of fresh fruits and vegetables in their diets and eat other foods that are good sources of potassium. Although sodium and chloride also are lost in the urine, it is not necessary to increase the intake of these electrolytes, as long as the individual is consuming a normal varied diet.

Potassium-sparing diuretics (e.g., spironolactone) also work to rid the body of excess fluids, but they do so without wasting potassium in the urine. Therefore, clients should be careful to avoid potassium-based salt substitutes so that they can avoid hyperkalemia (i.e., excessively high potassium levels in the blood).

Antipsychotics (e.g., phenothiazines, chlorpromazine) can cause a condition known as *psychogenic polydipsia.* People taking these drugs often experience dry mouth, and they will consume large amounts of water. If their fluid consumption exceeds his or her capacity for excretion, this can result in hyponatremia and water intoxication. Symptoms of water intoxication include vomiting, ataxia, agitation, seizures, and coma.

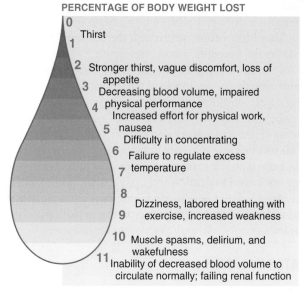

PERCENTAGE OF BODY WEIGHT LOST

0 — Thirst

1

2 — Stronger thirst, vague discomfort, loss of appetite

3 — Decreasing blood volume, impaired physical performance

4 — Increased effort for physical work, nausea

5 — Difficulty in concentrating

6 — Failure to regulate excess temperature

7

8

9 — Dizziness, labored breathing with exercise, increased weakness

10 — Muscle spasms, delirium, and wakefulness

11 — Inability of decreased blood volume to circulate normally; failing renal function

Figure 9.1 Adverse effects of progressive dehydration.

associated with risk factors for several adverse health conditions such as circulatory, urinary tract, gastrointestinal, and neurologic disorders.[6] In addition, dehydration may adversely influence cognitive function, fatigue, and mood at levels as low as 1% body mass loss.[7] Without correction, dehydration can advance to coma and death (Figure 9.1). A fluid loss of more than 10% of body weight typically requires medical assistance for a complete recovery.

Dehydration presents special concerns among elderly adults. The hypothalamus is the regulatory center for thirst, hunger, body temperature, water balance, and blood pressure. Age-associated physiologic changes to the hypothalamus and renal system, such as an increase in urine volume and decrease in fluid resorption, coupled with a decline in fluid intake, make this population vulnerable to chronic hypohydration.[8] Although elderly individuals exhibit an overall decreased thirst sensation and desire to consume fluid when they are dehydrated compared with younger adults, all mechanisms involved in perceptions of thirst are not yet clearly defined.[8] Although a reduced thirst sensation does not always constitute a state of dehydration, it does slow the process of rehydration.

WATER INTOXICATION

Although not common, water intoxication from overconsumption can happen. The excessive intake of plain water may result in the dangerous condition of hyponatremia (i.e., low serum sodium levels of less than 136 mEq/L). Under normal situations, increased urinary output rids the body of surplus water consumed, and this is not likely to pose a problem for a healthy person who is eating an otherwise typical diet. However, individuals with psychiatric disorders such as psychogenic **polydipsia** may consume an excess of water at such a rapid rate that the body cannot correct for the

Initial symptoms include thirst, headache, decreased urine output, dry mouth, and dizziness. As the condition worsens, symptoms can progress to visual impairment, hypotension, anorexia, muscle weakness, kidney failure, and seizures. Chronic or severe dehydration is

acute dilution of blood and ensuing hyponatremia. If the patient does not receive immediate medical attention, they may progress through the subsequent stages of delirium, seizures, coma, and death.[9,10]

As blood volume is diluted with excess water, the water moves to the intracellular fluid (ICF) spaces to reestablish equilibrium with sodium concentrations, thereby diluting ICF as well. This movement causes edema (Figure 9.2), lung congestion, and muscle weakness. Individuals who are most at risk for hyponatremia from water intoxication are infants and children (if they are forced to drink water), psychiatric patients with polydipsia, patients who are taking psychotropic drugs, and individuals who are participating in prolonged endurance events without electrolyte replacement.[2]

WATER BALANCE

BODY WATER: THE SOLVENT

Distribution

Body water content normally ranges from 45% to 75% of the total body weight. The relative amount of body water will change throughout the life cycle with the highest levels occurring during infancy and the lowest levels occurring during the advanced years (Table 9.2). Men usually have about 10% more body water than women do for an average of 60% and 50% of total body weight, respectively. Differences are generally attributable to a higher ratio of muscle to fat mass in males. Muscle contains significantly more water compared with adipose tissue. Thus, the more muscle mass and less fat mass a person has, the higher the person's total body water percentage will be. With that in mind, it is very possible that a muscular woman with low body fat would have a higher total body water content than a man of similar weight having less lean tissue and more fat mass.

There are two major compartments of total body water (Figure 9.3).

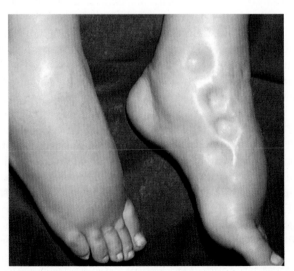

Figure 9.2 Edema. Note the finger-shaped depressions that do not rapidly refill after an examiner has exerted pressure. (From Bloom, A., & Ireland, J. [1992]. *Color atlas of diabetes* [2nd ed.]. St. Louis: Mosby.)

Extracellular fluid. *Extracellular fluid* (ECF) is the total body water outside of the cell. This water collectively makes up approximately 20% of the total body weight and 34% of the total body water. One fourth of the ECF is contained in the blood plasma or the intravascular compartment. The remaining ECF is composed of the following: (1) water that surrounds the cells and bathes the tissues (i.e., interstitial fluid); (2) water within the lymphatic circulation; and (3) water that is moving through the body in various tissue secretions (i.e., transcellular fluid).

Interstitial fluid circulation helps with the movement of materials in and out of body cells. Transcellular fluid is the smallest component of ECF (i.e., approximately 2.5% of total body water). Transcellular fluid consists of water within the gastrointestinal tract, cerebrospinal fluid, ocular and joint fluid, and urine within the bladder.

Intracellular fluid. *Intracellular fluid* is the total body water inside cells. This water collectively amounts to about twice the amount of water that is outside of the cells, thus making up approximately 35% to 45% of total body weight and two thirds of total body water.

Table 9.2 presents the relative amounts of water in the different body water compartments.

Overall Water Balance

Mechanisms such as thirst and hormone levels control how much water enters and leaves the body by various routes. The average adult metabolizes 2.5 to 3 L of water per day.

Water intake. Water enters the body in three main forms: (1) water in liquids; (2) water in foods; and (3) as

Table 9.2	Approximate Volumes of Body Fluid Compartments as a Percentage of Body Weight		
BODY FLUID	**INFANT**	**ADULT MALE**	**ADULT FEMALE**
Extracellular fluid			
Plasma	4	4	4
Interstitial fluid	26	16	11
Intracellular fluid	45	40	35
Total	**75**	**60**	**50**

(Copyright JupiterImages Corp.)

Reprinted from Patton, K. T., & Thibodeau, G. A. (2016). *Anatomy & physiology* (9th ed.). St. Louis: Mosby. Illustration copyright Rolin Graphics.

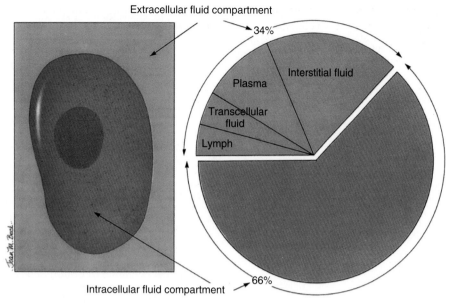

Figure 9.3   The distribution of total body water. (From Thibodeau, G. A., & Patton, K. T. [2010]. *Anatomy & physiology* [7th ed.]. St. Louis: Mosby.)

a product of cell oxidation when the body burns macronutrients for energy (i.e., metabolic water or "water of oxidation") (Figure 9.4). Table 9.3 provides the relative water content of a variety of foods.

Older adults are at higher risk for dehydration because of inadequate intake and the physiologic changes that are associated with aging. **Xerostomia** is one such physiologic condition that is more common in the geriatric population. A severe reduction in the flow of saliva negatively affects food intake as well as oral health in afflicted individuals. Xerostomia is also associated with the use of certain medications, with certain diseases or conditions, and with radiation therapy of the head and neck.[11] Conscious attention to adequate fluid intake is an important part of health maintenance and care. Fluid intake should not depend exclusively on thirst, because the thirst sensation is an indicator of present dehydration rather than an advanced warning.

Water output. Water leaves the body through the kidneys, skin, lungs, and feces (see Figure 9.4). Of these output routes, the largest amount of water exits through the kidneys. We must excrete some fluid daily as urine to rid the body of metabolic waste. This is referred to as *obligatory water loss,* because it is compulsory for survival. The kidneys may also process and release additional water each day, depending on body activities, needs, and intake. This additional water output varies in accordance with the climate, the physical activity level, and the individual's intake. On average, the daily water output from the body matches the intake of water (see Table 9.4).

SOLUTE PARTICLES IN SOLUTION

The solutes in body water are composed of a variety of particles in varying concentrations. Two main types of particles control water balance in the body: electrolytes and plasma proteins.

Electrolytes

Electrolytes are small inorganic substances (i.e., either single-mineral elements or small compounds) that can dissociate or break apart in solution and that carry an electrical charge. In any chemical solution, these *ions* are constantly in balance between cations and anions to maintain electrical neutrality.

Cations. Cations are ions that carry a positive charge (e.g., concentrations of sodium [Na^+], potassium [K^+], calcium [Ca^{2+}], and magnesium [Mg^{2+}]).

Anions. Anions are ions that carry a negative charge (e.g., concentrations of chloride [Cl^-], bicarbonate [HCO_3^-], phosphate [PO_4^{3-}], and sulfate [SO_4^{2-}]).

The constant balance between electrolytes—specifically sodium and potassium—maintains the electrochemical and cell membrane potentials. Because of their small size, electrolytes can freely diffuse across most membranes of the body, thereby maintaining a balance between the intracellular and extracellular electrical charge. Because the fluid and electrolyte balances are intimately related, an imbalance in one creates an imbalance in the other.

We measure electrolyte concentrations in body fluids in terms of milliequivalents (mEq). Milliequivalents

polydipsia excessive thirst and drinking.
xerostomia the condition of dry mouth that results from a lack of saliva; saliva production can be hindered by certain diseases (e.g., diabetes, Parkinson's disease) and by some prescription and over-the-counter medications.

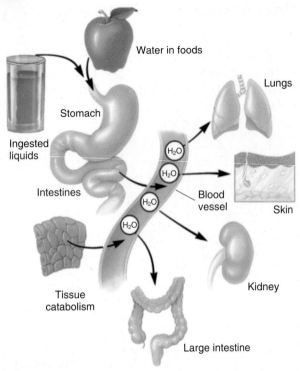

Figure 9.4 Sources of fluid intake and output. (From Thibodeau, G. A., & Patton, K. T. [2010]. *Anatomy & physiology* [7th ed.]. St. Louis: Mosby.)

Table 9.3	Water Content of Selected Food
FOOD	**WATER CONTENT (%)**
Apple, raw	86
Banana, raw	75
Bread, whole wheat	39
Broccoli, raw	89
Cantaloupe, raw	90
Carrots, raw	88
Cheese, cheddar, sharp	36
Chicken, roasted	64
Corn, cooked, drained	73
Grapes, raw	81
Lettuce, iceberg	96
Mango, raw	83
Orange, raw	87
Pasta, cooked	62
Peach, raw	89
Pickle	94
Pineapple, raw	86
Potato, baked	75
Squash, summer, cooked	94
Steak, tenderloin, , lean only, cooked	63
Sweet potato, boiled	80
Turkey, light meat, roasted	68

Data from Agricultural Research Service. (2019). *USDA Food Composition Databases*. U.S. Department of Agriculture. Retrieved February 27, 2019, from ndb.nal.usda.gov.

Table 9.4	Average Daily Adult Intake and Output of Water		
INTAKE		**OUTPUT**	
FORM OF WATER	**(mL/day)**	**BODY PART**	**(mL/day)**
Preformed		Lungs	350
In liquids	1500	Skin	
In foods	700	Diffusion	350
Metabolism (i.e., oxidation of food)	200	Sweat	100
		Kidneys	1400
		Anus	200
Total	**2400**	**Total**	**2400**

Modified from Thibodeau, G. A., & Patton, K. T. (2010). *Anatomy & physiology* (7th ed.). St. Louis: Mosby.

Table 9.5	Balance of Cation and Anion Concentrations in Extracellular Fluid and Intracellular Fluid[a]	
ELECTROLYTE	**EXTRACELLULAR FLUID (mEq/L)**	**INTRACELLULAR FLUID (mEq/L)**
Cation		
Na^+	142	35
K^+	5	123
Ca^{2+}	5	15
Mg^{2+}	3	2
Total	**155**	**175**
Anion		
Cl^-	104	5
PO_4^{3-}	2	80
SO_4^{2-}	1	10
Protein	16	70
CO_3^{2-}	27	10
Organic acids	5	
Total	**155**	**175**

[a]This balance maintains electroneutrality within each compartment.

represent the number of ionic charges or electrovalent bonds in a solution. We express the number of milli-equivalents of an ion in a liter of solution as mEq/L. Table 9.5 outlines the balance between cations and anions in the ICF and ECF compartments, which are exactly balanced.

Plasma Proteins

Plasma proteins—mainly in the form of albumin and globulin—are organic compounds of large molecular size. As such, they are too large to move easily across cell membranes the way that electrolytes do. Therefore, plasma proteins stay inside the blood vessels. Because the body has a constant drive for homeostasis, the proteins (primarily albumin) draw water into the vessels to reestablish equilibrium of the solute concentration between the fluid compartments. In this function, plasma proteins (called *colloids*) exert colloidal osmotic pressure (COP) to maintain the integrity of the blood volume. Without the presence of plasma proteins, fluid leaks from the capillaries and accumulates in the intercellular tissue spaces, causing edema (see Figure 9.2). Cellular proteins help guard ICF water in a similar manner.

Small Organic Compounds

In addition to electrolytes and plasma protein, there are other small organic compounds in body water. Their concentration is ordinarily too small to influence shifts of water. However, in some instances, uncharacteristically large concentrations will influence water movement. For example, glucose is a small particle that circulates in body fluids. In the event of uncontrolled diabetes mellitus, the glucose concentration is abnormally high, producing polyuria and body water loss.

SEPARATING MEMBRANES

Two types of membranes separate water throughout the body: capillary membranes and cell membranes.

Capillary Membranes

The walls of capillaries are thin and porous. Therefore, water molecules and small particles, including electrolytes and various nutrient constituents, can move freely through them. However, larger particles such as plasma protein molecules cannot pass through the small pores

---

colloidal osmotic pressure (COP) the fluid pressure that is produced by protein molecules in the plasma and the cell; because proteins are large molecules, they do not pass through the separating membranes of the capillary walls; thus, they remain in their respective compartments and exert a constant osmotic pull that protects vital plasma and cell fluid volumes in these areas.

polyuria excessive urination.

---

of the capillary membrane. These larger molecules remain in the capillary vessel and exert COP to bring water and small molecules back into the capillary.

Cell Membranes

Specially constructed cell membranes protect and nourish the cellular content. Although water is freely permeable, other molecules and ions use channels within the phospholipid bilayer for passage across the membrane. There is high specificity to the molecules allowed to pass through membrane channels. For example, sodium channels only allow sodium to pass, and chloride channels only allow chloride to pass.

FORCES MOVING WATER AND SOLUTES ACROSS MEMBRANES

The maintenance of dynamic equilibrium requires a variety of forces working cooperatively within the cell membrane.

Osmosis

Osmosis is the movement of water molecules from an area with a low solute concentration to an area with a high solute concentration. When solutions of different concentrations exist on either side of selectively permeable membranes, the osmotic pressure moves water across the membrane to help equalize the solutions on either side. Therefore, osmosis can also be defined as the force that moves water molecules from an area of greater concentration of water molecules (i.e., with fewer particles in solution) to an area of lesser concentration of water molecules (i.e., with more particles in solution). Figure 9.5 illustrates how water will move from the 10% glucose solution across the semipermeable membrane to the 20% glucose solution to equalize the solute concentrations. Because the membrane is permeable to glucose, the amount of glucose will also change on either side of the membrane to help establish equilibrium.

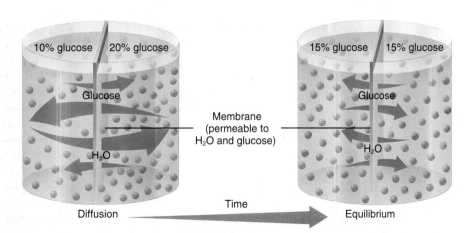

Figure 9.5 Osmosis and diffusion through a membrane. Note that the membrane that separates a 10% glucose solution from a 20% glucose solution allows both glucose and water to pass. The container on the left shows the two solutions separated by the membrane at the start of osmosis and diffusion. The container on the right shows the results of osmosis and diffusion after some time. (From Thibodeau, G. A., & Patton, K. T. [2007]. *Anatomy & physiology* [6th ed.]. St. Louis: Mosby.)

Diffusion

As osmosis applies to water molecules, diffusion applies to the particles in solution. Simple diffusion is the force by which particles move outward in all directions from an area of greater concentration of particles to an area of lesser concentration of particles (see Chapter 5). The relative movement of water molecules and solute particles by osmosis and diffusion effectively balances solution concentrations—and hence pressures—on both sides of the membrane. Again, refer to Figure 9.5, which demonstrates the two balancing forces of osmosis and diffusion.

Facilitated Diffusion

Facilitated diffusion follows the same principles of simple diffusion in that particles passively move down a concentration gradient. The only difference is that, with facilitated diffusion, membrane transporters assist particles with the crossing of the membrane. Some molecules (e.g., glucose) can diffuse across the cell membrane by either simple diffusion or facilitated diffusion, but they move much faster with the help of a transporter.

Filtration

Filtration is another form of a passive transport process in which water and molecules move down a hydrostatic pressure gradient. In this sense, the pores of capillary membranes filter both water and small permeable solute particles from an area of high hydrostatic pressure to an area of low hydrostatic pressure. As fluid pushes against the capillary membrane, the permeable membrane filters the small particles and allows them to cross through the pores. Meanwhile, the larger particles (e.g., protein) remain within the capillary. This way, water and small particles can move back and forth between capillaries and cells according to shifting pressures to establish homeostasis.

Active Transport

Particles in solution that are vital to body processes must move across membranes throughout the body at all times, even when the pressure gradients are against their flow. Thus, energy-driven active transport is necessary to carry these particles "upstream" across separating membranes. Such active transport mechanisms usually require a carrier to help ferry the particles across the membrane (see Chapter 5).

Pinocytosis

Sometimes large particles (e.g., proteins, fats) enter cells by the process of pinocytosis (see Chapter 5, Figure 5.8). In this process, large molecules attach themselves to the cell membrane, whereby the cell engulfs them encased in a vacuole. In this cavity, nutrient particles are carried across the cell membrane and into the cell. Once inside the cell, the vacuole opens, and cell enzymes metabolize the particles. Pinocytosis is one of the mechanisms by which fat is absorbed from the small intestine.

osmosis the passage of a solvent (e.g., water) through a membrane that separates solutions of different concentrations and that tends to equalize the concentration pressures of the solutions on either side of the membrane.
hydrostatic pressure the force exerted by a fluid pushing against a surface.
vacuole a small space or cavity that is formed in the protoplasm of the cell.

CAPILLARY FLUID SHIFT MECHANISM

We have covered the methods by which water and solutes cross membranes to nourish cells. We must now consider the driving force of order for this movement. The capillary fluid shift mechanism uses a combination of the membrane transport methods to perform a balancing act between opposing fluid pressures. It is one of the body's most important controls in maintaining homeostasis throughout the body.

Purpose

Water and other nutrients constantly circulate through the body tissues by way of blood vessels. However, to nourish cells, the water and nutrients must get out of the blood vessels (i.e., the capillaries) and into the cells. Water and cell metabolites, which are the products of metabolism that are leaving the cell, must then get back into the capillaries to circulate throughout the body. In other words, water, nutrients, and oxygen must leave the blood circulation and enter into the tissue circulation to distribute their goods within the cells; at this point, water and cellular waste products (metabolites and carbon dioxide) must leave the blood circulation for disposal through the kidneys and the lungs. The body maintains this constant flow of fluid through the tissues and carries materials to and from the cells by means of hydrostatic pressure and COP.

Process

When blood first enters the capillary system from the larger vessels that come from the heart (i.e., the arterioles), the greater blood pressure from the heart forces water and small particles (e.g., glucose) into the tissues to nourish the cells. This force of blood pressure is an example of hydrostatic pressure. However, plasma protein particles are too large to go through the pores of capillary membranes. When the circulating tissue fluids are ready to reenter the blood capillaries, the initial blood pressure has diminished. The COP of the concentrated protein particles that remain in the capillary vessel is now the greater influence. COP draws water and its metabolites back into the capillary circulation after having served the cells and carries them to larger vessels for circulation back to the heart. A small amount of normal turgor pressure from the resisting tissue of the capillary membrane remains the same and operates throughout the system.

Clinical application. This system is dependent upon adequate plasma protein to exert the required osmotic pressure. Without it, there would not be enough osmotic pressure to pull the fluid back into circulation. This is why protein-energy malnutrition results in edema (see Chapter 4).

ORGAN SYSTEM CIRCULATION

In addition to blood circulation, two other major organ systems help to protect the homeostasis of body water: gastrointestinal circulation and renal circulation.

Gastrointestinal Circulation

Fluid secretions involved with digestion and absorption include saliva, gastric juice, bile, pancreatic juice, and intestinal juice. Of these secretions, all but bile are predominantly water. In the latter portion of the intestine, we reabsorb most of the water and electrolytes into the blood to circulate repeatedly. *Gastrointestinal circulation* refers to the constant movement of a large volume of water and its electrolytes among the blood, the cells, and the gastrointestinal tract. The sheer magnitude of this vital gastrointestinal circulation, as shown in Table 9.6, indicates the significance of fluid loss from the upper or lower portion of the gastrointestinal tract. The body works continually to preserve the isotonicity of this circulation with the surrounding extracellular fluid.

Law of isotonicity. The gastrointestinal fluids and the blood in circulation are both part of the ECF compartments. These fluids are *isotonic,* which means that they are in a state of equal osmotic pressure from equivalent concentrations of electrolytes and other solute particles. For example, when a person drinks plain water without any solutes or accompanying food, electrolytes and salts enter the intestine from the surrounding blood supply to equalize the pressure and concentration. Likewise, ingesting a concentrated solution of food draws additional water into the intestine from the surrounding blood to dilute the intestinal contents. In each instance, water and electrolytes move among the parts of the ECF compartment to maintain solutions that are isotonic in the gastrointestinal tract with the surrounding fluid (see the Clinical Applications box, "Principles of Oral Rehydration Therapy").

Table 9.6	Approximate Total Volume of Digestive Secretions and Concentration of Electrolytes[a]
SECRETION	**VOLUME (mL)**
Saliva	1500
Gastric secretions	2500
Bile	500
Pancreatic secretions	700
Intestinal secretions	3000
Total	**8200**

[a]As produced over the course of 24 hours by an adult of average size.

Clinical Applications

Principles of Oral Rehydration Therapy

Diarrhea is frequently considered a minor problem in developed countries; however, it is the second leading cause of death worldwide among children younger than 5 years old (pneumonia is the leading cause).[1] Although the vast majority of the deaths from diarrhea are associated with fluid loss, the mere provision of water alone can be dangerous. The principles of electrolyte absorption dictate appropriate rehydration methods for children with diarrhea.

First introduced and proved successful in the 1940s, intravenous therapy provided sodium chloride (a base) and potassium in water.[2,3] Unfortunately, intravenous therapy is often not readily available to those who need it most. A large number of isolated, poor, rural families in both developed and developing countries do not have access to health care facilities. Fortunately, the World Health Organization has established a means of oral rehydration therapy that is much less expensive. If safe drinking water is available, a care provider can mix and administer the oral rehydration salt solution packet at home. The ingredients of the oral rehydration packets are based on the principles of sodium absorption in the small intestine and include the following[4]:

2.6 g of sodium chloride (table salt)
1.5 g of potassium chloride (or a salt substitute such as Diamond Crystal or Morton Salt Substitute)
2.9 g of trisodium citrate, dihydrate
13.5 g of glucose, anhydrous
Mixed with 1 L of safe water.
(A premade formula such as Pedialyte [Abbott Laboratories, Abbott Park, IL] is also appropriate.)

TRANSPORT OF METABOLIC COMPOUNDS

A number of metabolic compounds—principally glucose but also certain amino acids, dipeptides, and disaccharides—depend on sodium to allow them to cross the intestinal wall. Similarly, the rate at which sodium is absorbed depends on the presence of substances such as glucose or other protein metabolic products. The more substances that are present, the better will be the absorption of sodium and water.

FEEDING PRACTICES DURING DIARRHEAL DISEASE

In addition to oral rehydration therapy, infants and older children with acute diarrhea should continue to eat well-tolerated foods. Fasting practices based on the former belief that recovery is more effective if the bowel is at rest does not promote healing. To the contrary, feeding children their regular age-appropriate diets (i.e., breast milk, breast milk substitute, or solid foods), based on nutrient needs and deficits, helps restore health and promote recovery. Individual tolerance should guide food choices. The use of the BRAT diet (**b**ananas, **r**ice, **a**pplesauce, and **t**ea or **t**oast) does not encompass the variety of typical foods that infants and small children would consume and only worsens the energy and nutrient deficit.

REFERENCES

1. World Health Organization. (2019, May 17). *Diarrhoeal disease.* www.who.int/en/news-room/fact-sheets/detail/diarrhoeal-disease.
2. Darrow, D. C. (1946). The retention of electrolyte during recovery from severe dehydration due to diarrhea. *The Journal of Pediatrics, 28,* 515–540.

Continued

Clinical Applications—cont'd

Principles of Oral Rehydration Therapy

3. Darrow, D. C., et al. (1949). Disturbances of water and electrolytes in infantile diarrhea. *Pediatrics*, *3*(2), 129–156.
4. Department of Child and Adolescent Health and Development (CAH). (Ed.). (2006). *Oral rehydration salts: Production of the new ORS*. World Health Organization and UNICEF. Geneva, Switzerland: World Health Organization.

Clinical application. Because of the large amounts of water and electrolytes involved, fluid losses via the upper or lower gastrointestinal tract are the most common cause of clinical hydration and electrolyte complications. Such problems exist, for example, in cases of persistent vomiting or prolonged diarrhea in which the person is unable to replace losses through fluid and food ingestion. Diarrheal disease is the second leading cause of preventable child mortality and morbidity in the world.[12] It is not always possible to replace such losses without medical assistance.

Renal Circulation

The kidney's job is to help maintain appropriate levels of all constituents of the blood. To accomplish this task, the kidneys filter the blood, and then selectively reabsorb water and needed materials for transport throughout the body. The remaining waste products are concentrated and excreted as urine. This continual "laundering" of the blood by the millions of nephrons in the kidneys successfully maintains water and solute balance. When disease occurs in the kidneys and this filtration process does not operate normally, fluid and solute imbalances occur (see Chapter 21).

HORMONAL CONTROLS

Two hormonal systems help to maintain constant body water balance.

Antidiuretic Hormone Mechanism

The antidiuretic hormone (ADH) mechanism is a first-line defense against **hypovolemia**. The hypothalamus synthesizes ADH, also known as **vasopressin**, and the pituitary gland stores it for release when indicated. ADH conserves water by signaling the kidneys' nephrons to increase the reabsorption of water. In any stressful situation with a threatened or real loss of body water, release of this hormone will rapidly conserve body water to reestablish the normal blood volume and osmotic pressure (Figure 9.6).

Renin-Angiotensin-Aldosterone System

The renin-angiotensin-aldosterone system is a complex system that corrects for hypovolemia through a negative feedback mechanism. It works to increase blood volume slowly by reabsorbing sodium in the kidneys, which in turn increases water retention. There

are many checks and balances within this system to ensure activation is essential.

As blood flow volume through the kidneys drops below normal, the kidneys release the enzyme **renin** into the blood. Renin converts **angiotensinogen** to **angiotensin I**. As the blood flows through the lungs, an enzyme found on the capillaries, called **angiotensin-converting enzyme (ACE)**, converts angiotensin I into **angiotensin II**. Angiotensin II does several things: it increases the release of ADH from the pituitary gland, it leads to vasoconstriction, and it circulates to the adrenal glands (located on top of each kidney) where it triggers the release of **aldosterone**. Aldosterone then stimulates the kidneys' nephrons to reabsorb sodium (Figure 9.7). Therefore, the renin-angiotensin-aldosterone system is primarily a sodium-conserving mechanism, but it also exerts a secondary control over water reabsorption, because water follows sodium.

ACID-BASE BALANCE

Tight control of body fluid pH is critical for life. Chemical and physiologic buffer systems preserve this balance.

ACIDS AND BASES

The concept of acids and bases relates to hydrogen ion concentration. The abbreviation *pH* is a mathematical term that refers to the power of the hydrogen ion concentration denoting the level of acidity. A pH of 7 is the neutral point between an acid and a base. Because pH is a negative mathematic factor, the higher the

hypovolemia low blood volume.

vasopressin a hormone of the pituitary gland that acts on the distal nephron tubule to conserve water by reabsorption; also known as *antidiuretic hormone*.

renin an enzyme released from the kidney in response to hypovolemia; it converts angiotensinogen to angiotensin I.

angiotensinogen an inactive enzyme produced by the liver that circulates within the blood at all times.

angiotensin I an inactive peptide hormone that is the precursor to angiotensin II.

angiotensin-converting enzyme (ACE) the enzyme found on the capillary walls within the lungs that converts angiotensin I to angiotensin II. ACE is also present to a lesser extent in the endothelial cells and the epithelial cells within the kidneys.

angiotensin II an active hormone that constricts blood vessels and stimulates the release of aldosterone. Both actions lead to an increase in blood pressure.

aldosterone a hormone of the adrenal glands that acts on the distal nephron tubule to stimulate the reabsorption of sodium in an ion exchange with potassium; the aldosterone mechanism is essentially a sodium-conserving mechanism, but it also indirectly conserves water, because water absorption follows sodium resorption.

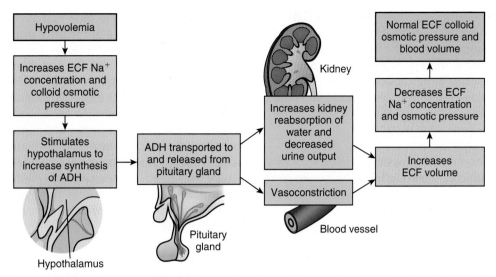

Figure 9.6 The antidiuretic hormone *(ADH)* mechanism. The ADH mechanism helps to maintain the homeostasis of extracellular fluid *(ECF)* colloid osmotic pressure by regulating its volume and electrolyte concentration.

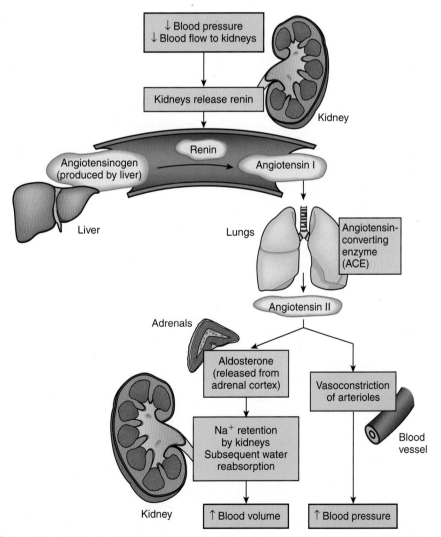

Figure 9.7 The renin-angiotensin-aldosterone mechanism. The renin-angiotensin-aldosterone mechanism restores normal extracellular fluid *(ECF)* volume when that volume decreases to less than normal by retaining sodium and water in the kidneys and by promoting vasoconstriction.

hydrogen ion concentration (i.e., the more acid), the lower the pH number. Conversely, the lower the hydrogen ion concentration (i.e., the less acid), the higher the pH number. Substances with a pH of less than 7 are acidic, and substances with a pH of more than 7 are alkaline. Box 9.1 lists various sources of acids and bases found in the body.

Acids

An acid is a compound that has more hydrogen ions and thus is capable of releasing extra hydrogen ions when it is in solution.

Bases

A base is a compound that has fewer hydrogen ions. Thus, in solution, it accepts hydrogen ions, thereby effectively reducing the solution's acidity.

Acids and bases are the normal by-products of nutrient absorption and metabolism. As such, mechanisms to reestablish equilibrium within the body are constantly at work.

BUFFER SYSTEMS

The body deals with degrees of acidity by maintaining buffer systems to handle an excess of either acid or base. The human body contains many buffer systems, because only a relatively narrow range of pH (i.e., 7.35 to 7.45) is compatible with life.

Chemical Buffer System

A chemical buffer system is a mixture of acidic and alkaline components. It involves an acid and a base partner that together protect a solution from wide variations in its pH. For example, with the addition of a strong acid to a buffered solution, the base partner reacts with the acid to form a weaker acid. If a solution gains a strong base, the acid partner combines with it to form a weaker base. The carbonic acid (H_2CO_3)/bicarbonate ($NaHCO_3$) buffer system is the body's main buffer system for the following reasons.

Available materials. The raw materials for producing carbonic acid (H_2CO_3) are readily available: these are water (H_2O) and carbon dioxide (CO_2).

Base-to-acid ratio. The bicarbonate buffer system is able to maintain this essential degree of acidity in the body fluids because the bicarbonate (base) is approximately 20 times more abundant than the carbonic acid. This 20:1 ratio is maintained even though the absolute amounts of the two partners may fluctuate during adjustment periods. Whether or not additional base or acid enters the system, as long as the 20:1 ratio is maintained, over time, the ECF pH is held constant.

Physiologic Buffer Systems

When chemical buffers cannot reestablish equilibrium, the respiratory and renal systems contribute to the efforts.

Respiratory control of pH. With every breath, CO_2 (an acid) leaves the body. Therefore, changes in respiration rates can either increase or decrease the loss of acids. Hyperventilation (i.e., increasing the depth and rate of breathing) increases the release of CO_2, thereby combating **acidosis**. Conversely, hypoventilation (i.e., slowing down the depth and pace of breathing) retains CO_2, which ultimately increases the acidity of blood to alleviate **alkalosis**.

Urinary control of pH. In the event that chemical buffer systems and the respiratory buffer system do not reestablish blood pH, the kidneys can adapt by excreting more or less hydrogen ions. If blood pH is too acidic, the kidneys will accept more hydrogen ions from the blood in exchange for a sodium ion. Because sodium ions are basic, blood is losing an acid (i.e., H^+) while gaining a base, thereby increasing blood pH back to normal.

Chemical and physiologic buffer systems are crucial for maintaining the blood pH within an acceptable range for life.

Box **9.1**   Sources of Acids and Bases

ACIDS
Carbonic acid and lactic acid: the aerobic and anaerobic metabolism of glucose
Sulfuric acid: the oxidation of sulfur-containing amino acids
Phosphoric acid: the oxidation of phosphoproteins for energy
Ketone bodies: the incomplete oxidation of fat for energy
Minerals: chlorine, sulfur, and phosphorus

BASES (CONSUMED IN DIET OR SUPPLEMENT FORM)
Sodium bicarbonate
Calcium carbonate
Minerals: potassium, calcium, sodium, and magnesium

---

acidosis a blood pH of less than 7.35; respiratory acidosis is caused by an accumulation of carbon dioxide (an acid); metabolic acidosis may be caused by a variety of conditions that result in the excess accumulation of acids in the body or by a significant loss of bicarbonate (a base).

alkalosis a blood pH of more than 7.45; respiratory alkalosis is caused by hyperventilation and an excess loss of carbon dioxide; metabolic alkalosis is seen with extensive vomiting, in which a significant amount of hydrochloric acid is lost and bicarbonate (a base) is secreted.

Putting It All Together

Summary

- The human body is approximately 45% to 75% water. The primary functions of body water are to provide the water environment that is necessary for cell work, to act as a transporter, to control body temperature, and to lubricate moving parts.
- Body water is distributed in two collective body water compartments: ICF and ECF. The water inside of the cells is the larger portion. The water outside of the cells consists of the fluid that is in spaces between cells (e.g., interstitial and lymph fluid), blood plasma, secretions in transit (e.g., the gastrointestinal circulation), and a smaller amount of fluid in cartilage and bone.
- Fluid intake and output maintains the overall water balance of the body.
- Electrolytes and plasma proteins are the two types of solute particles that control the distribution of body water. These solute particles influence the movement of water across cell or capillary membranes, thereby allowing for the tissue circulation that is necessary to nourish cells.
- The acid-base buffer system (primarily controlled by the lungs and kidneys) makes use of electrolytes and hydrogen ions to maintain a normal ECF pH of approximately 7.4. This pH level is necessary to sustain life.

Chapter Review Questions

See answers in Appendix A.

1. Elderly adults may be more at risk for dehydration than young adults because of a(n) _____.

   a. inability to dilute urine
   b. decreased serum glucose levels
   c. decreased thirst sensation
   d. poor intestinal fluid absorption

2. The easiest way to measure fluid loss during a day of hard physical labor in a hot climate is to _____.

   a. measure and compare fluid intake and urine output
   b. measure blood pressure throughout the day
   c. determine serum sodium levels before and after work
   d. measure body weight at the beginning and at the end of the day

3. A man with uncontrolled diabetes who is experiencing a high serum blood glucose level may present to the clinic with _____.

   a. polyuria
   b. anuria
   c. oliguria
   d. dysuria

4. Substances that work with electrolytes to help maintain body fluid balance include _____.

   a. dietary fiber
   b. plasma proteins
   c. blood hemoglobin
   d. vitamin C

5. The main electrolyte that surrounds the outside of the cells is _____.

   a. sodium
   b. calcium
   c. potassium
   d. calcium

Next-Generation NCLEX® Examination-style Case Study

See answers in Appendix A.

A 45-year-old female successfully completed a marathon last week. She trained for the race for 3 months. After the race, she began to feel lightheaded, vomited, and had a splitting headache. She visited a health care tent after the race. Her skin feels dry and her lips are chapped. She is currently taking an antidiuretic for hypertension, and Prozac for depression. She occasionally takes aspirin to manage pain and antacids for indigestion. Before the race, she weighed 125 lbs., but after the race, she weighed 121 lbs. She does not drink or eat before running because she gets too nervous. She drinks very little water during the race as well.

1. From the list below, select all factors that are of nutritional concern regarding the client.

   a. Medications
   b. Age
   c. Weight loss
   d. Fluid intake
   e. Food intake
   f. Exercise intensity

2. Choose the *most likely* options for the information missing from the statements below by selecting from the list of options provided.

   Diuretics and _____ increase the fluid needs of the client, and failure to consume enough fluids during exercise will mostly lead to _____.

OPTIONS	
antacids	hyponatremia
aspirin	dehydration
antidepressants	edema

3. Match the most appropriate nursing response option (provided below) to each client question.

CLIENT QUESTIONS	APPROPRIATE NURSE'S RESPONSE FOR EACH CLIENT QUESTION
"Where else in my diet can I get fluids?"	
"If I don't use the bathroom as much, I probably don't lose as much water. Is that true?"	
"Can I still exercise if I am taking diuretics and antidepressants?"	
"How often should I drink water?"	
"How much water should I drink two hours before exercise?"	
"How much water should I drink after exercise?"	
"Should I worry about dehydration if I lose a small amount of weight after a workout?"	

Nurse's Response Options

a. "5 to 10 ml/kg of fluid would be appropriate during that time."
b. "You should try to drink 20 to 24 oz for every pound of weight lost."
c. "You won't show symptoms of dehydration until losing more than 1% to 2% of regular body weight."
d. "It is important to drink water throughout the day, but especially before and after exercise to maintain fluid balance."
e. "Aside from liquids, foods such as smoothies, fruits, vegetables, and soups also contain fluids."
f. "You will lose fluids through the kidneys, as well as the skin, lungs, and feces."
g. "You will need to drink additional fluid throughout the day to maintain fluid balance while taking these specific medications."
h. "You should drink at least 2 gallons of water every day."
i. "Exercise should be avoided if you are on diuretics or antidepressants."
j. "Any amount of weight loss after a workout is strictly related to fat loss and does not relate to fluid loss."

4. Place an X under the appropriate column to identify health teachings that are <u>indicated</u> (appropriate or necessary) or <u>contraindicated</u> (could be harmful), or <u>nonessential</u> (is not necessary) for the client.

HEALTH TEACHING	INDICATED	CONTRAINDICATED	NONESSENTIAL
Drink 5 to 10 ml/kg of fluid 2 hours before working out and 20 to 24 ml per oz of body weight lost post workout.			
Utilize sports drinks with glucose and electrolytes if exercising for <60 minutes.			
Consume energy drinks that contain taurine, guarana, and gingko biloba during exercise.			
Consume sports drinks with at least 500% of the RDA of most, if not all, vitamins and minerals.			
Sports drinks may be beneficial if exercise is 90 minutes or more.			
Drink 3 to 4 liters of water in 30 minutes during physical activity.			

5. For each assessment finding, place an X under the appropriate column to indicate whether nursing and collaborative interventions were <u>effective</u> (helped to meet expected outcomes), <u>ineffective</u> (did not help to meet expected outcomes), or <u>unrelated</u> (not related to the expected outcomes).

ASSESSMENT FINDING	EFFECTIVE	INEFFECTIVE	UNRELATED
Lost ≤1% of body weight after exercising			
Urinates frequently			
Urine is light yellow			
Skin is moist and buoyant			
Muscles are sore after working out			
Feels sharp pain in foot			
Consumes water before and after race			
Does not consume electrolytes during exercise exceeding 60 minutes			

Additional Learning Resources

Please refer to this text's Evolve website for answers to the Case Study questions:

http://evolve.elsevier.com/Williams/basic/.

References and **Further Reading and Resources** in the back of the book provide additional resources for enhancing knowledge.

10 Nutrition During Pregnancy and Lactation

Stacie Wing-Gaia PhD, RDN

Key Concepts

- The mother's food habits and nutrition status before conception—as well as during pregnancy—influence the outcome of her pregnancy.
- Pregnancy is a prime example of physiologic synergism in which the mother, the placenta, and the fetus collaborate to sustain and nurture new life.

- Through the food that a pregnant woman eats, she provides the nourishment that is required to begin and support fetal growth and development.
- Through her diet and energy stores, a breastfeeding mother continues to provide nutrition to her nursing baby.

The tremendous growth of a baby from the moment of conception to the time of birth depends entirely on nourishment from the mother. The complex process of rapid human growth and lactation demands a significant increase in nutrients from the mother's diet.

This chapter explores the nutrient needs of pregnancy, as well as nutrition-related risk factors and complications. This chapter also discusses the physiologic process and nutrition demands of lactation. The health and wellness of a pregnant or lactating mother imparts a vital role in the health and development of an infant.

NUTRITION DEMANDS OF PREGNANCY

Historically, dietary practices during pregnancy were restrictive with little or no scientific basis. Early obstetricians sometimes recommended semi-starvation of the mother during pregnancy because low weight gain resulted in smaller babies and thus fewer complications associated with larger babies and higher weight gain (i.e., cesarean deliveries and toxemia). For these reasons, pregnant women were encouraged to select a diet that was restricted in kilocalories, protein, water, and salt.[1]

Developments in both nutrition and medical science have since refuted these past practices and have laid the foundation for the promotion of good nutrition in current maternal care. It is now known that both the mother's and the child's health depend on the pregnant woman eating a well-balanced diet with adequate essential nutrients. The 9 months between conception and the birth of a fully formed baby is an extraordinary period of rapid growth and intricate functional development. Such activities require increased energy and nutrient support. General guidelines for these nutrient

needs are provided in the comprehensive Dietary Reference Intakes (DRIs) issued by the National Academy of Sciences.[2–7]

The DRIs specify nutrition recommendations for the healthy populations. Women who are poorly nourished when becoming pregnant or those with additional health risks may require more nutrition support. The *Dietary Guidelines for Americans, 2020–2025* also outline specific recommendations for pregnant and lactating women (Box 10.1).[8] This chapter reviews the basic nutrition needs for the support of a normal pregnancy, with

---

Box 10.1 | *Dietary Guidelines for Americans, 2020–2025* for Specific Populations Regarding Pregnancy and Lactation

- Before becoming pregnant, women are encouraged to achieve and maintain a healthy weight.
- Pregnant women are encouraged to gain weight within the gestational weight gain guidelines.
- Follow the recommendations on the types of nutrient-dense foods and beverages that make up a healthy dietary pattern discussed in Chapter 1.
- Choose foods that supply more readily absorbed heme iron; additional iron sources; and enhancers of iron absorption, such as vitamin C–rich foods.
- Consume 400 to 800 mcg per day of synthetic folic acid from fortified foods or supplements in addition to food forms of folate from a varied diet.
- Ensure an adequate dietary intake of choline and iodine.
- Consume 8 to 12 ounces of seafood per week from a variety of seafood types that are lower in methylmercury. (The U.S. Environmental Protection Agency can advise on sources of seafood that are low in methylmercury.)
- Do not drink alcohol while pregnant.

From the U.S. Department of Agriculture and U.S. Department of Health and Human Services. (2020). *Dietary guidelines for Americans, 2020-2025* (9th ed.). www.dietaryguidelines.gov.

emphasis placed on critical energy and macronutrient requirements as well as on key micronutrient needs.

ENERGY NEEDS

Although most nutrient requirements increase with pregnancy, perhaps the most critical is the increase in daily energy needs. The metabolic cost of pregnancy is significant over the course of gestation. The exact energy requirement will vary greatly among women depending on their prepregnancy weight and height, body composition, health status, activity level, and stage of pregnancy.

Reasons for Increased Need

During the second and third trimesters of pregnancy, the mother needs more kilocalories for two general reasons: (1) to supply the increased fuel demanded by the metabolic workload for both the mother and the fetus; and (2) to spare protein for the added tissue-building requirements. Increases in fat and protein synthesis in addition to increased cardiovascular, respiratory, and renal workload result in a substantial increase in basal metabolic rate and need for more kilocalories. For these reasons, the mother must consider the nutrient and energy density of the food in her diet.

Amount of Energy Increase

It is important to understand that the energy required for pregnancy does not equate to "eating for two." In fact, the energy needs of pregnant women remain the same as nonpregnant women during the first trimester of pregnancy. However, energy needs increase by 340 kcal/day during the second trimester and approximately 452 kcal/day during the third trimester, an increase of approximately 15% to 20% above the energy needs of nonpregnant women. [6] It is important for health care professionals to counsel women on how to apply this information. For example, the increased energy needs of a woman during her second trimester of pregnancy can be met by one additional snack per day consisting of a medium banana (105 kcal), an 8-oz serving of whole milk yogurt (138 kcal), and ⅛ cup of mixed nuts (101 kcal). This snack provides 344 kcal, which meets the additional energy needs of the second trimester of pregnancy. Providing examples of exactly what "extra energy needs" means is important so that expecting mothers do not misunderstand the message and assume that they need to "eat for two." Increased complex carbohydrates, monounsaturated fats, and polyunsaturated fats are the preferred sources of energy, especially during late pregnancy and throughout lactation.

Active, large, teenage, or nutritionally deficient pregnant women may require more energy than the standard DRI guidelines. The emphasis should always be on adequate kilocalories to ensure the nutrient and energy needs of a rapidly growing fetus. Sufficient weight gain is vital to a successful pregnancy. Gestational weight gain is a predictor of infant birth weight, and birth weight is associated with body mass index (BMI) later in life (see back cover of text for BMI table).[9] This translates to each end of the spectrum; both too little and too much weight gain during gestation have implications for the overall health of the infant. Inadequate gestational weight gain increases the risk for preterm deliveries, and for low birth weight babies who have increased risks for poor outcome.[10] Conversely, excessive weight gain poses both short-term and potentially long-term complications for the mother and fetus.

CARBOHYDRATE NEEDS

In addition to daily energy needs, carbohydrate needs also increase during pregnancy, but to a lesser extent. The fetus relies primarily on glucose as a fuel source and is therefore important to the development and growth of the fetus. The Acceptable Macronutrient Distribution Range (AMDR) of carbohydrates is 45% to 65% total daily kilocalories, the same range as for nonpregnant adults. However, the absolute minimum daily carbohydrate requirement increases from 130 g/day to 175 g/d to provide additional glucose to fuel both the maternal and fetal brain.[6] Nutrition surveys indicate that pregnant women generally meet these carbohydrate intake requirements.[11] However, the source of the carbohydrates matter. Pregnant women should focus on consuming whole grains, legumes, fruits, and vegetables as their carbohydrate sources in lieu of processed foods with excessive added sugar. Observational studies indicate that women who regularly consume whole grains, fruit, and food sources high in selenium (e.g., legumes) and avoid processed sweets are less likely to have infants that are **small for gestational age (SGA)**.[12,13]

FAT NEEDS

Although the AMDR for fat remains the same during pregnancy (20% to 35% of total daily kilocalories), essential fatty acid requirements increase. The Adequate Intake (AI) for linoleic acid (an omega-6 fatty acid) increases from 12 g/d to 13 g/d and alpha-linolenic acid (ALA; an omega-3 fatty acid) increases from 1.1 g/d to 1.4 g/d.[6] These essential fatty acids are critical components of cell membranes and key regulators of inflammation. Most American diets are high in linoleic diets and low in ALA. Good sources of linoleic acid are corn, safflower, sunflower, and soy oil. Good sources of ALA are flax, chia, canola, walnut, and soybean oil.[14]

Reasons for Increased Need

Alpha-linolenic acid converts to docosahexaenoic acid (DHA) and eicosapentaenoic acid (EPA) within the body, which are necessary for fetal growth and development. EPA is important for regulating inflammation, blood vessel dilation, and blood clotting. DHA is a component of cell membranes and is important for fetal brain and retina development, especially during the third trimester of pregnancy when rapid brain growth occurs.[15] Studies suggest that maternal DHA may influence visual acuity and language development in the infant.[16,17] Only 9% of consumed ALA is converted to DHA and EPA during pregnancy.[18] Thus, pregnant (and lactating women) should regularly consume adequate EPA and DHA.

EPA and DHA Recommendations

The primary food sources of EPA and DHA are fish and seafood. Egg yolks and algae also contain DHA. Currently, there are no DRIs for either EPA or DHA, and recommendations vary between organizations. The Academy of Nutrition and Dietetics recommend adults consume 500 mg/d of EPA and DHA daily.[14] The *Dietary Guidelines for Americans, 2020–2025* and the Environmental Protection Agency recommend 8 to 12 ounces of low-methylmercury seafood per week.[8] Pregnant women should not eat seafood such as swordfish, king mackerel, tilefish, and shark because of high methylmercury levels. The Environmental Protection Agency advisory website contains the most current fish advisories: search "Eating Fish and Shellfish" at www.epa.gov. National Health and Nutrition Examination Survey (NHANES) data indicate that the majority of pregnant women do not meet recommendations for EPA and DHA with a mean intake of only 78.7 mg/d.[15] Pregnant women should therefore be encouraged to consume adequate low-methylmercury fish to meet recommendations and promote fetal growth and development.

PROTEIN NEEDS

Pregnancy is a period of extensive physiologic changes that require tissue accretion for both the mother and the fetus. Protein serves as the building block for this tremendous growth; thus, sufficient protein is necessary for the normal development of the placenta, maternal tissue, and the fetus.

Reasons for Increased Need

Development of the placenta. The placenta is the lifeline of the fetus to the mother. A mature placenta requires sufficient protein for its complete development as a vital and unique organ to sustain, support, and nourish the fetus.

Growth of maternal tissues. To support pregnancy and lactation, the increased development of uterine and breast tissue is required.

Increased maternal blood volume. The mother's plasma volume increases by 40% to 50% during pregnancy. More circulating blood is necessary to nourish the fetus and to support the increased metabolic workload. However, with extra blood volume comes a need for the increased synthesis of blood components, especially hemoglobin and albumin, which are proteins that are vital to pregnancy. An increase in hemoglobin helps to supply oxygen to the growing number of cells.

Meanwhile, albumin production increases to regulate blood volume through osmotic pressure (see Chapter 9). Most women (60% to 75%) will experience some level of edema during the latter part of gestation; however, adequate albumin helps prevent an excessive accumulation of water in tissues.

Amniotic fluid. Amniotic fluid, which contains various proteins, surrounds the fetus during growth and guards it against shock or injury.

Growth of the fetus. The mere increase in size from one cell to millions of cells in a 3.2-kg (7-lb) infant in only 9 months indicates the relatively large amount of protein that is required for such rapid growth.

Amount of Protein Increase

The protein DRI for nonpregnant women is approximately 46 g/day, and the DRI for pregnant women is approximately 71 g/day.[6] This represents an increase of 25 g/day more than the average woman's protein requirement. However, the average *nonpregnant* woman aged 20 to 39 years old in the United States already consumes 73 g of protein per day, which is sufficient for pregnancy.[11] Physically active or a high-risk pregnant women may need additional protein. Thus, individual nutrition counselling for both prepregnancy and pregnancy would be beneficial to help design personalized dietary advice.[19]

Food Sources

Complete protein foods of high biologic value include eggs, milk, beef, poultry, fish, pork, cheese, soy products, and other animal products (e.g., lamb, venison). Other incomplete proteins from plant sources such as legumes and grains contribute additional amounts of amino acids. Protein-rich foods also contribute other nutrients, such as calcium, iron, zinc, and fat-soluble vitamins. The sample food plan in Table 10.1 demonstrates the amount of food from each food group recommended to supply the daily needed nutrients. See Chapter 4 for more information on dietary sources of protein and protein quality.

KEY MICRONUTRIENT NEEDS

Pregnancy requires increased vitamins and minerals to meet the greater structural and metabolic requirements of gestation. The DRI tables are located in Appendix B. Although all nutrients are important for a successful pregnancy, this textbook will focus on only select micronutrients that pose a specific risk for deficiency during pregnancy.

Minerals

Many physiologic and metabolic changes take place during pregnancy. Contrary to popular beliefs, the mother must meet her nutrient needs *before* the placenta meets its nutrient needs and *before* the fetus meets its nutrient needs. Consequently, all nutrients are of

Table 10.1 Daily Food Plan for Pregnant Women[a,b]

	FIRST TRIMESTER *2200 KCAL*	SECOND TRIMESTER *2400 KCAL*	THIRD TRIMESTER *2600 KCAL*
Grains[c]	7 ounces	8 ounces	9 ounces
Vegetables[d]	3 cups	3 cups	3½ cups
Fruits	2 cups	2 cups	2 cups
Milk	3 cups	3 cups	3 cups
Meat and beans	6 ounces	6½ ounces	6½ ounces
Aim for at least this amount of whole grains per day	3½ ounces	4 ounces	4½ ounces
Aim for This Much Weekly			
Dark green vegetables	2 cups	2 cups	2½ cups
Red and orange vegetables	6 cups	6 cups	7 cups
Dry beans and peas	2 cups	2 cups	2½ cups
Starchy vegetables	6 cups	6 cups	7 cups
Other vegetables	5 cups	5 cups	5½ cups
Oils and Discretionary Calories			
Aim for this amount of oils per day	6 teaspoons	7 teaspoons	8 teaspoons
Limit extras (extra fats and sugars) to this amount per day	266 calories	330 calories	362 calories

[a]This particular food plan is based on the average needs of a pregnant woman who is 30 years old, who is 5 feet, 5 inches tall, whose prepregnancy weight was 125 pounds, and who is physically active between 30 and 60 minutes each day. Plans provided by the MyPlate.gov site are specific to each individual woman; however, this is an example for a woman of the described stature and activity level.
[b]These plans are based on 2200-, 2400-, and 2600-calorie food-intake patterns. The recommended nutrient intake increases throughout the pregnancy to meet changing nutrient needs.
[c]Make half of your grains whole.
[d]Vary your veggies.
From the Center for Nutrition Policy and Promotion. (n.d.). *USDA's MyPlate*. U.S. Department of Agriculture. Retrieved April 4, 2019, from www.choosemyplate.gov.

great importance in the maternal diet. **Teratogenic** effects may result from a maternal diet that is deficient in many of the minerals covered in Chapter 8 (e.g., Kestan disease, goiter, cretinism, fetal growth restriction). This text will cover the most common mineral deficiency concerns in the United States.

Calcium. A good supply of calcium—along with phosphorus, magnesium, and vitamin D—is essential for both maternal health and development of fetal bones and teeth. A diet that includes at least 3 cups of milk or milk substitute daily (e.g., calcium-fortified soy milk), calcium-fortified orange juice, generous amounts of green vegetables, and enriched or whole grains usually supplies enough calcium. During pregnancy, physiologic changes occur in the mother's absorption capacity to help meet the needs of some nutrients; for example, calcium absorption doubles during pregnancy.[20] This enhanced bioavailability helps the mother meet her calcium needs as well as those of the growing fetus. However, if calcium intake is insufficient, the mother's bone releases calcium.[20] Calcium supplements are appropriate for cases of poor maternal intake or pregnancies that involve more than one fetus. Because food sources of the two major minerals (i.e., calcium and phosphorus) are similar, a diet that is sufficient in calcium also provides enough phosphorus.

Iron. Iron is particularly important during pregnancy. Iron is essential for the increased hemoglobin synthesis that is required for the greater maternal blood volume as well as for the baby's prenatal storage of iron.

The average intake of iron for women of childbearing age in the United States is 14.5 g/day.[11] However, the current DRI for iron during pregnancy is 27 mg/day, which is significantly more than both a woman's nonpregnant DRI of 18 mg/day and the current average intake.[5] Food contains only small amounts of iron, which is typically not in a readily absorbable form. Similar to calcium, there is an increased absorptive capacity for iron during pregnancy. However, the maternal diet alone rarely meets requirements. Consuming foods that are high in vitamin C in addition to dietary sources of iron enhances the body's ability to absorb and use iron with a low bioavailability (i.e., plant sources of iron). In addition, it is helpful to avoid foods that inhibit iron absorption (e.g., whole-grain cereals, unleavened whole-grain breads, legumes, tea, and coffee) within meals that are high in iron to enhance absorption.

---

small for gestational age (SGA) infant is smaller than a sex-matched and gestational age–matched infant. Birth weight is below the 10th percentile.
teratogenic causing a birth defect.

Because the increased pregnancy requirement for iron is difficult to meet with the typical American diet, pregnant women often take a daily iron supplement. A standard prenatal vitamin contains the RDA for iron and is usually sufficient. Unless diagnosed with iron-deficiency anemia, pregnant women should take no more than the UL of 45 mg/d. Only pregnant women who are experiencing anemia should take a higher dose of iron because iron supplements appear to offer no benefit for women who are not deficient and increase the risk of gastrointestinal side effects. Although the U.S. Preventative Task Force did not find justification for routine iron supplementation or screening, they concluded that there was no harm in pregnant women taking an oral, low-dose (30 mg/day) supplement of iron such as that in a prenatal vitamin.[21] In the United States, Mexican American and non-Hispanic black women have a disproportionate prevalence of iron-deficiency anemia, for which the standard treatment is an oral dose of 60 to 120 mg/day of iron.[22] However, low socioeconomic status is associated with lower iron supplement use.[23] These data combined suggest that encouragement for African-American, Mexican-American, and low-income women to consume adequate iron through diet and supplementation during pregnancy is needed to benefit both the mother and the fetus.

As with most supplemental forms of nutrients, bioavailability is suboptimal compared with food sources; hence, the reinforcement of a balanced diet with ample iron is still important. See Table 8.5 for a list of foods that are high in iron.

Vitamins

The DRIs for pregnant women are slightly higher for most vitamins. As total energy intake increases, so do the nutrients contained in the foods consumed. Therefore, the selection of nutrient-dense foods generally provides the recommended intake for most vitamins.

As with the mineral section, the discussion here is limited to those vitamins that are of specific concern during pregnancy related to inadequate dietary intake. See Chapter 7 for more information on the function of each vitamin.

Folate. Folate is important for both mother and fetus throughout pregnancy. Tetrahydrofolic acid (TH_4) participates in DNA synthesis, cell division, and hemoglobin synthesis. It is particularly relevant during the early periconceptional period (i.e., from approximately 2 months before conception to week 6 of gestation) to ensure adequate nutrient availability in the endometrial lining of the uterus for embryonic tissue development. The neural tube forms during the critical period from 21 to 28 days' gestation, and it grows into the mature infant's spinal column and its network of nerves.

A neural tube defect (NTD) occurs when the neural tube fails to form properly. Full closure of the neural tube requires sufficient folate, possibly because of its role in methylation reactions and/or nucleotide biosynthesis.[24] Genetics and environment also play a role in the development of NTDs. Although folate intake alone does not guarantee a pregnancy will be NTD-free, there is enough evidence to support the use of folate supplements and/or food fortification to reduce the overall occurrence. As evidence, countries with mandatory folic acid fortification have lower NTD rates than countries with no or voluntary folic acid fortification policies.[25] NHANES data revealed that 50% of women who received folic acid only from enriched cereal grain products did not meet folic acid recommendations.[26] Thus, it is likely that a combination of foods high in folate, fortified foods, and folic acid supplements are necessary for women to meet folate recommendations to decrease the risk of NTDs.

Spina bifida and *anencephaly* are the two most common forms of NTDs, defined as any malformation of the embryonic brain or spinal cord. Spina bifida occurs when the lower end of the neural tube fails to close (see Figure 7.7). As a result, the spinal cord and backbone do not develop properly. The severity of spina bifida varies in accordance with the size and location of the opening in the spine. Disability ranges from mild to severe, with limited movement and function. Anencephaly occurs when the upper end of the neural tube fails to close. In this case, the brain fails to develop or is entirely absent. Pregnancies affected by anencephaly usually end in miscarriages or death soon after delivery.

The current DRIs recommend a daily folate intake of 600 mcg/day during pregnancy and 400 mcg/day for nonpregnant women during their childbearing years.[3] Women who are unable to achieve such dietary recommendations by eating foods that are fortified with folate may do so with a dietary supplement. All enriched flour and grain products, as well as fortified cereals, contain a well-absorbable form of folic acid. Other natural sources of folate include liver, legumes (e.g., pinto beans, black beans, kidney beans), orange juice, asparagus, and broccoli (see Table 7.11 for additional food sources of folate).

Vitamin D. As was mentioned in Chapter 7, vitamin D deficiency is a common worldwide problem, including among pregnant women. Vitamin D deficiency during pregnancy may be associated with adverse outcomes for both the mother and the fetus, including miscarriage, preeclampsia, gestational diabetes, and preterm birth. However, research studies investigating the connection between vitamin D deficiency and such pregnancy complications are contradictory.[27]

The current DRIs recommend pregnant and lactating women consume 15 mcg/d (600 IU) of vitamin D to ensure the absorption and use of calcium and phosphorus for fetal bone growth.[2] These needs can be met by the mother's intake of at least 3 cups of fortified milk (or milk substitute) in her daily food plan. Fortified milk contains 10 mcg (400 IU) of cholecalciferol (i.e., vitamin

D) per quart. The mother's exposure to sunlight increases her endogenous synthesis of vitamin D as well. Lactose-intolerant women or vegetarians can obtain adequate vitamin D from fortified soymilk or rice milk products (see Table 7.2 for additional food sources).

Choline. Although not technically a vitamin, choline is an essential water-soluble nutrient often grouped with the B-complex vitamins because of its various functions. The body makes choline, but only in small amounts. Therefore, it is required in the diet. Choline has many important functions, including phospholipid synthesis, neurotransmitter synthesis (acetylcholine), lipid transport, homocysteine metabolism, and gene expression.[28] Maternal choline intake plays an integral role in placental health, fetus neurodevelopment, and potential long-term cognitive effects (e.g., memory, attention span, and problem solving) through childhood.[28] Further, because of its role in single carbon metabolism (i.e., DNA methylation), insufficient choline is associated with NTDs independent of folate status.[28]

The current AI for choline during pregnancy is 450 mg/d with the AI increasing to 550 mg/d during lactation. Unfortunately, few Americans meet the recommendations, including only 8% of pregnant women.[29] This may be a function of inadequate knowledge regarding this important nutrient. One survey found that only 10% of health professionals and 6% of obstetricians and gynecologists knew about the importance of choline in pregnancy and lactation.[29] Pregnant women should be encouraged to incorporate choline-rich foods in their diet to ensure adequate amounts to support long-term cognitive health of the child. See Table 10.2 for foods rich in choline.

Registered dietitian nutritionists are an excellent resource for pregnant women who need help planning an individualized balanced diet.

WEIGHT GAIN DURING PREGNANCY

Amount and Quality

Appropriate weight gain is a positive reflection of good nutrition status and contributes to a successful pregnancy outcome. Table 10.3 provides an approximation of this weight distribution. The Institute of Medicine recommends setting weight gain goals that consider a woman's prepregnancy nutrition status and her BMI.[20] Table 10.4 provides the recommended total gestational weight gain as well as the average rate of weight gain relative to prepregnancy BMI. It is important to note that women with a high BMI still need to gain weight to support growth and development of the fetus.

Important considerations are the quantity and quality of weight gain as well as the foods consumed to achieve weight gain, which should consist of a nourishing, well-balanced diet. Inappropriate weight gain (i.e., too much or too little) is associated with adverse pregnancy outcomes. Based on a systematic review

Table 10.2	Select Food Sources of Choline	
ITEM	**QUANTITY**	**AMOUNT (MG)**
Beef liver, pan fried	3 oz	356
Egg (with yolk)	1 large	147
Beef top round, braised	3 oz	117
Soybeans, roasted	½ cup	107
Chicken breast, roasted	3 oz	72
Beef, ground, 93% lean meat, broiled	3 oz	72
Fish, cod, Atlantic, cooked	3 oz	71
Mushrooms, shiitake, cooked	½ cup	58
Potatoes, red, backed, flesh and skin	1 large	57
Wheat germ, toasted	1 oz	51
Beans, kidney, canned	½ cup	45
Quinoa, cooked	1 cup	43
Milk, 1% fat	1 cup	43
Yogurt, vanilla, nonfat	1 cup	38
Brussels sprouts, boiled	½ cup	32
Broccoli, chopped, boiled, drained	½ cup	31

Data from the Nutrient Data Laboratory. (2019). *USDA Food Composition Databases.* U.S. Department of Agriculture, Agricultural Research Service. Retrieved May 8, 2019, from ndb.nal.usda.gov/ndb/.

of weight gain in pregnancy, 23% of women gained weight below recommendations, which resulted in an increased risk of SGA and preterm infants. The study also found 47% of women gained more than the weight gain recommendations, which resulted in an increased risk of **macrosomia** and cesarean delivery.[10]

Severe caloric restriction during pregnancy is potentially harmful to the developing fetus and the mother. Such a restricted diet cannot supply all of the energy and nutrients that are essential to the growth process. Thus, it is inadvisable to attempt weight reduction during pregnancy. Special care for pregnant women who are suffering from eating disorders (e.g., anorexia nervosa, bulimia nervosa) is essential for the health of both the mother and the fetus.

Rate of Weight Gain

Approximately 1 to 2 kg (2 to 4 lb) is the average amount of weight gained during the first trimester of pregnancy. Thereafter, the rate of weight gain should be reflective of a woman's prepregnancy BMI. Women with a prepregnancy BMI between 18.5 and 24.9 kg/m^2 generally gain approximately 0.4 kg (14 oz) per week during the remainder of the pregnancy. The rate of weight gain for underweight women should be slightly more than the average. Overweight and

---

macrosomia an abnormally large baby.

Table **10.3**	Approximate Weight Gain Distribution During a Normal Pregnancy	
PRODUCT	**WEIGHT (LB)**	
Fetus	7.5	
Placenta	1.5	
Amniotic fluid	2	
Uterus	2	
Breast tissue	2	
Blood volume increase	3	
Maternal stores: fat, protein, water, and other nutrients	11	
Total	**29**	

9 Months

Full-term pregnant woman.

Reprinted from Lowdermilk, D. L., & Perry, S. E. (2012). *Maternity & women's health care.* (10th ed.). St. Louis: Mosby.

obese women should average a slower rate of weight gain (see Table 10.4).

It is important for health care providers to monitor unusual patterns of weight gain closely. For example, a sudden increase in weight after the 20th week of pregnancy may indicate abnormal edema and impending hypertension. Alternatively, an insufficient or low maternal weight gain is a predictor of SGA infants with increased risks for complications.

DAILY FOOD PLAN

General Plan

Ideally, a pregnant woman will have an individualized food plan established to meet her nutrition needs. This food plan should be a varied and balanced diet including all food groups designed to supply the essential nutrients (see Table 10.1).

Alternative Food Patterns

The food plan provided in Table 10.1 may be only a starting point for women with alternate food patterns. Such food patterns may occur among women with different ethnic backgrounds, belief systems, and lifestyles, thereby making individual diet counseling important. Specific nutrients (not specific foods) are obligatory for successful pregnancies. Eating a variety of foods provides these nutrients. Informed health care providers encourage pregnant women to use foods that meet both their personal and their nutrient needs. For example, vegans can meet their dietary protein needs using soy foods (e.g., tofu, soymilk, soy yogurt, soybeans) and complementary proteins (see Chapter 4 for additional information and resources that address planning a vegetarian diet).

Basic Principles of Diet and Exercise

Regardless the food pattern, two important principles govern the prenatal diet: (1) pregnant women should eat a sufficient quantity of high-quality, nutrient-dense food; and (2) pregnant women should eat regular meals and snacks and avoid fasting and skipping meals. In addition, pregnant women, even those sedentary before pregnancy, are encouraged to exercise. Historically, pregnant women were discouraged from exercising, but now women are encouraged to be physically active during pregnancy. There are numerous benefits to being active during pregnancy (Box 10.2). Pregnant women are encouraged to participate in at least 150 minutes of moderate-intensity aerobic activity spread throughout the week or 30 minutes of moderately intense exercise on most, if not all, days of the week (unless there is a medical reason that prohibits exercise).[19]

GENERAL CONCERNS

GASTROINTESTINAL PROBLEMS

Nausea and Vomiting

Nausea and vomiting affect approximately 50% to 80% of women during early pregnancy in the United States.[30] This can be distressing and disruptive to daily life. For the majority of women experiencing nausea and vomiting, these will persist throughout the entire day. Although often called "morning sickness" (i.e., nausea and vomiting limited to the morning hours), only a small percentage of women experience nausea and vomiting that is limited to the morning.[31] Nausea and vomiting are likely caused by hormonal adaptations to human chorionic gonadotropin (hCG) released from the placenta and elevated estradiol levels.[31] Nausea and vomiting most frequently occur during the first trimester between 6 to 12 weeks and resolve by 20 weeks. For approximately 20% of women, nausea and vomiting continue past 20 weeks but usually resolve by 22 weeks of gestation.[30] In most

Table 10.4   Recommendations for Total Weight Gain and Rate of Weight Gain During Pregnancy, by Prepregnancy BMI

PREPREGNANCY BMI	TOTAL WEIGHT GAIN		RATES OF WEIGHT GAIN[a] 2ND AND 3RD TRIMESTERS	
	RANGE IN KG	RANGE IN LB	MEAN (RANGE) IN KG/WEEK	MEAN (RANGE) IN LB/WEEK
Underweight ($<18.5\,kg/m^2$)	12.5-18	28-40	0.51 (0.44-0.58)	1 (1-1.3)
Normal weight ($18.5-24.9\,kg/m^2$)	11.5-16	25-35[b]	0.42 (0.35-0.50)	1 (0.8-1)
Overweight ($25.0-29.9\,kg/m^2$)	7-11.5	15-25	0.28 (0.23-0.33)	0.6 (0.5-0.7)
Obese ($\geq30.0\,kg/m^2$)	5-9	11-20	0.22 (0.17-0.27)	0.5 (0.4-0.6)

[a]Calculations assume a 0.5-2 kg (1.1-4.4 lb) weight gain in the first trimester.
[b]Normal weight women carrying twins: 37 to 54 lb.
From Rasmussen, K. M., & Yaktine, A. L. (Eds.). (2009). *Weight gain during pregnancy: Reexamining the guidelines.* Washington, DC: National Academies Press.

Box 10.2   Benefits of Exercise During Pregnancy

- Improves or maintains fitness
- Decreases excessive maternal weight gain
- Improves psychological well-being
- Decreases risk of gestational diabetes
- Decreases risk of preeclampsia
- Decreases postpartum recovery time

From the American College of Obstetricians and Gynecologists. (2015, reaffirmed 2017). *Physical activity and exercise during pregnancy and the postpartum period.* Committee Opinion. No. 650.

---

cases it is self-limiting and does not indicate further complication.

To date, there is inadequate evidence to support the efficacy of any particular pharmacologic or nonpharmacologic intervention for the treatment of nausea and vomiting during pregnancy.[30] Pregnant women often use alternative treatments (e.g., acupuncture, acupressure) for the relief of symptoms; however, these methods do not appear to be consistently effective for treating nausea and vomiting in this population. Some studies show improvements in symptoms with the use of ginger and vitamin B_6, although findings are inconsistent and high-quality research is limited.[30-33] Current guidelines from the American College of Obstetricians and Gynecologists recommend vitamin B_6 (pyridoxine) alone or vitamin B_6 plus doxylamine in combination for first-line pharmacotherapy in the treatment of nausea and vomiting associated with pregnancy.[31]

Although the data do not indicate any one treatment will be effective in all women, some dietary and lifestyle interventions may be beneficial. The following dietary actions *may* help with the relief of symptoms.[33]

- Avoid an empty stomach by eating small, frequent meals and snacks that are fairly dry and bland with low fat and low fiber.
- Drink liquids between (rather than with) meals.
- Avoid odors, foods, or supplements that trigger nausea.
- Try ginger (125 to 250 mg) or vitamin B_6 supplements (10 to 25 mg).

If nausea and vomiting persist and become severe and prolonged, an evaluation for **hyperemesis gravidarum** is necessary. This condition frequently requires medical treatment. Approximately 0.3% to 3% of pregnant women develop hyperemesis gravidarum.[33] Women who have experienced this condition with their first pregnancy are at a greater risk for recurrence during additional pregnancies.[33] Hyperemesis gravidarum is the leading cause of hospitalization for pregnant women in their first trimester.[33] Health care providers should closely monitor women with hyperemesis gravidarum for hydration, electrolyte balance, and appropriate weight gain. Compromised pregnancy outcome and fetal growth occur in pregnancies with persistent hyperemesis gravidarum that prevents adequate nutrition and weight gain. Prescription antiemetic medication may benefit some women in this situation (see the Drug-Nutrient Interaction box, "Antiemetic Medications").

 Drug-Nutrient Interaction

Antiemetic Medications

Hyperemesis gravidarum can compromise the nutrition status of both the mother and the fetus because of food aversions or inadequate nutrient intake. Dehydration and electrolyte imbalances are also major concerns. In severe cases, a physician may prescribe an antiemetic medication. Examples include metoclopramide, prochlorperazine, cyclizine, promethazine, and ondansetron. Some nutrition implications of taking antiemetics include dry mouth, loss of appetite, early satiety, diarrhea, abdominal pain, and constipation. Phenergan (promethazine) may increase the client's need for riboflavin.

Health care providers sometimes prescribe one of these same antiemetic medications, Reglan (metoclopramide), to stimulate the secretion of prolactin and thus increase the milk supply during lactation. However, the Food and Drug Administration has not approved Reglan for use during lactation and has published warnings regarding its use. The Academy of Pediatrics has approved a similar antiemetic drug, domperidone, for use during breastfeeding.

---

hyperemesis gravidarum a condition that involves prolonged and severe vomiting in pregnant women, with a loss of more than 5% of body weight and the presence of ketonuria, electrolyte disturbances, and dehydration.

Constipation

Although it is usually a minor complaint, constipation may occur during the latter part of pregnancy because of the increasing pressure of the enlarging uterus and the muscle-relaxing effect of progesterone on the gastrointestinal tract, thereby reducing normal peristalsis. Helpful remedies include adequate exercise, increased fluid intake, and consumption of high-fiber foods such as whole grains, vegetables, dried fruits (especially prunes and figs), and other fruits and juices. Pregnant women should avoid artificial and herbal laxatives.

Hemorrhoids

Hemorrhoids are enlarged veins in the anus that often protrude through the anal sphincter, and they are most common during the latter part of pregnancy. The increased weight of the baby and the downward pressure that this weight produces can cause vein enlargement. Hemorrhoids may cause considerable discomfort, burning, and itching; they may even rupture and bleed under the pressure of a bowel movement, thereby causing the mother anxiety. Dietary management for hemorrhoids is the same as that for constipation. Sufficient rest during the latter part of the day may also help to relieve some of the downward pressure of the uterus on the lower intestine. Hemorrhoids resolve spontaneously after delivery in many women, in which case long-term treatment is not necessary.

Heartburn

Pregnant women sometimes have heartburn or a "full" feeling. Heartburn occurs especially after meals from the pressure of the enlarging uterus crowding the stomach. Gastric reflux may occur in the lower esophagus, thereby causing irritation and a burning sensation. The full feeling comes from general gastric pressure, the lack of normal space in the area, a large meal, or the formation of gas. Dividing the day's food intake into a series of small meals and avoiding large meals at any time usually help to relieve these issues. Wearing loose fitting clothing may also help with comfort.

HIGH-RISK PREGNANCIES

Identifying Risk Factors

Pregnancy-related deaths claim 18 women out of every 100,000 live births in the U.S with the highest rates found in black women.[34] Therefore, identifying risk factors and addressing them early are critical to the promotion of a healthy pregnancy (see the Clinical Applications box, "Nutrition-Related Risk Factors in Pregnancy" for common nutrition-related risk factors).

To avoid the compounding results of poor nutrition during pregnancy, it is important to identify mothers who are at risk for complications as soon as possible. Health care professionals should not wait for clinical symptoms of poor nutrition to appear. The best approach is to identify poor food patterns and to prevent nutrition problems from emerging. Examples of inadequate dietary patterns for maternal and fetal nutrition are as follows: (1) insufficient food intake; (2) poor food selection; and (3) poor food distribution throughout the day.

 Clinical Applications

Nutrition-Related Risk Factors in Pregnancy

RISK FACTORS AT THE ONSET OF PREGNANCY
- Age: ≤18 years old or ≥35 years old
- Three or more pregnancies during a 2-year period
- History of poor obstetric or fetal outcomes (e.g., preterm birth)
- Poverty, food insecurity, or both
- Overly restrictive or unsafe food habits or eating disorder
- Abuse of tobacco, alcohol, or drugs
- Therapeutic diet that is required for a chronic disorder
- Poorly controlled preexisting condition (e.g., diabetes, hypertension)
- Weight: ≤85% or ≥120% of ideal body weight

RISK FACTORS DURING PREGNANCY
- Anemia: low hemoglobin level (i.e., less than 12 g/dL) or hematocrit level (i.e., less than 34%)
- Inadequate weight gain: any weight loss or weight gain of less than 1 kg (2 lb) per month after the first trimester
- Excessive weight gain: more than 1 kg (2 lb) per week after the first trimester
- Substance abuse (i.e., alcohol, tobacco, drugs)
- Gestational diabetes, hypertensive disorder of pregnancy, hyperemesis gravidarum, pica, or another pregnancy-related condition
- Poor nutrition status, especially involving folic acid, iron, or calcium
- Multifetal gestation

Teenage Pregnancy

Teenage pregnancy rates in the United States are at a record low with an annual rate of 18.8 pregnancies for every 1000 girls between the ages of 15 and 19 years.[35] Teen pregnancy is associated with a high risk for pregnancy complications and poor outcomes, with increased rates of low birth weight, preterm delivery, and infant mortality.[35]

The following problems *may* contribute to pregnancy complications with teens[36]: the physiologic demands of the pregnancy, which compromise the teenager's needs for her own unfinished growth and development; the psychosocial influences of a low income; inadequate diet; and experimentation with alcohol, smoking, and other drugs. Little or no access to appropriate prenatal care may also significantly contribute to a lack of support, including nutrition support, for the pregnancy. Early nutrition intervention is essential for positive pregnancy outcomes. Changes from inconsistent and often poor food patterns of teenagers may be difficult to achieve. Experienced and sensitive health care workers in teen clinics may provide supportive individual and group nutrition counseling for teen mothers.

Recognizing Special Counseling Needs

Every pregnant woman deserves personalized care and support during pregnancy. Women with risk factors such as those in the following discussion have distinct counseling needs. In each case, the clinician must work with the mother in a sensitive and supportive manner to help her develop a healthy food plan that is both practical and nourishing. Health care providers should identify harmful dietary practices (e.g., fad dieting, extreme macrobiotic diets, attempted weight loss) early to mitigate them. In addition to avoiding harmful practices, several topics require sensitive counseling, including those related to age and parity, poor lifestyle habits, and socioeconomic problems.

Age and parity. Pregnancies at either age extreme of the reproductive cycle carry special risks. Adolescent pregnancy has many emotional and nutrition-related risks. Sensitive counseling provides both helpful nutrition information and emotional support in addition to good prenatal care throughout pregnancy. Pregnant women who are 35 years old or older and are having their first child also require special attention. Pregnancy rates among women who are more than 35 years old continue to rise in the United States.[37] These women are at a higher risk for obstetric and perinatal complications such as preeclampsia, gestational diabetes, and cesarean delivery.[38] In addition, women with an extremely high parity rate (i.e., those who have had several pregnancies within a limited number of years) are at an increased risk for poor pregnancy outcomes[39] and additional physical and economic pressures of child care.

Obesity. Obesity presents health concerns at any stage of life, including pregnancy. High prepregnancy maternal BMI as well as excessive gestational weight gain increases the risk for adiposity in the offspring and perhaps the complications associated with obesity later in life.[40] Thus, individual and specific person-centered counseling for pregnant women is ideal to help improve overall pregnancy outcome.[19]

Alcohol. Alcohol use during pregnancy can lead to **fetal alcohol spectrum disorders (FASDs)**, of which **fetal alcohol syndrome (FAS)** is the most severe form (Figure 10.1). Fetal alcohol spectrum disorders comprise the leading causes of *preventable* mental retardation and birth defects in the United States. Despite health messages to avoid alcohol when pregnant, approximately 10% to 15% of women in North America consume alcohol during pregnancy and 3% binge

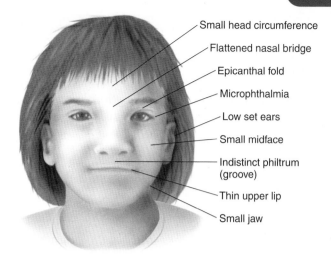

Figure 10.1 Fetal alcohol syndrome. (From Moore, M. [2009]. *Pocket guide to nutritional assessment and care* [6th ed.]. St. Louis: Mosby.)

drink.[41] It is difficult to determine the exact prevalence of FAS; however, one study estimated that 2 per 1000 live births in the United States are affected by FAS.[41] Alcohol is a potent and well-documented **teratogen.** FAS is 100% preventable by abstaining from alcohol during pregnancy.

Nicotine. An estimated 8.8% of pregnant women continue to smoke cigarettes during pregnancy.[42] Maternal cigarette smoking or exposure to secondhand smoke (also known as environmental tobacco smoke) during pregnancy is associated with placental complications (placenta previa and abruption), preterm delivery, fetal growth restriction, fetal brain development, congenital abnormalities, and child psychiatric disorders.[43-47] Maternal smoking is also the strongest modifiable risk factor for sudden infant death syndrome (SIDS).[48] Pregnancy is the leading cause of smoking cessation. Women who stop smoking at the onset of pregnancy have similar pregnancy outcomes as nonsmokers, meaning that they are able to avoid smoking-related complications for their infant by abstaining from smoking and avoiding smoke exposure.[49]

See the Clinical Applications box, "Low Birth Weight Baby" for more information regarding risk factors for fetal growth restriction.

---

fetal alcohol spectrum disorders (FASD) a group of physical and mental birth defects that are found in infants who are born to mothers who used alcohol during pregnancy; the physical and mental disabilities vary in severity; there is no cure.

fetal alcohol syndrome (FAS) a combination of physical and mental birth defects in infants who are born to mothers who used alcohol during pregnancy; this is the most severe of the fetal alcohol spectrum disorders; there is no cure.

teratogen a substance that causes a birth defect.

Low Birth Weight Baby

Infants who weigh less than 2500 g (5 lb, 8 oz) at birth often have medical complications and require special care in the newborn intensive care unit.

RISK FACTORS FOR LOW BIRTH WEIGHT BABIES
- Premature delivery
- Intrauterine growth restriction
- Health complications of the mother, including disease or infection
- Placenta complications
- Maternal use of cigarettes, alcohol, and drugs
- Maternal age (<18 or ≥35 years old)
- Inadequate maternal weight gain and/or poor dietary habits
- Poor socioeconomic factors
- Inadequate or late prenatal care

Drugs. Drug use, whether medicinal or recreational, presents problems for both the mother and the fetus, especially when it involves the use of illicit substances. Drugs cross the placenta and enter the fetal circulation, thereby creating a potential addiction in the unborn child. Globally, cocaine use and methamphetamine use are increasing in the general population.[50] The United States has reached a national crisis with prescription opioid abuse in the general population.[51] These drugs affect both the mother, fetus, and long-term health of the child. Maternal hypertension, placental abruption, preterm birth, cesarean section, mortality, and morbidity are highest with methamphetamine use followed by opioid and other illicit drugs. The effects of these drugs persist beyond pregnancy with impaired cognitive development and poor executive function occurring through adolescence.[50]

Neonatal abstinence syndrome (NAS) is a condition from which the infant suffers after birth because of the abrupt discontinuation of a drug chronically used throughout gestation. Substances that may result in NAS include opioids (heroin, methadone, buprenorphine, and prescription opioid medications), selective serotonin reuptake inhibitors (SSRIs), tricyclic antidepressants, methamphetamines, and inhalants.[51] Dangers come from the drugs themselves, the use of contaminated needles, and the impurities that are contained in illicit substances. Self-medication with over-the-counter drugs also may present adverse effects. Pregnant women should always check the label for safety notices of use during pregnancy or speak with their doctor or pharmacist regarding medications.

Medications made from vitamin A compounds (e.g., retinoids such as isotretinoin, prescribed for severe acne) have caused birth defects and spontaneous abortion of malformed fetuses by women who conceived during acne treatment.[52] Thus, the use of this medication without contraception is contraindicated. Despite the known risks, health care providers still sometimes prescribe these medications to pregnant women, resulting in unfavorable birth outcomes.[52]

Caffeine. Caffeine use is common during pregnancy. Caffeine crosses the placenta and enters fetal circulation. Studies on caffeine use and pregnancy risks have been controversial with conflicting results over the past several decades. The majority of studies support amounts of 300 mg/d or less of caffeine during pregnancy to decrease the risk for congenital malformations, growth restriction, preterm, or spontaneous abortion (miscarriage) associated with higher intakes of caffeine.[53] The use of caffeine and safety during pregnancy is understandably difficult to study.

Pica. Pica is the craving for and the purposeful consumption of nonfood items (e.g., chalk, laundry starch, clay). Pica is more common in children, pregnant women, women from minority racial populations, those malnourished, and those of low socioeconomic status.[54-56] Although the etiology is unknown, pica is significantly associated with iron-deficiency anemia as well as other contributing factors, such as poor zinc status, low calcium intake, hunger, and emotional stress.[56] The practice of eating nonfood substances can introduce pathogens (e.g., bacteria, worms) and inhibit micronutrient absorption, thereby resulting in various nutrient deficiencies. Most clients do not readily report the practice of pica; therefore, practitioners should always ask patients directly about their consumption of any nonfood substance.

Socioeconomic difficulties. Pregnant women who live in low-income situations may benefit from special counseling. Poverty places pregnant women at greater health risk because they often lack resources for adequate food, medical care, and shelter. Registered dietitian nutritionists and social workers on the health care team can provide specialized counseling and referrals. Community resources include programs such as the Special Supplemental Nutrition Program for Women, Infants and Children, known as *WIC*, which has helped to improve the health and well-being of many pregnant and lactating women and their children in the United States. In addition to food vouchers, WIC provides anthropometric and iron status assessment and nutrition education counseling regarding the nutrition needs of both the mothers and their babies (see Chapter 13 for more details).

COMPLICATIONS OF PREGNANCY

For the majority of pregnant women, gestation will progress without complication. However, for others, preexisting health conditions or health problems that develop during the pregnancy will present difficulties throughout gestation. One such example is *hyperemesis gravidarum,* discussed earlier in this chapter. Other issues may affect only the fetus, such as *neural tube defects.* Although there are a large number of conditions that may complicate pregnancy, the discussion here will focus on the more common conditions.

Anemia

Iron-deficiency anemia is the most common nutrient deficiency worldwide and is a risk factor for delivering low birth weight infants.[57-58] Adverse pregnancy outcomes associated with maternal anemia include higher risk of cesarean delivery, blood transfusion, maternal death, preterm birth, and retinopathy of prematurity.[57-59] Approximately 38.2% of pregnant women worldwide experience iron-deficiency anemia (Hb <110 g/dL), with the highest prevalence in (48.7%) in African regions.[60] Anemia is more prevalent among poor women, many of whom live on marginal diets that lack iron-rich foods, but it is not restricted to lower socioeconomic groups.

Improvement of adequate iron intake (through food and supplements) is necessary to avoid the long-term detrimental effects of iron deficiency on the fetus. As a result of the severe complications of iron-deficiency anemia, the World Health Organization currently recommends daily supplementation of 30 to 60 mg elemental iron for 3 consecutive months per year for menstruating women and adolescent girls where the prevalence of anemia is about 40%.[61] For women who are pregnant and non-anemic, the World Health Organization recommends supplementation of 120 mg elemental iron and 2800 mg of folic acid once per week throughout pregnancy.[62]

Intrauterine Growth Restriction

Women with high-risk pregnancies have an elevated risk of intrauterine growth restriction (IUGR). A fetus suffering from IUGR is at risk for fetal brain injury, neurologic disorders, stillbirth, preterm birth, low birth weight, and small for gestational age.[63,64] Approximately 4% of mothers in developed countries and as many as 30% of mothers in developing countries suffer from IUGR.[63] The primary cause of IUGR is placental insufficiency. Many factors contribute to IUGR, but low prepregnancy weight, inadequate weight gain during pregnancy, inadequate folate and iron status, and the use of cigarettes, alcohol, and other drugs are modifiable risk factors. Furthermore, infants who suffer from IUGR are at higher risk for the development of chronic diseases as adults, including cardiovascular disease and hypertension.[64]

Hypertensive Disorders of Pregnancy

The cause of hypertension during pregnancy is unknown, but it is a leading cause of pregnancy-related deaths worldwide. The definition of hypertension is a blood pressure of ≥140 mm Hg systolic or ≥90 mm Hg diastolic. Recently, the American College of Cardiology/American Heart Association Taskforce on Clinical Practice Guidelines for Hypertension lowered the diagnostic values for hypertension to a blood pressure of ≥130 mm Hg systolic and ≥80 mm Hg.[65] However, the newer guidelines exclude pregnancy. Hypertensive disorders of pregnancy include several classifications.[66]

- *Chronic hypertension:* Preexisting hypertension or hypertension that appears before 20 weeks' gestation or persists beyond 12 weeks after delivery. Affects approximately 1% to 5% of all pregnancies.
- *Gestational hypertension (pregnancy-induced hypertension):* High blood pressure diagnosed after 20 weeks' gestation without proteinuria or other diagnostic criteria for preeclampsia. Blood pressure returns to normal within 12 weeks' postpartum. Affects 6% to 17% of all pregnancies.
- *Preeclampsia*: Gestational hypertension with proteinuria (≥300 mg/d of protein in 24-hour urine collection) *or* end-organ dysfunction (e.g., thrombocytopenia, liver and/or renal impairment). Since 2013, proteinuria is not required for preeclampsia diagnosis. Affects 3% to 5% of all pregnancies.
- *Eclampsia:* Preeclampsia with seizures occurring from no other known cause. Eclampsia is most common after 28 weeks' gestation with up to 44% of cases occurring in the postpartum period.
- *Preeclampsia superimposed on chronic hypertension:* Preexisting hypertension with the development of proteinuria or end-organ dysfunction during gestation. Affects 20% to 25% of women with chronic hypertension.

Hypertension is the *silent disease* because it has no symptoms. However, pregnant women should consult with their health care provider if they experience symptoms such as severe headaches, blurred vision, chest pain, nausea, or a sudden weight gain (i.e., edema) because this may indicate hypertension. Specific treatment varies according to individual severity and presentation[67]; however, in any case, optimal nutrition is important, and prompt medical attention is required. Salt restriction is inappropriate because it does not prevent preeclampsia or help to treat the symptoms. An overall healthy diet before and during pregnancy with a high intake of plant foods, antioxidants, and high fiber is thought to be helpful.

Women with mild preexisting hypertension or gestational hypertension, without additional co-morbidities, are usually not at risk for poor pregnancy outcome.[66] Complications from severe hypertensive and preeclampsia/eclampsia often require hospitalization. Advanced cases require induced labor. Preeclampsia is a disorder of the placenta with no known cure. Preeclampsia/eclampsia is associated with poor fetal outcomes such as maternal and fetal morbidity and mortality, IUGR, low birth weight, and preterm delivery.[66] Thus, early and consistent prenatal care is imperative to identify symptoms early.

Gestational Diabetes

Gestational diabetes is glucose intolerance with onset occurring during pregnancy, and the definition

---

intrauterine growth restriction (IUGR) a condition that occurs when a newborn weighs less than 10% of predicted fetal weight for gestational age.

stillbirth the death of a fetus after the 20th week of pregnancy.

applies regardless of whether treatment is medication (e.g., oral hypoglycemic agents, insulin) or only diet modification. Women diagnosed with diabetes during the first trimester (usually by fasting or random blood glucose test) are assumed to have had undiagnosed diabetes before becoming pregnant and are therefore diagnosed with overt diabetes and not gestational diabetes.[68] The treatment for gestational diabetes follows a protocol similar to that for type 2 diabetes, with diet and exercise the first-line treatment.

Prenatal clinics routinely screen pregnant women between 24 and 28 weeks' gestation with either a "One-Step" or a "Two-Step" oral glucose tolerance test for diagnosis (see Chapter 20 for details). Screening is particularly important for women who are at higher risk for the development of gestational diabetes, including those who are 30 years old or older and are overweight (i.e., BMI of ≥ 25 kg/m^2) and who have a history of any of the following predisposing factors:

- Previous history of gestational diabetes
- Family history of diabetes
- Ethnicity associated with a high incidence of diabetes (Asian, Hispanic, African Americans, and Native Americans)
- Glucosuria
- Obesity
- Previous delivery of a large baby weighing 4.5 kg (10 lb) or more

Women with gestational diabetes are at higher risk for caesarean delivery and fetal damage such as birth defects, stillbirth, macrosomia, and neonatal hypoglycemia. Additionally, these women are 20 times more likely to develop type 2 diabetes, 2.8 times more likely to develop ischemic heart disease, and twice as likely to develop hypertension later in life.[69] Therefore, identifying and providing follow-up testing and treatment with a well-balanced diet, regular exercise, and medication (as needed) are important interventions.

Preexisting Disease

Preexisting diseases (e.g., cardiovascular diseases, hypertension, type 1 or type 2 diabetes, human immunodeficiency virus, eating disorders) can cause complications during pregnancy. Inborn errors of metabolism (e.g., phenylketonuria) and food allergies or intolerances (e.g., celiac disease, lactose intolerance) must also be taken into consideration and maintained under good control to mitigate any flare-ups or compromised nutrient intake/absorption.

Pregnant women may have any combination of preexisting conditions. In each case, a team of specialists manages a woman's pregnancy in accordance with the principles of care related to pregnancy and the particular disease involved. See Chapters 18 through 23 for major nutrition-related diseases that require medical nutrition therapy.

LACTATION

Breastfeeding is the ideal or "normal" food for the healthy growth and development of infants.[70] It is recommended to breastfeed for at least 1 year with iron-fortified solid foods added to the exclusive diet of breast milk at about 6 months of age.

TRENDS

Approximately 40% of infants worldwide are **exclusively breastfed** for the first 6 months of life, compared with only 25.6% in the United States.[71,72] Although rates are still low in the United States compared with other countries, breastfeeding has been on the rise in the last few decades (Figure 10.2). Breastfeeding initiation and continuation are highest among well-educated, older women (see the Cultural Considerations box, "Breastfeeding Trends in the United States").

The *Healthy People 2030* initiative lists specific goals to increase the prevalence and duration of breastfeeding in the United States[73]:

- Increase the proportion of infants who are breastfed at 1 year. Target: 54.1%
- Increase the proportion of infants who are breastfed exclusively through 6 months of age. Target: 42.4%

THE BABY-FRIENDLY HOSPITAL INITIATIVE

The World Health Organization and the United Nations Children's Fund launched the Baby-Friendly Hospital Initiative in 1991 to promote breastfeeding worldwide. The Baby-Friendly Hospital Initiative outlines the 10 steps for successful breastfeeding, found in Box 10.3. Almost all women who choose to breastfeed their infants can do so, provided they have the necessary information and support from their family, community, and health care system. Well-nourished mothers who exclusively breastfeed provide adequate

---

"One-Step" a method for diagnosing diabetes using a 75-g oral glucose tolerance test. The patient's fasting plasma glucose level is measured; then the patient drinks a solution with 75 mg of glucose and plasma glucose is measured again at 1-hour and 2-hour post consumption. Diagnostic criteria are based on the levels of plasma glucose at each measurement.

"Two-Step" a method for diagnosing diabetes using a two-step method of oral glucose tolerance test in a non-fasting patient. Step 1: Plasma glucose is measured 1 hour after the patient drinks a 50-g glucose solution. If the patient's plasma glucose level is ≥ 140 g/dL, then the patient must return for Step 2, which is a fasting 100-g glucose tolerance test.

exclusively breastfed feeding the infant only breast milk with no supplemental liquids or solid foods, other than necessary medications or vitamin/mineral supplements.

Percentage of U.S. Children Who Were Breastfed, by Birth Year[a,b]

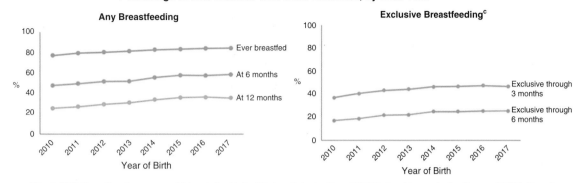

Figure 10.2 Breastfeeding among children in the United States. (Adapted from CDC National Immunization Survey. [2020]. *Breastfeeding among U.S. children born 2010-2017.* Centers for Disease Control and Prevention. Retrieved February 19, 2021, from www.cdc.gov/breastfeeding/data/nis_data/results.html.

[a]Data from 2010 to 2015 births were based on landline and cellular telephone sampling and data for 2016 births and onwards were based on cellular telephone sampling only. See Survey Methods for details and data prior to 2010 at Data, Trends, and Maps.

[b]Data from U.S. territories are excluded from national breastfeeding estimates to be consistent with the analytical methods for the establishment of Healthy People 2020 targets on breastfeeding.

[c]Exclusive breastfeeding is defined as ONLY breast milk—NO solids, water, or other liquids.

 Cultural Considerations

Breastfeeding Trends in the United States

Increasing the prevalence of breastfeeding continues to be a health goal both nationally and internationally. In the United States, 4 out of 5 infants (84.1%) initiate breastfeeding. However, breastfeeding rates at 1 year and exclusively breastfeeding at 6 months do not meet national goals (see map and table below). Breastfeeding is most common among women who have a higher socioeconomic and education level and are at least 30 years old. A higher prevalence of breastfeeding occurs among married women and in the Western states.[1,2]

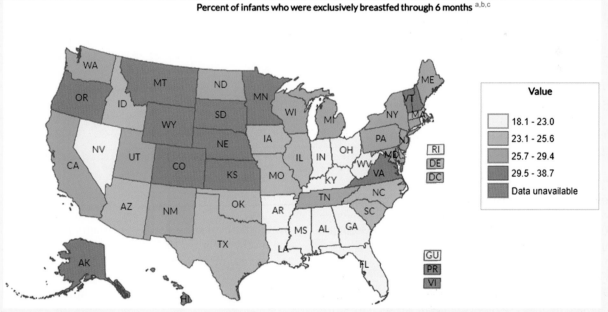

Percent of infants who were exclusively breastfed through 6 months [a,b,c]

Percent of infants exclusively breastfed through 6 months, 2017. (National Center for Chronic Disease Prevention and Health Promotion, Division of Nutrition, Physical Activity, and Obesity. [2021]. *Data, trends and maps.* Centers for Disease Control and Prevention. Retrieved February 19, 2021, from www.cdc.gov/nccdphp/dnpao/data-trends-maps/index.html.

[a]Exclusive breastfeeding is defined as ONLY breast milk—No solids, no water, and no other liquids.
[b]Breastfeeding rates through 2008 births are based on the National Immunization Survey's landline sampling frame. Starting with 2009 births, rates are based on the National Immunization Survey's dual-frame sample that includes respondents surveyed on landline or cellular telephones. If you would like more information about the sampling methodology and the impact of adding a sample of cellular telephone respondents to the National Immunization Survey, available at www.cdc.gov/breastfeeding/data/nis_data/survey_methods.htm.
[c]Only breastfeeding rates based on a dual-frame sample that includes respondents surveyed on landline or cellular telephones are included in trend graphics. If you would like more information about the sampling methodology and the impact of adding a sample of cellular telephone respondents to the National Immunization Survey, available at www.cdc.gov/breastfeeding/data/nis_data/survey_methods.htm.

Continued

🌐 Cultural Considerations—cont'd

Breastfeeding Trends in the United States

PREVALENCE OF BREASTFEEDING IN THE UNITED STATES[2]	
SELECTED CHARACTERISTICS OF MOTHER	PERCENTAGE *EXCLUSIVE* BREASTFEEDING THROUGH 6 MONTHS
Total	25.6
MOTHER'S AGE AT BABY'S BIRTH	
≤20 years	18.7
20 to 29 years	24.2
≥30 years	26.5
RACE OR ETHNICITY	
Non-Hispanic Asian	26.8
Non-Hispanic Black	21.2
Hispanic	21.5
Two or more races	26.6
Non-Hispanic White	28.7

PREVALENCE OF BREASTFEEDING IN THE UNITED STATES	
SELECTED CHARACTERISTICS OF MOTHER	PERCENTAGE *EXCLUSIVE* BREASTFEEDING THROUGH 6 MONTHS
EDUCATION	
Less than high school	17.1
High school graduate	21.5
Some college or technical school	23.3
Collage graduate	32.8
POVERTY INCOME RATIO[d]	
<100%	20.0
100% to 199%	23.8
200% to 399%	28.6
400% to 599%	29.3
≥600%	30.6

As a health care provider, be sure to note the perceived obstacles to the initiation and continuation of breastfeeding so that education and alternatives may be presented at the appropriate time (i.e., before delivery). The American Academy of Pediatrics notes the following potential obstacles[3]:

- Insufficient prenatal education about breastfeeding
- Disruptive hospital policies and practices
- Inappropriate interruption of breastfeeding
- Early hospital discharge in some populations
- Lack of timely routine follow-up care and postpartum home health visits
- Maternal employment (especially in the absence of workplace facilities that support breastfeeding)
- Lack of family and broad societal support
- Media portrayal of bottle-feeding as normal
- Commercial promotion of infant formula through the distribution of hospital discharge packs containing breast milk substitutes

- Coupons for free or discounted formula
- Misinformation about what medical conditions may be contraindications for breastfeeding
- Lack of guidance and encouragement from health care professionals

REFERENCES

1. National Center for Chronic Disease Prevention and Health Promotion, Division of Nutrition, Physical Activity, and Obesity. (2021). *Data, trends and maps.* Centers for Disease Control and Prevention. Retrieved February 19, 2021, from www.cdc.gov/nccdphp/dnpao/data-trends-maps/index.html.
2. National Immunization Survey. (n.d.). Rates of any and exclusive breastfeeding by sociodemographics among children born in 2017 *(percentage +/- half 95% confidence interval)*. Department of Health and Human Services, Centers for Disease Control and Prevention. Retrieved February 19, 2021, from www.cdc.gov/breastfeeding/data/nis_data/rates-any-exclusive-bf-sociodem-2017.html.
3. Gartner, L. M., et al. (2005). Breastfeeding and the use of human milk. *Pediatrics, 115*(2), 496–506.

[d]The poverty income ratio is the self-reported family income compared with the federal poverty threshold value. It depends on the number of people in the household.

nutrition to their infants, as well as other beneficial components (e.g., immunoglobulins, prebiotics).

PHYSIOLOGIC PROCESS OF LACTATION

Mammary Glands and Hormones

The female breasts are highly specialized secretory organs (Figure 10.3). Throughout pregnancy, the mammary glands are preparing for lactation. The mammary glands are capable of extracting certain nutrients from the maternal blood in addition to synthesizing other compounds. The combined effort results in nutrient-complete breast milk.

After the delivery of the baby, the two hormones **prolactin** and **oxytocin** stimulate milk production and secretion, respectively. The stimulation of the nipple from infant suckling sends nerve signals to the brain of the mother (Figure 10.4); this nerve signal then causes the release of prolactin and oxytocin. Let-down is the process of the milk moving from the upper milk-producing cells down to the nipple for infant suckling.

Supply and Demand

Milk production is a supply-and-demand procedure. The mammary glands are stimulated to produce milk each time that the infant feeds. Therefore, the more milk that is removed from the breast (during breastfeeding or pumping), the more milk the mother produces, thereby always meeting the infant's needs. Because of this supply-and-demand production, mothers of multiple infants (e.g., twins, triplets) are able to

Box 10.3 **Ten Steps to Successful Breastfeeding**

1. Have a written breastfeeding policy routinely communicated to all health care staff.
2. Train all health care staff in the skills that are necessary to implement this policy.
3. Inform all pregnant women about the benefits and management of breastfeeding.
4. Help mothers to initiate breastfeeding within 30 minutes after birth.
5. Show mothers how to breastfeed and maintain lactation, even if they may be separated from their infants.
6. Give newborn infants no food or drink other than breast milk unless medically indicated.
7. Practice rooming in: allow mothers and infants to remain together 24 hours a day.
8. Encourage breastfeeding on demand.
9. Give no artificial teats or pacifiers to breastfeeding infants.
10. Foster the establishment of breastfeeding support groups and refer mothers to these groups when discharged from the hospital or clinic.

From the United Nations Children's Fund. (n.d.). *The baby-friendly hospital initiative*. World Health Organization. Retrieved April 12, 2019, from www.unicef.org/programme/breastfeeding/baby.

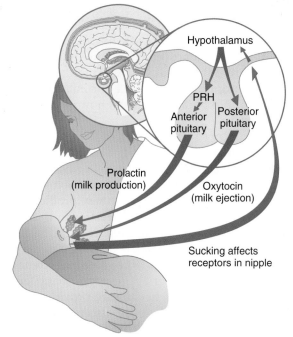

Figure 10.4 Physiology of milk production and the let-down reflex. *PRH*, Prolactin-releasing hormone. (Reprinted from Mahan, L. K., & Escott-Stump, S. [2012]. *Krause's food & nutrition therapy* [13th ed.]. Philadelphia: Saunders.)

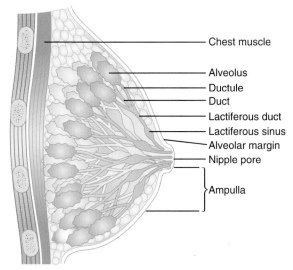

Figure 10.3 Anatomy of the breast. (Reprinted from Mahan, L. K., & Escott-Stump, S. [2008]. *Krause's food & nutrition therapy* [12th ed.]. Philadelphia: Saunders.)

produce more milk with the additional stimulation. The increase in milk supply is not immediate, and often mothers resort to supplementation. Supplementation, especially during early postpartum, disrupts the supply-and-demand process and results in early cessation of breastfeeding.[74,75] Some mothers of multiples choose to pump and then bottle-feed the infants the breast milk so that other members of the family can help with feedings.

Composition

Breast milk changes in composition to meet the specific needs of infants as they grow. **Colostrum** is the first milk that is produced beginning during the third trimester and through the first few days after birth. It is a yellowish fluid rich in antibodies, which gives the infant his or her first immune boost. It also acts as a laxative to remove the meconium (first bowel movement) from the infant. Because colostrum does not look like milk and a mother may not know the importance of colostrum, it is important to reassure the mother that colostrum is the perfect food for the newborn infant and to nurse frequently. Mature breast milk comes in within a few days after delivery but may be delayed more than 72 hours postpartum for women who are obese, used labor pain medications, or experienced a cesarean section.[76,77]

The terms *foremilk, midmilk,* and *hindmilk* reflect the changing milk composition throughout a feeding. Foremilk is high in lactose and low in fat. Too much foremilk from short, frequent feedings resulting in milk oversupply can cause gastrointestinal distress and symptoms similar to reflux in the

prolactin hormone released from the anterior pituitary gland that stimulates milk production.
oxytocin hormone released from the posterior pituitary gland that stimulates milk let-down.
colostrum fluid first secreted by the mammary glands for the first few days after birth, preceding the mature breast milk. Colostrum contains up to 20% protein, including a large amount of lactalbumin, more minerals, and immunoglobulins that represent the antibodies found in maternal blood. It has less lactose and fat than mature milk.

infant.[78] As the breast empties, the milk becomes more concentrated in fat. Hence, hindmilk is a good source of essential fatty acids. As you can see from Table 10.5, the composition of mature human milk is quite different from that of cow's milk. Cow's milk is an inappropriate food source for infants younger than 1 year old because of its high protein and electrolyte levels.

Complications

Although breastfeeding is a natural physiologic process, it is not without complications. Some women find breastfeeding difficult, and these problems rapidly lead to the cessation of breastfeeding. Several barriers to breastfeeding are reported in the literature. In addition to the barriers discussed in the Cultural Considerations box, "Breastfeeding Trends in the United States," hyperlactation, post-natal factors such as C-sections, and health care provider knowledge, attitudes, and beliefs are also factors in early breastfeeding cessation.[79-80]

Physiologic complications can also result from an infants' improper latch. These include sore or cracked nipples, engorgement, and plugged ducts. A trained lactation consultant can help women manage these complications. For the most part, women can avoid complications and successfully breastfeed by having prenatal breastfeeding education, family, and peer support.[81] A thorough understanding of the physiology of lactation and the psychosocial factors influencing the success of breastfeeding are imperative to effectively supporting a nursing mother.

NUTRITION AND LIFESTYLE NEEDS

The basic diet recommended for the mother during pregnancy continues through the lactation period. The MyPlate food guide system provides specific nutrient information for pregnant and lactating women (search "pregnant" or "breastfeeding" at www.choosemyplate.gov). The Daily Food Plan for Moms/Moms-to-be takes into account the mother's age, height, weight, and physical activity level; the infant's age; and the amount of breast milk the mom is producing to offer individualized recommendations. The website also provides help with menu planning for mothers with an easy-to-use interactive site.

Diet

Energy and nutrients. Lactation requires energy for both the process of milk production and the actual milk. The extra fat that is stored in the mother during pregnancy will meet some of the extra energy needs. The increased calorie recommendations are 330 kcal/day (plus 170 kcal/day from maternal stores) during the first 6 months of lactation and 400 kcal/day during the second 6 months of lactation above the woman's nonpregnant, nonlactating energy requirements. The requirement for protein during lactation is 25 g/day more than a woman's average need of 46 g/day, for a total of 71 g/day (approximately 1.1 g/kg body weight per day).[6]

Table 10.1 provides an example of a core food plan for meeting the nutrient needs of pregnant and lactating women. When considering the energy requirement for the development of a zygote to a 7.5-lb infant, it is no surprise that energy intake is a critical part of a healthy pregnancy. Likewise, providing that infant with enough nutrition through exclusive breastfeeding to double his or her birthweight in approximately 5 months will require a substantial amount of energy and nutrients provided by the mother through her diet and stored body fat.

Fluids. Because milk is a fluid, breastfeeding mothers need ample fluids for adequate milk production; their fluid intake should be approximately 3 L/day. Water and other sources of fluid such as juices, milk, and soup contribute to the fluid that is necessary to

| Table 10.5 | Nutrition Composition of Human Milk versus Cow's Milk[a] |

NUTRIENT	HUMAN MILK		COW'S MILK, WHOLE
	COLOSTRUM	MATURE	
Kilocalories	55	73	63
Protein (g)	2.0	1.07	3.25
Carbohydrate (g)[b]	7.4	7.2	4.95
Fat (g)	2.9	4.56	3.35
Fat-Soluble Vitamins			
A (IU)	296	221	167
D (IU)	—	3	53[c]
E (mg)	0.8	0.08	0.07
K (mcg)	—	0.3	0.3
Water-Soluble Vitamins			
Thiamin (mg)	0.02	0.015	0.05
Riboflavin (mg)	0.029	0.037	0.17
Niacin (mg)	0.075	0.18	0.09
Vitamin C (mg)	6	5.2	0
Folate (mcg)	0.05	5	5
Minerals			
Calcium (mg)	31	33	116
Phosphorus (mg)	14	15	87
Iron (mg)	0.09	0.03	0.03
Zinc (mg)	0.5	0.18	0.38
Magnesium (mg)	4.2	3	10
Sodium (mg)	48	18	44
Potassium (mg)	74	53	136

[a]Per 100 mL.
[b]Lactose.
[c]Fortified.

produce milk. Beverages that contain alcohol and caffeine should be limited or timed appropriately (i.e., after a feeding), because these substances pass into the breast milk.

Lifestyle

In addition to the increase in overall diet and fluid intake, lactating mothers require rest, moderate exercise, and relaxation. Because the production and let-down reflexes of lactation are hormonally controlled, negative environmental and psychologic factors may contribute to the early cessation of breastfeeding.[80] Such factors are called *prolactin inhibitors*, and they include stress, fatigue, medical complications, lack of support, poor self-efficacy, and irregular breastfeeding. A lactation specialist can help by counseling mothers about their new family situations and by helping them to develop a plan to meet their personal needs.

LONG-TERM IMPACTS OF FEEDING METHODS

Risks of Using Breast Milk Substitutes

Medical professionals agree that breastfeeding is the normal food for infants and that other feeding methods carry risks for the infant. For decades, the literature has presented many "benefits of breastfeeding." According to the Academy of Pediatrics, the many benefits of breastfeeding are only the normal expectations of infant feeding. In the Academy's view, breastfeeding is not a lifestyle choice, but a public health issue.[70]

Advantages of Breastfeeding

Many physiologic and practical advantages of breastfeeding provide favorable health outcomes for both the mother and infant. Consequently, suboptimal breastfeeding, which includes none, partial, or short-duration breastfeeding, is associated with several health risks for both infant and mother (Box 10.4).

Many of the positive infant outcomes of breastfeeding relate to decreased risk of infection and disease.[82] The antibodies in human milk that pass to the nursing infant make a significant contribution to the infant's immune system. This accounts for the reduced risk of many diseases and infections. In addition, research

indicates that breastfed infants have increased cognitive ability compared with formula-fed infants, despite differences in environments, with a positive relationship seen between the duration of breastfeeding and the intelligence quotient of the child.[82]

The mother receives many health benefits as well. Some noted advantages of breastfeeding for the mother are decreased bleeding; an earlier return to prepregnancy weight; and decreased risks of breast cancer, ovarian cancer, and osteoporosis.[83]

ADDITIONAL RESOURCES

The Academy of Nutrition and Dietetics and the American Academy of Pediatrics encourage and strongly support breastfeeding for all able mothers for the first 12 months of life and continued thereafter for as long as mutually desired.[70,83] The American Academy of Pediatrics keeps updated breastfeeding information available for the public at www.healthychildren.org. A multitude of additional resources about this topic is available from the World Health Organization: search "Breastfeeding" at www.who.int.

Box 10.4	**Risks Associated With Suboptimal Breastfeeding (None, Partial, or Short Duration)**

INFANTS	MOTHERS
• Acute otitis media • Nonspecific gastrointestinal infection • Upper and lower respiratory tract infection • Sudden infant death syndrome • Necrotizing enterocolitis (preterm, low birth weight infants) *Relationship established: further research needed* • Allergies • Cognitive development • Later overweight/obesity • Atopic dermatitis • Autoimmune disease (type 1 diabetes, celiac disease) • Comorbidities associated with excess weight	• Postpartum hemorrhage • Postpartum depression • Delayed ovulation *Relationship established: further research needed* • Hypertension • Postpartum weight status • Infant bonding • Pre- and post-menopausal breast cancer • Post-menopausal ovarian cancer • Comorbidities associated with excess weight

From Lessen, R., & Kavanagh, K. (2015). Position of the Academy of Nutrition and Dietetics: Promoting and supporting breastfeeding. *J Acad Nutr Diet*, 115(3), 444–449.

---

lactation specialist health care professionals with specialized knowledge and clinical expertise in breastfeeding and human lactation. Also known as a *lactation consultant.*

Putting It All Together

Summary

- Pregnancy involves the fundamental interaction of the following three distinct yet unified biologic entities: the mother, the placenta, and the fetus. Maternal needs also reflect the increasing nutrition needs of the placenta and the fetus.
- Optimal weight gain during pregnancy varies with the normal nutrition status and weight of the woman, with a goal of 25 to 35 lb for a woman of normal prepregnancy weight. Sufficient weight gain is important during pregnancy to support rapid growth. However, the overall quality of the diet is as significant as the quantity of weight gain.
- Common problems during pregnancy include nausea and vomiting associated with hormonal adaptations and, later, constipation, hemorrhoids, or heartburn that result from the pressure of the enlarging uterus. These problems are usually relieved without medication by simple and often temporary changes in the diet.
- Unusual or irregular eating habits, age, parity, inadequate weight gain, and low socioeconomic status are among the many related conditions that put pregnant women at risk for complications.
- The ultimate goal of prenatal care is a healthy infant and a healthy mother who can breastfeed her child. Breast milk provides essential nutrients in quantities that are uniquely suited for optimal infant growth and development.

Chapter Review Questions

See answers in Appendix A.

1. Complete protein sources that can help meet increased nutrient needs during pregnancy are _____.

   a. cow's milk and soymilk
   b. baked beans and green beans
   c. orange juice and grapefruit juice
   d. whole-grain cereal and whole-grain bread

2. An increase of 340 kcal/day is recommended during pregnancy throughout the _____.

   a. second trimester
   b. third trimester
   c. first and second trimesters
   d. second and third trimesters

3. It is important to counsel women of childbearing age to consume adequate amounts of folic acid to reduce the risk of _____.

   a. developing type 2 diabetes mellitus
   b. developing hyperemesis gravidarum
   c. malformation of the neural tube during gestation
   d. poor absorption of calcium and phosphorus during fetal bone growth

4. Benefits of breastfeeding include _____.

   a. more flexibility in the mother's schedule
   b. enhanced immune system in the infant
   c. reduced intelligence quotient in the infant
   d. decreased energy needs for the mother

5. Gestational diabetes is more common in women who have _____.

   a. anemia
   b. hyperemesis
   c. obesity
   d. hypertension

Next-Generation NCLEX® Examination-style Case Study

See answers in Appendix A.

A 30-year-old female is 21 weeks pregnant. She complains of fatigue, has pale skin, and has cravings to eat dirt when she is at the park with her 2-year-old. She takes her prenatal vitamins and iron supplements with breakfast, usually oatmeal or toast with almond butter and fruit. She follows a vegetarian diet. She read about the detriments of iron-deficiency anemia during pregnancy and is now concerned about her iron levels.

1. From the list below, select all of the factors that may increase the risk for iron deficiency anemia in the client.

   a. Increased iron needs in pregnancy
   b. Following a vegetarian diet
   c. Taking supplements with meals
   d. Taking prenatal vitamins
   e. Consuming iron in supplement form
   f. Consuming a balance of plant and animal foods

2. Choose the *most likely* options for the information missing from the statements below by selecting from the list of options provided.

   Although there are plant sources of iron in the client's diet, the _____ of iron is lower when compared to animal sources. Taking supplements with food can also lead to potential _____ interactions within the client.

OPTIONS	
amount	drug-nutrient
digestibility	allergic
bioavailability	drug-drug

3. Choose the *most likely* options for the information missing from the statements below by selecting from the list of options provided.

   The client consumes high-fiber foods containing _____ , which can bind to minerals, such as iron. This can make the minerals _____ for absorption.

OPTIONS	
amino acids	phytic acid
ascorbic acids	readily available
essential fatty acids	unavailable

4. Place an X under "effective" to identify methods that will help the client increase her iron status. Place an X under "ineffective" to identify methods that are not likely to improve her iron status.

METHODS	EFFECTIVE	INEFFECTIVE
Consume more plant proteins		
Consume enriched grains		
Consume more animal proteins		
Take iron supplements with small amounts of food.		
Take iron supplements with calcium supplements		
Take supplements with foods low in phytic acid		

5. From the list below, select all of the examples of foods that are typically enriched with iron.

a. Breakfast cereal
b. Orange juice
c. Pasta
d. Bread
e. Rice
f. Spinach
g. Ground beef

Additional Learning Resources

Please refer to this text's Evolve website for answers to the Case Study questions:
http://evolve.elsevier.com/Williams/basic/
References and **Further Reading and Resources** in the back of the book provide additional resources for enhancing knowledge.

Nutrition During Infancy, Childhood, and Adolescence

Stacie Wing-Gaia PhD, RDN

Key Concepts

- The normal growth of individual children varies within a relatively wide range of measures.
- Human growth and development require both nutrition and psychosocial support.

- Although basic nutrient needs change with each growth period, a variety of food patterns and habits supply the energy and nutrient requirements of normal growth and development.

In any culture, food nurtures both the physical and the emotional process of "growing up" for each infant, child, and adolescent. Food and eating during these significant years of childhood are an integral part of the overall process of psychosocial development and physical growth. The entire process plays a role in creating and shaping the whole person.

This chapter outlines the nutrition needs and food patterns of each age group and briefly discusses some of the more common health problems with nutrition implications.

GROWTH AND DEVELOPMENT

LIFE CYCLE GROWTH PATTERN

The normal human life cycle follows four general stages of overall growth, with individual variation. The nutrition needs of an individual will depend more on the person's biologic age than his or her chronologic age. For example, if two infants were born yesterday and one infant was 6 weeks premature and the other infant was born at full term, they will both be 1 day old but will have different nutrition needs relative to their physiologic development (i.e., their biologic age). The differences in nutrition needs, based on biologic age, are most important during key growth periods, during infancy, and the growth spurts surrounding puberty.

Infancy

Growth is rapid during the first year of life, with the highest rate of growth of the entire life cycle occurring within the first 6 months of life. Most infants more than double their birth weight by the time they are 6 months old, and they triple it by the time they reach approximately 12 to 15 months of age. Growth in length is not quite as rapid, but infants generally increase their birth length by 50% during the first year and double it by 4 years of age.

Childhood

Between infancy and adolescence, the childhood growth rate slows and becomes irregular. Growth occurs in small spurts, during which children have increased appetites and eat accordingly. Appetites usually taper off during periodic plateaus. Parents who recognize the ebb and flow of normal growth patterns during the latent period of childhood can relax and enjoy this time. Alternatively, unawareness of, or inexperience with, this normal flux in growth and appetite can result in stress and battles over food between parents and children.

Adolescence

The onset of puberty begins the second stage of rapid growth, which continues until adult maturity. Levels of growth hormone and sex hormones rise. This brings multiple and often overwhelming body changes to young adolescents. During this period, long bones grow quickly, sex characteristics develop, and fat and muscle mass increase significantly.

Adulthood

With physical maturity comes the final phase of a normal life cycle. Physical growth plateaus during adulthood and then gradually declines during old age. However, mental and psychosocial development lasts a lifetime.

MEASURING CHILDHOOD GROWTH

Individual Growth Rates

Children grow at widely varying rates. Therefore, the best counsel for parents is to recognize that children are individuals. A child's growth can be adequate even if the rate does not equal that of another child. Assessment of growth in children includes physical

---

biologic age age of the body relative to physiologic and maturity developmental standards.

chronologic age amount of time a person has lived.

development as well as mental, emotional, social, and cultural growth.

Physical Growth Measurement

Growth charts. Growth charts, such as those developed by the World Health Organization (WHO) and the Centers for Disease Control and Prevention (CDC), provide an assessment tool for measuring height and weight growth patterns for infants, children, and adolescents as well as head circumference for infants. Large numbers of well-nourished children who represent the national population are the basis of these charts. They serve as guides to follow an individual child's pattern of physical growth in relation to the standard growth curves of healthy children.

The current recommendation is for clinicians to use the WHO growth charts for infants from birth to 2 years old and the CDC growth charts for children who are more than 2 years old.[1] The combined use of the WHO and CDC growth charts allows practitioners to plot the growth patterns for height (or length), weight, and head circumference from birth to the age of 20 years. It is appropriate to use the BMI-for-age charts (BMI, body mass index) for children continuously from 2 years of age into adulthood. The BMI during childhood is an indicator of the adult BMI, allowing early identification of obesity risk.

It is not appropriate to use growth charts to identify "short" or "tall" children. Instead, growth charts are a method for continuous assessment of a child's growth rate. Plotting anthropometric measurements as a percentile of the population allows for child and population comparison. For example, if a child has a height-for-age at the 70th percentile, then 29% of age-matched and sex-matched children are taller, and 70% are shorter. With adequate nutrition and in the absence of disease, this child should continue to grow on about the 70th percentile curve.

There are specific growth charts for boys and girls. Figure 11.1 demonstrates two examples of growth charts. The Evolve site for this book includes a full set of the WHO and CDC growth charts, which are also available at www.cdc.gov/growthcharts. To assess a child's growth accurately, the following three things are essential: (1) an appropriate growth chart (girl vs. boy, appropriate age group, and WHO vs. CDC); (2) an accurate measurement; and (3) an accurate calculation of the child's age. Small errors in measurement can easily lead to a false alarm regarding a child's growth pattern. See the Clinical Applications box, "Use and Interpretation of Growth Charts," for step-by-step instructions on how to accurately use and interpret the standard charts.

Growth charts for children with special health care needs. Specialized growth charts are available for several conditions that affect standard childhood growth. Examples include low or very low birth weight infants, achondroplasia, Down syndrome, fragile X syndrome, Prader-Willi syndrome, sickle cell disease, and spastic quadriplegia. Specialty growth charts are developed by collecting anthropometric data of children with a particular condition and using that information to design a chart reflecting expected growth patterns. Although the amount of data used to create such charts is much less than that used to establish the standard CDC charts, these charts are usually still more appropriate to use for children with special health care needs. For example, children with Down syndrome are generally shorter in stature than age-matched controls. Thus, plotting them on a CDC growth chart will indicate that they are below average in height. On the other hand, plotting them on a specialized chart for children with Down syndrome allows comparison of their height to other age-matched children with the same condition and expected growth pattern. Specialized growth charts are not available for all special health care needs.

Psychosocial Development

There are various assessments available to measure mental, emotional, social, and cultural growth and development. Food closely relates to these aspects of psychosocial development as well as physical growth. The growing child should learn food attitudes and habits as a part of close personal and social relationships. Such relationships begin very early in life.

NUTRITION REQUIREMENTS FOR GROWTH

Growth requires an ample supply of macronutrients and micronutrients. Food intake must meet the daily demands of life and physical activity, while also providing for additional nutrients to build bones, supply tissues and organs, and increase the blood supply to match the growth.

ENERGY NEEDS

The demand for energy, as measured in kilocalories per kilogram (kg) of body weight per day (kcal/kg/d), is relatively large throughout infancy and childhood. During the first 3 years of life, children need between 80 and 120 kcal/kg/d to support rapid growth.[2] Although the exact energy needs of premature infants are highly variable and not well defined, estimated energy needs range from 110 to 135 kcal/kg/d.[3] To put the enormity of these energy needs into context, adults usually need between 30 and 40 kcal/kg/d.

The Dietary Reference Intake values (see Appendix B) present general recommendations for energy and protein needs at different ages. However, specific individual needs vary with biologic age and condition. As an example, the total daily energy expenditure distribution of an average 5-year-old child is as follows:

- Basal metabolism: 50%
- Physical activity: 25%
- Tissue growth: 12%
- Fecal loss: 8%
- Thermic effect of food: 5%

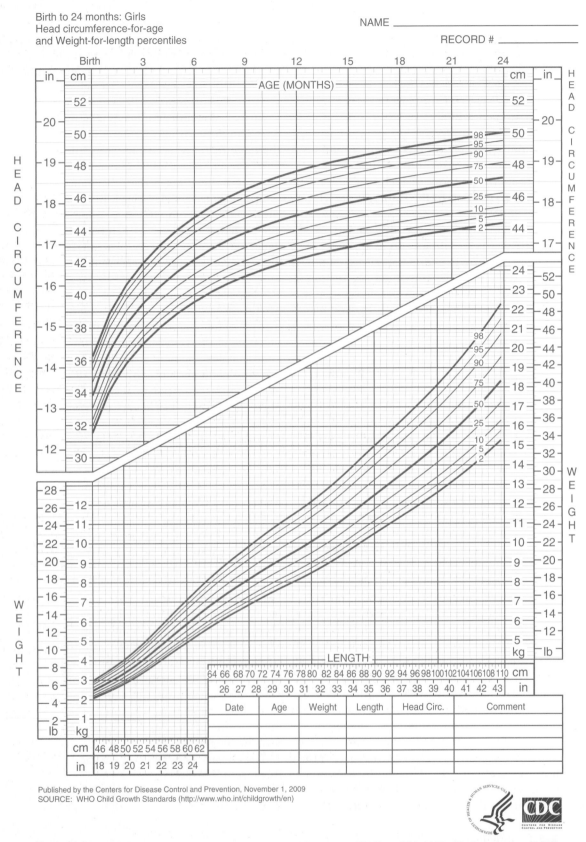

Birth to 24 months: Girls
Head circumference-for-age
and Weight-for-length percentiles

NAME _____

RECORD # _____

Published by the Centers for Disease Control and Prevention, November 1, 2009
SOURCE: WHO Child Growth Standards (http://www.who.int/childgrowth/en)

Figure 11.1 Example of a Centers for Disease Control and Prevention (CDC) and World Health Organization (WHO) growth chart. (Courtesy National Center for Health Statistics, National Center for Chronic Disease Prevention and Health Promotion, Hyattsville, MD.)

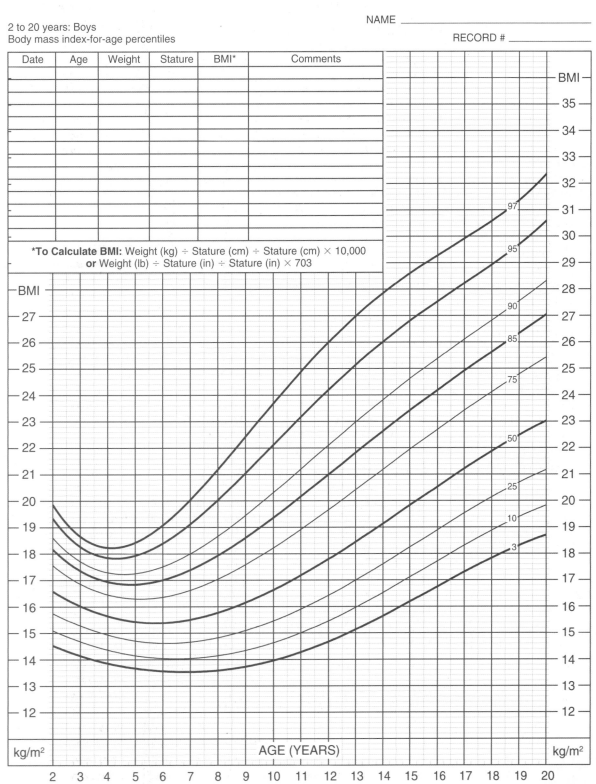

2 to 20 years: Boys
Body mass index-for-age percentiles

NAME _____

RECORD # _____

Date	Age	Weight	Stature	BMI*	Comments

*To Calculate BMI: Weight (kg) ÷ Stature (cm) ÷ Stature (cm) × 10,000
or Weight (lb) ÷ Stature (in) ÷ Stature (in) × 703

AGE (YEARS)

kg/m²

Published May 30, 2000 (modified10/16/00).
SOURCE: Developed by the National Center for Health Statistics in collaboration with
the National Center for Chronic Disease Prevention and Health Promotion (2000).
http://www.cdc.gov/growthcharts

SAFER · HEALTHIER · PEOPLE™

Figure 11.1, cont'd

Clinical Applications

Use and Interpretation of Growth Charts

PURPOSE

This guide instructs health care providers how to use and interpret the Centers for Disease Control and Prevention (CDC) and World Health Organization (WHO) growth charts. With the use of these charts, health care providers can assess growth in infants, children, and adolescents and compare it with a nationally representative reference based on children of all ages and ethnic groups.

During a routine screening, health care providers assess physical growth by using the child's weight, stature or length, and head circumference. When plotted correctly, a series of measurements offers important information about a child's growth pattern and possible nutrition risks. Contributing factors such as parental stature and the presence of acute or chronic illness should also be considered when making health and nutrition assessments.

STEP 1: OBTAIN ACCURATE WEIGHTS AND MEASURES

When weighing and measuring children, follow procedures that yield accurate measurements, and use well-maintained equipment.

STEP 2: SELECT THE APPROPRIATE GROWTH CHART

Select the growth chart to use according to the child's age and sex:

- Use the WHO growth standards to monitor growth for infants and children who are between the ages of birth and 2 years.
- Use the CDC growth charts for children who are ≥2 years old.

STEP 3: RECORD DATA

First, record information about factors obtained at the initial visit that may influence growth.

- Enter the child's name and the record number, if appropriate.
- Enter the mother's and father's statures, as reported.
- Enter the child's gestational age in weeks and date of birth.
- Enter the child's birth weight, length, and head circumference.
- Add any notable comments (e.g., breastfeeding, illnesses, unknown anthropometrics of biologic parent). Record information obtained during the current visit.
- Enter today's date.
- Enter the child's age.
- Enter the child's weight, stature, and head circumference (if appropriate) immediately after taking the measurement.
- Add any comments pertinent to measurements (e.g., child was not cooperative in getting measurements).

STEP 4: CALCULATE THE BODY MASS INDEX

Calculate the body mass index (BMI) by using weight and stature measurements (see below). The BMI-for-age chart compares a child's weight relative to stature with that of other age- and sex-matched children.

- Determine the BMI with the following calculation:
  BMI = Weight (kg)/Stature (m^2)
  Convert weight and stature measurements to the appropriate decimal value.

Example: 37 lb 4 oz = 37.25 lb; 41½ in. = 41.5 in.
Enter the BMI to one decimal place (e.g., 15.204 = 15.2).

STEP 5: PLOT THE MEASUREMENTS

On the appropriate growth chart, plot the measurements recorded in the data entry table for the current visit.

- Find the child's age on the horizontal axis. When plotting weight for length, find the length on the horizontal axis. Use a straight edge or a right-angle ruler to draw a vertical line up from that point.
- Find the appropriate measurement (i.e., weight, length, stature, head circumference, or BMI) on the vertical axis. Use a straight edge or a right-angle ruler to draw a horizontal line across from that point until it intersects the vertical line.
- Make a small dot where the two lines intersect.

STEP 6: INTERPRET THE PLOTTED MEASUREMENTS

- The curved lines on the growth chart show selected percentiles that indicate the rank of the child's measurement. For example, when plotting the dot on the 95th percentile for BMI-for-age, it means that 5% of age- and sex-matched children in the reference population have a higher BMI and 94% have a lower BMI.
  1. Determine the percentile rank.
  2. Determine if the percentile rank is indicative of nutrition risk. The cut-offs indicating nutrition or overall health concerns are the 2nd and 98th percentile. Measurements involving weight (BMI-for-age, weight-for-length/height, and weight-for-age) that are ≥85th and ≤97th percentiles indicate an *at risk status* that should be monitored.
  3. Compare today's percentile rank with the rank from previous visits to identify any major changes in the child's growth pattern and need for further assessment.

The WHO recommends screening children who fall outside the 2nd and 98th percentiles for potential health- or nutrition-related problems. Based on these parameters, classifications are as follows:

- Low weight-for-length: infants and children with a weight-for-length <2nd percentile
- Short stature: infants and children with a length-for-age <2nd percentile
- High weight-for-length: infants and children with a weight-for-length >98th percentile
- Children and adolescents with a BMI-for-age above the 85th percentile are at risk for being overweight as adults. The 95th percentile on the BMI-for-age charts correlates with a BMI of 30 kg/m^2 in adults, which indicates obesity. Because the BMI-for-age charts correlate with the adult BMI index, these charts are a useful assessment tool for chronic disease risk associated with obesity.

For additional information on the use and interpretation of growth charts, please see: World Health Organization Growth Chart Training, available at: www.cdc.gov/nccdphp/dnpao/growthcharts/who/index.htm.

From World Health Organization. (2008). *Training course on child growth assessment.* Geneva: WHO.

However, some children are more physically active than others are and consequently have a higher daily caloric expenditure. Likewise, a child who is experiencing a growth spurt has higher calorie needs to support tissue growth and a higher basal metabolism compared with a similar child who is not going through a growth spurt.

Carbohydrates are the preferred energy source of the body. Sufficient carbohydrates supply enough energy so that protein supports growth instead of providing energy. Fat is a backup energy source and supplies the essential fatty acids necessary for growth.

FAT NEEDS

Fat is an essential nutrient that provides energy, essential fatty acids, and aids in the absorption of fat-soluble vitamins. Infants require higher amounts of fat than adults do to support their rapid growth rate. The Acceptable Macronutrient Distribution Range (AMDR) for children 1 to 3 years old is 30% to 40% compared with 20% to 35% for adults. Fat requirements then decrease to 25% to 35% from age 4 to 18.[2]

Survey data indicate children get enough dietary fat, but not necessarily the right type of fat.[4] As with pregnancy and lactation, children and adolescents fall below the recommendations for docosahexaenoic acid (DHA) and eicosapentaenoic acid (EPA). Only 14% of 7- to 12-year-olds and 50% of 14- to 18-year-olds meet the Institute of Medicine's recommendations for DHA and EPA.[5,6] This may have long-term impacts on cognitive development and learning cognition.[5-7]

PROTEIN NEEDS

Protein is the fundamental tissue-building substance of the body. It supplies the essential amino acids for tissue growth and maintenance. As a child gets older and the growth rate slows, the protein requirements per kg of body weight gradually decline. For example, during the first 6 months of life, the protein requirements of an infant are 1.52 g/kg; however, the protein needs of an adult are only 0.8 g/kg.[2] A healthy, active, growing child usually eats enough of a variety of foods to supply the necessary protein and kilocalories for overall growth.

WATER REQUIREMENTS

Water is an essential nutrient that is second only to oxygen in its importance for life. Metabolic needs, especially during periods of rapid growth, demand adequate fluid intake. Infants require more water per unit of body weight than adults for the following three important reasons: (1) a greater percentage of the infant's total body weight is composed of water; (2) a larger proportion of the infant's total body water is in the extracellular spaces; and (3) infants have a larger proportional body surface area and metabolic rate compared with adults. In 1 day, an infant generally consumes an amount of water that is equivalent to 10% to 15% of his or her body weight, whereas an adult consumes a daily amount that is equivalent to 2% to 4% of his or her body weight. Table 11.1 provides a summary of the estimated daily fluid needs during the years of growth.

MINERAL AND VITAMIN NEEDS

All minerals and vitamins have important roles in tissue growth and maintenance as well as in overall energy metabolism. Positive childhood growth depends on adequate amounts of all essential nutrients. The following sections address the most common nutrients of concern. See Chapter 7 and Chapter 8 for more detailed information regarding essential vitamins and minerals.

Calcium

Approximately 99% of the body's calcium is in the human skeleton. Therefore, calcium is a necessary nutrient for proper bone growth. Genetics largely determine adult peak bone mass. However, lifestyle choices throughout the life cycle, including the in utero environment (i.e., maternal diet) account for approximately 20% to 40% of peak bone mass. The goal of nutrition is to provide essential nutrients such as calcium to achieve each person's genetic potential for bone mass. This is particularly true during periods of critical growth that occur during infancy, childhood, and adolescence.[8]

During the short period of adolescence, approximately 40% of adult peak bone mineral density is deposited, and 25% of this occurs the 2 years before puberty.[9] The development of good bone density requires an ample dietary supply of calcium, phosphorus, vitamin D, protein, and several other nutrients. Dairy foods provide all of these nutrients and are the main source of calcium for children. One study found that children consuming a diet high in dairy and whole grains had higher bone mineral density than their counterparts who consumed

Table 11.1	Approximate Daily Fluid Needs During Growth Years			
AGE	MALES AND FEMALES (L/DAY)	AGE	MALES (L/DAY)	FEMALES (L/DAY)
Birth to 6 months	0.7	9 to 13 years	2.4	2.1
7 to 12 months	0.8	14 to 18 years	3.3	2.3
1 to 3 years	1.3	>19 years	3.7	2.7
4 to 8 years	1.7			

Data from the Food and Nutrition Board. (2004). *Dietary Reference Intakes for water, potassium, sodium, chloride, and sulfate.* Institute of Medicine. Washington, DC: National Academies Press.

diets high in potatoes, rice, and vegetables or a diet high in refined grains, solid fat, and added sugar.[10] Currently, American children consume less dairy servings than the *Dietary Guidelines for Americans, 2020–2025* recommend.[11,12]

Unfortunately, the majority of children and adolescents fall below the calcium they need to form strong bones for life. Survey data indicate that 2- to 19-year-olds have calcium intakes averaging 979 mg/day, which fall below the Recommended Daily Allowance (RDA) of 1300 mg/d for 9- to 13-year-olds.[4] Those who do not consume dairy products consume even less calcium than their dairy-consuming peers do. Although parents may supplement their children with calcium to achieve recommendations, one meta-analysis found that calcium supplements had no effect on specific areas of bone (i.e., femoral neck and lumbar spine.) However, there was a small effect on total bone mineral content.[13] Because data are inclusive regarding calcium supplements, parents and caregivers should first strive to achieve calcium intakes through food to build lifelong healthy eating habits.

Iron

Iron is essential for hemoglobin formation and cognitive development during the early years of life. Infants and young children are at the greatest risk of iron-deficiency anemia at a time that corresponds with rapid brain growth. In addition, infants of mothers with iron-deficiency anemia during gestation are at risk for iron-deficiency anemia at birth. Iron deficiency during this critical time of brain growth is negatively associated with long-term cognitive performance in children.[14]

The iron content of breast milk is highly absorbable and fully meets the needs of an infant for the first 6 months of life.[15] At that point, the infant's nutrition needs for iron typically exceed that provided exclusively by breast milk, and the addition of solid foods (e.g., enriched cereal, egg yolk, meat) at approximately 6 months of age supplies additional iron. Infants who are not breastfed need an iron-fortified breast milk substitute.

The current average dietary intake of iron for children and adolescents between the ages of 2 and 19 years is 13.8 mg/d, which exceeds the recommended dietary allowance of 8 mg/d for males and 10 mg/d for children 4 to 8 years old.[11] However, female adolescents fall below their recommended 15 mg/d of iron, and one study estimated that as many as 15% of toddlers are iron deficient.[16] The Woman Infants and Children Supplemental Food Program targets iron as a key nutrient in their education and screening process. Only those with iron deficiency should supplement with iron. Iron supplementation in the absence of deficiency is associated with adverse short- and long-term effects such as diarrhea, changes to the gut microbiota, neurodegenerative diseases, and impaired growth.[17]

Vitamin Supplements

Approximately 32% of children in the United States regularly use dietary supplements, of which very few are under a health care provider's guidance.[18] The most commonly used dietary supplements are multivitamin/mineral supplements. Meanwhile, the American Academy of Pediatrics recognizes only two vitamins that may necessitate supplementation, which are vitamins K and D.[19]

Nearly all infants who are born in the United States and Canada receive a one-time prophylactic injection of 1 mg of vitamin K at birth. Vitamin K is critical for blood clotting. Bacterial production in the gut is the major contributor to the daily supply of vitamin K. Because infants are born without bacterial flora (i.e., we have a sterile gut at birth), their vitamin K synthesis and stores are minimal, thus warranting a vitamin K injection.

To prevent vitamin D deficiency, the American Academy of Pediatrics recommends breastfed infants receive oral vitamin D drops (400 IU) beginning at hospital discharge and continuing until the infant is drinking 16 oz of vitamin D–fortified milk, or dairy substitute, daily.[19] During pregnancy, vitamin D crosses the placenta so that the fetus gets approximately two-thirds of the mother's vitamin D concentration. After birth, breast milk vitamin D concentration correlates with maternal serum levels. Given the seasonal variation in vitamin D levels and the prevalence of suboptimal vitamin D intake, breast milk may not provide adequate vitamin D.[20,21] One study determined that breast milk provided less than 20% of the recommended vitamin D for infants.[20] It is possible to increase the vitamin D content in breast milk by (1) supplementing the mother during pregnancy or (2) supplementing the breastfeeding mother.[21,22] However, until consensus can be reached, caregivers are advised to supplement their breastfed infant with the recommended 400 IU/d. Formula-fed infants receive supplemental vitamin D in the breast milk substitute.

As with any supplement, it is possible to have too much. Toxicity in infants and children is possible. Excess amounts of vitamins A and D are of special concern in children (see Chapter 7). Lack of knowledge or inattention may result in excess intake over prolonged periods. Parents should provide only the amount that they are instructed to administer. Vitamins are similar to medication; caregivers should keep all vitamin supplements, including those in the form of gummy bears or other candy-type treat, out of children's reach.

NUTRITION REQUIREMENTS DURING INFANCY

Food is integral to each stage of development, which includes both physical growth and personal psychosocial development.

INFANT CLASSIFICATIONS

Maturity, gestational age, and weight determine the classification of an infant. Nutrient needs of the infant and feeding methods will vary accordingly to match these parameters.

Maturity

Term infants. Full-term infants are born between 37 and 42 weeks' gestation. Mature newborns have developed body systems and grow rapidly. Provided with adequate nutrition, they will gain approximately 168 g (6 oz) per week during the first 6 months.

Premature infants. Premature infants are born before 37 weeks' gestation. Special care is crucial for tiny premature babies to grow and develop. Weight or size for gestational age further categorizes premature infants.

Weight Classification

Although low birth weight can occur in both term and preterm infants, it is more common among premature infants. *Low birth weight* (LBW) infants weigh less than 2500 g (5 lb 8 oz); *very low birth weight* (VLBW) infants weigh less than 1500 g (3 lb 5 oz); *extremely low birth weight* (ELBW) babies weigh less than 1000 g (2 lb 3 oz). The lower the birth weight, the higher the risks for complications and poor infant outcome.

Size for Gestational Age Classification

This classification is relative to gestational age; therefore, medical terminology classifies infants who are born full term and preterm according to their expected size. The categories are as follows:

Appropriate for gestational age (AGA). The infant's weight, length, and head circumference are all within the normal range on a growth chart (i.e., between the 10th and 90th percentiles) relative to the infant's gestational age.

Large for gestational age (LGA). Birth weight is at the 90th percentile or higher for their age and sex, also known as *macrosomia*.

Small for gestational age (SGA). Birth weight is at the 10th percentile or less for their age and sex. This category includes two sub-classifications:

- *Proportionantly small for gestational age* (pSGA): Birth weight, length, and head circumference are all at the 10th percentile or less for age and sex.
- *Disproportionantly small for gestational age* (dSGA): Length and head circumference are of normal size, but weight is at the 10th percentile or less.

CONSIDERATIONS REGARDING FEEDING PREMATURE INFANTS

The feeding process is an important component of bonding between the parent and the infant. In the event that an infant is premature or otherwise experiences feeding complications, there are trained health care professionals who can assist parents in providing optimal nourishment for the child.

Physiologic Delays Relevant to Feeding

Premature infants are vulnerable to impaired growth and nutrient deficiencies. Because their bodies are not fully formed, premature infants differ from normal-weight term infants in the following ways:

1. They have more body water, less protein, and fewer mineral stores.
2. There is little subcutaneous fat to maintain body temperature.
3. They have poorly calcified bones.
4. Their nerve and muscle development is incomplete, resulting in weak or absent sucking reflexes.
5. They have a limited ability for digestion, absorption, and renal function.
6. Their immature livers lack developed metabolic enzyme systems and adequate iron stores.

To survive, these premature infants require special attention to their nutrition and feeding method.

Milk Content for Premature Infants

The American Academy of Pediatrics recommends the normal feeding of breast milk to premature and other high-risk infants. For infants of mothers who are not able to breastfeed, use of human milk from milk banks is encouraged.[19] Although milk composition is highly variable, mothers of preterm infants produce milk that is higher in immune factors, contributing to the higher protein in preterm milk.[23] Preterm infants miss the growth and nutrient storage that occurs during the third trimester of pregnancy. Therefore, to decrease the risk of sepsis and necrotizing enterocolitis and to provide additional nutrients, the American Academy of Pediatrics recommends adding a **human milk fortifier** to breast milk.[19] Because human milk composition is variable, recent research recommends individualizing milk fortification.[24]

Methods of Milk Delivery

For most premature infants, nursing or bottle-feeding can be successful with proper instruction and support. Infants who have not yet developed the sucking reflex, acquired between 32 and 34 weeks' gestation, can still benefit from breast milk. However, the mother must be willing and able to pump her breast milk and feed the baby by tube or cup. Breastfeeding mothers of premature infants often experience breastfeeding difficulties and high maternal stress. Evidence-based information and sensitive counseling will help these mothers successfully breastfeed their infants.[25]

If the infant cannot tolerate enteral feedings through the gastrointestinal tract, then peripheral or central vein feedings are required to nourish the infant directly through the vascular system. However, significant health risks are associated with parenteral nutrition in the infant. Therefore, it is avoided if possible.

WHAT, HOW, AND WHEN TO FEED THE MATURE INFANT

Breast Milk

Human milk is the ideal first food for infants, and it is the primary recommendation of pediatricians and registered dietitian nutritionists.[19,26] As the infant grows, breast milk adapts in composition to match the needs of the developing child, and the fat content of breast milk changes from the beginning to the end of a single feeding (see Chapter 10).

The newborn's **rooting reflex**, his or her oral needs for sucking, and basic hunger help to facilitate breast-feeding for healthy, relaxed mothers (Figure 11.2). Mothers who are away from their infant for several hours at a time and want to breastfeed their babies can do so by using manual expression or a breast pump while away. The milk can be stored and frozen in sealed plastic baby bottle liners for later use. Breastfeeding mothers can find support and guidance through local groups of La Leche League (www.llli.org), a community resource on breastfeeding, or professional certified lactation counselors. Refer to www.alpp.org/certifications/certifications-clc for local certified lactation counselors and training opportunities. See Chapter 10 for additional information about successful breastfeeding.

Breast Milk Substitute

If a mother chooses not to breastfeed or is unable to breastfeed, bottle-feeding of an appropriate breast milk substitute (i.e., infant formula) is an acceptable alternative. Research shows that product and water contamination and lack of adherence to recommended safety precautions when preparing infant formula increase the risk for infant food-borne illness and scalding.[27,28] The type of commercial infant formula chosen, sterile procedures in formula preparation, and the amount of formula consumed are some aspects that must be addressed to ensure the safety and health of the child.

Choosing a commercial infant formula. Most mothers who use breast milk substitutes use a standard commercial formula. In some cases of milk allergy or intolerance, a soy-based formula (not soy milk) is used. Mothers of infants who are allergic to cow's milk and soy-based formulas can use amino acid–based formulas for their infants. Examples include Nutramigen (Mead Johnson Nutrition, Evansville, IN), EleCare (Abbott Nutrition, Columbus, OH), and Neocate (Nutricia North America, Gaithersburg, MD). Table 11.2 compares the nutrient composition of breast milk with those of standard and specialty formulas.

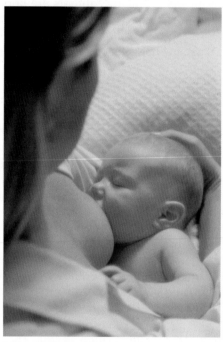

Figure 11.2 Breastfeeding the newborn infant. Note that the mother avoids touching the infant's outer cheek so as not to counteract the infant's natural rooting reflex at the touch of the breast. (Copyright JupiterImages Corp.)

Table 11.2 Nutrient Values of Human Milk and Breast Milk Substitutes

NUTRIENT COMPONENT PER LITER	HUMAN MILK, MATURE	STANDARD FORMULAS[a] ENFAMIL, WITH IRON, READY TO FEED	SPECIAL FORMULAS FOR INFANTS WHO ARE NOT BREASTFED OR WHO CANNOT TOLERATE STANDARD FORMULAS	
			NUTRAMIGEN (CASEIN HYDROLYSATE AND FREE AMINO ACIDS)	PURAMINO (FREE AMINO ACIDS)
Kilocalories	729	649	687	676
Protein (g)	10.7	14.2	19.05	18.9
Fat (g)	45.6	36	36.4	35.8
Carbohydrate (g)	71.7	74	70.9	71.7
Calcium (mg)	333	526	645	635
Phosphorus (mg)	146	361	437	351
Sodium (mg)	177	186	323	318
Potassium (mg)	533	732	750	743
Iron (mg)	0.31	12[b]	12.28[b]	12.17[b]

[a]Most standard formulas are very similar. This represents an average of Enfamil (Mead Johnson Nutrition, Evansville, Ind).
[b]With added iron.

Preparing the formula. With any commercial formula, the manufacturer's instructions for mixing concentrated or powdered formula with water should be precisely and consistently followed and refrigerated until use. Throughout the process, scrupulous cleanliness and accurate dilution are essential to prevent infection and illness. A ready-to-feed formula only requires a sterile nipple and bypasses many problems, but it is substantially more expensive. Heat bottles in a bowl of warm water (instead of a microwave) to prevent uneven heating and scalding the infant's mouth. Studies indicate mothers of low socioeconomic status are particularly vulnerable to inaccurate formula preparation. Furthermore, most mothers who bottle-feed do not receive detailed instructions on formula preparation from health care providers.[28] Clear instructions and feedback are necessary to ensure infants receive appropriate and safe nutrition.

Feeding the formula. Babies usually drink formula either cold or warm; they primarily want it to be consistent. Tilting the bottle to keep the nipple full of milk can prevent swallowing air, and the baby's head should be slightly elevated during feeding to facilitate the passage of milk into the stomach. Caregivers should be encouraged to never prop the bottle or leave the baby alone to feed, especially as a pacifier at sleep time. This practice deprives the infant of the cuddling that is a vital part of nurturing, and it allows milk to pool in the mouth, which can cause choking, earache, or **baby bottle tooth decay** (now known as early childhood caries, or ECC). Children should never sleep with a bottle of milk or fruit juice or any other caloric liquid that is capable of pooling in the mouth. Natural bacteria found in the mouth feed on carbohydrates, thereby producing enamel-damaging acid. Baby bottle tooth decay (Figure 11.3) is a serious and avoidable problem that results from this practice.

Cleaning bottles and nipples. Whether preparing a single bottle for each feeding or an entire day's batch, scrub, rinse, and sterilize all equipment with the use of the *terminal sterilization method*. Rinse bottles and nipples after each feeding with special bottle and nipple brushes that force water through nipple holes to prevent formula from crusting in them.

Weaning

Throughout the feeding process, observant parents quickly learn to recognize their baby's signs of hunger and satiety and to follow the baby's lead. Babies are individuals who set their own particular feeding schedule according to age, activity level, growth rate, and metabolic efficiency. A newborn has a very small stomach that holds only 1 to 2 fluid ounces (fl oz), but he or she will gradually take in more as his or her stomach capacity enlarges relative to overall body growth. The amounts of increased intake during the first 6 months vary and reflect growth patterns. By 6 to 9 months of age, if the infant eats increasing amounts of other foods and has the motor skills to use a cup, **weaning** from bottle-feeding takes place. The American Academy of Pediatrics recommends weaning infants from a bottle by 12 to 18 months.[29] For breastfed infants, it is possible to never use a bottle and go directly to a cup. For some children, growing physical capacities and the desire for independence lead to self-weaning, but many children need a little added encouragement from their parents.

Cow's Milk

Cow's milk is not an appropriate source of nutrition during the first year of life. Unmodified cow's milk provides too high of a solute load for the infant's gastrointestinal tract and renal system. Infants can drink cow's milk after 1 year of age. However, children between the ages of 1 and 2 years old should not be fed reduced-fat cow's milk (e.g., skim or low-fat milk), because insufficient energy is provided and because

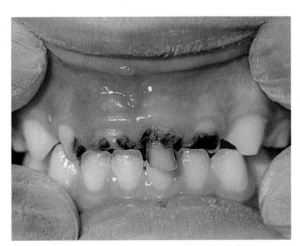

Figure 11.3 Baby bottle tooth decay. (From Swartz, M. H. [2006]. *Textbook of physical diagnosis, history, and examination* [5th ed.]. Philadelphia: Saunders.)

human milk fortifiers powder or liquid mixed with breast milk to increase the concentration of calories and protein in the milk for premature and low birth weight infants who need more kilocalories than provided in breast milk.

rooting reflex reflex that occurs when an infant's cheek is stroked or touched. The infant will turn toward the stimuli and make sucking (or rooting) motions in an effort to nurse.

baby bottle tooth decay also known as *early childhood caries* (ECC), the decay of the baby teeth as a result of inappropriate feeding practices such as putting an infant to bed with a bottle; also called *nursing bottle caries, bottle mouth,* and *bottle caries*.

weaning the process of gradually acclimating a young child to food other than the mother's milk or a breast milk substitute as the child's natural need to suckle wanes.

linoleic acid, which is the essential fatty acid for growth that is found in the fat portion of the milk, is lacking.

Solid Food Additions

When to introduce. Introduction of iron-fortified solid foods occurs at approximately 6 months of age. Introducing solid food before 4 months is associated with increased infant adiposity and childhood obesity.[30] Age is one of the basic indicators of readiness for solid foods. However, each infant will develop motor skills at his or her own rate. Other signs of readiness to begin solid foods include the following:

- The infant can hold up his or her head. Infants should have good head control before solid foods are introduced.
- The infant opens his or her mouth in anticipation of eating food. Infants ready for solid foods will show signs such as reaching for the food and eagerness for feeding.
- The infant can move the food from the spoon to his or her throat to swallow. The infant should have controlled movement of the tongue. The ability to swallow solids is a reflex that will develop when the infant is capable of this task. If the infant pushes food out of his or her mouth when served (tongue thrust), then he or she may not be ready for solids.
- The infant is large enough. Generally, infants should have doubled their birth weight before offering any solid foods.

The most effective prevention regimen against allergic disease is to provide breast milk and to avoid all solid foods and cow's milk until a minimum of 4 months of age. Although exclusively breastfeeding for the first 6 months is the recommendation, recent guidelines suggest that those infants at high risk for food allergies benefit from earlier exposure (i.e., between 4 and 6 months).[31] Thereafter, introduce one new food every 3 to 5 days as tolerated. It is equally important that parents and other caregivers are able to understand feeding cues from the infant (e.g., hunger, satiety) for a mutually pleasant experience.

What to introduce. Contrary to popular belief, there are no specific guidelines for the best sequence of food introductions. Some organizations promote the introduction of vegetables or meat before fruits or grains. This recommendation is based on the following two theories: (1) fruits are sweeter than vegetables, and infants may develop a preference for a sweet taste first and then not like the more bitter taste of vegetables (although this theory lacks strong support); and (2) infants who were given meat before cereal had better zinc intake.

Table 11.3 provides a general schedule for the introduction of solid foods, but individual needs, cultural preferences, and responses vary, and parents and caregivers should follow the suggestions of their individual practitioners regarding their specific child. Introduce foods one at a time (starting with iron-fortified cereal) and in small amounts so that if an adverse

Table 11.3	Guideline for Adding Solid Foods to an Infant's Diet During the First Year
WHEN TO ADD	**FOODS ADDED**[a]
6 months	Iron-fortified infant cereal made from rice, barley, or oats (these are offered one at a time) Pureed baby food (vegetables or strained fruit)
8 months	Whole-milk yogurt Pureed baby food (meats)
8 to 10 months	Introduce more grain products one at a time, including wheat, various crackers and breads, pasta, and cereal Add more vegetables and fruits in various textures (e.g., chopped, mashed, cooked, raw) Egg yolks, beans, and additional types of pureed meats Cottage cheese and hard cheeses (e.g., cheddar, Colby-Jack)
10 to 12 months	Infants should be able to tolerate a large variety of grain products and textures Chopped fruits and vegetables Finger foods
12 months	Whole eggs Whole milk

[a]Give semisolid foods immediately before milk feeding. Give 1 or 2 tsp at first. If the food is accepted and tolerated well, then increase the amount by 1 to 2 Tbsp per feeding.

reaction occurs, the offending food can be easily identified. It is appropriate to give highly allergenic foods (e.g., peanuts, tree nuts, and cow's milk) as complementary foods once the infant tolerates a few standard first foods (e.g., rice and oat cereal).

Commercial or homemade complementary foods. Some parents prefer to make their own baby food. Baby food is prepared at home by cooking, straining, and pureeing vegetables and fruits, freezing a batch at a time in ice cube trays, and then storing the cubes in plastic bags in the freezer. To feed the infant, simply reheat a single cube. Good food-safety practices are necessary at all times. A variety of commercial baby foods are also available and are now prepared without added sugar or unnecessary seasonings.

Throughout the early feeding period, regardless of the feeding plan, there are a few basic guiding principles: (1) essential nutrients—not any specific food or sequence—are needed; (2) food is a basis for learning; and (3) normal physical development guides an infant's feeding behavior (see the For Further Focus box, "How Infants Learn to Eat"). Good food habits begin early in life and continue as the child grows. By 8 or 9 months of age, infants should be able to eat soft table foods (i.e., cooked, chopped, and simply seasoned foods) without requiring special infant foods.

🔍 For Further Focus

How Infants Learn to Eat

Guided by reflexes and the gradual development of muscle control during their first year of life, infants learn many things about living in their particular environments. A basic need is food, which infants obtain through a normal developmental sequence of feeding behaviors during the process of learning to eat.

1 TO 3 MONTHS

Rooting, sucking, and swallowing reflexes are present at birth in term infants, along with the tonic neck reflex. Infants secure their first food, milk, with a suckling pattern in which the tongue is projected during a swallow. In the beginning, head control is poor, but it develops by the third month of life.

4 TO 6 MONTHS

The early rooting and biting reflexes fade. Infants now change from a suckling pattern with a protruded tongue to a mature and stronger suck with liquids, and a munching pattern begins. Infants are now able to grasp objects with a palmar grip, bring them to the mouth, and bite them.

7 TO 9 MONTHS

The gag reflex weakens as infants begin chewing solid foods. They develop a normal controlled gag along with control of the choking reflex. A mature munching increases their intake of solid foods while chewing with a rotary motion. These infants can sit alone, secure items, release and resecure them, and hold a bottle alone. They begin to develop a pincer grasp to pick up small items between the thumb and forefinger and put the items into the mouth.

10 TO 12 MONTHS

Older infants can now reach for a spoon. They bite nipples, spoons, and crunchy foods; they can grasp a bottle or food and bring it to the mouth; and, with assistance, they can drink from a cup. These infants have tongue control to lick food morsels from the lower lip, and they can finger-feed themselves with a refined pincer grasp. These normal developmental behaviors are the basis for the progressive pattern of introducing semisolid and table foods to older infants.

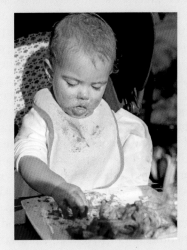

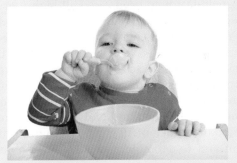

Copyright iStock Photo.

Summary Guidelines

The guidelines for infant feeding are as follows:

- *Breastfeed* for at least the first full year of life, and supplement with a vitamin K shot at birth and daily vitamin D drops.
- Use *iron-fortified formula* for any infant who is not breastfeeding.
- *Water and juice* are unnecessary for breastfed infants during the first 6 months of life.
- Introduce *solid foods* at approximately 6 months of age, after the extrusion reflex of early infancy disappears and the ability to swallow solid food is present.
- Introduce whole cow's milk, or milk substitute, at the end of the first year (if the infant is consuming one-third of his or her kilocalories as a balanced mixture of solid foods, including cereals, vegetables, fruits, and other foods). Provide whole milk, not reduced-fat or fat-free milk, until the age of 2 years.
- Do not give allergens such as wheat, egg white, citrus juice, and nuts as the first solid foods. Introduce them after the infant tolerates standard traditional solid foods. See Chapter 18 for more information about food allergies and intolerances.
- Do not give *honey* to an infant who is younger than 1 year old because of the risk of botulism spores. The immune system capacity of the young infant cannot resist this infection.
- Delay *foods with a high risk for choking and aspiration* such as hot dogs, nuts, grapes, carrots, popcorn, cherries, peanut butter, and round candy until the child is older.
- Beginning at age 6 months, provide fluoride supplementation to infants residing in communities where the fluoride concentration in the water is 0.3 ppm or less.[32]

Throughout the first year of life, breast milk or a breast milk substitute, a variety of solid food additions, and a loving and trusting relationship between the parents or caregivers and the child meet the requirements for physical growth and psychologic development of the infant.

NUTRITION REQUIREMENTS DURING CHILDHOOD

TODDLERS (1 TO 3 YEARS OLD)

During this stage of development, physical growth rate decreases and gross and fine motor skills increase. Children can now walk and explore more readily. As their environment expands so do language skills, social interactions, and independence. Appetite slows along with growth rates during the toddler years. Because parents are accustomed to the rapid growth and resulting appetite of the first year of life, they may be concerned when they see their toddler eating less food from both low appetite and susceptibility to distractions while eating. Increasing the variety of foods available helps children to develop good eating habits. The food preferences of young children grow directly from the frequency of a food's use in pleasant surroundings and the increased opportunity to become familiar with a number of foods. Reserving sweets for special occasions versus bribery or reward for good behavior helps reinforce good nutrition habits. The Ellyn Satter Institute provides many helpful tips and resources on feeding children: www.ellynsatterinstitute.org.

Energy and protein needs are still high (per kg of body weight) compared with adult needs. Toddlers have a wide range of energy needs during this time as determined by their velocity of growth and level of physical activity. Muscle mass, bone structure, and other body tissues continue to grow rapidly and require an adequate dietary supply of protein, minerals, and vitamins. The Food and Nutrition Board recommends a daily intake of 19 g of fiber to prevent constipation and to promote a healthy gastrointestinal tract.[2]

PRESCHOOL-AGED CHILDREN (3 TO 5 YEARS OLD)

Physical growth and appetite continue in spurts during this period while mental capacity expands. Children continue to form eating patterns, attitudes, and basic eating habits because of social and emotional experiences involving food. **Food jags** are common in this age group and a frequent source of concern and frustration for caregivers. A jag may last a few days or weeks, but they are usually self-limiting and of no major long-term health concern. Again, the key to happy and healthy eating is food variety, appropriately sized portions, and parental patience.

Group eating becomes a significant source of socialization. Children's food preferences generally reflect what their social group is eating. In such situations, a child learns a variety of food habits and establishes new relationships with food and with their mealtime companions. A solid foundation of healthy eating habits developed during this time with the supervision and encouragement from caregivers will set the stage for eating behaviors throughout childhood. Likewise, unhealthy habits established during this time may have long-term deleterious effects.

As with adults, MyPlate is a useful tool for meal planning in this age group. The U.S. Department of Agriculture published a child-friendly version of MyPlate, with dietary and physical activity recommendations and messages designed to appeal to young children (Figure 11.4). The USDA Food and Nutrition Information Center's "Lifecycle Nutrition" page has resources for educators, families, parents, and kids as well as much more information about improving the overall nutrition and health of children (search "Lifecycle Nutrition" at www.nal.usda.gov).

SCHOOL-AGED CHILDREN (5 TO 12 YEARS OLD)

During the early school years, a generally slow and irregular growth rate continues accompanied by overall body changes. Although physical growth slows, cognitive, emotional, and social growth occur extensively during this developmental state. By this time, body types are established, and growth rates vary widely. Development of girls usually bypasses that of boys during the latter part of this stage. With the stimulus of school and a variety of learning activities, children experience increasing mental and social maturity; they develop the ability to problem-solve and participate in competitive activities; and they discover a growing sense of autonomy.

Parental food habits continue to have the most influence on a child's eating behavior.[33] Although research is inconclusive regarding the most favorable parenting style to promote healthy eating, it is clear that parent modeling and dietary habits have a great influence on what a child eats and will eat as an adult.[33,34] In fact, parent or caregiver role modeling of healthy food choices (i.e., show children what to eat) may be an even greater indicator than actual parent dietary habits (i.e., what the parents actually eat).[35] Much research has focused on the family meal as an important component to healthy eating, particularly with increasing fruit and vegetable intake.[34,36] The benefits of the family meal extend beyond nutrition and include improved self-esteem, improved academic performance, decreased behavioral problems, decreased substance abuse, and decreased eating disorders.[37] Unfortunately, the family meal is often neglected because of busy schedules, lack of time, and poor planning. Box 11.1 provides tips to support family meals in today's busy lifestyle, an important aspect of overall well-being.

---

extrusion reflex the normal infant reflex to protrude the tongue outward when it is touched.

allergens food proteins that elicit an immune system response or an allergic reaction; symptoms may include itching, swelling, hives, diarrhea, and difficulty breathing as well as anaphylaxis in the worst cases.

food jag brief sprees or binges of eating one particular food.

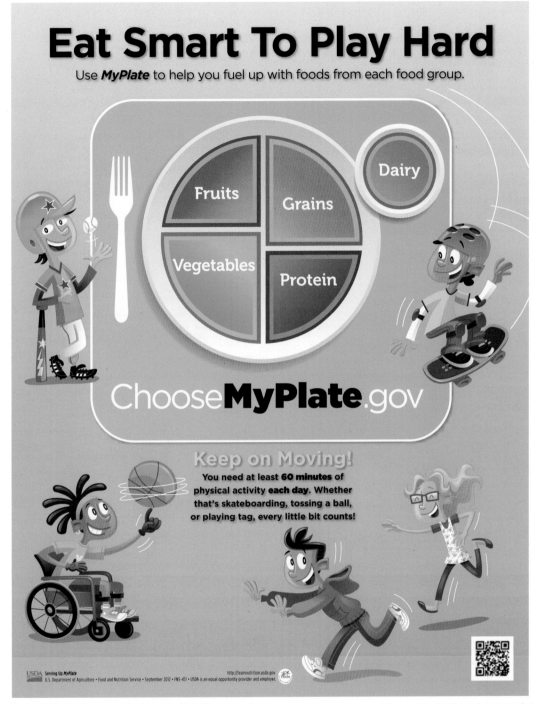

Figure 11.4 Eat Smart to Play Hard MyPlate Poster for Kids, which is targeted to meet the needs of children between the ages of 6 and 11 years. (Reprinted from the Food and Nutrition Service. [2012]. *Serving up MyPlate*. U.S. Department of Agriculture. Washington, DC: U.S. Government Printing Office. www.fns.usda.gov/tn/myplate.)

Although the family plays an integral role in building sound nutrition habits, the process of moving toward independence during this influential stage of life introduces other stimuli that affect food choices. One such persuasive factor is the amount and type of screen time to which children are exposed. Exposure of children to high amounts of screen time begins at an early age. Data from the CDC indicate that children aged 8 to 10 years old average 6 hours of screen time per day.[38] High-risk television behaviors are correlated to long-term negative effects on food habits (e.g., increased consumption of high-fat and high-sugar foods) and risk for obesity and insulin resistance.[39-41] Product marketing for foods with low nutrient value is commonplace in television advertisements.[41] One study concluded that every hour spent in front of a television was associated with a decrease in the overall quality of the child's diet (e.g., more junk food and less fruits and vegetables).[42] Although this is a powerful correlation, it is not causative. There are several factors and decisions involved, by both the child and the caregiver, when it comes

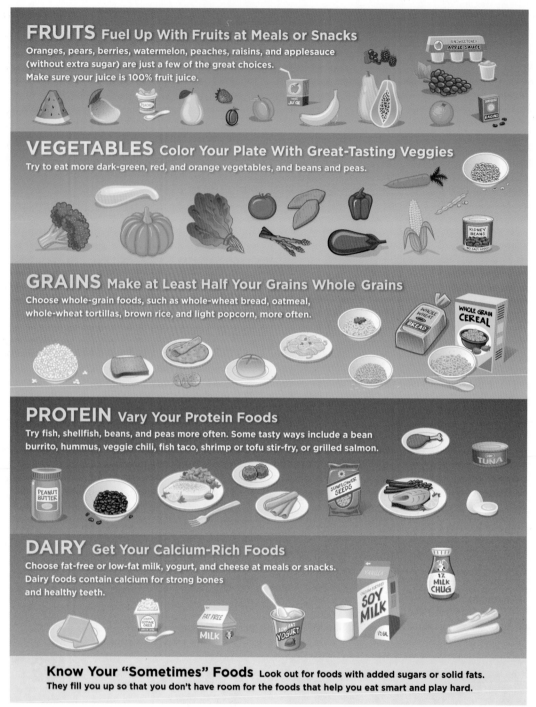

FRUITS Fuel Up With Fruits at Meals or Snacks

Oranges, pears, berries, watermelon, peaches, raisins, and applesauce (without extra sugar) are just a few of the great choices. Make sure your juice is 100% fruit juice.

VEGETABLES Color Your Plate With Great-Tasting Veggies

Try to eat more dark-green, red, and orange vegetables, and beans and peas.

GRAINS Make at Least Half Your Grains Whole Grains

Choose whole-grain foods, such as whole-wheat bread, oatmeal, whole-wheat tortillas, brown rice, and light popcorn, more often.

PROTEIN Vary Your Protein Foods

Try fish, shellfish, beans, and peas more often. Some tasty ways include a bean burrito, hummus, veggie chili, fish taco, shrimp or tofu stir-fry, or grilled salmon.

DAIRY Get Your Calcium-Rich Foods

Choose fat-free or low-fat milk, yogurt, and cheese at meals or snacks. Dairy foods contain calcium for strong bones and healthy teeth.

Know Your "Sometimes" Foods Look out for foods with added sugars or solid fats. They fill you up so that you don't have room for the foods that help you eat smart and play hard.

Figure 11.4, cont'd

Box 11.1   Implementing Family Meals in a Busy Lifestyle

- Model healthy eating
- Stock healthy food in the pantry
- Plan and make simple meals
- Have children help with meal preparation, in age-appropriate tasks
- Make a weekly meal plan before grocery shopping
- Prepare meals in bulk and freeze for later use
- Use a slow cooker (e.g., let the meal cook throughout the day and have a ready-to-eat meal that evening)
- Create a family eating space free from TVs and other electronic media
- Be flexible: "Family meals" can be any meal of the day
- Be realistic: "Family meals" may not happen every day, but strive for 3 times per week

to food consumption. In other words, turning on the TV does not put junk food into the hands of a child; someone had to purchase the food and make it available.

The Academy of Pediatrics previously set screen time limits as no screen time for children under age 2 years and 2 hours or less per day for children over 2 years.[43] In 2016 the Academy of Pediatrics revised guidelines to better reflect the use of educational screen time or "healthy media" related to a child's developmental state and parent modeling.[44] The Academy currently recommends personalized screen time limits to match the needs of each individual child. Check out the helpful family planning media screen time tool at www.healthychildren.org/MediaUsePlan.

Peer food habits and the school environment are two other examples of important factors that influence childhood eating behaviors. Some children bring their lunch to school, whereas others make food-purchasing decisions within the provisions available. Each school will provide a variety of healthy food options, but it is ultimately up to the child to decide what and how much to eat, which is why good food habits cultivated during the younger years are so important.

For some children the *School Breakfast and Lunch Programs* provide the only nourishing meals of their day. These federally assisted meal programs operate in public and nonprofit private schools as well as residential child-care institutions. The meals are free or at a low cost to the students and meet the childhood nutrition recommendations as outlined within the *Dietary Guidelines for Americans, 2020–2025*. Chapter 13 discusses the school breakfast and lunch programs and other community nutrition programs.

NUTRITION PROBLEMS DURING CHILDHOOD

There are several health problems that children may encounter during childhood, many of which have nutrition implications (e.g., diarrhea, vomiting, and fever). Although these issues are distressing for both children and caregivers, they usually do not have long-term health impacts. This chapter discusses select nutrition-related problems that have the potential for chronic health-related complications.

Failure to Thrive

The term *failure to thrive* describes infants, children, or adolescents who do not grow and develop normally. Failure to thrive most commonly affects young children between the ages of 1 and 5 years. Careful nutrition assessment is essential for identifying underlying feeding problems. The following factors may be involved:

- *Clinical disease:* central nervous system disorders, endocrine disease, congenital defects, or intestinal obstruction
- *Neuromotor problems:* poor sucking or abnormal muscle tone from the retention of primitive reflexes; eating, chewing, and swallowing problems
- *Dietary practices:* parental misconceptions or inexperience regarding normal infant feeding;

inappropriate formula-feeding or improper dilutions when mixing breast milk substitutes
- *Unusual nutrient needs or losses:* adequate diet for growth but inadequate nutrient absorption and thus excessive fecal loss; hypermetabolic state that requires increased dietary intake
- *Psychosocial problems:* family environment and relationships that result in neglect, abuse, or emotional deprivation of the child and require medical and nutrition intervention; similar problems also may occur between 2 and 4 years of age when parents and children have conflicts about normal changes caused by slowed childhood growth and energy needs that result in changing food patterns, food jags, erratic appetites, reduced milk intake, and disinterest in eating

A complex interaction of factors may lead to failure to thrive, and consequently there are no simple solutions. Thorough recording and evaluation of medical and diet history, supportive dietary guidance, and empathetic personal care are necessary to influence growth patterns in these infants or children. The careful and sensitive correction of the social and environmental issues that surround the problem is crucial for positive health outcomes.

Anemia

Iron fortification of cereals and breads has considerably reduced the cases of iron-deficiency anemia in the United States. However, anemia remains a concern for children with **food insecurity** and poor diets. Children should begin eating iron-rich foods at approximately 6 months of age. Milk anemia is a term that is sometimes used for toddlers (≥1 year old) who excessively consume cow's milk to the exclusion of other iron-rich foods. Although milk is an important source of several nutrients, it is a poor source of iron. Even if these children eat some iron-rich foods, their high calcium intake hinders the absorption of iron. Iron-deficiency anemia may delay cognitive development in children and have irreversible long-term effects.[45]

Obesity

Childhood and adolescent obesity began to rise in the United States in the 1970s and remains a significant health issue today (Box 11.2). The most recent data show that approximately 14% of 2- to 5-year-olds, 18% of 6- to 11-year-olds, and 21% of 12- to 19-year-olds are obese.[46] Overweight and obesity among children and adolescents is associated with a lower quality of life secondary to factors such as low self-esteem, bullying, depression, anxiety, and decreased physical functioning.[47] Furthermore,

---

screen time time spent in front of any electronic screen—television, computer, smart phone, DVD players, portable gaming devices, etc.

food insecurity limited or uncertain availability of nutritionally adequate and safe foods or limited or uncertain ability to acquire acceptable foods in socially acceptable ways.

| Box 11.2 | **Childhood Overweight and Obesity Facts** |

PREVALENCE OF OBESITY

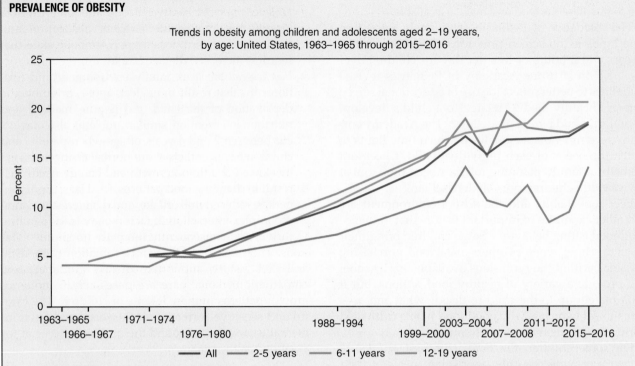

Trends in obesity among children and adolescents aged 2–19 years, by age: United States, 1963–1965 through 2015–2016

— All   — 2-5 years   — 6-11 years   — 12-19 years

Note: Obesity is body mass index (BMI) at or above the 95th percentile from the sex-specific BMI-for-age 2000 CDC Growth Charts.

Sources: NCHS, National Health Examination Surveys II (ages 6–11) and III (ages 12–17); National Health and Nutrition Examination Surveys (NHANES) I–III; and NHANES 1999–2000, 2001–2002, 2003–2004, 2005–2006, 2007–2008, 2009–2010, 2011–2012, 2013–2014, and 2015–2016.

CONTRIBUTING FACTORS
- Genetics
- Behavioral factors: excessive energy intake, low physical activity
- Environmental factors: parental role models, child-care environment, and lack of exposure to health, wellness, and nutrition at home and/or school

CONSEQUENCES
- Health risks: asthma, sleep apnea, hypertension, hyperlipidemia, metabolic syndrome, liver disease, type 2 diabetes, and polycystic ovarian syndrome

- Psychosocial risks: low self-esteem and social discrimination

The Centers for Disease Control and Prevention's website about childhood obesity (search "Childhood Obesity" at www.cdc.gov) has up-to-date information regarding the prevalence, current treatment recommendations, and information about state-based programs to help alleviate the health burden of childhood overweight and obesity.

medications used in the treatment of some conditions may cause, or worsen, the risk for undesirable weight gain (see the Drug-Nutrition Interaction box, "Antipsychotics and Nutrient Metabolism"). Although there are many issues involved, some factors during gestation and early infancy that increase the risk for childhood obesity include inadequate or excessive gestational weight gain, gestational diabetes, maternal smoking, and the use of breast milk substitutes (i.e., formula feeding).[48]

Both genetics and environment play major roles in the risk for obesity and are likely covariables.[48] Although overweight parents are more likely to have overweight children, there are modifiable risk factors that, if addressed, may reduce the risk for obesity for the entire family. Such factors include poor food selection, restrictive feeding practices that contribute to

bingeing behaviors, and physical inactivity. Infants and children are innately capable of recognizing satiety and self-regulating energy balance. However, this inherent awareness seems to decline between the ages of 3 and 5 years, when environmental factors (e.g., inappropriate portion sizes, encouragement to "clean the plate," caregivers using food as a reward) start to influence the amount of food eaten, despite satiety.

As stated earlier, attitudes and behaviors of parental figures are key determinants in the development of childhood eating habits. The following recommendations are helpful for guiding parents toward appropriate eating environments and for helping them to lower the risk of obesity in their children:

- Choose specific meal times.

Drug-Nutrient Interaction

Antipsychotics and Nutrient Metabolism

Children and adolescents with long-term health implications are receiving antipsychotic medications more frequently. The most common conditions for prescription are autism, schizophrenia, bipolar mania, Tourette syndrome, major depression, and for aggression associated with attention deficit hyperactivity disorder (ADHD). Boys with autism more frequently receive prescriptions for antipsychotics; and girls with depression and anxiety disorders more frequently receive prescriptions for antipsychotics.

Risperidone (generic for Risperdal) is one of the more common second-generation antipsychotic drugs. Nutrition-related side effects include weight gain, increased appetite, nausea, vomiting, constipation, and stomach pain. There is some concern that risperidone also increases blood glucose, blood pressure, cholesterol, and triglycerides. This combined with drug-associated weight gain may make children susceptible to metabolic syndrome and cardiovascular disease. One study evaluated the effects of second-generation antipsychotics on adolescents for 12 months. In 1 year, these adolescents had increased BMI, waist circumference, fasting blood glucose, and triglycerides and decreased HDL cholesterol.[1] There is some evidence risperidone negatively effects the gut microbiome, increasing inflammation and body weight.[2] More research is needed to understand the long-term effects of these drugs. However, health care providers should be aware of the increased risk for chronic disease and have clients work with registered dietitian nutritionists to attenuate risk factors (e.g., body weight).

REFERENCES

1. Sjo, C. P., Stenstrom, A. D., Bojesen, A. B., et al. (2017). Development of metabolic syndrome in drug-naive adolescents after 12 months of second-generation antipsychotic treatment. *Journal of Child and Adolescent Psychopharmacology, 27*(10):884–891.
2. Skonieczna-Żydecka, K., Łoniewski, I., Misera, A., et al. (2019). Second-generation antipsychotics and metabolism alterations: A systematic review of the role of the gut microbiome. *Psychopharmacology, 236*(5):1491–1512.

- Provide a wide variety of nutrient-dense foods (e.g., fruits, vegetables).
- Put cut-up vegetables in a lower level of the refrigerator so that children can help themselves to a healthy snack.
- Offer an age-appropriate portion size. Large servings can be overwhelming to picky eaters.
- Limit nonnutritive snacking and the use of juice or sugar-sweetened beverages.
- Encourage children to regulate their own food intake based on intuitive eating principles. Rather than saying, "Clean your plate," ask your child, "Are you full?"
- Have regular family meals to promote social interaction and to model healthy food-related behavior.
- Limit screen time.
- Make physical activity a daily family affair.

Physical activity is an important part of a healthy lifestyle from birth to death. Children aged 3 to 5 should be physically active throughout the day, and children/adolescents aged 6 to 17 should strive for at least 60 minutes of moderate to vigorous physical activity each day.[49] By developing an appreciation for, and an enjoyment of, regular physical activity during childhood, the risk for obesity and associated health problems later in life may be mitigated.

Lead Poisoning

Lead poisoning in children can be extremely damaging to the central nervous system, and it can negatively alter both cognitive and motor skills. The majority of lead exposure among children is the result of lead-based paint. Lead-containing paint chips from deteriorating buildings or renovations result in high levels of lead-contaminated dust. Children explore with their hands and mouths at this age, thereby making the oral intake and inhalation of lead highly likely. Chapter 13 covers lead poisoning in detail.

NUTRITION REQUIREMENTS DURING ADOLESCENCE (12 TO 18 YEARS OLD)

PHYSICAL GROWTH

Body Composition

The final growth spurt of childhood occurs with the onset of puberty. This rapid growth is evident in increasing body size and the development of sex characteristics in response to hormonal maturation. Because the velocity of growth and onset of puberty can vary greatly among individual boys and girls, biologic age is a better indicator of nutrition needs than chronologic age throughout adolescence.

There are distinct patterns of body composition changes. Girls store more subcutaneous fat in the abdominal area. The pelvis widens in preparation for future childbearing, and the size of the hips also increases, which can cause anxiety for many body-conscious young girls. In boys, increased muscle mass and long bone growth characterize growth. Initially, a boy's growth spurt is slower than that of a girl's, but he typically surpasses her in both weight and height.

Although the data are conflicting regarding boys, obese girls are likely to progress through puberty at an earlier age than normal-weight girls.[50] Early menarche is also associated with adult obesity and increased risk of cardiovascular disease.[51] Differences in biologic age, as defined by stage of puberty and body composition, are important when assessing growth on a growth chart (see the Cultural Considerations box, "Growth Charts: Can You Use Them for All Children?").

Bone Mineral Density

During childhood, bone mineral density accumulates slowly and then rapidly accelerates before puberty. The peak bone mineral accretion rate occurs on average at

Cultural Considerations

Growth Charts: Can You Use Them for All Children?

HUMAN MILK OR BREAST MILK SUBSTITUTES

Breastfed infants have a slightly different growth curve than infants fed a breast milk substitute (i.e., infant formula). Breastfed infants grow slightly more rapidly than formula-fed infants do during the first 2 months of life, and then the rate of growth declines to a level that is slower than that of infants receiving breast milk substitutes. Because formula-fed infants were the basis for the original CDC growth charts, it is not appropriate to use these charts for children under the age of 2 years.

The WHO charts used infants who were exclusively breastfed (the standard for normal infant nutrition) in accordance with feeding recommendations (i.e., breastfeed for at least 12 months, with solid foods introduced between 4 and 6 months) to obtain the standard growth curves. All health care providers should plot infants on the WHO growth charts, regardless of feeding method.

GROWTH CHARTS IN RELATION TO VARIATIONS IN SEXUAL MATURATION

When charting the growth patterns of an adolescent, practitioners should be aware of the differences in the timing of sexual maturation and how that relates to overall weight and body fat. Obesity and ethnicity influence the timing of puberty. For example, obese females begin menarche before girls of normal weight.[1] Black girls and boys begin the process of sexual maturity before Mexican-American or white children do.[2,3] Such differences are important when assessing growth on a growth chart. More sexually mature children are expected to be taller and heavier than their less mature peers.

USING GROWTH CHARTS FOR VARIOUS RACES

Ideally, growth charts would be available for various ethnicities. Currently, there are not enough available data to do this. Therefore, the CDC and the WHO promote the use of the standard growth charts for all racial and ethnic groups. Future studies will determine if significant differences exist and warrant the development of charts that are specific to different racial and ethnic backgrounds.

REFERENCES

1. Li, W., Liu, Q., Deng, X., Chen, Y., Liu, S., & Story, M. (2017). Association between obesity and puberty timing: A systematic review and meta-analysis. *International Journal of Environmental Research and Public Health*, *24*(10), 14.
2. Ramnitz, M. S., & Lodish, M. B. (2013). Racial disparities in pubertal development. *Seminars in Reproductive Medicine*, *31*(5), 333–339.
3. Hoyt, L. T., Deardorff, J., Marceau, K., et al. (2018). Girls' sleep trajectories across the pubertal transition: Emerging racial/ethnic differences. *Journal of Adolescent Health*, *62*(4), 496–503.

12.5 years in girls and 14 years in boys. Approximately 95% of adult bone is completed within the 4 years before and 4 years after peak bone accretion.[8] Linear growth reaches its peak at about 16 years of age for females and 21 years of age for males. Adolescents consuming a balanced diet with calcium-containing dairy or dairy substitutes achieve higher peak bone mass and linear growth than do their counterparts who do not eat a balanced diet. As discussed previously, adolescents often fall short on dairy and calcium intake.[4,11] The long-term benefits of maximizing bone growth during adolescence are paramount for healthy bones throughout the remainder of life.

EATING PATTERNS

Rapid growth as well as self-consciousness and peer pressure influence adolescent eating habits. Teens tend to skip meals, to snack, to eat at fast-food restaurants regularly, and to eat any kind of food at any time of day (e.g., pizza for breakfast). Furthermore, meal patterns and habits established in early adolescence through parental guidance and modeling are indicative of meal patterns that will be maintained through late adolescence and early adulthood, thus highlighting the importance of establishing well-balanced healthy meals and eating schedules during the childhood and early adolescence years.[52] This is also a time when some teenagers begin to experiment with alcohol. Even a mild form of alcohol abuse in combination with the elevated nutrition demands of adolescence can easily undermine a teen's nutrition status. Boys usually fare better than girls do in overall nutrition. Their larger appetite and the sheer volume of food consumed usually ensure an adequate intake of nutrients. Alternatively, because girls are frequently under a greater social pressure for thinness, they may tend to restrict their food and have an inadequate nutrient intake.

EATING DISORDERS

Social, family, and body image pressures strongly influence many young girls and an increasing number of young boys. As a result, they sometimes follow unwise self-imposed crash diets for weight loss. In some cases, clinical eating disorders such as anorexia nervosa and bulimia nervosa may develop. Psychologists have traditionally identified mothers as the main source of family pressure to remain thin. However, fathers may also contribute to the problem if they are emotionally distant and do not provide important feedback to build self-worth and self-esteem in their young children. Parents and caregivers must help their children to see themselves as loved no matter what they weigh so that these children are not as vulnerable to social influences that equate extreme thinness with beauty.

Eating disorders involve a distorted body image and a morbid and irrational pursuit of thinness. Such disordered eating often begins during the early adolescent years, when many girls see themselves as fat even though their average weight is often below the normal weight for their height. The longer the duration of the illness, the less likely a person is to achieve a full recovery. Thus, early detection and intervention are critical for overall health. Please see Chapter 15 for the warning signs, diagnostic criteria, treatment options, and preventive measures for eating disorders.

Putting It All Together

Summary

- The growth and development of healthy children depends on optimal nutrition support. Conversely, good nutrition depends on many social, psychologic, cultural, and environmental influences that affect individual growth potential throughout the life cycle.
- The nutrition needs of children change with each unique growth period.
- Social and cultural factors influence the developing food habits of all children and these habits often last a lifetime.
- Infants experience the most rapid growth in the life cycle. Human milk is the natural first food, with solid foods introduced at approximately 6 months of age, when digestive and physiologic processes have matured.
- Toddlers, preschoolers, and school-aged children experience slowed, irregular growth compared with infancy. During this period, their energy demands are lower per kilogram of body weight compared with that of infancy, but they require a well-balanced diet for continued growth and health.
- Adolescents undergo a large growth spurt during puberty. This rapid growth involves both physical and sexual maturation. A well-balanced diet should supply adequate nutrients to support the large amount of bone mineralization and tissue growth that occurs at this time.
- There are several nutrition-related health concerns that affect children and adolescents; obesity is the most common.

Chapter Review Questions

See answers in Appendix A.

1. Which of the following foods would most likely be appropriate for an 8-month-old infant?

   a. Whole milk
   b. Scrambled egg
   c. Chopped apples
   d. Regular yogurt

2. Which food is not an appropriate first solid food for an infant?

   a. Infant oat cereal
   b. Egg white
   c. Pureed carrots
   d. Applesauce

3. Which of the following feeding tips would be appropriate to convey to parents of toddlers?

   a. Season food more than usual so that the child will eat.
   b. Offer a variety of foods but do not force the child to eat.
   c. Serve small portions and ensure that the child finishes them.
   d. Do not allow children to serve themselves small portions.

4. Parents can help school-age children develop healthy eating habits by _____.

   a. teaching how to restrict food intake to avoid weight gain
   b. leading by example and eating a diet that provides nutrient-dense foods
   c. ensuring that children never eat high-fat or energy-dense snack foods
   d. encouraging children not to adopt parents' unhealthy eating habits

5. Teenage girls more often respond to social and peer pressure to restrict food intake and control weight, which can lead to _____.

   a. obesity
   b. epilepsy
   c. disordered eating
   d. type 1 diabetes mellitus

Next-Generation NCLEX® Examination-style Case Study

See answers in Appendix A.

A 7-month-old male infant was born weighing 4 lbs., 8 oz. His parents are bottle feeding him with cow's milk. The parents position the baby and the bottle appropriately, but the baby is always fussy and frequently has diarrhea. They give him daily vitamin D drops (400 IU) and have been introducing him to scrambled egg whites. Currently, the infant's growth chart shows that his weight is at the 9th percentile, his length is at the 50th percentile, and his head circumference is at the 52nd percentile. The mother is concerned about the infant's growth and frequent bouts of prolonged crying.

1. Of the history and assessment findings listed below, select all that require follow-up.

   a. Birth weight of 4 lbs., 8 oz.
   b. Bottle feeding cow's milk
   c. Length at 50th percentile
   d. Head circumference at 52nd percentile
   e. Weight at 9th percentile
   f. Introducing infant to scrambled eggs
   g. Diarrhea
   h. Vitamin D drops
   i. Feeding positioning

2. Choose the *most likely* options for the information missing from the statement below by selecting from the list of options provided.

   Cow's milk is insufficient in _____ and _____ , which may hinder normal growth in the infant.

OPTIONS	
calories	vitamin D
protein	calcium
carbohydrates	riboflavin
essential fatty acids	

3. Match the most appropriate nursing response option (provided below) to each client question.

CLIENT QUESTIONS	APPROPRIATE NURSE'S RESPONSE FOR EACH CLIENT QUESTION
"How long should infants be breastfed?"	
"What do I use to feed my 7-month-old infant if I don't want to breastfeed?	
"Can I feed my 7-month-old infant water and juice?"	
"When can infants drink cow's milk?"	

Nurse's Response Options

a. "You can use an iron-fortified breast milk substitute, if necessary."
b. "Infants can be introduced to cow's milk during the first 6 months of life."
c. "Infants can be introduced to cow's milk at the end of the first year."
d. "Those options are unnecessary for infants during the first 6 months of life."
e. "You should breastfeed for at least the first full year of life."
f. "After the first 6 months, you don't need to breastfeed anymore."
g. "You can use any type of milk."
h. "You should avoid cow's milk until the child is 5 years old."

4. From the list below, select all of the foods that would be appropriate to introduce to an infant who is just starting solid foods.

   a. Citrus juice
   b. Nuts
   c. Soft fruit
   d. Egg whites
   e. Wheat
   f. Soft vegetables
   g. Yogurt

5. For each assessment finding, place an X under the appropriate column to indicate whether nursing and collaborative interventions were <u>effective</u> (helped to meet expected outcomes), or <u>ineffective</u> (did not help to meet expected outcomes).

ASSESSMENT FINDING	EFFECTIVE	INEFFECTIVE
Infant is happy and cries less		
Normal bowel movements 1-2 times per day		
Weight increased 2 percentiles		
Parents feed infant peanuts and hotdogs		
Infant is getting iron-fortified breast milk substitute if the mother is not breastfeeding		
Parents leave infant with a bottle of juice propped into the infant's mouth to feed		

Additional Learning Resources

Please refer to this text's Evolve website for answers to the Case Study questions:

http://evolve.elsevier.com/Williams/basic/

References and **Further Reading and Resources** in the back of the book provide additional resources for enhancing knowledge.

Nutrition for Adults: The Early, Middle, and Later Years

Key Concepts

- Gradual aging throughout the adult years is a unique process that reflects an individual's genetic heritage and life experience.

- Aging is a total life process that involves biologic, nutrition, social, economic, psychologic, and spiritual aspects.
- Nutrition requirements change along with progressive physiologic changes of the body.

The rapid growth and development of adolescence leads to physical maturity as adults. Physical growth in bone structure levels off, but the constant cell growth and regeneration that are necessary to maintain a healthy body continue. Other aspects of growth and development—mental, social, psychologic, and spiritual—continue for a lifetime.

Food and nutrition continue to provide essential sustenance during the adult aging process. **Life expectancy** continues to rise throughout most areas of the world; thus, health promotion and disease prevention are even more important to ensure quality of life throughout these extended years.

This chapter explores the ways in which positive nutrition can help adults lead healthier, disease-free lives.

ADULTHOOD: CONTINUING HUMAN GROWTH AND DEVELOPMENT

COMING OF AGE IN AMERICA

Americans are experiencing tremendous change in the composition of the population. The *Healthy People* initiative represents a national effort to maintain health at all ages by supporting people in their ability to make informed, evidence-based decisions about their well-being. One of the primary goals set for the United States is to attain high-quality, longer lives that are free of preventable disease, disability, injury, and premature death by improving the five key social determinants of health (Figure 12.1).[1] Achieving this goal requires proper nutrition, among other healthy lifestyle habits, throughout life to enjoy vitality in the advanced years.

Population and Age Distribution

The U.S. Census Bureau predicts that the demographics of the U.S. population will change dramatically in the next couple of decades. Specifically, the percentage of the population qualifying as "older" will increase significantly during this period, while the percentage of children in the population will decline. In fact, the U.S. Census Bureau forecasts that by the year 2035 older adults (over 65 years) will outnumber children (under 18 years) for the first time in U.S. history (Figure 12.2).[2] The median age will increase from 38 years old to 43 years old by 2060, with women outnumbering men in the eldest groups. Growth rates for various ethnic subgroups continue to rise as well (see the Cultural Considerations box, "The Aging Composition of the U.S. Population"). A shifting age distribution in the population obliges changes in the health care system as well as job demands in geriatric health care. Healthy nutrition and lifestyle factors adopted early in life (e.g., not smoking, maintaining a healthy weight, and normal blood pressure) promote disease-free years at this end of the life spectrum.[3,4]

Life Expectancy and Quality of Life

Life expectancy has dramatically increased during the past century, from only 47 years in 1900 to a projected average of 85.6 years in 2060 (84 years for men and 87.1 for women).[5] However, there are notable differences in life expectancy among various population groups and among those with different household incomes and living environments.[6] Americans consistently value health-related quality of life, which is one's personal sense of physical and mental health and ability to act within the environment. Quality of life is a major focus of the *Healthy People* initiative.[1]

---

life expectancy the number of years that a person of a given age may expect to live; this is affected by environment, lifestyle, sex, and race.

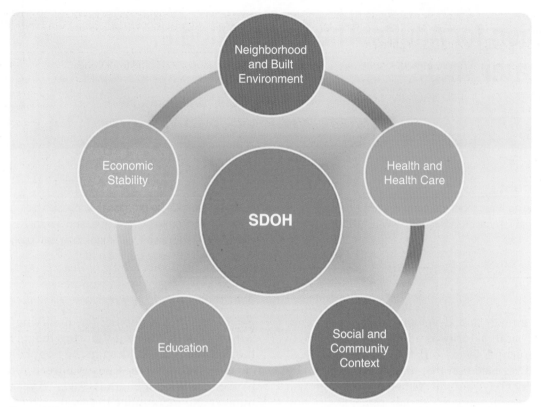

Figure 12.1 Social determinants of health. (From U.S. Department of Health and Human Services. [2010]. *Healthy People 2030*. health.gov/healthypeople. Published 2020. [Accessed 28 April, 2021].)

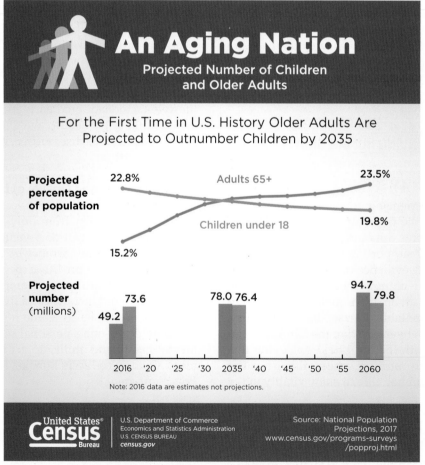

Figure 12.2 An aging nation: projected number of children and older adults by 2035. (From U.S. Census Bureau, Population Division. [2018]. *Projected age groups and sex composition of the population: Main projections series for the United States, 2017-2060*. Washington, DC: U.S. Government Printing Office.)

🌐 Cultural Considerations

The Aging Composition of the U.S. Population

Shifting racial and ethnic patterns continue to reshape the American population as a whole, particularly in the older segment of the population. Although all racial and ethnic groups will increase in absolute numbers, the fraction of each group will change extensively in the coming decades. Currently, non-Hispanic white adults make up about 77% of the population living in the United States that are older than age 65. By the year 2060, this segment of the senior population will decrease to 55%, while the percentage of Hispanic or Latino elderly will grow from 8% to 21%.[1]

2016 race and Hispanic origin age 65 years and older

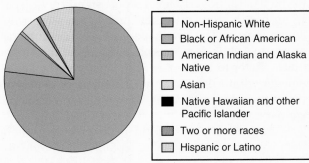

- Non-Hispanic White
- Black or African American
- American Indian and Alaska Native
- Asian
- Native Hawaiian and other Pacific Islander
- Two or more races
- Hispanic or Latino

2060 race and Hispanic origin age 65 years and older

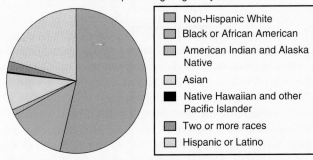

- Non-Hispanic White
- Black or African American
- American Indian and Alaska Native
- Asian
- Native Hawaiian and other Pacific Islander
- Two or more races
- Hispanic or Latino

(From U.S. Census Bureau, Population Division. [2018]. *Race and Hispanic origin by selected age groups: Main projections series for the United States, 2017-2060.* Washington, DC: U.S. Government Printing Office.)

Life expectancy varies among groups. For example, the current life expectancy for Hispanics is the longest at 82.1 years, whereas it is 80.7 years for Caucasians, and 77 years for African Americans.[2] Living arrangements, household income, educational attainment, type of medical insurance, and many other variables fluctuate among population groups, all of which influence life expectancy.

Health care providers should recognize and address the cultural and ethnic needs of an elderly individual when providing nutrition education. All areas of social, socioeconomic, and available health care provisions affect the best plan of care. Cookie-cutter meal plans for one ethnic group are not particularly useful for another culturally diverse population. Given the rapidly changing ethnic diversity of the elderly population in the United States, it is increasingly important to appreciate and practice cultural sensitivity.

In addition, the growth structure of the population presents specific concerns with regard to health, medical, and financial dependency. The population participating in the workforce contributes directly to benefit programs through income taxes that support dependent populations (i.e., individuals under age 18 and over age 65). Only 15% of the population was over age 65 and eligible for services such as social security and Medicare in 2016. By 2060, that percentage will increase to 23.4%.[3] Meanwhile, the working class population (aged 18 to 64 years) will decrease from 62% to 56.7%. Essentially, there will be a larger responsibility on the working age population to support the increasing numbers of elderly dependents. Healthy aging will be imperative to sustain the health care system.

REFERENCES

1. U.S. Census Bureau, Population Division. (2018). *Race and Hispanic origin by selected age groups: Main projections series for the United States, 2017-2060.* Washington, DC: U.S. Government Printing Office.
2. U.S. Census Bureau, Population Division. (2014). *Projected life expectancy at birth by sex, race, and Hispanic origin for the United States: 2015 to 2060.* Washington, DC: U.S. Government Printing Office.
3. U.S. Census Bureau, Population Division. (2018). *Projected age groups and sex composition of the population: Main projections series for the United States, 2017-2060.* Washington, DC: U.S. Government Printing Office.

Impact on Health Care

Career opportunities in the fields of disease prevention and health promotion are at an all-time high. Community and private classes focused on healthy lifestyles and nutrition target the prime concerns for a growing adult population. Weight management and diabetes management are two of the most popular topics. Dietitians, nurses, life coaches, personal trainers, psychologists, and other members of the health care team may be involved at various levels of such programs. A dire need exists for individuals to adopt healthy lifestyles in an effort to safeguard their health. It will be difficult for the current health care system in America to continuing financing the increasing expense of disease treatment, particularly when most chronic diseases are preventable.

SHAPING INFLUENCES ON ADULT GROWTH AND DEVELOPMENT

Human aging has the unique potential for growth and fulfillment at every stage. The periods of adulthood (i.e., the young, middle, and older years) are no exception. Many individual and group events mark the course; however, at each stage, the basic areas of adult life—physical, psychosocial, socioeconomic, and nutritional—shape general growth and development possibilities.

Physical Growth

Genetic potential governs the overall physical growth and maturity of the human body, which level off during the early adult years. Physical growth is no longer a process of increasing numbers of cells; rather, it involves the vital growth of new cells to replace old ones. After physical maturity is established, energy requirements decrease. Adjustment to a gradually declining metabolic rate, and thus the need for fewer kilocalories, is important for weight management. At older ages, individual vigor reflects the health status of the preceding years.

Psychosocial Development

Human personality development continues throughout the adult years. Three unique stages of personal psychosocial growth progress through the young, middle, and older years. The exact chronologic age at which an adult enters each stage varies. For example, the designation of "older adults" as aged 65 years old or older is an estimation. Individuals will progress through each stage at their own rate and may not consider themselves an "older adult" until they are well into their 80s or even 90s.

Young adults (20 to 44 years old). With physical maturity, young adults become increasingly independent. They form many new relationships; adopt new roles; and make many choices about continued education, career, jobs, commitments, and family. Young adults often experience considerable stress but also significant personal growth. These are years of professional development, establishing a home community, and deciding whether to expand their family, all of which are part of early personal struggles to make their way in the world. Sometimes health problems relate to these early demanding periods. The firm establishment of healthy lifestyle behaviors during this period (e.g., engaging in regular exercise, choosing balanced meals that promote and preserve health) is important for maintaining long-term quality of life.

Middle adults (45 to 64 years old). The middle years often present an opportunity to expand personal growth. In many cases of middle-aged adults who raised children, their children have grown and are beginning to make their own lives, and parents may have a sense of "it's my turn now." This also is a time of coming to terms with what life has offered with a refocusing of ideas, life directions, and activities. Early evidence of chronic disease appears in some middle-aged adults. Wellness, health promotion, and the reduction of disease risks continue to be major focuses of health care.

Older adults (65 years old and older). Adults vary widely with regard to their personal and physical resources for dealing with older age. They may have a sense of wholeness and completeness, or they may increasingly withdraw from life. If the outcome of their life experiences is positive, they arrive at an older age rich in the wisdom of their years; they are more likely to enjoy life and health and enrich the lives of those around them. However, some elderly people arrive at these years poorly equipped to deal with the adjustments associated with aging and the health problems that may arise. As this population continues to grow, the subdivisions of young-old (65 to 74 years old), elderly (75 to 84 years old), and old-old (85 years old and older) are a general way to characterize subgroups of older adults. Many factors that influence perceived and actual quality of life are integrally associated with nutrition status.

Socioeconomic Status

Social and economic variables considerably influence quality of life and health status in the elderly population. Adults with a family income of less than 200% of the federal poverty level report significant disparity in health relative to their higher-income–earning counterparts.[7] This trend persists despite universal access to Medicare-funded health care in the United States. Refer to Figure 12.1; how many of the key elements within the social determinants of health are directly or indirectly associated with socioeconomic status?

Sometimes social and financial pressures, along with a decreasing sense of acceptance and productivity, diminish the self-esteem and perceived value of the elderly. For example, economic insecurity may negatively affect nutrition status and necessitate the reliance on food assistance programs (Figure 12.3). Depression is a clinical syndrome that is not part of normal aging. Studies show that individuals suffering from depression are also more likely to have poor overall health, increased health care costs, poor financial resources, feelings of loneliness, and increased mortality.[8-10] Elderly clients with declining health are particularly susceptible to depression, which is a leading cause of **unintentional weight loss**.[11-13] *Failure to thrive* in the geriatric population, which is generally multifactorial and caused by a combination of chronic diseases, is associated with impaired physical function, malnutrition, depression, and cognitive impairment.[14] All people need a sense of belonging, achievement, and self-worth. Unfortunately, many elderly people suffer from meager financial resources, loneliness, uncertainty, and depression, all of which increase mortality in a vicious cycle.

An increasing number of retirement-age adults are continuing to contribute to the workforce in their advanced years. These individuals are redefining what it means to be a senior citizen and report significantly higher psychologic and physiologic well-being status than retirees.[15,16] Improved socioeconomic status, physical activity, social networks, and cognitive function may all be protective effects of continued employment.

unintentional weight loss weight loss of 5% of body weight over a 6- to 12-month period that is not intentional.

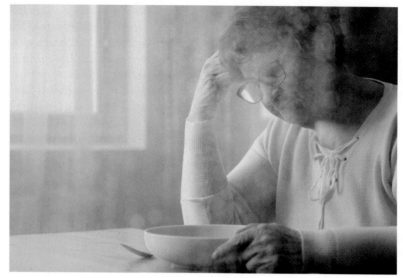

Figure 12.3 The food intake of elderly individuals may be negatively impacted by social and financial pressures. (Copyright iStock Photo; Credit: KatarzynaBialasiewicz.)

Nutrition Needs

The energy and nutrient needs of individual adults in each age group vary in accordance with living and working situations. The Dietary Reference Intake (DRI) recommendations for healthy adults meet most needs, but the aging process influences individual nutrition requirements. Only in the most recent DRIs have scientists distinguished the nutrient needs of the 50- to 70-year-old adults from those who are over 70 years old. In previous publications of the DRIs there was not a large enough population of healthy elderly adults to study their nutrient requirements. With the aging of the population in recent decades, there are enough data on nutrient requirements of the elderly to warrant a separate category for those older than 70 years.

THE AGING PROCESS AND NUTRITION NEEDS

GENERAL PHYSIOLOGIC CHANGES

Biologic Changes

Throughout life, every experience makes an imprint on one's individual heritage. Everyone ages in different ways, depending on his or her personal makeup and available resources.

Metabolism. Beginning at about the age of 30 years, a gradual loss of functioning cells begins, which results in reduced cell metabolism and changes in body composition. This change in metabolic rate reflects both lean muscle mass loss as well as a loss of high metabolically active organ tissues such as the brain, liver, heart, and kidneys.[17,18] The rate of this decline accelerates during the later years. Not all skeletal muscle mass loss is mandatory, though. A contributing factor to **sarcopenia** is inadequate dietary protein metabolism and physical activity.[19,20]

Regular physical activity helps to maintain muscle mass, the metabolic rate, and overall health. However, 28% of Americans aged 50 and over do not participate in any leisure-time physical activity.[21] The current *Physical Activity Guidelines for Americans* recommend 150 to 300 minutes of moderate-intensity physical activity (or 75 to 150 minutes of vigorous-intensity physical activity) per week to reduce the risk of chronic disease (see Chapter 16).[22]

Hormones. Hormonal changes during the aging process have many repercussions in general health. The common decline in insulin production or insulin sensitivity results in elevated blood glucose levels and diabetes. Decreases in the level of **melatonin** may interfere with normal sleep cycles. Parts of the normal changes in body composition are attributable to decreases in the levels of growth hormone and the sex hormones estrogen and testosterone. **Menopause** involves the cessation of estrogen and progesterone production by the ovaries. This dramatic change in a woman's life, which usually occurs between the ages of 45 and 55 years, represents the most significant hormonal change associated with age. Menopause is accompanied by an increase in body fat, a decrease in lean tissue, and an increase in the risk of chronic disease (specifically heart disease and osteoporosis). Despite these changes, women today are better equipped than ever before with both social and medical support to embrace this period of life and to maintain health for many decades to come.

Effect on Food Patterns

Some of the physical changes of aging affect food patterns. For example, the secretion of digestive juices lessens, and the motility of gastrointestinal muscles gradually

---

sarcopenia loss of lean tissue mass associated with aging.
melatonin the hormone responsible for regulating body rhythms.
menopause the end of a woman's menstrual activity and capacity to bear children.

weakens, which together cause diminished absorption and bioavailability of nutrients. Decreased taste, smell, thirst, and vision also affect appetite and reduce food and fluid intake. Some conditions that can negatively influence food intake in the elderly are not so obvious. For example, decreased hand function can reduce hand-eye coordination and the ability to prepare and cook food. Older people may experience increased concern about body functions, more socioeconomic stress, personal losses, and fewer opportunities to maintain self-esteem; all of these concerns can alter the pleasure and priority of healthy dietary habits. A lack of sufficient nourishment is a chief nutrition problem for older adults.

Individuality of the Aging Process

The stages of biologic change related to **senescence** are generally similar for aging individuals. However, each person is unique: people may show a wide variety of individual responses depending on their genetic heritage and the health and nutrition resources of their prior years. For example, some individuals are in the best shape of their lives after retirement when given the extra time to eat and exercise freely and without stressful time constraints. Meanwhile, other adults respond to retirement in just the opposite manner by becoming less active and adopting poor dietary habits. Thus, specific nutrition needs vary with functional ability.

NUTRITION NEEDS

Macronutrients and Fluids

The basal metabolic rate declines an average of 1% to 2% per decade, with a more rapid decline occurring at approximately 40 years of age for men and 50 years of age for women.[23] This correlates with a gradual loss of functioning body cells and reduced physical activity, as discussed earlier. The mean energy expenditure for women who are between the ages of 51 and 70 years and have an ideal body mass index (BMI) between 18.5 to 25 kg/m² is 2066 kcal/day; for women who are older than 70 years, it is substantially lower at 1564 kcal/day. For men of the same age and BMI status, energy expenditure averages are 2469 kcal/day and 2238 kcal/day, respectively.[23] These values reflect the averages of the population, assuming a 5% decrease in metabolic activity during the middle and older years. Actual kilocalorie needs will vary greatly among individuals as a reflection of their physical and health status and living situations. Not all adults are intuitive about their declining energy needs. Failure to reduce energy intake compatibly with reduced energy needs leads to weight gain. Sarcopenia coupled with obesity throughout the adult years increases the prevalence of disability.[24,25] Thus, health promotion that includes weight control, physical activity, and disease prevention is an important aspect of healthy living throughout the entire life span.

The basic fuels that are necessary to supply energy needs for the adult are the same as they are for all stages of life: primarily carbohydrate, along with moderate fat.

Carbohydrate. A well-designed diet contains enough carbohydrates to meet 45% to 65% of total kilocalorie needs, with an emphasis on complex carbohydrates (e.g., whole grains, vegetables). The simple sugars (i.e., the mono- and disaccharides in soft drinks, candy, and sweets) may also be used for energy, but they should be consumed in limited amounts and make up no more than 10% of total kilocalorie intake. As a person's metabolic rate declines, so does the room for empty calories (i.e., simple sugars).

Fat. High-quality dietary fat provides a backup energy source, important fat-soluble vitamins, and essential fatty acids. A balanced diet consists of about 30% fat, with an emphasis on monounsaturated and polyunsaturated fat sources. Dietary fat enhances taste, aids appetite, and in some cases provides needed kilocalories to prevent unintentional weight loss.

Protein. The DRIs recommend a protein intake of 0.8 g per kilogram of body weight for adults. Thus, a man weighing 154 lb would use approximately 56 g of protein daily. The average-weight woman (127 lb) would use approximately 46 g of protein per day. A balanced diet provides 10% to 35% of the total kilocalories in the form of protein (see Chapter 4).[23] The average adult in the United States consumes approximately 1.5 times this amount of protein on any given day.[26]

Older adults (≥65 years) need slightly more protein per kilogram of body weight in response to decreased metabolic performance, changes in gut microbiota, and sarcopenia. In addition, the requirement for protein may rise during illness or convalescence or in the presence of a wasting disease. In any case, protein needs are related to two basic factors: (1) the protein quality (i.e., the quantity and ratio of its amino acids) and (2) an adequate number of total kilocalories in the diet. The current protein recommendations for adults 65 years old and older are to consume between 1.0 and 1.5 g of protein/kg/day depending on their health status (Table 12.1).[27,28]

Fluid. Water needs (relative to total energy needs) do not decline with age. See Table 9.1 for fluid intake recommendations for adults.

Micronutrients and Health Concerns

A diet that includes a variety of foods should supply adequate amounts of most vitamins and minerals for healthy adults. However, some essential nutrients may require special attention because of medication

Table 12.1   Dietary Protein Recommendations for Adults

HEALTH STATUS	PROTEIN (G/KG/DAY)
Healthy adults ≤65 years old	0.8
Healthy adults ≥65 years old	1.0 to 1.2
Older adults with acute or chronic illness	1.2 to 1.5

interactions and their relationship with possible morbidity in the aging adult.

Bone health. Vitamin D and calcium are essential nutrients for the growth and maintenance of healthy bone tissue (among many other physiologic functions). Osteoporosis (porous bone) is a disorder in which bone mineral density is low and bones become brittle, with a high risk of breaking (see Figure 8.1). The prevalence of **osteopenia** and osteoporosis, along with resultant disability, increases dramatically with age. Recent reports show that 59% of adults over the age of 50 years in the United States have at least one clinical risk for an osteoporotic fracture, and 23% of adults exhibit two or more risk factors.[29] Race and sex are also influential in overall bone health (see the Cultural Considerations box, "Bone Health in Sex and Racial Groups," in Chapter 8). Contributing factors to poor bone health for all populations include the following: (1) inadequate calcium and vitamin D intake; (2) physical inactivity; (3) smoking and alcohol use; (4) decreased estrogen level after menopause in women; (5) thin body frame; (6) certain disease states; and (7) the use of medications that alter mineral bioavailability and bone turnover. See Chapters 7 and 8 for good food sources of calcium and vitamin D.

Food safety. Safe food handling practices are important throughout the life cycle. In the event that an elderly individual begins to lose eyesight, hand-eye coordination, or taste and smell acuity, the risk for food-borne illness increases. The loss of such skills alters the ability to taste and smell spoiled food, see properly to prepare food, or have the coordination necessary to cut and chop food—all of which pose a potentially dangerous health risk. Chapter 13 covers specific food-borne illnesses and food safety practices at length.

Nutrient Supplementation

The use of dietary supplements by elderly adults—usually on a self-prescribed basis—is common, although not necessarily always warranted. For some nutrients, the normal physiologic changes associated with aging compromise availability. For example, there is a reduction in the bioavailability of vitamin B_{12} and the endogenous synthesis of vitamin D with advancing age. Therefore, dietary intake from food alone may not provide an adequate intake of certain nutrients.

Vitamin B_{12}. The DRIs specify that individuals who are 50 years old or older should consume vitamin B_{12} in supplemental form or through fortified foods because of the high risk of deficiency that results from decreased gastric acid production.[30] Gastric mucosal cells secrete hydrochloric acid, which is necessary for vitamin B_{12} digestion, along with intrinsic factor (see Figure 7.8). However, as people age, the production and secretion of hydrochloric acid often decrease and may result in inadequate vitamin

senescence the process or condition of growing old.
osteopenia a condition that involves low bone mass and an increased risk for fracture.

B_{12} absorption. In this case, oral supplements would not overcome the lack of hydrochloric acid and/or intrinsic factor. Thus, subcutaneous vitamin B_{12} injections, which bypass the digestive tract and are not dependent on such factors for absorption, are necessary.

Vitamin D. Some researchers believe that about half of the elderly population worldwide is deficient in vitamin D and warrants supplementation.[31-33] However, the true prevalence of vitamin D deficiency is unknown.[34,35] As discussed in Chapter 7, there are no universally accepted measurement tools for assessing vitamin D status nor parameters for normal versus suboptimal blood levels. The current U.S. consensus is that vitamin D deficiency screening in elderly individuals is not justified in asymptomatic adults.[36] Individuals with known risk factors for vitamin D deficiency may benefit from vitamin D evaluation to determine the need for supplementation. Known risk factors include obesity, low bone density (osteopenia or osteoporosis), living in nursing homes or other situations with little to no sunlight exposure, and avoiding dairy products (which are a good source of vitamin D).

The DRIs for vitamin D are 600 IU/day for individuals who are between 1 and 70 years old and 800 IU/day for individuals who are older than 70 years of age.[37] To meet the dietary recommendation for vitamin D, elderly individuals can consume foods that are fortified with vitamin D to overcome the reduced ability to endogenously synthesize the hormone. Current evidence-based guidelines do not recommend the routine supplementation of vitamin D in adults without known risk factors.[38] Supplementing with vitamin D in older or institutionalized adults *may* reduce the risk of falls, although not necessarily the risk of fracture, but other health benefits are inconclusive.[39] As with all fat-soluble vitamins, there is a risk of toxicity from excessive supplementation of vitamin D.[37]

Excess supplementation. Too much nutrient supplementation is counterproductive. The subset of the population that is most likely to take dietary supplements is older, white, educated, active women who do not smoke and have annual incomes above the poverty line.[40,41] Not coincidentally, the adults most likely to take dietary supplements are also the ones who are likely to have the best overall diet and healthy lifestyle. Most people do not talk to their primary care physicians about what and how much of a dietary supplement they take, unless specifically asked. Although it is rare that a multivitamin/mineral supplement, or the previously mentioned individual supplements of vitamins B_{12} or D, would result in toxicity alone, it is always prudent to report and discuss the use of dietary and herbal supplements to health care providers.

CLINICAL NEEDS OF THE ELDERLY

Clinical needs of the elderly, as with all stages of life, fall into distinct areas of focus. We generally categorize these as either health promotion, disease prevention, or disease treatment.

HEALTH PROMOTION AND DISEASE PREVENTION

Reducing Risk for Chronic Disease

The emphasis of adult health care is on reducing individual risks for chronic disease through healthy lifestyle choices. The development of the *Dietary Guidelines for Americans* and the national health objectives in the *Healthy People* initiative used this approach (see Chapter 1, Figures 1.1 and 1.5). The guidelines draw attention to individual needs, good eating habits founded on moderation and variety, and continued participation in physical activity at every stage of life.

Nutrition Status

Many of the health problems experienced by elderly adults result from the physiologic changes of aging and progressive states of malnutrition. Malnutrition is multifactorial. Some of the potential causes of malnutrition are listed below.

- Poor food habits due to:
  - Lack of appetite or loneliness and not wanting to eat alone
  - Lack of food availability as a result of economic or social issues
- Poor oral health due to:
  - Missing teeth
  - Poorly fitting dentures
- General gastrointestinal problems due to:
  - Declining salivary secretions and dry mouth, with diminished thirst and taste sensations
  - Inadequate hydrochloric acid secretion in the stomach
  - Decreased enzyme and mucus secretion in the intestines
  - Decline in gastrointestinal motility

Individual medical symptoms range from vague indigestion or irritable colon to specific diseases such as peptic ulcer or diverticulitis (see Chapter 18). The Mini Nutritional Assessment—Short Form (MNA-SF) is one of the standard assessment tools routinely used to evaluate nutrition risk in elderly individuals (Figure 12.4).[42,43] The MNA-SF is a reliable tool that is highly sensitive and can detect the risk of malnutrition early. Other assessment tools that health care providers may prefer to use in the geriatric population include the Mini Nutritional Assessment (standard form), the Nutritional Risk Screening 2002, the Malnutrition Universal Screening Tool, the Subjective Global Assessment, and the Geriatric Nutritional Risk Index.

Dental health. Poor oral health is indicative of reduced overall health and quality of life in the elderly, both of which increase the risk for malnutrition.[44,45] The number of healthy teeth remaining; the ability to chew food; the presence of xerostomia (dry mouth), periodontal disease, or dental caries; the degree of taste perception; the ability to swallow; and the perception of oral health are all important aspects in one's ability to eat, speak, and socialize comfortably. Elderly individuals who are institutionalized and have no remaining teeth (i.e., edentulous) have a specific need for individualized nutrition care (see the Clinical Applications box, "Feeding Older Adults With Sensitivity").

Dehydration. Dehydration, which can be a problem in any age group, is common in the elderly population. Physiologic changes in the hypothalamus naturally occur with age, and, as a result, elderly individuals exhibit an overall decreased thirst sensation and reduced fluid intake compared with younger adults.[46] In addition, other physiologic changes associated with aging, such as diminishing kidney function and altered hormonal

---

⌂ Clinical Applications

Feeding Older Adults With Sensitivity

Many older adults have eating and/or feeding problems that could lead to malnutrition. Each person is a unique individual with particular needs requiring sensitive support to meet his or her nutrient and personal necessities. Below are general guidelines and suggestions for compassionately assisting elderly individuals to support a positive eating experience.

BASIC GUIDELINES

- *Analyze food habits carefully.* Learn about the attitudes, situations, and desires of the older person relative to his or her cultural, socioeconomic, and physiologic needs. A variety of foods can meet nutrition needs, so make suggestions in a practical, realistic, and supportive manner.
- *Never moralize.* Never say, "Eat this because it is good for you." This approach has little value for anyone, especially for those who are struggling to maintain their personal integrity and self-esteem in a youth-oriented, age-fearing culture.
- *Encourage food variety.* New tastes and seasonings often encourage appetite and increase interest in eating. Many people think that a bland diet is best for all elderly persons, but this is not necessarily true. The decreased taste sensitivity of aging necessitates added attention to variety and seasoning. Smaller amounts of food and more frequent meals may also encourage better nutrition.

ASSISTED FEEDING SUGGESTIONS

When physically assisting an individual of any age with the feeding process, keep the following guidelines in mind.

- Make no negative remarks about the food.
- Identify all food served.
- Allow the person to have at least three bites of the same food before going on to another food to allow time for the taste buds to become accustomed to the food.
- Give sufficient time for the person to chew and swallow.
- Give liquids throughout the meal and not just at the beginning and end.
- Keep attention focused on the client. Do not carry on a conversation with another person, read, use a cell phone, or otherwise disrespect the person who is relying on you for support.

Mini Nutritional Assessment

MNA®

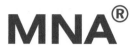

**Nestlé
NutritionInstitute**

Last name:		First name:		
Sex:	Age:	Weight, kg:	Height, cm:	Date:

Complete the screen by filling in the boxes with the appropriate numbers. Total the numbers for the final screening score.

Screening

A Has food intake declined over the past 3 months due to loss of appetite, digestive problems, chewing or swallowing difficulties?
0 = severe decrease in food intake
1 = moderate decrease in food intake
2 = no decrease in food intake ☐

B Weight loss during the last 3 months
0 = weight loss greater than 3 kg (6.6 lbs)
1 = does not know
2 = weight loss between 1 and 3 kg (2.2 and 6.6 lbs)
3 = no weight loss ☐

C Mobility
0 = bed or chair bound
1 = able to get out of bed / chair but does not go out
2 = goes out ☐

D Has suffered psychological stress or acute disease in the past 3 months?
0 = yes   2 = no ☐

E Neuropsychologic problems
0 = severe dementia or depression
1 = mild dementia
2 = no psychological problems ☐

F1 Body Mass Index (BMI) (weight in kg) / (height in m[2])
0 = BMI less than 19
1 = BMI 19 to less than 21
2 = BMI 21 to less than 23
3 = BMI 23 or greater ☐

IF BMI IS NOT AVAILABLE, REPLACE QUESTION F1 WITH QUESTION F2.
DO NOT ANSWER QUESTION F2 IF QUESTION F1 IS ALREADY COMPLETED.

F2 Calf circumference (CC) in cm
0 = CC less than 31
3 = CC 31 or greater ☐

Screening score ☐☐
(max. 14 points)

12-14 points: Normal nutritional status
8-11 points: At risk of malnutrition
0-7 points: Malnourished

Ref.   Vellas B, Villars H, Abellan G, et al. *Overview of the MNA® - Its History and Challenges*. J Nutr Health Aging 2006;10:456-465.

Rubenstein LZ, Harker JO, Salva A, Guigoz Y, Vellas B. *Screening for Undernutrition in Geriatric Practice: Developing the Short-Form Mini Nutritional Assessment (MNA-SF)*. J. Geront 2001;56A: M366-377.

Guigoz Y. *The Mini-Nutritional Assessment (MNA®) Review of the Literature - What does it tell us?* J Nutr Health Aging 2006; 10:466-487.

Kaiser MJ, Bauer JM, Ramsch C, et al. *Validation of the Mini Nutritional Assessment Short-Form (MNA®-SF): A practical tool for identification of nutritional status.* J Nutr Health Aging 2009; 13:782-788.

® Société des Produits Nestlé, S.A., Vevey, Switzerland, Trademark Owners

For more information: www.mna-elderly.com

Figure 12.4 Mini Nutritional Assessment—Short Form. (Copyright Nestle USA, Inc., Glendale, CA 2009.)

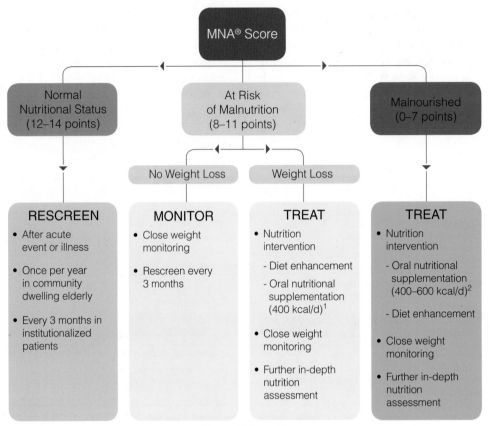

Figure 12.4, cont'd

responses to hypovolemia (e.g., compromised response to vasopressin and the renin-angiotensin-aldosterone system) may exacerbate losses of body fluid.[47] Although this combination does not necessarily guarantee dehydration in elderly adults, it does lead to slower rates of rehydration. Added sickness, such as vomiting, diarrhea, or fever, could push an elderly person into a state of dehydration. Another example would be a person choosing to avoid fluids because he or she needs assistance with getting water or getting to the bathroom, thus rationalizing, "It's just easier to not drink much."

Weight status. Unintentional weight loss and weight gain can be signs of malnutrition. Many of the same depressed living situations and emotional factors that result in unhealthy weight loss also may lead to excessive weight gain. Overeating or undereating are frequently used coping mechanism for stressful life conditions throughout all of the adult years. Obesity among adults has been on the rise in all subgroups of the population for decades (see Chapter 15).[48] Not surprisingly, so have obesity-related chronic diseases.

Physical Activity

Regular physical activity and adequate dietary protein intake should be a part of life through the adult and elderly years to maintain lean tissue and anabolic processes.[28] Physical activity is a major factor in aspects of healthy aging, such as weight management, the preservation of strength and cognitive function, and overall quality of life.[49-51] The *Physical Activity Guidelines* and the *Dietary Guidelines for Americans* specifically note the long-term benefits of regular cardiovascular and strength-training exercises in adults.[22,52] As the population continues to age, health care facilities are adapting to the increased need for aerobic and balance classes aimed specifically at older adults. Box 12.1 lists some of the benefits of physical activity.

One specific example of how exercise can help prevent disease is with type 2 diabetes. Decreased glucose tolerance is the *prediabetes syndrome,* in which the insulin response to glucose in the bloodstream is inadequate to maintain euglycemia but blood glucose levels are not high enough for a diagnosis of diabetes (more detail provided in Chapter 20). Weight management through regular physical activity along with balanced meals and snacks can help individuals to avoid

---

Box 12.1	Benefits of Physical Activity

- Help maintain weight control
- Reduce the risk of cardiovascular disease, type 2 diabetes, and some forms of cancer
- Strengthen bones and muscles
- Improve mental health and mood
- Improve one's ability to perform daily activities of living and prevent falls, especially among older adults
- Increase the chance of living longer

Centers for Disease Control and Prevention. (n.d.). *Physical activity basics.* Retrieved March 26, 2019, from www.cdc.gov/physicalactivity/.

hyperglycemia and potentially delay or avoid the onset of type 2 diabetes.[53] The reason physical activity is important in this equation is that exercise increases the skeletal tissue glucose uptake independent of insulin. Thus, even though insulin sensitivity is declining with age, regular exercise improves blood glucose levels by shuttling glucose from the blood into the tissues by way of muscle contraction–stimulated transporters.

Individual Approach

Effective health promotion and disease prevention requires individualized and realistic planning. All personalities and problems are unique, and specific needs vary widely. An adult suffering from malnutrition or any of the chronic diseases discussed later will need a sensitive person-centered approach addressing all aspects of health and well-being (see the Clinical Applications box, "Case Study: Situational Problem of an Elderly Woman").

⬖ Clinical Applications

Case Study: Situational Problem of an Elderly Woman

Mrs. Johnson, a recently widowed 78-year-old woman, lives alone in a three-bedroom house in Atlanta, Georgia. A fall 1 year ago resulted in a broken hip, and she now depends on a walker for limited mobility. Her only child, a daughter, lives in Portland, Oregon, and is not capable of financially helping her mother. Mrs. Johnson's only income is a monthly Social Security check for $1332. Her monthly mortgage payment, property taxes, insurance payments, utility, and phone bills amount to $1127.

A recent medical examination revealed that Mrs. Johnson has iron-deficiency anemia and that she has lost 12 pounds during the past 3 months. Her current weight is 80 pounds, and she is 5 feet, 2 inches tall. Mrs. Johnson states that she has not been hungry, and her daily diet is repetitious: broth, a little cottage cheese and canned fruit, saltine crackers, and hot tea. She lacks energy, she rarely leaves the house, and she appears to be emaciated and generally distraught.

QUESTIONS FOR ANALYSIS

1. Identify Mrs. Johnson's personal problems and describe how they might be influencing her eating habits and food intake?
2. What nutrition improvements could she make in her diet (include food suggestions), and how are these related to her physical needs at this stage of her life?
3. What practical suggestions do you have for helping Mrs. Johnson to cope with her physical and social environment? What resources, income sources, food, and companionship can you suggest? How do you think these suggestions would benefit her nutrition status and overall health?
4. Revisit Figure 12.1, the social determinants of health. Considering what you know about Mrs. Johnson, what aspects of her life may compromise the key determinants of her quality of life and overall health?

CHRONIC DISEASES OF AGING

Chronic diseases of aging (e.g., hypertension, heart disease, stroke, emphysema, diabetes, cancer, arthritis, asthma) occur more frequently with advancing age, but they may occur at a younger age in individuals with a strong family history of disease. Health experts believe that chronic disease is not necessarily a normal consequence of aging. Rather, a handful of lifestyle improvements could prevent the majority of chronic diseases. The Centers for Disease Control and Prevention recommends the following lifestyle changes to promote health and prevent chronic disease in adulthood: (1) stop smoking and exposure to secondhand smoke; (2) improve diet by increasing intake of fruits and vegetables and reducing intake of sodium and saturated fat; (3) participate in regular physical activity; and (4) limit alcohol intake.[54]

Diet Modifications

In the presence of chronic disease, diet modifications and nutrition support are an important part of therapy. Chapters 17 through 23 cover the details of modified diets for common diseases. In any situation, individualized food plans that are sensitive to cultural norms, personal preference, and socioeconomic availability are essential for successful therapy.

Medications

Because people are living longer (many with one or more chronic diseases), older adults may be taking several prescription drugs in addition to over-the-counter medications. **Polypharmacy** may compromise nutrition status when drug-nutrient interactions occur (see Chapter 17). Medications commonly used by the elderly (e.g., blood pressure medication, antacids, anticoagulation medications, laxatives, diuretics, decongestants) can directly affect fluid balance, appetite, and the absorption and use of nutrients, thereby possibly contributing to malnutrition or dehydration. When questioning clients about medication use, health care providers should specifically ask about the use of dietary supplements and herbs. Toxicities from supplements, whether touted as "natural" or not, can be dangerous. Careful evaluation of a client's drug use and instructions about how to take medications in relation to meals are important parts of the overall health care plan (see the Drug-Nutrient Interaction box, "Medication Use in the Adult").

---

polypharmacy the use of multiple medications by the same person.

Drug-Nutrient Interaction

Medication Use in the Adult

Polypharmacy is pervasive in the United States. Ninety percent of seniors take at least one prescription medication and 41% take five or more prescription drugs regularly.[1] The most commonly prescribed medications in the United States for seniors are cardiovascular agents (to treat high blood pressure, high cholesterol level, and heart disease), diuretics, proton pump inhibitors (to treat gastric reflux and ulcers), antidiabetic agents, anticoagulants, analgesics, and antidepressants.[1]

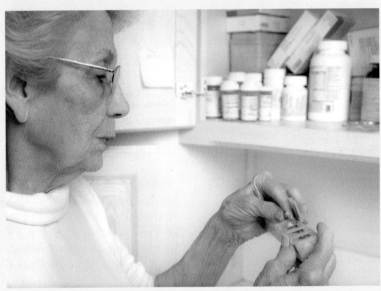

(Copyright iStock Photo; Credit: dszc.)

In addition to prescription drugs, nonprescription (i.e., over-the-counter) medications, dietary supplements (i.e., vitamins and minerals), and herbal supplements are often used by the same individual. There is a great potential for drug-nutrient interactions with frequently used medications, particularly with antidepressants, antihyperlipidemics, hypertensive medications, nonsteroidal anti-inflammatory drugs, and antihistamines. Because such a high percentage of individuals are taking at least one medication, practitioners must be conscious of the risk for deleterious interactions.

Medications can have side effects that alter appetite, weight, or the ability to absorb nutrients from food. Residents in long-term care facilities are at high risk for polypharmacy and nutrition-related complications. Multidisciplinary teams that openly communicate with their patients about changes in appetite, eating habits, and medication regimen are more likely to identify potential risks. Listed below are general guidelines to avoid food-drug interactions when taking certain medications.

REFERENCE
1. National Center for Health Statistics. (2018). Health, United States. In *Health, United States, 2017: With special feature on mortality*. Hyattsville, MD: National Center for Health Statistics (US).

DRUG CLASS	HOW TO AVOID FOOD-NUTRIENT INTERACTIONS[a]
Certain antidepressants (i.e., monoamine oxidase inhibitors)	Avoid tyramine-containing foods such as tap beer, red wine, aged cheese, sauerkraut, cured meats, fermented food, soy products (e.g., soy sauce, miso soup, tofu), caviar, and herbal products containing ginseng and St. John's wort. Carefully check for interactions with other medications. Drink 2 to 3 L of water per day and take with food.
Antihyperlipidemics	Take with the evening meal (e.g., lovastatin) and avoid more than one alcoholic drink per day. Decrease dietary intake of fat and cholesterol. Include rich sources of fat-soluble vitamins, folate, B_{12}, and iron in the diet. Avoid St. John's wort and grapefruit juice.
Antihypertensives	Avoid licorice, high-potassium salt substitutes, herbal products containing ginseng, and tyramine-containing foods (examples provided above). Ensure a balanced diet complete with all vitamins and minerals. Avoid taking with grapefruit juice.
Nonsteroidal anti-inflammatory drugs	Limit alcohol intake. Increase intake of foods that are high in vitamin C and iron. Take with food and water.
Antihistamines	Avoid alcohol and grapefruit juice.

[a]These are general interactions for a few select medications. It is imperative that all clients taking prescription medications consult with their health care team for potential interactions.

COMMUNITY RESOURCES

GOVERNMENT PROGRAMS FOR OLDER AMERICANS

Adults who are living below the national poverty level have a higher incidence of multiple chronic diseases than any other socioeconomic group.[55] Health care providers must be aware of community resources and refer clients when appropriate. Many older adults who are at risk for malnutrition and who are eligible for nutrition assistance programs are not partaking in the available services. In many cases, a personal advocate who is willing to assist in completing the program application and help set up the initial involvement can improve participation.

Older Americans Act

Under the Older Americans Act of 1965, the Administration on Community Living (formerly known as the Administration on Aging) of the U.S. Department of Health and Human Services manages several programs for older adults. Nutrition Services Incentive Programs provide cash and/or commodities to supplement meals offered at congregate and home-delivered nutrition programs. The focus of these programs is to reach elderly individuals with the greatest social and economic need. Take a moment to familiarize yourself with the services available in your community at the Administration for Community Living's website, acl.gov/programs/health-wellness/nutrition-services. The likelihood of successfully making a referral depends on whether you are equipped with the appropriate resources at the point of patient care.

Congregate nutrition services. This program provides adults who are older than 60 years of age and their caregivers (particularly those with low incomes and at risk for institutional care) with nutritionally sound meals in senior centers and other public or private community facilities. In these settings, older adults can gather for a hot midday meal and have access to both wholesome food and social support. In addition to meals, some facilities provide other services, including nutrition screening, education, assessment, and counseling, as needed. On a recent survey, 77% of participants reported eating healthier and improved overall health because of this lunch program.[56]

Home-delivered nutrition services. For those older adults who are unable to travel to the community centers, meals are delivered by couriers to their homes (i.e., Meals on Wheels). This service helps meet the nutrition needs of the frail, homebound, and isolated elderly while providing human contact and support. The couriers are usually concerned volunteers and are often the only person a participant will interact with during the day. The average age of participants is 79 years old. This service allows many older adults to remain living in their own homes far longer than they would otherwise be able to do.[56]

United States Department of Agriculture

The U.S. Department of Agriculture provides both research and services for older adults. See the Further Reading and Resources at the back of this book for the websites of each of the programs listed here.

Research centers. The U.S. Department of Agriculture supports research centers for aging throughout the country. For example, the Human Nutrition Research Center on Aging at Tufts University in Boston is one of the largest research facilities in the world dedicated to the study of nutrition needs in aging. Studies there involve research on topics such as nutrition and its interactions with cardiovascular disease, Alzheimer's disease, cancer, inflammation, immunity, obesity, and the microbiome. Providing better care for older adults depends, in part, on gaining additional knowledge about the nutrition requirements of this population.

Extension services. The U.S. Department of Agriculture operates agricultural extension services in **state land grant universities**, including food and nutrition education services. Community partners educate the public on topics such as affordable and accessible food, food resource management, food recovery, food donations, and emergency food assistance programs. The education opportunities incorporate the principles of the *Dietary Guidelines for Americans*, the *Physical Activity Guidelines for Americans*, the MyPlate guidelines, and the *Healthy People* objectives. They also provide education services focused on the specific nutrition needs of the elderly.

Supplemental Nutrition Assistance Program. Supplemental Nutrition Assistance Program (SNAP), previously known as the Food Stamp Program, is a federally funded program focused on preventing hunger in low-income families. SNAP-Education (SNAP-Ed) is an optional education program that provides nutrition education and obesity prevention interventions. Households with a monthly income of 130% or less of the national poverty line are financially eligible for SNAP benefits, but other state-specific requirements may vary. Participants receive electronic benefits transfer cards (similar to debit cards) to purchase approved food items at authorized food retail outlets. About 40 million low-income individuals benefit from SNAP services every month. Elderly adults (≥60 years old) have the lowest participation rates in SNAP with only 45% of those eligible for services participating. This is significantly less than other age groups, whose participation rates approach 100%.[57] SNAP promotes the

---

state land grant universities an institution of higher education that has been designated by the state to receive unique federal support as a result of the Morrill Acts of 1862 and 1890.

consumption of fruits, vegetables, whole grains, fat-free or low-fat milk products, lean meats, poultry, and fish.

Commodity supplemental food program. Individuals who are older than 60 years of age with a household income of 130% or less of the federal poverty line are also eligible for assistance in the form of food packages. These food packages supplement the diet with foods that are high in the nutrients that are typically lacking in the diet of an elderly person. Providing a complete diet is not the intention of the program.

Senior farmers' market nutrition program. This is a grant-based program that provides low-income older adults (i.e., 60 years of age or older with an income that is 185% or less of the federal poverty income guidelines) with coupons that they can exchange for fresh fruits, vegetables, honey, and herbs obtained from farmers' markets, community-supported agriculture programs (CSAs), and roadside stands. This program has increased the average servings of fruits and vegetables among participants, and it helps support local farmers.

Public Health Departments

Public health departments throughout the United States are an outreach division of the U.S. Department of Health and Human Services. Skilled health professionals work in the community through local and state public health departments. Public health nutritionists are important members of this health care team; they provide nutrition counseling and education, and they help with various food assistance programs.

PROFESSIONAL ORGANIZATIONS AND RESOURCES

National Groups

The American Geriatrics Society and the Gerontological Society of America are national professional organizations of physicians, nurses, dietitians, and other interested health care workers. These socie-ties publish journals and promote community and government efforts to meet the needs of aging individuals.

Community Groups

Senior centers in local communities are valuable resources for well and disabled adults. Local medical societies, nursing organizations, and dietetic associations sponsor various programs to help meet the needs of elderly people. Local senior centers often host such programs on site. The Commission on Dietetics offers a board certification as a Specialist in Gerontological Nutrition. Other health care professional licensing bodies offer similar certifications. There are registered dietitian nutritionists in private practice in most communities, and they can supply a variety of individual and group services as well.

Volunteer Organizations

Many volunteer activities of health organizations (e.g., the American Heart Association, the American Diabetes Association, the Alzheimer's Association) relate to the needs of older people and may serve as both rewarding opportunities for young-old adults and important sources of health-sustaining activities and information for old-old adults.

Chapter 13 discusses additional resources for nutrition assistance.

ALTERNATIVE LIVING ARRANGEMENTS

There are multitudes of alternative living arrangements for seniors of all levels of independence. For example, independent living facilities are for independently functioning individuals who do not need medical attention and who enjoy recreational and social events with other seniors. Other housing options provide more services, may be staffed with health care workers, and provide different levels of care in accordance with needs. Examples include congregate care, continuing care retirement communities, and assisted living facilities. Fully staffed nursing homes have medical professionals that are able to provide most medical needs in the absence of an acute illness requiring hospitalization. The next sections of this chapter discuss only the types of alternative living arrangements that provide food and health care. See the Further Reading and Resources section at the back of the book for organizations that provide helpful information about alternative living arrangements for seniors.

CONGREGATE CARE ARRANGEMENTS

Congregate care arrangements help keep the elderly living in their own homes for as long as possible with outside assistance available to meet particular needs. We previously covered some congregate care services: congregate community meals, nutrition education through extension services, and home-delivered meals. Other services include personal care aides, adult day services, transportation, respite care, and more. Personal care aides may shop for groceries, cook, and help with feeding and other activities of daily living, as indicated.

The emphasis on modified diets in such settings varies. Congregate meals and home-delivered meals are not likely to be specific to diets for individuals with highly particular needs. For example, individuals with diabetes who count carbohydrates, those with food intolerances or allergies, or those who have difficulty swallowing certain food consistencies (e.g., individuals with dysphagia) may require further assistance. Regulation for most congregate care programs is at the state level. Public programs (e.g., those that offer congregate meals and home-delivered meals) are required to offer meals that meet the *Dietary Guidelines for Americans,* and each meal should provide one-third of the DRIs for key nutrients.

CONTINUING CARE RETIREMENT COMMUNITIES

Continuing care retirement communities provide a continuum of residential long-term care, from independent living with community-organized events to nursing care facilities. Dietary assistance varies by the needs of the resident. Seniors can move into the community as independent living residents and participate in community activities and meals as they choose. When their functional statuses indicate, seniors receive more care. Continuing care retirement communities usually have assisted living facilities and nursing homes in a campus-style setting. The following sections of this chapter cover the nutrition-related involvement in each type of facility within this continuum-of-care approach.

ASSISTED LIVING FACILITIES

Assisted living facilities are known by several names, including *board and care, domiciliary care, sheltered housing, residential care,* and *personal care.* Assisted living arrangements may also exist within continuing care communities. Individual state governments regulate licensure for assisted living facilities. Most assisted living facilities provide meals and snacks; housekeeping; laundry; and help with dressing, bathing, and personal hygiene. Some facilities provide social activities, limited transportation, and basic medication administration, but they may not provide medical or nursing care. Living areas vary from full apartments with kitchens, to studio-type apartments with small kitchenettes, to rooms with baths. The functional status of the individual helps to determine the most appropriate setting.

Meal settings vary from room service–delivered meals to cafeteria or restaurant settings. Some facilities provide menus with several options at each meal, and others serve a set menu for all residents. Most assisted care facilities cater to basic dietary requests and the therapeutic diet needs based on disease diagnosis of their residents. States vary widely with regard to regulations and standards for nutrition policies and services. Most states require that a registered dietitian nutritionist review and approve the meal plans annually.

NURSING HOMES

Nursing homes, or long-term care facilities, provide the most medical, nursing, and nutrition support of the alternative living arrangements. Many nursing homes also provide a residential rehabilitation site outside of the hospital for patients to recover from injuries, acute illnesses, and operations. Most individuals in nursing homes need help with activities of daily living (e.g., bathing, toileting, transferring), and many need assistance with eating.

Nursing homes have dietitians on staff who are able to design meal plans to meet the individualized dietary requirements of the residents. However, much less emphasis on therapeutic diets is given for this population, because a less-restrictive diet model is thought to be more beneficial at this life stage.[58] Malnutrition is a common concern for nursing home residents, and there is a direct link between food intake, risk for malnutrition, and quality of life. Efforts at increasing food and nutrient intake by improving the ambiance and physical seating options, staff training in feeding assistance (see the Clinical Applications box, "Feeding Older Adults with Sensitivity"), the quality of modified textured foods (i.e., pureed foods), and personalization of the meals may benefit some at-risk residents.[59]

Putting It All Together

Summary

- Meeting the nutrition needs of adults—especially older adults—may present a challenge for several reasons. Current and past social, economic, and psychologic factors influence needs, and the biologic process of aging differs widely among individuals.

- Updates to research and recommendations regarding the nutrition needs of an aging population reflect the continual increase in life expectancy.

- Health promotion and disease prevention during early adulthood are key for sustaining functionality throughout the later years of life.

- Individual supportive guidance and patience from health care professionals are necessary when administering nutrition resources and support.

- A variety of assisted living arrangements and nutrition services are available for seniors of all functional levels.

Chapter Review Questions

See answers in Appendix A.

1. The best way for older adults to maintain their muscle mass and metabolic rate is _____.

   a. ensuring ample carbohydrate intake
   b. engaging in regular physical activity
   c. using multivitamin/multimineral supplements
   d. maintaining adequate fluid intake

2. Maintaining a diet with adequate amounts of _____ may reduce the risk of osteoporosis.

   a. protein and vitamin C
   b. vitamins B_{12} and B_6
   c. iron and zinc
   d. calcium and vitamin D

3. A 56-year-old woman has been taking her antihistamine medication with a glass of grapefruit juice each morning. The health care professional should encourage her to _____.

   a. continue this practice
   b. replace the grapefruit juice with water
   c. take the medication at bedtime with grapefruit juice
   d. take the medication with only a half glass of grapefruit juice

4. A typical physiologic change in older adults that can alter nutrient intake is _____.

   a. an increase in metabolism requiring more calories to meet energy needs
   b. an increase in intestinal motility that can lead to constipation
   c. less hydrochloric acid secretion in the stomach
   d. a general increase in appetite, especially toward the end of the day

5. The Older American Act provides programs for older adults for meal assistance that include _____.

   a. support groups with counselors who eat meals together
   b. delivery of groceries to participants at home
   c. home-delivered meals and congregate meals
   d. vouchers for purchasing energy-dense foods

Next-Generation NCLEX® Examination-style Case Study

See answers in Appendix A.

A 67-year-old man (height, 5'5"; weight, 145 lbs.) is quarantined at home during the COVID-19 pandemic. His daughter, an ER nurse, usually stops by every day to check on him, keep him company, and make sure he is taking his medications safely. Now she works extra hours and is unable to see him in person because of social distancing safety precautions. He is financially stable, owns a car, and can prepare food for himself, but he does not feel safe leaving the house to go to the grocery store. He eats 3 meals per day and has no issues chewing and swallowing. He is taking multiple medications, including an antidepressant, antihyperlipidemic, antihypertensive, nonsteroidal anti-inflammatory drugs (e.g., ibuprofen), and antihistamines on occasion.

1. From the list below, select all of the nutrition concerns regarding the client's history.

   a. Polypharmacy
   b. Food preparation skills
   c. Dysphagia
   d. Dyspnea
   e. Appetite
   f. Food access

2. From the list below, identify all potential nutrition interventions that are appropriate for the client.

   a. Drug-nutrient interaction education
   b. Meals on Wheels
   c. SNAP
   d. Commodity supplemental food program
   e. Senior farmers market nutrition program
   f. WIC

3. Match the most appropriate recommendation (provided below) to each drug class to reduce the risk of an adverse drug-nutrient interaction.

DRUG CLASS	APPROPRIATE RECOMMENDATION
Antihypertensives	
Antihistamines	
Antihyperlipidemic	
Nonsteroidal anti-inflammatory drugs	
Antidepressants	

Recommendation Options

a. Avoid tyramine-containing foods. Carefully check for interactions with other medications. Drink 2 to 3 L of water per day and take with food.
b. Take with the evening meal and avoid more than 1 alcoholic drink per day. Lower intake of dietary fat and cholesterol. Include rich sources of fat-soluble vitamins, folate, vitamin B_{12}, and iron in the diet. Avoid St. John's wort and grapefruit juice.
c. Avoid licorice, high-potassium salt substitutes, herbal products, and tyramine-containing foods. Ensure a balanced diet and avoid taking with grapefruit juice.
d. Limit alcohol intake. Increase intake of foods that are high in vitamin C and iron. Take with food and water.
e. Avoid alcohol and grapefruit juice.

Additional Learning Resources

Please refer to this text's Evolve website for answers to the Case Study questions:
http://evolve.elsevier.com/Williams/basic/.
References and **Further Reading and Resources** in the back of the book provide additional resources for enhancing knowledge.

Community Food Supply and Health

Key Concepts

- Modern food production, processing, and marketing have both positive and negative influences on food safety.
- A variety of organisms in contaminated food can transmit disease.

- Poverty often prevents individuals and families from having adequate access to their community food supply.
- There are several aid programs available to help individuals secure food for themselves and their families.

The health of a community largely depends on the safety of its available food and water supply. The American system of government control agencies and regulations, along with local and state public health officials, works diligently to maintain a safe food supply. The food supply in the United States has undergone dramatic changes during the past several decades.

This chapter explores the factors that influence the safety of food. Potential health problems related to the food supply can arise from several sources, such as the lack of sanitation, food-borne disease, and poverty.

FOOD SAFETY AND HEALTH PROMOTION

Keeping the enormous food supply in the United States safe is a huge job. Several federal agencies help to ensure food safety and quality. In addition to the agencies listed in Table 13.1, multiple other federal, state, and local agencies participate in education and research to promote the safety of the food supply.

U.S. FOOD AND DRUG ADMINISTRATION

Although several agencies are involved in the overall food safety of products sold in the United States, we will cover only the diverse roles of the U.S. Food and Drug Administration (FDA) here because they are responsible for the majority of the food supply.

Enforcement of Federal Food Safety Regulations

The U.S. Congress charged the FDA with ensuring that the United States' food supply is safe. The agency enforces federal food safety regulations through various activities that ensure the safety of most food products, including the following: (1) enforcing food sanitation and quality control; (2) governing food additives; (3) regulating the movement of foods across state lines; (4) supervising the nutrition labeling of foods; and (5) ensuring the

safety of public food service. The agency's methods of enforcement are recall, seizure, injunction, and prosecution. The use of recall is the most common method, followed by seizures of contaminated food. Injunction involves a court order to stop the sale and production of a food item. This procedure is not common, and it generally occurs in response to a claim that a food item is potentially harmful or that it has not undergone appropriate testing or acquired adequate approval for sale.

Consumer Education and Research

The FDA's Center for Food Safety and Applied Nutrition maintains an electronic reading room with informative materials intended for educators, health professionals, and the public. Pamphlets, publications, and other materials are available to download, distribute, or print from their website. Food Safety.gov (www.foodsafety.gov) is an organization that serves as the liaison between the public and all government agencies that are involved in food safety.

Along with the U.S. Department of Agriculture's (USDA) Agricultural Research Service, the FDA scientists continually evaluate foods and food components through their own research. Some of the current research projects involving nutrition include the following: impact of diet and activity factors on maternal, child, and adolescent development; risk and safety assessment of high-risk foods and food contaminants; and safe and sustainable practices for food production. The FDA is also involved in the *Healthy People* initiative by guiding goals and objectives associated with food safety (see Figure 1.1 in Chapter 1).

FOOD LABELS

Early Development of Label Regulations

During the mid-1960s, the FDA established "truth in packaging" regulations that dealt mainly with food

Table 13.1	Agencies Involved in Food Safety Regulation
AGENCY	**RESPONSIBILITIES**
U.S. Food and Drug Administration (FDA)	Primary governing body of the American food supply, with the exception of commercial meat, poultry, and egg products. Also governs dietary supplements, bottled water, food additives, and breast milk substitute infant formulas
Food Safety and Inspection Service of the U.S. Department of Agriculture (USDA)	Responsible for the food safety of both domestic and imported meat, poultry, and processed egg products
National Oceanic and Atmospheric Administration (NOAA) Seafood Inspection Program	Governs the safety of seafood and fisheries
Environmental Protection Agency	Regulates the use of pesticides and other chemicals and ensures the safety of public drinking water
Federal Trade Commission	Regulates the advertising and truthful marketing of food products
Centers for Disease Control and Prevention	Monitors and investigates cases of food-borne illness, and is proactive with regard to education and prevention

standards of identity. As food processing advanced and the number of available food items grew, the labels included nutrition information as well.

Food standards. The basic standards of identity require that labels on foods that do not have an established reference standard (e.g., an orange doesn't need a label stating that it is an orange) must list all of the ingredients in order of relative amount found in the product. Other food standard information on labels relates to food quality, fill of container, and enrichment or fortification. Food labels must note major food allergens, although some exceptions apply. For example, a container of milk does not have to include a notice of "this product contains milk." The FDA defines the following foods as major allergens: milk, egg, fish, crustacean shellfish, tree nuts, peanuts, wheat, and soybeans.[1]

Nutrition information. The FDA developed a labeling system that describes a food's nutritive value after the adoption of regulations in 1973. Some producers added information beyond the requirements to meet market demand. Many people were concerned that nutrition labeling was inadequate, but the real difficulty was what and how much was on the label and in what format. Information about nutrients and food constituents that consumer groups believed should be listed on labels included the amount of macronutrients and their total energy value, the key micronutrients (e.g., calcium, iron, vitamin A), and the levels of sodium, cholesterol, trans fat (as of 2006), and saturated fat. Concerned public and professional groups also want nutrients identified in terms of percentages of the current Dietary Reference Intake standards per defined portion.

The use of food label information varies relative to health orientation. One-third to one-half of shoppers consult the food label, review the ingredients list, or read the health claims printed on the food package before purchasing a food product. However, individuals already making healthy food choices (e.g., low intake of sugar-sweetened beverages, high intake of fruits and vegetables) are the ones most likely to read and make food-purchasing decisions based on label information.[2-5] Women with advanced education and higher income are the most likely demographic to use the food label to aid in purchasing decisions.[6,7] Although there are many factors beyond food labels that contribute to healthy dietary choices, if the labels are to invoke a positive influence on the dietary selections of the population as a whole, the presentation and information must be clear, concise, and easily understandable to all.

Background of Present Label Regulations

Two factors have fueled rapid progress toward better food labels: (1) an increase in the variety of food products entering the U.S. marketplace; and (2) changing patterns of American eating habits. Both factors led many health-conscious consumers and professionals alike to refer to nutrition labeling to help attain health goals.

Despite the initial regulations, a number of labeling problems persisted, such as misleading health claims, varying serving sizes, and vague terms such as "natural." These problems indicated a need to reorganize the entire food-labeling system. Three landmark reports that related nutrition and diet to national health goals reinforced this need: the *Surgeon General's Report on Nutrition and Health*, the *National Research Council's Diet and Health Report*, and the national health goals and objectives described in the Public Health Service's *Healthy People* initiative. Based on these reports, the Institute of Medicine of the National Academy of Sciences established a Committee on the Nutrition Components of Food Labeling to study and report on the scientific issues and practical needs involved in food-labeling reform. The committee's report provided basic guidelines for the rule-making process conducted by the FDA, the USDA, and the U.S. Department of Health and Human Services for submission to Congress to achieve the needed reforms.[8] Three areas formed the basis of the recommendations from the Institute of Medicine: (1) foods for mandatory regulations; (2) the format of label information; and (3) the education of consumers. This report became the basic guideline for the Nutrition Labeling and Education Act of 1990.

Current Food Label Format

Nutrition Facts Label. Figure 13.1 represents the current FDA-approved Nutrition Facts Label. There are significant changes from previous versions, including the following:

- *Serving sizes* reflect typical consumption. For example, a 20-oz soda is one serving instead of 2.5 servings (previously 8 oz = 1 serving).
- A larger font size to draw attention to the *calories per serving.*
- No longer including *calories from fat* below the total calories.
- Including *added sugars*, and the respective percent daily value (% DV), to distinguish between naturally occurring sugar in a food from added sugar.
- *Vitamin D and potassium* will replace *vitamin A and vitamin C* as required nutrients on the label. Current research indicates that vitamins A and C are no longer of public health concern as nutrient deficiencies,

whereas vitamin D and potassium intake are generally inadequate.

- The *Daily Reference Values* now reflect the current DRI values.

Displaying this label on the side or on the back of the food package is the most common location. The serving size (i.e., customarily consumed amount of the food at one time) must be expressed in household measures and metric weight. Providing the nutrients listed on the label in Figure 13.1 meets the minimum requirement for nutrition information on the food packaging. Manufacturers may voluntarily include additional information, such as amounts of polyunsaturated fat, monounsaturated fat, soluble and insoluble fiber, sugar alcohol (e.g., sorbitol), other carbohydrates, other vitamins and minerals, and caffeine.[9]

The FDA established 2000 calories as the reference amount for calculating the *percent daily value* (% DV), although individuals may vary greatly with regard to their specific needs. As a reference tool, the % DVs reflect the overall value of a specific nutrient in the food (see the For Further Focus box, "Glossary of Terms for Nutrition Facts Labels"). For example, if the % DV for fiber in one serving of whole-grain bread is 10%, a person eating the bread acquires one-tenth of the recommended total fiber intake for his or her day.

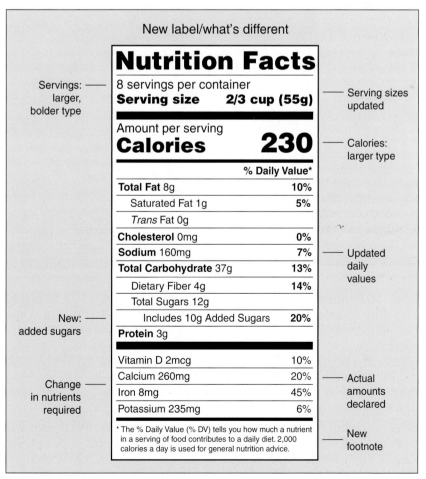

Figure 13.1 The Nutrition Facts Label approved by the U.S. Food and Drug Administration. (Courtesy U.S. Food and Drug Administration, Washington, DC.)

Glossary of Terms for Nutrition Facts Labels

To improve communication between producers and consumers, all producers must use the standard wording on their food labels as indicated by the U.S. Food and Drug Administration (FDA). All producers must use the commonly accepted terms, whether these terms appear in the Nutrition Facts box or elsewhere as part of the manufacturer's product description. The following is a sampling of these terms.

NUTRITION FACTS BOX
Daily Values

Daily values (DVs) are reference values that relate the nutrition information to a total daily diet of 2000 kcal, which is appropriate for most women and teenage girls as well as for some sedentary men. The footnote indicates the daily values for a 2500-kcal diet, which meets the needs of most men, teenage boys, and active women. Figure 13.1 provides an example of what nutrients must appear on the label to help consumers determine how a food fits into a healthy diet. Manufacturers may choose to list other vitamins and minerals as well, but this is not required.

Daily Reference Value

As part of the DVs listed, the daily reference values are a set of dietary standards for the following nutrients: total fat; saturated fat; cholesterol; sodium; total carbohydrate; dietary fiber; added sugar; vitamin D; calcium; iron; and potassium. No % DV is provided for trans fat, total sugar, or protein. There is no recommendation or need to include sugar or trans fat in the diet and protein is not a public health concern because most individuals consume enough protein daily.

Descriptive Terms on Products

The FDA has specifically defined many terms. Manufacturers must follow these definitions if they use these terms on their product. The following are examples:

- *Fat free:* Less than 0.5 g of fat per serving.
- *Low cholesterol:* ≤20 mg of cholesterol per serving and per 100 g; 2 g of saturated fat or less per serving. Any food containing more than 2 g of saturated fat per serving may not make a label claim about low cholesterol, regardless of the cholesterol content.
- *Light* or *Lite:* At least a one-third reduction in kilocalories. If fat contributes 50% or more of total kilocalories, fat content must be reduced by 50% compared with the reference food.
- *Reduced/less sodium:* At least a 25% reduction; 140 mg

or less per reference amount per serving.
- *High:* 20% or more of the DV per serving.
- *Reduced saturated fat:* At least 25% less saturated fat than an appropriate reference food.
- *Lean:* Applied to meat, poultry, and seafood; less than 10 g of fat, 4 g of saturated fat, and 95 mg of cholesterol per serving.
- *Extra lean:* Applied to meat, poultry, and seafood; less than 5 g of fat, 2 g of saturated fat, and 95 mg of cholesterol per serving.

For more information, search "Nutrition Facts Label" and "Nutrition Labeling and Education Act Requirements" on the FDA website (www.fda.gov).

HEALTH CLAIMS

The FDA guidelines indicate that substantial scientific evidence must support any health claim on a label. The following are examples of approved claims:

Cancer
- Low dietary fat intake and a reduced risk of cancer
- High fruit and vegetable intake and a lowered risk of cancer
- A diet high in fiber-containing grain products, fruits, and vegetables and a reduced risk of cancer

Heart Disease and Hypertension
- Low dietary cholesterol and saturated fat intake and a reduced risk of coronary heart disease
- Regular consumption of soy protein and a reduced risk of coronary heart disease
- A diet high in grain products and fruits and vegetables that contain fiber, especially soluble fiber, and the prevention of coronary heart disease
- Regular ingestion of stanols/sterols and a reduced risk of coronary heart disease
- A diet low in sodium and the prevention of hypertension

Other: Neural Tube Defects, Osteoporosis, Dental Caries
- Adequate folate/folic acid intake and the prevention of neural tube defects
- A diet containing adequate calcium and vitamin D and the prevention of osteoporosis
- The use of noncariogenic carbohydrate sweeteners may reduce the risk of dental caries

For more information, search "Authorized Health Claims" on the FDA website (www.fda.gov).

Front-of-package labeling. Many food manufacturers use front-of-package labeling to broadcast nutrition information. Figure 13.2 presents several examples of such labels in use around the world. Currently, there are few U.S. federal regulations in place to standardize front-of-package labels. Ideally, front-of-package labels would be symbolic (instead of text-heavy) and visually easy to interpret. Such icons should be understandable despite education level or native language. Studies indicate that using graded summary labels such as the multiple traffic light labels, Nutri-Score labels, or the 5-Color Nutrition Label (see Figure 13.2) are the most well accepted and comprehensive way to help individuals identify healthier food options.[10-13]

Because front-of-package and shelf-tag labeling is voluntary and at the discretion of the food manufacturer, there are many limitations with this method of consumer nutrition education. Consumers may be confused and frustrated with the inconsistencies of nutrition information printed on processed food packages. Much to the chagrin of nutrition professionals and the public in general, the labels food manufacturers choose to use on their products may or may not be helpful in deciphering the foods that are the most wholesome. Although various attempts at developing nutrient profile systems to "grade foods" are underway, the inherit problem is that there is not a uniformly accepted method for defining a food's

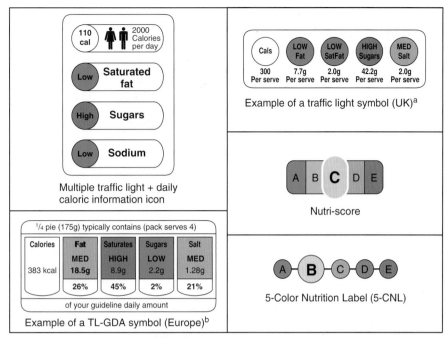

[a]%GDA symbol reprinted with permission from the Food and Drink Federation, United Kingdom.
[b]TL-GDA symbol reprinted with permission from the Food Standards Agency, United Kingdom.

Figure 13.2 Examples of front-of-packaging labels. (Hersey, J. C., et al. [2013]. Effects of front-of-package and shelf nutrition labeling systems on consumers. *Nutr Rev, 71*[1], 1–14; Roberto, C. A., et al. [2012]. Evaluation of consumer understanding of different front-of-package nutrition labels, 2010-2011. *Prev Chronic Dis, 9,* E149; Egnell, M., et al. [2018]. Objective understanding of Nutri-Score Front-Of-Package nutrition label according to individual characteristics of subjects: Comparisons with other format labels. *PLoS One, 13*[8], e0202095; Ducrot, P., et al. [2016]. Impact of different front-of-pack nutrition labels on consumer purchasing intentions: A randomized controlled trial. *Am J Prev Med, 50*[5], 627–636.)

overall *diet quality*.[14-16] The fluctuation of these messages tends to discredit the intent instead of instill trust in the public.

Health claims. The FDA strictly regulates health claims that link nutrients or food groups with a risk for disease. To make an association between a food product and a specific disease, the FDA must approve both the claim and the wording used on the package. Additionally, the food must meet the criteria set forth for that specific claim. Health claims may appear on the front, side, or back of a food package.

The For Further Focus box entitled "Glossary of Terms for Nutrition Facts Labels" provides an approved list of nutrients and the specific diseases with which they are associated (for use in the United States). An example of such a health claim would be the link between a diet that is low in saturated fat and cholesterol and a reduced risk of coronary heart disease. For a food to carry this label, it must be low in saturated fat, low in cholesterol, and low in total fat. If the food is fish or game meat, it must be "extra lean." The specific wording of this example claim must include the following: *saturated fat and cholesterol, coronary heart disease,* or *heart disease;* there must also be a physician's statement about the claim that defines high or normal total cholesterol level. The FDA also provides model claim statements from which food producers may choose. For this specific claim, one model statement is

as follows: *"Although many factors affect heart disease, diets low in saturated fat and cholesterol may reduce the risk of this disease."*[17]

FOOD TECHNOLOGY

America's food supply has radically changed over the years. These changes, which have swept the food marketing system, are rooted in widespread social changes and scientific advances. The agricultural and food processing industries have developed various methods and compounds to increase and preserve the food supply. However, critics voice concerns about how these changes have affected food safety and the overall environment. Such concerns frequently focus on pesticide use and food additives.

AGRICULTURAL PESTICIDES

Reasons for Use

Large American agricultural corporations as well as individual farmers use a number of chemicals to improve their crop yields. These materials have made possible the advances in food production to feed a growing population. For example, farmers use certain substances to control a wide variety of destructive insects that reduce crop yield. Growing produce without certain pesticides limits yield and is more labor intensive. The consumer then assumes the additional expense to overcome these production costs.

Controversy

Concerns and confusion continue regarding the use and effects of such substances. The four general areas of concern are as follows: (1) pesticide residues on foods; (2) the gradual leaching of the chemicals into groundwater and surrounding wells; (3) the increased exposure of farm workers to these chemicals; and (4) the increased amount of chemicals necessary as insects develop tolerance. Over time, the use of some chemicals has created a pesticide dilemma, and there is currently no clear answer regarding what to do in the face of conflicting interests. Thousands of pesticides are in use, and assessing the risks of specific pesticides is an important but complicated task.

Alternative Agriculture

An increasing number of concerned farmers, with help from soil scientists, are turning away from heavy pesticide use toward alternative agricultural methods.

Organic farming. Organic plant foods grow without synthetic pesticides, fertilizers, sewage sludge, genetically modified organisms, or ionizing radiation. Organic meat, poultry, eggs, and dairy products are from animals raised without antibiotics or growth hormones. In 2002 the USDA enacted a set of nationally recognized standards to identify certified organic food. For a food to carry the USDA Organic Seal (Figure 13.3), the farm and processing plant where the food was grown and packaged must have undergone government inspections and met the USDA organic standards (see the For Further Focus box, "Organic Food Standards").[18] Not all foods produced organically display the Organic Seal because it is a voluntary program. Companies that use the label on their food without certification face a large fine. Sales of organic foods continue to grow, and an increasing number of farmers—especially in California, which is the major supplier of U.S. fruits and vegetables—are using organic farming.

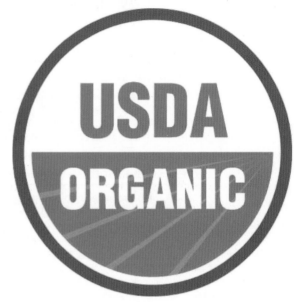

Figure 13.3 Official U.S. Department of Agriculture Organic Seal. (Courtesy National Organic Program, Agricultural Marketing Service, U.S. Department of Agriculture, www.ams.usda.gov/about-ams/programs-offices/national-organic-program, Washington, DC.)

For Further Focus

Organic Food Standards

The National Organic Program, which is a constituent of the U.S. Department of Agriculture (USDA), ensures the standards for organic foods. In response to the growing market, the National Organic Program has set strict standards for the growth, production, and labeling of organic foods. Although the USDA deems many methods prohibited by the organic standards safe (e.g., irradiation, genetic modification), these methods of farming are banned in certified organic foods because of public concern. Consumers of organic foods cite varied reasons for choosing organically produced foods over conventionally produced foods. The most common reasons include reduced exposure to contaminants, increased nutrient value, animal welfare, and environmental concerns (e.g., soil and water quality, biodiversity, greenhouse gas emissions).[1]

Organic foods have four labeling categories with specific guidelines for each, as follows:

1. *100% organic:* Products that carry this label must be made or produced exclusively with certified organic ingredients, and they must have passed a government inspection. These products may use the USDA Organic Seal on their labels and advertisements.

2. *Organic:* Products labeled as *organic* must contain at least 95% organic ingredients and must have passed a government inspection. The National Organic Program must approve all other ingredients for use as nonagricultural substances or as products not commercially available in organic form. These products may also use the USDA Organic Seal with the percentage of organic ingredients listed.

3. *Made with organic:* Products made with at least 70% certified organic ingredients may state on the product label *"made with organic ingredients"* and list up to three ingredients or food groups. These foods also must meet the National Organic Program guidelines for growth or production without synthetic pesticides, fertilizers, sewage sludge, bioengineering, or ionizing radiation. The products may not display the USDA Organic Seal or use it in any advertising.

4. *Specific organic ingredients:* Foods made with less than 70% certified organic ingredients may not use the USDA Organic Seal or make any organic claims on the front panel of the package. They can list the specific organic ingredients on the side panel of the package.

All food products made with at least 70% organic ingredients must also supply the name and address of the government-approved certifying agent on the product. For more information about the USDA organic standards, search "National Organic Program" from the USDA website (www.usda.gov).

REFERENCE

1. Brantsaeter, A. L., et al. (2017). Organic food in the diet: Exposure and health implications. *Annual Review of Public Health, 38,* 295–313.

Organic foods are less likely to contain pesticide residues and may be better for the environment and animals. However, there is not yet enough evidence to determine whether organic foods are more safe or nutritious for human consumption than conventionally produced foods.[19-21] Many studies have compared the specific nutrient parameters of individual foods grown either in an organic or in a conventional manner. Unfortunately, poor study design, conflicting results, marginal differences reported, and varying methods used for evaluating nutritive value do not allow for confidence when determining the overall human health significance.[19] Future research with well-controlled subjects and long-term exposure will provide insight to this ongoing debate.

Organic farmers can still use natural pesticides and fertilizers; therefore, they are not producing pesticide-free foods. Other common points of confusion are with the use of the following terms: *natural, hormone free,* and *free range.* These terms are not synonymous with *organic.* Truthful terms about the production of a food can appear on the food label, but they do not mean that the product is organic. The term *natural* may be used on products that contain no artificial ingredients (e.g., coloring, chemical preservatives) and if the product and its ingredients are only minimally processed. The Food Safety and Inspection Service of the USDA does not approve use of the terms *hormone free* or *antibiotic free.* Instead, manufacturers may use the phrases *raised without added hormones* and *raised without added antibiotics,* if the producer is able to supply an affidavit that attests to the production practices used to support the claim. One important note about the use of hormones is that beef and lamb are the only animal products that may use hormones. Therefore, including any such claim on a poultry product also requires the following statement on the food label: "Federal regulations prohibit the use of hormones in poultry."

Organic farming may be more beneficial for the environment and safer for the agricultural workers. However, organic farming has lower crop yields, requires more land, and is more expensive than conventionally grown crops. Nevertheless, the consumer demand for organic food in the United States continues to thrive and provides encouragement for the development of sustainable systems to support organic agriculture.

Biotechnology. Biotechnology is a broad term that has application in human nutrition, medications, agriculture, and environmental sciences. Biotechnology is the use of biologic processes or organisms to make or modify products. In its most basic form, selective breeding of plants or animals with desired traits is an example of biotechnology that has been in use for many millenniums. Two commonly used medications produced through means of biotechnology are insulin and penicillin. Two examples of biotechnology in agriculture are the development of corn that expresses a specific protein that serves as an insecticide and the synthesis of rice with increased levels of β-carotene.

Although various genetic manipulations have improved crop yields for thousands of years, most U.S. consumers are unaware of the extent to which these foods have entered the marketplace. In the United States, 94% of soybean crop acreage and 92% of corn crops are genetically modified (GM) varieties (Figure 13.4).[22] Thus, most people in the United States have

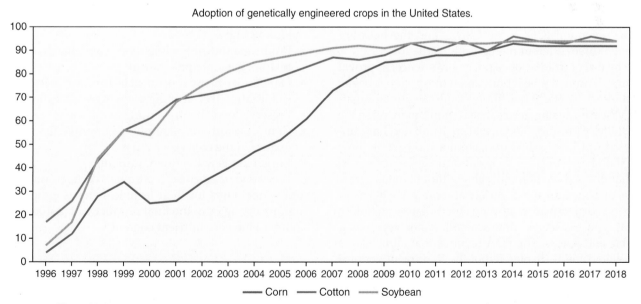

Figure 13.4 Adoption of genetically engineered crops in the United States. (Source: USDA, Economic Research Service using data from Fernandez-Cornejo and McBride [2002] for the years 1996-1999; National Agricultural Statistics Service. [2000-2018]. *Adoption of genetically engineered crops in the U.S.* Washington, DC: U.S. Department of Agriculture, Economic Research Service.)

consumed some form of GM foods (also referred to as genetically engineered [GE] foods) because corn and soy are omnipresent in grocery store products.

Plant physiologists have developed strains of plants that reduce the need for toxic pesticide and herbicide application to protect against virus infections and insects. Development of other GM products includes qualities such as drought resistance; enhanced protein, oil, or vitamin content; and viral/fungal resistance. At this time, there are 10 GM plants approved for commercial production in the United States, which are soybean, corn, canola, cotton, alfalfa, sugar beets, squash, papaya, apple, and potato. The National Institutes of Health, the Animal Plant Health Inspection Service of the USDA, the FDA, and the Environmental Protection Agency are all involved in the regulation of GM foods in commercial use, which are the most heavily regulated foods available. These agencies monitor the composition, safety, and environmental effects of GM crops.

Such forms of agriculture remain controversial around the world because of many unknown factors regarding the long-term effects on the environment and overall human health. Although the research in this area is still relatively new and sparse, the data available thus far indicate that consumption of GM foods poses no known adverse health effects to humans with regard to allergenicity or nutrient adequacy.[23] Additional long-term research will be important for all types of GM crops to ensure safety and acceptability.

Irradiation. Food irradiation is the use of ionizing radiation to kill bacteria and parasites that are on food after harvest. Irradiation helps to prevent food-borne illness caused by *Escherichia coli, Salmonella, Campylobacter, Listeria, Shigella,* and *Salmonella* spp. The World Health Organization, the Centers for Disease Control and Prevention (CDC), the USDA, and the FDA approved three different methods of irradiation.

The use of irradiation is not a new science; approval for irradiation of wheat flour and white potatoes began in the early 1960s. In addition to reducing or eliminating disease-causing germs, irradiation can increase the shelf life of produce. Foods that are irradiated have unaltered nutritive value; they are not radioactive, they have no harmful substances introduced because of irradiation, and are not noticeably different in taste, texture, or appearance.[24] A variety of foods have been approved for irradiation in the United States, including meat, poultry, seeds, some seafood, fruits, vegetables, herbs, and spices. The FDA requires that all labels on irradiated foods display either the Radura symbol for irradiation (Figure 13.5) or a written description noting the food's exposure to irradiation.

Consumer rejection in the United States and around the world is mainly due to fear of the unknown long-term effects of irradiation on human health. The U.S. government continues to support the use and safety of such foods; however, without consumer acceptance,

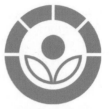

Figure 13.5 Radura symbol of irradiation. (Courtesy Food Safety and Inspection Service, U.S. Department of Agriculture, Washington, DC.)

companies that are using such procedures have limited success.

FOOD ADDITIVES

The use of food additives (i.e., intentionally added chemicals that prevent spoilage and extend shelf life) is not new to the food industry, either. Table 13.2 lists examples of food additives. The two most common additives are sugar and salt, although consumers often do not acknowledge these basic ingredients as *food additives*. Using additives for food preservation has been around for centuries, especially salt in cured meats. The phrase *generally recognized as safe* denotes additives in foods that do not require FDA approval.

Over the past few decades, the number and variety of additives in the food supply have increased; the current variety of food market items would be impossible without them. Scientific advances have created processed food products, and the changing society has created a market demand. The expanding population, a larger workforce, and more complex family life have increased the desire for more variety and convenience in foods as well as better safety and quality. Food additives help to achieve these desires, and they serve many other purposes, such as the following:

- Produce uniform qualities (e.g., color, flavor, aroma, texture, general appearance)
- Standardize many functional factors (e.g., thickening, stabilization [i.e., keeping parts from separating])
- Preserve foods by preventing oxidation
- Control acidity or alkalinity to improve flavor and texture of the cooked product
- Enrich foods with added nutrients

Processed foods use a number of micronutrients and antioxidants for their technical effects either during processing or in the final product, not just for their ability to increase nutrient content.

> **organic farming** the use of farming methods that employ natural means of pest control and that meet the standards set by the National Organic Program of the U.S. Department of Agriculture; organic foods are grown or produced without the use of synthetic pesticides or fertilizers, sewage sludge, genetically modified organisms, or ionizing radiation.

Table 13.2   Examples of Food Additives

The following summary lists the types of common food ingredients, the reasons they are used, and some examples of the names listed on product labels referring to them. Some additives have more than one purpose.

TYPES OF INGREDIENTS	WHAT THEY DO	EXAMPLES OF USES	NAMES FOUND ON PRODUCT LABELS
Preservatives	Prevent food spoilage from bacteria, mold, fungi, or yeast (antimicrobials); slow or prevent changes in color, flavor, or texture and delay rancidity (antioxidants); maintain freshness	Fruit sauces and jellies, beverages, baked goods, cured meats, oils and margarines, cereals, dressings, snack foods, packaged fruits, and vegetables	Ascorbic acid, citric acid, sodium benzoate, calcium propionate, sodium erythorbate, sodium nitrite, calcium sorbate, potassium sorbate, BHA, BHT, EDTA, tocopherols (vitamin E)
Sweeteners	Add sweetness with or without extra calories (nutritive or nonnutritive)	Beverages, baked goods, confections, tabletop sugar, sugar substitutes, many processed foods	Sucrose (sugar), glucose, fructose, sorbitol, mannitol, corn syrup, high fructose corn syrup, saccharin, aspartame, sucralose, acesulfame potassium (acesulfame-K), neotame
Color additives	Offset color loss resulting from exposure to light, air, temperature extremes, moisture and storage conditions; correct natural variations in color; enhance colors that occur naturally; provide color to colorless foods	Many processed foods, (candies, snack foods, margarine, cheese, soft drinks, jams and jellies, gelatins, pudding and pie fillings)	FD&C Blue Nos. 1 and 2, FD&C Green No. 3, FD&C Red Nos. 3 and 40, FD&C Yellow Nos. 5 and 6, Orange B, Citrus Red No. 2, annatto extract, β-carotene, grape skin extract, cochineal extract or carmine, paprika oleoresin, caramel color, fruit and vegetable juices, saffron (NOTE: Exempt color additives are not required to be declared by name on labels but may be declared simply as colorings or color added)
Flavors and spices	Add specific flavors (natural and synthetic)	Pudding and pie fillings, gelatin dessert mixes, cake mixes, salad dressings, candies, soft drinks, ice cream, BBQ sauce	Natural flavoring, artificial flavor, and spices
Flavor enhancers	Enhance flavors already present in foods (without providing their own separate flavor)	Many processed foods	Monosodium glutamate (MSG), hydrolyzed soy protein, autolyzed yeast extract, disodium guanylate or inosinate
Fat replacers (and components of formulations that are used to replace fats)	Provide expected texture and a creamy "mouth-feel" in reduced-fat foods	Baked goods, dressings, frozen desserts, confections, cake and dessert mixes, dairy products	Olestra, cellulose gel, carrageenan, polydextrose, modified food starch, microparticulated egg white protein, guar gum, xanthan gum, whey protein concentrate
Nutrients	Replace vitamins and minerals lost in processing (enrichment), add nutrients that may be lacking in the diet (fortification)	Flour, breads, cereals, rice, macaroni, margarine, salt, milk, fruit beverages, energy bars, instant breakfast drinks	Thiamine hydrochloride, riboflavin (vitamin B$_2$), niacin, niacinamide, folate or folic acid, β-carotene, potassium iodide, iron or ferrous sulfate, α-tocopherols, ascorbic acid, vitamin D, amino acids (L-tryptophan, L-lysine, L-leucine, L-methionine)
Emulsifiers	Allow smooth mixing of ingredients, prevent separation, keep emulsified products stable, reduce stickiness, control crystallization, keep ingredients dispersed, and help products dissolve more easily	Salad dressings, peanut butter, chocolate, margarine, frozen desserts	Soy lecithin, mono- and diglycerides, egg yolks, polysorbates, sorbitan monostearate

Continued

Table 13.2	Examples of Food Additives—cont'd		
TYPES OF INGREDIENTS	**WHAT THEY DO**	**EXAMPLES OF USES**	**NAMES FOUND ON PRODUCT LABELS**
Stabilizers, thickeners, binders, and texturizers	Produce uniform texture, improve "mouth-feel"	Frozen desserts, dairy products, cakes, pudding and gelatin mixes, dressings, jams and jellies, sauces	Gelatin, pectin, guar gum, carrageenan, xanthan gum, whey
Leavening agents	Promote rising of baked goods	Breads and other baked goods	Baking soda, monocalcium phosphate, calcium carbonate
Anti-caking agents	Keep powdered foods free-flowing, prevent moisture absorption	Salt, baking powder, confectioner's sugar	Calcium silicate, iron ammonium citrate, silicon dioxide
Humectants	Retain moisture	Shredded coconut, marshmallows, soft candies, confections	Glycerin, sorbitol
Yeast nutrients	Promote growth of yeast	Breads and other baked goods	Calcium sulfate, ammonium phosphate
Dough strengtheners and conditioners	Produce more stable dough	Breads and other baked goods	Ammonium sulfate, azodicarbonamide, L-cysteine
Firming agents	Maintain crispness and firmness	Processed fruits and vegetables	Calcium chloride, calcium lactate
Enzyme preparations	Modify proteins, polysaccharides and fats	Cheese, dairy products, meat	Enzymes, lactase, papain, rennet, chymosin
Gases	Serve as propellant, aerate, or create carbonation	Oil cooking spray, whipped cream, carbonated beverages	Carbon dioxide, nitrous oxide

Reprinted from International Food Information Council and U.S. Food and Drug Administration. (2010). *Food ingredients and colors*. Retrieved May 2019 from www.fda.gov/downloads/Food/IngredientsPackagingLabeling/ucm094249.pdf.

FOOD-BORNE DISEASE

Tracking the prevalence, food origin, and pathogen responsible for food-borne illness is an extremely difficult task. The symptoms of food-borne illness are often difficult to distinguish from other forms of illness and are frequently mistaken as a "stomach bug" or the "flu." Furthermore, most forms of food-borne illness are short-lived and self-limiting, and the victim may not visit a physician. Even if the person does see a physician, identifying the pathogen responsible is challenging. The CDC tracks, investigates, and reports the incidence of food-borne illness in the United States, but their ability to do so is dependent upon the victim reporting the illness. Local, state, and tribal health departments voluntarily report food-borne illness to the CDC. Reporting **outbreaks of food-borne illness** to the CDC is more likely than the reporting of individual instances of illness. Thus, the estimated cases of food-borne illness are extrapolations of actual reported cases.

---

outbreak of food-borne illness the occurrence of two or more similar illnesses resulting from ingestion of a common food.

PREVALENCE

The CDC estimates that 1 in 6 people get sick each year from food-borne illness. Many disease-bearing organisms inhabit the environment and can contaminate food and water. The last century saw exceptional advances in knowledge about the pathogens that commonly contaminate food and water and about ways to prevent food-borne illness outbreaks. However, lapses in control still occur, and these can result in high incidences of illness and hospitalization as well as economic burden. The estimated annual incidence of food-borne illness continues to be a public health concern as rates are well above the *Healthy People* targets.[25,26] Of the identified causes of food-borne illness in the United States, 52% are due to bacteria, 46% are due to viruses (of which the vast majority are norovirus), 1% are the result of chemical or toxic agents, and 1% are due to parasites.[27] Figure 13.6 shows the relative incidence of foodborne illness for the most common forms of bacteria.

FOOD SAFETY

Buying and Storing Food

The control of food-borne disease focuses on strict sanitation measures and rigid personal hygiene. First, the food itself should be of good quality and not defective

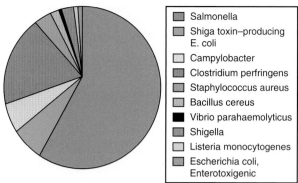

Most common bacterial outbreak-associated illnesses

- Salmonella
- Shiga toxin–producing E. coli
- Campylobacter
- Clostridium perfringens
- Staphylococcus aureus
- Bacillus cereus
- Vibrio parahaemolyticus
- Shigella
- Listeria monocytogenes
- Escherichia coli, Enterotoxigenic

Figure 13.6 Incidence of the most common forms of bacterial-associated food-borne illness. (Source: Dewey-Mattia, D., et al. [2018]. Surveillance for foodborne disease outbreaks—United States, 2009-2015. *MMWR Surveill Summ*, 67[10], 1–11.)

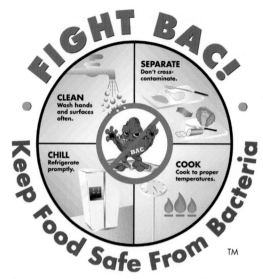

Figure 13.7 The Partnership for Food Safety Education developed the "Fight BAC!" (i.e., bacteria) campaign to prevent food-borne illness. (Campaign graphics are available at www.fightbac.org. Courtesy Partnership for Food Safety Education, Washington, DC.)

or diseased. Second, dry or cold storage should protect it from deterioration or decay, which is especially important for products such as refrigerated convenience foods; this is the fastest growing segment of the convenience food market, and it is potentially the most dangerous because these foods are not sterile. These vacuum-packaged or modified-atmosphere chilled food products are only minimally processed and not sterilized, and they are at risk of temperature abuse. Home refrigerator temperatures are safest at 40° F or colder. At temperatures 45° F or higher, any precooked or leftover foods are potential reservoirs for bacteria that survive cooking and that can then recontaminate cooked food. Food safety depends on the following critical actions (Figure 13.7):

- *Clean:* Wash hands and surfaces often.
- *Separate:* Do not cross-contaminate.
- *Cook:* Cook to proper temperatures.
- *Chill:* Refrigerate promptly.

Carefully clean all food preparation areas, utensils, and dishes; wash and clean produce well. Follow cooking procedures and temperatures as directed. Store leftover food and reheat appropriately or discard (Table 13.3). Do not cool food to room temperature before refrigerating; this practice allows food to sit in a temperature range that is perfect for bacterial growth. Refrigerate leftovers within 2 hours. Contain and dispose of garbage in a sanitary manner. Safe methods of food handling, cooking, and storage are simple and mostly common sense; however, they often are neglected, and this may lead to food-borne illness.

The Food Safety and Inspection Service website (www.fsis.usda.gov) provides safety publications for all types of foods and populations.

Preparing and Serving Food

All people who handle food—especially those who work in public food services—should follow strict measures to prevent contamination. For example, washing hands properly and wearing clean clothing, gloves, and aprons are imperative. Basic rules of hygiene apply to all people who are handling food, whether they work in food processing and packaging plants, process and package foods in markets, or prepare and serve food in restaurants. In addition, people with infectious diseases should have limited access to direct food handling.

When cooking the following foods, make sure to meet these minimal internal temperatures:

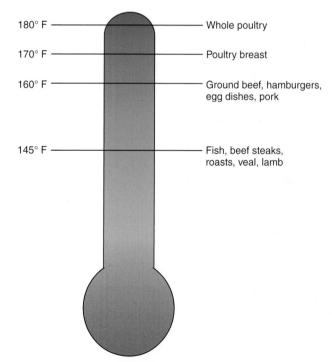

180° F	Whole poultry
170° F	Poultry breast
160° F	Ground beef, hamburgers, egg dishes, pork
145° F	Fish, beef steaks, roasts, veal, lamb

Thermometer showing minimal temperatures for specific foods in cooking.

The Hazard Analysis & Critical Control Point (HACCP) food safety system focuses on preventing food-borne illness by identifying critical points and

Table **13.3**   **Cold Storage**

PRODUCT	REFRIGERATOR (40° F)	FREEZER (0° F)
Eggs		
Fresh, in shell	3 to 5 weeks	Do not freeze
Raw yolks and whites	2 to 4 days	1 year
Hard cooked	1 week	Does not freeze well
Liquid Pasteurized Eggs, Egg Substitutes		
Opened	3 days	Does not freeze well
Unopened	10 days	1 year
Mayonnaise, Commercial		
Refrigerate after opening	2 months	Do not freeze
Frozen Dinners and Entrees		
Keep frozen until ready to heat	—	3 to 4 months
Deli and Vacuum-Packed Products		
Store-prepared (or homemade) egg, chicken, ham, tuna, and macaroni salads	3 to 5 days	Does not freeze well
Hot Dogs and Luncheon Meats		
Hot Dogs Opened package	1 week	1 to 2 months
Unopened package	2 weeks	1 to 2 months
Luncheon Meat Opened package	3 to 5 days	1 to 2 months
Unopened package	2 weeks	1 to 2 months
Bacon and Sausage		
Bacon	7 days	1 month
Sausage, raw—from chicken, turkey, pork, beef	1 to 2 days	1 to 2 months
Smoked breakfast links, patties	7 days	1 to 2 months
Hard sausage—pepperoni, jerky sticks	2 to 3 weeks	1 to 2 months
Summer Sausage Labeled "Keep Refrigerated"		
Opened	3 weeks	1 to 2 months
Unopened	3 months	1 to 2 months
Corned Beef		
Corned beef, in pouch with pickling juices	5 to 7 days	Drained, 1 month
Ham, Canned, Labeled "Keep Refrigerated"		
Opened	3 to 5 days	1 to 2 months
Unopened	6 to 9 months	Do not freeze
Ham, Fully Cooked		
Vacuum sealed at plant, undated, unopened	2 weeks	1 to 2 months
Vacuum sealed at plant, dated, unopened	"Use-By" date on package	1 to 2 months
Whole	7 days	1 to 2 months
Half	3 to 5 days	1 to 2 months
Slices	3 to 4 days	1 to 2 months
Hamburger, Ground, and Stew Meat		
Hamburger and stew meat	1 to 2 days	3 to 4 months

Table 13.3   **Cold Storage—cont'd**

PRODUCT	REFRIGERATOR (40° F)	FREEZER (0° F)
Ground turkey, veal, pork, lamb, and mixtures of them	1 to 2 days	3 to 4 months
Fresh Beef, Veal, Lamb, and Pork		
Steaks	3 to 5 days	6 to 12 months
Chops	3 to 5 days	4 to 6 months
Roasts	3 to 5 days	4 to 12 months
Variety meats—tongue, liver, heart, kidneys, chitterlings	1 to 2 days	3 to 4 months
Pre-stuffed, uncooked pork chops, lamb chops, or chicken breasts stuffed with dressing	1 day	Do not freeze well
Soups and stews, vegetable or meat added	3 to 4 days	2 to 3 months
Fresh Poultry		
Chicken or turkey, whole	1 to 2 days	1 year
Chicken or turkey, pieces	1 to 2 days	9 months
Giblets	1 to 2 days	3 to 4 months
Cooked Meat and Poultry Leftovers		
Cooked meat and meat casseroles	3 to 4 days	2 to 3 months
Gravy and meat broth	3 to 4 days	2 to 3 months
Fried chicken	3 to 4 days	4 months
Cooked poultry casseroles	3 to 4 days	4 to 6 months
Poultry pieces, plain	3 to 4 days	4 months
Poultry pieces in broth, gravy	3 to 4 days	6 months
Chicken nuggets, patties	3 to 4 days	1 to 3 months
Other Cooked Leftovers		
Pizza, cooked	3 to 4 days	1 to 2 months
Stuffing, cooked	3 to 4 days	1 month

Reprinted from Food Safety and Inspection Service. (n.d.). *Basics for handling food safely*. Retrieved May 2019 from www.fsis.usda.gov/wps/portal/fsis/topics/food-safety-education/get-answers/food-safety-fact-sheets/safe-food-handling/basics-for-handling-food-safely/ct_index.

eliminating hazards. Many organizations, including the USDA and the FDA, use the HACCP standards. For more information about HACCP, visit www.fda.gov/Food/GuidanceRegulation/HACCP.

FOOD CONTAMINATION

Food-borne illness usually begins with flu-like symptoms, but it can advance to a lethal illness. Not all bacteria found in foods are harmful, and some are even beneficial (e.g., the bacteria in yogurt). Bacteria that are harmful to people are referred to as *pathogens*. Age and physical condition increase the risk for food-borne illness in certain subgroups of the population. Groups with the highest risks are young children, pregnant women, elderly individuals, and people with compromised immune systems.

Food-borne illness generally results from the ingestion of bacteria, viruses, or parasites. Bacteria cause illness through either infection or by the accumulation of bacteria-produced toxins. All types of foods can be carriers of food-borne illness. Figure 13.8 shows the relative existence of food-borne illness resulting from various food sources.

Bacterial Food Infections

Bacterial food infections result from eating food that is contaminated by large colonies of bacteria. Specific diseases result from specific bacteria (e.g., salmonellosis, shigellosis, listeriosis).

Salmonellosis. *Salmonella typhi* and *Salmonella paratyphi* are the common species of salmonella that cause the food-borne infection salmonellosis. The American veterinarian pathologist Daniel Salmon (1850–1914), first isolated and identified the species; thus, the given name. The gastrointestinal tracts of most animals, including humans and birds, contain *Salmonella* spp. These organisms readily grow in raw or unpasteurized milk or foods containing raw or undercooked eggs, poultry, or meat. Seafood from polluted waters—especially shellfish such as oysters and clams—may also be a source of infection. The unsanitary handling of foods and utensils can spread the bacteria.

Number of outbreak-associated illnesses by food category

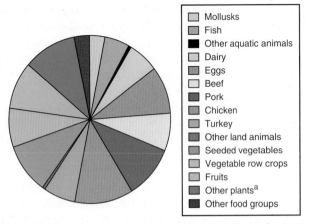

☐	Mollusks
☐	Fish
■	Other aquatic animals
☐	Dairy
☐	Eggs
☐	Beef
☐	Pork
☐	Chicken
☐	Turkey
☐	Other land animals
☐	Seeded vegetables
☐	Vegetable row crops
☐	Fruits
☐	Other plantsª
■	Other food groups

Figure 13.8 Number of outbreak-associated illnesses by food category. ªOils, sugars, fungi, sprouts, root vegetables, herbs, grains, beans, nuts, seeds. (Source: Dewey-Mattia, D., et al. [2018]. Surveillance for foodborne disease outbreaks—United States, 2009-2015. *MMWR Surveill Summ*, 67[10], 1–11.)

Resulting cases of gastroenteritis may vary from mild to severe diarrhea. Immunization, pasteurization, and sanitary regulations that involve community water and food supplies as well as food handlers help to control outbreaks.

More than 46,000 cases of salmonellosis are reported in the United States each year, although thousands of other cases likely go unreported.[28] Because the incubation and reproduction of the bacteria take time after the food is eaten, symptoms of food infection develop relatively slowly (i.e., up to 48 hours later). Symptoms include diarrhea, fever, vomiting, and abdominal cramps. The illness usually lasts 4 to 7 days, with most affected individuals recovering completely. Severe dehydration from diarrhea and vomiting may require intravenous fluids.

Shigellosis. The bacteria *Shigella* causes Shigellosis. Kiyoshi Shiga (1870–1957), a Japanese physician, first discovered the main species of the organism, *Shigella dysenteriae*, during a dysentery epidemic in Japan in 1898. *Shigella* is in the feces of infected individuals and can infect other people or food through means of poor hygiene. Boiling water or pasteurizing milk kills the organisms, but unsanitary handling of the food or milk may easily result in reinfection. Similar to the spreading of salmonella, feces, flies, and foods unsanitarily handled transmit the disease. Shigellosis, similar to salmonellosis, is more common during the summer, and it most often occurs in young children.

Nearly half a million cases of food-borne illness per year are attributed to shigellosis.[29] Shigellosis, usually confined to the large intestine, may vary from a mild, transient intestinal disturbance in adults to fatal dysentery in young children. Symptoms appear within 4 to 7 days and include cramps, diarrhea, fever, vomiting, and blood or mucus in the stool. Because of the long incubation period, it is exceptionally difficult to identify the food source.

Listeriosis. The bacterial *Listeria* causes listeriosis. The English surgeon Baron Joseph Lister (1827–1912), for whom the bacteria is named, first applied knowledge of bacterial infection to the principles of antiseptic surgery in a benchmark 1867 publication that led to "clean" operations and the development of modern surgery. However, only within the past 30 years has knowledge of bacteria's role as a direct cause of food-borne illness increased and the major species to cause human illness, *Listeria monocytogenes*, been identified. Before 1981, scientists believed that listeria was an animal disease and only transmitted to people by direct contact with infected animals. However, this organism occurs widely in the environment and in high-risk individuals, such as the elderly, pregnant women, infants, and clients with suppressed immune systems.

Listeriosis can produce a rare but fatal illness with severe symptoms such as diarrhea, flu-like fever and headache, pneumonia, sepsis, meningitis, and endocarditis. Pregnant women have suppressed T-cell immunity, which increases their risk for listeriosis substantially more than any other segment of the population.[30] There have been traces of listeriosis in a variety of foods, including soft cheese, poultry, seafood, raw milk, refrigerated raw liquid whole eggs, and meat products (e.g., pâté). *Listeria* spp. are capable of growing in some foods despite being refrigerated.

Escherichia coli. Theodor Escherich (1857–1911), a German pediatrician and bacteriologist, discovered the rod-shaped bacteria *Escherichia coli* in 1885. It went unrecognized as a human pathogen until almost a century later in 1982. There are many types of *E. coli*, and not all types are harmful to humans. In fact, some strains are part of the healthy gut flora that survive in the intestines and produce a valuable supply of vitamin K. *E. coli* spreads most commonly through fecal contamination (e.g., contaminated foods, not properly washing hands after changing diapers), undercooked meat, and unpasteurized foods (e.g., milk, apple cider, soft cheeses).

Shiga toxin–producing strains of *E. coli* cause significant illness in the United States annually, and approximately 43% of those cases are from the O157 strain.[31] Drug-resistant strains of *E. coli* are most dangerous to populations with compromised or immature immune systems (see the Drug-Nutrient Interaction box, "Drug-Resistant *Escherichia coli*"). Most cases of infection involve diarrhea, stomach cramps, and low-grade fevers that start within 2 to 8 days after ingestion and that usually resolve within 7 days. About 5% to 10%

of individuals infected with *E. coli* will develop **hemolytic uremic syndrome**, which is a potentially deadly condition.

Drug-Nutrient Interaction

Drug-Resistant *Escherichia coli*

Animal food production practices frequently use low-dose antimicrobial drugs to improve growth and reduce disease in livestock. Coupled with the excessive use of antibiotics in humans, this widespread, extended use of antimicrobials and antibiotics has resulted in drug-resistant strains of common food-borne and environmental pathogens. Multidrug-resistant strains of *Escherichia coli* bacteria are prevalent in the current food supply, particularly in retail chicken products.[1] Resistance to first-line antibiotics by these bacteria represents a major cause of illness, failed treatments, death, and increased health care costs.[2,3]

Populations that are at risk for infection with drug-resistant strains of bacteria include children, elderly adults, and those who are immunocompromised. Infections with drug-resistant *E. coli* frequently are seen as either a gastrointestinal illness or urinary tract infection. The routine use of antibiotics in children increases their subsequent risk for antimicrobial-resistant infections.[4] Elderly individuals living in nursing homes experience significantly more drug-resistant infections compared to their community-dwelling peers.[5] Individuals with compromised immune systems, from any number of causes, suffer greatly from infections of such resistant, difficult to treat illnesses on top of their primary illness.

In health care settings, proper food safety practices, infection prevention, and antibiotic stewardship are especially important. Drug-resistant strains of bacteria necessitate the long-term use of powerful antibiotics. Antibiotics destroy the natural gut flora commonly leading to nausea, vomiting, and diarrhea. Some antibiotics such as ciprofloxacin (Cipro) can bind to calcium, magnesium, iron, and zinc, thereby interfering with their absorption. Thus, the long-term use of this antibiotic can result in poor bioavailability of these minerals.

Animal food producers, veterinary medicine, and human health care practitioners must all work together to reduce the global burden of drug-resistant forms of pathogens.

REFERENCES

1. Johnson, J. R., et al. (2017). Extraintestinal pathogenic and antimicrobial-resistant *Escherichia coli*, including sequence type 131 (ST131), from retail chicken breasts in the United States in 2013. *Applied and Environmental Microbiology*, 83(6).
2. Poolman, J. T., & Wacker, M. (2016). Extraintestinal pathogenic Escherichia coli, a common human pathogen: Challenges for vaccine development and progress in the field. *The Journal of Infectious Diseases*, 213(1), 6–13.
3. Mukherjee, S., et al. (2017). Antimicrobial drug-resistant Shiga toxin-producing *Escherichia coli* infections, Michigan, USA. *Emerging Infectious Diseases*, 23(9), 1609–1611.
4. Bryce, A., et al. (2016). Global prevalence of antibiotic resistance in paediatric urinary tract infections caused by Escherichia coli and association with routine use of antibiotics in primary care: Systematic review and meta-analysis. *BMJ*, 352, i939.
5. Pulcini, C., et al. (2019). Antibiotic resistance of Enterobacteriaceae causing urinary tract infections in elderly patients living in the community and in the nursing home: A retrospective observational study. *Journal of Antimicrobial Chemotherapy*, 74(3), 775–781.

> **hemolytic uremic syndrome** a condition that results most often from infection with *Escherichia coli* and that presents with a breaking up of red blood cells (i.e., hemolysis) and kidney failure.

Vibrio. Filippo Pacini (1812–1883) first isolated microorganisms that he called "vibrions" from cholera patients in 1854. The Vibrionaceae pathogen causes vibriosis and cholera. A salt-requiring organism, it inhabits the saltwater regions of North America. Transmissions occur for most individuals via water-related activities in contaminated water (86%) with a much lower frequency by food-borne infection from contaminated seafood. The coastal states, particularly in the Gulf Coast region, report the vast majority (96%) of *Vibrio*-related illnesses.[32] Immunocompromised individuals are most susceptible to *Vibrio* infection, which commonly is seen as skin or ear infections. Thoroughly cooking seafood—especially shellfish such as oysters—reduces the risk of infection.

Bacterial Food Poisoning

Ingesting foods contaminated with toxins from specific types of bacteria causes *food poisoning*. Consuming the powerful toxin directly leads to rapid development of symptoms. Staphylococcal and clostridial bacterial food poisoning are the most common.

Staphylococcal food poisoning. Staphylococcal food poisoning is primarily due to *Staphylococcus aureus,* a round bacterium that forms masses of cells. *S. aureus* releases powerful toxins in the contaminated food that rapidly produce illness (i.e., 1 to 6 hours after ingestion). The symptoms appear suddenly, and they include severe cramping and abdominal pain with nausea, vomiting, and diarrhea, usually accompanied by sweating, headache, fever, and sometimes prostration and shock. However, recovery is rapid, and symptoms ordinarily subside within 1 to 3 days. The amount of toxin ingested and the susceptibility of the individual eating it determine the degree of severity.

The source of the food contamination could be something as minor as a small, or even unnoticed, staphylococcal infection on the hand of a worker preparing the food. Foods that are particularly effective carriers of staphylococci and their toxins include custard or cream-filled bakery goods, processed meats, ham, tongue, cheese, ice cream, potato salad, sauces, chicken and ham salads, and combination dishes such as spaghetti and casseroles. The victim has no warning of the toxin's presence, as it causes no change in the normal appearance, odor, or taste of the food (see the Case Study box, "A Community Food Poisoning Incident"). Collecting a careful food history and portions of food for testing (if possible) helps to determine the source of the poison. The actual bacteria may no longer exist in food samples because sufficient heat kills the organisms but does not destroy the bacteria-produced toxins.

NEXT-GENERATION NCLEX® EXAMINATION-STYLE UNFOLDING CASE STUDY
Food Poisoning Incident

A wife and husband agreed that their lodge dinner had been the best they had ever had, especially the dessert: custard-filled cream puffs. The husband had eaten two of them and thought that may have caused him to feel ill shortly after they arrived home. His wife's stomach felt a little upset, too, so they both took some antacid pills, thinking that their "stomach-aches" were from eating more rich food than they were accustomed to eating. They went to bed early. At 11:00 PM, the wife woke up alarmed. Her husband was vomiting, and he had diarrhea and increasingly severe stomach cramps. He complained of a headache, fever, and his pajamas were wet with sweat. His wife began to have similar pains and symptoms, although they were not as severe as her husband's symptoms.

1. **Select all of the indicators that may suggest foodborne illness.**

   a. Illness 1-6 hour after ingestion of cream puffs
   b. Consuming multiple custard-filled cream puffs
   c. Age
   d. Severe abdominal cramps
   e. Nausea and vomiting
   f. Diarrhea
   g. Fever
   h. Headache

2. **Choose the *most likely* options for the information missing from the statements below by selecting from the list of options provided**

   The couple's food-borne illness was most likely caused by the ingestion of _____, _____, or _____.

OPTIONS	
bacteria	parasites
fungi	mold
viruses	dirt

The lodge where they had dinner imports the cream puffs from a local bakery. Their friends that had dinner at the lodge were also experiencing similar symptoms. Later that night, the husband starting vomiting more frequently and lay prostrate on the ground.

   After reporting the incident, an investigation was held. The local health department found that an employee had an infected cut on his finger. There was also a report of the delivery truck breaking down for 3 hours that day. A server at the event stated that the cream puffs were also sitting out (not refrigerated) for an extended period since they were served at the same time as dinner.

3. **Choose the *most likely* options for the information missing from the statements below by selecting from the list of options provided**

   The agent that most likely caused the couple's illness was _____, a form of food _____.

OPTIONS	
poisoning	giardia
infection	additive
clostridium	appendicitis
staphylococcus	urinary tract infection
E. coli	

4. **Select all of the actions that the driver and food-service staff should have done to keep food safe.**

   a. Wash hands/surfaces before preparing cream puffs
   b. Wear same gloves during different tasks while preparing cream puffs
   c. Keep cream puffs refrigerated at 40 degrees F or below
   d. Refrigerate cream puffs within 2 hours of sitting out
   e. Use different spatula to prepare cream puffs and raw meat
   f. Keep apron on, even when leaving the food prep area

5. **Use an X to identify the education topics to provide to the food service staff at the bakery that are <u>indicated</u> (appropriate or necessary) or <u>contraindicated</u> (could be harmful).**

ACTION	INDICATED	CONTRAINDICATED
Cool food to room temperature before storing		
Refrigerate food within 2 hours of serving		
Reheat leftovers until warm		
Storing leftovers in open containers		
Disposing trash and garbage appropriately		
Refrigerate food after 2 hours of serving		
Reheat leftovers to specific temperature depending on the food		

6. **From the information provided, select all of the food safety regulations that the food service staff did not follow when preparing the cream puffs.**

   a. Food sanitation
   b. Quality control
   c. Food additives
   d. Regulating food across state lines
   e. Food labeling
   f. Food safety regarding time and temperature control

Clostridial food poisoning. *Clostridium perfringens* and *Clostridium botulinum* are spore-forming, rod-shaped bacteria that can release powerful toxins in infected foods and result in clostridial food poisoning.

C. perfringens spores are widespread in the environment, including soil, water, dust, and refuse. This organism is frequently located on raw meat and poultry, and it multiplies rapidly in foods held at temperatures between 109° F and 117° F for extended periods. In many cases, cooked meat is improperly prepared, refrigerated, or reheated. Control depends on careful preparation and adequate cooking of meats, prompt service, and immediate refrigeration at sufficiently low temperatures. Once ingested, the bacteria produce toxins within the gastrointestinal tract, resulting in poisoning and illness.

The bacterium *C. botulinum* causes a more serious type of food poisoning than *C. perfringens* but occurs much less frequently. Food-borne botulism results from the ingestion of food that contains the powerful paralyzing toxin produced from this strain of *Clostridium*. Depending on the dose of toxin consumed and the individual response, symptoms will appear within 18 to 36 hours. Nausea, vomiting, weakness, blurred vision, and slurred speech are typical initial symptoms. The toxin progressively irritates motor nerve cells and blocks the transmission of neural impulses at the nerve terminals, thereby causing a gradual paralysis. In severe cases, a sudden respiratory paralysis with airway obstruction may end in death.

C. botulinum spores are widespread in soil throughout the world and may accompany harvested food to the food processing plant. Canned foods are a high-risk food for botulism contamination. Like all *Clostridia*, this species is **anaerobic**, or nearly so. The relatively air-free can and canning temperatures (≥27° C [80° F]) provide good conditions for toxin production. The development of high standards in the commercial canning industry has predominantly eliminated this source of botulism. Home-canned foods are more susceptible to contamination. Boiling food for 10 minutes destroys the toxin, although not the spore. Therefore, all home-canned food—no matter how well preserved it is considered to be—should be boiled for at least 10 minutes before it is eaten.

Viruses

Food-borne disease outbreaks resulting from norovirus contamination are the most common cause of food-borne illness in the United States.[33] However, norovirus is much less likely to cause hospitalization than other forms of food-borne illness such as *Salmonella* or *E. coli* contamination. Other viral forms of food-borne illness include **hepatitis** A and rotavirus. Hepatitis A is much less common in the United States and other areas that routinely use hepatitis A vaccines than in less developed countries. Again, the stringent control of community water and food supplies as well as the personal hygiene and sanitary practices of food handlers are essential for the prevention of food-borne disease.

> **anaerobic** without oxygen; a microorganism that can live and grow in an oxygen-free environment.
>
> **hepatitis** the inflammation of the liver cells; symptoms of acute hepatitis include flu-like symptoms, muscle and joint aches, fever, nausea, vomiting, diarrhea, headache, dark urine, and yellowing of the eyes and skin; symptoms of chronic hepatitis include jaundice, abdominal swelling and sensitivity, low-grade fever, and ascites.

Parasites

Giardiasis (from the parasite *Giardia lamblia*) is the most common form of parasitic food-borne illness in the United States. Water, food, person-to-person, and animal-to-person contact are all viable methods of transmission. *Giardia* lives in the intestines of infected individuals and spreads to others through their feces. *Giardia* can live outside of the body for a long time (weeks or even months) and thus reinfection is a risk. Symptoms begin 1 to 3 weeks after the individual becomes infected and include gastrointestinal disturbances such as diarrhea, stomach cramps, gas, and greasy stools.

Two types of parasitic worms are of concern in relation to food: (1) roundworms, such as the *trichina (Trichinella spiralis)* worm found in pork; and (2) flatworms, such as the common tapeworms found in beef and pork. The following control measures are essential: (1) laws controlling hog and cattle food sources and pastures to prevent the transmission of the parasites to the meat produced for market; and (2) the avoidance of rare beef and undercooked pork as an added personal precaution. Table 13.4 summarizes examples of common food contamination.

Environmental Food Contaminants

Lead. Heavy metals such as lead may contaminate food and water as well as the air and environmental objects. Lead toxicity (defined as a blood lead level ≥5 mcg/dL) contributes to neurologic disorders in children and all-cause mortality, particularly cardiovascular disease, in adults.[34-36] Some studies indicate that lead toxicity, especially when coupled with iron deficiency, is associated with behavior problems, such as hyperactive/impulse and defiant/hostile behaviors, in children, which could contribute to poor learning capacity.[37-39] Although lead poisoning in the United States has dramatically declined since the removal of lead from gasoline and paint, it continues to plague certain subgroups of the population (see the Cultural Considerations box, "The Continued Burden of Lead Poisoning"). Eliminating high blood lead levels in children remains one of the *Healthy People* initiative goals.[26]

Of all sources of lead, lead paint (banned in the United States in 1978) is the most problematic source of contamination for children. Lead-based paints are still in production in many countries in the world (China, India, several other Asian and African

Table 13.4 Examples of Food-Borne Disease

ORGANISM	COMMON NAME OF ILLNESS	ONSET TIME AFTER INGESTING	SIGNS AND SYMPTOMS	DURATION	FOOD SOURCES
Bacillus cereus	*B. cereus* food poisoning	10 to 16 hours	Abdominal cramps, watery diarrhea, nausea	24 to 48 hours	Meats, stews, gravies, vanilla sauce
Campylobacter jejuni	Campylobacteriosis	2 to 5 days	Diarrhea, cramps, fever, and vomiting; diarrhea may be bloody	2 to 10 days	Raw and undercooked poultry, unpasteurized milk, contaminated water
Clostridium botulinum	Botulism	12 to 72 hours	Vomiting, diarrhea, blurred vision, double vision, difficulty swallowing, muscle weakness; can result in respiratory failure and death	Variable	Improperly canned foods, especially home-canned vegetables; fermented fish, baked potatoes in aluminum foil
Clostridium perfringens	Perfringens food poisoning	8 to 16 hours	Intense abdominal cramps, watery diarrhea	Usually 24 hours	Meats, poultry, gravy, dried or precooked foods, time- and/or temperature-abused foods
Cryptosporidium	Intestinal cryptosporidiosis	2 to 10 days	Diarrhea (usually watery), stomach cramps, upset stomach, slight fever	May be remitting and relapsing over weeks to months	Uncooked food or food contaminated by an ill food handler after cooking, contaminated drinking water
Cyclospora cayetanensis	Cyclosporiasis	1 to 14 days, usually at least 1 week	Diarrhea (usually watery), loss of appetite, substantial loss of weight, stomach cramps, nausea, vomiting, fatigue	May be remitting and relapsing over weeks to months	Various types of fresh produce (imported berries, lettuce, basil)
Escherichia coli producing toxin	*E. coli* infection (common cause of "travelers' diarrhea")	1 to 3 days	Watery diarrhea, abdominal cramps, some vomiting	3 to 7 or more days	Water or food contaminated with human feces
Escherichia coli O157:H7	Hemorrhagic colitis or *E. coli* O157:H7 infection	1 to 8 days	Severe (often bloody) diarrhea, abdominal pain and vomiting; usually little or no fever is present; more common among children 4 years old or younger; can lead to kidney failure	5 to 10 days	Undercooked beef (especially hamburger), unpasteurized milk and juice, raw fruits and vegetables (e.g., sprouts), contaminated water
Hepatitis A	Hepatitis	28 days average (15 to 50 days)	Diarrhea, dark urine, jaundice, flu-like symptoms (i.e., fever, headache, nausea, abdominal pain)	Variable, usually 2 weeks to 3 months	Raw produce, contaminated drinking water, uncooked foods and cooked foods that are not reheated after contact with an infected food handler, shellfish from contaminated waters

Table 13.4   Examples of Food-Borne Disease—cont'd

Organism	Disease	Onset/Incubation	Symptoms/Signs	Duration	Food Sources
Listeria monocytogenes	Listeriosis	9 to 48 hours for gastrointestinal symptoms, 2 to 6 weeks for invasive disease	Fever, muscle aches, and nausea or diarrhea; pregnant women may have a mild flu-like illness, and infection can lead to premature delivery or stillbirth; elderly or immunocompromised patients may develop bacteremia or meningitis	Variable	Unpasteurized milk, soft cheeses made with unpasteurized milk, ready-to-eat deli meats
Noroviruses	Variously called viral gastroenteritis, winter diarrhea, acute non-bacterial gastroenteritis, food poisoning, and food infection	12 to 48 hours	Nausea, vomiting, abdominal cramping, diarrhea, fever, headache; diarrhea is more prevalent among adults, vomiting is more common among children	12 to 60 hours	Raw produce, contaminated drinking water, uncooked foods and cooked foods that are not reheated after contact with an infected food handler; shellfish from contaminated waters
Salmonella	Salmonellosis	6 to 48 hours	Diarrhea, fever, abdominal cramps, vomiting	4 to 7 days	Eggs, poultry, meat, unpasteurized milk or juice, cheese, contaminated raw fruits and vegetables
Shigella	Shigellosis or bacillary dysentery	4 to 7 days	Abdominal cramps, fever, diarrhea; stools may contain blood and mucus	24 to 48 hours	Raw produce, contaminated drinking water, uncooked foods and cooked foods that are not reheated after contact with an infected food handler
Staphylococcus aureus	Staphylococcal food poisoning	1 to 6 hours	Sudden onset of severe nausea and vomiting, abdominal cramps; diarrhea and fever may be present	24 to 48 hours	Unrefrigerated or improperly refrigerated meats, potato, and egg salads; cream pastries
Vibrio parahaemolyticus	*V. parahaemolyticus* infection	4 to 96 hours	Watery (occasionally bloody) diarrhea, abdominal cramps, nausea, vomiting, fever	2 to 5 days	Undercooked or raw seafood, such as shellfish
Vibrio vulnificus	*V. vulnificus* infection	1 to 7 days	Vomiting, diarrhea, abdominal pain, blood-borne infection, fever, bleeding within skin, ulcers that require surgical removal; can be fatal to persons with liver disease or weakened immune systems	2 to 8 days	Undercooked or raw seafood, such as shellfish (especially oysters)

Reprinted from U.S. Food and Drug Administration. (2018). *What you need to know about foodborne illness*. U.S. Department of Health and Human Services. Retrieved May 2019 from www.fda.gov/food/consumers/what-you-need-know-about-foodborne-illnesses.

The Continued Burden of Lead Poisoning

Lead toxicity continues to burden populations all around the world, including populations within the United States. Among all age groups, children between the ages of 1 and 5 years have the highest risk, and subsequent long-term consequences, of elevated blood lead levels (BLLs). Among racial groups, non-Hispanic black children have the highest incidence of lead toxicity in the United States. Additionally, the burden among children living in households with low socioeconomic status is significantly higher than children living in households without such financial constraints.[1]

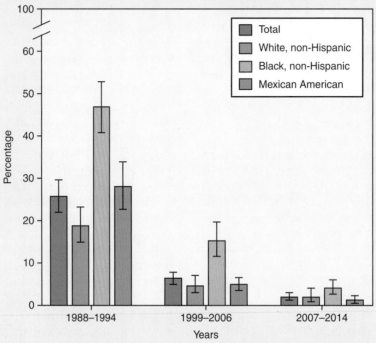

Percentage of children aged 1 to 5 years with elevated blood lead levels, by race/ethnicity. (Source: Centers for Disease Control and Prevention. [2016]. Percentage of children aged 1–5 years with elevated blood lead levels, by race/ethnicity—National Health and Nutrition Examination Survey, United States, 1988–1994, 1999–2006, and 2007–2014. *MMWR Morb Mortal Wkly Rep, 65,* 1089.)

The accumulation of lead in the blood results in oxidative stress and interferes with the normal physiologic functions of calcium, zinc, and iron. In addition to neurologic damage, prolonged elevated lead in the body can cause anemia, kidney damage, seizures, encephalopathy, and eventually paralysis. In January 2012 the CDC's Advisory Committee on Childhood Lead Poisoning recommended that an elevated BLL in children be defined as ≥5 mcg/dL (down from the previously defined level of ≥10 mcg/dL). However, a Canadian study found that boys with very low prenatal lead exposure (as little as 0.6 mcg/dL cord blood) still suffer compromised cognitive function.[2] Thus, many researchers believe that no levels of lead in the blood are safe. However, there are still more than 75,000 children under 5 years of age in the United States with elevated blood lead levels.[3]

The figure depicted above illustrates the BLLs of children by race beginning in 1988. Note the successful decrease in severely affected children over time. The disparity in elevated blood lead levels among black/non-Hispanic children and children residing in low-income households remains a public health concern in the United States.

REFERENCES
1. Tsoi, M. F., et al. (2016). Continual decrease in blood lead level in Americans: United States national health nutrition and examination survey 1999-2014. *The American Journal of Medicine, 129*(11), 1213–1218.
2. Desrochers-Couture, M., et al. (2018). Prenatal, concurrent, and sex-specific associations between blood lead concentrations and IQ in preschool Canadian children. *Environment International, 121*(Pt 2), 1235–1242.
3. Raymond, J., & Brown, M. J. (2017). Childhood blood lead levels in children aged <5 years—United States, 2009-2014. *MMWR Surveill Summ, 66*(3), 1–10.

countries) and are available for international trade.[40] Additionally, toys for children produced in these same countries still contain excessive levels of lead-based paint.[41] Millions of homes in the United States have lead in their paint surfaces. Children living in these homes face lead exposure because of breathing airborne particles of paint dust created by disturbed or deteriorating walls or by abrasive paint removal before remodeling. Drinking water may be another important source of lead in high-risk households with water that comes through lead pipes or passes through lead-soldered plumbing joints. Current Environmental Protection Agency rules for public drinking water have helped lower this source of lead exposure.

The costs of lead toxicity during childhood last a lifetime. Long-term consequences include poorer intellectual performance, hand-eye coordination, short-term memory, attention span, and socioeconomic attainment as adults.[36,42,43] This same high-risk population group is also at risk for iron deficiency. Iron-deficiency anemia has a similar deleterious effect on neurology, and it can further complicate lead toxicity and long-term neurologic damage.[44]

Natural toxins. Plants and microorganisms that produce toxins also contaminate the food and water supply. Bacteria convert mercury, which is a by-product of human production and a natural element in the environment, to methyl mercury. Methyl mercury is a toxin that contaminates large bodies of water and the fish living within that water. This contamination can pass through the food chain to people who regularly consume large fatty fish (e.g., tilefish, swordfish, shark, mackerel, tuna, orange roughy, marlin, grouper, bluefish). Fungi produce aflatoxin, which is another natural toxin. It may contaminate foods such as peanuts, tree nuts, corn, and animal feed.

Other food contaminants and pollutants that may pose a risk to human health come from a variety of sources (e.g., factories, sewage, pesticides, fertilizers) but end up leaching into the ground, thereby contaminating food production areas and the water supply.

FOOD NEEDS AND COSTS

HUNGER AND MALNUTRITION

Worldwide Malnutrition

Hunger, famine, and death exist in many countries of the world today. Lack of sanitation, cultural inequality, overpopulation, and economic and political structures that do not appropriately use resources are all factors that may contribute to malnutrition. Figure 13.9 demonstrates the complicated interaction of the many factors leading to malnutrition.

Chronic food or nutrient shortages within a population perpetuate the cycle of malnutrition, in which undernourished pregnant women give birth to low birth weight infants. These infants are then more susceptible to infant death or growth retardation during childhood. Unmet nutrient needs throughout childhood and adolescence exacerbate the incidence of malnourished or growth-stunted adults with shorter life expectancies and reduced work capacities. Figure 13.10 illustrates the two drastically different outcomes that occur depending on whether a child has access to education, financial needs, and health care. Malnutrition may result from total kilocalorie deficiency or single-nutrient deficiencies. The most common deficiencies in the world today are iron-deficiency anemia, protein-energy malnutrition, vitamin A deficiency, and iodine deficiency.

The United Nations Committee on World Food Security attempts to address the issue of 821 million people worldwide who do not have enough food to meet their basic nutrition requirements. The long-term goals of this committee are to eliminate world hunger by raising the level of overall nutrition, improving agricultural productivity, and enhancing the lives of the rural populations.[45,46] The plan is composed of several commitments to stabilize the social, economic, and environmental production and distribution of

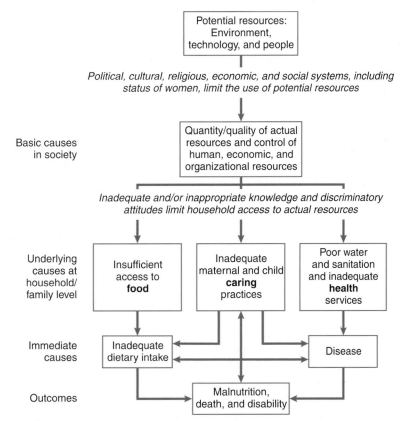

Figure 13.9 Multiple causes of malnutrition. (Adapted from United Nations Children's Fund. [1998]. *The state of the world's children*. New York: UNICEF/Oxford University Press.)

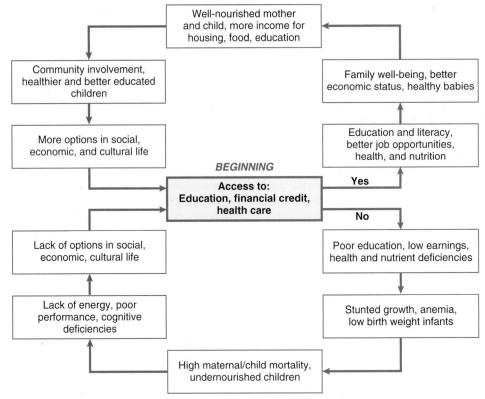

Figure 13.10 Differences in life outcomes when education, financial credit, and health care are accessible. (Modified from Cohen, M. J., et al. [1994]. *Hunger 1995: Causes of hunger: The state of world hunger*. Silver Spring, MD: Bread for the World Institute.)

nutritionally adequate food. The following website provides information and updates about the progress of this committee: www.fao.org/publications/sofi/en/.

Malnutrition in America

In the United States, which is one of the wealthiest countries on earth, hunger and malnutrition among the poor persist. More than 37 million individuals (11.5% of the U.S. noninstitutionalized population) experience **food insecurity** regularly.[47] Households with the highest risk for food insecurity are those with young children (particularly those headed by a single adult), those with incomes below 185% of the poverty threshold, those headed by a black non-Hispanic or Hispanic adult, and households in central city areas.[47] At both the government and the personal levels of any society, food availability and use involve money and politics. There are many contributing factors, such as land management practices, water distribution, and food production and distribution policies.

FOOD ASSISTANCE PROGRAMS

In situations of economic stress and natural disasters, individuals and families may need help with acquiring resources, including food. Many people experience hunger every day. Dietitians, nurses, social workers, and other health care providers must be aware of the available food assistance programs to make appropriate and timely referrals. Box 13.1

provides the websites for each food assistance program covered next in this chapter.

Commodity Supplemental Food Program

Under the Commodity Supplemental Food Program (CSFP), the USDA purchases food items that are good sources of nutrients but that are often lacking in the diets of the target population (i.e., low-income elderly ≥60 years old). The USDA then distributes the food to state agencies and tribal organizations. Local agencies (e.g., departments of health, social services, education, or agriculture) then evaluate eligibility, provide nutrition education, and disperse food to designated individual recipients. This program is not currently available in every state. The most recent report noted that an average of 630,000 people participate in the CSFP services each month.[48]

Box 13.1	Food Assistance Programs

Commodity Supplemental Food Program (CSFP): www.fns.usda.gov/csfp

Supplemental Nutrition Assistance Program (SNAP): www.fns.usda.gov/snap

Special Supplemental Food Program for Women, Infants, and Children (WIC): www.fns.usda.gov/wic

School Meals Program: www.fns.usda.gov/nslp/national-school-lunch-program

Nutrition Services Incentive Program: acl.gov/programs/health-wellness/nutrition-services

Supplemental Nutrition Assistance Program

Supplemental Nutrition Assistance Program (SNAP) began during the late depression years of the 1930s and expanded during the 1960s and 1970s. This program has helped many people to purchase food, the majority of whom are children and elderly adults. The USDA estimates that 40.3 million people participated in SNAP services in the United States monthly at an annual cost of $65.3 billion.[49] With this program, the primary care provider of the household receives electronic benefits transfer cards. These cards work in a way that is similar to a debit card in approved retail stores to supplement the household's food needs for 1 month. Households must have a monthly income that is below the program's eligible poverty limit to qualify. SNAP is a federal program and operates in all states and U.S. territories. Administration is at the local level.

Special Supplemental Food Program for Women, Infants, and Children

The Special Supplemental Food Program for Women, Infants, and Children (WIC) provides nutrition supplementation, education, and counseling in addition to referrals for health care and social services to women who are pregnant, postpartum, or breastfeeding and to their infants and children who are younger than 5 years old. WIC has established criteria for participation, and each applicant must be income-eligible and determined to be at nutrition risk. The food packages provided through WIC meet the *Dietary Guidelines for Americans* and promote the consumption of fruits, vegetables, and whole grains. The average monthly food cost is currently about $41 per participant.[50] Participants receive vouchers that increase the purchasing power for foods such as milk, eggs, cheese, juice, fortified cereals, fruits, and vegetables at participating retailers. These foods supplement the diet with rich sources of protein, iron, and certain vitamins to help reduce risk factors such as poor growth patterns, low birth weight, prematurity, preeclampsia, miscarriage, and anemia.

Established in 1972, WIC currently has almost 7 million participants. WIC offices are in every state and U.S. territory. Approximately half of all participants are children between the ages of 1 and 5 years.[51]

School Meals Program

The school breakfast and lunch programs provide meals that meet the *Dietary Guidelines for Americans* recommendations for many children who otherwise would lack balanced meals. There are several programs available to assist low-income children with receiving healthy food while at school. Current programs in the United States include the National School Lunch, Fresh Fruit and Vegetable, School Breakfast, Special Milk, and Summer Food Service programs. The National School Lunch program includes subprograms for children from low-income families that provide nutritionally balanced meals and snacks after school and during the summer months, when school is not in session. The USDA supports the program by reimbursing schools for each meal served and by donating food from surplus agricultural stocks.

> **food insecurity** limited or uncertain availability of nutritionally adequate and safe foods or limited or uncertain ability to acquire acceptable foods in socially acceptable ways.
>
> **school breakfast and lunch programs** federally assisted meal programs that operate in public and nonprofit private schools and residential child-care institutions; these programs provide nutritionally balanced, low-cost, or free meals to children each school day.

Children eat free or at reduced rates, and these meals often make up their main food intake for the day. The meals provided must fulfill approximately one-third of a child's Recommended Dietary Allowance for protein, vitamin A, vitamin C, iron, calcium, and calories, and it must meet the *Dietary Guidelines for Americans*, which call for diets that are lower in total fat and that contain more fruits, vegetables, and whole grains.[52] The Special Milk Program provides milk to children who do not have access to the other meal programs.

Nutrition Services Incentive Program

The U.S. Department of Health and Human Services Administration for Community Living administers the Nutrition Services Incentive Program. The purpose of the program is to promote socialization, health, and well-being for older individuals by reducing hunger and food insecurity.

This program provides cash or commodities from the USDA for the delivery of nutritious meals to the elderly. Regardless of income, all people who are older than 60 years of age can eat hot lunches at a community center under the Congregate Meals Program. If they are ill or disabled, they can receive meals at home by using the services of the Home-Delivered Meals Program. The act specifies that economically and socially needy people be given priority. Both programs accept voluntary contributions for meals.

FOOD BUYING AND HANDLING PRACTICES

Many American families struggle to cover food costs with limited available funds. Even on a low-cost plan for food purchasing, an average family of four can expect to spend $724 to $852 per month on food alone.[53] Shopping for food can be complicated, especially when each item in a supermarket's overabundant supply shouts, "Buy me!" Food marketing is big business, and producers compete for prize placement and shelf space. A large supermarket stocks many thousands of different food items. A single food item may be marketed a dozen different ways at as many different prices. The following wise shopping and handling practices help with the provision of healthy foods as well as with controlling food costs.

Plan Ahead

Use sales circulars in newspapers, plan general menus, and keep a checklist of basic pantry supplies. Make a list ahead of time according to the location of items in a regularly used grocery store. Such planning controls impulse buying and reduces extra trips. Plan a time to food shop without children in tow.

Buy Wisely

Understanding packaging, carefully reading labels, and watching for sale items help to improve purchasing power. Only buy in quantity if it results in real savings and if the food can be adequately stored or used. Be cautious when selecting "convenience foods"; the time saved may not be worth the added cost. For fresh foods, try alternative food sources such as farmers' markets, community-supported agriculture (CSAs), and local gardens.

Store Food Safely

Control food waste and prevent illness caused by food spoilage or contamination. Conserve food by storing items in accordance with their nature and use. Use dry storage, covered containers, and correct-temperature refrigeration as indicated. Keep opened and partly used food items at the front of the shelf for timely use. Avoid waste by preparing only the amount needed. Use leftovers in creative ways or freeze for quick meals later.

Cook Food Well

Use cooking processes that retain maximal food value and that maintain food safety. Cooking vegetables for shorter periods (e.g., stir-frying, steaming, microwaving) and with as little water as possible helps to retain their vitamin and mineral nutritive quality. Prepare food with imagination and good sense. Give zest and appeal to dishes with a variety of seasonings, combinations, and serving arrangements. No matter how much they know about nutrition and health, people usually eat because they are hungry and because the food looks and tastes good, not necessarily because it is healthy.

Putting It All Together

Summary

- Common public concerns about the safety of the community food supply focus on the use of chemicals such as pesticides and food additives. These substances have produced an abundant food supply, but they have also raised public concerns.
- The FDA is the main government agency responsible for maintaining safety in the food supply. It conducts activities related to areas such as food safety, food labeling, food standards, consumer education, and research.
- Numerous organisms such as bacteria, viruses, and parasites that can contaminate food may cause food-borne disease. Rigorous public health measures control the sanitation of food handling areas and the personal hygiene of food handlers. The same standards should apply to food prepared and stored at home.
- Individuals and families under economic stress may benefit from food resource and financial assistance programs. There are many programs available in the United States.
- Cost-saving and competent food storing practices are important aspects of safe and efficient food use.

Chapter Review Questions

See answers in Appendix A.

1. When purchasing packaged foods, consumers with food allergies should pay particular attention to _____.

   a. the Nutrition Facts Label
   b. any health claims
   c. symbols on the package
   d. the list of ingredients

2. The most common form of food-borne illness in the U.S. is from _____.

   a. norovirus
   b. shigellosis
   c. listeriosis
   d. giardiasis

3. One of the most important ways to prevent contamination while handling food is to _____.

   a. wash hands and wear disposable gloves
   b. let leftovers cool to room temperature before storing in the refrigerator
   c. cook all meat and egg dishes to 120° F
   d. always remove peelings from fruit

4. Jenny finds some leftover pizza that has been in the refrigerator for 7 days. She is wondering if it is still safe to eat. Your response should be _____.

   a. yes, as long as she reheats it thoroughly
   b. yes, as long as it does not have an odor or mold
   c. no, discard it after 3 to 4 days
   d. no, discard it after 24 hours

5. Improperly home-canned green beans can result in _____.

   a. tapeworms
   b. botulism
   c. listeriosis
   d. rotavirus

Next-Generation NCLEX® Examination-style Case Study

See answers in Appendix A.

A mother with a 1-year-old baby girl recently lost her job, making it financially difficult to purchase food. Her husband's income covers utilities and rent, but there is not enough funds left over to support the household's need for food. At her baby's last well-baby check-up, the nurse plotted the infant's height and weight on the growth charts and recorded her at the 8th percentile. The mother reports that her daughter feeds appropriately and is starting to eat solid foods, but they only have enough breast milk substitute to feed her 4 oz. twice per day. A 1-year-old should be drinking 8 oz. two to three times per day. She noticed that the baby only has one bowel movement about every other day.

1. From the list below, select all of the items from the client's history that put her at nutrition risk.

   a. Height and weight at 8th percentile
   b. Food insecurity
   c. Housing
   d. Nutrient intake
   e. Feeding skills
   f. Constipation

2. Choose the *most likely* options for the information missing from the statement below by selecting from the list of options provided.

   The infant's _____ and _____ suggests that she is not getting enough nutrients through her feedings.

OPTIONS	
poor growth	feeding skills
diarrhea	breast milk substitute
constipation	anorexia

3. From the list below, select all of the appropriate nutrition programs that the health care team should recommend to the client.

   a. WIC
   b. SNAP
   c. National School Lunch Program
   d. Meals on Wheels
   e. National School Breakfast Program

4. Use an X for the health teachings below that are <u>indicated</u> (appropriate or necessary) or <u>contraindicated</u> (could be harmful) regarding food buying and handling practices.

HEALTH TEACHING	INDICATED	CONTRAINDICATED
Look for sales in newspapers and online.		
Make a list of food and supplies before going to the grocery store.		
Read food labels.		
Store dry food in closed containers in a dry place and cool food to appropriate temperatures.		
Cook food to appropriate temperatures and use separate cutting boards for ready-to-eat foods.		
Go down every aisle of the grocery store when shopping.		
Thaw raw chicken on the counter before cooking.		

5. For each assessment finding, use an X to indicate whether nursing and collaborative interventions were <u>effective</u> (helped to meet expected outcomes), <u>ineffective</u> (did not help to meet expected outcomes), or <u>unrelated</u> (not related to the expected outcomes).

ASSESSMENT FINDING	EFFECTIVE	INEFFECTIVE	UNRELATED
Parents use WIC vouchers to buy fruits, vegetables, and whole grains.			
Infant's height and weight are at the 15th percentile and continue to increase.			
Infant continues to have bowel movements every other day.			
Parents are able to purchase enough food to meet their needs.			
Infant is a picky eater when it comes to solid foods.			

Additional Learning Resources

Please refer to this text's Evolve website for answers to the Case Study questions:
http://evolve.elsevier.com/Williams/basic/.
References and **Further Reading and Resources** in the back of the book provide additional resources for enhancing knowledge.

Food Habits and Cultural Patterns

Kary Woodruff PhD, RDN, CSSD

Key Concepts

- Personal food habits develop as part of a person's social and cultural heritage as well as his or her lifestyle and environment.

- Social and economic changes may alter food practices.
- Many different cultures influence American eating patterns.

Why do people eat what they eat? Food is necessary to sustain life and health, and although good health and nutrition are important considerations, there is a multitude of influences on individual food selection. There are physiologic, emotional, social, economic, and cultural influences on individual food selection.[1]

Our values, beliefs, and individual ways of life all relate intimately to our food habits. Sometimes these food patterns change over time along with exposure to other cultural patterns.

SOCIAL, PSYCHOLOGIC, AND ECONOMIC INFLUENCES ON FOOD HABITS

SOCIAL IMPACT

Human behavior reflects activities, processes, and structures that make up social life. Economic status, education, residence, occupation, and family structure are examples of factors that may influence social group formation in any society. Thus, values and practices differ among groups. Subgroups also develop based on region, religion, age, sex, social class, health issues, special interests, ethnic backgrounds, politics, and other common traits such as group affiliations. Like any other form of human behavior, influences from every direction gradually form our food habits.

Food is a symbol of acceptance, warmth, and friendliness in social relationships. People tend to accept food or food advice from friends, acquaintances, and people whom they view as trusted authorities readily. This guidance is especially prominent in family relationships. Food habits that are closely associated with family sentiments often stay with people throughout their lives. During adulthood, certain foods may even trigger a flood of childhood memories and are valued for reasons apart from any nutrition-related importance.

FACTORS THAT INFLUENCE PERSONAL FOOD CHOICES

A biopsychosocial model proposes three main influences on individual food choices. There are (1) biologic or genetically based factors; (2) the impact of the social/psychologic and behavioral environment that includes the family relationships; and (3) the wider environmental, societal, and cultural influences.[2] Included in the latter category are ethnic and regional cultural practices influencing the establishment of food traditions early in life, which may positively or adversely affect food consumption patterns (e.g., globalization of the food supply). Box 14.1 provides a summary of factors that are frequently involved in personal food choices. Review the list and consider what other factors influenced what you ate today. How might those factors differ from what influenced your classmates' food choices?

Biologic and Genetic influences

Biologic and genetic factors greatly influence food selection. Hunger and satiety are important drivers of what and how much individuals eat and have a strong biologic basis. Even the sensory experiences of eating, including the concept of taste, are innate traits. Humans have an inherent preference for sweet and salty foods and a natural avoidance of bitter and sour tastes. Differences between individuals' taste preferences have a genetic origin and may ultimately influence the development of diet-related diseases.[3]

Food and Psychosocial Development

Emotional maturity grows along with physical development throughout the life span. Food habits are part of both physical and psychosocial growth at each stage of human development. For example, a 2-year-old toddler who is taking his first steps toward independence may learn to manipulate his parents or caretakers through food by refusing to eat at meal times

Box **14.1**	Factors Influencing Personal Food Choices

PHYSICAL FACTORS	PHYSIOLOGIC FACTORS
Available food supply	Allergies
Food technology	Disability
Geography, agriculture, and distribution	Health and disease status
Sanitation and housing	Heredity
Season and climate	Nutrient and energy needs
Storage and cooking facilities	Therapeutic diets
SOCIAL AND ECONOMIC FACTORS	**PSYCHOLOGIC FACTORS**
Advertising and marketing	Habits
Culture	Preferences
Education	Emotions
Nutrition literacy	Mood
Income	Cravings
Food cost	Attitudes about food
Political and economic policies	Personal food acceptance
Religion and social class	Positive or negative experiences and associations
Social problems, poverty, alcoholism, and drug abuse	

or otherwise being a picky eater. Alternatively, **food neophobia** may be the trigger for such behaviors. This normal developmental trait may be an instinct from the evolutionary past that protected children from eating harmful foods when they were starting to become independent from their mothers. Other psychologic factors are also rooted in childhood experiences. For example, when a child is hurt or disappointed, parents may offer a cookie or a piece of candy to distract the child. As an adult, this individual may turn to similar comfort foods to help him or her cope. Certain foods, particularly sweets and other pleasurable flavors, stimulate "feel good" body chemicals in the brain called *endorphins* that give a mild "high" that may help ease the sensation of pain.[4]

Environmental and Marketing Influences

Television, radio, magazines, and other social media messages also manipulate personal food habits. Influences from peers, availability of convenience items, marketing at the local grocery store, and many other factors sway the decision-making process for food choices throughout life. Advertising strategies that use brand mascots and cartoon media characters on food packages greatly affect children's eating patterns by increasing the preference for products bearing the familiar character logo.[5] Because fresh fruits and vegetables are not processed or packaged, healthier snack items rarely include such logos. Foods commonly advertised on American television are generally energy dense and nutrient poor. These products contain food components discouraged by the dietary guidelines (i.e., saturated fat, added sugar, and sodium).[5,6]

Marketing trends and media also influence what a culture views as beautiful. The American culture values a thin female figure. Such provocations may adversely influence food choices, lifestyle behaviors, and body-image expectations. See Chapter 15 for more information on body image, disordered eating behaviors, and clinical eating disorders.

Economic Influences

Many American families live under socioeconomic pressures, especially during periods of recession and inflation. As discussed in Chapter 13, over 37 million Americans face food insecurity, of which poverty is a leading cause.[7] (See the section headed "Malnutrition in America" in Chapter 13 for additional information.)

The cost of a healthy diet composed of whole grains, lean meats, fruits, vegetables, and low-fat dairy is difficult to achieve for some families who are living at or below the federal poverty line. The dietary patterns that are recommended by the U.S. Department of Agriculture are nutrient dense but more costly than the typical American diet.[8] Thus, it is not surprising that there is a disparity in the burden of unnecessary illness and malnutrition for people with a lower socioeconomic status. Individuals struggling with food insecurity have poorer physical and mental health outcomes and experience higher rates of chronic diseases; consequently, these individuals also face greater health care costs.[9,10]

To make healthy food more affordable, some organizations have suggested additional taxation on selected foods with little or no nutrient quality as a means of subsidizing the cost of healthy choices, such as fruits and vegetables. Such taxation would thereby make "junk food" a more expensive option than buying fruits and vegetables. Initial studies looking at taxation on sugar-sweetened beverages (i.e., soda) indicates that if the tax is substantial enough, then consumption of these drinks does decrease.[11]

CULTURAL DEVELOPMENT OF FOOD HABITS

Each society that identifies itself with a common denominator (e.g., ethnicity, religion, geographic location, lifestyle) has unique cultural and culinary patterns. Historically, geographic and ethnic boundaries preserved these food cultures. Globalization and the increased flow of technology, information, goods, and people across borders have resulted in the spread of various culture-specific elements. The increased availability of various ethnic food markets and restaurants exemplify this cultural expansion. However, globalization has also caused a dilution of traditional food patterns as younger generations may opt for more diverse cuisines. Lifestyles have also changed globally such that individuals have less time for traditional food preparation practices and thus must rely on more convenient and quick preparation methods. Although long-established food cultures persist, modernization and globalization continue to shift daily food patterns around the world.

STRENGTH OF PERSONAL CULTURE

Culture involves much more than the major and historical aspects of a person's communal life (e.g., language, religion, politics, location). It also develops from the habits of everyday living and family relationships, including preparing and serving food. In a gradual process of conscious and unconscious learning, cultural values, attitudes, customs, and practices become a deep part of individual lives. Although elements of this heritage may be revised or rejected as adults, people are ultimately responsible for shaping their own lives and passing traditions on to the subsequent generations as they see fit. A world of cultural diversity has shaped Americans' broad range of food habits.

Food habits are among the oldest and most deeply rooted aspects of a culture. An individual's cultural background largely determines what, how, and even why an individual eats. Countless customs, whether rational, irrational, beneficial, or injurious, exist throughout the world. Foods take on symbolic meanings related to major life events such as birth, death, and weddings. From ancient times, food has played an essential role in sacred ceremonies and religious rites. Food gathering, preparing, and serving have followed specific customs, many of which remain intact today.

TRADITIONAL CULTURE-SPECIFIC FOOD PATTERNS

America's diversity can be recognized and even celebrated as a foundation for its national strength. America's broad cultural food availability highlights this diversity. Although some individuals may refer to the United States as a "melting pot" of ethnic and racial groups, this image is an inaccurate reflection of this cultural phenomenon. The "melting pot" assumes the belief of cultural assimilation, whereby society expects minority cultural groups to give up their values and norms and adopt those of the dominant white culture. Instead, individuals should recognize their own cultural heritage that they bring with them. This self-awareness allows individuals to connect more deeply with others and to understand different cultural values.[12] Cultural awareness extends beyond just learning a list of a group's traditional patterns and customs; rather, cultural literacy requires an understanding of the beliefs and values that underlie these behaviors.

American family and community life integrate diverse cultural food patterns. These patterns have contributed particular dishes or modes of cooking to American eating habits. These influences have resulted, in turn, in the Americanization of many of these cultural food habits. Older members of the family may rely on traditional foods more regularly, with younger members of the family adopting them on special occasions or holidays. Nevertheless, traditional foods carry deep meaning and bind families and cultural communities in close fellowship.

The following sections discuss some of the specific cultural food patterns that have shaped the American food supply. These descriptions are not intended to provide an overly simplistic stereotype of different cultural groups; we cannot lump any one person into one identity with others of an ethnic group.[12] Instead, we should appreciate the individuality and differences of each person. For example, a Mexican-American may engage in a variety of food practices and may or may not enjoy eating traditional Mexican food. Instead of making assumptions about individual dietary patterns, we can recognize that a variety of unique, traditional foods provides a rudimentary foundation of cultural food behaviors. Such an understanding of various cultural food patterns is valuable when providing dietary guidance as a health care professional.

Hispanic Influences

People often use the term Hispanic interchangeably with Mexican; this may be because 63% of the Hispanic population in the United States is of Mexican origin.[13] However, the Hispanic population also includes individuals of Cuban, Puerto Rican, and South and Central American descent. Together, this population represents the fastest growing population in the United States. Because this ethnic group includes individuals from more than 20 countries, the food patterns and practices are equally distinct and diverse. Each Latin American country has food traditions and cultural practices that represent unique customs and histories.

Mexican. Mexican and Central American dishes center on corn, tomatoes, squashes, chilies, avocados, rice, legumes/beans, and various fruits. The Spanish settlers also brought with them Asian, European, and African influences. Traditional meal patterns focus on lunch as the largest meal of the day, with a lighter breakfast and dinner. The Mexican diet is generally high in complex carbohydrates, including tortillas, rice, beans, and bread, and is sufficient in protein foods, which include eggs, beans, fish, and meat. Lard is the fat used most commonly in meal preparation. See Table 14.1 for representative foods from each food group within a traditional Mexican cuisine.

Although Mexican food is popular in the United States, these dishes do not necessarily reflect the traditional foods habitually consumed in Mexico. Mexican Americans, in general, consume more dairy products and use less lard than in traditional Mexican diets and tend to follow American eating patterns, which include

food neophobia the fear of new food.
assimilation the process in which a minority ethnic group or culture acquires the values, beliefs, and behaviors of a dominant ethnic or cultural group.

Table 14.1	Historical Dietary Patterns of Hispanic and Native American Cultures

ETHNIC GROUP	BREAD, CEREAL, AND RICE GROUP	VEGETABLE GROUP	FRUIT GROUP	MILK, YOGURT, AND CHEESE GROUP	MEAT, POULTRY, FISH, DRY BEANS, EGGS, AND NUTS GROUP	FATS, OILS, AND SWEETS GROUP
Mexican	Corn and related products, taco shells, corn or flour tortillas, rice, white bread	Chili peppers, tomatoes and salsa, squash, jicama, onions, garlic, prickly pear cactus, yuca root (cassava or manioc)	Avocado, guacamole, citrus fruits, bananas	Cheese, flan, sour cream, and aged cheese	Black or pinto beans, refried beans, Mexican sausage (chorizo), beef, chicken, pork, goat, eggs	Lard
Caribbean persons (includes Puerto Rican and Cuban individuals)	Rice, sweet potatoes, chayote squash, plantains (usually fried)	Beets, eggplant, corn, tubers (yuca), white yams (boniato)	Tropical fruits, avocado, coconut, citrus, mango	Flan, hard cheese (queso de mano)	Chicken, fish, pork, legumes, sausage (chorizo)	Lard, olive and peanut oil
Native American (each tribe may have specific foods; commonly consumed foods are listed here)	Blue corn flour used to make cornbread, mush dumplings; fruit dumplings (walakshi); fry bread (biscuit dough deep fried); ground sweet acorns; tortillas; wheat or rye used to make cornmeal and flour	Cabbage, carrots, cassava, dandelion greens, eggplant, milkweed, onions, pumpkin, squash, sweet and white potatoes, turnips, wild tullies (a tuber), yellow corn	Dried wild cherries and grapes; wild bananas, berries, and yuca	Not heavily used in traditional dishes	Duck, eggs, fish eggs, geese, venison, beef, pork, chicken, turkey, elk, mutton, smoked or processed meat, wild rabbit, dried beans, lentils, nuts (all)	Lard and shortening

Modified from Grodner, M., Roth, S., & Walkingshaw, B. (2012). *Nutritional foundations and clinical applications: A nursing approach* (5th ed.). St. Louis: Mosby.

dinner as the largest meal of the day. **Acculturation** to the typical Western diet of Americans is a significant concern for Hispanic and Latino immigrants. Adopting such dietary habits is associated with reduced quality of life due to chronic disease (see the Cultural Considerations box: Acculturation to an American Diet).

Puerto Rican. The second largest Hispanic population in the United States comes from the Caribbean country of Puerto Rico. The Puerto Rican people share a common heritage with many Hispanic Caribbean countries, so many of their food patterns are similar (Figure 14.1). However, Puerto Ricans add more tropical fruits and vegetables, including starchy vegetables such as plantains and green bananas. As seen with Mexican-American diets, Puerto Rican Americans have adopted dinner as the largest meal of the day in contrast to the traditional meal pattern of lunch being most substantial (see Table 14.1).

Native American Influences

The Native American population of American Indians and Alaska Natives is composed of 573 federally recognized distinct tribal groups sometimes live in small rural communities, in metropolitan cities, and on reservations.[14] Despite the diversity of each tribe, these varied

acculturation the process of an individual or group of people adopting the behaviors and lifestyle habits of a new culture.

groups share a spiritual attachment to the land and a determination to retain their culture. Food has great religious and social significance in these groups. Serving food is an integral part of celebrations, ceremonies, and everyday hospitality. Foods may be prepared and used according to regional differences. The food that Native Americans grow locally, harvest, or hunt on the land or fish from its rivers determines the variation in cuisine and reflects what is available in food markets (see Table 14.1).

Among the American Indian groups of the Southwest United States, one example is the Navajo people, whose reservation extends over a 25,000–square mile area at the junction of New Mexico, Arizona, and Utah. The Navajos learned to farm and established corn and other crops as staples. They later learned to herd from the Spaniards, which made sheep and goats available for food and wool. Some families also raise chickens, pigs, and cattle. Other Native American tribes in the United States have their unique heritage and distinct dietary habits relative to customs and the regions in which they live.

🌐 Cultural Considerations

Acculturation to an American Diet

Acculturation occurs when immigration from one part of the world to another part of the world accompanies social, psychologic, and cultural changes while individuals adapt to the new culture. Several studies have evaluated the changes that occur over time, specifically with Hispanic or Latino immigrants, because this population represents the fastest-growing ethnic group in the United States. One such systematic review evaluated the relationship between ethnicity, acculturation, and overall diet quality among Latinos who were living in the United States. Researchers found that Latinos who exhibited more acculturation consistently scored worse in overall diet quality, fruit and vegetable intake, sodium intake, and intake of empty calories than their less acculturated counterparts (i.e., those Latinos who maintained their cultural diet rather than adopting poor dietary habits in America). Interestingly, those who were more acculturated scored better on whole and refined grains.[1]

Researchers have linked acculturation to an increased risk for chronic diseases such as diabetes, obesity, and cardiovascular disease in Hispanic/Latino populations.[2-4] The risk of diabetes in this population is increased, even when controlling for demographic factors, socioeconomic status, and BMI, although it appears that education status (i.e., obtaining higher levels of education) may play a protective role.[5] The management of diabetes and other cardiometabolic diseases also must include a focus on sociocultural factors. For example, researchers examining compliance with the American Diabetes Association's (ADA) dietary recommendations for diabetes management found that overall adherence was low. However, Hispanic individuals who were less acculturated tended to follow dietary patterns that were more compliant with the ADA's guidelines for saturated fat, sodium, fiber, and cholesterol intake levels.[1] Health care practitioners can help Hispanic populations identify healthy food options that are familiar with traditional food patterns and that are accessible in American society.

REFERENCES

1. Yoshida, Y., et al. (2017). Role of age and acculturation in diet quality among Mexican Americans—findings from the national health and nutrition examination survey, 1999-2012. *Preventing Chronic Disease, 14,* E59.
2. Anderson, C., et al. (2016). Acculturation and diabetes risk in the Mexican American mano a mano cohort. *American Journal of Public Health, 106*(3), 547–549.
3. Divney, A. A., et al. (2019). Hypertension prevalence jointly influenced by acculturation and gender in US immigrant groups. *American Journal of Hypertension, 32*(1), 104–111.
4. Florez, K. R., & Abraido-Lanza, A. (2017). Segmented assimilation: An approach to studying acculturation and obesity among Latino adults in the United States. *Family & Community Health, 40*(2), 132–138.
5. Van Hook, J., et al. (2016). It is hard to swim upstream: Dietary acculturation among Mexican-origin children. *Population Research and Policy Review, 35*(2), 177–196.

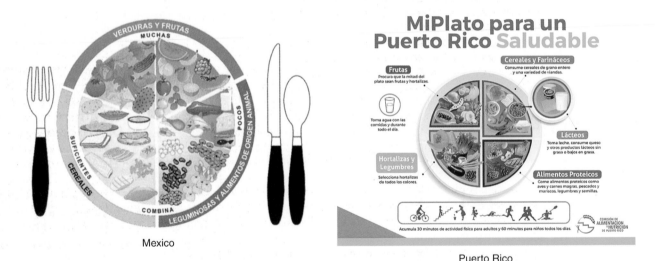

Figure 14.1 National food guides for Mexico and Puerto Rico. (Mexican national food guide: reprinted from Painter, J., Rah, J. H., & Lee, Y. K. [2002]. Comparison of international food guide pictorial representations. *J Am Diet Assoc, 102,* 483–489, with permission from the Academy of Nutrition and Dietetics; and Puerto Rico's national food guide: alimentacionynutricionpr. org/mi-plato-saludable/.)

Today, Native American food habits combine traditional dietary staples (e.g., corn/maize, beans, squash, and rice) with modern food products from available supermarkets and fast-food restaurants (Figure 14.2). However, health concerns are growing because of the increased reliance on modern convenience and snack foods that are high in fat, sugar, calories, and sodium. These dietary patterns, along with socioeconomic and genetic factors, have resulted in the highest rates of type 2 diabetes seen among the American Indian population and is a pressing public health issue.[15]

Influences of the Southern United States

Black or African American. Black or African-American individuals make up the second largest minority group in the United States. According to the U.S. Census, 12.6% of Americans are black or African American.[16] The majority of black people in the United States arrived from West Africa through enslavement during the 1600s and 1700s. Slave traders sold approximately 12.5 million Africans into slavery, with nearly 6% of those individuals ending up in the United States (the remaining individuals went to the Caribbean and South America).[17]

Dairy Group
1 cup low-fat, skim, or acidophilus milk
1 cup low- or non-fat yogurt
1 1/2 ounces natural cheese (or 2 ounces processed), low- or non-fat preferred

*Breast milk for babies, goat's milk, bone soup, fish head soup, or canned salmon with bones

Vegetable Group
1 cup raw leafy greens
1/2 cup other vegetables, cooked or raw
3/4 cup vegetable juice, green beans, squash, kale, broccoli, or zucchini

*Sprouts or new shoots, wild mushrooms, nopalitos, wild onion, amaranth leaves (wild spinach), fresh or dried squash, lambsquarter (kappa), wild mustard, peeled stems, purslane or jicama

Bread Group
1 6-inch corn tortilla
1 7 1/2-inch flour tortilla**
4-6 crackers**
1 slice bread**
1/2 hamburger bun**
1/2 cup cooked cereal**
1 ounce ready-to-eat cereal**
1/2 cup rice or pasta (cooked)**

*Indian biscuits (bannock bread), popcorn, Indian wheat or psyllium (plantago), barley, wild oats, wild rice, amaranth and mesquite flour, popped amaranth seeds, wild peas, or corn (fresh, frozen or cooked)

Fats & Sweets
Very small amounts, if any

Fats & Sweets
Butter or margarine, lard, gravy, fried foods, mayonnaise, ranch dressing, chips, sugar, candy, jelly, desserts, soda pop, sports drinks, or fruit flavored juice.

*Fry bread, animal fat, fish oil, honey, chucata (mesquite gum), atole (sweetened liquid corn or mesquite), or Mexican cheese

Meat Group
2-3 ounces cooked meat, poultry, or fish
Count as one ounce of meat:
   1 medium egg or 1 low-fat hotdog
   1/2 cup cooked dried beans, peas or tuna
   2 Tbsp peanut butter, nuts or seeds

*Deer, rabbit, squirrel, pigeon, lamb, mariscos, fish (fresh or frozen), fowl, quail, eggs of birds or salmon, chia seeds, garbanzo or tepary beans, wild acorns, hazelnuts, or pine nuts

Fruit Group
1/2 - 3/4 cup 100% fruit juice
1 small piece fresh fruit
1/2 cup canned or fresh chopped fruit or melon
1/4 cup dried fruit

*Blueberries, huckleberries, or blackberries, choke cherries, wild crabapples, wild black cherries, prickly pear or saguaro fruit, strawberries, plums, melons

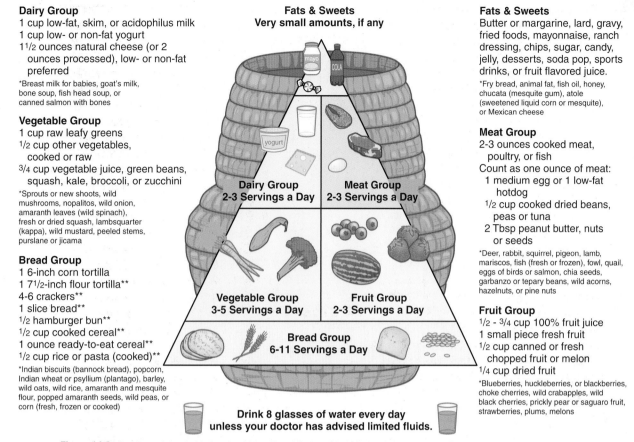

Dairy Group
2-3 Servings a Day

Meat Group
2-3 Servings a Day

Vegetable Group
3-5 Servings a Day

Fruit Group
2-3 Servings a Day

Bread Group
6-11 Servings a Day

Drink 8 glasses of water every day
unless your doctor has advised limited fluids.

Figure 14.2 Southern Arizona Native American Food Guide: Choices for a Healthy Life. *Traditional foods. **Whole-grain products recommended. (Osterkamp, L. K., & Longstaff, L. [2004]. Development of a dietary teaching tool for American Indians and Alaskan Natives in Southern Arizona. *Nutr Educ Behav, 36,* 272–274.)

Although the majority of black people in the United States have African heritage, some individuals came later from the Caribbean and Central America. Thus, not all Americans with black or brown skin are African Americans.

African-American cultures, especially in the Southern states, have contributed a rich heritage to American food patterns, particularly to Southern cooking as a whole. The food patterns of Southern African Americans developed through a creative ability to turn staples at hand into memorable food. The term "soul food," in fact, introduced during the Civil Rights movement in the 1960s, describes wholesome food that uses everything available. Although regional differences exist within the basic food patterns, Table 14.2 outlines the representative uses of foods from the basic food groups. Unique foods such as spoonbread (a soufflé-like dish of cornmeal with beaten eggs) and "Hoppin John" (black-eyed peas served over rice, traditionally served on New Year's Day to bring good luck for the new year) are two examples of foods specific to this region. African Americans have a high prevalence of lactose intolerance. Consequently, meals may include some cheese but not much milk. Pork, corn, green leafy vegetables, and fried foods are common staples in traditional meals. Sunday dinner feasts provide time for social and family gathering, where traditional comfort foods are in high demand (particularly in the southern states).

French American. The **Cajun** people living in the southwestern coastal waterways of Louisiana have contributed a unique cuisine to America's rich and varied fare. This culinary pattern continues to provide a distinct paradigm for the rapidly expanding forms of American ethnic food. The Cajuns are descendants of the early French colonists of Acadia (present-day Nova Scotia), a peninsula on the eastern coast of Canada. A group of the impoverished Acadians settled in the bayou country of what is now Louisiana after the British deported them in the mid-1750s. To support themselves, they developed their distinctive food pattern from the available seafood and from what they could grow and harvest. Over time, Cajuns blended their French culinary background with the Creole (descendants from the Spanish and French colonists) cooking that they found in their new homeland around New Orleans.

Cajun and Creole foods have strong and spicy flavors, with the abundant seafood as a base and usually cooked as a stew and served over rice. The well-known hot chili sauce Tabasco, made from crushed and fermented red chili peppers blended with spices and vinegar, is still made by generations of a Cajun family on Avery Island on the coastal waterway of southern Louisiana. Other popular seasonings include cayenne pepper, crushed black pepper, white pepper, bay leaves, thyme, and **filé powder**. The most popular shellfish native to the region is the crawfish, grown commercially

Table 14.2	Historical Dietary Patterns of the African-American and Cajun-American Cultures					
ETHNIC GROUP	BREAD, CEREAL, RICE, AND PASTA GROUP	VEGETABLE GROUP	FRUIT GROUP	MILK, YOGURT, AND CHEESE GROUP	MEAT, POULTRY, FISH, DRY BEANS, EGGS, AND NUTS GROUP	FATS, OILS, AND SWEETS GROUP
African American (particularly in the southern states)	Biscuits, cornbread as spoonbread, cornpone, or hush puppies; grits	Leafy greens (dandelion greens, kale, mustard greens, collard greens), butter beans, cabbage, corn, green beans, okra, sweet and white potatoes, tomatoes, turnips	Peaches, bananas, watermelon, melon, fruit juice	Buttermilk	Eggs, ground beef, pork and pork products (chitterlings, bacon, pig's feet, pig ears), poultry, organ meats, venison, rabbit, catfish, buffalo fish, flounder, legumes, peanuts	Lard, shortening, and vegetable oils; pies and cakes
French/Cajun	French bread, hushpuppies, cornbread muffins, cush-cush (cornmeal mush cooked with milk), grits, rice	Onions, bell peppers, celery, okra, parsley, shallots, tomatoes, yams	Ambrosia (freshly peeled orange segments and orange juice with sliced bananas and freshly grated coconut), blackberries, lemons, limes, strawberries	Not heavily used in traditional dishes	Catfish, red snapper, shrimp, blue crab, oysters, crawfish, chicken, pork sausage, legumes	Poultry fat; pies, bread pudding, pecan pralines

Cajun a group of people with an enduring tradition whose French-Catholic ancestors established permanent communities in southern Louisiana after being expelled from Acadia (now Nova Scotia, Canada) by the reigning English during the late 18th century; they developed a unique food pattern from a blend of native French influence and the Creole cooking that they found in the new land.

filé powder a substance made from ground sassafras leaves; it seasons and thickens the dish into which it is added.

crawfish boil traditional Louisiana Cajun festive meal. Typically includes crawfish, crab, shrimp, small ears of corn, new potatoes, onions, garlic and seasonings such as cayenne pepper, hot sauce, salt, lemons, and bay leaf. Smoked sausage links are occasionally added. All ingredients are added to a large pot and boiled. The contents are then spread out on newspaper-covered tables for everyone to eat from directly.

in the fertile rice paddies of the bayou areas. The low-country boil, or **crawfish boil,** originated from this region. Gumbo, jambalaya, and crawfish étouffée are other popular spicy Cajun dishes. See Table 14.2 for other representative foods.

Wine is a staple for drinking and cooking for the Cajuns and French Canadians, because of its French heritage. Figure 14.3 presents the Canadian Food Guide, which does not necessarily demonstrate specific French inclinations. Note how Canada's Food Guide has similar plate proportions as the MyPlate recommendations from the United States (see Figure 1.4).

Asian Food Patterns

There are many distinct cultures and food patterns throughout Asia. China, Japan, some of the Southeastern Asian countries (Vietnam, Korea, and the Philippines), as well as India, have strongly influenced Asian cultural food patterns most commonly encountered in the United States.

Chinese. China includes many different regions with varied and distinct landscapes. Thus, its culinary practices are equally diverse. Traditional Chinese cooks select the freshest foods possible, including plentiful fruits and vegetables, hold them for the shortest time possible, and cook them quickly at a high temperature in a *wok* (a round-bottom pan) with small amounts of fat and liquid. The wok controls the amount of heat produced, and a quick stir-frying method preserves the natural flavor, color, and texture. The Chinese prefer to cook their vegetables just before eating so that they are still crisp and flavorful when served. Grains, particularly rice, are a staple in most traditional meals. Chinese cuisine includes meat in small amounts in combined dishes, rather than as a single main entree. Chinese dishes use only a small amount of milk, and eggs and soybean products (e.g., tofu) to add other sources of protein. Foods that are dried, salted, pickled, spiced, candied, or canned serve as garnishes or relishes to mask some flavors or textures or to enhance others. The traditional beverage is unsweetened green tea. Seasonings include soy sauce, ginger, almonds, and sesame seeds. Peanut oil is

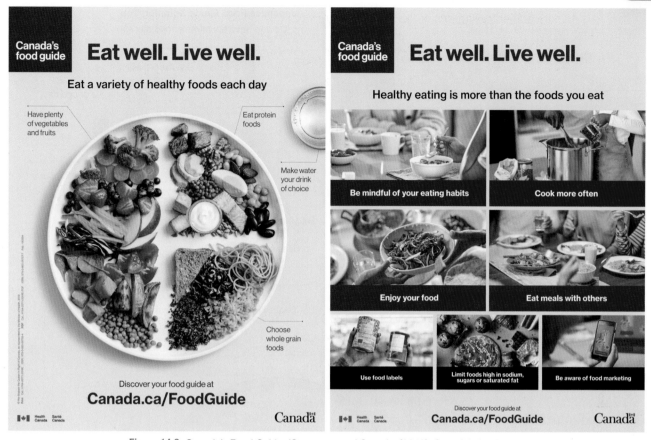

Figure 14.3 Canada's Food Guide. (Government of Canada. [2019]. *Canada's food guide*. food-guide.canada.ca/en/.)

the main cooking fat. Figure 14.4 illustrates the pictorial food guides for China, Japan, and Korea. Table 14.3 provides representative foods from each culture.

Japanese. In many ways, Japanese food patterns are similar to those of the Chinese. Rice is the basic grain served at meals, soy sauce provides seasoning, and tea serves as the main beverage. The Japanese diet contains more seafood, especially in the form of sushi, than the Chinese diet does (see Table 14.3). The term *sushi* does not mean raw fish. Sushi dishes include small amounts of short-grain sticky rice mixed with vinegar and a little sugar served with garnishes such as fish, egg, vegetables, and fruits. Japanese dishes include many varieties of fish, shellfish, and fish eggs. Vegetables are often steamed or pickled. Japanese cuisine focuses on fresh, seasonal fruit, and a tray of fruit is a typical dessert after the main meal. Soybean products are common in the Japanese diet, as is the use of seaweed. Aesthetic appeal is an important part of food preparation and presentation in Japanese culture. Both lunch and dinner meals typically include a bowl of soup. The overall Japanese diet is high in sodium content and low in milk products because of the high prevalence of lactose intolerance.

South and East Asian. Aside from China and Japan, the largest Asian ethnic groups in the United States come from the Philippines, Korea, Vietnam, and India.

As a whole, the food patterns from the various Southeast Asian countries (including the Philippines, Korea, and Vietnam) share similar characteristics and have influenced American diet and agriculture. Asian grocery stores throughout the country stock many traditional Asian food items. The Southeast Asian food pattern uses rice (both long-grain and glutinous) as a base for its cuisine and serves rice at almost all meals. The Vietnamese customarily eat their rice plain in a separate rice bowl not mixed with other foods, whereas other Southeast Asians may eat rice in mixed dishes. Meals often include soup, along with many fresh fruits and vegetables, fresh herbs and other seasonings such as chives, spring onions, chili peppers, ginger root, coriander, turmeric, and fish sauce. These dietary patterns include many kinds of seafood (i.e., fish and shellfish), chicken, duck, and pork, and only small quantities of red meat (see Table 14.3). In a traditional Asian diet, nuts and legumes, including soy, are the primary sources of protein. Stir-frying in a wok with a small amount of lard or peanut oil is a common method of cooking.

Third- and fourth-generation immigrants and refugees have largely acculturated to American food choices. These changes include the use of more eggs, beef, pork, dairy products, candy and other sweet snacks, bread, fast foods, soft drinks, butter, margarine, and coffee.

Asian Indians represent the third largest ethnic group of Asian Americans, and their dietary practices are as

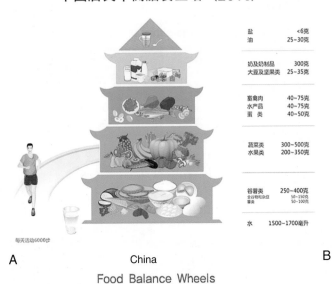

中国居民平衡膳食宝塔（2016）

盐	<6克
油	25~30克
奶及奶制品	300克
大豆及坚果类	25~35克
畜禽肉	40~75克
水产品	40~75克
蛋类	40~50克
蔬菜类	300~500克
水果类	200~350克
谷薯类	250~400克
全谷物和杂豆	50~150克
薯类	50~100克
水	1500~1700毫升

每天活动6000步

A China

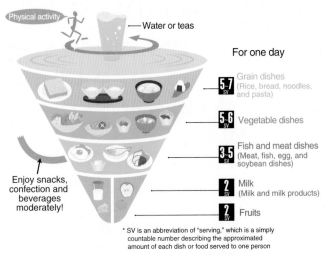

Japanese Food Guide Spinning Top
Do you have a well-balanced diet?

Physical activity

Water or teas

For one day

5-7 SV Grain dishes (Rice, bread, noodles, and pasta)

5-6 SV Vegetable dishes

3-5 SV Fish and meat dishes (Meat, fish, egg, and soybean dishes)

2 SV Milk (Milk and milk products)

2 SV Fruits

Enjoy snacks, confection and beverages moderately!

* SV is an abbreviation of "serving," which is a simply countable number describing the approximated amount of each dish or food served to one person

Decided by Ministry of Health, Labour and Welfare and Ministry of Agriculture, Forestry and Fisheries.

B

Food Balance Wheels

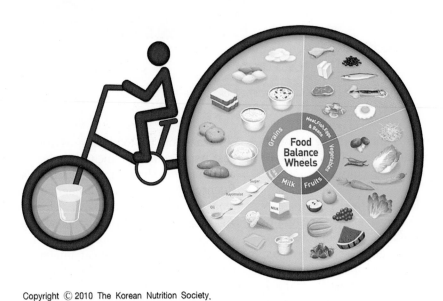

C

Korea

Figure 14.4 National food guides. (A) China; (B) Japan; (C) Korea. (China's National Food Guide: dg.cnsoc.org/article/0 4/8a2389fd5520b4f30155be01beb82724.html. Yoshiike, N., Hayashi, F., Takemi, Y., et al. [2007]. A new food guide in Japan: The Japanese food guide Spinning Top. *Nutr Rev, 65*[4], 149–154. Lee, M., Chae, S. W., Cha, Y. S., et al. [2013]. Development of a Korean Diet Score [KDS] and its application assessing adherence to Korean healthy diet based on the Korean Food Guide Wheels. *Nutr Res Pract, 7*[1], 49–58.)

diverse as the various regions on the expansive Indian subcontinent. Grains such as wheat and rice, tropical fruits and vegetables, leafy vegetables, tubers, legumes, beans, and dairy products make up the bulk of dietary patterns of traditional Indian dishes. Indian cuisine includes small quantities of meats (most often chicken), eggs, and seafood. Nuts and legumes are common protein sources. Herbs and spices representing regional differences flavor the cuisine, such as the popular dishes of curry and dal. Flavorful fruit- and herb-infused

chutneys often accompany meals. There are increasing numbers of Asian Indian ethnic grocery stores available in the United States, allowing individuals to retain traditional practices. As with other ethnic groups, however, adoption of Western dietary practices has resulted in an increased risk of diet-related chronic diseases.[18]

Mediterranean Influences

Although the Mediterranean region includes several countries with varied cultural practices, the general

Table 14.3   Cultural Dietary Patterns of Asian Influence

ETHNIC GROUP	BREAD, CEREAL, RICE, AND PASTA GROUP	VEGETABLE GROUP	FRUIT GROUP	MILK, YOGURT, AND CHEESE GROUP	MEAT, POULTRY, FISH, DRY BEANS, EGGS, AND NUTS GROUP	FATS, OILS, AND SWEETS GROUP
Chinese	Rice, noodles, wheat products, stuffed noodles (wonton), filled buns (boa); stuffed dumplings	Asparagus, bamboo shoots; bean sprouts, cabbage, Chinese celery, Chinese parsley (coriander), Chinese turnips (lo bok), cucumbers, dry fungus (black Judas ear), leafy green vegetables, Chinese broccoli (gai lan), lotus tubers, okra, snow peas, taro root, white radish	Kumquats	Not heavily used in traditional dishes	Fish, seafood, legumes, nuts, organ meats, pigeon eggs, pork and pork products, tofu	Peanut, soy, sesame, and rice oil; lard
Japanese	Short-grain rice and rice products, rice flour (mochiko), noodles (somen, soba)	Artichokes, bamboo shoots, broccoli, beets, burdock (gobo), cabbage, dried mushrooms (shiitake), eggplant, horseradish (wasabi), ginger, green onion, Japanese parsley (seri) lotus root (renkon), mustard greens, pickled vegetables, seaweed, white radish	Pear-like apples (nasi), dates, figs, persimmons, plums, pineapple	Not heavily used in traditional dishes	Fish and shellfish including dried fish with bones, raw fish (sashimi), fish cake (kamaboko); soybeans and soybean products (tofu), red beans (adzuki)	Soy and rice oil
Filipino	Noodles, rice, rice flour (mochiko), stuffed noodles (wonton), white bread	Bamboo shoots, dark green leafy vegetables (malunggay and saluyot), eggplant, sweet potatoes, okra, palm, peppers, turnips, root crop, pickled vegetables	Avocado, banana, bitter melon (ampalaya), breadfruit, guavas, jackfruit, limes, mango, papaya, pod fruit (tamarind), pomelos, rhubarb, tangelo (naranghita), strawberries, pickled fruits	Custards, evaporated milk	Fish in all forms; dried fish (dilis); egg roll (lumpia); fish sauce (alamang, bagoong); legumes, organ meats, pork with chicken in soy sauce (adobo), pork sausage, tofu	None
Southeastern Asians (i.e., Laos, Cambodia, Thailand, Vietnam, Korea, the Hmong, and the Mien)	Rice (long and short grain) and related products such as noodles; Hmong cornbread or cake	Artichoke, bamboo shoots, beans, broccoli, Chinese parsley (coriander); cabbage (such as kimchi), Chinese chard and radish, Korean radish, mustard greens, mushrooms, peppers, pickled vegetables, water chestnuts, Thai chili peppers	Apple pear (Asian pear), bitter melon, dates, durian, figs, grapefruit, guava, jackfruit, mango, papaya	Sweetened condensed milk	Beef, chicken, duck, eggs; fish and shellfish, legumes, peanuts, soybeans, organ meats, pork, tofu, dog meat	Lard, peanut and sesame oil
Asian Indians	Rice, white potatoes, wheat products (such as naan), amaranth, barley	Tomatoes, cucumbers, cabbage, spinach, zucchini, snake gourd, carrots, turnip, chilies	Guava, bananas, papayas, oranges, sugar apple, Buddha's hand, pineapple	Milk (including condensed milk), yogurt (such as a lassi drink), cheese (such as paneer)	Peanuts, lentils, pulses, kidney beans, chicken, mutton, fish	Peanut, coconut, sesame, and vegetable oils; ghee (clarified butter)

With materials modified from Grodner, M., Roth, S., & Walkingshaw, B. (2012). *Nutritional foundations and clinical applications: A nursing approach* (5th ed.). St. Louis: Mosby.

dietary patterns of this region may have protective qualities against the development of certain chronic diseases (see the Clinical Applications box, "Mediterranean Diet and Heart Disease"). We only focus on the influences that have the largest impact within the United States and those that are most closely associated with the Mediterranean Diet Pyramid (Figure 14.5).

As with any study involving dietary patterns and disease, it remains difficult to elucidate the specific factors of the Mediterranean Diet that provide cardioprotective benefits. Nevertheless, observational studies have established that individuals and populations following a Mediterranean-type diet and lifestyle have a reduction in the risk of cardiovascular disease.[19] Consuming a diet rich in plant foods provides ample antioxidants, phytochemicals, fiber, vitamins, and minerals. Avoiding processed foods also reduces the intake of trans fats,

added sugar, and high-glycemic foods. Low to moderate intake of red wine provides antioxidant polyphenols that are protective against atherogenesis. A high intake of olive oil and low consumption of animal products provide a favorable unsaturated to saturated lipid ratio. The diet is anti-inflammatory and palatable and easily followed long term. Thus, health care providers often recommend the Mediterranean approach as an effective method for cardiovascular disease prevention.

Italian. Italian life centers on the sharing of food. Families and friends celebrate special occasions with meals, and food may serve as a form of artistic expression. Although there are distinct regional differences in food preparation and patterns, there are commonalities as well. Bread and pasta are the basic ingredients of most meals, although some regions in Italy focus on potato

---

Clinical Applications

Mediterranean Diet and Heart Disease

The Mediterranean Diet reflects the traditional dietary patterns of the cultures surrounding the Mediterranean Sea. There are many variations on what specifically constitutes the Mediterranean Diet because the region encompasses many countries (see map) and diverse cultural food traditions. In general, however, it is a diet high in fruits, vegetables, legumes, nuts, whole grains, fatty fish, and olive oil; moderate in dairy products and wine; and low in meat, processed and packaged foods, and added sugars. The resultant dietary pattern is one that is high in heart-healthy mono- and polyunsaturated fats, vitamins, minerals, fiber, and antioxidants. Consequently, individuals following a Mediterranean food pattern have a lower risk of overall mortality, neurodegenerative diseases, overall

cancer incidence, diabetes, and cardiovascular diseases.[1] The United States dietary guidelines promote the Mediterranean Diet as a healthy dietary pattern that is palatable and easy to follow. Individuals may use this approach not only for the management of chronic diseases but as a preventive approach as well.[2]

REFERENCES
1. Dinu, M., et al. (2018). Mediterranean diet and multiple health outcomes: An umbrella review of meta-analyses of observational studies and randomised trials. *European Journal of Clinical Nutrition*, *72*(1), 30–43.
2. U.S. Department of Agriculture and U.S. Department of Health and Human Services. (2020, December). *Dietary guidelines for Americans, 2020-2025* (9th ed.). www.dietaryguidelines.gov.

Countries that border the Mediterranean Sea

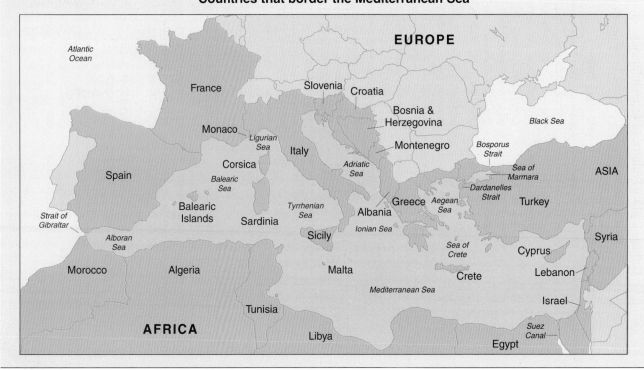

and rice dishes. Cheese is a favorite dairy food, with many popular varieties available. Italians prepare meats, poultry, and fish in many ways, and the varied Italian sausages and cold cuts are famous worldwide. Italian cuisine highlights vegetables by themselves, mixed in main dishes, or added to soups, sauces, and salads. Seasonings include herbs and spices, garlic, wine, olive oil, tomato puree, and salted pork. Although Italian dishes generally include few ingredients, the quality of those ingredients is valued most. Italy is famous for its export of wine, and Italians themselves drink wine with most meals. Italians often consume fresh fruit as a dessert or as a snack (Table 14.4).

Greek. Greek cuisine has strong Ottoman and Roman influences and reflects the values of fresh, wholesome ingredients and dishes. Everyday meals are simple, but Greek holiday meals are occasions for serving many delicacies. Bread is the center of every meal, and most dishes are prepared using olive oil. Greek individuals seldom use milk as a beverage but instead serve it in the cultured form of yogurt. Cheese is a favorite food, especially *feta*, which is a white cheese made from sheep's milk and preserved in brine. Lamb is the preferred meat, but Greek cuisine includes other sources of protein, especially chicken and fish. Eggs are sometimes a main dish, but they are rarely a breakfast food. This dietary pattern includes plentiful portions of vegetables and frequently serves them as the main entree, cooked with broth, tomato sauce, onions, olive oil, and herbs such as parsley. Meals often include a typical salad of thinly sliced raw vegetables and feta cheese, dressed with olive oil and vinegar; the traditional Greek salad is a favorite at many American restaurants. Wheat and barley are the most common grains found in the diet. Fruit is an everyday dessert, but Greek celebrations may include rich pastries such as *baklava* (see Table 14.4).

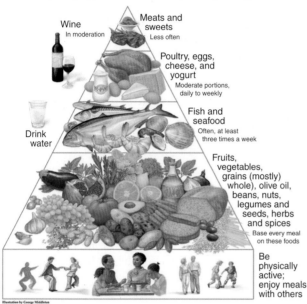

Mediterranean Diet Pyramid
A contemporary approach to delicious, healthy eating

© 2009 Oldways Preservation and Exchange Trust • www.oldwayspt.org

Figure 14.5 Mediterranean Diet Pyramid. (Copyright 2009, Oldways Preservation & Exchange Trust, Boston, Mass; www.oldwayspt.org/mediterranean-diet-pyramid.)

Table 14.4   Historical Dietary Patterns of the Mediterranean

ETHNIC GROUP	BREAD, CEREAL, RICE, AND PASTA GROUP	VEGETABLE GROUP	FRUIT GROUP	MILK, YOGURT, AND CHEESE GROUP	MEAT, POULTRY, FISH, DRY BEANS, EGGS, AND NUTS GROUP	FATS, OILS, AND SWEETS GROUP
Italian	Bread, pasta, polenta, risotto (rice)	Artichokes, asparagus, cabbage, capers, chicory, corn, eggplant, endive, fennel, garlic, golden onion, green leafy vegetables, mushrooms, peppers, potatoes, radicchio, tomatoes, truffles	Apricots, cherries, dates, figs, grapes, pomegranates, oranges	Many rich cheeses made from cow's, sheep, and goat milk such as asiago, mozzarella, Taleggio, gorgonzola, ricotta, provolone, Ragusano	Beef, goat, lamb, pork (prosciutto, salami, sausage), poultry, fish (including anchovies, sardines, and a variety of other seafood and shellfish), legumes (chickpeas, fava beans, lentils)	Olive oil, lard
Greek	Bread, pita bread, barley, rice	Artichokes, beets, Brussels sprouts, cabbage, cucumber, eggplant, garlic, green beans, leeks, bell peppers, spinach, stuffed grape leaves, tomatoes, zucchini	Apricots, avocado, cherries, currants, dates, figs, grapes, pomegranates, oranges, olives, jams and chutneys are popular	Buttermilk, cream, yogurt, a variety of cheeses made from goat, sheep, and cow's milk such as feta, graviera, kefalotyri myzithra, and manouri	Lamb, beef, veal, rabbit, poultry, eggs, snails, legumes (chickpeas, fava beans, lentils, red beans), seafood (fish eggs, mussels, squid, octopus); meat pies are popular	Olive oil, honey

RELIGIOUS DIETARY LAWS

The dietary practices within Christianity (e.g., Catholic, Protestant, and Latter Day Saints churches), Judaism, Hinduism, Buddhism, and Islam fluctuate according to each follower's understanding and interpretation of what constitutes a healthy and proper diet. Such dietary laws may determine what, how, and when its adherents may consume, or avoid specific foods. Some dietary laws are applicable at all times (e.g., no pork at any time for Islamic followers), whereas other laws apply only during religious ceremonies (e.g., abstaining from meat on Fridays during Lent for Roman Catholics). Following are examples of two such religions and their dietary laws.

Jewish

Basic food pattern. All Jewish festivals are religious in nature and have historical significance, but the observance of Jewish food laws differs among the three most common groups within Judaism: (1) orthodox, with strict observance; (2) conservative, with less strict observance; and (3) reform, with less ceremonial emphasis and minimal general use. Jewish dietary laws are known as *kashrut* as established in the Torah. Foods selected and prepared in alignment with these rules are *kosher*, from the Hebrew word meaning "fit, proper." These laws originally had special ritual significance. Current Jewish dietary laws govern the slaughter, preparation, and serving of meat; the combining of meat and milk; and the use of fish and eggs. The following are some of the Jewish food restrictions:

- *Meat:* Appropriate meats should come from animals that chew their cud and that have cloven hooves. Individuals following a kosher diet avoid pork, rabbits, and birds of prey at all times and thoroughly cleanse meat of any blood.
- *Meat and milk:* Although the kosher Jewish diet includes both meat and milk products, adherents to kosher laws cannot consume meat and milk products at the same meal or prepared with the same dishes. Orthodox homes maintain two sets of regular dishes: one for serving meat and the other for meals that contain dairy products. These homes may also maintain an additional two sets of dishes specifically for use during Passover.
- *Fish:* Kosher law only allows its followers to consume fish with fins and scales and restricts the consumption of shellfish and crustaceans.
- *Eggs:* Individuals adhering to kosher laws may consume eggs with either dairy or meat, but they may not consume eggs containing a blood spot.

Representative foods and influence of festivals. Many traditional Jewish foods relate to festivals of the Jewish calendar that commemorate significant events in Jewish history; examples include the Sabbath, Rosh Hashanah, Yom Kippur, Sukkot, Hanukkah, Purim, and Passover. A few representative foods, mostly of Eastern European influence, include the following:

- *Bagels:* Doughnut-shaped hard yeast rolls
- *Blintzes:* Thin, filled, rolled pancakes
- *Borscht (borsch):* A soup of meat stock, beaten egg or sour cream, beets, cabbage, or spinach served hot or cold
- *Challah:* A Sabbath loaf of white bread that the baker shapes as a twist or coil; individuals serve this bread at the beginning of the meal after the Kiddush, which is the blessing over the wine
- *Gefüllte (gefilte) fish:* From a German word meaning "stuffed fish," this is usually the first course of the Sabbath evening meal. The cook prepares *gefüllte* by chopping and seasoning fish filets and then stuffing them back into the skin or rolled into balls
- *Kasha:* Buckwheat groats (hulled kernels) used as a cooked cereal or as a potato substitute with gravy
- *Knishes:* Pastries filled with ground meat or cheese
- *Lox:* Smoked and salted salmon
- *Matzo:* Flat, unleavened bread
- *Strudel:* A thin pastry filled with fruit and nuts, which is rolled and baked

Muslim

Basic food pattern. The Islamic teachings found in the Quran guide Muslim dietary laws and serve as the foundation for the restriction or prohibition of some foods and the promotion of others. The laws are binding, and Muslims must follow them at all times, even during pregnancy, hospitalization, and travel. In the most strict and observant areas, these laws are also binding for visitors in the host Muslim region. Islamic dietary law outlines foods that are permissible, or *halal*, based on what it is and how individuals obtain and prepare the food. Foods forbidden by Islamic dietary law are *haram*. Haram foods include pork and birds of prey, meats not slaughtered in the proper way, blood, and alcohol in any form, and other intoxicating drugs unless medically necessary. Most other foods are halal.

The Quran mentions certain foods as being of special value to physical and social health, including figs, olives, dates, honey, milk, and buttermilk. Individuals may consume foods that Muslim dietary laws prohibit when no other sources of food are available.

Representative foods in the Middle East. Specific food choices will reflect not only the Muslim dietary law but also the geographic region in which people live. Following are several typical foods and dishes commonly used as appetizers, main dishes, snacks, or salads for individuals in the Middle East:

- *Bulgur (or burghel):* Partially cooked and dried, cracked wheat that is available in a coarse grind as a base for pilaf or in a fine grind for use in tabouli and kibbeh
- *Falafel:* A "fast food" made from a seasoned paste of ground, soaked beans that are formed into shapes and fried
- *Fatayeh:* A snack or appetizer that is similar to a small pizza, with toppings of cheese, meat, or spinach

- *Kibbeh:* A meat dish made of a cracked wheat shell filled with small pieces of lamb and fried in oil
- *Pilaf:* Sautéed and seasoned bulgur or rice that is steamed in a bouillon, sometimes with poultry, meat, or shellfish
- *Pita:* A flat circular bread torn or cut into pieces and stuffed with sandwich fillings or used as a scoop for a dip such as *hummus,* made from chickpeas
- *Tabouli:* A salad made from soaked bulgur that has been combined with chopped tomatoes, parsley, mint, and green onion and then mixed with olive oil and lemon juice

Influence of festivals. Fasting is the fourth pillar of Islam as commanded by the Quran. Muslin people observe a 30-day period of daylight fasting during **Ramadan**. Ramadan represents the sacred fast when Muhammad received the first of the revelations that subsequently formed the Quran; it is the month when Muhammad's followers first drove their enemies from Mecca in 624 C.E. (COMMON ERA) During the month of Ramadan, Muslims all over the world fast daily by taking no food or drink from dawn until sunset. These individuals traditionally break the daily fast by eating an odd number of dates and having a glass of water or other beverage, followed by the family's "evening breakfast," or the iftar. At the end of Ramadan, a traditional feast that lasts up to 3 days concludes the observance known as Eid-al-Fitr (see the Cultural Considerations box, "Eid al-Fitr: The Post-Ramadan Festival"). Eid-al-Adha is a 3-day celebration of the pilgrimage to Mecca.

Muslims past the age of puberty observe the fast of Ramadan. Individuals with diabetes, who are taking

> **Ramadan** the ninth month of the Muslim year, which is a period of daily fasting from sunrise to sunset.

certain medications, who are pregnant or breastfeeding, or with other medical contraindications, may experience complications during this time and thus may abstain from fasting. These individuals may make up the days of fasting before the next Ramadan fast if it is appropriate to do so. Health care professionals must be sensitive to such religious practices when counseling clients.

Table 14.5 outlines other common religions with specific dietary practices and their food or beverage restrictions.

CHANGING AMERICAN FOOD PATTERNS

The stereotype of the all-American family of two parents and two children eating three meals a day with no snacks in between is no longer the norm. Extensive changes have occurred regarding Americans' lifestyles and, subsequently, their food habits. Modifying one's personal eating patterns is difficult enough; helping clients and patients to make necessary changes for positive health reasons can be even more challenging. Such guidance requires a culturally sensitive and flexible understanding of the complex factors that are involved.

HOUSEHOLD DYNAMICS

The typical American household has changed dramatically over the past several decades. Family structures are changing, and that which constitutes a family continues to evolve. Beginning in the 1960s, the number of women in the workforce rose rapidly, a trend evidenced among all social, economic, and ethnic groups. Currently, women make up nearly 47% of the workforce in the United States, and 70% of women with children younger than 18 years old are employed.[20] Women are also the primary or sole earners in 40% of U.S. household families.[21] Working parents increasingly rely on food items and cooking methods that save time, space, and labor. Americans are spending less time preparing and cooking meals and are eating out more frequently than 50 years ago; in fact, approximately 32% of calories in the American adult diet come from food prepared outside of the home.[22]

WITH WHOM AND WHERE WE EAT

Rarely do families regularly sit down to eat meals together anymore, particularly for breakfast and lunch meals. However, research shows that family meals are consistently associated with increased fruit and vegetable intake, a decreased intake of unhealthful foods, a decreased risk of disordered eating, and a lower risk of obesity in adulthood. Family meals may be protective against alcohol and substance use among children and other behavioral problems, and family meals are

Cultural Considerations

Eid al-Fitr: The Post-Ramadan Festival

Muslims worldwide conclude the month of prayer and fasting, known as Ramadan, with a festival lasting 1 to 3 days. The Islamic prophet Muhammad originated this celebration, known as the festival Eid al-Fitr.

Over the years, Muslims serve many delicacies that symbolize the joy of returning from fasting and the heightened sense of unity, goodwill, and charity that the fasting experience has brought to the people. Although the dishes served are reflective of the country and locality, it is common to find many sweet offerings. The foods served may include chicken or veal sautéed with eggplant and onions, slowly simmered in pomegranate juice, and spiced with turmeric and cardamom seeds. The highlight of the meal is usually *kharuf mahshi,* which is a whole lamb (i.e., a symbol of sacrifice) stuffed with a rich dressing made of dried fruits, cracked wheat, pine nuts, almonds, and onions and seasoned with ginger and coriander. Cooks bake the stuffed lamb in hot ashes for many hours so that it is tender enough to pull it apart and eat it with their fingers.

As the meal concludes, individuals enjoy rich pastries and candies flavored with spices or flower petals. Muslims may take some of the sweets home and savor them for as long as possible as a reminder of the festival.

Table 14.5   Religious Dietary Practices

	SEVENTH-DAY ADVENTIST	BUDDHIST	EASTERN ORTHODOX	HINDU	JEWISH	MORMON	MUSLIM	ROMAN CATHOLIC
Beef		Avoided by most devout		Prohibited or strongly discouraged				
Pork	Prohibited or strongly discouraged	Avoided by most devout		Avoided by most devout	Prohibited or strongly discouraged		Prohibited or strongly discouraged	
All meat	Avoided by most devout	Avoided by most devout	Permitted but some restrictions apply	Avoided by most devout	Permitted but some restrictions apply		Permitted but some restrictions apply	Permitted but some restrictions apply
Eggs, dairy	Permitted but avoided at some observances	Permitted but avoided at some observances	Permitted but some restrictions apply	Permitted but avoided at some observances	Permitted but some restrictions apply			
Fish	Avoided by most devout	Avoided by most devout	Permitted but some restrictions apply	Permitted but some restrictions apply	Permitted but some restrictions apply		Permitted but some restrictions apply	
Shellfish	Prohibited or strongly discouraged	Avoided by most devout	Permitted but avoided at some observances	Permitted but some restrictions apply	Prohibited or strongly discouraged			
Meat and dairy at same meal					Prohibited or strongly discouraged			
Leavened foods					Permitted but some restrictions apply			
Ritual slaughter of animals					Practiced		Practiced	
Alcohol	Prohibited or strongly discouraged	Avoided by most devout		Avoided by most devout		Prohibited or strongly discouraged	Prohibited or strongly discouraged	
Caffeine	Prohibited or strongly discouraged					Prohibited or strongly discouraged	Avoided by most devout	

Modified from Kittler, P. G., Sucher, K. P., & Nahikian-Nelms, M. (2012). *Food and culture* (6th ed.). Belmont, CA: Brooks/Cole.

positively associated with improved academic performance.[23] Public health efforts to overcome barriers to family meal practices may significantly improve the health of individual family members.

HOW OFTEN AND HOW MUCH WE EAT

Frequency

Food habits have also changed regarding when we eat. Americans, on average, eat approximately three meals and two snacks per day. However, the percentage of individuals who follow such structured meal times has declined over the past 40 years.[24,25] Although the number of snacks that Americans consume has remained relatively stable, the percentage of calories coming from snacks is increasing at a faster rate as compared with the increase in calories coming from meals. The increase in calories from snacks may be problematic given that snacks tend to be nutrient poor; specifically, they are higher in added sugar, sodium, and fats (see the For Further Focus box, "Snacking: An All-American Food Habit").[24]

For Further Focus

Snacking: An All-American Food Habit

The snack market in the United States continues to grow. Although consumer spending on all foods has increased, the proportion of money spent on snacks is especially large. Snacks also contribute to the increasing energy intake of Americans; over a 35-year period from 1977 to 2012, there was a 50% increase in the calories coming from snack foods. On average, Americans consume about 500 calories a day in snacks. Unfortunately, these calories tend to represent nutrient-poor choices. Grain-based desserts (i.e., cookies, cakes) are the most common source of snack-derived calories, followed by salty snacks, other desserts and sweets, and sugar-sweetened beverages.[1]

Many of the snacks that Americans consume provide significant amounts of sodium, added sugars, and saturated fats. Snacking behaviors contribute to the increase in overweight and obesity incidence in the United States, particularly when individuals consume energy-dense snacks (i.e., high-calorie snacks).[2] It is important to recognize that snacks also provide an opportunity to consume more nutrient-dense options, including fruits, vegetables, whole grains, and low-fat/nonfat dairy foods. Thus, healthier snack choices can help Americans increase their intake of key nutrients of concern, such as fiber, iron, calcium, vitamin A, and potassium, among other important vitamins and minerals.

Snacks are relatively significant contributors to overall daily energy intake. Snacking—or grazing, as some people do, which involves more frequent nibbling—is a significant component of food behavior. Not all snack foods are junk food, and snacking is not inherently problematic. Rather than rule against the practice, health providers should promote snack foods that enhance nutrition well-being using a culturally sensitive approach.

REFERENCES

1. Dunford, E. K., & Popkin, B. M. (2017). Disparities in snacking trends in US adults over a 35 year period from 1977 to 2012. *Nutrients, 9*(8).
2. Larson, N. I., et al. (2016). Adolescent snacking behaviors are associated with dietary intake and weight status. *Journal of Nutrition, 146*(7), 1348–1355.

Portion Sizes

Growing portion sizes are a concerning trend in typical American meals and snacks. Portion sizes of processed foods that are nutrient poor have increased substantially over the past several decades, and so has consumption of these foods.[26,27] A 2019 study compared the changes in fast-food menu items over a 30-year period (from 1986 to 2016) from 10 major fast-food restaurants. Researchers found that the energy content of entrees, sides, and desserts increased significantly over the 30-year period. The sodium content also increased significantly, as did the portion sizes for both entrees and desserts.[27] These changes to menu offerings are highly problematic, given the frequency with which Americans dine at fast-food restaurants.

The U.S. Department of Health and Human Services created an interesting Portion Distortion Quiz that depicts serving size changes over a 20-year period. It is worth checking out this resource as an educational tool and a revelation (www.nhlbi.nih.gov/health/educational/wecan/eat-right/portion-distortion.htm).

Despite the many warnings regarding portion size effects, serving sizes remain unnecessarily large, and most consumers continue to eat and drink relative to the amount of food and beverage served, instead of in response to their actual hunger and energy needs.[28] The mechanisms underlying the portion size effect are complex and emphasize the impact that environmental cues have on eating behaviors. Even individuals trained in portion control strategies consume more food and additional energy when presented with larger portion sizes, highlighting the challenging nature of this issue.[29]

Healthy eating patterns include portion size control. However, education alone is an insufficient intervention for combatting the portion size effect. Greater changes on a policy level are required to address the adverse health effects resulting from larger portion sizes.

ECONOMIC BUYING

In an effort to save money on food expenditures, many Americans are turning to alternatives to grocery stores for their purchases. Americans' purchases of packaged foods at warehouse clubs, mass merchandisers, and convenience stores have risen significantly, while expenditures at grocery stores have decreased.[30] Warehouse club stores, such as bulk-food chains such as Costco and Sam's Club, significantly reduce overhead costs, and storeowners can pass those savings on to consumers. Buying in bulk (i.e., economy size or family size) can save money, but only if consumers use the quantity efficiently; shoppers lose the cost savings benefits if the food is improperly stored or not eaten before it spoils. Unfortunately, foods purchased at these retailers tend to be lower in nutrients while higher in added sugars, sodium, saturated fat, and overall calories.[30] Food retailers often provide cost-per-unit pricing on the shelves to make comparing the prices of similar foods in different-sized containers or packages easier for the consumer.

Tempting advertisements often lure consumers into ordering or purchasing more food than they need at restaurants and grocery stores. Deals such as "two for one" and "value meals" could be a great bargain, but they supply more food than is necessary for one person. Educating clients on understanding proper portion sizes, buying in bulk, and knowing how to properly store food for later use (see Chapter 13) help promote a healthy lifestyle for them and their family.

Putting It All Together

Summary

- Individuals live in a social setting. Each person inherits a culture and a particular social structure, complete with its food habits and attitudes about eating.
- The effects that major social and economic shifts have on health—as well as the current social forces, including cultural, religious, and psychologic—influence how and why people make dietary changes.
- America's dietary patterns continue to evolve and reflect the process of globalization. People who live fast-paced, complex lives are increasingly reliant on new forms of convenience food.
- Foods consumed away from the home that include fast foods and packaged foods continue to increase energy intake and oversized portions.

Chapter Review Questions

See answers in Appendix A.

1. A client who abides by the kashrut would be least likely to consume _____.

   a. chicken noodle soup
   b. tofu and broccoli stir-fry
   c. salmon tacos with coleslaw
   d. ham and cheese sandwich with pickles

2. Individuals of American Indian heritage would most likely follow a dietary pattern based on which of the following foods?

   a. Corn, squash, and dried beans
   b. Fish, pasta, and Brussels sprouts
   c. Dumplings, bean sprouts, and rice
   d. Falafel, hummus, and pita bread

3. A menu that included items such as pilaf, bulgur, and tabouli is most likely to be found at a restaurant serving food from which geographic region?

   a. Southeast Asia
   b. Western Europe
   c. Northern Europe
   d. Middle East

4. Which European country commonly consumes foods that are consistent with a Mediterranean dietary pattern?

   a. Germany
   b. Belgium
   c. Italy
   d. Austria

5. Which factor is most likely to influence the nutrition habits of children?

   a. A decrease in the physical education curriculum provided at school
   b. An evening news program that highlights the dangers of fast-food consumption
   c. Cereal packaging that includes a popular cartoon figure
   d. Soda products that include cane sugar as a primary ingredient

Next-Generation NCLEX® Examination-style Case Study

See answers in Appendix A.

A 23-year-old woman (height, 5'4"; weight, 155 lbs.) works full-time as a medical assistant while also going to nursing school and helping take care of her niece. She is physically and mentally stressed, and at her last physical exam, her doctor mentioned that her blood pressure was higher than normal (130/90 mm Hg). In addition, she had gained 10 lbs. since her last annual appointment. At work, she eats a multitude of processed snack foods, such as chips, cookies, and candy. She consumes fast food about once per week. Instead of meals, she consumes snacks frequently throughout the day. The client provided the following 24-hour dietary recall:

   8 AM: frozen peanut butter and jelly sandwiches (2)
   9 AM: small bags of chips (2) and soda (12 oz.)
   11 AM: frozen meat-lovers Pizza Pocket (1)
   12 PM: Mott's fruit-flavored gummy snacks soda (12 oz.)
   3 PM: frozen bean, beef, and cheese burritos (2)
   5 PM: small bag of potato chips (1) and medium-sized brownies (2)

1. From the list below, select all of the items provided in the client's history that put her at nutrition risk.

   a. Frequent snacking and grazing
   b. Frequency of fast food consumption
   c. Portion sizes
   d. High intake of energy-dense foods
   e. High intake of nutrient-dense foods

2. From the list below, identify all nutrients that are most likely consumed in excess by the client based on the food recall provided.

   a. Vitamin A
   b. Sodium
   c. Iron
   d. Vitamin K
   e. Saturated fat
   f. Calcium
   g. Sugar
   h. Fiber
   i. Potassium

3. Choose the *most likely* options for the information missing from the statements below by selecting from the list of options provided.

The client's snacking increases overall calorie intake, and consuming _____ snacks increases the risk for overweight and obesity. In addition, the client's increased consumption of _____ might contribute to _____.

OPTIONS	
nutrient-dense	fiber
energy-dense	diabetes
fruits	hypertension
vegetables	obesity
sodium	

4. From the list below, select all of the appropriate nutrition interventions for the client.

a. Selecting healthier food choices
b. Decreasing frequency of snacks
c. Following a strict diet
d. Reducing portion sizes
e. Planning meals ahead of time
f. Eliminating food groups, such as carbohydrates and fats

5. Use an X for the health teaching below that is <u>indicated</u> (appropriate or necessary) or <u>contraindicated</u> (could be harmful).

HEALTH TEACHING	INDICATED	CONTRAINDICATED
Aim to consume a meal pattern including 3 meals and 2 snacks.		
Increase your fruit and vegetable intake by trying to eat a fruit and vegetable at each meal.		
Consuming low-fat dairy and whole-grain foods will provide more nutrients than processed foods.		
Identify individual serving sizes on food labels.		
Consume the serving sizes served at restaurants because they are likely appropriate.		
Consume high amounts of fruit juices to increase fiber and nutrients.		
Skip meals at work if you forgot to pack a lunch.		

6. For each assessment finding, use an X to indicate whether the nursing and collaborative interventions were <u>effective</u> (helped to meet expected outcomes) or <u>ineffective</u> (did not help to meet expected outcomes).

ASSESSMENT FINDING	EFFECTIVE	INEFFECTIVE
Blood pressure changed from 130/90 mm Hg to 120/80 mm Hg		
Client lost 5 lbs. in the last 2 weeks		
Client skips breakfast and lunch 2 days out of the week		
Client snacks less during the day		
Client consumes fast food 3 times per week		
Client consumes at least 2 servings of fruit and vegetables every day		

Additional Learning Resources

Please refer to this text's Evolve website for answers to the Case Study questions:
http://evolve.elsevier.com/Williams/basic/.
References and **Further Reading and Resources** in the back of the book provide additional resources for enhancing knowledge.

Weight Management

Theresa Dvorak MS, RDN, CSSD, ATC

Key Concepts

- A host of various genetic, environmental, and psychologic factors contribute to individual cases of obesity.
- Short-term food patterns or fads often stem from food misinformation that appeals to various human psychologic needs; however, these fads do not necessarily meet physiologic needs.

- Realistic weight management focuses on individual needs and health promotion, including meal pattern planning and regular physical activity.
- Severe underweight carries physiologic and psychologic risk to the body.

Excess body weight in the United States threatens the health of many Americans. Currently 71.6% of adults are overweight, of which approximately 40% are obese and 7.7% are extremely obese. This epidemic, which results in large part from poor diet, physical inactivity, and genetics, is not limited to adults: 18.5% of children and adolescents between the ages of 2 and 19 years old are also obese.[1] The variety of weight-loss diets is abundant. So too are the philosophical methods implored to shed unwanted pounds. This variety often leads to confusion about sound weight-loss methods and expectations. Despite an apparent obsession with weight and the multibillion-dollar industry of weight-loss diets and products, Americans continue to grow in undesirable directions (Figure 15.1). This chapter examines the problem of weight management and seeks a more positive and realistic health model that recognizes personal needs and sound weight goals.

OBESITY AND WEIGHT CONTROL

BODY WEIGHT VERSUS BODY FAT

Obesity develops from many interwoven factors—including personal, physical, psychologic, and genetic. *Obesity* is a clinical term used in the traditional medical sense for people who are at least 20% above their desired weight for height, denoting excess body fat. Interchangeably using the terms *overweight* and *obese* is common practice, but they technically have different meanings. *Overweight* denotes a body weight that is above a population weight-for-height standard. Meanwhile, the word *obese* is a more specific diagnostic term that refers to the degree of fatness (i.e., the relative excess amount of fat in the total **body composition**). Over the past 5 decades, the percentage of obese adults (i.e., those with a **body mass index [BMI] of ≥30 kg/m²**) has almost tripled.[1,2] Although the relative prevalence of overweight and obesity among adults in America has remained steady over the past decade, it remains at epidemic proportions.

Box 15.1 provides the classifications of BMI, and the BMI chart is located on the inside back cover of the textbook. Body fat percentages relate to BMI measurements for most individuals (Figure 15.2). The Centers for Disease Control and Prevention growth charts allow for the tracking of BMI from childhood to adulthood (see Chapter 11). BMI is a reliable method of predicting the relative risk of becoming an overweight adult based on the presence or absence of excess body weight at various times throughout childhood. Children and adolescents who are overweight or obese are significantly more likely to continue to suffer from obesity as they age.[3]

Every person is different, and normal weight ranges vary in healthy people. Until recently, health practitioners overlooked the important factor of age for setting a reasonable body weight. With advancing age, body weight usually increases until approximately the age of 50 years for men and the age of 70 years for women, after which it usually declines.

The exclusive use of BMI to define obesity has undergone criticism because it does not measure body fat per se but rather total body weight relative to height. This method classifies a few individuals as obese when they do not actually have excess body fat. For example, a football player in peak condition can be extremely "overweight" according to standard height/weight

> **body composition** the relative sizes of the four body compartments that make up the total body: lean body mass (muscle mass), fat, water, and bone.
> **body mass index (BMI)** the body weight in kilograms divided by the square of the height in meters (i.e., kg/m²).

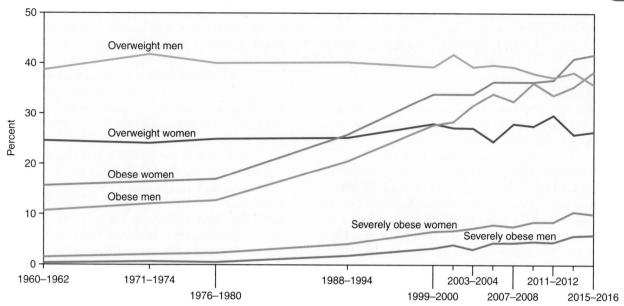

Figure 15.1 Trends in overweight, obesity, and severe obesity among men and women aged 20 to 74: United States, 1960 through 2015-2016. Overweight is defined as BMI of 25 to 29.9 kg/m²; obesity is defined as BMI of 30 to 39.9 kg/m²; severe obesity is defined as BMI of 40 kg/m² or greater. (From National Center for Health Statistics. [2018]. *Prevalence of overweight, obesity, and severe obesity among adults aged 20 and over: United States, 1960-1962 Through 2015-2016.* Hyattsville, MD: U.S. Government Publishing Office).

Box 15.1 Body Mass Index Classifications

BODY MASS INDEX RANGE (KG/M²)	CLASSIFICATION
18.5 to 24.9	Normal weight
25 to 29.9	Overweight
30 to 35	Obese
>35	Clinically or extremely obese

charts. In other words, he can weigh considerably more than the average person of the same height, but much more of his weight is likely lean muscle mass rather than excess fat. Thus, for individuals with significantly more muscle mass than the average person, BMI may not be the ideal means of assessing health risks associated with weight. To increase accuracy of assessing chronic disease and mortality risk, the use of waist circumference is included because the greater the amount of adipose tissue stored within the abdominal region, the higher the risk for disease and all-cause mortality.[4]

WAIST CIRCUMFERENCE AND INCREASED RISK

Men: ≥40 inches

Women: ≥35 inches

BODY COMPOSITION

Body composition is not always easy to measure in clients. Therefore, the recommended standard for assessing health relative to weight is the BMI and waist circumference measurements used together. However, body composition assessment provides an additional measure of overall health and fitness. Health professionals can measure body composition with a variety of methods:

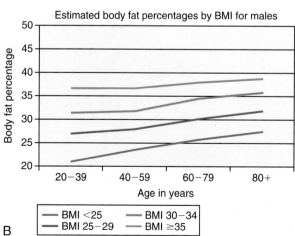

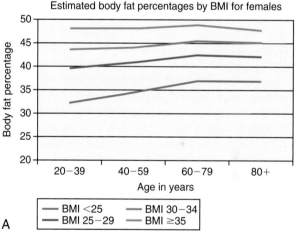

Figure 15.2 Body fat percentage as it correlates with body mass index (BMI): (A) females; (B) males. (Modified from Li, C., Ford, E. S., Zhao, G., et al. [2009]. Estimates of body composition with dual-energy x-ray absorptiometry in adults. *Am J Clin Nutr, 90*[6], 1457–1465.)

- *Skin fold calipers* measure the width of skin folds at precise body sites, because we deposit most of the body fat in layers just under the skin (Figure 15.3). Importing the data from the skin fold measurements into a specific formula provides an estimated body fat percentage. Calipers are an easy, portable, inexpensive, and noninvasive way to measure body fat. However, the reliability of the test depends on the accuracy of locating the correct anatomic location, the quality of the calipers, and the skill of the technician.

- *Hydrostatic weighing* is a more precise method and is often used in athletic programs and research studies; although with advancing technologies, it is not used as frequently now. Hydrostatic weighing requires the complete submersion of an individual in water. For an accurate reading, the person must exhale as much air as possible and then remain as still as possible underwater for a few seconds. Although this method is relatively accurate, it is not easy, portable, or inexpensive, and many clients are not willing or able to perform the test.

- *Bioelectrical impedance analysis* (BIA) is an easy, portable, inexpensive, and noninvasive body composition measurement tool. One type, a foot-to-foot analyzer, requires that the person stand on a modified scale with bare feet while an undetectable electrical current travels through his or her body (Figure 15.4). The analyzer calculates the individual's body fat percentage based on sex, age, height, weight, total body water, and the rate at which the electrical current travels. Fat impedes the current; therefore, a lower total body fat composition results in a faster travel time of the current. Such analyzers have both a standard adult setting and an athletic setting. Although this method does not require any special skill on either the client's part or the technician's part, there are discrepancies between total body fat percentages as measured by bioelectrical impedance versus dual-energy x-ray absorptiometry in some populations (such as surgical, oncology, or critically ill patients).[5-7] Although the use of BIA is promising, there is a need for the development and validation of predictive equations for diverse populations. Bioelectrical impedance machines that use a multiple-frequency bioelectrical impedance analysis with eight-point tactile electrodes have the least error and the highest correspondence to reference amounts of body fat.[8]

- *Air displacement plethysmography* using a BOD POD machine (Life Measurement, Inc., Concord, CA) is a reliable method of assessing body composition that does not rely on technical expertise or radiation (Figure 15.5). However, it is expensive and not portable. This measurement requires the individual to sit in an egg-shaped device wearing tight-fitting clothes. The BOD POD calculates the percentage of body fat using weight, body volume, thoracic lung volume, and body density. The BOD POD is not for individuals over 500 pounds or those with a fear of confined spaces. The BOD POD is a reliable measurement tool for most individuals; however, it may overestimate body fat percentage in underweight individuals and overestimate in overweight/obese individuals.[9] Child-specific fat-free mass density values are required when using the BOD POD to assess body composition in children.[10]

- *Dual-energy x-ray absorptiometry* (DEXA) is a highly accurate way to assess body composition using radiation to distinguish bone mineral, fat-free mass, and fat

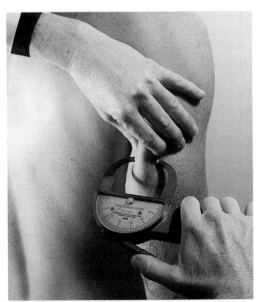

Figure 15.3 Assessment tools include skin fold calipers, which measure the relative amount of subcutaneous fat tissue at various body sites. (Reprinted from Mahan, L. K., & Escott-Stump, S. [2011]. *Krause's food & nutrition therapy* [13th ed.]. Philadelphia: Saunders.)

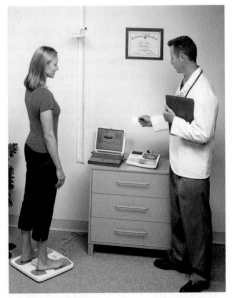

Figure 15.4 Tanita bioelectrical impedance body composition measurement tool. (Courtesy Tanita Corp., Arlington Heights, Ill.)

A body fat content within the range of 21% to 26% of total body weight (typically equivalent to a BMI of ≤25 kg/m²) is usually associated with the lowest risk of chronic disease for adult men. For adult women, the range is somewhat higher: 34% to 38%.[11] Body fat percentages vary between sex, race/ethnicity, and through the life span. At a BMI of 25 kg/m² adult non-Hispanic black men have a lower percentage body fat compared with non-Hispanic white and Mexican-American men. This relationship is similar in adult women as well (Figure 15.7).[11] Older individuals (at least 70 years old) may have a decrease in fat-free mass and an increase in fat mass at the same BMI equivalent.[11,12] Given these variations within the population, current research has not identified an ideal body fat percentage for a given BMI that corresponds with specific disease risks among varying races/ethnicities or across the life span.

MEASURES OF WEIGHT MAINTENANCE GOALS

Standard Height/Weight Tables

Height/weight tables are only general population guides and not the sole diagnostic tool for an individual. One of the standard tables used in the United States is the Metropolitan Life Insurance Company's ideal weight-for-height chart. Life expectancy information gathered since the 1930s from the company's population of life insurance policyholders formed the basis of these charts. Many people have questioned how well these tables represent the total current population, because the data are based on such a select group of individuals (most of whom were white, middle- to

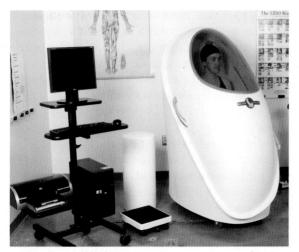

Figure 15.5 The BOD POD uses air displacement technology to measure body composition. (Courtesy Life Measurements, Inc., Concord, Calif.)

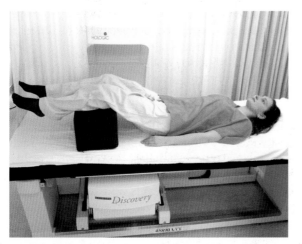

Figure 15.6 Dual-energy x-ray absorptiometry. (Courtesy University of Utah, Division of Nutrition and Integrative Physiology, Salt Lake City, Utah.)

mass (Figure 15.6).[5] Although this measurement tool is less intimidating than hydrostatic weighing or BOD POD for some people, it is substantially more expensive than other methods. Currently, DEXA is the gold standard to validate all other body composition analysis methods. It is difficult to measure individuals whose body mass extends beyond the range of the scanner.

The aforementioned methods of measuring body composition are valuable assessments for determining a person's body fatness. However, there is inherent error within all of them and to date there are insufficient data to determine population norms. Even within the same method of analysis, different results may be obtained by (1) using different settings (e.g., athlete vs. nonathlete), (2) using the same machine but with a different manufacturer, (3) using different technicians (for some methods), or (4) administrator error. Thus, maintaining the same testing protocol for longitudinal measurements is the best way to determine body composition changes accurately.

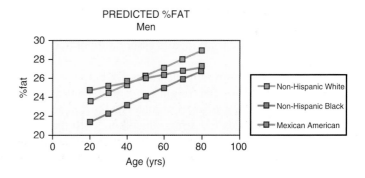

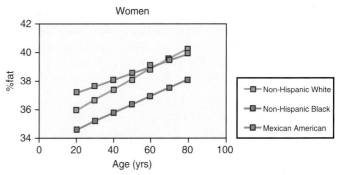

Figure 15.7 Body fat percentage by age: (A) males; (B) female. (Modified from Heymsfield, S. B., et al. [2016]. Why are there race/ethnic differences in adult body mass index-adiposity relationships? A quantitative critical review. *Obes Rev, 17*[3], 262–275.)

upper-class men for the first few decades of data gathering) and may not consider the wide variety of individuals who are found within a diverse community.

More recent height/weight tables rely on BMI calculations from the National Research Council data for weight and health, the current *Dietary Guidelines for Americans,* and recent medical studies. These guidelines directly relate height and weight ranges to relative risks for chronic diseases (see the BMI table on the inside back cover). Within each age group, obesity is significantly associated with higher all-cause mortality rates.[13]

Healthy Weight Range

The Hamwi method is a basic calculation for determining a healthy or ideal weight goal relative to sex and height:

- *Men:* 106 lb for the first 5 feet, then add or subtract 6 lb for each inch above or below 5 feet, respectively. A range of +/− 10% accounts for small and large body frames.
- *Women:* 100 lb for the first 5 feet, then add or subtract 5 lb for each inch above or below 5 feet, respectively. A range of +/− 10% accounts for small and large body frames.

For example, a 5-foot 6-inch tall woman would have an ideal body weight range of 100 lb + (6 in × 5 lb) = 130 ± 10%. Therefore, her ideal body weight is 130 lb with an acceptable range of 117 to 143 lb.

As with BMI, this calculation does not account for usual changes that are associated with age (i.e., a loss of stature and slight increases in weight) or for individuals with very high muscle mass. A person's ideal weight may give him or her an approximate number for a healthy weight goal. Relying on ideal body weight calculations must include consideration of the following: frame size, variation, and essentiality of body fat.

Body frame. We can estimate a person's body frame size by dividing his or her height (in centimeters) by their wrist circumference (in centimeters). For an accurate measurement, flex the arm at the elbow with the palm facing up and the hand relaxed. With a flexible measuring tape, measure the wrist circumference at the joint distal (i.e., toward the hand) to the styloid process (i.e., the bony wrist protrusion). Individuals with a small frame size would have an ideal body weight at the lower end of their ideal body weight range and vice versa for individuals with a large frame size. The following example indicates the standards for body frame size, which are useful for interpreting ideal body weight:

Height: 5 ft, 4 in = 64 in × 2.54 cm / in = 162.56 cm
Wrist circumference = 15.8 cm
162.56 / 15.8 = 10.29 = Medium frame

FRAME SIZE	MALE RATIO	FEMALE RATIO
Small	>10.4	>10.9
Medium	10.4 to 9.6	10.9 to 9.9
Large	<9.6	<9.9

Individual variation. Ideal weight varies with time and circumstance throughout life. A person's ideal weight depends on many factors, including sex, age, body shape, metabolic rate, genetics, physical activity, and overall well-being. Just as everyone varies in shoe size, so too do we vary in body weight.

Necessity of body fat. Some body fat is essential for survival. Every cell membrane in the body has fat molecules within it. Fat provides insulation, temperature regulation, the cushioning of vital organs, and many other functions. The estimated essential body fat level (i.e., the minimal amount required for health) is approximately 3% for men and 12% for women. These are *minimal* amounts of body fat and not optimal levels. Health and hormonal regulation decrease with inadequate body fat and severe caloric restriction.[14,15]

OBESITY AND HEALTH

Weight Extremes

Clinically severe or significant obesity is a health hazard and creates other medical problems by placing strain on all body systems. Both extremes of weight—extreme adiposity and extreme thinness—pose health problems.

Overweight and Health Problems

Obesity increases the risk of related conditions such as hypertension, type 2 diabetes, heart disease, arthritis, and certain types of cancer.[16-18] Weight loss can reduce elevated blood glucose levels and blood pressure in obese people.[19,20] In turn, these improvements reduce risks related to heart disease and diabetes.

CAUSES OF OBESITY

Energy Imbalance

How does a person become overweight? Although some people have congenital obesity, a major contributor to obesity is physical inactivity. Weight loss interventions that include physical activity can help to reach optimal body weight, BMI, waist circumference, blood pressure, lipid profiles, and insulin sensitivity among people independent of changes to dietary intake.[21] Regular exercise has a significant effect on increasing lean body mass and reducing the risk of the chronic diseases associated with obesity.

Energy imbalance (e.g., more energy intake from food and drink than energy output through physical activity and basal metabolic needs) results in excess weight accumulation. Excess intake of macronutrients is stored in the body as fat. Approximately 3500 kcal is stored in each 1 lb (0.45 kg) of body fat. A minor daily imbalance in which energy intake exceeds output by a mere 100 kcal (approximately 14 almonds) can result in a significant weight gain in 1 year, as follows:

100 kcal / day × 365 days / year = 36,500 extra kcal / year
36,500 kcal ÷ 3500 kcal / lb = 10.4 lb / year

However, some overweight people only eat moderate amounts of food relative to some people of average weight who eat much more but never seem to gain unwanted pounds. Because many individual differences exist, we know that factors other than energy balance are involved in maintaining a healthful weight.

Hormonal Control

Leptin. A research group at Rockefeller University first reported the "obesity gene" in an overweight strain of laboratory mice. Soon thereafter, these researchers located the human equivalent of the same gene.[22] This gene encodes for the hormone leptin. The researchers named the hormone *leptin* from the Greek word *leptos,* meaning "thin or slender." The initial theory was that leptin released from adipose tissue controlled satiety in people by serving as a negative feedback mechanism against the overconsumption of total energy. Plasma leptin levels rise after weight gain and drop after weight loss.[23] Recent findings show that the brain produces leptin and that it is involved in many diverse functions in the body, such as blood pressure control, cardiac function, immune function, autonomic regulation, reproduction and bone formation. Obesity is associated with leptin resistance; however, much like insulin resistance, it often depends on the brain region and/or cell type functions.[23] Some individuals with severe **early onset obesity** lack the leptin receptor, thereby receiving no negative feedback regarding energy intake.[24-26] Even so, only 3% of individuals with early onset obesity lack a leptin receptor. The exact role that leptin plays in the neurobiology of human obesity remains unclear.

Ghrelin. The counterpart to leptin is the enteric peptide ghrelin. Ghrelin is an appetite stimulant that the stomach secretes to activate the **appetite-regulating network**. Ghrelin increases food intake and seems to promote lipogenesis.[23,27] Certain forms of ghrelin increase during fasting; however, other forms of ghrelin do not change. Despite years of research, many questions remain unanswered about the roles of leptin and ghrelin and with regard to why some individuals do not respond to fluctuations of these substances in their plasma levels.

Genetic and Environmental Factors

Genetic inheritance probably influences a person's chances of obesity more than any other factor. Family food and lifestyle patterns provide an environment that allows this genetic trait to present itself (see the Cultural Considerations box, "Genetics and the Predisposition for Obesity").[16]

Genetic control. Obesity, for the most part, is a polygenic disease, meaning that there are multiple variants accounting for a person's susceptibility. More than 200

Hamwi method a formula for estimating the ideal body weight based on sex and height.

clinically severe or significant obesity a BMI of 40 kg/m² or more or a BMI of 35 to 39 kg/m² with at least one obesity-related disorder; also referred to as *extreme obesity* and *morbid obesity*.

congenital obesity the excessive accumulation and storage of fat in the body that is present during infancy and/or childhood and is considered monogenetic.

early onset obesity a genetically associated obesity that occurs during early childhood.

appetite-regulating network a hormonally controlled system of appetite stimulation and suppression.

genetic variants linked to obesity and body weight have been identified.[3] Epigenetic research indicates that maternal and paternal obesity, as well as the prenatal environment, may also affect long-term growth and metabolism in the offspring.[28,29] This is not to say that a person has no control over his or her own body weight: the genetic influence is the predisposing factor but not the determining factor. The daily life, environment, and habits that a person chooses influence the expression of this genetic trait (Figure 15.8). In a review of genetic and epigenetic influences on obesity, researchers concluded that nutrition modifications, changes in fat mass as well as fat-free mass, and exercise interventions could counteract acquired epigenetic programming.[30]

Family reinforcement. Families exert social pressure and teach children habits and attitudes toward food. Establishing inappropriate family food patterns at this age can reinforce an individual's genetic predisposition for increased body fat. We know that overweight and obese children are at significant risk for remaining overweight or obese as adults.[3,31] Thus, the development of healthy eating and physical activity habits during childhood and teenage years are highly encouraged to establish balanced food and lifestyle patterns. The Academy of Nutrition and Dietetics' nutrition guide for healthy children recommends an emphasis on increasing the nutrient-density (as opposed to energy-density) of foods, healthful food choices (such as fruits and vegetables), and physical activity.[32]

Physiologic factors. The amount of body fat that a person carries correlates to the number and size of fat cells in the body. Critical periods for becoming obese occur during early growth periods, when cells are multiplying rapidly throughout childhood and adolescence. After the body has added extra fat cells for more fuel storage, these cells remain for a person's lifetime and can store varying amounts of fat. Basal metabolic rate, physical activity, and lean muscle mass are major physiologic factors for determining individual fat storage. Women store more fat during pregnancy and after menopause in response to hormonal changes.

Cultural Considerations

Genetics and the Predisposition for Obesity

When comparing the prevalence of obesity among various racial and ethnic groups in the United States, researchers have found significant differences with regard to the risk for obesity in men and women of varying race/ethnicities (see figure).[1] There also appears to be a significant difference between non-Hispanic black, non-Hispanic Asian, and Hispanic men when compared with women of the same race and Hispanic origin.

Hispanic black and Hispanic youth compared with non-Hispanic white and non-Hispanic Asian children.[1]

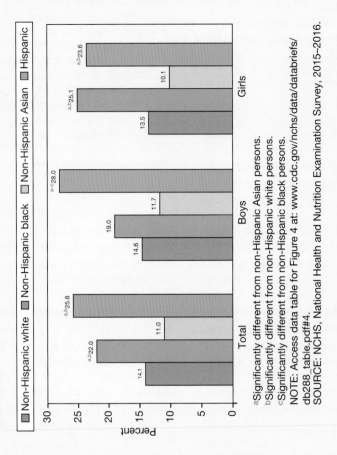

■ Non-Hispanic white ■ Non-Hispanic black □ Non-Hispanic Asian ■ Hispanic

[a] Significantly different from non-Hispanic Asian persons.
[b] Significantly different from non-Hispanic white persons.
[c] Significantly different from non-Hispanic black persons.
NOTE: Access data table for Figure 4 at: www.cdc.gov/nchs/data/databriefs/db288_table.pdf#4.
SOURCE: NCHS, National Health and Nutrition Examination Survey, 2015–2016.

Although genetics does play a role in the prevalence of and predisposition for obesity, such influences cannot explain such an increase in obesity among the entire population. These data also show that there may be many cultural, ethnic, environmental, and socioeconomic factors that must be addressed when attempting to slow or even reverse the alarming trends in obesity.

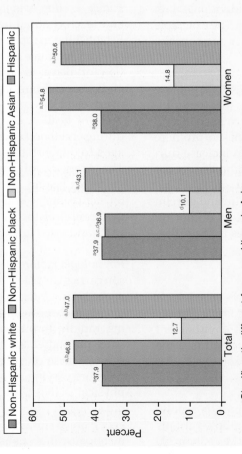

■ Non-Hispanic white ■ Non-Hispanic black □ Non-Hispanic Asian ■ Hispanic

[a] Significantly different from non-Hispanic Asian persons.
[b] Significantly different from non-Hispanic white persons.
[c] Significantly different from Hispanic persons.
[d] Significantly different from women of same race and Hispanic origin.
Notes: All estimates are age adjusted by the direct method to the 2000 U.S. census population using the age groups 20–39, 40–59, and 60 and over.
Access data table for Figure 2 at: www.cdc.gov/nchs/data/databriefs/db288_table.pdf#2.
Source: NCHS, National Health and Nutrition Examination Survey, 2015–2016.

Another dramatic difference was noted when looking at the data for prevalence of childhood (2–19 years old) obesity among various racial and ethnic groups (see figure). The numbers show a significantly higher prevalence of obesity in both sexes among non-

REFERENCE

1. Hales, C. M., Carroll, M. D., Fryar, C. D., & Ogden, C. L. (2017). *Prevalence of obesity among adults and youth: United states, 2015–2016. NCHS data brief, no.288.* Hyattsville, MD: National Center for Health Statistics.

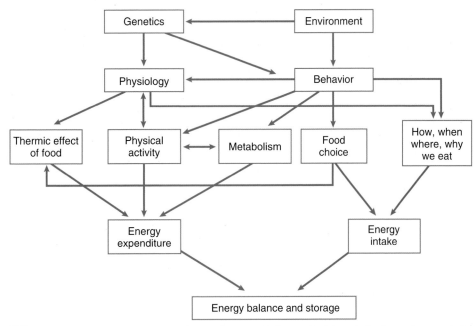

Figure 15.8 Interwoven influence among genetics, environmental effects, physiology, behavior, and energy balance.

Psychologic factors. Work, family, and social environments may cultivate emotional stress, which many people respond to by eating "comfort foods." Media messages and societal pressures to maintain the cultural "ideal" thin body type contribute to the strain of constant dieting. These messages are often dichotomous (e.g., good versus bad food; eat this, not that) and convey negative and oversimplified ideas, which in turn can perpetuate the chronic dieters' dilemma of yo-yo dieting (e.g., weight loss followed by weight gain) and cause deleterious reductions in metabolic rate and lean body mass.

Other environmental factors. Many environmental factors add to the ever-increasing problem of obesity. The following are only a few examples related to food: an increase in energy-dense food availability, low-cost fast and convenient foods, increase in portion sizes, and a decrease in food preparation time and skills. Environmental factors related to lifestyle that contribute to energy imbalances include a decrease in physical activity, increase in screen time (e.g., television, computer, video games), less active leisure time, and decreased physical requirements for activities of daily living (e.g., domestic appliances such as washing machines, vacuum cleaners, and dishwashers; central heating, cars, delivery services, elevators).

INDIVIDUAL DIFFERENCES AND EXTREME PRACTICES

Individual Energy Balance Levels
Several factors influence a person's energy balance. Estimating energy requirements is a useful starting point for practitioners to assess an individual's calorie needs.

Energy out. Factors such as the basal metabolic rate (BMR), body size, lean body mass, age, sex, and physical activity influence the total daily calorie expenditure (see Chapter 6). Some people have more genetic-based metabolic efficiency (i.e., the ability to "burn" energy more readily than others do).

Energy in. When a person's energy intake is calculated, Nutrition Facts labels (see Chapter 13) and dietary analysis software provide only an estimated value. Reported food and drink values represent the averages of many similar samples of that type of food. Thus, determining the exact amount of kilocalories consumed by a person throughout the day is difficult.

Extreme Practices
Desperate attempts to lose weight may drive people to extreme measures, which sometimes worsen health risks.

Fad diets. A constant array of diet books and weight-loss supplements that promise to "melt the fat away" continue to flood the American market (Table 15.1). These books and supplements usually sell briefly and then fade away, largely because their quick fixes either do not work or are not sustainable. They lead individuals to believe that weight loss is easy and effortless, when the reality is very different. Such a complex problem has no simple answers. Most of the fad diets fail on the following two counts:

1. *Scientific inaccuracies and misinformation:* Fad diets and supplements are often nutritionally inadequate and based on false claims.

2. *Failure to address the necessity of changing long-term habits and behaviors:* People are often set up for failure regarding the maintenance of a healthy weight. The complexity of changing food and exercise habits to develop a new lifestyle is often unrecognized.

With some diets, the degree of energy restriction is impossible to maintain long term. Many fad dieters find themselves caught in a vicious cycle of **chronic dieting syndrome** and its harmful physical and psychologic effects.

Table 15.1   Comparison of Select Common Weight-Loss Diets

DIET	PHILOSOPHY	FOODS TO EAT	FOODS TO AVOID	DIET COMPOSITION (AVERAGE FOR 3 DAYS)	RECOMMENDED SUPPLEMENTS	HEALTH CLAIMS SCIENTIFICALLY PROVEN?	PRACTICALITY	LOSE AND MAINTAIN WEIGHT?
Atkins[a]	Eating too many carbohydrates causes obesity and other health problems; ketosis leads to decreased hunger; carbohydrates prevent your body from burning fat	Meat, fish, poultry, eggs, cheese, high-fiber vegetables, butter, oil, nuts, seeds	Carbohydrates, specifically bread, pasta, most fruits and high-carbohydrate vegetables, milk, alcohol	Protein: 27% Carbohydrates: 5% Fat: 68% (saturated, 26%)	Atkins supplement that includes chromium picolinate, carnitine, co-enzyme Q10	No long-term validated studies published	Limited food choices; difficult to eat in restaurants, because only plain protein sources and limited vegetables and salads allowed	Yes, but initial weight loss is mostly water; does not promote a positive attitude toward food groups; difficult to maintain for the long term because the diet restricts food choices
hCG[b]	Daily injections of human chorionic gonadotropin hormone keep the body in an anabolic state and reduce appetite; combined with a very low calorie diet that promotes weight loss	500 calories per day Breakfast: Tea or coffee without sugar Lunch and Dinner: 100 g of lean meat, vegetable, breadstick, and either an apple, an orange, or ½ a grapefruit	Oils, butter, dressing Also avoid cosmetics, lotions, medications, massages	Protein: 53% Carbohydrates: 36% Fat: 11%	125 IU of hCG administered daily	No long-term validated studies published to support the claim Studies have found dangers such as thromboembolism, hypothyroidism, bone mineral loss, and anxiety	Very limited food choices and caloric intake	Yes, by caloric restriction; limited food choices are not practical for the long term; diet is only meant to be followed for 26–40 days
Intermittent Fasting[c,d]	Partial to complete fast 1–2 days per week with no restriction on other days. Partial fast versions allow for 500–600 kcal every other or 2 days per week with no restriction on the other days	All foods are allowed	Only total kcals is limited on fasting days	Not applicable (dependent on individual choices)	None	Evidence exists for short-term weight loss, lack of long-term maintenance studies	May be very difficult due to extreme decrease in kcals on fasting days	Possibly if weekly caloric intake is lower than output

DIET	PHILOSOPHY	FOODS TO EAT	FOODS TO AVOID	DIET COMPOSITION (AVERAGE FOR 3 DAYS)	RECOMMENDED SUPPLEMENTS	HEALTH CLAIMS SCIENTIFICALLY PROVEN?	PRACTICALITY	LOSE AND MAINTAIN WEIGHT?
Paleo[e]	Eating the diet we are genetically adapted to based on our hunter-gatherer ancestry; high-protein, low-carbohydrate intake will reduce risk of chronic disease and promote weight loss	Meat, seafood, fruits, vegetables, eggs, nuts, seeds, plant oils	Grains, legumes, dairy, refined sugars, potatoes, processed foods, salt	Protein: 46% Carbohydrates: 28% Fat: 28%	None	No; theories and long-term results not validated	Deficient in calcium and vitamin D	Possibly if caloric intake is less than output
The South Beach Diet[f]	Switching to the "right" carbohydrates stops insulin resistance, reduces cravings, and causes weight loss	Seafood, chicken breast, lean meat, low-fat cheese, nut oils, most vegetables, low-fat dairy; later, most whole grains and beans	Fatty meats, full-fat cheese, refined grains, sweets, juice, potatoes	Phase 1: Protein: 34% Carbohydrates: 14.8% Fat: 50%	Multivitamins and omega-3 fatty acids; Metamucil recommended during phase 1	Evidence does exist to link the avoidance of saturated fats with the reduced risk of heart disease	First phase is more difficult; later phases are mostly healthy foods and more practical	Yes, although initial weight loss is mostly water; sustained weight loss through reduced calorie intake
Weight Watchers[g]	Promotes wellness and weight loss through diet, exercise, supportive community, and behavior change. Based on a points system, each food and activity has an associated point value.	Focus on lean protein (poultry and fish), beans, legumes, fruits, vegetables	No food is off limits and can be budgeted for in the daily point system	Protein: 10%–35% Carbohydrates: 45%–65% Fat 10%–35% (saturated, <10%)	Recommends a multivitamin	Evidence does support that it produces weight loss up to 1 year.	Various types of programs available depending on cost and level of support from health coaches. Depending on accessibility it may be difficult to have direct support.	Yes if caloric intake is less than output

Continued

Table 15.1   Comparison of Select Common Weight-Loss Diets—cont'd

DIET	PHILOSOPHY	FOODS TO EAT	FOODS TO AVOID	DIET COMPOSITION (AVERAGE FOR 3 DAYS)	RECOMMENDED SUPPLEMENTS	HEALTH CLAIMS SCIENTIFICALLY PROVEN?	PRACTICALITY	LOSE AND MAINTAIN WEIGHT?
Whole30[h]	Eliminating processed foods for a 30-day period allows your metabolism to reset and rebalances hormone levels	Meat, seafood, eggs, vegetables, some fruit	Added sugars, alcohol, grains, legumes, dairy	Protein: 53% Carbohydrates: 30% Fat: 19%	None	No long-term validated studies published	Not practical for long term; difficult to eat in restaurants because of restrictions	Possibly, if caloric intake is less than output
Zone 1-2-3 Program[i]	Eating the right combination of foods leads to a metabolic state at which the body functions at peak performance and stabilizes hormonal communication, thereby leading to decreased hunger, increased weight loss, increased energy, and increased control of cellular inflammation	Protein, fat, and carbohydrates in exact proportions only (40/30/30); alcohol in moderation	Fruit (some types), saturated fats	Protein: 34% Carbohydrates: 36% Fat: 29% (saturated, 9%) Alcohol: 1%	200IU of vitamin E	No; theories and long-term results not validated	Food must be eaten in required proportions of protein, fat, and carbohydrates; menus are plain and unappealing; vegetable portions are very large; difficult to calculate portions	Yes, by caloric restriction; could result in weight maintenance if carefully followed; diet is rigid and difficult to maintain

IU, International units.

[a]Atkins, R. C. (1999). *Dr. Atkins' new diet revolution.* New York: Avon Books.
[b]Simeons, D. A. (2010). *Pounds & inches: A new approach to obesity.* Rome, Italy: Popular Publishing. Goodbar, N., Foushee, J., Eagerton, D., Haynes, K., & Johnson, A. (2013). Effects of the human chorionic gonadotropin diet on patient outcomes. *Ann Pharmacother. 47,* E23–E23.
[c]Carter, S., Clifton, P. M., & Keogh, J. B. (2018). Effect of intermittent compared with continuous energy restricted diet on glycemic control in patients with type 2 diabetes: A randomized noninferiority trial. *JAMA Netw Open, 1*(3), e180756.
[d]Leicht, L. (2018). Intermittent fasting. WebMD LLC. Retrieved April 8, 2019, from www.webmd.com/diet/a-z/intermittent-fasting.
[e]Cordain, L. (n.d.). *The Paleo Diet™—live well, live longer.* Retrieved December 3, 2014, from thepaleodiet.com/.
[f]Agatston, A. (2003). *The South Beach Diet.* Emmaus, PA: Rodale.
[g]Weight Watchers International, Inc. (n.d.). *Weight Watchers.* Retrieved April 8, 2019, from www.weightwatchers.com/us/.
[h]Hartwig, M., & Hartwig, D. (2014). *It starts with food.* Riverside, NJ: Victory Belt Publishing.
[i]Sears, B. (1995). *The zone.* New York: HarperCollins.

Very low–calorie diets. The drastic approach of very low–calorie diets (e.g., <800 kcal/day) requires constant medical supervision. Possible effects of a very low–calorie diet include acidosis, low blood pressure, electrolyte imbalance, a loss of lean muscle mass, and decreased BMR. Long-term maintenance has deleterious effects on health. Many people discontinue these diets because of the extreme nature and the high medical cost.[19] When individuals resume normal eating after following a very low–calorie diet, they frequently gain back more fat mass than lost initially.[33]

Specific macronutrient restrictions. Avoiding any food group or macronutrient (e.g., carbohydrates, fats, or proteins) as a means for weight loss is unfounded. Such diets that are extremely low fat or extremely low in carbohydrates are usually too restrictive to maintain for extended periods, and they also carry health risks.

Clothing and body wraps. Special "sauna suits" and body wrapping claim to help weight loss in certain body areas or to reduce cellulite tissue. Some people endure mummy-like body wrapping in an attempt to reduce body size. However, the resulting small weight loss is a result of temporary water loss. Fat mass cannot be melted away; the stored energy must be used (i.e., burning the calories) in the **adipocytes**.

Weight-loss drugs. Because of potentially fatal complications, diuretics and exogenous hormones used to alter body weight or lean tissue mass require strict medical necessity and supervision. Various amphetamine compounds were once popular for the medical treatment of obesity; however, there are dangerous health consequences and they are no longer used. Common over-the-counter drugs include phenylpropylamine (Accutrim, Dexatrim), which is a stimulant that is similar to amphetamine; and ephedra, which is currently banned in the United States. In addition, many herbal products claim weight-loss benefits. The U.S. Food and Drug Administration (FDA) maintains an updated list of contaminated and potentially dangerous over-the-counter drugs and supplements on its website (search "drug information for consumers" at www.fda.gov).

A pair of related weight-loss drugs—fenfluramine and phentermine—were previously prescribed together in the popular "fen-phen" combination for weight loss. Shortly thereafter, physicians found that one in eight clients who were using fen-phen developed valvular regurgitation, which can be fatal.[34] The FDA, with the support of the medical community, quickly removed these drugs from the market in 1997. Likewise, in 2010 the FDA withdrew sibutramine (Meridia) from the U.S. market because of an increased risk of heart attack and stroke with its use. Sibutramine was another weight-loss medication that worked by reducing appetite and increasing energy expenditure. Although the pursuit of pharmacotherapy for the treatment of obesity is intense, few safe options are currently available.

Prescription medications that treat obesity generally work in one of the following four ways:
1. Reducing energy intake by suppressing the appetite
2. Increasing energy expenditure by stimulating the BMR
3. Reducing the absorption of food in the gut
4. Altering lipogenesis and lipolysis

The FDA approved orlistat (Alli, Xenical) for the treatment of clinically significant obesity in 1999. Orlistat inhibits dietary fat absorption. Orlistat has been successful with weight loss, but reports indicate that maximal benefits occur only when it is combined with lifestyle changes that induce a **negative energy balance**.[35] As with many medications, unpleasant side effects are associated with this medication, including diarrhea, gas, and abdominal pain (see the Drug-Nutrient Interaction box, "Orlistat: An Over-the-Counter Weight-Loss Aid").

 Drug-Nutrient Interaction

Orlistat: An Over-the-Counter Weight-Loss Aid

In February 2007 the U.S. Food and Drug Administration approved the drug orlistat (Alli) as an over-the-counter weight-loss aid for overweight adults. When combined with a low-fat, decreased calorie diet, the drug can be an effective adjunct to a weight-loss program. Orlistat works by inhibiting the absorption of fat in the intestine by up to a one-third of what is consumed, thereby reducing the caloric impact of food.[1]

As a result of its mechanism of action, orlistat also inhibits the absorption of fat-soluble vitamins. A multivitamin taken at least 2 hours before or after a dose of orlistat is recommended to prevent the suboptimal absorption of vitamins A, D, E, and K.[2] In addition, orlistat can cause uncomfortable gastrointestinal side effects such as flatulence and loose stools. Eating large amounts of fat can increase these side effects, whereas fiber supplements that contain psyllium may help to reduce them.[3]

Currently, orlistat is the only anti-obesity drug approved for use by adolescents 12 to 19 years of age, because it may aid in reduced BMI and waist circumference. However, it is contraindicated for people with absorptive disorders (e.g., pancreatitis, gall bladder disorders) and for those who are not overweight. Orlistat should not be taken for longer than 2 years. Because this drug is now available over the counter, clients may take orlistat irresponsibly. It is important for clinicians to inquire about all medications and dietary supplements that their clients are taking so that they may accurately advise these individuals about potential interactions and negative health consequences.

REFERENCES
1. Rosa-Goncalves, P., & Majerowicz, D. (2019). Pharmacotherapy of obesity: Limits and perspectives. *American Journal of Cardiovascular Drugs*, 19(4), 349–364.
2. Paccosi, S., Cresci, B., Pala, L., et al. (2020). Obesity therapy: How and why? *Current Medicinal Chemistry*, 27(2),174–186.
3. Sumithran, P., & Proietto, J. (2014). Benefit-risk assessment of orlistat in the treatment of obesity. *Drug Safety*, 37(8), 597–608.

---

chronic dieting syndrome a cyclic pattern of weight loss by dieting followed by rapid weight gain; this abnormal psychophysiologic food pattern becomes chronic, changing a person's natural body metabolism and relative body composition to the abnormal state of a metabolically obese person of normal weight.
adipocytes fat cells.

The FDA approved two other drugs in 2012 primarily for use in obese and/or clients with type 2 diabetes; these drugs were lorcaserin (Belviq) and phentermine/topiramate (Qsymia). Lorcaserin affects certain serotonin receptors to enhance satiety, thus decreasing caloric intake. Phentermine/topiramate reduces caloric intake by slowing gut emptying.[35] In 2014 the FDA approved the use of liraglutide (Saxenda) and naltrexone/bupropion (Contrave) for weight loss. Similar to Belviq and Qsymia, these drugs were originally developed and approved for treatment of non–weight-related conditions. Liraglutide causes weight loss by an increase in satiety and thus a decrease in calorie consumption. However, it is very expensive and requires injection of the drug, resulting in a very small client pool for whom it is suitable for use. The combined effect of naltrexone and bupropion also enhances the satiety signals in the body, which leads to a decrease in food intake and body weight. Contrave has adverse side effects, such as nausea, constipation, vomiting, headache, dizziness, dry mouth, and changes in blood pressure. Contrave is contraindicated in individuals with uncontrolled hypertension and cardiovascular disease.[35] Thus, even though the above drugs aid in weight loss, they are unsafe for many people, and long-term studies are required to determine broad-use safety. When a client discontinues the medication, weight regain is likely without adequate nutrition and lifestyle changes.

Surgery. Surgical techniques are a treatment option for severely obese clients who have not had success with other methods of long-term weight loss. Studies show that bariatric surgery provides significant and sustained weight loss and a reduced relative risk of death because of a decrease in several conditions and co-morbid diseases associated with obesity.[19] Although surgery historically has been the most successful method of permanent weight loss among clients with severe obesity, it is not without risks and complications.

There are two primary types of surgical procedures for weight loss: restrictive (e.g., making the stomach smaller) and combination restrictive and malabsorptive procedures (e.g., making the stomach smaller and inducing malabsorption). Gastric restriction surgeries reduce the client's appetite and food intake by creating a small stomach pouch that only allows for tiny amounts of food at any given time. For gastric banding, a surgeon places an adjustable gastric band on a client's stomach during laparoscopic surgery. Using a small port, the band is subcutaneously adjusted as needed (Figure 15.9A). Malabsorptive procedures rearrange the small intestine to decrease the length and efficiency of the gut for nutrient absorption. The most commonly performed is the Roux-en-Y bariatric procedure (Figure 15.9B). This procedure restricts the stomach to about 20 to 30 mL, reconfigures the small intestine, and may lead to neuron and hormone changes within the gut. Because of the reconfiguration of the small intestine, the client needs vitamin and mineral supplements for the remainder of his or her life. The most common nutrient deficiencies include iron, calcium, vitamin D, and vitamin B_{12}. The inherent risks of surgery and postsurgical malnutrition are critical issues for the client.[36,37]

Weight-loss surgeries require a skilled team of specialists, nutrition care, careful client selection, and continuous follow-up in partnership with the client and his or her family. Following any surgical procedure, counseling by a registered dietitian nutritionist (RDN) is important to avoid complications such as **dumping syndrome**. The RDN will counsel on the importance of decreasing simple carbohydrate intake, avoiding fluid with food, and determining portion size and an eating plan, while providing instruction on how to avoid malnutrition. Long-term success is dependent on the client being able to maintain nutrition, physical activity, and behavioral changes to support health.

A more limited type of cosmetic surgery developed during the 1980s is a form of local fat removal, called **lipectomy** or *liposuction*. Lipectomy removes fat deposits under the skin in places of cosmetic concern, such as the stomach, hips, or thighs. A thin tube enters through a small incision in the skin and suctions out the desired amount of fat. This procedure can be painful, and it carries risks such as infection, large disfiguring skin depressions, and blood clots that can lead to dangerous circulatory problems or even kidney failure. Any surgical procedure carries risk and may cause other problems and side effects.

---

negative energy balance more total energy is expended than consumed.

dumping syndrome condition in which there is a quick emptying of the stomach of a hyperosmolar content into the small intestine, causing fluid to shift into the intestinal lumen from the intravascular compartment.

lipectomy the surgical removal of subcutaneous fat by suction through a tube that is inserted into a surface incision or by the removal of larger amounts of subcutaneous fat through a major surgical incision.

Adjustable gastric band   **Roux-en-Y gastric bypass**

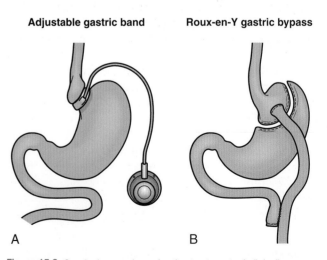

A   B

Figure 15.9 Surgical procedures for the treatment of clinically severe obesity: (A) gastric banding; (B) Roux-en-Y.

A SOUND WEIGHT-MANAGEMENT PROGRAM

ESSENTIAL CHARACTERISTICS

There are no shortcuts to successful long-term weight control or weight loss. Weight loss requires hard work and strong individual motivation. Weight management requires a personalized intensive lifestyle intervention that focuses on lifestyle, food, and exercise behaviors. Choices that build a healthy mental and physical state with ample positive social support are desirable. The most recent position paper by the Academy of Nutrition and Dietetics regarding weight management states that "successful treatment of overweight and obesity in adults requires the ability of adopting and maintaining lifestyle behaviors, which contribute to both sides of the energy-balance equation. Lifestyle behaviors are influenced by several factors at differing levels of the socioecological model, which include factors at the intrapersonal, community, organizational, government, and public level."[36]

BEHAVIOR MODIFICATION

Basic Principles

Food behavior is rooted in many human experiences. Behavior-oriented therapies assist individuals in changing patterns that contribute to excessive weight and can help empower them to plan constructive actions to meet personal health goals. This behavioral approach must begin with a detailed examination of the following three basic aspects of each undesirable eating behavior:

1. *Cues or antecedents:* What stimulates the behavior?
2. *Response:* What happens during the eating or sedentary behavior after the cue?
3. *Consequences:* What happens after the response to the eating or sedentary behavior that reinforces it?

Strategies and Actions

A successful program of personal behavior modification for weight management focuses on the following: (1) management of the eating behavior (e.g., a food diary that includes when, where, why, how, and how much); (2) the promotion of physical activity to increase energy output; and (3) the pursuit of emotional (stress), social, and psychologic health. Three progressive actions follow for the planning of individual strategies as outlined here.

Defining problem behavior. Specifically define the problem behavior, potential barriers to the new behavior, and the desired behavior outcome. This process clearly establishes goals and contributing objectives.

Recording and analyzing baseline behavior. Record eating and exercise behavior, and carefully analyze it in terms of physical setting and people involved. What types of patterns emerge? How often do these patterns occur? What conditions seem to trigger desirable and undesirable behaviors? What consequent events seem to maintain the habits (e.g., time, place, people, social responses, hunger before and after, emotional state, other factors)?

Planning a behavior management strategy. Set up controls of the external environment that involves the situational forces related to each of the three behavior areas involved: (1) the stimulus that occurs before the behavior; (2) the response to the behavior; and (3) the results of the behavior. The goal is to break the identified links to old and undesirable behaviors and to recondition them to the desired new eating and exercise behaviors. The Clinical Applications box entitled "Breaking Old Links: Strategies for Changing Food Behavior" provides a few examples of reconditioning personal food and exercise habits to more positive behaviors.

DIETARY MODIFICATION

Basic Principles

The central dietary approach in a weight-management program designed to achieve lasting success includes the following five characteristics:

1. *Realistic goals:* Goals must be realistic in terms of overall weight loss and rate of loss, averaging ½ to 1 lb per week (or no more than 2 lb per week for clinically severe obese clients). Reviews and guidelines based on the available literature state that even minor amounts of weight loss (e.g., 3% to 10% of body weight) can reduce the health risks that are associated with obesity.[36,38] Therefore, clients do not need to focus on achieving their *ideal* body weight but rather a relative weight loss based on their current weight.
2. *Negative energy balance:* The most important factor that affects weight loss is the establishment of a negative energy balance with a reduction of about 500 kcal/day.[36] The best approach to negative energy balance is through a combination of reduced energy intake and increased energy output.
3. *Nutrient adequacy:* The diet must be nutritionally adequate. Consuming less food requires conscious choices of nutrient-dense foods. In addition, the ratio of macronutrients should have an appropriate balance with a wide variety of food sources.
4. *Cultural appeal:* The food plan must be similar enough to an individual's cultural eating patterns to form the basis for a permanent alteration of eating habits.
5. *Energy readjustment to maintain weight:* Once clients have achieved the desired weight, they adjust their kilocalorie intake in accordance with maintenance needs.

Energy Balance Components

The two sides of the energy balance equation are energy intake in the form of food and drink and energy output in the form of metabolic work and physical activity. Manipulation of either or both sides of the equation aid in successful weight reduction.

---

intensive lifestyle intervention lifestyle intervention delivered at high intensity (≥14 sessions in 6 months).

Clinical Applications

Breaking Old Links: Strategies for Changing Food Behavior

Old habits die hard. They are never easy to change, but the effort is worthwhile in the case of undesirable eating behaviors that contribute to excess body fat and are harmful to health. Following are some practical behavioral suggestions.

1. Manage Behavioral Cues

Minimize as many cues for the problem behavior as possible. Anticipate situations that are associated with problem foods, and then put temptation out of reach, and make the problem behavior as difficult as possible to perform. Freeze leftovers, remove problem food items from the kitchen or store them in hard-to-reach places, or take a route home other than by the familiar bakery or fast-food restaurant.

Suppress the cues that cannot be entirely eliminated. Control social situations that maintain the behavior, reward the alternate desired behavior, have a trusted person help keep you accountable for your behavior changes, manage stress without the use of food, minimize contact with excessive food, use smaller plates to make smaller food portions appear larger, and make use of positive non-food "treat" activities (e.g., hiking, bowling, or a massage).

Strengthen cues for desirable behaviors. Set SMART goals: Specific, Measurable, Attainable, Realistic, and Timely. Do not set your goals too high. Keep them focused. Follow the MyPlate guidelines and the *Dietary Guidelines for Americans* for appropriate food choices and amounts. Do not be an obsessive calorie counter. Instead, learn the general values of some of your home-prepared meals, modify recipes or make occasional substitutes, and read labels often. Use food behavior aids (e.g., records, a diary or journal). Distribute appropriate foods among meal and snack patterns. Avoid the common pattern of no breakfast, little or no lunch, and a huge dinner. Make desirable food behavior as attractive and as enjoyable as possible. For home meals try to avoid making a separate menu for yourself (or another person on a weight-loss program). Adapt your needs to the family meal, and then adjust the seasonings or method of preparation to involve fewer kilocalories, especially by reducing or omitting fat. Everyone deserves to be healthy. When eating away from home, watch your portions. When you are a guest, limit extras such as sauces and dressings, and trim your meat well. In restaurants, select singly prepared items rather than combination dishes. Avoid items with heavy sauces or fat seasonings as well as fried foods. Select fruit or sherbet for dessert rather than pastries. Focus more on the social aspect rather than the food.

2. Manage Actual Food Behavior in Response to Cues

Slow the pace of eating. Take one bite at a time, and place the utensil on the plate between bites. Chew each bite slowly. Sip water. Consciously plan conversation with meal companions for between bites. Visualize eating in slow motion. Enhance the social aspect of eating.

Savor the food. Eat slowly, and sense the taste, smell, and texture of the food. Develop and practice these sensory feelings to the extent that they can be described and brought to mind afterward. Look for food seasonings and combinations that will enhance this process and bring to mind positive feelings about the food experience.

Do not be discouraged if you binge. Individuals who have previously struggled with binge eating behavior may have an occasional setback. Try to keep these binges infrequent and, when possible, plan ahead for special occasions. Adjust the following day's diet or the remainder of the same day accordingly. Changing binge eating behavior is not easy. The assistance of psychologic and nutrition experts may be helpful.

Avoid eating in response to stress; eating because of stress may cause guilt and added calories while doing nothing for the stressor. Instead try doing a combination of things to better cope: write in your journal, talk to someone, go for a walk, hug a friend, do a hobby, take 10 deep breaths, or drink a glass of water.

3. Manage the Follow-up Behavior

Decelerate the problem behavior. Slow down its frequency, and respond neutrally when it occurs rather than with negative talk or thoughts. Give social reinforcement to the decreasing number of times that the problem behavior occurs. Acknowledge the ultimate consequences of the undesirable behavior in the development of health problems.

Accelerate the desired behavior. Update the progress records or personal journal daily. Respond positively to all desired behavior, and provide material reinforcement for positive behavior. Provide social reinforcement by enlisting the help of close friends or family for constructive efforts to modify behavior. Staying focused on "Why is this change important to me?" Or, "Why do I want to make this change?" You will be able to find intrinsic motivation for when it gets really hard. Some find it helpful to repeat it as a mantra daily.

Such a program requires patience, motivation, and work. Continuously evaluate progress toward desired behavior while maintaining a realistic goal and then plan individual or group maintenance and support activities during an extended follow-up period.

Energy input: food behaviors. Clinicians should not assign arbitrary serving sizes and numbers of servings without knowledge of the client's actual eating patterns. Food diaries are helpful for establishing the client's normal food choices, the amounts typically eaten, and the distribution of meals throughout the day. From this baseline information, clinicians can help to identify minor changes to initiate, such as eating smaller portions, replacing sugar-sweetened beverages with water, decreasing the overall energy density of foods consumed, and encouraging clients to eat slowly to savor the food's taste and to improve satiety.[36,39] Emphasize whole foods and minimize processed foods. Ideally, the distribution of calories is even throughout the day. The use of fat, sugar, salt, and fiber should be quantified and modified, if necessary, to meet the *Dietary Guidelines for Americans*. Table 15.2 provides suggested servings of the food groups and subgroups to meet recommended nutrient intakes at various kilocalorie levels. These guides can serve as a focal point for sound nutrition education. The Clinical Applications box "Breaking Old Links: Strategies for Changing Food Behavior" provides some additional suggestions.

Table 15.2   Healthy U.S.-Style Dietary Pattern for Ages 2 and Older, With Daily or Weekly Amounts From Food Groups, Subgroups, and Components

CALORIE LEVEL OF PATTERN[a]	1000	1200	1400	1600	1800	2000	2200	2400	2600	2800	3000	3200
FOOD GROUP OR SUBGROUP[b]	Daily Amount[c] of Food From Each Group											
	(Vegetable and protein foods subgroup amounts are per week.)											
Vegetables (cup eq/day)	1	1½	1½	2	2½	2½	3	3	3½	3½	4	4
Vegetable Subgroups in Weekly Amounts												
Dark-Green Vegetables (cup eq/wk)	½	1	1	1½	1½	1½	2	2	2½	2½	2½	2½
Red and Orange Vegetables (cup eq/wk)	2½	3	3	4	5½	5½	6	6	7	7	7½	7½
Beans, Peas, Lentils (cup eq/wk)	½	½	½	1	1½	1½	2	2	2½	2½	3	3
Starchy Vegetables (cup eq/wk)	2	3½	3½	4	5	5	6	6	7	7	8	8
Other Vegetables (cup eq/wk)	1½	2½	2½	3½	4	4	5	5	5½	5½	7	7
Fruits (cup eq/day)	1	1	1½	1½	1½	2	2	2	2	2½	2½	2½
Grains (ounce eq/day)	3	4	5	5	6	6	7	8	9	10	10	10
Whole Grains (ounce eq/day)[d]	1½	2	2½	3	3	3	3½	4	4½	5	5	5
Refined Grains (ounce eq/day)	1½	2	2½	2	3	3	3½	4	4½	5	5	5
Dairy (cup eq/day)	2	2½	2½	3	3	3	3	3	3	3	3	3
Protein Foods (ounce eq/day)	2	3	4	5	5	5½	6	6½	6½	7	7	7
Protein Foods Subgroups in Weekly Amounts												
Meats, Poultry, Eggs (ounce eq/wk)	10	14	19	23	23	26	28	31	31	33	33	33
Seafood (ounce eq/wk)[e]	2-3[f]	4	6	8	8	8	9	10	10	10	10	10
Nuts, Seeds, Soy Products (ounce eq/wk)	2	2	3	4	4	5	5	5	5	6	6	6
Oils (grams/day)	15	17	17	22	24	27	29	31	34	36	44	51
Limit on Calories for Other Uses (kcal/day)[g]	130	80	90	100	140	240	250	320	350	370	440	580
Limit on Calories for Other Uses (%/day)	13%	7%	6%	6%	8%	12%	11%	13%	13%	13%	15%	18%

NOTE: The total dietary pattern should not exceed *Dietary Guidelines* limits for added sugars, saturated fat, and alcohol; be within the Acceptable Macronutrient Distribution Ranges for protein, carbohydrate, and total fats; and stay within calorie limits. Values are rounded.

aPatterns at 1000, 1200, and 1400 kcal levels are designed to meet the nutritional needs of children ages 2 through 8 years. Patterns from 1600 to 3200 kcal are designed to meet the nutritional needs of children 9 years and older and adults. If a child 4 through 8 years of age needs more energy and, therefore, is following a pattern at 1600 calories or more, his/her recommended amount from the dairy group should be 2½ cup eq per day. Amount of dairy for children ages 9 through 18 is 3 cup eq per day regardless of calorie level. The 1000 and 1200 kcal patterns are not intended for children 9 and older or adults. The 1400 kcal level is not intended for children ages 10 and older or adults.

bFoods in each group and subgroup are:

Vegetables

Dark-Green Vegetables: All fresh, frozen, and canned dark-green leafy vegetables and broccoli, cooked or raw: for example, amaranth leaves, basil, beet greens, bitter melon leaves, bok choy, broccoli, chamnamul, chrysanthemum leaves, chard, cilantro, collards, cress, dandelion greens, kale, lambsquarters, mustard greens, poke greens, romaine lettuce, spinach, nettles, taro leaves, turnip greens, and watercress.

Red and Orange Vegetables: All fresh, frozen, and canned red and orange vegetables or juice, cooked or raw: for example, calabaza, carrots, red chili peppers, red or orange bell peppers, pimento/pimiento, sweet potatoes, tomatoes, 100% tomato juice, and winter squash such as acorn, butternut, kabocha, and pumpkin.

Beans, Peas, Lentils: All cooked from dry or canned beans, peas, chickpeas, and lentils: for example, black beans, black-eyed peas, bayo beans, brown beans, chickpeas (garbanzo beans), cowpeas, edamame, fava beans, kidney beans, lentils, lima beans, mung beans, navy beans, pigeon peas, pink beans, pinto beans, split peas, soybeans, and white beans. Does not include green beans or green peas.

Starchy Vegetables: All fresh, frozen, and canned starchy vegetables: for example, breadfruit, burdock root, cassava, corn, jicama, lotus root, lima beans, immature or raw (not dried) peas (e.g., cowpeas, black-eyed peas, green peas, pigeon peas), plantains, white potatoes, salsify, tapioca, taro root (dasheen or yautia), water chestnuts, yam, and yucca.

Other Vegetables: All other fresh, frozen, and canned vegetables, cooked or raw: for example, artichoke, asparagus, avocado, bamboo shoots, bean sprouts, beets, bitter melon (bitter gourd, balsam pear), broccoflower, Brussels sprouts, cabbage (green, red, napa, savoy), cactus pads (nopales), cauliflower, celeriac, celery, chayote (mirliton), chives, cucumber, eggplant, fennel bulb, garlic, ginger root, green beans, iceberg lettuce, kohlrabi, leeks, luffa (Chinese okra), mushrooms, okra, onions, peppers (chili and bell types that are not red or orange in color), radicchio, sprouted beans (e.g. sprouted mung beans), radish, rutabaga, seaweed, snow peas, summer squash, tomatillos, turnips, and winter melons.

Fruits

All fresh, frozen, canned, and dried fruits and 100% fruit juices: for example, apples, Asian pears, apricots, bananas, berries (e.g., blackberries, blueberries, cranberries, currants, dewberries, huckleberries, kiwifruit, loganberries, mulberries, raspberries, and strawberries); citrus fruit (e.g. calamondin, grapefruit, kumquats, lemons, limes, mandarin oranges, pomelos, tangerines, and tangelos); cherries, dates, figs, grapes, guava, jackfruit, lychee, mangoes, melons (e.g., cantaloupe, casaba, honeydew, and watermelon); nectarines, papaya, passion fruit, peaches, pears, persimmons, pineapple, plums, pomegranates, prunes, raisins, rhubarb, sapote, soursop, starfruit, and tamarind.

Grains

Whole Grains: All whole-grain products and whole grains used as ingredients: for example, amaranth, barley (not pearled), brown rice, buckwheat, bulgur, millet, oats, popcorn, quinoa, dark rye, triticale, whole-grain cornmeal, whole-wheat bread, whole-wheat chapati, whole grain cereals and crackers, and wild rice.

Refined Grains: All refined-grain products and refined grains used as ingredients: for example, white breads, refined-grain cereals and crackers, corn grits, cream of rice, cream of wheat, barley (pearled), masa, pasta, and white rice. Refined-grain choices should be enriched.

Dairy

All fluid, dry, or evaporated milk, including lactose-free and lactose-reduced products and fortified soy beverages (soy milk), buttermilk, yogurt, kefir, frozen yogurt, dairy desserts, and cheeses (e.g., brie, camembert, cheddar, cottage cheese, colby, edam, feta, fontina, goat, gouda, gruyere, limburger, Mexican cheeses [queso anejo, queso asadero, queso chihuahua], monterey, mozzarella, muenster, parmesan, provolone, ricotta, and Swiss). Most choices should be fat-free or low-fat. Cream, sour cream, and cream cheese are not included due to their low calcium content.

Protein Foods

Meats, Poultry, Eggs: Meats include beef, goat, lamb, pork, and game meat (e.g., bear, bison, deer, elk, moose, opossum, rabbit, raccoon, squirrel). Poultry includes chicken, Cornish hens, dove, duck, game birds (e.g., ostrich, pheasant, and quail), goose, and turkey. Organ meats include brain, chitterlings, giblets, gizzard, heart, kidney, liver, stomach, sweetbreads, tongue, and tripe. Eggs include chicken eggs and other birds' eggs. Meats and poultry should be lean or low-fat.

Seafood: Seafood examples that are lower in methylmercury include: anchovy, black sea bass, catfish, clams, cod, crab, crawfish, flounder, haddock, hake, herring, lobster, mackerel, mullet, oyster, perch, pollock, salmon, sardine, scallop, shrimp, sole, squid, tilapia, freshwater trout, light tuna, and whiting.

Nuts, Seeds, Soy Products: Nuts and seeds include all nuts (tree nuts and peanuts), nut butters, seeds (e.g., chia, flax, pumpkin, sesame, and sunflower), and seed butters (e.g., sesame or tahini and sunflower). Soy includes tofu, tempeh, and products made from soy flour, soy protein isolate, and soy concentrate. Nuts should be unsalted.

Beans, Peas, Lentils: Can be considered part of the protein foods group as well as the vegetable group, but should be counted in one group only.

cFood group amounts shown in cup equivalents (cup eq) or ounce equivalents (ounce eq). Oils are shown in grams. Quantity equivalents for each food group are:

Vegetables, Fruits (1 cup eq): 1 cup raw or cooked vegetable or fruit; 1 cup vegetable or fruit juice; 2 cups leafy salad greens; ½ cup dried fruit or vegetable.

Grains (1 ounce eq): ½ cup cooked rice, pasta, or cereal; 1 ounce dry pasta or rice; 1 medium (1 ounce) slice bread, tortilla, or flatbread; 1 ounce of ready-to-eat cereal (about 1 cup of flaked cereal).

Dairy (1 cup eq): 1 cup milk, yogurt, or fortified soymilk; 1½ ounces natural cheese such as cheddar cheese or 2 ounces of processed cheese.

Protein Foods (1 ounce eq): 1 ounce lean meats, poultry, or seafood; 1 egg; ¼ cup cooked beans or tofu; 1 tbsp nut or seed butter; ½ ounce nuts or seeds.

dAmounts of whole grains in the Patterns for children are less than the minimum of 3 ounce-eq in all Patterns recommended for adults.

eThe U.S. Food and Drug Administration (FDA) and the U.S. Environmental Protection Agency (EPA) provide joint advice regarding seafood consumption to limit methylmercury exposure for women who might become or are pregnant or breastfeeding, and children. Depending on body weight, some women and many children should choose seafood lowest in methylmercury or eat less seafood than the amounts in the Healthy US-Style Eating Pattern. For more information, see the FDA and EPA websites FDA.gov/fishadvice; EPA.gov/fishadvice.

fIf consuming up to 2 ounces of seafood per week, children should only be fed cooked varieties from the "Best Choices" list in the FDA/EPA joint "Advice About Eating Fish," available at FDA.gov/fishadvice and EPA.gov/fishadvice. If consuming up to 3 ounces of seafood per week, children should only be fed cooked varieties from the "Best Choices" list that contain even lower methylmercury: flatfish (e.g., flounder), salmon, tilapia, shrimp, catfish, crab, trout, haddock, oysters, sardines, squid, pollock, anchovies, crawfish, mullet, scallops, whiting, clams, shad, and Atlantic mackerel. If consuming up to 3 ounces of seafood per week, many commonly consumed varieties of seafood should be avoided because they cannot be consumed at 3 ounces per week by children without the potential of exceeding safe methylmercury limits; examples that should not be consumed include: canned light tuna or white (albacore) tuna, cod, perch, black sea bass. For a complete list please see: FDA.gov/fishadvice and EPA.gov/fishadvice.

gFoods are assumed to be in nutrient-dense forms, lean or low-fat and prepared with minimal added saturated fat, added sugars, refined starches, or salt. If all food choices to meet food group recommendations are in nutrient-dense forms, a small number of calories remain within the overall limit of the pattern (i.e., limit on calories for other uses). The amount of calories depends on the total calorie level of the pattern and the amounts of food from each food group required to meet nutritional goals. Calories up to the specified limit can be used for added sugars, added refined starches, saturated fat, alcohol, or to eat more than the recommended amount of food in a food group.

From U.S. Department of Agriculture and U.S. Department of Health and Human Services. (2020, December). *Dietary guidelines for Americans, 2020-2025* (9th ed.). Retrieved from www.dietaryguidelines.gov.

Energy output: exercise behaviors. Increasing energy output through physical activity helps clients to achieve a negative energy balance. For someone who has no planned physical activity, a regular daily exercise schedule that starts with simple walking for approximately a half hour each day and building up to a brisk pace is a great way to begin. It is ideal to include both aerobic exercise (e.g., swimming, running, biking) and resistance exercise to a successful weight-management program (see the For Further Focus box, "Benefits of Aerobic Exercise in Weight Management"). An exercise class may be helpful to maintain motivation. Encourage clients to experiment with various activities until they find one that they enjoy and that they feel they can maintain for the long term. Following are current recommendations by the *Dietary Guidelines for Americans*, regarding exercise and weight maintenance or weight loss[40]:

- Choose a healthy eating pattern at an appropriate calorie level to help achieve and maintain a healthy body weight, support nutrient adequacy, and reduce the risk of chronic disease.
- Increase the amount of physical activity engagement each week.
- Limit the amount of time spent in sedentary situations.

Chapter 16 covers specific physical activity recommendations.

A Sound Food Plan

A careful diet history (see Chapter 17) can be the basis for a sound personalized food plan that involves the principles of energy and nutrient balance, distribution balance and portion control, a food guide, and a preventive approach.

Energy balance. Under normal circumstances, when a person enters a state of negative energy balance, weight loss occurs. Because 1 lb of fat is equal to approximately 3500 kcal, an energy deficit of 500 kcal/day results in a weight loss of about 1 lb per week and a deficit of 250 kcal equals a ½-lb weight loss per week (Box 15.2). Determining an individual's current total energy needs is the first step in making a personalized food plan (Box 15.3). Modifications to energy intake and energy output can then yield a negative energy balance. As discussed throughout this text, individual energy needs vary greatly. Therefore, assuming that all people on a weight-loss program should limit caloric intake to 1400 kcal/day (or any other prefabricated amount) is not appropriate. For a person who normally consumes 2000 kcal/day, the ideal scenario is a deficit of approximately 500 kcal/day. Those 500 kcal should not all come from diet, though. Reducing calorie intake by 25% (2000 × 25% = 500 kcal) would likely leave a person hungry and constantly thinking about food. Instead, the weight-loss program could include a 250-kcal reduction in energy intake and a 250-kcal increase in energy expenditure for a total deficit of 500 kcal (see the Case Study box, "Energy Balance and Weight-Management Plan").

For Further Focus

Benefits of Aerobic Exercise in Weight Management

The goal of weight management is to achieve and maintain a healthy body composition. However, when a person tries to lose weight to reach a weight goal merely by reducing food intake, he or she will not only lose excess body fat but may also lose lean body mass (muscle).

To achieve optimal body composition, consider the combination of diet management and aerobic exercise. Aerobic exercise consists of activities sustained long enough to draw on the body's fat reserve for fuel while oxygen intake increases (thus the term *aerobic*). Lean body tissue burns fats in the presence of oxygen. Therefore, aerobic activity is best suited for achieving the ideal balance of high lean body mass and low fatty tissue in the body.

The benefits of aerobic exercise to an overweight person in a weight-management program include the following:
- Suppressed appetite
- Reduced total body fat
- Higher BMR
- Increased circulatory and respiratory function
- Increased energy expenditure
- Retention of tissue protein and building of lean body mass levels

Some individuals complain about the slow rate of weight loss, difficulty in controlling appetite, and consistent "flabbiness" despite continuing diet management. These individuals may welcome the suggestion of aerobic activity to help manage weight loss. Suggestions include a brisk daily walk, jumping rope, swimming, bicycling, jogging, running, aerobic or spinning classes, or another activity that increases the heart rate enough to maintain an aerobic effect for 20 to 30 minutes. Carefully note the physical stress this activity may place on individuals who have not exercised for some time or who have medical problems related to exertion. These individuals should have a medical check-up before beginning such a program on their own or at a fitness center. Then the program should start slowly and incrementally increase in time and intensity.

Box 15.2 | **Kilocalorie Adjustment Necessary for Weight Loss**

To lose 454 g (1 lb) per week there needs to be a 500-kcal energy deficit per day.

BASIS OF ESTIMATION
1 lb of body fat = 454 g
1 g of pure fat = 9 kcal
1 g of body fat = 7.7 kcal (differences because of water in fat cells)
454 g × 7.7 kcal/g = 3496 kcal/454 g of body fat (or ≈3500 kcal)
500 kcal energy deficit × 7 days = 3500 kcal = 454 g of body fat = 1 lb

Nutrient balance. Basic diet components for nutrient balance are as follows:
- *Carbohydrate:* Approximately 45% to 65% of the total kilocalories, with emphasis on complex forms such as whole grains, fruits, and vegetables that are good sources of fiber. Limit simple sugars.

Box 15.3 Estimation of Adult Energy Needs

MIFFLIN-ST. JEOR EQUATION

Men

Total Energy Expenditure (kcal/day) = (Weight [kg] × 10 + Height [cm] × 6.25 – Age × 5 – 5) × Physical activity coefficient

Women

Total Energy Expenditure (kcal/day) = (Weight [kg] × 10 + Height [cm] × 6.25 – Age × 5 – 161) × Physical activity coefficient

Physical Activity Coefficient

1.200 = Sedentary (little or no exercise)

1.375 = Lightly active (light exercise or sports 1 to 3 days per week)

1.550 = Moderately active (moderate exercise or sports 3 to 5 days per week)

1.725 = Very active (hard exercise or sports 6 to 7 days per week)

1.900 = Extra active (very hard exercise or sports and physical job)

- *Protein:* Approximately 10% to 35% of the total kilocalories, with emphasis on lean foods and small portions.
- *Fat:* Approximately 20% to 35% of the total kilocalories, with emphasis on essential fatty acids from plant foods and minimal animal and trans fats.
- The food plan should meet the recommendations of the *Dietary Guidelines for Americans* (see Figure 1.5 in Chapter 1).

The use of special "diet foods" is not necessary. All foods can fit into a sound weight-loss plan with moderation and be put into the context of the overall plan.

Distribution balance and portion control. Spreading food evenly throughout the day with four to five meals or snacks, including breakfast, and avoiding the practice of skipping meals ensure healthy food behaviors.[36] Hunger usually peaks every 4 to 5 hours. If an individual has certain "problem times" of the day, planning simple snacks for those periods helps to maintain balance. Long periods without refueling can result in low blood glucose level and intense hunger followed by subsequent

---

NEXT-GENERATION NCLEX® EXAMINATION-STYLE UNFOLDING CASE STUDY
Energy Balance and Weight-Management Plan

See Answers in Appendix A.

A 27-year-old female accountant lives a sedentary life because of her long work hours and 2-year-old son at home. She weighs 170 lbs., and is 5 ft., 6 in. tall. Her average food intake is approximately 2400 kcal/day.

QUESTIONS FOR ANALYSIS

1. Select her current energy needs using the Mifflin-St. Jeor equation.
   Total Energy Expenditure (kcal/day) = (Weight [kg] × 10 + Height [cm] × 6.25 – Age × 5 – 161) × Physical activity coefficient

   a. 1830 kcals/day
   b. 1720 kcals/day
   c. 1900 kcals/day
   d. 1550 kcals/day
   e. 2000 kcals/day

2. Choose the *most likely* options for the information missing from the statements below by selecting from the list of options provided.

   Comparing her estimated energy needs using Mifflin-St. Jeor to her current energy needs, the patient is currently in _____ energy balance, resulting in weight _____.

OPTIONS	
positive	gain
sustained	negative
loss	maintenance

She was a college athlete and never struggled with her weight until now. She wants to lose weight in a healthy, long-term way by adjusting her energy balance. She wants to lose fat but is concerned about losing muscle mass.

3. Select the amount of calorie deficit that she should strive for each day (without adding exercise) in order to lose 1 lb. per week.

   a. 250 kcals
   b. 1200 kcals
   c. 500 kcals
   d. 350 kcals
   e. 400 kcals
   f. 100 kcals

4. Use an X to identify effective and ineffective practices that could help her reduce her calories to create a negative energy balance.

PRACTICES	EFFECTIVE	INEFFECTIVE
Increase physical activity		
Increase caloric deficit >500 kcals/day		
Follow healthy eating patterns consuming a variety of foods		
Eat in front of the TV		
Increase sedentary behavior		
Create moderate calorie deficit ≤500 kcals/day		
Consume calorie dense foods		
Consume less calories then expended		
Increase exercise		

5. Choose the *most likely* options for the information missing from the statements below by selecting from the list of options provided.

Based on the patient's concerns, she should consider ____1____ exercise for longer periods to increase use of ____2____ for fuel instead of lean body mass.

OPTION 1	OPTION 2
anaerobic	fat
resistance	glycogen
aerobic	ketones

6. Select the best assessment tools to measure the efficiency of the weight loss plan and the patient's progress.
   a. BMI, body composition, waist circumference
   b. Body composition, weight, percent body fat
   c. Waist circumference, height, age
   d. Weight, age, height
   e. BMI, weight, age
   f. Body composition, percent body fat, percent lean body mass

periods of overeating, usually of quick and accessible foods, which is often energy-dense "junk foods." Balanced meals and healthful snacks require the foresight of planning and preparation.

Inappropriately large portion sizes continue to contribute to the energy intake imbalance for many people. Meals eaten both at home and away from home may be problematic, so try to use smaller plates and cups, order a half serving, or pack half of the entrée to go at the start of the meal. Portion sizes and portion control are important factors in a sound food plan.

Food guide. The Academy of Nutrition and Dietetics published a book titled *Choose Your Foods: Food Lists for Weight Management* with food exchange lists that follow the general *Dietary Guidelines for Americans* (found through online booksellers). This basic food exchange system is a good general reference guide for comparative food values and portions, variety in food choices, and basic meal planning. Table 15.2 provides examples of food plans that meet nutrient needs at 12 different calorie levels. The MyPlate guidelines (see Figure 1.4 in Chapter 1) also provide tips on making healthful food and beverage choices. The overall food guide should consist of plenty of fruits and vegetables, whole grains, and lean proteins, while reducing the energy density of foods eaten, with water as the ideal beverage. Given the complexity of the variables associated with weight loss and maintenance, it is most effective for the RDN to create an individualized food plan collaboratively with the client.

Preventive approach. Prevention of excess weight gain is the most effective means of healthy weight management. Supporting young parents and children in healthy lifestyle choices before obesity develops can help to prevent many problems later in adulthood. This support and guidance should include early nutrition counseling and education, which can help to build positive health habits, especially in the forms of healthful eating behaviors and increased exercise through active play and physical activities for the entire family. Many programs for young children—such as Head Start, school breakfast and lunch programs, and the Special Supplemental Nutrition Program for Women, Infants and Children (WIC) (see Chapter 13)—address obesity issues through education and prevention for parents and children.

FOOD MISINFORMATION AND FADS

A fad is a widely shared fashion or pursuit. Food fads are scientifically unsubstantiated beliefs about certain foods that may persist for a short time in a given community or society. The word *fallacy* means "a deceptive, misleading, or false notion or belief." Food fallacies are false or misleading beliefs that underlie food fads. The jargon term *quack* is a shortened form of *quicksalver*, a term from centuries ago in which the Dutch described the pseudophysician or pseudoprofessor who sold worthless salves, magic elixirs, and cure-all tonics. He proclaimed his wares in a patter that skeptical people compared with the quacking of a duck. In medicine, nutrition, and allied health fields, a quack is a fraudulent pretender who claims to have skill, knowledge, or qualifications that he or she does not truly possess. The motive for such quackery is usually money, and the quack uses a hoax to feed on the physical and emotional needs of his or her victims.

Unscientific statements about food often mislead consumers and contribute to poor food habits. False information may come from folklore or fraud. However, empowering individuals to recognize misinformation helps them make sound food choices according to evidence-based nutrition guidelines from responsible nutrition professionals.

FOOD FADS

Types of Claims

Food faddists make exaggerated claims about certain types of food. These claims generally fall into the following four basic groups:
1. *Food cures:* Certain foods cure specific conditions.
2. *Harmful foods:* Certain foods cause harm if eaten.
3. *Food combinations:* Special food combinations restore health and are effective for reducing weight.
4. *Natural foods:* Only "natural" foods can meet body needs and prevent disease. The term *natural* often describes unprocessed or minimally processed products that contain no artificial ingredients, coloring ingredients, or chemical preservatives. However, there is no universally recognized definition of what constitutes "natural" in food terms. Some people consider all processed foods unhealthy, including those that are enriched or fortified.

Erroneous Claims

Erroneous claims require careful examination. On the surface, they seem to be simple statements about food and health. However, further observation reveals that they focus on a food itself and not on the specific nutrients that are in the food, which are the actual physiologic agents of life and health. Some individuals may be allergic to specific foods and should avoid them. In addition, certain foods may supply relatively large amounts of individual nutrients and therefore are good sources of those nutrients. Remember that people require specific nutrients and not necessarily specific foods.

Dangers

Why should health care workers be concerned about food fads and their effect on food habits? What harm do food fads cause? Food fads generally involve four possible negative effects.

Danger to health. Responsibility for one's health is fundamental. However, self-diagnosis and self-treatment can be dangerous, especially when such action follows questionable sources. By following such a course, people with real illness may fail to seek appropriate medical care. Fraudulent claims of cures have misled many ill and anxious people and have postponed proven effective therapy.

Cost. Some foods and supplements used by faddists are harmless, but many are expensive. Money spent for useless items is wasted. When dollars are scarce, a family may neglect to buy foods that fill basic needs in an attempt to purchase a "miracle cure."

Lack of sound knowledge. Misinformation hinders the development of individuals and society and ignores scientific progress. The perpetuation of certain superstitions can counteract sound teaching about health.

Distrust of the food market. People should be watchful of their food environment, but a blanket rejection of all modern food production is unwarranted. People must develop intelligent concerns and rational approaches to meet their nutrition needs.

WHAT IS THE ANSWER?

How can one counter food habits that are associated with food fads, misinformation, or even outright deception? The basis of helpful instruction is personal conviction, practice, and enthusiasm. The following are approaches to positive teaching.

Using Reliable Sources

Sound background knowledge is essential and should include the following strategies:

- Know the product being pushed and the people or company behind it.
- Know how human physiology and biochemistry work.

- Know the scientific method of problem solving (e.g., collect the facts, identify the problem, determine a reasonable solution or action, carry it out, and evaluate the results).

Sound community resources include the following:

- Extension educators work in the community through state and county Extension Service offices and direct highly successful community nutrition activities, such as their Expanded Food and Nutrition Education Program. These specialists develop many food and nutrition guides, especially for those with limited education or who speak English as a second language. Search "Expanded Food and Nutrition Education Program" at usda.gov for additional information.
- The FDA and U.S. Department of Agriculture (USDA) produce many free educational materials related to food and nutrition (see Chapter 13). Search "Resources for Various Cultural and Ethnic Groups" at usda.gov.
- Public health nutritionists and RDNs located in county and state public health offices and as part of special programs (e.g., WIC) can provide information. Search "WIC state agencies" at usda.gov.
- RDNs in local medical care centers who serve hospitalized patients, outpatient clinics, and private practice also are valuable resources. Find an expert at the Academy of Nutrition and Dietetics nationwide nutrition network (www.eatright.org/find-an-expert).

Recognizing Human Needs

Consider the emotional needs that food and food rituals help to fulfill. These needs are a part of life, and they can be positive influencers in nutrition teaching. Even if a person is using food as an emotional crutch, the emotional need is still real. Never take away crutches without offering a better and wiser form of support. Food and all the associations that go along with it compose a basic enjoyment of life. Maintaining a balance between food as entertainment and food as fuel is the challenge of identifying the role of food in relation to human needs. The establishment of a healthy diet must consider all such human needs; it may involve specialized help, such as that provided by behavioral therapists.

Use any opportunity that arises to present sound nutrition and health information, whether formally or informally. Learn about the available resources described previously. Develop communication skills, avoid monotony, and use a well-disciplined imagination.

Thinking Scientifically

Even very young children can use the problem-solving approach to explore everyday food behavior choices. Children are naturally curious. With their eternal questioning—"Why?"—they often seek evidence to support the statements that they hear. Three basic questions help with the evaluation of claims in any situation: (1) "What do you mean?" (2) "How do you know?" (3) "What is your evidence?"

Box 15.4 **The Food and Nutrition Science Alliance's 10 Red Flags of Junk Science**

1. Recommendations that promise a quick fix
2. Dire warnings of danger from a single product or regimen
3. Claims that sound too good to be true
4. Simplistic conclusions drawn from a complex study
5. Recommendations based on a single study
6. Dramatic statements that are refuted by reputable scientific organizations
7. Lists of "good" and "bad" foods
8. Recommendations made to help sell a product
9. Recommendations based on studies published without peer review
10. Recommendations from studies that ignore differences among individuals or groups

Reprinted from the Food and Nutrition Science Alliance (FANSA). (1995). *10 Red flags of junk science*. Chicago: FANSA.

The Food and Nutrition Science Alliance is a partnership of seven professional scientific societies that have joined to disseminate sound nutrition information. This organization issued a list of 10 red flags to help guide consumers toward making educated decisions about nutrition and health issues (Box 15.4). This list is an excellent guide when evaluating reports and claims about various diets, supplements, and other nutrition-related fads.

Knowing Responsible Authorities

The FDA is legally responsible for controlling the quality and safety of food and drug products marketed in the United States. However, this is a tremendous task requiring public help. Other government, professional, and private organizations can provide additional resources (see the Further Reading and Resources list at the back of the book).

UNDERWEIGHT

GENERAL CAUSES AND TREATMENT

Extremes in underweight—just as in overweight—can pose health problems. Although general malnutrition and excessive thinness is a less-common problem in developed nations than overweight and obesity, it does occur, and it is usually associated with poor living conditions or long-term disease. An underweight person is someone who is more than 10% below the average weight for height and age; someone who is ≥20% below the average weight has cause for significant health concerns. Physiologic and psychologic effects may occur, especially among young children (e.g., compromised immunity, strength, and overall health).

Causes

Underweight is associated with conditions that cause general malnutrition, including the following:
- *Wasting disease:* Long-term disease with chronic infection and fever that raise the BMR
- *Poor food intake:* Diminished food intake that results from psychologic factors that cause a person to refuse to eat, loss of appetite, or personal poverty and limited access to food
- *Malabsorption:* Poor nutrient absorption that results from chronic diarrhea, a diseased gastrointestinal tract, the excessive use of laxatives, or drug-nutrient interactions
- *Hormonal imbalance:* Hyperthyroidism or a variety of other hormonal imbalances that increase the caloric needs of the body
- *Low energy availability:* Inadequate energy intake relative to energy needs. May result from greatly increased physical activity without a corresponding increase in food or a lack of available food supply
- *Poor living situation:* An unhealthy home environment that results in irregular and inadequate meals, where eating is considered unimportant, and where an indifferent attitude toward food exists

Dietary Treatment

Special nutrition care to rebuild body tissues and to regain health is necessary for underweight and undernourished clients. Food plans should be adapted to each person's unique situation, whether it involves his or her personal needs, living situation, economic needs, or any underlying disease. The dietary goal, in accordance with each person's tolerance, is to increase energy and nutrient intake, with adherence to the following needs:
- *Energy and nutrient-dense diet:* Above the standard requirements relative to age and sex standards
- *High protein:* To rebuild tissues
- *High carbohydrate:* To provide the primary energy source in an easily digested form
- *Moderate fat:* To provide essential fatty acids and add energy without exceeding tolerance limits
- *Good sources of vitamins and minerals:* Provided by a variety of nutrient-dense foods and dietary supplements when individual deficiencies require them

Nourishing meals and snacks composed of favorite foods as well as a high variety of foods attractively served may help to revive the appetite and increase the desire to eat more. A basic aim is to help build good long-term food habits for improved nutrition and weight status. Residents in long-term care facilities are especially vulnerable to weight-loss problems, and they have special needs (see the Clinical Applications box, "Problems of Weight Loss among Older Adults in Long-Term Care Facilities"). This rehabilitation process requires creative counseling for the client and the family along with practical guides and support. In some cases, tube feeding or intravenous feeding (e.g., parenteral nutrition) may be necessary (see Chapter 22).

Ideal weight gain includes lean and fat tissue. To gain muscle, physical exercise must be part of the treatment. Resistance training increases lean tissue and, in turn, boosts appetite. A variety of weight-lifting and strength-training programs, depending on the desires of the individual, are encouraged as an important part of healthy weight gain.

⌂ **Clinical Applications**

Problems of Weight Loss Among Older Adults in Long-Term Care Facilities

The population of adults who are 65 years old and older is rapidly increasing. The most rapid population increase over the next decade will be among those who are older than 85, and many of these elderly people will require long-term care in nursing homes.

One of the problems encountered among elderly residents is low body weight and rapid unintentional weight loss. These conditions can become serious health problems, and they are a sensitive indicator of malnutrition that can contribute to illness and death. Because weight loss is such a strong predictor of morbidity and mortality in clinical settings, early and continuing observation to assess needs is important, especially in relation to factors that contribute to weight loss.

In general, the following can cause weight loss in this population: (1) the physical effects of the metabolic changes of aging; (2) the physical effects of disease; or (3) certain factors that alter the amount and type of food eaten. Physical disease (e.g., cancer) can cause extreme weight loss because of metabolic abnormalities, taste changes, loss of appetite, nausea, and vomiting. Other diseases that affect weight include gastrointestinal problems, uncontrolled diabetes, cardiovascular disorders (e.g., congestive heart failure), pulmonary disease, infection, and alcoholism. Psychologic factors or psychiatric disorders may also contribute to malnutrition and weight loss from depression, dementia, disorientation, apathy, and appetite disturbance. Nutrient deficiencies (e.g., low levels of folate and B-complex vitamins) as well as protein-energy malnutrition can cause altered mental states. Specific nutrition support can correct these conditions.

The following additional physiologic, psychologic, and social factors may influence food intake and body weight and thus contribute to malnutrition among elderly people:

- *Body composition changes:* Height and body weight gradually decline as people age. Body weight usually peaks between the ages of 34 and 54 years in men and between 55 and 75 years in women, and it generally decreases thereafter. Body fat losses are largely insignificant. One cause of weight loss is a decline in body water, in part by the weakening of the normal thirst mechanism. Therefore, to maintain fluid status clinicians and caregivers must offer water and encourage drinking often because thirst does not secure adequate water intake. Constant attention to fluid intake also helps with the common problem of xerostomia (i.e., dry mouth) in older adults. Xerostomia results from inadequate salivary secretions, which makes eating difficult, thereby contributing to malnutrition. Lean body mass also declines with age, and this results in a lower basal metabolic rate and decreased physical activity and energy requirements. Thus, any possible increase in physical activity and the use of nutrient-dense foods are encouraged.
- *Taste changes:* The regeneration of taste buds slows with age, but the extent and effect on food intake vary widely. The sense of smell also declines with age and may negatively affect taste. Thus, it is helpful to use more seasoning and flavoring in food preparation.
- *Dentition:* About half of Americans have lost some or all of their teeth by the age of 65 years. Many have dentures, but chewing problems are often present. Nursing home residents frequently report chewing, biting, and swallowing problems that interfere with eating and adequate food intake. The assessment of specific needs and dental care solutions helps to correct eating problems.
- *Gastrointestinal problems:* Delayed gastric emptying may contribute to distention and lack of appetite. A decrease in gastric secretions, including hydrochloric acid, may hinder the absorption of protein, vitamin B_{12}, folate, and iron, thereby contributing to anemia and a loss of appetite. Constipation is a common complaint that often leads to laxative dependence and that results in interference with nutrient absorption. An increase in dietary fiber, liquids, and physical activity can help to provide a more natural approach to establishing normal bowel movements.
- *Drug-nutrient interactions:* Elderly people often take a number of prescribed and over-the-counter medications, some of which are the direct cause of anorexia, nausea, and vomiting. Other drugs are indirect causes in that they induce nutrient malabsorption; this leads to deficiencies that in turn cause anorexia and weight loss. Drug therapy for elderly clients should involve constant medical, nutrition, and nursing attention to ensure appropriate use.
- *Functional disabilities:* Difficulty with eating may prevent or alter the capacity of elderly people to take in sufficient food. These problems may vary from more difficult functional disabilities that interfere with putting food into the mouth and swallowing (e.g., problems that often require a trained therapist) to dependence on feeding assistance provided by sensitive nursing care.
- *Social problems:* Socioeconomic problems are often involved in the care of the elderly. A specially trained geriatric social worker can help to secure possible sources of financial assistance. A sense of social isolation can also lead to decreased food intake. Family support, sensitive contact with nursing home staff and residents, and as much involvement as possible in group activities are helpful.

Health care workers in geriatric settings need continuing education and sensitization to the potential dangers of low body weight and unintentional weight loss among their clients. Older individuals with acute and chronic illnesses and functional disabilities are at the greatest risk for nutrition-related problems. These clients require continual nutrition assessment and the monitoring of their body weight. Some of the restrictions of "special diets" should be relaxed or discontinued when the risk of malnutrition is evident, with the goal of increasing nutrient intake and making eating as enjoyable as possible.

DISORDERED EATING

To discuss disordered or abnormal eating, we must first define "normal eating." Normal eating is when an individual is capable of the following:

- Eating when he or she is hungry and stopping when full
- Demonstrating moderate restraint with regard to food selection
- Recognizing that overeating and undereating are sometimes acceptable and trusting his or her body to establish a balance
- Having the ability to be flexible with his or her eating schedule

Disordered eating is an eating pattern that is abnormal, and it can include a variety of subclinical problems. This type of eating or thought pattern can range from infrequent episodes, to more often such as with **other specified feeding or eating disorder**, or persistent enough to meet diagnostic criteria for an eating disorder. Disordered eating can range from an insurmountable fear of eating fat to an inability to eat in public. Family and personal tensions as well as social pressures for thinness may result in serious body image disturbances and eating problems that push the disordered eating behavior to the point of becoming a clinical eating disorder. The three most common eating disorders are **anorexia nervosa**, **bulimia nervosa**, and **binge eating disorder** (Box 15.5).

Box 15.5   **Diagnostic Criteria for Eating Disorders**

ANOREXIA NERVOSA

Individuals exhibiting some or all of the following characteristics meet the diagnostic criteria for anorexia nervosa:

A. They restrict their energy intake to significantly lower than what their body requires. This restriction leads to a body weight significantly lower than what health care providers would expect for their age, sex, developmental state, and physical health.

B. They have an extreme fear of gaining weight or becoming fat; or they persistently behave in a way that prevents weight gain, despite their current weight status, which is significantly lower than minimally expected.

C. They experience one or more of the following: disturbances in the way in which they perceive their body weight or shape, their body shape and weight unjustifiably influences their self-evaluation, or they continue to deny the gravity of their current low body weight.

Within the diagnosis of anorexia nervosa, health care providers may further classify the patient as one of the following two types:

1. *Restricting type:* Individuals in this category establish and maintain a very low body weight by means of energy restriction and/or excessive exercise (i.e., they have *not* regularly engaged in binge eating or purging behaviors within the previous 3 months).

2. *Binge eating/purging type:* Individuals within this category have regularly engaged in repetitive binge eating or purging behaviors over the previous 3 months.

BULIMIA NERVOSA

Individuals exhibiting some or all of the following characteristics meet the diagnostic criteria for bulimia nervosa:

A. They experience recurrent episodes of binge eating that are characterized by the following:

- They consume, during a discrete period (e.g., within any 2-hour period), a quantity of food that is greater than most people would consume in a similar situation or amount of time.
- They feel a lack of control while eating during the binge episode (e.g., a feeling that they cannot stop eating or control what or how much they consume).

B. They repetitively use inappropriate compensatory behaviors to prevent weight gain, such as self-induced vomiting; the misuse of laxatives, diuretics, or other medications; fasting; or excessive exercise.

C. They experience both binge eating episodes and inappropriate compensatory behaviors an average of once a week for 3 months.

D. Their body shape and weight unjustifiably influences their self-evaluation.

E. They do not experience these disturbances exclusively during episodes of anorexia nervosa.

BINGE EATING DISORDER

Individuals exhibiting some or all of the following characteristics meet the diagnostic criteria for binge eating disorder:

A. They experience recurrent episodes of binge eating that are characterized by the following:

- They consume, during a discrete period (e.g., within any 2-hour period), a quantity of food that is greater than most people would consume in a similar situation or amount of time.
- They feel a lack of control while eating during the binge episode (e.g., a feeling that they cannot stop eating or control what or how much they consume).

B. The American Psychiatric Association describes *binge eating* as an episode that is associated with at least three of the following traits:

- The individual eats until they are uncomfortably full.
- The individual eats large amounts of food even though they are not physically hungry.
- The individual eats faster than normal.
- The individual eats alone because they are embarrassed by how much they are consuming.
- They experience feelings of disgust, depression, or guilt after overeating.

C. They experience distress regarding their binge eating episodes.

D. They experience binge eating episodes an average of once a week for 3 months.

OTHER SPECIFIED FEEDING OR EATING DISORDER

This diagnosis is appropriate for individuals who experience disordered eating behaviors but do not meet the diagnostic criteria for any other specified eating disorder. For example:

A. They meet all of the diagnostic criteria for anorexia nervosa, except that their weight remains within, or above, a normal weight range (regardless of significant weight loss).

B. They meet all of the diagnostic criteria for bulimia nervosa, except that the binge eating and inappropriate compensatory mechanisms occur less frequently than once a week or for a duration of less than 3 months.

C. They meet all of the diagnostic criteria for binge eating disorder, except that the binge episodes occur less frequently than once a week or for a duration of less than 3 months.

D. They regularly use inappropriate compensatory behaviors but do not experience binge eating episodes.

E. They repeatedly experience *night eating syndrome,* in which they consume large amounts of food after the evening meal or upon waking from sleep.

Modified from the American Psychiatric Association. (2013). *Diagnostic and statistical manual of mental disorders* (5th ed., text revision). Washington, DC: American Psychological Association Press.

The Academy of Nutrition and Dietetics describes eating disorders as psychiatric disorders with diagnostic criteria based on psychologic, behavior, and physiologic characteristics.[41] Anorexia nervosa has the highest premature death rates of any psychiatric disorder. Individuals with anorexia are 2.8 times more likely to die from all-cause mortality and 3.1 times more likely to die by suicide than other females in the general population.[42] Studies also show that eating disorder clients who are suffering from additional psychiatric co-morbidities, especially those related to substance abuse, have more pronounced rates of death.[42,43] Eating disorders are secretive in nature and surveys often have small sample sizes; therefore, establishing a true estimate of population prevalence is difficult. Research indicates that eating disorders occur less frequently among males than females and often involve a muscularity-oriented body image and disordered eating patterns aimed to achieve a muscular ideal rather than the thin-ideal common among females.[44] There are often misunderstandings about the nature of eating disorders as well as the impact on the person with the eating disorder and those around her or him. Box 15.6 lists nine truths about eating disorders.

Most clinical eating disorders have similar risk factors, all of which have genetic and/or environmental factors. These risk factors include the following:

- *Sociocultural influences:* Idealization of thinness, perceived pressure for thinness, thin-ideal internalization, and denial of thin-ideal costs[45]
- *Personality traits:* Negative emotionality (anxiety, anger), perfectionism; overeating, dieting, negative urgency/impulsivity especially when distressed in clients specifically with bulimia nervosa and binge eating disorder [45,46]

- *Neurocognitive processes:* Decreased cognitive flexibility (inability to move between multiple tasks), motor or cognitive inhibitory control, and serotonin disturbances[47,48]
- *Child maltreatment:* All types of child maltreatment are associated with an increased risk of eating disorders. Sexual abuse and physical neglect have the strongest relationships in males, whereas sexual abuse and emotional abuse were the strongest among females[49]

Anorexia Nervosa

The estimated lifetime prevalence of anorexia nervosa is 0.8% (0.12% among men and 1.4% among women).[50] This complex psychologic disorder results in self-imposed starvation. In addition to the diagnostic criteria provided in Box 15.5, Table 15.3 outlines some clinical signs that are associated with both anorexia nervosa and bulimia nervosa. Some of the features of anorexia nervosa include the following[51,52]:

- Low body weight
- Restriction of calories
- Fear of weight gain
- **Body dysmorphic disorder**
- Anxiety and/or depression
- Social withdrawal
- Perfectionism
- Low self-esteem

All forms of eating disorders require an interdisciplinary team for treatment success. Restoring a healthy weight and normalizing eating patterns are key nutrition therapy goals that are specific to anorexia nervosa.

Bulimia Nervosa

The estimated lifetime prevalence of bulimia nervosa is 0.28% (0.08% in men, and 0.46% in women).[50] Bulimia

---

| Box 15.6 | Nine Truths About Eating Disorders |

1. Many people with eating disorders look healthy yet may be extremely ill.
2. Families are not to blame and can be the clients' best allies in treatment.
3. An eating disorder diagnosis is a health crisis that disrupts personal and family functioning.
4. Eating disorders are not choices, but serious biologically influenced illnesses.
5. Eating disorders affect people of all sexes, ages, races, ethnicities, body shapes and weights, sexual orientations, and socioeconomic statuses.
6. Eating disorders carry an increased risk for both suicide and medical complications.
7. Genes and environment play important roles in the development of eating disorders.
8. Genes alone do not predict who will develop eating disorders.
9. Full recovery from an eating disorder is possible. Early detection and intervention are important.

From Schaumberg, K., et al. (2017). The science behind the Academy for Eating Disorders' nine truths about eating disorders. *Eur Eat Disord Rev, 25*(6), 432–450.

---

other specified feeding or eating disorder subthreshold disordered eating that is not consistent with the diagnostic criteria for bulimia nervosa or anorexia nervosa.

anorexia nervosa an extreme psychophysiologic aversion to food that results in life-threatening weight loss; a psychiatric eating disorder that results from a morbid fear of fatness, in which a person's distorted body image is reflected as fat when the body is malnourished and extremely thin as a result of self-starvation.

bulimia nervosa a psychiatric eating disorder related to a person's fear of fatness in which cycles of gorging on large quantities of food are followed by compensatory mechanisms (e.g., self-induced vomiting, the use of diuretics and laxatives) to maintain a "normal" body weight.

binge eating disorder a psychiatric eating disorder that is characterized by the occurrence of binge eating episodes at least twice a week for a 6-month period.

body dysmorphic disorder an obsession with a perceived defect of the body.

Table 15.3	Presenting Signs and Symptoms Associated With Eating Disorders
General	Significant weight loss or fluctuation, cold intolerance, weakness, fatigue/lethargy, dizziness, fainting, hot flashes or sweating episodes
Oral and Dental	Oral trauma/ lacerations, perimyolysis and dental caries, parotid glad enlargement
Cardiorespiratory	Chest pain, heart palpitations, orthostatic tachycardia/ hypotension, dyspnea, edema
Gastrointestinal	Epigastric discomfort, abdominal bloating, early satiety, gastroesophageal reflux, hematemesis, hemorrhoids and rectal prolapse, constipation
Endocrine	Amenorrhea or oligomenorrhea, low sex drive, stress fractures, low bone mineral density, infertility
Neuropsychiatric	Depressive/anxious/obsessive/compulsive symptoms and behaviors, memory loss, poor concentration, insomnia, self-harm, seizures, suicidal thoughts, plans or attempts
Dermatologic	Lanugo hair, hair loss, carotenoderma, calluses or scars on the back of the hand from self-induced vomiting, dry brittle hair and nails

Modified from Academy for Eating Disorders' Medical Care Standards Committee. (2016). *Eating disorders: A guide to medical care* (3rd ed.). Reston, VA: Academy for Eating Disorders.

is an eating disorder that involves repeated episodes of binge eating followed by one or more compensatory mechanisms to rid the body of excess calories. Compensatory mechanisms include self-induced vomiting, laxative abuse, insulin misuse, diet pills, strict dieting or fasting, and excessive exercise. The constituents of a binge will vary among clients, but it generally involves the consumption of excessive quantities of food during a short period. Oral and dental problems from the purging behavior may involve oral mucosal irritation, decreased salivary secretions (xerostomia), and irreversible tooth enamel erosion. Table 15.3 provides other clinical signs and symptoms.

Individuals with bulimia nervosa often go unnoticed and undiagnosed compared with individuals with anorexia nervosa. Their body weights are generally within a normal range, but they may fluctuate. Some features of bulimia nervosa include the following[53]:
- Negative self-evaluation
- Parental influences such as comments about weight
- Parental obesity
- Childhood obesity
- High use of escape-avoidance coping
- Social anxiety
- Childhood sexual or physical abuse
- Depressive symptoms

Eliminating episodes of binging and purging are the key nutrition therapy goals for clients with bulimia nervosa.

Binge Eating Disorder
The estimated lifetime prevalence of binge eating disorder is 0.85% (0.42% for men and 1.25% for women).[50] This eating disorder involves binging episodes without compensatory behaviors. This type of binge often follows stress or anxiety as an emotional eating pattern to soothe or relieve painful or tense feelings or experiences. Clients with binge eating disorder are frequently overweight or obese and often have other chronic diseases.[54] Some features of binge eating disorder include the following[55]:

- High levels of concern about shape, weight, and eating
- Negative self-evaluation
- Perfectionism
- Childhood obesity
- Greater hedonic hunger and motivation to eat for pleasure without caloric need
- Depression, anxiety, or attention-deficit/hyperactivity disorder
- Substance abuse disorders
- Physical and sexual abuse

Eliminating binge-eating episodes is the key nutrition therapy goal for clients with binge eating disorder. Therapy may involve psychotherapy, behavioral weight-loss treatment, and psychopharmacology.

Treatment
These psychologic disorders require therapy from a team of skilled professionals, including physicians, psychologists, and RDNs. Even with the best of care, recovery is slow, and the word *cure* is seldom used. Many clients with eating disorders have persistent food and weight preoccupations throughout their lives.

Clients with eating disorders often have neurologic disturbances. The initial theory was that these chemical disturbances were the cause of disordered eating behavior. However, when a normal weight and eating pattern returns in the client, often the neurologic chemistry also returns to normal. Therefore, one of the first issues to address for the treatment of an eating disorder is establishing a healthy weight in the client. Psychologic therapy is more successful when the client has fewer neurologic disturbances. Next, the team of professionals must work together to restore eating habits and attitudes toward food, to optimize physical and mental health, and to heal intrapersonal and interpersonal problems. Continuing support groups that include friends, family, and health care professionals are critical for long-term treatment.

Putting It All Together

Summary

- In the traditional medical model, obesity is an illness and a health hazard, which may be true in some cases. Modern approaches use person-centered positive health modules that emphasize the important aspects of whole-body health.
- Planning a weight-management program for either an overweight or an underweight person must involve the metabolic and energy needs of the individual. This plan also accounts for personal food choices and habits as well as considering the fatty tissue needs during different stages of the life cycle.
- Important aspects of a weight-reduction program include changing food behaviors and increasing physical activity.
- Food fads and misinformation are increasingly popular within all facets of society. Identifying harmful practices and providing accurate information are basic functions of the health care provider.
- Excessive thinness is a cause for health concern. A variety of medical and psychologic conditions may result in malnutrition and underweight.
- Eating disorders require professional team therapy that includes medical, psychologic, and nutrition care.

Chapter Review Questions

See answers in Appendix A.

1. An ideal weight range for a female who is 5 feet, 3 inches tall is

   _____.

   a. 90 to 100 lb
   b. 100.5 to 115.2 lb
   c. 103.5 to 126.5 lb
   d. 126.5 to 136.8 lb

2. Casey is about 20 lb overweight and wants to lose 10 lb of body weight for her high school reunion. When should she begin to change her diet and exercise habits to promote healthy weight loss and reach her goal?

   a. At least 2 months before the reunion
   b. At least 10 weeks before the reunion
   c. At least 4 weeks before the reunion
   d. At least 10 days before the reunion

3. A sound weight-management program includes _____.

   a. gradual weight loss and adequate nutrient intake
   b. periods of fasting to cleanse the body of toxins
   c. minimal carbohydrate intake
   d. use of portion-controlled commercial products

4. Reducing excess body fat and the ability to build lean body mass are benefits of _____.

   a. a low-carbohydrate diet
   b. aerobic exercise
   c. protein supplements
   d. bariatric surgery

5. A meal plan for a client who is underweight as a result of malabsorption incorporates _____.

   a. high-protein, high-fat foods
   b. high-protein, low-carbohydrate foods
   c. high-protein, energy-dense foods
   d. low-protein, high-fat foods

Next-Generation NCLEX® Examination-style Case Study

See answers in Appendix A.

A 22-year-old woman is finishing her first semester of graduate school. She prioritizes her 4.0 GPA and her body image. She makes sure that she is making healthy food choices and going to the gym 5 days per week for an hour per day. While hanging out with friends, they notice that she is eating smaller amounts of food and obsessing over counting calories. At one of her gym sessions, she feels a lot of pain in her foot and is diagnosed with a stress fracture. The nurse notes that the client has not menstruated in the last 4 months and that her current weight is 15% below the average weight for height and age. Her mother states that she has been weighing herself a lot the past few months. A dietary recall illustrates that she consumes approximately 1200 calories per day.

1. From the list below, select all factors from the client's history that put her at elevated nutrition risk.

   a. Body weight
   b. Calorie intake
   c. Exercise patterns
   d. Menstrual cycle
   e. Injuries
   f. Social patterns
   g. Perfectionism
   h. Portion sizes
   i. Food choices

2. Based on the information provided, the nurse anticipates that the client is at risk for _____.

   a. bulimia nervosa
   b. binge eating disorder
   c. anorexia nervosa
   d. orthorexia
   e. other specified feeding or eating disorder

3. Use an X to identify which health professionals would be <u>necessary</u> and <u>unnecessary</u> for referral of the client.

HEALTH PROFESSIONAL	NECESSARY	UNNECESSARY
Physician		
Physical trainer		
Health coach		
Registered dietitian nutritionist		
Psychologist		
Chiropractor		
Nutritionist		

4. Place an X under the appropriate column to identify health teachings that are <u>indicated</u> (appropriate or necessary) or <u>contraindicated</u> (could be harmful) for the client.

HEALTH TEACHING	INDICATED	CONTRAINDICATED
Consume a diet rich in energy and nutrients to establish a healthy weight.		
Consume foods, such as eggs, lean meat, legumes, and soy, to rebuild tissues.		
Focus on specifically eating foods that you have been avoiding.		
Focus on drinking liquid supplements like Ensure so that you don't have to think about eating.		
Choose foods, such as pasta, rice, and cereal, to provide quick digesting energy.		
You should eat a diet high in fat to provide essential fatty acids and boost calorie intake.		
Focus on eating a variety of foods and be sure to include your favorite foods.		
You should avoid any foods that are high in saturated fat and added sugar like chips and cookies.		
You should restrict carbohydrates, such as rice, bread, and pasta.		

5. For each assessment finding, use an X to indicate whether nursing and collaborative interventions were <u>effective</u> (helped to meet expected outcomes) or <u>ineffective</u> (did not help to meet expected outcomes).

ASSESSMENT FINDING	EFFECTIVE	INEFFECTIVE
Gained 5 lbs. after 2 weeks of treatment		
Consumes 3 meals per day		
Consumes a variety of fruits and vegetables		
Feels distress after consuming large meals		
Weighs herself twice per day		
Purges after consuming dessert-like foods		
Avoids foods, such as sour cream, oil, avocado, and cheese		
Goes to the gym twice per day, 7 times per week		
Started journaling her emotions in a notebook		
Eats meals with family and friends		

Additional Learning Resources

Please refer to this text's Evolve website for answers to the Case Study questions:
http://evolve.elsevier.com/Williams/basic/.
References and **Further Reading and Resources** in the back of the book provide additional resources for enhancing knowledge.

Nutrition and Physical Fitness

Kary Woodruff PhD, RDN, CSSD

Key Concepts

- Regular physical activity is an important part of a healthy lifestyle throughout the life span.
- Sedentary lifestyles are a contributing factor to poor health and chronic diseases.
- A healthy personal exercise program combines both strengthening and aerobic activities.
- Different levels of physical activity draw on a variety of body fuel sources.

This chapter demonstrates that balanced nutrition and physical fitness are essential interrelated components of an overall healthy lifestyle. Both reduce risks associated with chronic diseases, and both are important therapies for the treatment of chronic conditions. Health care providers should provide their clients with sound guidelines for nutrition and physical fitness while role modeling healthy behaviors.

PHYSICAL ACTIVITY RECOMMENDATIONS AND BENEFITS

GUIDELINES AND RECOMMENDATIONS

Technology is rapidly reducing the necessity for physical activity as part of everyday life. Many modern conveniences (e.g., escalators, electronic messaging) contribute to sedentary lifestyles and the overall health issues that accompany them. Only 23% of Americans are meeting the recommended guidelines for aerobic and muscle-strengthening activity, and only 53% of adults participate in 150 minutes of moderate physical activity each week, which is the minimum recommendation.[1]

Increased participation in regular physical activity is a national health goal. The U.S. Department of Health and Human Services has set nutrition and physical fitness goals for Americans—among many other health-related goals—in its *Healthy People 2030* initiative. The targets for participation in physical activity are listed in Box 16.1.[2] In addition to these goals, the *Physical Activity Guidelines for Americans* the *Dietary Guidelines for Americans, 2020-2025;* the MyPlate guidelines; and the Dietary Reference Intakes address the need to participate in regular physical activity.

Physical activity differs from exercise according to the following definition[3]:

- *Physical activity:* Bodily movement produced by the contraction of skeletal muscles that substantially increases energy expenditure above the basal level.

- *Exercise:* A subcategory of physical activity that is planned, structured, repetitive, and with the purpose of improving or maintaining one or more component of physical fitness.

The *Physical Activity Guidelines for Americans* are based on the following four components[3]:

- *Intensity:* How hard a person works to do the activity.
  - Moderate intensity is equivalent in effort to brisk walking.
  - Vigorous intensity is equivalent in effort to running or jogging.
- *Frequency:* How often a person performs aerobic activity.
- *Duration (specific to aerobic exercise):* How long a person performs an activity during any one session.
- *Sets and repetitions (specific to muscle-strengthening activity):* How many times a person does the muscle-strengthening activity, such as lifting a weight.

The *Physical Activity Guidelines for Americans* are as follows[3]:

- *Children and adolescents:* Preschool-aged children ages 3 to 5 years should be physically active throughout the day. Children and adolescents ages 6 to 17 years should engage in 60 minutes or more of physical activity each day.
  - *Aerobic:* Most of the 60 or more minutes per day should be either moderate- or vigorous-intensity aerobic physical activity and should include vigorous-intensity physical activity at least 3 days a week.
  - *Muscle strengthening:* As part of their 60 or more minutes of daily physical activity, children and adolescents should include muscle-strengthening physical activity on at least 3 days of the week.
  - *Bone strengthening:* As part of their 60 or more minutes of daily physical activity, children and adolescents should include bone-strengthening physical activity on at least 3 days of the week.

| Box 16.1 | *Healthy People 2030* Physical Activity Objectives |

ADULTS

- Reduce the proportion of adults who engage in no leisure-time physical activity. Target: 21.2%.
- Increase the proportion of adults who meet current physical activity guidelines for aerobic physical activity and for muscle-strengthening activity.
  - Increase the proportion of adults who engage in aerobic physical activity to meet the current minimum guidelines for substantial health benefits (i.e., moderate intensity for at least 150 minutes/week, or at least 75 minutes/week of vigorous intensity, or an equivalent combination.) Target: 59.2%.
  - Increase the proportion of adults who engage in aerobic physical activity at a level needed for more extensive health benefits (i.e., moderate intensity for more than 300 minutes per week, more than 150 minutes per week of vigorous-intensity exercise, or an equivalent combination). Target: 42.3%.
  - Increase the proportion of adults who perform muscle-strengthening activities on two or more days of the week. Target: 32.1%.
  - Increase the proportion of adults who meet the minimum guidelines for aerobic physical activity and muscle-strengthening activity. Target: 28.4%.

ADOLESCENTS

- Increase the proportion of adolescents (grades 9 through 12) who meet current physical activity guidelines for aerobic physical activity and for muscle-strengthening activity.
  - Increase the proportion of adolescents who meet the current aerobic physical activity guideline (i.e., physically active for at least 60 minutes on all 7 days of the week). Target: 30.6%.
  - Increase the proportion of adolescents who participate in muscle-strengthening activity on 3 or more days of the week. Target: 56.1%.
  - Increase the proportion of adolescents who meet the minimum guidelines for aerobic physical activity and muscle-strengthening activity. Target: 24.1%.

From U.S. Department of Health and Human Services. (2020). *Healthy People 2030*. Retrieved February 21, 2021, from health.gov/healthypeople.

- *Adults:* Adults should move more and sit less throughout the day. Some physical activity is better than none, and adults who participate in any amount of physical activity gain some health benefits.
  - For substantial health benefits, adults should perform at least 150 to 300 minutes a week of moderate-intensity aerobic physical activity, 75 to 150 minutes a week of vigorous-intensity aerobic physical activity, or an equivalent combination of moderate- and vigorous-intensity aerobic activity. Spreading aerobic activity throughout the week is ideal.
  - Engaging in physical activity beyond the equivalent of 300 minutes a week of moderate-intensity aerobic activity provides more extensive health benefits.
  - Adults should also perform moderate- or high-intensity muscle-strengthening activities that involve all major muscle groups on 2 or more days

a week, because these activities provide additional health benefits.

- *Older adults:* The guidelines given for adults also apply to older adults. In addition, the following guidelines are specific to older adults:
  - As part of weekly physical activity, older adults should focus on physical activity that includes balance training as well as aerobic and muscle-strengthening activities.
  - Older adults should determine their level of effort for physical activity relative to their level of fitness.
  - Older adults with chronic conditions should understand whether and how their conditions affect their ability to perform regular physical activity safely.
  - When older adults cannot perform 150 minutes of moderate-intensity aerobic activity a week because of chronic conditions, they should be as physically active as their abilities and conditions allow.

Figure 16.1 provides suggestions on how to incorporate recommended activities into daily life.

HEALTH BENEFITS

All people can develop healthy lifestyles using personalized programs designed to meet individual needs. Developing a regular exercise routine supports consistency of activity. Water aerobics, walking, and other low-impact workouts are popular and enable more people to participate (e.g., those who cannot lift heavy weights or participate in high-intensity aerobic activities). Many new members of fitness clubs are older adults who have health problems that may improve with moderate exercise. Regular exercise helps with the management of health, reduces the risk of chronic disease, promotes independence, and increases quality of life (Box 16.2).

For most people, physical activity should not pose a health problem or hazard. The Exercise Pre-participation Health Screening Questionnaire for Exercise Professionals is designed to identify the small number of adults for whom physical activity may be inappropriate or those who should have medical clearance regarding the type of activity that is most suitable for them (Figure 16.2).[4] It is the responsibility of all health care practitioners to understand and operate within their scope of practice for exercise recommendations and prescriptions. This chapter discusses general recommendations. Much like in the field of dietetics, in which the registered dietitian nutritionists (RDNs) are the recognized nutrition experts, exercise scientists, physiologists, and certified personal trainers are the experts in exercise.

The sense of fitness achieved by exercise helps people to feel good physically, emotionally, and psychologically. In addition to this general sense of well-being, exercise (especially aerobic exercise) has particular benefits for people with certain health problems, such as those that follow.

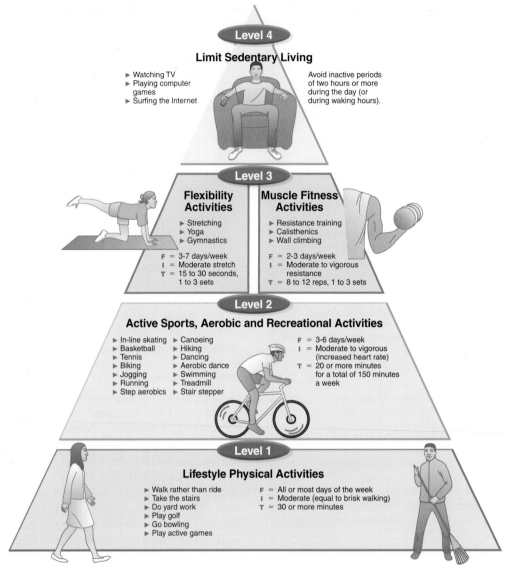

Accumulate moderate activity from the pyramid on all or most days
of the week, and vigorous activity at least three days a week.

Eating well helps you stay active and fit.

Figure 16.1 Physical activity pyramid. *F*, frequency; *I*, intensity; *T*, time.

Coronary Heart Disease

Exercise reduces the risk for heart disease in several ways, including improved heart function, decreased blood cholesterol levels, and improved oxygen transport.

Heart muscle function. The heart is a four-chambered organ that is approximately the size of an adult fist. Exercise—especially aerobic conditioning—strengthens the heart muscle, thereby enabling it to pump more blood per beat (i.e., stroke volume). A heart strengthened by exercise has an increased **aerobic capacity;** in other words, the heart can pump more blood per minute without an undue increase in heart rate. Therefore, exercises relying primarily on the aerobic oxygen system for energy (e.g., walking, jogging, exercise using cardiopulmonary exercise machines) improve heart function.

Blood lipid levels. Resistance training programs may improve blood lipid profiles by significantly lowering the total cholesterol level, the low-density lipoprotein level, the total cholesterol to high-density lipoprotein ratio, and the triglyceride level.[5] Additionally, moderate intensity aerobic exercise has been shown to increase high-density lipoprotein levels, and when intensity level is increased, low-density lipoprotein and triglyceride levels were lowered.[6] Both exercise effects (i.e., improved heart function and cholesterol profile) lower the risk for diseased arteries.

Oxygen-carrying capacity. Exercise also strengthens the circulatory system by increasing the oxygen-carrying capacity of the blood. As training continues, a person's efficiency of oxygen use and uptake (VO_2) will improve and can increase one's overall level of fitness.

Box 16.2	Health Benefits Associated With Regular Physical Activity[a]

CHILDREN AND ADOLESCENTS
Strong or Moderate Evidence

- Improved weight management (ages 3 through 17 years)
- Improved bone health (ages 3 through 17 years)
- Increased cardiorespiratory and muscular fitness (ages 6 through 17 years)
- Improved cardiometabolic health biomarkers (ages 6 through 17 years)
- Reduced symptoms of depression (ages 6 through 17 years)
- Improved cognition (ages 6 through 17 years)

ADULTS AND OLDER ADULTS
Strong Evidence

- Lower risk of early death
- Lower risk of cardiovascular disease and related mortality
- Lower risk of high blood pressure
- Lower risk of adverse blood lipid profile
- Decreased risk of type 2 diabetes
- Lower risk of certain cancers (bladder, breast, colon, endometrium, esophagus, kidney, lung, stomach)
- Reduced weight gain
- Weight loss, particularly when combined with reduced calorie intake
- Improved weight maintenance after weight loss
- Improved cardiorespiratory and muscular fitness
- Prevention of falls
- Reduced depression
- Reduced anxiety
- Better cognitive function
- Lower risk of dementia
- Improved sleep
- Better functional health
- Increased bone density
- Decreased risk for fall-related injuries
- Improved quality of life

[a]*NOTE:* The Advisory Committee rated the evidence of health benefits of physical activity as strong, moderate, or weak. To do so, the Committee considered the type, number, and quality of studies available, as well as the consistency of findings across studies that addressed each outcome. The Committee also considered evidence for causality and dose response in assigning the strength-of-evidence rating.
From U.S. Department of Health and Human Services. (2018). *Physical activity guidelines for Americans* (2nd ed.). Washington, DC: DHHS.

Hypertension

Cardiovascular complications increase with rising blood pressure levels. According to the American Heart Association, nearly half (46%) of Americans have **hypertension.**[7] Blood pressure reduction resulting from exercise appears to be greater among hypertensive individuals, although individuals with blood pressure in the normal range see modest reductions as well.[8] Exercise, a nonpharmacologic therapy, is a first line of defense for individuals with elevated blood pressure and is an adjunct therapy for blood-pressure lowering medications for those with hypertension.[9]

Normal rises in blood pressure occur during both aerobic and resistance-type exercises; and both forms of exercise are beneficial for individuals with hypertension.

However, exercisers with diagnosed hypertension should avoid excess exertion to prevent severe stress on the cardiovascular system. An example would be holding your breath during the exertion phase of the exercise, such as with the lifting of heavy weights.

Diabetes

Physically active lifestyles are especially beneficial for individuals with type 2 diabetes to improve overall health and to reduce the risk of the chronic complications associated with diabetes.[10] Exercise improves the action of a person's naturally produced insulin by increasing the sensitivity of insulin receptor sites. Exercise also enhances glucose uptake without requiring insulin through the process of skeletal muscle cells clearing glucose from the blood. When an individual is managing type 1 diabetes mellitus, balancing food intake and insulin injections with the type of exercise and timing helps prevent reactions caused by drops in blood glucose levels (see Chapter 20 for a more detailed discussion of diabetes).[10]

Weight Management

Although exercise alone is typically insufficient to promote significant weight loss, regular exercise in conjunction with a reduced caloric intake can support body weight loss (see Chapter 15). Combining aerobic exercise and resistance exercise can result in greater reductions in fat mass while maintaining or increasing lean body mass.[11] Aside from weight loss, obese individuals receive important health benefits from exercise training, including improvements outlined above (e.g., improvements in blood pressure, blood lipid levels, insulin sensitivity) as well as improved physical fitness and quality of life.

Bone Disease

Weight-bearing exercises (e.g., walking, running) help to strengthen bones by increasing **osteoblast** activity. The weight-bearing load increases calcium deposits in bone, thereby increasing bone density and reducing the risk for osteoporosis. Although the benefits of exercise on bone density are most notable during the peak bone growth periods of adolescents and young adults, older adults are encouraged to engage in weight-bearing exercise regularly to prevent further decreases in bone mineral density. However, excessive forms of training can have a destructive effect, in which bone density is lost because of overtraining or undernutrition, or both.

---

aerobic capacity a state in which oxygen is required to proceed; milliliters of oxygen consumed per kilogram of body weight per minute as influenced by body composition.
hypertension chronically elevated blood pressure; systolic blood pressure is consistently 130 mm Hg or more or diastolic blood pressure is consistently 80 mm Hg or more.
osteoblast cells that are responsible for the mineralization and formation of bone.

Exercise Pre-participation Health Screening Questionnaire for Exercise Professionals

Asses your client health needs by marking all true statements.

Step 1

SYMPTOMS
Does your client experience
__ chest discomfort with exertion
__ unreasonable breathlessness
__ dizziness, fainting, blackouts
__ ankle swelling
__ unpleasant awareness of a forceful, rapid or irregular heart rate
__ burning or cramping sensations in the lower legs when walking short distance

If you **did** mark any of the statements under the symptoms, **STOP**; your client should seek medical clearance before engaging in or resuming exercise. Your client may need to use a facility with a **medically qualified staff.**

If you **did not** mark any symptoms, continue to steps 2 and 3.

Step 2

CURRENT ACTIVITY
Does your client currently perform planned, structured physical activity at least 30 min at moderate intensity on at least 3 days per week for at least the last 3 months?

Yes ☐   No ☐

Continue to Step 3

Step 3

MEDICAL CONDITIONS
Has your client had or do they currently have:
__ a heart attack
__ heart surgery, cardiac catheterization, or coronary angioplasty
__ pacemaker/implantable cardiac defibrillator/rhythm disturbance
__ heart valve disease
__ heart failure
__ heart transplantation
__ congenital heart disease
__ diabetes
__ renal disease

Evaluating Steps 2 and 3:

- If you **did not mark any of the statements in Step 3**, medical clearance is not necessary.
- If you marked Step 2 **"yes"** and **marked any of the statements in Step 3**, your client may continue to exercise at light to moderate intensity without medical clearance. Medical clearance is recommended before engaging in vigorous exercise.
- If you marked Step 2 **"no"** and **marked any of the statements in Step 3**, medical clearance is recommended. Your client may need to use a facility with a **medically qualified staff.**

Figure 16.2 Exercise Pre-participation Health Screening Questionnaire for Exercise Professionals. (From Magal, M., & Riebe, D. [2016]. New preparticipation health screening recommendations. *ACSM Health Fit J, 20*[3], 22–27.)

Mental Health

Exercise can improve mood through physiologic and biochemical mechanisms. For example, exercise stimulates the production of *endorphins,* natural chemicals that decrease pain and improve mood, and may include an exhilarating type of "high." Recent studies have shown that exercise can improve the management of stress, anxiety, and depression. As individuals age, physical activity is associated with a lower risk of cognitive decline and dementia, while improving sleep quality and overall quality of life.[12]

TYPES OF PHYSICAL ACTIVITY

A well-balanced exercise program incorporates resistance training, aerobic activities, flexibility and balance exercises, in addition to an assortment of activities of daily living. This regimen can include various enjoyable activities that effectively reduce the risk of many chronic diseases.

Resistance Training

Resistance training creates and maintains muscle and bone strength, improves blood pressure in prehypertensive/hypertensive individuals, and increases insulin sensitivity. An ideal resistance program should include 8 to 10 separate exercises (with at least 8 to 12 repetitions of each) focusing on all major muscle groups and that are performed 2 to 3 days per week. A more progressive model incorporates gradual load increases to stimulate muscle overload, greater muscle specificity and variation, and a training regimen of 4 to 5 days per week.[13] For an individual whose primary goal is to gain strength and power, the repetitions should be of high intensity, with fewer than six repetitions before muscle fatigue occurs. For improved endurance, a lower weight should be used that will allow at least 15 repetitions before muscle fatigue occurs.

Table **16.1** Aerobic Exercises for Physical Fitness

TYPE OF EXERCISE	AEROBIC FORMS
Ball playing	Handball
	Racquetball
	Tennis
Bicycling	Stationary biking
	Touring or mountain biking
Dancing	Aerobic routines
	Ballet
	Zumba
Jumping rope	Brisk pace
Running or jogging	Brisk pace
Skating	Ice skating
	Roller skating
Skiing	Cross country
Swimming	Steady pace
Walking	Brisk pace

Aerobic Exercise

Forms of exercise that involve moving the body's large muscles in a rhythmic manner for a sustained period of time include activities such as swimming, running, jogging, bicycling, aerobic dancing routines, and similar workouts (Table 16.1). Perhaps the simplest and most popular form of aerobic exercise is walking. Figure 16.3

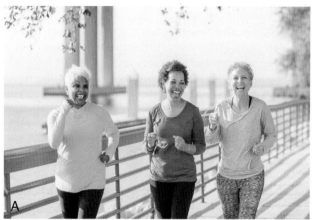
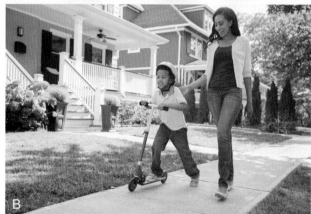
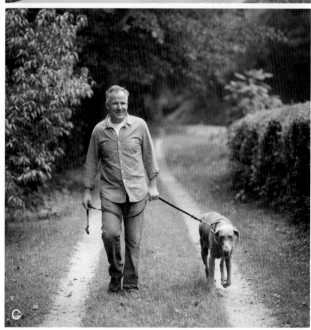

Figure 16.3 Aerobic walking is an exercise that can fit into almost anyone's lifestyle. (*Left to right:* Copyright iStock Photos; A, Credit:kali9; B, Credit:monkeybusinessimages; and C, Credit:stevecoleimages.)

illustrates how aerobic walking can fit into almost anyone's lifestyle. If the pace is fast enough to elevate the pulse rate, then walking can be an excellent form of aerobic exercise. It is convenient, and it requires no equipment other than good walking shoes. Table 16.2 provides information about energy expenditure per hour for various activities at a given body weight.

Weight-Bearing Exercise

Both aerobic and resistance-type exercises may fit into this category. Weight-bearing exercises such as walking, jogging, aerobic dancing, and jumping rope are important for bone structure and strength. In these exercises, muscles are working against gravity. The load put on bones during weight-bearing exercises increases the bone density and decreases the risk of falls, which can be debilitating for aging individuals.

Activities of Daily Living

Many activities of daily living do not reach aerobic levels (e.g., walking to work or to the store, walking the dog, playing with children on the playground) but are enjoyable and are important parts of daily life. The likelihood of an activity becoming beneficial and sustainable depends on the enjoyment obtained from it. Activities of daily living create opportunities to be active throughout the day regardless of structured exercise while maintaining strength and agility and decreasing time spent in sedentary behavior.

Sedentary Behavior

Sedentary behavior is any waking behavior characterized by a low level of energy expenditure and includes sitting, reclining, or lying. Americans are sedentary for an average of 8 hours/day. The harmful effects of excessively sedentary lifestyles, such as an increased risk for all-cause and cardiovascular disease mortality and increased incidence of type 2 diabetes, are well known.[14,15] These risks persist independent of the amount of exercise in which one engages. Only those engaging in high amounts of moderate-to-vigorous physical activity may offset some of this increased risk. The key message for Americans is that they need to sit less and move more!

MEETING PERSONAL NEEDS

Health Status and Personal Gains

When planning a personal exercise program, first assess an individual's health status, present level of fitness, personal needs, and resources necessary for equipment and related costs. Seeking advice and guidance from a certified personal trainer or an exercise physiologist will be of great benefit. Several different organizations certify personal trainers, but some are more reputable than others. The American College of Sports Medicine is one of the leading authorities for certifying professionals as health fitness specialists, certified personal trainers, clinical exercise specialists, and registered clinical exercise physiologists (visit www.acsm.org).

The exercise that is chosen should be something that is both enjoyable and of aerobic value. In addition, the individual should start slowly and build gradually to avoid burnout and injury. Moderation and regularity are the chief guides.

Achieving Aerobic Benefits

To build aerobic capacity, the level of exercise must raise the pulse rate to within 60% to 90% of an individual's maximal heart rate. An acceptable way to estimate the maximal heart rate is to subtract the person's age from 220. Achieving aerobic benefits requires a total of 150 minutes per week of exercise at 70% of maximal heart rate for most people (Table 16.3). Check the resting pulse rate before starting the exercise period and then again during and immediately afterward to monitor progress toward the target exercising heart rate and aerobic capacity. Heart rate monitors are a convenient way to monitor and keep track of the heart rate.

Exercise Preparation and Care

Whatever the choice of exercise, preparation and continuing care are important. It is not in the scope of this nutrition text to explore the details of various exercise programs. However, some very basic guidelines include warming up the muscles to prevent stress or injury and taking time to cool down after exercising. Do not go beyond tolerance limits; instead, listen to the body. Rest when tired and stop when hurting. Contact a physician if symptoms do not subside. When you are ready for a greater challenge, you can gradually increase the exercise level by number of repetitions, weight intensity, or endurance—not all three at the same time.

Table **16.2**	Approximate Energy Expenditure Per Hour During Various Activities
ACTIVITY	**KILOCALORIES PER HOUR**[a]
Sleeping	67
Typing, sitting	90
Standing	175
Walking slowly (24 min/mile)	210
Circuit training, moderate effort	300
Water aerobics	385
High-impact aerobics	420
Football, flag or touch	560
Walking quickly (12 min/mile)	580
Bicycling, mountain	595
Stair, treadmill	630
Swimming, vigorous effort	686
Running (8 min/mile)	826

[a]For an adult who weighs 70 kg (154 lb).
Modified from Ainsworth, B. E., Haskell, W. L., Hermann, S. D., et al. (2011). 2011 Compendium of physical activities: A second update of codes and MET values. *Med Sci Sports Exerc, 43*(8), 1575–1851.

Table 16.3	Target Zone Heart Rate According to Age to Achieve Aerobic Physical Effect of Exercise		
	MAXIMAL ATTAINABLE	TARGET ZONE	
AGE (YEARS)	HEART RATE (PULSE = 220 − AGE)	70% MAXIMAL RATE	85% MAXIMAL RATE
20	200	140	170
25	195	136	166
30	190	133	161
35	185	129	157
40	180	126	153
45	175	122	149
50	170	119	144
55	165	115	140
60	160	112	136
65	155	108	132
70	150	105	127
75	145	101	124

DIETARY NEEDS DURING EXERCISE

MUSCLE ACTION AND FUEL

Structure and Function

The synchronized action of millions of specialized cells that make up our skeletal muscle mass makes all forms of physical activity possible. A finely coordinated series of small bundles within the muscle fibers produce a smooth symphony of action through simultaneous and alternating contraction and relaxation. This muscular activity requires oxygen and energy.

Oxygen

Without an increase in oxygenated blood delivered to the working muscle, exercise could only last a few minutes. Aerobic, or oxidative, metabolism uses carbohydrates and fats as energy for working muscles during extended periods. Although there are many factors that determine the body's ability to transport and use oxygen, the fitness of the cardiovascular system as well as an individual's relative and absolute muscle mass are important determinants of oxygen use during exercise.

Cardiovascular fitness. Aerobic capacity, which defines cardiovascular fitness, depends on the body's ability to deliver and use oxygen in sufficient quantities to meet the demands of increasing levels of exercise. Oxygen uptake increases with exercise intensity until either meeting the demand or exceeding the ability to supply it. The maximum rate at which the body can take in oxygen (i.e., aerobic capacity) is the **VO₂max**. This capacity is a determinant of the intensity and duration of exercise that a person can perform.

Body composition. Body composition is a reflection of the four body compartments that make up the total body weight: lean body mass, fat, water, and bone (see Chapter 15). Lean body mass is more metabolically active (i.e., requires more fuel pound for pound) than other body tissues such as adipose tissue. Thus, the amount of lean body mass (relative to total fat mass) influences a person's fitness level and oxygen use.

Fuel Sources

The fuel sources required for energy are the basic energy nutrients: primarily carbohydrate (glucose and glycogen) and fat. The body only oxidizes protein in very small quantities during exercise, and it is not an ideal or a significant energy source under normal circumstances.

The relative use of stored fat for energy during exercise depends on the level of fitness of the person and the intensity of the exercise. Trained endurance athletes are more efficient at using fat for energy than are their untrained counterparts. Regardless of training status, as exercise intensity increases, so does reliance upon carbohydrate as a fuel source. Think of it as a dimmer switch. Sustained, low-intensity exercises (i.e., 25% to 65% VO₂max) rely primarily on muscle fat stores for energy through the aerobic pathway and use relatively smaller amounts of carbohydrate.[16] As intensity increases, so does the relative contribution of carbohydrate for energy. When exercise intensity exceeds approximately 65% VO₂max, carbohydrate becomes the predominant fuel source and fat contributes less, although this percentage may vary according to training status and dietary factors. This is due in part to the relative rate in which each macronutrient is broken down to render adenosine triphosphate (ATP). Because fat is a more dense nutrient, fat metabolism is slower and requires more oxygen than does the metabolism of carbohydrate (Table 16.4).

Table 16.4	Source of Energy for Varying Exercise Intensity
EXERCISE INTENSITY	FUEL USED BY MUSCLE
<30% VO₂max (easy walking)	Mainly muscle fat stores
40% to 65% VO₂max (jogging, brisk walking)	Fat and carbohydrate in similar proportions
75% VO₂max (running)	Mainly carbohydrate
>80% VO₂max (sprinting)	Nearly 100% carbohydrate

VO₂max, Peak oxygen uptake.

VO₂max the maximal uptake volume of oxygen during exercise; this is used to measure the intensity and duration of exercise that a person can perform.

GENERAL TRAINING DIET

All individuals who regularly participate in physical activity must apply the general principles of exercise and energy balance (previously described). At what point does a person who regularly exercises become an athlete? It is often difficult to determine exactly when someone's nutrient needs require additional attention. From a nutrition standpoint, a major difference in an athlete's diet compared with that of the general public is that athletes have greater fluid and energy needs related to their training demands. However, optimal nutrition strategies enhance physical activity, athletic performance, and exercise recovery for everyone.[17]

Failure to meet the increased energy and fluid needs can have significant consequences for these individuals. The extreme demands placed on the bodies of athletes involved in heavy training renders them more susceptible to immunosuppression. A well-balanced diet with adequate calories, macronutrients, and micronutrients from a variety of foods helps to prevent exercise-induced malnutrition and the risk for injury and infection.[18,19]

Recommendations for adults may not apply to child and adolescent athletes. Nutrient and energy needs of this population are specific to their current developmental requirements. A Certified Specialist in Sports Dietetics (CSSD) can customize nutrient recommendations for these athletes.

Energy and Nutrient Stores

Exercise increases energy requirements and helps regulate appetite to meet this need. See Table 16.2 for some examples of the amount of kilocalories expended by general activities. For athletes and other active individuals, proper dietary choices are essential to achieve daily energy needs, nutrient reserves, and optimal performance. Without adequate energy during prolonged exercise, nutrient levels fall too low to sustain the body's continued demands. Fatigue follows, and exhaustion may result.

This chapter covers the energy and nutrient needs for most individuals who participate in physical activity under the next heading. Specific dietary recommendations for meeting energy needs and maximizing nutrient stores for high-performing athletes is outside of the scope of this text; these individuals are encouraged to work individually with certified sports dietitians.

Fluid and Energy Needs

Fluid. Blood is primarily water, and thus fluid status directly affects the body's ability to distribute oxygen and nutrients to working muscle cells. Dehydration of 2% or more of one's body weight will impair athletic performance, particularly in hot and humid climates.[20] The extent of dehydration depends upon the intensity and duration of the exercise, the environmental conditions, rehydration strategies, fitness level, and the pre-exercise hydration status. With continued

exercise, the body temperature rises in response to the release of heat during energy production. To control this temperature rise, the body sends as much heat as possible to the skin through blood, where heat escapes in sweat that evaporates on the skin. Over time—and especially in hot weather—excessive sweating can lead to dehydration. If dehydration continues, athletes may experience problems such as cramps, delirium, vomiting, hypothermia, or hyperthermia. Fluid replacement strategies implemented during exercise may prevent many of these problems.

Planning for fluid intake is important for all types of athletes for whom there will be considerable fluid loss. Athletes who are engaged in longer and more demanding endurance events (i.e., more than 60 to 90 minutes), especially in a warm environment, may benefit from an electrolyte and glucose sports drink that has optimal gastric emptying and intestinal absorption times (see the Chapter 9 For Further Focus box, "Hydrating with Water, Sports Drink, or Energy Drink").[20]

Total energy. When exercise levels rise from mild or moderate amounts up to strenuous levels, caloric needs also rise to supply adequate fuel. Exact energy needs vary depending on sex, age, body size, genetics, body composition, environmental conditions, medications, and phase of menstrual cycle for women. Additionally, the type and volume of training alters energy needs, which may vary on a day-to-day basis. Adequate total energy intake allows athletes to maintain appropriate weight and body composition while maximizing performance.[17] Chapter 6 covers the various methods for calculating basic energy needs. The Cunningham (Box 16.3) or Harris-Benedict equations can estimate total energy needs, which are then multiplied by an activity factor correlated to an individual's specific daily energy expenditure. A CSSD can assess an athlete's energy needs based upon the details of an athlete's training and competition needs and provide appropriate energy recommendations. Consuming a variety of foods best meets an athlete's nutrient and energy needs, as represented by the MyPlate guidelines (see Figure 1.4).

Macronutrient and Micronutrient Recommendations

Carbohydrate. Carbohydrate is the preferred fuel and critical energy source for an active person before and during exercise and fuels the recovery period. Complex carbohydrates sustain energy needs and supply necessary fiber, vitamins, and minerals. Carbohydrate

---

Box 16.3	Cunningham Equation[1]

$$\text{kcal/day} = 500 + 22 \times \text{FFM (kg)}$$

REFERENCE

1. Phillips, S. M. (2014). A brief review of critical processes in exercise-induced muscular hypertrophy. *Sports Medicine*, 44(Suppl. 1), S71–77.

fuels come from two sources: circulating blood glucose and glycogen stored in muscle and liver tissue. Complex carbohydrates (i.e., starches) are preferable to simple carbohydrates (i.e., monosaccharides and disaccharides) when consumed as part of the diet. Starches break down gradually, help to maintain blood glucose levels more evenly (thus avoiding **hypoglycemia**), and maintain glycogen stores as a constant primary fuel.

Diets that are too low in carbohydrate are unable to meet energy demands and result in poor performance and increased fatigue, especially during prolonged bouts of intense exercise.[21] A low-carbohydrate diet decreases the body's capacity for work, which intensifies over time. Physically active individuals on low-carbohydrate diets are susceptible to fatigue, ketoacidosis, and dehydration. Conversely, a diet with sufficient carbohydrate intake enhances muscle glycogen concentrations and exercise performance.[21] In addition, consuming small amounts of carbohydrates during longer bouts of exercise improves whole-body carbohydrate oxidation and metabolic efficiency, especially if the individual did not consume a high-carbohydrate meal before exercise.[21] Therefore, eating foods with adequate carbohydrates before and during exercise helps to maintain the glucose concentrations that are necessary to exercise strenuously and delay fatigue.

Athletes who are competing in prolonged endurance events should increase their energy intake from carbohydrates. Consuming 3 to 7 g of carbohydrate per kg of body weight per day usually meets general training needs, although this amount varies according to training and competition schedules. Endurance athletes have higher needs of 7 to 10 g/kg body weight per day, with ultra-endurance athletes requiring up to 12 g/kg body weight per day.[17]

Fat. Dietary recommendations for fat intake to support physical activity do not vary from standard guidelines. In the presence of oxygen, fatty acids serve as a fuel source from stored fat tissue. There is insufficient evidence to support improved physical performance with a dietary fat intake of more than 30% of the total daily energy intake. However, an extremely low fat intake can be dangerous if the diet is deficient in the essential fatty acids (i.e., linoleic and α-linolenic acids). A moderate level of fat is necessary in the diet to ensure the adequate intake of the essential fatty acids and the absorption of fat-soluble vitamins.

Dietary fat is needed to meet energy needs, to supply essential fatty acids, and to maintain weight. No performance benefit occurs from consuming a diet that is less than 20% or greater than 35% of calories in the diet coming from fat. See the For Further Focus box, "High-Fat Diets and Athletic Performance."

Protein. Adequate dietary protein is essential for tissue repair and remodeling, protein turnover, and for metabolic adaptation. The intensity, duration, and type of exercise as well as sex, age, energy intake, and carbohydrate availability dictate protein requirements.[22]

For Further Focus

High-Fat Diets and Athletic Performance

The athletic community has not been immune to the recent popularity of low-carbohydrate, high-fat diets, of which the ketogenic diet is one example. Although there are various iterations of these diets, they are typically low in carbohydrate (less than 50 g a day), high in dietary fat (70% to 80% of calories), and moderate in protein. Proponents of this diet claim that even very lean athletes have plentiful lipid stores compared with having a limited storage of carbohydrate. Diets high in fat induce adaptations that increase the release, transport, uptake, and utilization of fat by the muscle.[1,2] Such adaptations help to spare an athlete's reliance upon carbohydrate as an energy source, which otherwise can limit exercise capacity.

Indeed, studies on athletes adapted to a low-carbohydrate, high-fat diet demonstrate the metabolic adaptations that allow them to oxidize fat at higher rates. Currently, however, there is insufficient evidence to indicate that this translates to a performance benefit for the athlete.[1] Rather, performance of those following a low-carbohydrate/high-fat diet is impaired when exercising at higher intensities, a context that applies to most competitive athletes.[3]

Research is investigating whether a low-carbohydrate, high-fat diet may help achieve improvements in body composition (i.e., an increase in lean body mass and/or a decrease in fat mass). However, the athlete must weigh this potential benefit with the understanding that this dietary approach may have adverse effects on athletic performance. Appropriate timing and provision of adequate carbohydrates support optimal performance during key training and competitive situations.

REFERENCES

1. Burke, L. M. (2015). Re-examining high-fat diets for sports performance: Did we call the 'nail in the coffin' too soon? *Sports Medicine*, 45(Suppl. 1), S33–S49.
2. Spriet, L. L. (2014). New insights into the interaction of carbohydrate and fat metabolism during exercise. *Sports Medicine*, 44(Suppl. 1), S87–S96.
3. Burke, L. M., et al. (2017). Low carbohydrate, high fat diet impairs exercise economy and negates the performance benefit from intensified training in elite race walkers. *Journal of Physiology*, 595(9), 2785–2807.

For endurance and strength-trained athletes, protein requirements range from 1.2 to 2.0 g/kg/day.[17] Dietary intake alone can usually meet protein needs, even for vegetarians and highly trained athletes (see the For Further Focus box, "The Vegetarian Athlete"). For example, a 160-lb (72.7-kg) male track athlete may have protein needs of 1.6 g/kg body weight: 72.7 kg × 1.6 g of protein/kg = 116 g of protein per day. The average daily protein intake by U.S. men and women who are 20 years old and older is nearly 100 g and 70 g per day, respectively.[23] Thus, even for an athlete who incorporates resistance exercise into his training, a slight increase of 16 g of protein per day over the average American intake would meet his needs. Some athletes choose to consume protein supplements to help meet increased protein needs. Consumption of small to moderate amounts of these products may be safe. Although

For Further Focus

The Vegetarian Athlete

There are numerous forms of vegetarian diets varying in the amounts and types of omitted animal foods (see Chapter 4). Growing numbers of athletes are adopting these dietary approaches, largely owing to the associated health and environmental benefits. Questions arise if these athletes are able to meet their increased nutrient needs.

The most common concern is whether this dietary approach can provide an athlete with sufficient protein. In fact, a balanced vegetarian diet that includes a variety of plant-based protein sources consumed consistently throughout the day can easily meet the protein needs of all active individuals. An intentional, thought-out meal plan can achieve this goal, and vegetarian athletes may benefit from specific nutrition education. One recent study that analyzed the protein intake of vegetarian and omnivore (meat-consuming) athletes saw no significant differences in total protein consumption and found that both groups met their respective protein recommendations.[1] Depending upon the degree of dietary restriction, additional nutrients of concern for this population may include energy, iron, zinc, vitamin B_{12}, iodine, calcium, vitamin D, and n-3 fatty acids.[2] A sports dietitian can assess a vegetarian athlete's diet for adequacy to identify if there are any specific nutrients of concern.

Overall, the nutrient quality of vegetarian diets seems to score higher compared with omnivorous diets.[3] Although the research connecting a vegetarian diet to athletic performance is limited, it appears that a vegetarian diet may not necessarily improve outcomes, but it does not hinder performance either.[4] Active individuals can adequately fuel their athletic endeavors while consuming a vegetarian diet.

REFERENCES

1. Lynch, H. M., Wharton, C. M., & Johnston, C. S. (2016). Cardiorespiratory fitness and peak torque differences between vegetarian and omnivore endurance athletes: A cross-sectional study. *Nutrients, 8*(11).
2. Thomas, D. T., Erdman, K. A., & Burke, L. M. (2016). Position of the Academy of Nutrition and Dietetics, Dietitians of Canada, and the American College of Sports Medicine: Nutrition and athletic performance. *Journal of the Academy of Nutrition and Dietetics, 116*(3), 501–528.
3. Clarys, P., et al. (2014). Comparison of nutritional quality of the vegan, vegetarian, semi-vegetarian, pesco-vegetarian and omnivorous diet. *Nutrients, 6*(3), 1318–1332.
4. Craddock, J. C., Probst, Y. C., & Peoples, G. E. (2016). Vegetarian and omnivorous nutrition-comparing physical performance. *International Journal of Sport Nutrition and Exercise Metabolism, 26*(3), 212–220.

higher-protein diets may not be dangerous in otherwise healthy individuals, athletes should not displace sufficient carbohydrate and fat intake with excess protein.

Vitamins and minerals. Energy production does not oxidize vitamins and minerals. However, vitamins and minerals are essential as catalytic cofactors in enzyme reactions (see Chapter 7 and Chapter 8). Increased physical exertion during exercise does not require a greater intake of vitamins and minerals beyond currently recommended intakes. A well-balanced diet supplies adequate amounts of vitamins and minerals. Because athletes have an increased dietary need for energy, a larger kilocalorie intake from nutrient-dense foods would automatically boost their general intake of vitamins and minerals.

Multivitamin and mineral supplementation does not improve physical performance in healthy people who are eating well-balanced diets. However, athletes who restrict their energy intake, eliminate one or more food groups from their diet, or who consume nutrient-poor diets may consume insufficient amounts of micronutrients and require supplementation. Additionally, therapeutic iron supplements may be necessary for some individuals who are experiencing iron-deficiency anemia. Health care providers may also consider assessing vitamin D status in indoor athletes or athletes with limited sun exposure. In addition, amenorrheic female athletes need assessment of their nutrient-energy status. Chronic negative energy balance is not uncommon among athletes such as gymnasts, ballet dancers, and runners, who may also suffer from disordered eating. Disordered eating patterns may include low calcium, protein, and energy intake, which can have serious consequences for bone development (see the Clinical Applications box, "The Female Athlete Triad: How Performance and Social Pressure Can Lead to Low Bone Mass and Menstrual Dysfunction").

---

hypoglycemia an abnormally low blood glucose level that may lead to muscle tremors, cold sweat, headache, and confusion.
amenorrheic the absence or abnormal cessation of the menses.

🔖 **Clinical Applications**

The Female Athlete Triad: How Performance and Social Pressure Can Lead to Low Bone Mass and Menstrual Dysfunction

The female athlete triad (Triad) is a medical condition comprising three interrelated components faced by physically active women: (1) low energy availability with or without disordered eating; (2) menstrual dysfunction; and (3) low bone mineral density (BMD). Each component of the Triad can be highly variable and must be considered along a spectrum. At the "healthy" end of the continuum, there is adequate energy availability, ovulatory menstrual cycles, and normal bone mineral density. At the other end of the continuum,

we identify clinical endpoints of low energy availability with or without disordered eating, amenorrhea, and osteoporosis. The goal of the practitioner is early attention and intervention to prevent any of the Triad's components from advancing to pathologies exhibited at the clinical end of the spectrum.

We define energy availability as the amount of dietary energy remaining after subtracting the energy required for exercise training.[1] Adequate energy is required for all metabolic processes; if, after exercise is accounted for, the remaining

Clinical Applications—cont'd

The Female Athlete Triad: How Performance and Social Pressure Can Lead to Low Bone Mass and Menstrual Dysfunction

energy balance is too low, normal metabolism suffers. Low energy availability results from an inadequate dietary intake to meet both the training and the physiologic needs of the female athlete. This may be the result of restrained eating, dieting, disordered eating/eating disorder behaviors (see Chapter 15), or simply the athlete's lack of knowledge regarding increased energy requirements. Regardless of the cause, prolonged low energy availability may ultimately lead to menstrual dysfunction. The combination of a hypoestrogenic environment and energy deficiency play a causal role in low bone mineral density.[2]

Women who participate in competitive endurance sports (e.g., cycling, long-distance running), who are judged partially on physical appearance (e.g., ice skating, diving, or dancing), or who compete in weight class events (rowing, martial arts) are more likely to experience pressures to maintain a low body weight. Societal and competitive pressures to be thin may exacerbate the situation. Athletes often believe that a low body weight enhances performance, and some are willing to take significant health risks to achieve this body image ideal. Such pressures may lead some women to restrict energy intake leading to inadequate energy availability, particularly when combined with high energy expenditure. Performance may deteriorate as the athlete loses focus and concentration and as she becomes fatigued. Some women develop psychologic eating disorders, which in turn may progress to additional health problems, including depression, low self-esteem, seizures, cardiac arrhythmia, myocardial infarction, and other health complications.

Chronic inadequate caloric intake can cause menstrual irregularity. Amenorrhea is the cessation of previously regular menses for 3 months; primary amenorrhea is the repression of all menstrual cycles until the age of 15 years. In the most competitive circles, young female gymnasts may experience this condition if they strive to delay the onset of puberty to maintain their small, prepubescent physiques. Some women may experience oligomenorrhea, which are sporadic cycles occurring 3 to 9 times a year. Metabolism, intensive exercise, dieting, and stress alter the levels of estrogen and progesterone that regulate menses.

Bone density reaches its peak before the age of 30 years; therefore, young women must strive for dense bones during early adulthood to achieve healthy bone density later in life. Osteopenia results when bone density diminishes early; if it is severe enough, this is a risk for future osteoporosis. In fact, female athletes at moderate to high risk of the Triad are 2 to 4 times more likely to sustain a bone stress injury.[3] There is also increased incidence of bone stress injuries among male

athletes with low energy availability.[4] Bone stress injuries contribute to compromised bone mineral density later in life.

Weight-bearing activities (e.g., gymnastics) can improve BMD and may help to prevent decreases in bone density later in life. The concern for female athletes who eat improperly is that the rate of BMD decline intensifies with continued erratic menstrual cycles. Without monitoring diet and exercise levels, weight-bearing sports will not overcome the tendency toward low BMD. In today's weight-conscious society, the emphasis must not be on a perfect image or body size, but rather on the balance of health and training.

The primary treatment for the Triad is to address the underlying cause, that is, low energy availability. Increasing dietary intake and modification of exercise training helps to normalize energy status.[2] Ensuring sufficient energy availability is the most effective way to support resumption of menses and improve bone health. The cause of inadequate intake must be assessed—if it is due to lack of knowledge, athlete education is required; if there is concurrent disordered eating/eating disorders, then psychologic treatment must be included as well.

Male athletes are not immune to the effects of low energy availability. The term *relative energy deficiency of sports* (RED-S) identifies impaired physiologic functioning resulting from low energy availability in male and female athletes. RED-S includes disturbances in metabolic rate, bone health, immunity, protein synthesis, and cardiovascular health and extends to all athletes.[5] The need to educate trainers, athletes, and health professionals about the consequences of neglected nutrition is imperative so that all athletes can achieve lifelong health and well-being.

REFERENCES
1. De Souza, M. J., et al. (2014). 2014 female athlete triad coalition consensus statement on treatment and return to play of the female athlete triad: 1st International conference held in San Francisco, California, May 2012 and 2nd International conference held in Indianapolis, Indiana, May 2013. *British Journal of Sports Medicine, 48*(4), 289.
2. Daily, J. P., & Stumbo, J. R. (2018). Female athlete Triad. *Primary Care, 45*(4), 615–624.
3. Tenforde, A. S., et al. (2017). Association of the female athlete triad risk assessment stratification to the development of bone stress injuries in collegiate athletes. *The American Journal of Sports Medicine, 45*(2), 302–310.
4. Kraus, E., et al. (2019). Bone stress injuries in male distance runners: Higher modified female athlete triad cumulative risk assessment scores predict increased rates of injury. *British Journal of Sports Medicine, 53*(4), 237–242.
5. Mountjoy, M., et al. (2018). International Olympic Committee (IOC) consensus statement on relative energy deficiency in sport (RED-S): 2018 Update. *International Journal of Sport Nutrition and Exercise Metabolism, 28*(4), 316–331.

ATHLETIC PERFORMANCE

There are unique nutrition-related implications for athletes and those who are highly physically active. The following sections highlight topics addressing concerns for individuals with higher levels of physical activity.

CARBOHYDRATE LOADING

To prepare for an endurance event, athletes sometimes follow a dietary process called *carbohydrate* or *glycogen loading*. The current practice takes place the week before the event and is most appropriate for endurance athletes. The protocol includes a moderate and gradual tapering of exercise while increasing total carbohydrate intake in the diet to ensure maximal glycogen stores. See Table 16.5 for an example of a carbohydrate loading regimen.

PREGAME MEAL

The ideal pregame meal depends on the tolerance of the athlete, as well as the type and duration of the activity

Table 16.5 Example of a Precompetition Program for Carbohydrate Loading

DAY(S)	EXERCISE	DIET
1	90-minute period at 70% VO_2max	Mixed diet; 5 g of carbohydrate/kg body weight
2 and 3	Gradual tapering of time and intensity: <40-minute period	Same as day 1
4 and 5	Continuation of tapering: <20-minute period	Mixed diet; 10 g of carbohydrate/kg body weight
6	Complete rest	Same as days 4 and 5
7	Day of competition	High-carbohydrate pre-event meal

to be completed. It usually is a light to moderate meal eaten 2 to 4 hours before the event. This meal should be sufficient in carbohydrate (approximately 1 to 4 g of carbohydrate per kilogram of body weight), low in fat and fiber, and moderate in protein; it should also provide sufficient fluid and be familiar to the athlete.[24] Fat, fiber, and protein slow the rate of emptying in the stomach and thus are not beneficial in high quantities immediately before a workout or competition.

This schedule gives the body time to digest, absorb, and transform the meal into stored glycogen. Appropriate food choices include pasta, bread, rice, granola bars, and cereal with nonfat milk. Box 16.4 outlines a sample pregame meal. Of most importance, however, is planning the pregame meal in accordance with what works well for the specific athlete.

NUTRITION DURING EXERCISE

For activities lasting 1 hour or less, most athletes do not require dietary sources of energy during the exercise period. However, the interval consumption of carbohydrate enhances performance during longer endurance or higher-intensity events. For high-intensity or endurance exercise lasting more than 1 hour, recommendations include 30 to 60 g of carbohydrate per hour; for ultra-endurance events longer than 2.5 hours, individuals may need up to 90 g of carbohydrate per hour.[25] Consuming equal amounts of the preferred food or drink at regular intervals (i.e. every 15 to 20 minutes) throughout the event is ideal compared with consuming the entire amount at once. Athletes should experiment with various forms of carbohydrate before a competition to determine what they tolerate best. Athletes can choose from a large variety of sports drinks, gels, and other forms of carbohydrates. The food of choice should provide simple carbohydrates with little or no fat, protein, or fiber.

Box 16.4 Sample Pregame Meal

This sample pregame meal includes approximately 209 g of carbohydrates; it is high in complex carbohydrates and low to moderate in protein, fat, and fiber:

- 1 blueberry bagel (270 kcal, 52 g of carbohydrate)
- 1 tbsp raspberry jam (50 kcal, 13 g of carbohydrate)
- 1 banana, medium (105 kcal, 27 g of carbohydrate)
- 1.5 cups low-fiber cereal (240 kcal, 50 g carbohydrate)
- 1 cup nonfat milk (80 kcal, 12 g carbohydrate
- 16 ounces of apple juice (220 kcal, 56 g of carbohydrate)

NUTRITION AFTER EXERCISE: RECOVERY

Proper nutrition in the recovery period is essential for the body to replenish depleted fuel sources and to allow continued adaptation and growth after the exercise stimulus. Consuming carbohydrate-containing foods and beverages as soon as possible after exercise (and no later than 2 hours after exercise) maximizes glycogen resynthesis.[21] Consuming 1 to 1.2 g of carbohydrate per kilogram of body weight per hour, for up to 4 hours, provides sufficient amount of carbohydrate, particularly for athletes completing exhaustive exercise or those with less than 24 hours to recover before their next exercise bout. Carbohydrate-containing foods should be spread out over several meals and snacks instead of consuming one large meal at one time. To maximize muscle protein synthesis, athletes should consume 15 to 25 g of high-quality protein within the first few hours after exercise and continue to consume protein-containing foods every 3 to 5 hours.[26] Examples of food choices that combine carbohydrate and protein include fruit and yogurt, a turkey and vegetable sandwich, chocolate milk with an apple, and a peanut butter and banana sandwich.

HYDRATION BEFORE, DURING, AND AFTER EXERCISE

Adequate hydration is an important consideration for athletes. Fluid needs depend on the following: (1) the intensity and duration of the exercise; (2) the surrounding temperature, altitude, and humidity; (3) the individual's fitness level, body size and composition, and metabolic rate; and (4) preexercise hydration status. The thirst mechanism may not be an accurate gauge for fluid replacement; therefore, athletes should make a specific plan for fluid intake relative to their individualized needs. In addition to water loss, which can be as much as 2.4 L/h in extreme conditions, sweat also contains sodium and small amounts of other minerals (e.g., potassium, magnesium, chloride), which may have to be replaced depending upon the amount of sweat lost.

The following list provides recommendations to maximize performance and to avoid the complications of dehydration:

- *Before exercise:* Establish euhydration 2 to 4 hours before exercise by drinking 5 to 10 mL/kg body weight of water or a sports beverage. Void excess fluid before competition, and do not attempt hyperhydration.

- *During exercise:* Drink during exercise to avoid excessive water loss (defined as a loss of more than 2% of body weight from water). The amount of fluid that is necessary to accomplish this will be highly individualized.
- *After exercise:* Replace fluid loss after the completion of exercise by drinking 16 to 24 oz of fluid for every pound of body weight that is lost.[20]

A number of sports drinks with added sugar, electrolytes, and flavorings are available, but questions have been raised about their use or misuse (see the For Further Focus box, "Hydrating with Water, Sports Drink, or Energy Drink" in Chapter 9). Except for endurance events that last more than 1 hour, plain water usually is the rehydration fluid of choice. For events that last longer than 60 to 90 minutes, beverages with 6% to 8% carbohydrate concentrations and selected electrolytes may be beneficial.

ERGOGENIC AIDS AND MISINFORMATION

Since ancient times, athletes have been seeking and experimenting with "magic" substances or treatments to gain a competitive edge. Nutrient supplements and **ergogenic** aids are highly prevalent in the athletic world, although very few of these substances have demonstrated even a slight increase in performance, and several are questionable with regard to safety. Most of the marketed ergogenic aids do not work as claimed, but they are relatively harmless (see the Drug-Nutrient Interaction box, "Nutrition and Ergogenic Supplements").

The use of anabolic-androgenic steroids is of great concern; it is dangerous, and, in competitive sports, it is illegal. Steroid use is widespread among elite athletes and bodybuilders, although its use is most prevalent among recreational athletes. Some athletes start experimenting with steroids as young as junior high school.[27] Steroids are synthetic sex hormones that have two actions: (1) anabolic (i.e., tissue growth) and (2) androgenic (i.e., **masculinization**). Athletes have taken steroids in megadoses of 10 to 30 times their normal body hormonal output to increase muscle size, strength, and performance. However, the physiologic side effects can be devastating, including masculinization and **gynecomastia**; liver abnormalities such as dysfunction, tumor, and hepatitis; an increased risk of atherosclerosis; and the atrophy of the testicles and decreased sperm production. Psychologic effects vary from mood swings to depression and mania or hypomania.

Athletes and their coaches are particularly susceptible to claims and myths about foods and dietary supplements. All athletes, particularly those who are involved in highly competitive sports, constantly search for the competitive edge. Knowing this, manufacturers sometimes make distorted or false claims about their products. Athletes should know that there are no quick fixes. Regarding supplements and ergogenic aids, there are five questions to ask: Is it safe? Is it legal? Is it ethical? Is it pure? Is it effective? Health care providers should be familiar with common fads and myths that are circulating in the community so that they can approach these individuals and know what to recommend as effective alternatives.

---

ergogenic the tendency to increase work output; various substances that increase work or exercise capacity and output.

masculinization a condition marked by the attainment of male characteristics (e.g., facial hair) either physiologically as part of male maturation or pathologically by either sex.

gynecomastia the excessive development of the male mammary glands, frequently as a result of increased estrogen levels.

 Drug-Nutrient Interaction

Nutrition and Ergogenic Supplements

Dietary supplements comprise a wide range of products, including essential vitamins and minerals, sports foods (e.g., protein powders and sports drinks), and products targeted for health and performance optimization. Ergogenic aids are popular among competitive athletes and other individuals who seek to gain a performance edge. Research indicates that only a limited number of supplements may have a small benefit to performance, whereas a far greater amount may pose adverse health or performance risks. Athletes should heed caution when it comes to supplements and consider the potential risks and benefits before use. We can classify ergogenic aids according to the amount of available scientific support: established, equivocal or developing, as well as banned substances in organizations such as the World Anti-Doping Agency (WADA) and the National Collegiate Athletic Association (NCAA) (see list below).

ESTABLISHED PERFORMANCE SUPPLEMENTS

- *Creatine* loading can have acute performance benefits in sports involving high-intensity exercise, as well as long-term benefits with resistance training programs, by enhancing the rate of ATP resynthesis. Weight gain after creatine loading is common because of increased water retention and may not benefit athletes in weight class sports or endurance sports.[1]
- *Caffeine* is a stimulant with established performance benefits across numerous exercise modalities, including endurance sports and short-term, repeated sprint tasks.[2] Higher doses do not appear to enhance performance benefits and will likely increase the risk of negative side effects such as nausea, insomnia, anxiety, and restlessness.

Continued

Drug-Nutrient Interaction—cont'd

Nutrition and Ergogenic Supplements

- *Nitrate (NO3.)* is a popular supplement that enhances the body's nitric oxide production, thus increasing exercise efficiency and economy. A nitrate bolus benefits acute performance within 2 to 3 hours. Prolonged supplementation of 3 days augments these benefits. It appears that trained individuals have less of a response to nitrate supplementation compared with untrained individuals.[3] Supplementation may cause GI upset in susceptible athletes and should therefore be experimented with before use in competition.
- *Beta-alanine* enhances the intracellular buffering capacity during muscle contraction and thus may reduce fatigue, particularly in untrained individuals. Chronic consumption with doses split throughout the day may increase buffering capacity and reduce potential side effects such as sins rash and/or transient paresthesia.[4]
- *Sodium bicarbonate* acts as an acute extracellular blood buffer for contracting muscles, reducing the fatigue associated with high-intensity exercise. Not all individuals respond to supplementation, and experimenting with different dosages at various time points before commencing exercise is important.[5] GI distress is often associated with supplementation but co-ingestion of a small, carbohydrate-rich meal or split-dosing strategies can minimize this distress.

EQUIVOCAL PERFORMANCE SUPPLEMENTS
- *Sodium citrate*, similar to sodium bicarbonate, acts as a blood buffer by increasing the extracellular pH of the environment. However, further investigation is needed to clarify the efficacy of supplementation.[6]
- *Phosphate* supplementation may have ergogenic benefits that include enhanced rates of ATP resynthesis and increased buffering capacity during high rates of anaerobic glycolysis.[7] Supplement protocols need additional research before recommendations for performance gains are established.
- *Carnitine* is located predominantly within skeletal muscle and plays a critical role in energy production, specifically fat oxidation. Additional research is needed to substantiate potential ergogenic effects.[6]

DEVELOPING PERFORMANCE SUPPLEMENTS
- Probiotics, vitamins C and D, omega 3-fatty acids, and anti-inflammatories such as food polyphenols (e.g., quercetin, curcumin, and anthocyanin) are just a few developing supplements that show ergogenic potential but require further research before conclusive recommendations can be made regarding their use.[7]

SUBSTANCES BANNED BY THE WORLD ANTI-DOPING AGENCY	SUBSTANCES BANNED BY THE NATIONAL COLLEGIATE ATHLETIC ASSOCIATION
• Anabolic androgenic steroids • Peptide hormones, growth factors and mimetics • Beta-2 agonists (albuterol) • Stimulants (amphetamines) • Diuretics and masking agents • Narcotics • Beta blockers • Glucocorticoids • Cannabinoids • Erythropoietin	• Stimulants • Anabolic agents • Alcohol and beta blockers (for rifle only) diuretics and other masking agents • Street drugs • Peptide hormones and analogues • Anti-estrogens • Beta-2 agonists

Modified from www.wada-ama.org/sites/default/files/wada_2019_english_prohibited_list.pdf; and www.ncaa.org/2018-19-ncaa-banned-drugs-list.

REFERENCES
1. Kreider, R. B., et al. (2017). International Society of Sports Nutrition position stand: Safety and efficacy of creatine supplementation in exercise, sport, and medicine. *Journal of the International Society of Sports Nutrition, 14,* 18.
2. Maughan, R. J., et al. (2018). IOC consensus statement: Dietary supplements and the high-performance athlete. *International Journal of Sport Nutrition and Exercise Metabolism, 28*(2), 104–125.
3. Van De Walle, G. P., & Vukovich, M. D. (2018). The effect of nitrate supplementation on exercise tolerance and performance: A systematic review and meta-analysis. *Journal of Strength and Conditioning Research, 32*(6), 1796–1808.
4. Saunders, B., et al. (2017). Beta-alanine supplementation to improve exercise capacity and performance: A systematic review and meta-analysis. *British Journal of Sports Medicine, 51*(8), 658–669.
5. McNaughton, L. R., et al. (2016). Recent developments in the use of sodium bicarbonate as an ergogenic aid. *Current Sports Medicine Reports, 15*(4), 233–244.
6. Peeling, P., et al. (2018). Evidence-based supplements for the enhancement of athletic performance. *International Journal of Sport Nutrition and Exercise Metabolism, 28*(2), 178–187.
7. Burke, L. M. (2017). Practical issues in evidence-based use of performance supplements: Supplement interactions, repeated use and individual responses. *Sports Medicine, 47*(Suppl.1), 79–100.

With contributions from Corinna Coffin.

Putting It All Together

Summary

- Many muscle fibers and cells work together to make physical activity possible. Carbohydrate, mainly in the form of complex-carbohydrate foods or starches, is the primary fuel for energy to run this system.

- Carbohydrate metabolism yields circulating blood glucose and stored glycogen in muscles and the liver for fuel. Stored body fat supplies additional fuel as fatty acids, whereas protein provides insignificant energy for exercise. Vitamins and minerals are important parts of coenzymes for the process of energy production.

- Activities of daily living, aerobic exercise, and resistance training have many benefits that increase with practice. Excellent aerobic exercises include sustained fast walking, cycling, jogging, swimming, and aerobic dancing or similar workouts. Resistance training increases muscle strength, which has a direct influence on metabolic rate and bone density. Weight-bearing exercise is also important for maintaining bone density.

- Individual macronutrient needs of athletes vary depending upon the sport type, and the frequency and amount of training in which they engage. In general, athletes have higher needs for protein, carbohydrates, energy, and fluids. Water is generally the best way to avoid dehydration. The next meal will typically replace electrolytes that are lost in sweat.

- Athletes benefit from strategically timing their fluids, meals, and snacks such that the nutrients they consume appropriately fuel their workouts, as well as allow for effective recovery from exercise. It is not just what an athlete eats that matters, but rather when and how much they are consuming that is equally important.

Chapter Review Questions

See answers in Appendix A.

1. Which type(s) of exercise may be beneficial in lowering blood pressure in a hypertensive individual?

   a. Aerobic exercise
   b. Resistance exercise
   c. Aerobic and resistance exercise
   d. Balance and flexibility exercises

2. An older male adult with a chronic disease is not able to meet the recommended 150 minutes of moderate-intensity aerobic physical activity. He should be encouraged to _____.

   a. engage in 75 to 150 minutes a week of resistance exercise
   b. be as physically active as his abilities allow
   c. focus on yoga or other stretching exercises
   d. refrain from exercise altogether

3. The type of exercise that primarily uses fat as an energy source is _____.

   a. high-intensity aerobic exercise
   b. low-intensity aerobic exercise
   c. high-intensity resistance exercise
   d. low-intensity resistance exercise

4. Which of the following snacks would be the most appropriate for recovering from exercise?

   a. A bagel with jam and a banana
   b. A protein supplement containing 50 g of whole protein
   c. Greek yogurt mixed with assorted fruit
   d. Whole wheat toast with mashed avocado

5. The most appropriate recovery fluid for an athlete going out for a 40-minute run in 50-degree weather would be _____.

   a. an energy drink
   b. a sports drink
   c. diluted apple juice
   d. water

Next-Generation NCLEX® Examination-style Case Study

See answers in Appendix A.

A 20-year-old male triathlete (height, 5'5"; weight, 125 lbs.) recently injured his calf muscle. He trains 5 days out of the week. Although he gets 7 to 8 hours of sleep, he still feels exhausted sitting in his college classes. He is stressed about school after missing a few days because of a recent bout of strep throat. He noticed his muscles feel tired during his workouts. A dietary recall was collected:

Breakfast: eggs (2), bacon (3 strips), and water
Snack: string cheese (1), carrots (¼ c.), and ranch (2 Tbsp.)
Lunch: chicken patty, medium apple, celery (¼ c.), and peanut butter (2 Tbsp.)
Snack: beef jerky (2 oz.)
Dinner: salmon (3 oz.), asparagus (½ c.), and cauliflower rice (½ c.)
Snack: mixed nuts (½ c.)

1. From the list below, select all factors from the client's history that are a nutritional concern.

   a. Exercising 5 days per week
   b. Sore muscles
   c. Falling asleep during class
   d. Injured calf muscle
   e. Meal frequency
   f. Hours of sleep
   g. Strep throat

2. Choose the *most likely* options for the information missing from the statement below by selecting from the list of options provided.

   The client's dietary intake indicates inadequate ____1____ intake, which is the preferred source of energy during the athlete's ____2____ exercise.

OPTION 1	OPTION 2
protein	glycolytic
fat	resistance
vitamins	endurance
minerals	high-intense
carbohydrate	anaerobic

3. Choose the *most likely* options for the information missing from the statement below by selecting from the list of options provided.

A few days before the triathlon, this client would benefit from ____1____ to ensure maximal ____2____ stores.

OPTION 1	OPTION 2
protein packing	triglyceride
carbohydrate counting	amino acid
fat supplementation	glycogen
carbohydrate loading	cholesterol

4. Use an X to indicate the health teaching below that is <u>indicated</u> (appropriate or necessary) or <u>contraindicated</u> (could be harmful) for the athlete.

HEALTH TEACHING	INDICATED	CONTRAINDICATED
Consume carbohydrate foods 2 to 4 hours before exercise.		
Consume foods containing high amounts of fat, fiber, and protein 1 to 4 hours before exercise.		
Consume carbohydrate during exercise lasting longer than 1 hour.		
Avoid consuming carbohydrate foods after exercise.		
Consume foods with fat, protein, and fiber during exercise.		

5. For each assessment finding, use an X to indicate whether nursing and collaborative interventions were <u>effective</u> (helped to meet expected outcomes) or <u>ineffective</u> (did not help to meet expected outcomes).

ASSESSMENT FINDING	EFFECTIVE	INEFFECTIVE
Consumes cereal with non-fat milk 3 hours before exercise.		
Consumes sports drinks during training that lasts 45 minutes.		
Consumes fruit chews during exercise lasting 2 hours.		
Consumes chicken and broccoli 2.5 hours after exercise.		
Able to complete his workouts with fewer breaks.		

Additional Learning Resources

Please refer to this text's Evolve website for answers to the Case Study questions:
http://evolve.elsevier.com/Williams/basic/.
References and **Further Reading and Resources** in the back of the book provide additional resources for enhancing knowledge.

Nutrition Care

Key Concepts

- Centering nutrition support on the patient/client and his or her individual needs is the most effective form of health care.
- A team of health professionals and support staff best provides comprehensive health care.
- A personalized health care plan, evaluation, and follow-up care guide actions to promote healing and health.
- Drug-nutrient interactions can create significant medical complications.

People face acute illness or chronic disease and treatment in a variety of settings and locations. Nutrition support is fundamental for the successful treatment of disease, and it is often the primary therapy. To meet individual needs, a broad knowledge of nutrition status, requirements, and ways of meeting the identified needs is essential. Each member of the health care team plays an important role in developing and maintaining a person-centered health care plan.

This chapter focuses on the comprehensive care of the client's nutrition needs as provided by the registered dietitian nutritionist (RDN). Nurses are intimately involved in the care process and often identify nutrition needs within the nursing diagnosis. An effective care plan involves all health care team members as well as the client, the family, and his or her support system.

THERAPEUTIC PROCESS

SETTING AND FOCUS OF CARE

Nutrition support may take place in a variety of settings and in a variety of forms. For example, individuals may seek and receive nutrition support in a private practice, outpatient facility, hospital, long-term care facility, rehabilitation center, public health community setting, or at home. The ultimate goal of nutrition support is to establish energy and nutrient balance according to the specific needs of the individual.

Modern hospitals are a marvel of medical technology, but medical advances sometimes bring confusion and anxiety to clients, whose illnesses place them in the midst of a complex system of care. Various members of the medical staff interact with hospitalized clients on vastly different timetables from one another. Sometimes the day's intended schedule does not proceed as planned because of modifications in team member communications or treatment necessities. Clients need personal advocates. Health care providers such as the nurse and the dietitian can provide essential support and personalized care for these clients.

The type of, and requirement for, nutrition support comes in many different forms. Nutrition support can range from help with balancing daily meal plans to providing nutrition therapy through intravenous feedings. A client's individual needs and a person-centered approach must drive the foundation of effective nutrition care. Figure 17.1 demonstrates the Nutrition Care Process model, in which personal interactions define the relationship between the client, the nutrition professional, and the client's care plan. The clients' nutrition status always determines their immediate needs, and this may change frequently, requiring constant monitoring and adjustment. Such personalized care demands great commitment from the health care team. Despite all of the methods, tools, and technologies described in this text and elsewhere, remember this basic fact: the therapeutic use of the self is the most healing tool that a person will ever use. This is a simple yet profound truth, because the human encounter is where health care workers bring themselves and their skills.

HEALTH CARE TEAM

In the area of nutrition care, the RDN, also known as a registered dietitian (RD), carries the major responsibility of medical nutrition therapy. The For Further Focus box titled "Qualifications of a Registered Dietitian Nutritionist" outlines the requirements for becoming an RDN. Working closely with the physician, the dietitian determines individual nutrition therapy needs and a plan of care. Team support is essential throughout this process. Nurses are in a unique position to provide additional nutrition support by referring clients to the dietitian when necessary. Of all the health care team members, nurses are in the closest continuous contact with hospitalized clients and their families. Such a connection is important to ensure the most beneficial health care approach and timely response to changing client needs.

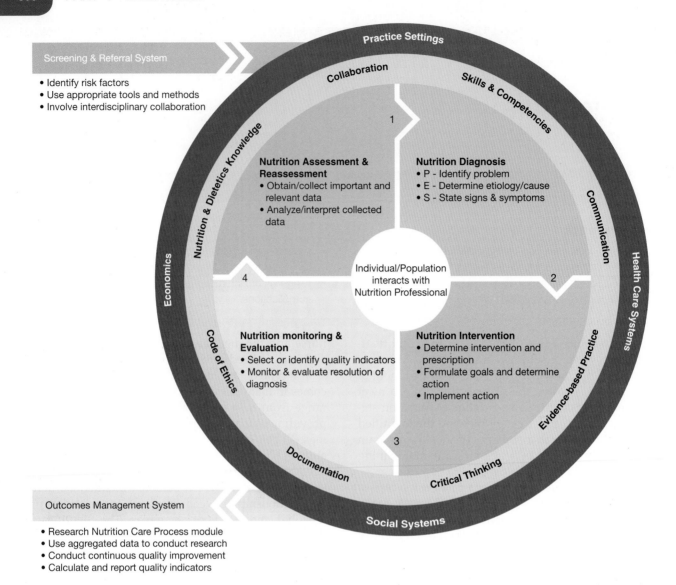

Screening & Referral System

- Identify risk factors
- Use appropriate tools and methods
- Involve interdisciplinary collaboration

Nutrition Assessment & Reassessment
- Obtain/collect important and relevant data
- Analyze/interpret collected data

Nutrition Diagnosis
- P - Identify problem
- E - Determine etiology/cause
- S - State signs & symptoms

Individual/Population interacts with Nutrition Professional

Nutrition monitoring & Evaluation
- Select or identify quality indicators
- Monitor & evaluate resolution of diagnosis

Nutrition Intervention
- Determine intervention and prescription
- Formulate goals and determine action
- Implement action

Outcomes Management System

- Research Nutrition Care Process module
- Use aggregated data to conduct research
- Conduct continuous quality improvement
- Calculate and report quality indicators

Figure 17.1 The Nutrition Care Process model. (Reprinted from Swan, W. I., et al. [2017]. Nutrition Care Process and model update: Toward realizing people-centered care and outcomes management. *J Acad Nutr Diet, 117*[12], 2003–2014.)

For Further Focus

Qualifications of a Registered Dietitian Nutritionist

WHAT IS A REGISTERED DIETITIAN NUTRITIONIST?

A registered dietitian nutritionist (RDN) is a food and nutrition expert who has met academic and professional requirements, including the following:

- Earned a bachelor's degree with coursework approved by the Academy of Nutrition and Dietetics Accreditation Council for Education in Nutrition and Dietetics (ACEND) (www.eatright.org/ACEND); coursework typically includes nutrition sciences, biochemistry, physiology, microbiology, chemistry, sociology and communication, food service systems management, business, and computer science. NOTE: Beginning on January 1, 2024, potential RDNs must hold a minimum of a master's degree to qualify for sitting the national registration board exam.
- Completed an ACEND-accredited, supervised practice internship (usually between 6 and 12 months). Typical internships are either combined with a bachelors or master's degree or at a health care facility or community agency.

- After completing the requirements, a potential RDN must pass a national board examination administered by the Commission on Dietetic Registration (www.cdrnet.org).
- RDN's must keep professionally current by completing 75 hours of approved continuing educational requirements on a 5-year cycle.

Some RDNs also hold additional certifications in specialized areas of practice, such as pediatric nutrition, renal nutrition, nutrition support, diabetes education, weight management, and sports nutrition. The Commission on Dietetic Registration provides the required training for, and grants, these certifications.

HOW IS A REGISTERED DIETITIAN NUTRITIONIST DIFFERENT FROM A "NUTRITIONIST"?

- The "RDN" or "RD" (if preferred) credential is a legally protected title. Only authorized practitioners (by the Commission on Dietetic Registration of the Academy of Nutrition and Dietetics) may use the title.

Qualifications of a Registered Dietitian Nutritionist

- Some RDNs may call themselves "nutritionists," but not all nutritionists are registered dietitians. The definition and requirements for the term *nutritionist* vary. Some states have licensure laws that define the scope of practice for someone who is using the designation, but, in other states, virtually anyone can call himself or herself a "nutritionist," regardless of education or training, or lack thereof.

  To find out more about what services RDNs provide and what the qualifications are for Nutrition and Dietetics Technician, Registered, please visit www.eatright.org. Go to the *About Us* page.

Reference: Academy of Nutrition and Dietetics. (2019). *About us.* Retrieved June 4, 2019, from www.eatrightpro.org/resources/about-us.

Physician and Support Staff

Headed by the physician, the health care team also may include several other allied health professionals, depending on the needs of the client. The team may include some or all of the following members: nurse, dietitian, physical therapist, occupational therapist, speech-language pathologist, psychiatrist, respiratory therapist, radiologist, physician assistant, **kinesiotherapist**, pharmacist, and social worker. When developing this team relationship, all involved parties rely on one another's expertise for a successful outcome serving the client's needs.

Roles of the Nurse and the Dietitian

Successful nutrition care specifically depends on the close collaboration of the dietitian, the nurse, and the client. The dietitian determines the nutrition needs, plans and manages nutrition therapy, evaluates the plan of care, and documents results. Throughout this entire process, the nurse helps to develop, support, and carry out the plan of care. This teamwork is particularly vital for clients with strict or complicated nutrition requirements. A dietitian may only see a client once or twice during a hospital stay, whereas the nurse will have constant contact with the client and will often be the person dealing with immediate nutrition-related questions because of his or her frequent contact.

The *nursing process* is a specific process by which nurses deliver care to clients and includes the following steps: assessment, diagnosis, outcome/planning, implementation, and evaluation. The nursing diagnosis is the nurse's clinical judgment about a client's response to actual or potential health conditions or needs.[1] A nursing diagnosis may include several issues that are nutrition related, such as diarrhea, malnutrition, failure to thrive, and fluid-volume deficit. Although covering the nursing process is not within the scope of this text, an appreciation of the interconnected work of the nurse and the dietitian on the health care team is important.

A skilled nurse is the thread that bonds each member of the health care team together. Nurses are skilled multitaskers, and they carry a heavy load of the overall responsibilities in a clinical setting. When necessary, nurses may also serve the client as essential coordinators, advocates, interpreters, teachers, and counselors.

Coordinators and advocates. Nurses usually work more closely with clients than any other health care provider does. They are best able to coordinate the client's required services and treatments, and they can consult and refer the client to other practitioners as needed. For example, malnutrition is common in hospital settings, and there are many factors involved (e.g., pain or medicine-induced anorexia, surgery, and emotional or psychologic distress). However, sometimes clients have reduced food intake because of conflicts with medical procedures, appointments during mealtime, or unmet culture/religious dietary customs with the routine hospital diet. The nurse may be able to help resolve such conflicts by coordinating specific meals or meal-delivery times with consideration for the client's wishes and scheduled procedures.

---

nursing diagnosis "[a] clinical judgment about an individual, family, or community experiences/responses to actual or potential health problems/life processes. Nursing diagnoses provide the basis for selection of nursing interventions to achieve outcomes for which the nurse has accountability," as defined by the North American Nursing Diagnosis Association.

Nutrition Care Process model a systematic approach to providing high-quality individualized nutrition care. The model consists of the following steps: assessment, diagnosis, intervention, and monitoring and evaluation.

medical nutrition therapy a specific nutrition service and procedure that is used to treat an illness, injury, or condition; it involves an in-depth nutrition assessment of the client, nutrition diagnosis, nutrition intervention (which may include diet therapy, counseling, and/or the use of specialized nutrition supplements), and nutrition monitoring and evaluation.

kinesiotherapist a health care professional who treats the effects of disease, injury, and congenital disorders through the application of scientifically based exercise principles that have been adapted to enhance the strength, endurance, and mobility of individuals with functional limitations or for those clients who require extended physical conditioning.

Interpreters. The nurse can help to reduce a client's anxiety with the use of careful, brief, and easily understood explanations about various treatments and plans of care. This may include reinforcement of a prescribed therapeutic diet and the resulting food choices to sustain compliance. These activities may be difficult with uninterested clients, but efforts to understand such client behaviors are paramount to bridging the gap. A client's psychologic and emotional status has a strong influence on his or her overall ability to deal with the medical problem at hand and to adhere to the treatment protocol. Discharged clients who do not possess a proper interpretation of their prognosis or plan of continued care may be noncompliant and experience unnecessary stress, confusion, medical complications, and hospital readmission. A nurse can usually help answer questions about a client's nutrition plan of care, but if that is not the best option, the nurse can also refer the client to the dietitian for additional explanation.

Teachers and counselors. Basic teaching and counseling skills are essential in nursing. Many opportunities exist during daily care for conversations about sound medical and nutrition principles, which will reinforce the care plan with the client. Learning about health care needs (including nutrition) should begin with the client's hospital admission or initial contact, carry through the entire period of care, and continue in the home environment, with the support of community resources as needed.

PHASES OF THE CARE PROCESS

The Academy of Nutrition and Dietetics has developed a standardized Nutrition Care Process for RDNs (see "Nutrition Care Process" at www.ncpro.org). The Nutrition Care Process is "a systematic method that nutrition and dietetics practitioners use to provide nutrition care."[2] It is composed of the following four distinct and interrelated steps: (1) assessment; (2) diagnosis; (3) intervention; and (4) monitoring and evaluation. The Nutrition Care Process provides a consistent structure and framework for nutrition professionals to use to provide individualized care for clients. Use of this process is appropriate for patients, clients, and groups that have identified nutrition risk factors and that need assistance to achieve or maintain health goals. You can learn more about each category of the Nutrition Care Process at www.andeal.org/ncp.

NUTRITION ASSESSMENT

The purpose of the nutrition assessment step is to collect, classify, and synthesize as much information as possible about the client's situation to assess his or her nutrition status. Family and medical history questionnaires are useful methods of gathering pertinent information on admission or during the initial office visit. Appropriate care considers the client's nutrition status, food habits, and living situation as well as his or her needs, desires, and goals. The client and his or her family are the primary sources of this information. Other sources include the client's medical chart, oral or written communication with hospital staff, and related research. Although the Nutrition Care Process begins with this step, the nutrition assessment phase is actually a dynamic process that includes recurrent reassessment and analysis of the client's status.[2] The following sections describe each of the five categories of data collected during the nutrition assessment phase of the Nutrition Care Process, which are the following:

- Food and nutrition-related history
- Anthropometric measurements
- Biochemical data, medical tests, and procedures
- Nutrition-focused physical findings
- Client history

Food- and Nutrition-Related History

In most cases, the RDN is responsible for evaluating the client's diet. Knowledge of the client's basic eating habits may help to identify possible nutrition deficiencies. The Clinical Applications box entitled "Nutrition History: Activity-Associated Food Pattern of a Typical Day" shows an example of a general guide for gathering a nutrition history. Sometimes the dietitian will use a 3-day (and sometimes longer) food record to obtain a more specific food history; this involves clients recording everything that they eat and the amounts and methods of preparation for 3 full days. A more extended view of the diet may reveal additional information about food habits or problems as they relate to the individual's socioeconomic status, food access, family, living situation, and general support system.

Clinicians should be aware that underreporting energy intake is common in children and adults and that this may affect dietary assessment and recommendations.[3-7] A variety of methods are used to collect dietary intake, all of which have strengths and weaknesses (Table 17.1). Clients often do not volunteer information regarding dietary supplement intake (see the Drug-Nutrient Interaction box, "Dietary Supplement Use"). Thus, direct questions about supplement use (e.g., vitamins, minerals, multivitamin/mineral combinations, herbs) are more likely to yield accurate answers and to provide insight into overall nutrient consumption. Noting allergies and intolerances guides alternative recommendations to meet nutrient needs without causing negative reactions.

Physical activity logs are similar to dietary intake logs in that a client records all activity throughout the day in an effort to calculate energy expenditure. Similar to diet logs, physical activity questionnaires tend to be inaccurate and overestimate actual energy expenditure when compared with the gold standard of doubly labeled water method.[8,9] Less subjective measurement tools such as pedometers, accelerometers, motion sensors, and heart rate monitors may predict energy expenditure more accurately than questionnaires, but some devices still vary considerably compared with the doubly labeled water method.[10-12] Dietitians must consider the accuracy of the method used to estimate total energy expenditure when providing nutrition recommendations.

Clinical Applications

Nutrition History: Activity-Associated Food Pattern of a Typical Day

Name: _____ Date: _____

Height: _____ Weight (lb): _____ /(kg): _____ Body mass index: _____ kg/m²

Ideal weight: _____ Usual weight: _____

Referral:

Diagnosis:

Diet order:

Allergies/intolerances:

Occupation:

Recreation, physical activity:

Present food intake:

TIME/LOCATION	FOOD (AND METHOD OF PREPARATION)	SERVING SIZE	TOLERANCE/COMMENTS
Breakfast			
Snack			
Lunch			
Snack			
Dinner			

Summary: Total servings of foods in each category:

Breads/grains: ____ Vegetables: ____ Fruits: ____ Dairy: ____ Meat: ____ Fat/sugar: ____

Dietary supplements, herbs, complementary/alternative medications:

Name of supplement: _____ Dose per day: _____

Table **17.1**   Strengths and Limitations of Techniques Used to Measure Dietary Intake

TECHNIQUE	BRIEF DESCRIPTION	STRENGTHS	LIMITATIONS
24-hour food recall	A trained interviewer asks the respondent to recall, in detail, all food and drink consumed during the previous 24 hours	Fast, inexpensive, and easy to administer; Can provide detailed information about the types of foods consumed; Low respondent burden; Is not dependent on respondent's level of education, literacy, or writing skills; Does not alter respondent's usual intake	One 24-hour recall cannot illustrate typical dietary intake; Underreporting and overreporting are common; Depends on respondent's memory; Accuracy is somewhat dependent upon the skill of the interviewer; Omissions of sauces, dressings, and beverages can lead to low estimates of energy intake
Multiple-day food record	The respondent records, at the time of consumption, the types and amounts of all foods and beverages consumed for 3 to 7 days	Does not rely on memory because the participants record intake immediately after consumption; Can provide detailed intake data; Multiple-day data are more representative of usual intake; Reasonably valid for up to 5 days	Requires high degree of cooperation; Client must be literate and able to write; Takes more time to obtain data; Analysis is labor intensive; Act of recording food intake often alters usual intake; Underreporting and inaccurately estimating portion sizes are common; Respondent burden can result in low response rates

Continued

Table 17.1   Strengths and Limitations of Techniques Used to Measure Dietary Intake—cont'd

TECHNIQUE	BRIEF DESCRIPTION	STRENGTHS	LIMITATIONS
Food frequency questionnaires	The respondent indicates how many times a day, week, month, or year that he or she usually consumes specific foods by using a questionnaire consisting of hundreds of foods or food groups	Can be self-administered Machine readable Relatively inexpensive May be more representative of usual intake over longer periods of time than a few days of diet records Does not alter respondents' usual intake	Modest demand on respondent May not represent usual food or portion sizes typically chosen by respondent Cultural/ethnic specific foods are often not included Intake data can be compromised when multiple foods are grouped within single listings Requires literacy and good long-term memory Not effective for monitoring short-term dietary changes
Diet history	A trained nutrition professional interviews the client about the number of meals eaten per day; his or her appetite and food dislikes; the presence or absence of gastrointestinal distress; the use of dietary supplements; and other lifestyle choices	Assesses usual nutrient intake Can detect seasonal changes Data about all nutrients can be obtained Can correlate well with biochemical measures	Lengthy interview process Requires highly trained interviewers May overestimate nutrient intake Requires the cooperation of a respondent with the ability to recall his or her usual diet Difficult and expensive to code for group analysis

 Drug-Nutrient Interaction

Dietary Supplement Use

Dietary supplements include vitamins, minerals, amino acids, fatty acids, herbs, botanicals, and other substances that have physiologic effects in the body. As noted in the Drug-Nutrient Interaction boxes throughout this textbook, dietary supplements can interact with one another and with medications resulting in either beneficial or detrimental effects on the body. Nutrient intake from food combined with high doses of micronutrients from supplements and from fortified foods and beverages may result in a habitual intake above the Upper Tolerable Limit (UL) for many vitamins and minerals. Exceeding the UL (see Appendix B) may manifest as gastrointestinal symptoms or overt signs of toxicity in some individuals.

The use of complementary and alternative medicine (CAM), such as vitamin, mineral, and herbal supplement use, is popular in the United States. One-half of the U.S. adult population and one-third of children take some form of dietary supplement on a regular basis (49% of men, 59% of women, 32% of children).[1,2] Yet, only half (53.7%) of CAM users report their use to their primary health care provider, and only 34% of hospitalized patients report their CAM use to the hospitalist.[3,4] This oversight may be because clients are unaware of potential interactions with drugs or other therapies or because clients simply forgot about their supplements. On the other hand, it may be because health care providers failed to ask specifically about the client's use of CAM. Without full disclosure, it is not possible for the health care team to assess the potential for drug-nutrient interactions or offer alternative solutions.

Many clients need more education about the importance of talking to their health care providers about the use of vitamin, mineral, and herbal supplements. Additionally, health care providers may need further training to elicit information about dietary supplement use from their clients, particularly for hospitalized clients. As a health care provider, ensure that you are objective about CAM use when speaking with clients or their care provider. In addition, always encourage clients to discuss supplementation with a physician or pharmacist to avoid potential drug-nutrient interactions.

REFERENCES

1. Cowan, A. E., et al. (2018). Dietary supplement use differs by socioeconomic and health-related characteristics among U.S. adults, NHANES 2011-2014. *Nutrients, 10*(8).
2. Jun, S., et al. (2018). Dietary supplement use among U.S. children by family income, food security level, and Nutrition Assistance Program participation status in 2011-2014. *Nutrients, 10*(9).
3. Yeo, Y., et al. (2016). Use of electronic personal health records (PHRs) for complementary and alternative medicine (CAM) disclosure: Implications for integrative health care. *Complementary Therapies in Medicine, 26,* 108–116.
4. Ben-Arye, E., et al. (2017). Mind the gap: Disclosure of dietary supplement use to hospital and family physicians. *Patient Education and Counseling, 100*(1), 98–103.

Anthropometric Measurements

All providers responsible for taking **anthropometric measurements** should practice taking correct measurements to avoid errors and maintain proper equipment and careful technique. Height, weight, and body mass index (BMI) are the most common anthropometric measurements that are used in clinical practice to predict basic nutrition risk parameters. In some situations, the RDN may take body composition and waist circumference measurements as well.

Height. The health care provider or technician will measure height using a wall-mounted measuring tape, if possible, or the moveable measuring rod on a platform clinic scale. For the most accurate results, the technician will have the person stand as straight as possible, without shoes or a hat. The technician will measure children who are younger than 2 years old while they are lying down with a stationary headboard and a movable footboard (Figure 17.2). Alternative measures for nonambulatory clients provide estimates for people who cannot stand up straight, have lower-body amputations, or are unable to get out of bed (Box 17.1).

Weight and body mass index. For accurate results, weigh the client at consistent times (e.g., early morning after the bladder is emptied and before breakfast) while wearing the same, or similar, clothing (e.g., an examination gown). Ask the client about his or her usual body weight and compare it with standard BMI tables (see BMI chart located inside the back cover of this book). Inquire about recent weight loss (e.g., how much over what period). Rapid unintentional weight loss, particularly in elderly clients, is significantly associated with increased health risks and mortality.[13] Health care providers should refer any clients who have lost ≥5% of their body weight in 1 month or ≥10% of their body weight in any amount of time for unknown reasons to an RDN for a thorough evaluation (see Table 22.1 for malnutrition diagnostic criteria). Noting recent weight gain is equally important. Understanding the client's general weight history over time (e.g., peaks and lows at what ages) will give a broad view of ordinary weight fluctuations for the individual.

The BMI, calculated by using both weight and height measurements, is a helpful assessment tool throughout the life cycle.

Body composition and waist circumference. The dietitian may measure various aspects of body size and composition to determine relative levels of lean tissue compared with fat mass. Chapter 15 covers several different methods for estimating body composition. Some methods include a skin fold thickness measurement with calipers, hydrostatic weighing, bioelectrical

---

> ### Box 17.1   Alternative Measures for Nonambulatory Clients
>
> **TOTAL ARM SPAN**
> - With a flexible metric tape, measure the client's full arm span from fingertip to fingertip across the front of the clavicles.
> - For clients with limited movement in one arm, measure from the fingertip to the midpoint of the sternum on the dominant hand, and then double the measurement.
>
> **KNEE HEIGHT**
> - With the client lying on his or her back, bend his or her knee and ankle to a 90-degree angle.
> - Using a knee height caliper, measure the left knee-to-floor height from the outside bony point just under the kneecap (i.e., the fibular head) and down to the floor surface to the nearest 0.1 cm.
> - Use the following equations to calculate total body height from knee height:
>   - Men: 64.19 – (0.04 × age in years) + (2.02 × knee height in centimeters)
>   - Women: 84.88 – (0.24 × age in years) + (1.83 × knee height in centimeters)
> - The answer will be an estimate of height in centimeters. Convert centimeters to inches: 1 in = 2.54 cm
>
> **RECUMBENT BED LENGTH**
> - Align the body so that the lower extremities, trunk, shoulders, and head are in a straight line.
> - Mark on the bed sheet the position of the base of the heels and the top of the crown.
> - Measure the distance with a tape measure.
>
> **SEGMENTAL HEIGHT MEASUREMENT**
> - Measure four segments of body while the person is lying on his or her side on a firm surface.
> - Measure the following segments with a flexible measuring tape: top of head to base of neck, base of the neck to the tailbone, greater trochanter to knee, and the knee to base of heel (foot flexed).
> - Add the segment measurements together.

Reference: Academy of Nutrition and Dietetics. (2019). *Nutrition care manual.* Chicago, IL: Academy of Nutrition and Dietetics.

---

doubly labeled water method gold standard for measuring energy expenditure. Participants ingest water labeled with a known concentration of isotopes of hydrogen and oxygen. Technicians measure the elimination of the isotopes to predict the energy expenditure and metabolic rate.

anthropometric measurements the physical measurements of the human body that are used for health assessment, including height, weight, skin fold thickness, and circumference (i.e., of the head, hip, waist, wrist, and mid-arm muscle).

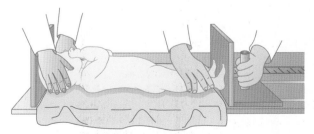

Figure 17.2 Measuring height in an infant. (Reprinted from Mahan, L. K., & Escott-Stump, S. [2012]. *Krause's food & nutrition therapy* [13th ed.]. Philadelphia: Saunders.)

impedance analysis, dual-energy x-ray absorptiometry, and the BOD POD body composition tracking system (COSMED, USA, Concord, CA). Mid-arm muscle circumference and triceps skin fold are two easy and fast anthropometric measurements frequently used in clinical settings for assessing body composition changes.

BMI and body composition measurements indicate the risk for overweight and obesity (i.e., body fatness), but they do not evaluate where excess fat is stored or relative fitness levels of the client. The location of body fat is an important factor in nutrition assessment, because not all body fat carries the same risks. Individuals who store body fat in the abdominal region have significantly more health risks than their counterparts of the same weight who store fat in the hip and thigh regions. The Clinical Practice Guidelines for Medical Care of Patients with Obesity note that, for a lowered health risk, waist circumference should be less than 102 cm for men and less than 88 cm for women (and even lower in some Asian populations).[14] Waist circumference assessment and waist-to-height ratio are important considerations for both overweight and normal-weight individuals, because they indicate the risk for chronic diseases (e.g., type 2 diabetes, cardiovascular disease, hypertension, certain types of cancer, overall mortality), even among individuals of normal weight.[15-20]

Biochemical Data, Medical Tests, and Procedures

Laboratory data and radiographic tests may be helpful in assessing a client's nutrition status. Such reports generally are available in the client's medical chart. Examples of biochemical tests pertinent to nutrition include, but are not limited to, the following:

- Blood urea nitrogen and serum electrolytes: evaluate renal function
- Complete blood count: evaluate for anemia
- Creatinine height index: evaluate protein tissue breakdown
- Fasting glucose: evaluate for hyper- and hypoglycemia
- Lipid profile: evaluate blood lipid and lipoprotein levels
- Liver enzymes: evaluate liver function
- Plasma proteins: serum albumin and prealbumin indicate protein status
- Total lymphocyte count: evaluate immune function
- Urinary urea nitrogen excretion: estimate nitrogen balance

The medical tests that are used for nutrition assessment are generally reliable for people of any age; however, when reviewing laboratory values, keep in mind that some conditions may interfere with test results. For example, hydration status, the presence of chronic diseases, changes in organ function, time from last meal, and certain medications can alter test results. The necessity of additional medical tests or procedures depends on the client, such as the following:

- *Gastrointestinal function:* Medical procedures are also useful to evaluate function, disease, or malfunction along the gastrointestinal tract (e.g., disturbances in gastric emptying time, peptic ulcer disease, inflammatory bowel disease).
- *Skeletal system integrity:* Several tests can assess the risk for osteopenia or osteoporosis, especially with older clients; x-rays, dual-energy x-ray absorptiometry, and bone scans can help determine the status of bone integrity.
- *Resting metabolic rate:* Evaluating a client's resting metabolic rate helps to establish total energy needs. Chapter 6 covers both direct and indirect measurement methods.

Nutrition-Focused Physical Findings

The careful observation of various areas of the client's body may reveal signs of poor nutrition. Table 17.2 provides examples of clinical signs relevant to a client's nutrition status. In addition, other members of

Table 17.2 Signs That Suggest Nutrient Imbalance

AREA OF CONCERN	POSSIBLE DEFICIENCY	POSSIBLE EXCESS
Hair		
Dull, dry, and brittle	Protein	
Easily plucked, with no pain	Protein	
Hair loss	Protein, zinc, biotin	Vitamin A
Flag sign (i.e., loss of hair pigment in strips around the head)	Protein, copper	
Head and Neck		
Bulging fontanel (in infants)		Vitamin A
Headache		Vitamins A, D
Epistaxis (i.e., nosebleed)	Vitamin K	
Thyroid enlargement	Iodine	
Eyes		
Conjunctival and corneal xerosis (i.e., dryness)	Vitamin A	
Pale conjunctiva	Iron	
Blue sclerae	Iron	
Corneal vascularization	Vitamin B_2	

Table **17.2**   **Signs That Suggest Nutrient Imbalance—cont'd**

AREA OF CONCERN	POSSIBLE DEFICIENCY	POSSIBLE EXCESS
Mouth		
Cheilosis or angular stomatitis (i.e., lesions at the corners of the mouth)	Vitamin B$_2$	
Glossitis (i.e., red, sore tongue)	Niacin, folate, vitamin B$_{12}$, and other B vitamins	
Gingivitis (i.e., inflamed gums)	Vitamin C	
Hypogeusia or dysgeusia (i.e., poor sense of taste or distorted taste)	Zinc	
Dental caries	Fluoride	
Mottling of teeth		Fluoride
Atrophy of papillae on tongue	Iron, B vitamins	
Skin		
Dry or scaly	Vitamin A, zinc, essential fatty acids	Vitamin A
Follicular hyperkeratosis (resembles gooseflesh)	Vitamin A, essential fatty acids, B vitamins	
Eczematous lesions	Zinc	
Petechiae or ecchymoses	Vitamins C, K	
Nasolabial seborrhea (i.e., greasy, scaly areas between the nose and lip)	Niacin, vitamins B$_{12}$, B$_6$	
Darkening and peeling of skin in areas exposed to sun	Niacin	
Poor wound healing	Protein, zinc, vitamin C	
Nails		
Spoon shaped	Iron	
Brittle and fragile	Protein	
Heart		
Enlargement, tachycardia, or failure	Thiamin	
Small heart	Energy	
Sudden failure or death	Selenium	Potassium
Arrhythmia	Magnesium, potassium, selenium	
Hypertension	Calcium, potassium	Sodium
Abdomen		
Hepatomegaly	Protein	Vitamin A
Ascites	Protein	
Musculoskeletal Extremities		
Muscle wasting (especially in the temporal area)	Energy	
Edema	Protein, thiamin	
Calf tenderness	Thiamin, vitamin C, biotin, selenium	
Beading of ribs or "rachitic rosary" in a child	Vitamins C, D	
Bone and joint tenderness	Vitamins C, D, calcium, phosphorus	
Knock knees, bowed legs, or fragile bones	Vitamin D, calcium, phosphorus, copper	
Neurologic		
Paresthesias (i.e., pain and tingling or altered sensation in the extremities)	Thiamin, vitamins B$_6$, B$_{12}$, biotin	
Weakness	Thiamin, vitamins C, B$_6$, B$_{12}$, energy	
Ataxia and decreased position and vibratory senses	Thiamin, vitamin, B$_{12}$	
Tremor	Magnesium	
Decreased tendon reflexes	Thiamin	
Confabulation or disorientation	Thiamin, vitamin B$_{12}$	
Drowsiness and lethargy	Thiamin	Vitamins A, D
Depression	Thiamin, vitamin B$_{12}$, biotin	

the health care team (e.g., physician, nurse, physical therapist) may record their own findings from physical examinations in the medical chart that add to the data analysis in making a nutrition assessment.

Client History

Guided questioning helps clients to identify and remember elements of their personal, family, and medical histories that may be pertinent to their assessment. As stated previously, clients frequently forget to mention their use of dietary supplements such as herbs. Direct questioning during this stage helps to identify the use of other complementary and alternative medicine. Many elements of a client's personal history can affect his or her current nutrition status and help to guide the plan of care; such elements include socioeconomic status, religion, culture, ethnicity, family interactions, education level, food security, and employment status. Economic needs are paramount for many people in high-risk populations. Health care providers who are cognizant of the personal and cultural needs of their clients will be more effective when helping a client plan for immediate and long-term nutrition requirements.

Psychologic and emotional problems can weigh heavily on the overall outcome of a client's prognosis and well-being. For example, elderly clients in long-term health care facilities disproportionately suffer from depression and malnutrition, which are compounding problems when individuals are already in poor health.[21-23] Although poor nutrition status and unintentional weight loss are associated with depression, it is not always clear if depression is the cause or consequence of poor nutrition. Thus, inquiry into a client's psychologic well-being during this step may help to identify and address some contributing modifiable factors.

At the conclusion of the data-gathering process, health care providers must distinguish relevant from irrelevant data, validate the data, and then determine whether there is a need to obtain additional information before moving to the next phase. As stated earlier, the assessment phase of the nutrition care plan is ongoing, and health care providers continually reassess the client's status throughout their care.

NUTRITION DIAGNOSIS

A nutrition diagnosis involves the "identification and labeling of an existing nutrition problem that the nutrition and dietetics professional is responsible for treating."[2] Examining all of the information gathered thus far reveals the client's basic needs. Other needs develop and guide the care plan as the hospitalization or consultation continues. The following list includes each of the categories addressed during the nutrition diagnosis phase of the Nutrition Care Process.

- *Intake*: e.g., How much is the client consuming relative to their needs?
- *Clinical*: e.g., What nutrition problems may the client have related to his or her diagnosis?

- *Behavioral and Environmental*: e.g., How does the client's knowledge, beliefs, and physical and socioeconomic environment affect his or her access to food?

A nutrition diagnosis statement will have three distinct and concise elements: *Problem*, *Etiology*, and the *Signs/symptoms*. We refer to this as a *PES statement*.

Problem

Assigning a nutrition diagnostic category follows the careful assessment of nutrition indices and analysis of the data. The nutrition diagnostic statement identifies nutrition problems, which may include nutrient deficiencies (e.g., iron-deficiency anemia) or underlying disease that requires a modified diet (e.g., renal disease, liver disease). Such a diagnosis sets realistic and measurable outcome goals. This then allows for the identification of appropriate interventions and a means for tracking the progress toward attaining the specified outcome.

Etiology

The causes or contributing risk factors are identifiable factors that directly lead to the stated problem. The Academy of Nutrition and Dietetics defines etiology as "a factor gathered during the nutrition assessment that contributes to the existence or the maintenance of pathophysiological, psychosocial, situational, developmental, cultural, and/or environmental problems."[2] Correctly identifying the etiology is the only way to design an intervention plan adequately. The words *related to* precedes the etiology within the nutrition diagnostic PES statement.

Signs and Symptoms

Signs and symptoms of nutrition problems are an accumulation of subjective and objective changes in the client's health status that indicate a nutrition problem and that are the results of the identified etiology. The nutrition diagnosis will evolve as the client's nutrition needs change. The words *as evidenced by* precede the signs and symptoms within a nutrition diagnostic PES statement. The following is an example of a nutrition diagnostic PES statement:

Excessive caloric intake (problem) related to frequent consumption of energy-dense meals (etiology) as evidenced by average intake of calories exceeding recommended amount by 350 kcal/day and a 10-pound weight gain during the past 15 months (signs).

NUTRITION INTERVENTION

After completing the assessment and diagnosis, the dietitian should be ready to plan and implement the most suitable form of nutrition intervention. Nutrition interventions are "purposefully planned action(s) designed with the intent of changing a nutrition-related behavior, risk factor, environmental condition, or aspect of health status."[2] The goal is to resolve the nutrition-related etiology and/or diagnosis. Objectives of the care plan are client driven, thus focusing attention on personal needs and goals as well as on the identified requirements of medical care for the client. The dietitian must work collaboratively with the client to establish suitable and realistic actions to carry out the personal care plan. Such activities ideally include family members, caretakers, and any necessary interdisciplinary providers. The following sections describe each of the categories addressed during the nutrition intervention phase of the Nutrition Care Process, which are the following:

- Food and nutrient delivery
- Nutrition education and counseling
- Coordination of nutrition care

Food and/or Nutrient Delivery

Personal adaptation. Personalizing the diet to meet individual needs is necessary for successful nutrition therapy. This requires active planning with the client and his or her family/friends who are intimately involved in the client's daily life. The RDN must explore the following four areas with the client:

1. *Personal needs:* What is required to meet personal/cultural desires, concerns, goals, or life situation needs?
2. *Diagnosis:* How does the client's disease or condition affect the body and its normal metabolic functions?
3. *Nutrition therapy:* Prioritize diagnoses based on urgency, impact, and resources. How and why must the diet change to meet the needs created by the client's particular disease or condition? What are the current medical nutrition therapy evidence-based guidelines relative to the client's situation?
4. *Food plan:* How do these necessary nutrient modifications affect daily food choices? Focusing on the etiology, the dietitian will write a nutrition intervention plan to meet these specific needs.

Mode of feeding. Clients' normal nutrition requirements dictate the primary principle of diet therapy, and their condition guides the amount of modification required. The following three components demonstrate common modifications to the oral diet:

1. *Energy:* An increase or decrease in the total energy value of the diet, expressed in kilocalories
2. *Nutrients:* Modification in amount or form to one or more of the essential nutrients (i.e., protein, carbohydrate, fat, minerals, vitamins, and water)
3. *Texture:* Modification to the texture or seasoning of the diet (e.g., liquid and low-residue diets)

In the event that nutrient needs are not adequately satisfied through oral intake, the RDN will explore other methods of nutrient delivery. When a client's gastrointestinal tract is functioning, but he or she cannot or will not consume food orally, **enteral** feedings are an option. Administering enteral feedings by a tube makes use of the digestion and absorption functions of the gastrointestinal tract at some point below the mouth. Exact placement of the feeding tube depends on the point within the gastrointestinal tract where a client is able to tolerate introduction of food or nutrients. The tube may pass through the nasal cavity down the esophagus to the stomach or small intestine for short-term feedings. Surgical placement of the tube directly into the GI tract to avoid the nasal cavity allows for long-term enteral feedings. Chapter 22 covers details about when enteral feedings are used, placement of tubes, and types of formula.

If clients are unable to tolerate any nutrient delivery into the gastrointestinal tract, health care providers must consider **parenteral** nutrition therapy. Because it is administered intravenously, parenteral nutrition therapy carries risks associated with its invasive nature. However, it is an effective way of meeting the nutrient needs of a client whose gastrointestinal tract is not functioning. Chapter 22 also covers parenteral nutrition therapy.

Nutrition Education and Counseling

Communicating with a client about his or her specific nutrition intervention plan is a critical step in the potential success of the treatment. Clients and families who understand the necessary changes to food or nutrient delivery methods are able to appreciate the benefit from such adjustments and are more likely to remain compliant. Education may be a one-on-one experience with the dietitian, or it may occur in a group setting. Initial education and counseling interactions during inpatient stays can continue through outpatient appointments, when necessary.

Nutrition intervention plans are generally long-term lifestyle modifications designed to promote and improve health. Some clients have more changes to make than others, and they will need continued nutrition counseling support to reach one goal at a time. Establishing a long-term plan to make such changes takes a commitment to education, counseling, and both professional and personal support. Modifications to the plan of care over time reflect the client's response to intervention.

Coordination of Nutrition Care

Several health care providers may be involved in a nutrition intervention plan. For example, enteral tube feedings require the coordination of dietitians, nurses, the prescribing physician, and the clinical pharmacist. Interdisciplinary connections within health care make the coordination of nutrition care possible and more

---

enteral a mode of feeding that makes use of the gastrointestinal tract through oral or tube feeding.

parenteral a mode of feeding that does not make use of the gastrointestinal tract but that instead provides nutrition support via the intravenous delivery of nutrient solutions.

effective. In addition, family, friends, care providers, and other members of the client's personal support group may be helpful during the coordination of the client's care. This step includes all professional and personal resources and referrals necessary to carry out and maintain the intervention.

NUTRITION MONITORING AND EVALUATION

The fourth step of the Nutrition Care Process is nutrition monitoring and evaluation. In this step, the RDN identifies the clients' progress toward their goals. The three components of this process are as follows: (1) monitor progress, (2) measure outcomes, and (3) evaluate outcomes.[2]

The organization of outcome measures for this step of the Nutrition Care Process falls into the same categories as the nutrition assessment categories, excluding client history, as listed below:

- Food and nutrition-related history
- Anthropometric measurements
- Biochemical data, medical tests, and procedures
- Nutrition-focused physical findings

In this phase, nutrition professionals will collect data pertinent to the identified client goals and then compare these data with the client's previous status from the nutrition assessment phase to assess progress. To accurately and meaningfully evaluate the nutrition intervention strategies put into place, the RDN must identify quality indicators that reflect progress toward a specific goal. For example, if the goal is for the client to consume 74 g of high biologic protein per day through enteral feedings, then measuring body weight change does not reflect progress toward meeting the identified goal. Rather, analyzing feeding schedules and enteral formula delivery records in the client's medical chart would be a more appropriate method of evaluating the client's progress toward meeting their goal.

Assessing the efficacy of the nutrition intervention plan will guide necessary changes. If changes are not necessary and the client's goals have been satisfied, the dietitian may discharge the client from nutrition services at this point. If the client's goals have not yet been satisfied, the dietitian will work collaboratively with clients to revisit their diagnosis and renew their intervention strategy. The nutrition and dietetic professionals then continue to monitor and evaluate the clients' progress within their nutrition care plan.

DIET-DRUG INTERACTIONS

There are a variety of diet-drug interactions, and they have varying degrees of clinical significance for clients. Note that you may see *diet-drug interactions* expressed in several ways, such as drug-diet interactions, food-medication interactions, drug-nutrient interactions, and drug-food interactions. In most cases throughout this text, and elsewhere, we use the expression *"drug-nutrient interaction."* In this section, the term *diet-drug interaction* is appropriate because we are discussing more than single nutrient interactions with medications.

Many negative reactions are possible with polypharmacy, especially among elderly clients, who may also take dietary supplements and herbal products.[24-26] Almost half of the U.S. population takes at least one prescription drug per day, 21.5% take three or more, and 10.9% take five or more prescription drugs every day.[27] The majority of people taking multiple prescriptions per day are over the age of 65. Clients may experience different diet-drug interaction reactions from one another. Such reactions can vary depending on normal dietary habits, nutrition status, disease type and severity, compliance, and other medications or supplements that they are currently taking. Figure 17.3 demonstrates mechanisms by which diet-drug interactions may alter a client's outcome.

Gathering information about all medication use is essential to the care process; this includes over-the-counter medications, prescribed medications, dietary supplements, alternative/complimentary medications, as well as alcohol and recreational drugs. Because diet-drug interactions involve medications prescribed by a physician, dispensed by a pharmacist, and food or nutrients consumed by clients, the responsibility for knowledge of such interactions extends to the physician, pharmacist, dietitian, and the client. The nurse must be particularly familiar with diet-drug interactions as well because nurses most commonly administer both items to the client. The bottom line is that all members of the health care team should be aware of potential diet-drug reactions and communicate regularly.

Diet-drug interactions are often categorized using the distinctions listed below[25,28]:

- Class 1: Effect of obesity and malnutrition on drug action
- Class 2: Effect of nutrition on drug action
- Class 3: Effect of specific nutrients or dietary supplements on drug action
- Class 4: Effects of drugs on nutrition status
- Class 5: Effects of drugs on nutrient status

It is not within the scope of this textbook to cover extensively the many possible diet-drug interactions. There are Drug-Nutrient Interaction boxes throughout the text to highlight common interactions of interest within each chapter. Box 17.2 provides a brief list of resources for well-known diet-drug interactions. The following sections describe the different types of diet-drug interactions.

DRUG-FOOD INTERACTIONS

Interactions in which food increases or decreases the effect of a drug can adversely influence the health of a client. Certain foods may affect the absorption, distribution, metabolism, or elimination of a drug, thereby altering the intended dose response (see Figure 17.3). The timing, size, and composition of meals relative to medication administration are all common causes of drug-food interactions. For example, a high-fat meal increases the absorption of some drugs that are

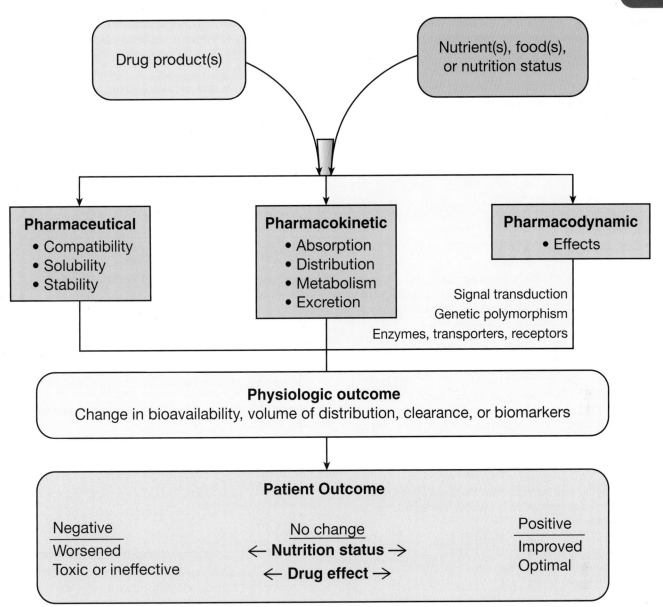

Figure 17.3 Mechanisms of drug-nutrient interactions that influence a patient's outcome. (Reprinted from Boullata, J. I., & Hudson, L. M. [2012]. Drug-nutrient interactions: A broad view with implications for practice. *J Acad Nutr Diet, 112*[4], 506–517.)

Box 17.2 **Resources for Diet-Drug Interactions**

- Asher, G. N., Corbett, A. H., & Hawke, R. L. (2017). Common herbal dietary supplement-drug interactions. *Am Fam Physician, 96*(2), 101–107.
- Little, M. O. (2018). Updates in nutrition and polypharmacy. *Curr Opin Clin Nutr Metab Care, 21*(1), 4–9.
- Mohn, E. S., et al. (2018). Evidence of drug-nutrient interactions with chronic use of commonly prescribed medications: An update. *Pharmaceutics, 10*(1).
- Peter, S., et al. (2017). Public health relevance of drug-nutrition interactions. *Eur J Nutr, 56*(Suppl. 2), 23–36.
- Spanakis, M., et al. (2019). PharmActa: Empowering patients to avoid clinical significant drug-herb interactions. *Medicines (Basel), 6*(1).
- A Pocket Guide to Food-Medication Interactions: www.foodmedinteractions.com.
- U.S. Food and Drug Administration: Search "Avoiding Drug Interactions" at www.fda.gov.

lipophilic (i.e., "fat loving"), whereas a high-fiber meal may bind other drugs and reduce their absorption.

The interaction of grapefruit juice and several medications has been under critical evaluation for many years. A substance called *furanocoumarin* in grapefruit juice can dramatically alter the bioavailability of certain drugs to a toxic level.[29] The anticoagulation medication warfarin is a commonly prescribed drug for clients with heart disease. It is also one of the most highly interactive medications with certain foods, specifically with those that are high in vitamin K, such as green, leafy vegetables. Many clients are not familiar with high-vitamin K foods, thus they may not realize the potential for interaction when choosing such foods. Other examples of drug-food interactions include: (1) medications that interfere with the appetite because of changes in taste or smell sensations (e.g., amitriptyline, metronidazole) and (2) medications that stimulate the appetite (e.g., antihistamines, steroids). Over time, these alterations in appetite may affect nutrition status.

DRUG-NUTRIENT INTERACTIONS

Taking medications along with over-the-counter vitamin and mineral supplements may result in deleterious drug-nutrient interactions (see the Case Study box, "Drug-Nutrient Interaction"). Table 17.3 provides some potential drug-nutrient interactions and their known risk factors. As a health care provider, always ask clients what other medications they are taking, specifically their vitamin, mineral, and herbal supplement use. Drug-nutrient interactions may result in the depletion of a nutrient, or the nutrient may induce a change in the rate of metabolism of the drug. The Cultural Considerations box entitled "Prescription Medication and Dietary Supplement Use" discusses the prevalence and common demographic traits of clients who are taking both dietary supplements and prescription medications.

NEXT-GENERATION NCLEX® EXAMINATION-STYLE UNFOLDING CASE STUDY
Drug Nutrient Interaction

See Answers in Appendix A.

A 26-year-old woman reported to her doctor with symptoms that included fatigue; headaches; muscle, joint, and bone pain; dry, flaking skin; hair loss; nausea and vomiting; and weight loss. After a physical examination and laboratory work, she was determined to have liver damage. The only prescription medication that she takes is isotretinoin for acne. Isotretinoin is 13-*cis*-retinoic acid, and it is a vitamin A–related compound. She also reported taking several dietary supplements, including a multivitamin, a vitamin E supplement, and a vitamin D supplement, each of which contains 500% of the Recommended Dietary Allowance of its respective vitamin; an antioxidant liquid mix that contains β-carotene; and an occasional high-antioxidant supplement containing vitamins A, C, and E, zinc, and selenium.

1. Choose the *most likely* options for the information missing from the statements below by selecting from the list of options provided

   The Registered Dietitian Nutritionist (RDN) determines that the client's symptoms are most likely caused by surpassing the ____1____, causing vitamin ____2____.

OPTION 1	OPTION 2
tolerable upper intake level	deficiency
recommended dietary allowance	mobility
adequate intake	toxicity
estimated average requirement	activation

2. Select the compound that is most likely related to the client's signs and symptoms.

   a. Vitamin D
   b. Vitamin C
   c. Zinc
   d. Copper
   e. Vitamin A
   f. Vitamin E

3. Choose the *most likely* options for the information missing from the statements below by selecting from the list of options provided.

   The client's vitamin ____1____ is related to her liver damage because the liver is the main site of vitamin ____2____.

OPTION 1	OPTION 2
deficiency	deactivation and excretion
activation	excretion and removal
toxicity	absorption and digestion
mobility	storage and metabolism

4. Use an X to identify each item that is considered <u>safe</u> or <u>contraindicated</u> (should be avoided) when taking isotretinoin.

ITEM	SAFE	CONTRAINDICATED
broccoli		
alcohol		
sweet potato		
multivitamins		
vitamin A supplements		
carrots		
antioxidant supplements		

   The woman mentions that she is trying to get pregnant. The nurse gives her recommendations regarding her medication and supplements.

5. Select all of the recommendations that are appropriate for this client.

   a. Keep taking medications/supplements as is
   b. Avoid all food containing vitamin A
   c. Stop taking isotretinoin immediately
   d. Speak to your physician regarding drug-nutrient interactions during pregnancy
   e. Stop taking supplements, but it is safe to continue taking isotretinoin
   f. Avoid large doses of vitamin A from supplements at this time

6. Select the best measures to assess the client's liver function.

   a. Blood urea nitrogen
   b. Complete blood count
   c. Fasting blood glucose
   d. Aspartate aminotransferase
   e. Alanine aminotransferase
   f. White blood cell count

DRUG-HERB INTERACTIONS

Interactions that involve prescription drugs and herbs are the least well-defined drug interactions. Scientists have studied the herb-drug interactions of the most commonly taken herbs, such as St. John's wort (*Hypericum perforatum*) and *Ginkgo biloba*, extensively.[30,31] The exact mechanism by which herbs interact with medications varies. St. John's wort has an extensive list of drug-herb interactions, some of which are clinically severe, but not all of which are unfavorable.[32] Medication groups that have documented adverse reactions when taken with St. John's wort include anticancer medications, antihistamines, antimicrobials bronchodilators, cardiovascular medications, corticosteroids, hypoglycemic agents, immunosuppressants, lipid-lowering medications, nonsteroidal antiinflammatory medications, opioids, oral contraceptives, and drugs that act on the gastrointestinal tract.[33,34] Some experts recommend that clients avoid taking St. John's wort concurrently with *any* other over-the-counter or prescription medication.[32]

Other commonly used herbs that are involved in drug interactions include ginkgo (*Ginkgo biloba*), ginger (*Zingiber officinale*), ginseng (*Panax ginseng*), and garlic (*Allium sativum*).[35] Many herbs also have clinically documented medicinal properties. The health care team should evaluate a client's use of herbal products on an individual basis to determine their appropriateness with the client's current dietary habits and medications.

Table 17.3   Potential Drug-Nutrient Interactions With Known Risk Factors

DRUG CATEGORY	NAME	NUTRIENT	EFFECT ON NUTRIENT STATUS OR FUNCTION	RISK FACTORS
Acid-Suppressing Drugs	Proton Pump Inhibitors	Vitamin B_{12} Vitamin C Iron Calcium Magnesium Zinc β-Carotene	Decrease Decrease Decrease Decrease Decrease Decrease Decrease	Advanced age *H. pylori* infection Genetics (slow metabolizers) Low dietary intake (vegetarians) Pre-existing iron deficiency Women Duration of drug use
Non-Steroidal Anti-Inflammatory Drugs	Aspirin	Vitamin C Iron	Decrease Decrease	Absence of cold virus Advanced age *H. pylori* infection
Anti-Hypertensives	Diuretics (loop, thiazide) Diuretics (potassium-sparing) Angiotensin-Converting Enzyme Inhibitors Calcium Channel Blockers	Calcium Magnesium Thiamin Zinc Potassium Folate Iron Folate	Decrease (loop) Increase (thiazide) Decrease (loop and thiazide) Decrease (loop) Decrease (thiazide) Decrease (thiazide) Increase N/A Decrease	Dose/duration of drug use Form of loop diuretic Advanced age Heart failure Low magnesium intake Alcohol use Low dietary thiamin intake Gastrointestinal disorders Renal disease Low dietary zinc intake Form of thiazide used Low folate status Impaired liver function Liver cirrhosis (alcoholics) Use of captopril Renal disease Diabetes mellitus Potassium supplement use Presence of dental plaque Poor oral hygiene Concurrent use of beta-blockers
Hypercholesterolemics	Statins	Coenzyme Q10 Vitamin D Vitamin E/β-Carotene	Decrease Increase/Decrease Increase/Decrease	Dose Advanced age Statin-associated myopathy Heart disease Vitamin D deficiency
Hypoglycemics	Biguanides (Metformin) Thiazolidinediones	Vitamin B_{12} Calcium/ Vitamin D	Decrease Decrease	Dose/duration of drug use Advanced age Vegetarians Women Low calcium/vitamin D intake

Continued

Table 17.3 Potential Drug-Nutrient Interactions With Known Risk Factors—cont'd

DRUG CATEGORY	NAME	NUTRIENT	EFFECT ON NUTRIENT STATUS OR FUNCTION	RISK FACTORS
Corticosteroids	Glucocorticoids (oral)	Calcium/Vitamin D Sodium Potassium Chromium	Decrease Increase Decrease Decrease	Low calcium/vitamin D intake At risk for bone fracture/loss
Bronchodilators	Corticosteroids (inhaled)	Calcium/ Vitamin D	Decrease	Presence of COPD Smoking At risk for bone fracture/loss Low calcium/vitamin D intake
Antidepressants	Selective Serotonin Reuptake Inhibitors	Folate Calcium/Vitamin D	Increase Decrease	Low folate intake Genetics (MTHFR variants) Alcoholism At risk for bone fracture/loss Low calcium/vitamin D intake
Oral Contraceptives	Estrogen and /or Progesterone	Vitamin B_6 Vitamin B_{12}/Folate Calcium Magnesium Vitamin C/Vitamin E	Decrease Decrease Increase/ decrease Decrease Decrease	Vegetarians Low folate intake Genetics (folate metabolism) Duration of drug use Physical activity level Low calcium intake Age at first use Race Type of combined oral contraceptive used

Modified from Mohn, E. S., et al. (2018). Evidence of drug-nutrient interactions with chronic use of commonly prescribed medications: An update. *Pharmaceutics, 10*(1).

Cultural Considerations

Prescription Medication and Dietary Supplement Use

The concurrent use of prescription medications and dietary supplements is common in the United States. About half of adults report regular use of dietary supplements.[1] Meanwhile, about half of the adult population is also regularly taking prescription medications.[2] The use of both prescription medication and dietary supplements increases along with age precipitously (see figure).

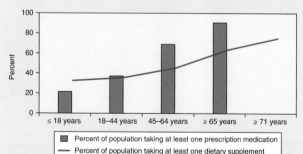

Concurrent use of prescription medication and dietary supplements

- ■ Percent of population taking at least one prescription medication
- — Percent of population taking at least one dietary supplement

(Source: National Center for Health Statistics. [2018]. Health, United States. In *Health, United States, 2017: With special feature on mortality*. Hyattsville, MD: National Center for Health Statistics [US]; Cowan, A. E., et al. [2018]. Dietary supplement use differs by socioeconomic and health-related characteristics among U.S. adults, NHANES 2011-2014. *Nutrients, 10*[8]; Jun, S., et al. [2018]. Dietary supplement use among U.S. children by family income, food security level, and nutrition assistance program participation status in 2011-2014. *Nutrients, 10*[9].)

Because of the significant risk of drug-nutrient interactions, nondisclosure of supplement use presents a problem for both health care providers and clients, particularly when they are simultaneously taking prescription medications. It is helpful for health care providers to appreciate the high use of supplements among certain demographic groups so that they may provide extra attention to the matter when working with these clients. Although there are always exceptions, some common demographic traits of adults in the United States who take some form of dietary supplements are as follows[1]:

- Female
- ≥50 years old
- Non-Hispanic white
- Higher education
- Higher income
- Food secure

With a significant portion of the adult population using *both* dietary supplements and prescription medications, it is imperative for health care providers to ask clients specifically about their use of complementary and alternative medication.

REFERENCES

1. Cowan, A. E., et al. (2018). Dietary supplement use differs by socioeconomic and health-related characteristics among U.S. adults, NHANES 2011-2014. *Nutrients, 10*(8).
2. National Center for Health Statistics. (2018). *Health, United States. In Health, United States, 2017: With special feature on mortality.* Hyattsville, MD: National Center for Health Statistics (US).

Putting It All Together

Summary

- The basis for effective person-centered nutrition care begins with the client's nutrition needs and must involve the client and his or her family or care providers.
- The careful assessment of factors that influence nutrition status requires a broad foundation of pertinent information (e.g., physiologic, psychosocial, medical, cultural, personal).
- Nutrition therapy reflects the personal and physical needs of the client. Successful therapy requires close collaboration among nutrition and dietetic professionals, medical, and nursing staff in the health care facility. The nurse is in a unique position to reinforce the nutrition principles of the diet with the client and his or her family or care providers.
- Drug interactions with nutrients, foods, or other medications can cause complications with client care. Careful questioning to determine all prescription and over-the-counter supplements and medication use will help to guide the client's education needs.

Chapter Review Questions

See answers in Appendix A.

1. A simple anthropometric measurement that can help indicate risk for chronic disease, even in normal weight individuals, is _____.

   a. waist circumference
   b. serum albumin level
   c. knee height
   d. hemoglobin level

2. A client recently diagnosed with type 2 diabetes needs help to determine a healthy energy intake. The most appropriate member of the health care team to help with this is the _____.

   a. registered nurse
   b. physician
   c. registered dietitian nutritionist
   d. pharmacist

3. The correct order of the four steps included in the Nutrition Care Process are _____.

   a. planning, intervention, diagnosis, monitoring, and evaluation
   b. planning, intervention, monitoring, follow-up, and evaluation
   c. assessment, diagnosis, intervention, and monitoring and evaluation
   d. assessment, diagnosis, planning, follow-up, and discharge

4. Warfarin can specifically interact with certain types of foods that are high in _____.

   a. vitamin K
   b. vitamin B
   c. potassium
   d. iron

5. With regard to nutrition intervention, the role of the nurse on the health care team for a client who has just been diagnosed with chronic kidney disease is to _____.

   a. assess protein, calorie, and fluid requirements required each day
   b. reinforce the nutrition principles of the diet with the client and family
   c. develop a meal plan that will be the most satisfying to the client
   d. determine the most appropriate dietary supplement regimen for the client

Next-Generation NCLEX® Examination-style Case Study

See Answers in Appendix A.

A 60-year-old male (Ht.: 5'6" Wt.: 140 lbs.) is experiencing gastrointestinal symptoms such as stomach pain, nausea, and diarrhea. He has no prior medical history. The client reports recently adding a new dietary supplement to his existing supplement regimen and that is when his symptoms started. He could not remember the name of the supplements as his memory is "not what it used to be". His medical record indicates that he is not currently taking any prescription but takes Tylenol occasionally. The doctor thinks there may be a potential food-drug interaction. When asked about his diet, he struggled to remember what he ate the day before.

1. From the list below, select all factors from the client's history that require a follow up.

   a. BMI
   b. Stomach pain, nausea, and diarrhea
   c. Medications
   d. Dietary supplements
   e. Diet history
   f. Medical history

2. From the list below, identify the best method(s) to collect dietary intake information from the client.

   a. 24-hour recall
   b. Multiple-day food record
   c. Food frequency questionnaire
   d. Diet history
   e. Dual-energy x-ray absorptiometry
   f. BOD-POD

3. Place an X under the appropriate column to identify interventions that are <u>indicated</u> (appropriate or necessary) or <u>contraindicated</u> (could be harmful) for the client.

INTERVENTIONS	INDICATED	CONTRAINDICATED
Plans out dietary supplement use around mealtimes.		
Educate the client on the effects and use of his supplements and		
Educate the client on proper dosing and timing of his supplements.		
Avoid coordinating with other health care professionals if possible.		
Educate the client with a one-day strict meal plan that will avoid any drug-nutrient interactions.		
Schedule meals and intake before considering the client's lifestyle.		

Gastrointestinal and Accessory Organ Problems

Key Concepts

- Diseases of the gastrointestinal tract and its accessory organs interrupt the body's normal cycle of digestion, absorption, and metabolism.
- Food allergies result from an inappropriate immune response to certain proteins found in food.
- Underlying genetic diseases may cause metabolic defects that block the body's ability to handle specific foods.

We often take for granted the body's highly organized and intricate system for handling food. However, when something goes wrong with the system, the whole body is affected. The gastrointestinal (GI) tract is a sensitive mirror, directly and indirectly, of the individual human condition.

This chapter looks at the system that manages food and its nutrients. The digestive process works as a series of cascading events throughout the GI tract. Secretions from the accessory organs (i.e., pancreas, liver, and gallbladder) are instrumental in the process. Effective medical nutrition therapy for disorders involving the GI tract must reflect the functioning of this finely integrated network and the person whose life it affects.

Diseases may affect the GI tract anywhere from the mouth to the anus. This chapter covers the most commonly affected areas of the GI tract under the headings that state where the primary problems begin or exist.

UPPER GASTROINTESTINAL TRACT

MOUTH

Dental Problems

Dental caries (i.e., cavities) result from the combined effect and presence of bacteria and fermentable carbohydrates. When bacteria ferment carbohydrates, they produce acids that erode the tooth structure. An increased use of fluoridated public water and toothpaste, as well as better dental hygiene, has decreased the incidence of dental caries in recent decades. Fluoride toothpastes are effective for preventing dental caries at fluoride concentrations of 1000 ppm.[1] However, untreated tooth decay still plagues some 20% of children and 32% of adults in the United States.[2]

Elderly individuals who are missing teeth or have ill-fitting dentures are prone to compromised nutrition status due, in part, to avoiding certain types of food that are painful or difficult to eat.[3-5] Specifically, people without healthy teeth frequently avoid foods such as whole fruits, vegetables, meats, and other high-fiber foods and opt for energy-dense, easy-to-chew foods instead. About 43% of adults over age 50 in the United States have tooth loss to the point of nonfunctional dentition (i.e., <21 teeth remaining), and there is great disparity for those with lower socioeconomic standing (see the Cultural Considerations box, "Social Disparities and Dental Status").[6] Sometimes a mechanical soft diet is helpful for individuals who are lacking teeth. For such a diet, all foods are soft cooked, and meats are ground and mixed with sauces or gravies so that less chewing is necessary.

Surgical Procedures

A fractured jaw or other surgeries that involve the mouth and neck pose obvious eating problems. The client must receive nutrients, which may be in the form of high-protein, high-caloric liquids. Other prepared commercial formulas are also available and discussed in Chapter 22. As healing progresses, adding soft foods that require little chewing effort helps the individual with progression to a full diet in accordance with his or her personal tolerance.

Oral Tissue Inflammation

Tissues of the mouth often reflect a person's overall nutrition status. Malnutrition—especially severe states—causes the deterioration of the oral tissues, which may result in local infection or injury that brings pain and difficulty with eating. The following conditions of the oral cavity can contribute to malnutrition:

- *Gingivitis:* Inflammation of the gums that involves the mucous membrane and its supporting fibrous tissue surrounding the base of the teeth (Figure 18.1A).

Cultural Considerations

Social Disparities and Dental Status

Oral health is an indicator of overall health. Untreated dental caries and missing teeth are a common problem worldwide and negatively influence well-being and oral health-related quality of life.[1,2] When a person has no remaining natural teeth, he or she is edentulous. Edentulism is of significant nutrition concern because teeth are an important part of mechanical digestion. However, dental health care is not a mandatory coverage for most health care policies, and supplemental medical insurance policies can be cost prohibitive for many individuals and families, particularly the elderly population and low-income individuals.

Untreated dental problems and loss of teeth are highly associated with older age, race/ethnicity, lower income, and education level.[3–6] The image below portrays the disparity in edentulism relative to socioeconomic status. The majority of individuals with no remaining teeth are also the ones who can ill-afford dentures.

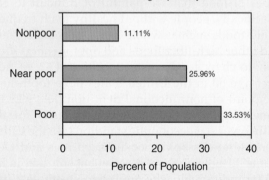

Prevalence of edentulism in the U.S. among people 65 years and older according to poverty status

- Nonpoor: 11.11%
- Near poor: 25.96%
- Poor: 33.53%

Percent of Population

Poor: <100% federal poverty guideline; near poor: 100%–199% federal poverty guideline; nonpoor: ≥200% federal poverty guideline. (Source: Dye, B. A., Weatherspoon, D. J., Lopez, G., & Mitnik G. [2019]. Tooth loss among older adults according to poverty status in the United States from 1999 through 2004 and 2009 through 2014. *J Am Dent Assoc, 150*[1], 9–23.e3.)

There are strong public health implications regarding which population subgroups policies and health care providers should target for education and intervention to decrease tooth loss. Although addressing means to overcome poverty is not a typical responsibility of most health care workers, education for oral hygiene is relatively easy and quick to address. Even without twice-yearly dental visits, the act of brushing with fluoride-based toothpaste and flossing teeth regularly greatly reduces tooth loss in all socioeconomic sects of the population.

Given the health care implications and morbidity associated with the loss of teeth, improving oral hygiene and retention of healthy teeth is a reasonable goal for improving overall health.

REFERENCES

1. Ferreira, R. C., et al. (2019). Is reduced dentition with and without dental prosthesis associated with oral health-related quality of life? A cross-sectional study. *Health Qual Life Outcomes, 17*(1), 79.
2. GBD 2016 Disease and Injury Incidence and Prevalence Collaborators (2017). Global, regional, and national incidence, prevalence, and years lived with disability for 328 diseases and injuries for 195 countries, 1990-2016: A systematic analysis for the Global Burden of Disease Study 2016. *Lancet, 390*(10100), 1211–1259.
3. Dye, B. A., Weatherspoon, D. J., Lopez, G., & Mitnik, G. (2019). Tooth loss among older adults according to poverty status in the United States from 1999 through 2004 and 2009 through 2014. *J Am Dent Assoc, 150*(1), 9–23.e3.
4. Elani, H. W., et al. (2017). Social inequalities in tooth loss: A multinational comparison. *Community Dentistry and Oral Epidemiology, 45*(3), 266–274.
5. Gupta, N., et al. (2018). Disparities in untreated caries among children and adults in the U.S., 2011-2014. *BMC Oral Health, 18*(1), 30.
6. Hybels, C. F., et al. (2016). Trends in decayed teeth among middle-aged and older adults in the United States: Socioeconomic disparities persist over time. *J Public Health Dent, 76*(4), 287–294.

- *Stomatitis:* Inflammation of the oral mucous lining of the mouth (Figure 18.1B).
- *Glossitis:* Inflammation of the tongue (Figure 18.1C).
- *Cheilosis:* A dry, scaling process at the corners of the mouth that affects the lips and the corner angles, thereby making opening the mouth to eat uncomfortable (Figure 18.1D).

Mouth ulcers may develop from infectious sources, such as: (1) the herpes simplex virus, which causes mouth sores on the inside mucous lining of the cheeks and lips or on the external portion of the lips, where they are commonly called *cold sores* or *fever blisters;* (2) *Candida albicans,* which is a fungus that causes similar sores on the oral mucosa and results in a condition called *candidiasis* or *thrush;* and (3) hemolytic *Streptococcus,* which is a bacteria that causes the mucosal ulcers that we commonly call *canker sores.* Mouth ulcers are usually self-limiting and short lived. Other causes

include simple toothbrush abrasions and allergies. Clients with an underlying illness such as cancer or human immunodeficiency virus (HIV)—both of which diminish the body's immune system—often have mouth ulcers. Chemotherapy and radiation treatment to the mouth destroy the fast-replicating cells in the oral tissue and can result in painful mouth sores (see Chapter 23).

In these situations, eating may be painful. Clients can usually tolerate progressing from nutrient-dense liquids that are high in protein and calories to soft foods (e.g., nonacidic and bland to avoid irritation). They may prefer to avoid temperature extremes as well. Room-temperature soft or liquid foods are usually better accepted. For a person suffering from mouth pain, a mouthwash that contains a mild topical local anesthetic before meals helps to relieve the irritation caused by eating. In severe cases or cases that last more than 7 to 10 days, a dietitian may perform a full nutrition assessment to ensure that the client is receiving adequate nutrients to satisfy needs.

Salivary Glands

Disorders of the salivary glands in the mouth (Figure 18.2) also affect eating and related nutrition status. Problems may arise from infection, such as the mumps virus that attacks the parotid gland. Other problems arise from mucous cysts (i.e., mucoceles) and obstructed salivary ducts, typically on the lower lip or the insides of the cheeks. Both excess salivation

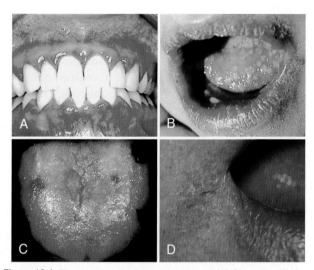

Figure 18.1 Tissue inflammation of the mouth. (A) Gingivitis. (B) Stomatitis. (C) Glossitis. (D) Cheilosis. ([A] Reprinted from Murray, P. R., Rosenthal, K. S., & Pfaller, M. A. [1994]. *Medical microbiology* [2nd ed.]. St Louis: Mosby. [B] Reprinted from Doughty, D. B., & Broadwell-Jackson, D. [1993]. *Gastrointestinal disorders*. St Louis: Mosby. [C] Reprinted from Hoffbrand, A. V., & Pettit, J. E. [Eds.]. [1988]. *Sandoz atlas of clinical hematology*. London: Gower Medical. [D] Reprinted from Lemmi, F. O., & Lemmi, C. A. E. [2000]. *Physical assessment findings* [CD-ROM]. Philadelphia: Saunders.)

and inadequate salivation can interfere with eating and salivary gland function. Numerous disorders that affect the nervous system, local mouth infections, injuries, and drug reactions cause excess salivation. Conversely, a dry mouth from a lack of salivation may be temporary and caused by fear, infection, or a drug reaction. *Xerostomia* (chronic dry mouth) is often associated with rheumatoid arthritis or radiation therapy, or it may occur as a side effect from many chronically used medications. Xerostomia causes swallowing and speaking difficulties, taste interference, and tooth decay.

The addition of more liquid food items to regular meals such as beverages, soups, stews, juicy fruits, and gravies or sauces may facilitate the eating process. Spraying an artificial saliva solution inside the mouth may relieve extreme mouth dryness. Some clients find that chewing sugar-free gum or sucking on sugar-free hard candy between meals helps improve their flow of saliva.

Swallowing Disorders - dysphagia

Swallowing is not as simple an act as it may seem. It involves highly integrated actions of the mouth, the **pharynx**, larynx, and the esophagus; in addition, after swallowing has begun, it is beyond voluntary control. Swallowing difficulty is a common problem with a variety of causes. It may be only temporary (e.g., a piece of food lodged in the back of the throat), and **abdominal thrusts** may be appropriate first aid. However, **dysphagia** is a chronic problem in some clients, and it is particularly common among those with neurologic disorders such as Alzheimer's disease, Parkinson's disease, and stroke complications.[7] Other common causes of dysphagia are head and neck cancer, tooth loss, xerostomia, neurodegenerative and neuromuscular disorders, post-intubation trauma, and muscular weakness of the larynx. An individual with dysphagia may have an impairment in one or more of the

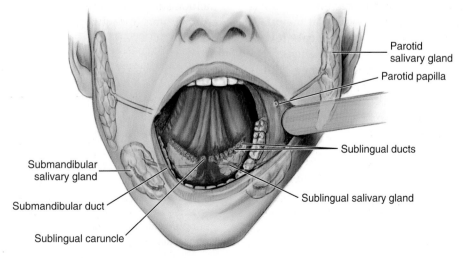

Parotid salivary gland

Parotid papilla

Sublingual ducts

Submandibular salivary gland

Submandibular duct

Sublingual caruncle

Sublingual salivary gland

Figure 18.2 Location of the salivary glands. (Reprinted from Fehrenbach, M. J., & Herring, S. W. [2007]. *Illustrated anatomy of the head and neck* [3rd ed.]. St Louis: Saunders.)

stages of swallowing, which are the oral, pharyngeal, and esophageal phases. To treat dysphagia effectively, a **speech-language pathologist** identifies if the problem is a mechanical obstruction or a neuromuscular disorder and diagnoses the situation accordingly.

Symptoms of dysphagia include an unexplained drop in food intake or repeated episodes of aspiration-related pneumonia. The presence of dysphagia significantly increases a patient's length of stay in the hospital, medical expenses, medical complications, risk for mortality, and risk for malnutrition when compared with similar individuals without dysphagia.[8,9] All health care personnel should watch for warning signs of dysphagia. These signs may include the reluctance to eat certain food consistencies or any food at all, very slow chewing or eating, fatigue from eating, frequent throat clearing, complaints of food "sticking" in the throat, pockets of food held in the cheeks, painful swallowing, regurgitation, and coughing or choking during attempts to eat. Clients with dysphagia do not always exhibit overt signs such as coughing when food enters the airway. Silent aspiration, or aspiration that occurs without a cough, is a common cause of complications.

A team of interprofessional specialists that includes a physician, a nurse, a registered dietitian nutritionist (RDN), a speech-language pathologist, and an occupational therapist work collectively to treat clients with dysphagia. The speech-language pathologist may recommend swallowing techniques that help prevent aspiration, such as sitting in an upright position when eating, chin-down positioning when consuming liquids, and clearing the pharyngeal cavity with dry swallows. Thin fluids (e.g., water) are generally the most problematic to swallow properly. Thus, in addition to employing swallowing techniques, the standard practice is to adapt the diet to individual needs in stages of thickened liquids and pureed foods. Pureed foods are generally the consistency of mashed potatoes or pudding. Care providers may use a food processor to puree regular table food to achieve the desired consistency. Several manufacturers produce pureed foods or various meat- or vegetable-shaped food molds. However, the efficacy, acceptance, and compliance of using thickened liquids and modified textured foods are controversial.[10-12] See the For Further Focus box, "Thickened Liquids and Modified Texture Food for Dysphagia," for additional information.

ESOPHAGUS

Central Tube

The esophagus is a long, muscular tube that extends from the throat to the stomach. Circular muscles or sphincters bind both ends of the esophagus and act as valves to control the passage of food. The upper sphincter muscle remains closed except during swallowing, thereby preventing airflow into the esophagus

and the stomach. The sphincter automatically opens when swallowing and then closes immediately afterward. Various disorders along the tube may disrupt normal swallowing, including muscle spasms or uncoordinated contractions as well as the stricture or narrowing of the tube caused by scar tissue from a previous injury, the ingestion of caustic chemicals, a tumor, or **esophagitis**. These problems hinder eating and require medical attention through stretching procedures or surgery to widen the tube in addition to drug therapy to heal the inflammation. The diet during such problems ranges from liquid to soft in texture, depending on the extent of the problem and individual tolerance.

Lower Esophageal Sphincter

Functional defects of the lower esophageal sphincter (LES) may come from changes in the smooth muscle itself or from the nerve, muscle, and hormone control of peristalsis (see Chapter 5). Spasms occur when the LES maintains an excessively high muscle tone, even while resting, thereby failing to open normally when the person swallows. This condition is medically termed **achalasia** because of its tense muscle state, but we commonly refer to it as *cardiospasm* because of its proximity to the heart (although unrelated to the heart). Symptoms include difficulty swallowing, frequent vomiting,

---

mechanical soft diet a meal plan that consists of foods that have been chopped, blended, ground, or prepared with extra fluid to make chewing and swallowing easier.

parotid glands the largest of the three pairs of salivary glands; the parotid glands lie, one on each side, above the angle of the jaw and below and in front of the ear; they continually secrete saliva, which passes along the duct of the gland and into the mouth through an opening in the inner cheek that is level with the second upper molar tooth.

pharynx the muscular membranous passage that extends from the mouth to the posterior nasal passages, the larynx, and the esophagus.

abdominal thrusts (previously referred to as the Heimlich maneuver) a first-aid maneuver that is used to relieve a person who is choking from the blockage of the breathing passageway by a swallowed foreign object or food particle; to perform the maneuver, when standing behind the choking person, clasp the victim around the waist, place one fist just under the sternum (i.e., the breastbone), grasp the fist with the other hand, and then make a quick, hard, thrusting movement inward and upward to dislodge the object.

dysphagia difficulty swallowing.

speech-language pathologist a specialist in the assessment, diagnosis, treatment, and prevention of speech, language, cognitive communication, voice, swallowing, fluency, and other related disorders.

esophagitis inflammation of the esophagus.

achalasia a disorder of the esophagus in which the muscles of the tube fail to relax, thereby inhibiting normal swallowing.

For Further Focus

Thickened Liquids and Modified Texture Food for Dysphagia

The use of modified texture foods and thickened liquids has been the accepted customary care for individuals with dysphagia for many decades. However, until recently there were not any universally accepted names or definitions of food consistencies or viscosity of thickened liquids. Subsequently, standardization of a modified texture diet in accordance with the intended diet order was difficult, if not impossible. The International Dysphagia Diet Standardization Initiative (IDDSI) has recently set forth a descriptive framework for testing and clearly categorizing each of the seven food and liquid consistencies within a dysphagia diet.[1]

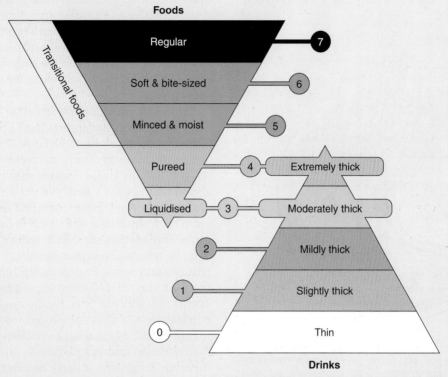

International Dysphagia Diet Standardization Initiative framework. (From Cichero, J. A., et al. [2017]. Development of international terminology and definitions for texture-modified foods and thickened fluids used in dysphagia management: The IDDSI framework. *Dysphagia, 32*[2], 293–314.)

The official launch date in the United States for using the IDDSI framework was May 1, 2019. Trained health care providers should be able to use simple tools such as a syringe, fork, or spoon to test the food consistency or liquid viscosity precisely to confirm compliance with the diet order. Recent studies have questioned the use of modified textured foods because patients are not accepting or compliant with the diet, nor has it consistently or significantly improved the overall health outcome of patients.[2–4] However, researchers collected data for these studies before the ISDDI framework implementation. Follow-up studies after adopting the standardized food and liquid consistencies on patient acceptance and compliance, dysphagia complications, quality of life, and overall health outcome will determine the continued use of this protocol.

See iddsi.org/framework/ for details on the IDDSI framework.

REFERENCES

1. Cichero, J. A., et al. (2017). Development of international terminology and definitions for texture-modified foods and thickened fluids used in dysphagia management: The IDDSI framework. *Dysphagia, 32*(2), 293–314.
2. O'Keeffe, S. T. (2018). Use of modified diets to prevent aspiration in oropharyngeal dysphagia: Is current practice justified? *BMC Geriatrics, 18*(1), 167.
3. Painter, V., Le Couteur, D. G., & Waite, L. M. (2017). Texture-modified food and fluids in dementia and residential aged care facilities. *Clinical Interventions in Aging, 12*, 1193–1203.
4. Seshadri, S., Sellers, C. R., & Kearney, M. H. (2018). Balancing eating with breathing: Community-dwelling older adults' experiences of dysphagia and texture-modified diets. *Gerontologist, 58*(4), 749–758.

a feeling of fullness in the chest, weight loss, malnutrition, and pulmonary complications and infections caused by the aspiration of food particles, especially during sleep. Surgical treatment of achalasia involves dilating or cutting (*esophageal myotomy*) the LES muscles. Both procedures can improve the relaxation of the LES, but neither improves the process of normal peristalsis.

The postoperative medical nutrition therapy (MNT) starts with oral liquids and progresses to a regular diet within a few days, depending on tolerance. Avoiding very hot or cold foods, citrus juices, and highly spiced foods may help prevent irritation. It is also helpful for clients to eat frequent small meals as tolerated, eat slowly, take small bites, and thoroughly chew their food.

Gastroesophageal Reflux Disease

Gastroesophageal reflux disease (GERD) is one of the most common GI problems for adults. Clients often describe it as "acid setting up shop" in the esophagus. It occurs when contents from the stomach reflux back into the esophagus because of LES incompetence (Figure 18.3). Unlike the stomach, mucus does not protect the esophageal tissue from the hydrochloric acid and pepsin secreted in the stomach. The constant regurgitation of acidic gastric contents into the lower part of the esophagus results in erosive esophagitis. Impaired esophageal peristalsis, prolonged or spontaneous LES relaxation, use of certain medications (e.g., anticholinergics, selective serotonin reuptake inhibitor antidepressants), hiatal hernias, **scleroderma**, and obesity are common contributors to chronic GERD.[13,14] Typical symptoms include frequent and severe heartburn within an hour after eating, dysphagia, and excessive belching. The pain sometimes moves into the neck or jaw or down the arms. Long-term complications include aspiration and pneumonia, stenosis (i.e., a narrowing or stricture of the esophagus), esophageal ulcer or perforation, adenocarcinoma, and **Barrett's esophagus**.

Table 18.1 provides conservative measures and dietary suggestions for improving LES competency and reducing the symptoms of GERD. GERD symptoms and medication necessity decrease congruently with weight loss in obese individuals (particularly with abdominal obesity), thus weight-reduction strategies are an important aspect of MNT in overweight clients.[15,16] Individuals with GERD frequently use antacids and medications that reduce acid production (e.g., histamine-2 receptor agonist) prophylactically to reduce symptoms. Proton pump inhibitors (PPIs) are the mainstay of pharmacologic treatment for GERD symptoms and are effective in most clients.[13,17] **Fundoplication** is a surgical procedure that restores LES function and esophageal peristalsis, thereby treating the condition and not just the symptoms. This procedure has long-term success and improves the quality of life in clients whose management with PPI therapy is unsuccessful.[18]

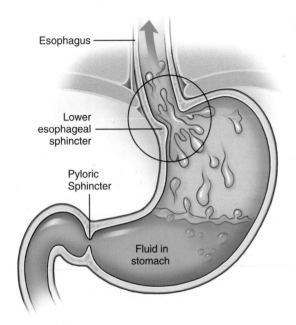

Figure 18.3 Reflux of gastric acid up into the esophagus through the lower esophageal sphincter in a client with gastroesophageal reflux disease. (Reprinted from Thibodeau, G. A., & Patton, K. T. [2010]. *Anatomy & physiology* [7th ed.]. St Louis: Mosby.)

Labels in figure: Esophagus; Lower esophageal sphincter; Pyloric Sphincter; Fluid in stomach

Table 18.1	Medical Nutrition Therapy for Gastroesophageal Reflux Disease

The health care provider should initiate evidence-based interventions (noted below with an [a]) for all clients with GERD and suggest a trial of other lifestyle and dietary modifications to assess if additional modifications are beneficial.

GOAL	ACTION
Increase lower esophageal sphincter pressure	Avoid medications that reduce LES pressure (e.g., anticholinergics, calcium channel blockers, opiates, progesterone). Some individuals find it helpful to avoid excessive high-fat meals (e.g., fried foods, high-fat meats, cream), peppermint, and spearmint-containing food products.
Decrease reflux frequency and volume	Achieve and maintain an appropriate body weight.[a] Avoid eating at least 3 to 4 hours before going to bed.[a] Raise the head of the bed 6 to 9 inches.[a] Some individuals may find it helpful to eat small, frequent meals; sip small amounts of liquid with meals; drink mostly between meals; avoid constipation by consuming adequate fiber and water; and to participate in regular physical activity (e.g., at least 30 minutes per day on most days of the week).
Clear food from the esophagus	Sit upright while eating. Do not recline for at least 2 hours after eating.[a] Some individuals also find it helpful to wear loose-fitting clothing (especially after a meal) and to eat while seated in a calm environment.
Decrease esophageal irritation	Individuals with esophagitis may find it beneficial to avoid common irritants such as alcohol, smoking, coffee, strong tea, chocolate, carbonated beverages, tomato and citrus juices, and spicy foods.

[a]Indicates the evidence-based lifestyle strategies for improving GERD symptoms.

scleroderma hardening and tightening of the skin and connective tissue.

Barrett's esophagus complication of severe gastroesophageal reflux disease in which the squamous cell epithelium of the esophagus changes to resemble the tissue lining the small intestine; increases the risk of esophageal adenocarcinoma.

fundoplication a surgery that is used to treat gastroesophageal reflux disease; the upper portion of the stomach (i.e., the fundus) is wrapped around the esophagus and sewn into place so that the esophagus passes through the muscle of the stomach; this strengthens the esophageal sphincter to prevent acid reflux.

Hiatal Hernia

The lower end of the esophagus normally enters the chest cavity through an opening in the diaphragm called the *hiatus* (Figure 18.4A). A hiatal hernia occurs when a portion of the upper stomach also protrudes through this opening, as shown in Figure 18.4B and C. Hiatal hernias are more common in obese adults, for whom weight reduction is essential to treatment.

Health care providers advise clients with hiatal hernias to eat small amounts of food at a time, to avoid lying down after meals, and to sleep with the head of the bed elevated to prevent the reflux of acidic stomach contents. The presence of acid, enzymes, and food mixture can irritate the lower esophagus and the upper herniated area of the stomach. The frequent use of antacids helps to control the symptoms of heartburn. Large hiatal hernias or smaller sliding hernias typically require surgical repair.

STOMACH AND DUODENUM: PEPTIC ULCER DISEASE

The mucosal lining of the stomach and duodenum protects the organ tissue from corrosive gastric acid and enzymatic secretions (both of which are necessary for food digestion). Damage to the tissue may result if the mucosa is weakened or disturbed and cannot provide adequate protection against acidic gastric contents. The general term *peptic ulcer* refers to an eroded mucosal lesion in the central portion of the GI tract. Lesions can occur in the lower esophagus, the stomach, or the duodenum (i.e., the duodenal bulb). Ulcers are common in the duodenal bulb because the gastric contents emptying there are the most concentrated. A peptic ulcer is a crater-like lesion in the wall of the stomach or duodenum resulting from the continuous erosion of the tissue through the mucosal layers down to the muscular layers (Figure 18.5A). In extreme cases, the ulcer can perforate with relatively high rates of mortality.

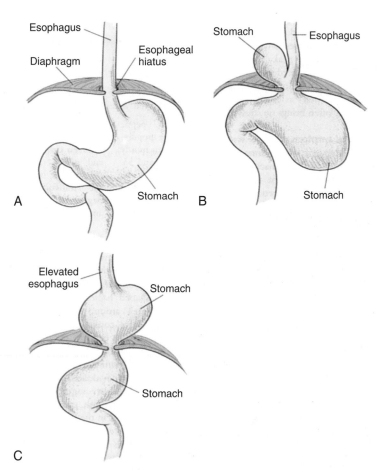

Figure 18.4 Hiatal hernia compared with normal stomach placement. A, Normal stomach. B, Paraesophageal hernia, with the esophagus in its normal position. C, Esophageal hiatal hernia, with an elevated esophagus. (Courtesy Bill Ober.)

Etiology

Before scientists discovered that the bacteria *Helicobacter pylori* is the major causative organism of peptic ulcer disease (PUD) in 1982, the disease was thought to be the result of excess stress, acid, and spicy food. Although these factors may still exacerbate the disease, we now know that infection with *H. pylori* causes the majority of duodenal and gastric ulcers; the long-term use of nonsteroidal antiinflammatory drugs (NSAIDs) is responsible for most of the remaining cases. Lesions generally result from an imbalance among the ulcerative factors and the protective factors of the gastric mucosa. Some or all of the following three factors are involved: (1) the amount of gastric acid and pepsin secretions; (2) the extent of *Helicobacter pylori* infection; and (3) the degree of tissue resistance and mucosal integrity.

Helicobacter pylori. *H. pylori* are common, spiraling, rod-shaped bacteria that inhabit the GI area around the pyloric valve (Figure 18.5B). This muscular valve connects the lower part of the stomach with the duodenal bulb. Acidic environments are favorable for *H. pylori* colonization. Infection by *H. pylori* is a major determinant of chronic active gastritis, and it is a critical ingredient, along with gastric acid and pepsin, in the ulcerative process. *H. pylori* infection affects more than one-half of the adult population worldwide, but not all people with the bacteria will develop an ulcer.[19]

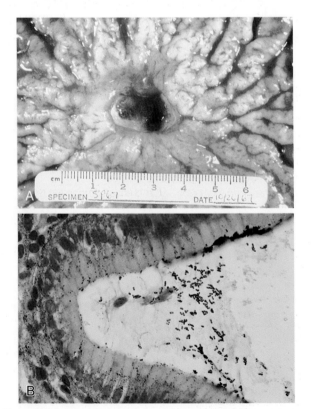

Figure 18.5 A, Gastric ulcer. B, *Helicobacter pylori (black particles)* infecting the stomach mucosa. (Reprinted from Patton, K. T., & Thibodeau, G. A. [2016]. *Anatomy & physiology* [9th ed.]. St Louis: Mosby.)

Because of aggressive treatment for *H. pylori* infection, the incidence rate of PUD has decreased during recent years.[20-22] The transmission mechanism by which *H. pylori* infection spreads is not yet known; however, it is believed to transfer from person to person through the fecal-oral or oral-oral routes.

Nonsteroidal antiinflammatory drugs. NSAIDs are widely used medications. This drug class includes ibuprofen (Advil, Motrin) and aspirin (acetylsalicylic acid). Prolonged or excessive use of NSAIDs damages the gastric mucosa at both the local and systemic level, decreases the mucosal integrity, and may result in erosion, ulceration, and bleeding.[22] The NSAIDs, including at least a dozen antiinflammatory drugs, are so named to distinguish them from steroid drugs, which are synthetic variants of natural adrenal hormones.

Psychologic factors. Both physiologic and psychologic factors are involved in the overall environmental risk for ulceration. The influence of psychologic factors in the development of PUD varies, and no distinct personality type is free from the disease. Individuals with highly stressful lives (whether actual or perceived) or mental vulnerability are significantly more likely to develop an ulcer, independent of other known risk factors such as *H. pylori* infection or the use of NSAIDs.[23-25]

The health effects resulting from the brain and the gut microbiota relationship (i.e., brain-gut axis) are vast and can influence GI health and predisposition for disease.[26-31] A recent study of approximately 467,000 participants found that the stress of unwanted and unpleasant nighttime environmental noise was significantly associated with the prevalence of PUD.[32] Of course, correlation is not causation, but it is an interesting finding given the size of the study and the indication for stress on the GI tract. Several neurologic and physiologic changes that result from severe or long-term stress have negative effects on the GI tract. Such changes include alterations in gut motility, gastric secretions, mucosal permeability, microbiota diversity, and barrier function; changes in visceral sensitivity; compromised recovery from injured mucosa; and reduction in blood flow.[33]

Clinical Symptoms

General symptoms of PUD include abdominal pain and a burning sensation. Symptoms vary significantly among patients and the location of the ulcer. The amount and concentration of hydrochloric acid secretions are higher in patients with duodenal ulcers, whereas the secretions may be normal in those with gastric ulcers. Some clients will have increased pain after a meal, whereas others experience relief from the presence of food in the GI tract. Hemorrhage may be one of the first clinical symptoms for some individuals. Inadequate dietary intake, iron-deficiency anemia, and unintentional weight loss indicate nutrition risk associated with PUD.[14] Radiographs and visualization with **gastroscopy** can confirm diagnosis.

Medical Intervention

Physiologic trauma and emotional stress can lead to excess acid secretions in the stomach. For individuals who are already infected with *H. pylori* bacteria, that may be the missing link for creating a perfect environment for rapid growth and inflammation that ultimately results in an ulcer. Therefore, the treatment of peptic ulcers must focus on eliminating the cause (i.e., bacteria or drugs) and focus on the environmental cues that are involved in the promotion of excessive acidic secretions and compromised gut health.

There are four basic goals for the treatment PUD: (1) alleviate or minimize the symptoms; (2) promote healing; (3) eliminate the cause; and (4) prevent complications.

Drug therapy. Advances in knowledge and therapy have provided physicians with the following four types of drugs for the management of PUD[34,35]:

1. Antibiotics, which address the *H. pylori* infection (e.g., amoxicillin, clarithromycin, tetracycline, metronidazole). See the Drug-Nutrient Interaction box titled "Tetracycline and Mineral Absorption" for more information about potential nutrient interactions with tetracycline.
2. Antacids, which counteract or neutralize the acid. Bismuth (Pepto-Bismol) and magnesium-aluminum compounds (e.g., Mylanta, Maalox) are typical antacids used for the treatment of PUD symptoms.
3. Hydrochloric acid secretion controllers:
   - Histamine H2-receptor antagonists (H2-blockers) reduce hydrochloric acid production and secretion. These medications are available over the counter and include cimetidine (Tagamet), ranitidine (Zantac), famotidine (Pepcid), and nizatidine (Axid).
   - PPIs reduce hydrochloric acid production by inhibiting the hydrogen ion secretion that is necessary to produce hydrochloric acid. These drugs include lansoprazole (Prevacid), omeprazole (Prilosec), esomeprazole (Nexium), pantoprazole (Protonix), and rabeprazole (AcipHex).
4. Mucosal protectors, which deactivate pepsin and produce a gel-like substance to cover the ulcer and to protect it from acid and pepsin while it heals itself (e.g., bismuth subsalicylate [Pepto-Bismol], sucralfate [Carafate]).

Maintenance drug therapy is helpful in preventing ulcer recurrence. A continuous low-dose drug therapy usually follows initial treatment. Some individuals will use the same medications that treated the initial ulcer infection for intermittent full-dose rescue treatment or symptomatic self-care, as needed. The

 Drug-Nutrient Interaction

Tetracycline and Mineral Absorption

Tetracycline is a broad-spectrum antibiotic that health care providers prescribe to treat stomach ulcers as well as other conditions such as respiratory tract infections, acne, and infections of the skin. Minerals with a 2+ charge—including magnesium, calcium, and iron—bond with tetracycline to form a non-bioavailable compound. Thus, the body eliminates both the medication and the nutrient via feces. Any amount of calcium, in particular, significantly reduces the availability of tetracycline absorption. Thus, tetracycline is less effective, and mineral absorption is poor.

To ensure optimal absorption of both the medication and the essential minerals, health care providers should instruct clients to avoid high-calcium foods (e.g., milk), calcium or iron dietary supplements, or antacids or laxatives that contain magnesium for at least 1 to 2 hours before and 2 to 3 hours after taking tetracycline.

regular use of PPIs, H2-blockers, or sucralfate will help most individuals remain in remission after successful treatment of the ulcer. Success rates depend on the relative risk factors that influence recurrence (Box 18.1).

Lifestyle factors. As noted earlier, there is a connection between mentally stressful situations and GI disorders. Although we do not yet completely understand the relationship between psychologic stress and the development of PUD, such stressed-induced GI changes and lifestyles may exacerbate the development of gastric ulcer disease in susceptible persons. Adequate

---

Box 18.1   Risk Factors for Recurring Peptic Ulcer

HIGH RISK
Medical/Physical
- *Helicobacter pylori* infection
- Previous peptic ulcer with complications
- Hypersecretion of gastric acid
- Family history of peptic ulcer disease among close relatives
- Use of bisphosphonates to prevent osteoporosis

Behavioral
- Failure to maintain prescribed diet and drug therapy
- Frequent use of aspirin and other nonsteroidal antiinflammatory drugs
- Smoking

MODERATE RISK
Medical/Physical
- Age of 50 years old or older

Behavioral/Emotional
- Alcohol consumption
- Poor dietary habits
- Continuous and unrelieved emotional stress

rest, relaxation, and sleep have long been the foundation of general care to enhance the body's natural healing process. Thus, incorporating positive coping and relaxation skills into daily life may help clients to better deal with personal psychosocial stress factors. Clients should also eliminate habits that contribute to ulcer development (e.g., smoking, alcohol use), and avoid irritating drugs (e.g., NSAIDs).

Medical Nutrition Therapy for Peptic Ulcer Disease

In the past, doctors advised a highly restrictive bland diet for PUD patients. A bland diet has long since proved to be ineffective and lacking in adequate nutrition support for the healing process. Such a restrictive diet is unnecessary today, because more effective medication regimens are available to control acid secretions and to assist with healing. Thus, the dietitian will create a personalized MNT protocol using information provided by clients regarding their physical response to various foods. As part of the nutrition support for medical management, two basic goals guide food habits.

Eating a well-balanced and healthy diet. The availability of nutrients and a person's oxidative status (among other things) modulates their epithelial tissue regeneration potential.[36] Therefore, the primary focus of nutrition therapy is to supply a well-balanced, regular, healthy diet to improve antioxidant intake, maintain a healthy gut microbiota, increase tissue healing and maintenance, and to restore any nutrient deficiencies.[14] A hearty intake of dietary antioxidants and phytonutrients (provided by whole fruits and vegetables), coupled with avoidance of foods and behaviors known to increase oxidative stress (e.g., trans fats, smoking, high alcohol intake) helps to restore GI well-being, microbiota diversity, and reduce the inflammatory response.[37] The Dietary Reference Intakes (see Appendix B) outlines nutrient needs and the MyPlate.gov guidelines (see Figure 1.4) expresses dietary needs as food choices. The goals of the *Dietary Guidelines for Americans, 2020-2025* (see Figure 1.5) provide further focus.

Avoiding acid stimulation. Individuals with PUD should avoid behaviors that stimulate excess gastric acid secretion, which irritates the gastric mucosa. The following few food-related habits affect acid secretion:

- *Food quantity:* To avoid stomach distention, do not eat large quantities at meals. Avoid eating immediately before going to bed, because food intake stimulates acid output.
- *Irritants:* Individual tolerance is the rule, but some food seasonings such as hot chili peppers, black pepper, and chili powder may irritate an already weakened mucosal layer. Caffeine, coffee (regular and noncaffeinated), chocolate, tea, and alcohol may increase acid secretions or prevent healing in some individuals. Clients will need to determine which foods they can tolerate and which foods worsen symptoms independently.
- *Smoking:* Complete smoking cessation is best, because smoking provokes GI mucosal injury, reduces the diversity of healthy microbiota in the gut, and hinders ulcer healing in several biochemical and physiologic pathways.[38,39] Smoking also affects gastric acid secretion, induces oxidative stress, and hinders the effectiveness of drug therapy.

LOWER GASTROINTESTINAL TRACT

SMALL INTESTINE DISEASES

Diseases within the small intestine generally result in malabsorption because of the impaired function of the organ. A defect in the absorption of one or more of the essential nutrients characterizes malabsorption syndromes. Malabsorption results from a disturbance in the normal digestive process or absorptive pathway, and the defect may include any of the following processes:

- *Digestion of macronutrients:* Carbohydrates, proteins, and fats are broken down in the small intestines into their basic building blocks (i.e., monosaccharides and disaccharides, amino acids, and fatty acids and glycerol, respectively) with the help of enzymes, hydrochloric acid, and bile acid.
- *Terminal digestion at the brush border mucosa:* Disaccharidases and peptidases hydrolyze disaccharides and peptides for the final step of digestion.
- *Absorption:* The products of macronutrient digestion, micronutrients (i.e., vitamins and minerals), and water are absorbed across the epithelium of the small intestine into the general or lymphatic circulation.

Malabsorption disorders affect several organ systems and functions. Chronic deficiencies of vitamins, minerals, and macronutrients can lead to several forms of anemia (e.g., iron, folate, vitamin B_{12}), nutrient-specific diseases (e.g., osteopenia, osteoporosis); and other musculoskeletal, endocrine, and nervous system abnormalities. The most common symptoms of malabsorption disorders are chronic diarrhea and **steatorrhea**.

This section reviews two specific conditions triggering malabsorption—cystic fibrosis (CF) and inflammatory bowel disease. Table 18.2 includes a list of other malabsorption syndromes. Diarrhea is usually a symptom of a disease or disorder rather than a disease itself. However, we will cover it in this section because diarrhea pertains to most malabsorption disorders.

Table 18.2	Major Malabsorption Syndromes
SYMPTOMS	**ETIOLOGY**
Defective Intraluminal Digestion	
Defective digestion of fats and proteins	Pancreatic insufficiency from pancreatitis or cystic fibrosis Zollinger-Ellison syndrome,[a] with inactivation of pancreatic enzymes by excess gastric acid secretion
Solubilization of fat as a result of defective bile secretion	Ileal dysfunction or resection with decreased bile salt uptake Cessation of bile flow from obstruction or hepatic dysfunction
Nutrient preabsorption or modification	Bacterial overgrowth
Primary Mucosal Cell Abnormalities	
Defective terminal digestion	Disaccharidase deficiency (e.g., lactose intolerance) Bacterial overgrowth with brush border damage
Defective epithelial transport	Abetalipoproteinemia[b] Primary bile acid malabsorption that results from mutations in the ileal bile acid transporter
Reduced small intestinal surface area	Bariatric surgery Cancer Celiac disease Crohn's disease Distal ileal resection or bypass Partial or total gastrectomy Short bowel syndrome
Lymphatic obstruction	Lymphoma Tuberculosis and tuberculous lymphadenitis
Infection or Inflammation	Acute infectious enteritis Parasitic infestation Radiation enteritis Small intestine bacterial overgrowth Whipple's disease

[a]Rare disorder that causes tumors in the pancreas and duodenum and ulcers in the stomach and duodenum. The tumors secrete a hormone called gastrin that causes the stomach to produce too much hydrochloric acid, which in turn causes stomach and duodenal ulcers.
[b]An inherited disorder of fat metabolism from the inability to synthesize β lipoproteins.
From the National Institute of Diabetes and Digestive and Kidney Diseases. (n.d.). *Zollinger-Ellison syndrome*. Retrieved July 6, 2019, from www.niddk.nih.gov/health-information/digestivediseases/zollinger-ellison-syndrome?dkrd=hispt0292; and Kumar, V., Fausto, N., & Abbas, A. (2005). *Robbins & Cotran pathologic basis of disease* (7th ed.). Philadelphia: Saunders.

---

gastroscopy an examination of the upper intestinal tract using a flexible tube with a small camera on the end; the tube is approximately 9 mm in diameter, and it takes color pictures as well as biopsy samples, if necessary.

steatorrhea fatty diarrhea; excessive amount of fat in the feces, which is often caused by malabsorption diseases.

Cystic Fibrosis

CF is a common fatal genetic disease. In the United States it occurs in approximately 1 in 2500 to 3500 Caucasian births, 1 in 17,000 African-American births, and 1 in 31,000 Asian Americans.[40] Although we characterize the disease as a pulmonary disease, CF is a multisystem disorder that has a profound impact on the GI tract. Because pulmonary diseases are outside of the scope of this text, this chapter focuses on the nutrition implications of CF.

Disease process. CF is an autosomal recessive genetic disease. The metabolic defect disrupts the normal function of chloride channels, which, in turn, disrupt the movement of chloride and water in body tissues. Chloride ions trapped in cells cause thick, sticky mucus to accumulate. This abnormal mucus clogs ducts and passageways, leading to multiple complications throughout the organ systems, most notably the respiratory and digestive systems.

Previously, children with CF only lived a few years, dying from complications such as damaged airways and lung infections as well as fibrous pancreas and malnutrition. However, the discovery of the CF gene and the underlying metabolic defect has improved the management of the disease and helped extend the life expectancy into adulthood.

The characteristic CF symptoms include the following:

- *Thick mucus in the lungs:* Causes damaged airways, more difficult breathing, persistent coughing, and pulmonary infections (e.g., bronchitis, pneumonia).
- *Pancreatic insufficiency:* Leads to a lack of normal pancreatic enzymes (see Chapter 5) to digest macronutrients and a progressive loss of insulin-producing β-cells and eventual diabetes mellitus in approximately 50% of adults with CF.[41]

- *Malabsorption:* Food is left undigested and unabsorbed, with consequential diarrhea, steatorrhea, malnutrition, failure to thrive, stunted growth, and delayed puberty.
- *Liver and gallbladder disease:* Clogged bile ducts lead to a progressive degeneration of functional liver tissue.
- *Elevated sweat chloride concentration:* Salt depletion through excess sweating.

Medical nutrition therapy for cystic fibrosis. The following practices augment any form of treatment: (1) newborn screening and diagnosis; (2) early initiation of nutrition management; (3) patient education regarding nutrition needs; and (4) nutrient and pancreatic enzyme replacement as indicated by pancreatic insufficiency. MNT is a critical component of the treatment regimen for CF, and it can have a significant impact on successful growth, pulmonary function, and survival. One of the MNT goals is to maintain an age-appropriate growth rate for infants and children and to maintain appropriate BMI and lean tissue in adults (as measured by weight- and length-for-age percentiles in infants; weight-, length-, and BMI-for-age percentiles for children; and BMI for adults).[42] To achieve this goal, individuals must meet their nutrient needs.

Adequate enzyme replacement is the foundation that makes aggressive diet therapy a possibility for meeting growth needs when a patient's own pancreas cannot provide the necessary enzymes to support macronutrient digestion. Enzyme-replacement products (e.g., pancrelipase) contain the normal pancreatic enzymes for each energy nutrient (primarily lipase for fat digestion and proteases for protein digestions). Pharmaceutical companies process these enzymes into very small enteric-coated capsules or microspheres. The capsules do not open or dissolve until they reach the alkaline medium of the duodenum. The client takes these enzyme-replacement capsules, which vary with his or her age, weight, and symptoms, just before eating each meal or snack.

Individuals with CF may require significantly more energy and nutrients than the Dietary Recommended Intakes (DRIs) for their age, depending on the severity of the disease, presence of inflammation, and level of pancreatic insufficiency. The consensus guidelines recommend frequent nutrition status assessment (every 3 to 6 months) and energy intake adjustments to achieve and maintain normal growth and nutrition status.[42] Accurately determining energy needs is the first step in designing an appropriate diet to meet nutrient needs. A high-energy, nutritionally adequate diet is required and may necessitate oral or enteral nutrition supplementation to maintain weight and prevent malnutrition. Nutrition therapy for CF includes diet modifications to support nutrient needs, prevent malnutrition, and mitigate CF-related diseases with nutrient related consequences (e.g., osteoporosis, diabetes, GI complications); behavioral counseling to support healthy dietary habits and body image; and nutrition support (oral or enteral) as indicated.[42] Box 18.2 outlines the current standards of nutrition care for the management of CF. Try applying these principles of care while completing the Case Study box, "Cystic Fibrosis."

Box 18.2 **Medical Nutrition Therapy for Cystic Fibrosis**

EVIDENCE-BASED RECOMMENDATIONS

1. Maintain optimal ranges of weight-for-age and stature-for-age for children and of body mass index (BMI) for adults to support better lung function. Focus on maintenance of lean tissue.
   Optimal ranges:
   - Children up to the age of 20 years: ≥50th percentile recommended
   - Women: minimum BMI of 18.5 kg/m^2, goal BMI of 22 kg/m^2
   - Men: minimum BMI of 18.5 kg/m^2, goal BMI of 23 kg/m^2
2. Increase energy intake to 110% to 200% of the standards for the healthy population to achieve and maintain nutrition status.
3. Treat pancreatic insufficiency with pancreatic enzyme replacement therapy.
4. Evaluate biochemical markers of micronutrients, particularly the fat-soluble vitamins, and correct suboptimal levels with nutrient supplementation.
5. Regularly monitor for CF-associated complications with nutrition implications such as diabetes, bone disease, liver disease, and iron-deficiency anemia. Modify dietary intake or implement nutrition support as indicated.
6. Regularly evaluate the need for, or continuation of, oral nutrition supplements.

GENERAL DIETARY PRINCIPLES

1. Include at least three meals and two to three snacks per day.
2. Encourage high-fat foods and additives without dietary restriction.
3. Encourage a variety of whole grains, nuts, fruits, and vegetables to maintain adequate vitamin and mineral intake.
4. Provide nutrition counseling to discuss ideas for high-energy boosters, based on the client's usual intake and preferences, to meet energy needs.
5. Provide high-salt nutrition therapy to replace the electrolytes lost through sweat.

WHEN ORAL INTAKE IS INADEQUATE AND NOT EXPECTED TO IMPROVE

1. The health care team should consider enteral nutrition for clients with a BMI <18.5 kg/m^2 and when weight gain is not achieved after initial attempts at intervention.
2. Nocturnal feedings through gastrostomy tubes allow the patient to eat meals during the day and supplement with additional nutrients throughout the night.
3. Individualize high-energy density enteral formulas to the patient. Semi-elemental formulas are also appropriate.
4. Continue providing pancreatic enzyme replacement with supplemental nutrition support.

Academy of Nutrition and Dietetics. (2019). *Nutrition care manual*. Chicago.
Turck, D., et al. (2016). ESPEN-ESPGHAN-ECFS guidelines on nutrition care for infants, children, and adults with cystic fibrosis. *Clin Nutr, 35*(3), 557–577.

NEXT-GENERATION NCLEX® EXAMINATION-STYLE UNFOLDING CASE STUDY
Cystic Fibrosis

See answers in Appendix A.

A 16-year-old girl with cystic fibrosis is currently in the hospital because of pneumonia and is experiencing significant difficulty with breathing. She is currently 5 feet 2 inches tall and weighs 95 lbs. She has a decent appetite but tires easily while eating. Her stools are large and frequent, and they contain undigested food material.

1. Of the nutritional concerns listed below, which are related to the patient's condition?

   a. Increased energy needs
   b. Malabsorption
   c. Inadequate digestive enzymes
   d. Increased needs for water soluble vitamins
   e. Excessive weight gain
   f. Malnutrition

2. Use letters to match the patient's assessment data with the *most likely* cause.

ASSESSMENT DATA	ASSOCIATED CAUSE ANSWERS
Increased calorie needs	
Undigested stool	
Inadequate calorie intake	
Underweight	

   Cause Options

   a. Inadequate intake
   b. Lack of digestive enzymes
   c. Tires easily while eating
   d. Difficulty breathing

The patient has been increasing her dietary intake with the use of oral supplements (e.g., Ensure, Boost) but is still struggling to gain weight and meet her recommended nutrient needs.

3. From the options provided, choose the *most likely* answer for the information missing from the statements below.

   Although the patient has increased her nutrient intake, she may not be gaining weight due to _____ insufficiency. She would most likely benefit from _____ replacement therapy.

OPTIONS	
lymphatic	hormone
bile	enzyme
pancreatic	gallbladder

4. Select the vitamins that the registered dietitian nutritionist should be most concerned about for this patient.

   a. Vitamin A
   b. Vitamin B₁
   c. Vitamin D
   d. Vitamin E
   e. Vitamin C
   f. Vitamin K

The patient is assessed before she is discharged from the hospital. She is wondering what she should do to increase her total energy intake to avoid losing weight and becoming malnourished again.

5. Use an X to identify <u>effective</u> and <u>ineffective</u> strategies for weight gain for this patient.

STRATEGIES	EFFECTIVE	INEFFECTIVE
Three meals with two to three snacks per day		
High fat foods		
Restrict foods high in fat		
Restrict foods high in sodium		
Encourage a variety of foods from each food group		
Utilize oral supplements if needed		
Discourage use of calorie dense foods		

6. For each assessment finding, use an X to indicate whether nutrition and nursing interventions were <u>effective</u> (helped to meet expected outcomes), <u>ineffective</u> (did not help to meet expected outcomes), or <u>unrelated</u> (not related to the expected outcomes).

ASSESSMENT	EFFECTIVE	INEFFECTIVE	UNRELATED
BMI increased to 18.9			
Regular bowel movements			
Fat present in stool			
Consumes at least 75% of meals			
Has difficulty breathing			
Has increased nutrient needs			

Inflammatory Bowel Disease

Inflammatory bowel disease (IBD) is a general term that describes chronic inflammation of the GI tract and the persistent activation of the mucosal immune system against the normal healthy gut flora. Chronic inflammation disrupts the protective epithelial barrier. This may lead to ulceration of the mucosal surface and destruction of segments within the GI tract. Because of lesions, portions of the GI tract are not functional, which causes malabsorption. Long-term complications of IBD (e.g., osteoporosis, iron deficiency anemia, kidney stones) relate to malnutrition from chronic malabsorption of macro- and micronutrients.[43,44] Iron-deficiency anemia is a particularly common co-morbidity for individuals with IBD.[45] **Short-bowel syndrome** may result if repeated surgical removal of parts of the small intestine is necessary due to disease progression.

In addition to genetics, scientists believe that there is a multitude of environmental exposures, beginning at birth, which increase the risk for IBD. Two important exposures during childhood that increase the risk for IBD are the lack of breastfeeding and the overuse of antibiotics.[46,47] Exposures in adulthood that increase the risk for IBD include the use of oral contraceptives and NSAIDs, suffering from bacterial gastroenteritis or dysbiotic gut microbiota, eating a Western diet, and smoking.[46,48,49]

IBD is more common in Europe and North America than in other areas of the world. However, incidence rates are increasing worldwide, along with industrialization, suggesting environmental risk factors. In North America, the prevalence of IBD ranges from 96 to 319 cases per 100,000 persons. The prevalence of IBD is as high as 505 cases per 100,000 people in areas of northern Europe such as Norway.[50] Crohn's disease and ulcerative colitis are the two most common forms of inflammatory bowel disease. These **idiopathic** diseases share many symptoms and management strategies, but they differ with regard to their clinical manifestations (Table 18.3).

Crohn's disease. Crohn's disease may affect any portion of the GI tract from the esophagus to the anus. Most commonly, lesions occur in the ileum and colon. Inflammation may skip sections of the GI tract and affect more than one section at a time (Figure 18.6). Symptoms vary, depending on the location of the inflammation, but they most commonly include the following: abdominal pain, fever, fatigue, anorexia, weight loss, and diarrhea. Clients may experience long asymptomatic periods between flare-ups, or they may experience continuous and progressive attacks. Complications from chronic inflammation such as bowel obstruction, strictures, fistulas, and abscesses, may cause severe bowel damage and disability. In addition to the risks mentioned above for IBD, individuals with Jewish ancestry are specifically susceptible to Crohn's disease.

Malnutrition and increased micronutrient requirements are common with Crohn's disease because of malabsorption and poor food intake. Confirmed nutrient deficiencies necessitate supplementation and/or nutrition support. Nutrient needs are high during periods of healing, but compromised nutrient bioavailability is often problematic at the same time. Surgical removal of portions of the GI tract and drug-nutrient interactions further exacerbate malabsorption and complications. For example, long-term corticosteroid use further increases the risk for osteoporosis.[43] Malnutrition decreases quality of life, and it can have long-term negative consequences; thus, screening, early detection, and aggressive medical nutrition therapy are important parts of disease management.

Ulcerative colitis. Ulcerative colitis (UC) is an inflammatory disease that is limited to the colon and rectum. However, we will cover it along with Crohn's disease under the section Small Intestine Diseases because both diseases are IBDs with similar manifestations. Symptoms include bloody diarrhea, abdominal pain, nausea/vomiting, weight loss, and fever. The inflammation does not skip sections of the bowel; rather, it is progressive from the anus (see Figure 18.6). Severe complications associated with UC are **megacolon** and disease advancement to the point of requiring a total colectomy.

With the exception of iron-deficiency anemia and vitamin K deficiency, UC is not associated with as many micronutrient deficiencies as Crohn's disease because of the location of the inflammation.[44] However, as pain or inflammation increase, food intake decreases and additional deficiencies may occur. All inflammatory bowel conditions can have severe and often devastating nutrition ramifications, as more and more of the absorbing surface area becomes involved or surgical removal is required. Malnutrition can exacerbate an attack and hinder the healing process. Restoring positive nutrition is a basic requirement for tissue healing and health.

Medical nutrition therapy for inflammatory bowel disease. Current studies and clinical practice indicate the benefit of a regular nourishing diet that reflects individual tolerances and disease status for IBD clients. A close working relationship among the physician, the RDN, and the nurse is essential. The client's appetite often is poor, but adequate nutrition intake is imperative. The health care team will explore a range of feeding modes, including enteral and parenteral nutrition support as needed, to achieve the nutrition care that is necessary.

---

short-bowel syndrome malabsorption disordered caused by a lack of functional small intestine.
idiopathic of unknown cause.
megacolon abnormally enlarged colon.

Table 18.3   Clinical Manifestations of Crohn's Disease and Ulcerative Colitis

MANIFESTATION	COMMON TO BOTH INFLAMMATORY BOWEL DISEASES	
Etiology	Unknown	
Genetics	Over 200 genetic loci are positively associated with IBD. Genetic predisposition is the most important risk factor for IBD	
Gut flora	Intestinal gut flora plays a role, but there is no specific microbe that is the underlying causative factor	
Immune response	Linked to inappropriate T-cell activation or too little control by regulatory T lymphocytes	
Symptoms	Abdominal pain, diarrhea, and weight loss	
Complications	Malnutrition, osteoporosis, dermatitis, ocular symptoms, liver and gallbladder complications, and kidney stones	
	SPECIFIC TO TYPE OF INFLAMMATORY BOWEL DISEASE	
	CROHN'S DISEASE	**ULCERATIVE COLITIS**
Incidence[a]	96 to 319 per 100,000 persons	140 to 286 per 100,000 persons
Additional risk factors	Jewish ancestry and smoking	Former smokers are at higher risk than current smokers and those that have never smoked
Bowel region affected	Ileum and colon	Colon only
Distribution	Skip lesions	Continuous from rectum
Inflammation and Ulceration	Mucosa and all underlying tissue layers	Mucosa and submucosal layers only
Fat-soluble vitamin malabsorption	Yes, if lesions are in ileum	No
Response to surgery	Poor to fair	Good
Long-term complications	Fibrosing strictures, fistulas to other organs, cancer, malabsorption of vitamin B_{12} and bile salts, thereby causing pernicious anemia and steatorrhea, bowel obstruction, polyarthritis, sacroiliitis, ankylosing spondylitis, erythema nodosum, and clubbing of the fingertips	Perforation and toxic megacolon; these patients also have a high risk for cancer

[a]Prevalence in North America. Prevalence varies greatly worldwide. See reference 50 for prevalence details on other regions.

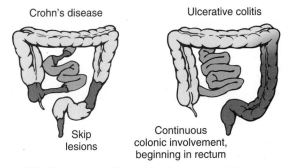

Crohn's disease — Skip lesions

Ulcerative colitis — Continuous colonic involvement, beginning in rectum

Figure 18.6 Comparison of the distribution pattern of Crohn's disease and ulcerative colitis. (Reprinted from Kumar, V., Fausto, N., & Abbas, A. [2005]. *Robbins & Cotran pathologic basis of disease* [7th ed.]. Philadelphia: Saunders.)

Principles of continuing dietary management of IBD include the following[14]:

During periods of inflammation:

- Use enteral nutrition support, if necessary. Enteral feedings of either **polymeric formula** or **elemental formula** may help restore nutrient balance and induce remission (see Chapter 22). The medical management guidelines recommend exclusive enteral nutrition therapy as the first-line treatment for pediatric patients.[51]
- If the patient's symptoms, tolerance, and GI function do not tolerate enteral feedings, use parenteral nutrition support.

- Progress to low-fat, high-protein, high-kilocalorie, small, frequent meals when returning to a normal diet, as tolerated.
- The diet should be low in fiber only during acute attacks or with strictures. Otherwise, the client can gradually increase fiber intake.
- Vitamin and mineral supplementation should include vitamin D, zinc, calcium, magnesium, folate, vitamin B_{12}, and iron.

During periods of remission:

- Meet energy and protein needs that are specific for weight, and replenish nutrient stores.
- In the presence of **hyperoxaluria**, individuals with Crohn's disease should avoid foods that are high in oxalates (see Box 21.3 in Chapter 21 for a list of high-oxalate foods).
- Increase antioxidant intake, and consider supplementation with omega-3 fatty acids and glutamine.
- Consider the use of **probiotics** and **prebiotics**.

Diarrhea

Diarrhea typically is not a disease of the small or large intestine but rather a symptom or result of another underlying condition. In some cases, diarrhea may result from intolerance to specific foods or nutrients, such as in lactose intolerance (see Chapter 2) or acute food poisoning from a specific food-borne organism or toxin (see Chapter 13). A variety of bacteria (e.g., *Campylobacter, Clostridium difficile, Escherichia coli, Listeria monocytogenes, Salmonella enteritidis, Shigella*), parasites (e.g., *Giardia lamblia, Cryptosporidium parvum, Cyclospora cayetanensis, Entamoeba histolytica*), and viral infections (rotavirus, norovirus) are known causes of diarrhea. We frequently blame irregular meals, unfamiliar foods, and travel tensions for traveler's diarrhea, a well-known GI disturbance. However, bacterial infections are the cause of the majority of cases (i.e., approximately 90%), of which *E. coli* is the most common. Norovirus and rotavirus are the cause of up to 10% of the remaining cases.[52]

Chronic diarrhea (i.e., diarrhea lasting ≥4 weeks) is a significant cause of global mortality, especially for children ≤5 years old and elderly ≥70 years old Although the prevalence of death from diarrheal diseases has decreased substantially in the past two decades, they are still the fifth most frequent reason globally for years of life lost.[53] Improvements in sanitation and access to safe drinking water are responsible for reducing the burden of this largely preventable cause of morbidity and mortality.

In addition to determining and treating the underlying cause of diarrhea, rehydration and restoring electrolyte and acid-base balance are critical elements for recovery. Some individuals are able to restore euhydration by drinking oral rehydration solutions such as Pedialyte, CeraLyte, and Rehydralyte. Others may require intravenous fluid and electrolyte replacement to regain balance. Other general goals of MNT are to slow the rate of movement through the GI tract with thicker stool consistency and to repopulate the GI tract with healthy and varied flora.[14] As soon as the client tolerates it, he or she should resume a regular refeeding schedule to avoid malnutrition. Additional patient-based nutrition interventions depend on the causative agent, duration of diarrhea, degree of electrolyte and acid-base imbalance, and nutrition status.

The health care provider should carefully monitor the resumption of nutrient intake in severely malnourished clients. **Refeeding syndrome** is a potentially fatal metabolic disturbance that involves fluid and electrolyte imbalances and that can result in cardiac failure. When a malnourished client begins a feeding schedule that is too aggressive, sudden shifts in electrolytes leave low serum levels of phosphate, potassium, magnesium, glucose, and thiamine. Malnourished patients require a measured reintroduction to nutrients and close monitoring.

LARGE INTESTINE DISEASES

Diverticular Disease

The presence of small pouches along the mucosal lining in the colon characterizes diverticular disease. Normally, segmental circular muscle contractions methodically move waste down the colon to form feces for elimination. However, abnormal gut motility increases colonic pressure. When this happens in a segment of the colon with weakened bowel walls, small **diverticula** may "pop out" or herniate (Figure 18.7).

If the diverticula become infected with trapped fecal matter, a condition called **diverticulitis**, localized pain and tenderness intensify in the lower left side of the abdomen. GI bleeding, diarrhea, and fever are other common symptoms that the patient may experience. Severe complications include abscess, sepsis, and perforation and may require surgical intervention.

The commonly used term that refers to both diverticulosis and diverticulitis is *diverticular disease*. Diverticular disease is multifactorial and one of the most common GI disorders in the U.S., accounting for nearly 2 million health care visits annually.[54] The presence of diverticula is particularly common among older people in Western societies. However, the majority of people remain asymptomatic without complications. Only 10% to 20% of individuals with diverticular disease experience symptomatic acute diverticulitis.

Scientists have not found one specific cause for diverticular disease. However, recent studies have noted several common genetic variants in people with diverticular disease that may give rise to intestinal neuromuscular, smooth muscle, and connective tissue dysfunction.[55,56] Such genetic predisposition may increase the risk for abnormal intestinal motility and the potential for diverticula formation through the weakened connective tissue. In addition to the genetic risks and abnormal gut motility, there is evidence that the underlying age-related pathogenesis of diverticular disease is associated with an abnormal immune response, **microbiome** shifts, and visceral hypersensitivity.[57]

---

polymeric formula a nutrition support formula that is composed of complete protein, polysaccharides, and fat as medium-chain fatty acids.

elemental formula a nutrition support formula that is composed of simple elemental nutrient components that require no further digestive breakdown and are thus readily absorbed; these formulas include protein as free amino acids and carbohydrate as the simple sugar glucose.

hyperoxaluria excess oxalates in the urine.

probiotic a food that contains live microbials, which are thought to benefit the consumer by improving intestinal microbial balance (e.g., lactobacilli in yogurt).

prebiotic nondigestible foods that promote the growth of beneficial microorganisms within the gut.

refeeding syndrome a potentially lethal condition that occurs when severely malnourished individuals are fed high-carbohydrate diets too aggressively; a sudden shift in electrolytes and fluid retention and a drastic drop in serum phosphorus, potassium, and magnesium levels cause a series of complications that involve several organs.

diverticula small protruding pouches, or herniations, in the colonic mucosa through the muscular layer.

diverticulitis the inflammation of pockets of tissue (i.e., diverticula) in the lining of the mucous membrane of the colon.

microbiome microorganisms living in a specific environment.

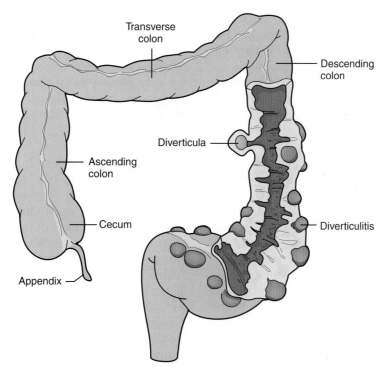

Figure 18.7 Diverticula formation in the colon.

In acute cases of diverticulitis with bloody diarrhea, the health care team may restrict patients to *nothing by mouth* (nil per os, or NPO) or clear liquids until they can progress slowly to a normal, nutritionally adequate diet. The patient will include only low-fiber foods until inflammation and bleeding resolve. The dietary management of diverticulosis includes increasing dietary fiber (particularly insoluble fiber) to 26 to 45 g/day along with adequate fluid intake.[14] Although historically recommended, there is little evidence that avoiding certain foods (e.g., nuts, seeds) that can accumulate in the small diverticula pouches is truly protective against inflammation. Emerging therapies include the use of probiotic and prebiotic food sources to encourage a healthy gut microbiome. Antibiotics treat underlying inflammation.

Irritable Bowel Syndrome

Irritable bowel syndrome (IBS) is the most commonly diagnosed GI disorder. The exact prevalence is hard to determine because the definitions of IBS have varied throughout epidemiologic studies. Many people with symptoms do not seek medical attention, and it often overlaps other GI-associated and non-GI disorders (e.g., depression, anxiety, hypochondriasis, fibromyalgia, chronic fatigue syndrome).[58,59] IBS is a functional bowel disorder in which abdominal pain is associated with defecation or a change in bowel habits.[59,60] IBS displays three major types of symptoms: (1) chronic and recurrent pain in the lower abdomen; (2) small-volume bowel dysfunction that varies from constipation or diarrhea to a combination of both; and (3) excess gas formation with increased distention and bloating.

Currently, there is no universal agreement on the cause for IBS. It is a multicomponent disorder involving a genetic predisposition, altered sensation and motility of the GI tract, infection, inflammation, dietary intolerances, altered intestinal permeability, **dysbiosis**, and altered gut-brain axis function.[14,61] Because symptoms and triggers vary among individuals with IBS, so too are the approaches to management. Treatment options focus on minimizing the symptoms and may include medications, diet and lifestyle (e.g., exercise) interventions, as well as psychologic/behavior therapy.[59]

A highly individualized approach to nutrition care is essential. Guided by personal food preferences and symptom patterns, the dietitian can formulate a reasonable food plan with the client. In general, the food plan should give attention to the following basic principles[14]:

- Follow a regular diet with an optimal energy and nutrient composition.
- Eliminate food allergens and intolerances. Along with any known allergens or intolerances, the health care provider may evaluate the client's tolerance to foods that contain the following: fermentable oligosaccharides, disaccharides, and monosaccharides and polyols (FODMAPs).
- Omit foods that increase gas and flatulence. Some foods are recognized gas formers because of known constituents (e.g., indigestible short chains of glucose [oligosaccharides] as in the case of legumes). Others may cause gaseous discomfort on an individual basis.
- Consider the use of probiotics and prebiotics.
- Consider the use of food diaries. Tracking nutrient intake, environment, emotions, activity, and symptoms may help to narrow instigating factors for future avoidance.

Clients are highly individualized with regard to the symptoms that they most often experience. For example, the predominant symptom may be diarrhea, constipation, lower abdominal pain, excessive gas, or bloating (but not necessarily all of them). Therefore, the dietary recommendations are equally as individualized. Experienced practitioners have learned that, when helping clients to manage IBS, an honest and creative relationship is essential. Lifestyle and diet are highly personal, and wise nutrition management involves realistic counseling toward a healthier life.

Constipation

Adults spend a significant amount of health care resources each year on problems associated with constipation. Clinical diagnostic criteria for constipation require that the individual experience symptoms (e.g., <3 defecations/week, difficulty in defecating) for at least 3 months, do not have loose stools without the use of laxatives, and do not meet the criteria for IBS. Constipation may result from various conditions or diseases such as pregnancy, colorectal cancer, neurologic or neuromuscular diseases, or metabolic disturbances. Additionally, it could be a side effect from medications, anesthesia, frequent laxative use, low-fiber diets, anxiety, and sedentary behaviors.

The most important aspect of the treatment and prevention of constipation is risk assessment to identify the potential causes of constipation. Improved diet, exercise, and bowel habits may help remedy the situation. Clients should avoid laxative or enema dependency. There are a variety of over-the-counter medications and prescription medications available, with varying degrees of efficacy and cost.[62] Medical nutrition therapy for constipation includes adequate fiber intake (particularly from fruits, vegetables, bran, and whole-wheat products) and adequate fluid intake (at least 64 oz/day). Additionally, clients should participate in physical activity daily and may benefit from pro/prebiotics.[14] Constipation occurs at all ages, and a personalized approach to management is fundamental.

FOOD INTOLERANCES AND ALLERGIES

Several conditions may cause food allergies or intolerances. Intolerances—unlike allergies—are not life threatening, and they are not immunologic. The underlying problem of an allergic reaction is the body's immune system reacting to a protein as if it were a threatening foreign object and then launching a powerful attack against it. In the case of celiac disease, the body initiates an autoimmune response when exposed to an offending protein.

FOOD INTOLERANCES

Food intolerances are adverse reactions to foods or food constituents and are not immune mediated. The most common worldwide food intolerance is to the disaccharide lactose. The intolerance is a result of inadequate production of the *lactase* enzyme to properly digest and absorb the carbohydrate found in milk products into its two monosaccharide components: glucose and galactose (see Chapter 2). Food intolerances may present as GI disturbance, hives, flushing, or headache. Individuals can prevent adverse reactions by avoiding the offending food products.

FOOD ALLERGIES

The word **allergy** comes from two Greek words that mean "altered reactivity," and it refers to the abnormal reactions of the immune system to a number of substances in the environment and within food. The Centers for Disease Control and Prevention reports that 5.8% of children under the age of 18 years old in the United States likely have food allergies, and the incidence decreases into adulthood.[2] Worldwide prevalence of food allergies in adults is around 3.5%. Reported cases of food allergies have increased over the past several decades. However, exact prevalence is difficult to determine because self-reported food allergies typically overestimate true allergies, as do frequently used methods for assessing allergies such as skin-prick and atopy patch test.[63-65] Experts believe that both genetic and environmental factors are involved in the etiology of food allergies (Figure 18.8).[65]

Common Food Allergens

The most common food allergens include the proteins found in hen's eggs, cow's milk, peanuts, tree nuts, shellfish, wheat, fish, and soy.[64] Children will often outgrow allergies to milk, egg, soy, and wheat but are less likely to outgrow allergies to peanuts and tree nuts. Although it is more common for food allergies to present during the first 2 years of life, allergies may begin at any age.

Signs and symptoms. Symptoms of food allergies can vary widely and may involve the skin or the GI, respiratory, or cardiovascular systems. Frequently reported symptoms include hives, itching in the mouth, throat, or eyes, nausea, diarrhea, abdominal pain, and wheezing. **Anaphylactic shock** is the most severe form of allergic reaction, and it can result in death relatively quickly. Individuals who are in anaphylactic shock have swelling of the face and throat, difficulty breathing, anxiety, increased heart rate, and, if not treated,

---

dysbiosis imbalance of the intestinal microbiome.

allergy a state of hypersensitivity to particular substances in the environment that works on body tissues to produce problems in the functioning of the affected tissues; the agent involved (i.e., the allergen) may be a certain food that is eaten or a substance (e.g., pollen) that is inhaled or touched.

anaphylactic shock a severe and sometimes fatal allergic reaction that results from exposure to a protein that the body perceives as foreign and that elicits a systemic response that involves multiple organs.

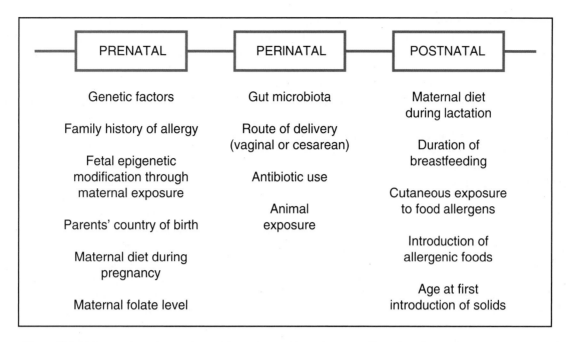

PRENATAL	PERINATAL	POSTNATAL
Genetic factors	Gut microbiota	Maternal diet during lactation
Family history of allergy	Route of delivery (vaginal or cesarean)	Duration of breastfeeding
Fetal epigenetic modification through maternal exposure	Antibiotic use	Cutaneous exposure to food allergens
Parents' country of birth	Animal exposure	Introduction of allergenic foods
Maternal diet during pregnancy		Age at first introduction of solids
Maternal folate level		

Figure 18.8 Major genetic and environmental determinants of food allergy risk. (From Oria, M. P., & Stallings, V. A. [Eds.]. [2016]. *Finding a path to safety in food allergy: Assessment of the global burden, causes, prevention, management, and public policy*. National Academies of Sciences, Engineering, and Medicine. Washington, DC: National Academies Press [US]. Copyright 2017 by the National Academy of Sciences. All rights reserved: Washington, DC.)

decreased blood pressure and loss of consciousness. The person's throat, lips, and tongue swell to the point of blocking the airway, ultimately suffocating the individual. Peanut, tree nut, and seafood allergies carry the highest risk of anaphylaxis.

Diagnostics. Currently, there is not a simple *and* reliable laboratory test to assess food allergies. Skin or blood tests alone are insufficient for a proper food allergy diagnosis, and many physicians incorrectly use and interpret "positive" skin-prick and blood test.[66,67] The expert committee on food allergies recommends that all individuals with suspected food allergies undergo diagnostic confirmation because a vast number of presumed food allergies are not real allergies. Unnecessarily avoiding foods, or food groups, is burdensome and reduces food and nutrient variety. Furthermore, without clear diagnostic confirmation individuals who are experiencing symptoms consistent with food allergies could be avoiding the wrong food and thus put themselves at risk for serious and unsuspecting complications when they encounter the actual allergen.[65] If a client shows signs of an allergic reaction, experts recommend using a combination of the following methods as diagnostic measures in conjunction with a medical history and physical exam: elimination diet, a food-specific skin-prick test, food-specific serum IgE immunoassay, and an oral food challenge. The pathophysiology of the allergy (e.g., IgE mediated or not) will help guide the most appropriate tests to use. There is not a universally accepted diagnostic algorithm for food allergy testing, and it is usually not necessary to perform all available tests, but a single test is insufficient for proper diagnosis.[65,68]

The National Academy of Sciences book titled *Finding a Path to Safety in Food Allergy: Assessment of the Global Burden, Causes, Prevention, Management, and Public Policy* is an excellent resource for food allergies. The book provides expert recommendations for diagnosing and managing food allergies and the pros and cons of various diagnostic tests currently in use. The full text is free to download at www.nap.edu.

Medical nutrition therapy for food allergies. There are two objectives involved in MNT for food allergies: (1) avoid offending foods and (2) substitute nutritionally appropriate alternatives for the excluded foods.[14] Referring a person with food allergies to an RDN to provide family support, education, and counseling may be helpful. Guidance regarding food substitutions or special food products and modified recipes to maintain nutrition needs for growth is sometimes necessary. Children tend to become less allergic as they grow older, but cooking guides and family education that address the deciphering of food labels are essential from the beginning. Furthermore, if anaphylaxis is a known risk, clients should be under the care of a physician for the provision of self- or family-administered emergency medications if anaphylaxis occurs.

Although many risk factors for the development of food allergies are not modifiable, some dietary factors during pregnancy and early life may help reduce the risk of food allergies in infants. Current recommendations for preventing food allergies are as follows[14,65,69]:

- Pregnant women should strive for a well-balanced healthy diet and not avoid any specific allergens during gestation (unless she has allergies).

- Exclusively breastfeed infants for a minimum of 4 to 6 months. The mother should not avoid eating food allergens during lactation (unless she has allergies). For infants on breast milk substitutes, do not feed a soy-based formula unless specifically advised by a health care provider because of confirmed allergy or intolerance.
- Introduce solid foods, including allergenic foods, to infants between 4 and 6 months of age. Avoid early and late solid food introductions (see Chapter 11).

Celiac Disease

Celiac disease is an autoimmune and inflammatory disease, rather than strictly an allergy. We are covering celiac disease in this section because the MNT approach is very similar to that for an allergy.

The global prevalence of celiac disease (CD) is approximately 1% of the population. It affects slightly fewer people in the United States (0.8%), of which the majority are non-Hispanic whites.[70,71] About 40% of the population have the genetic polymorphism that leads to CD, but only 2% to 3% of people with this genetic predisposition will develop CD, thereby signifying the influence of environmental factors and potentially other genetic factors as well.[72]

Disease process. The pathology of CD is an autoimmune response to a specific sequence of amino acids found in wheat, barley, and rye proteins. We collectively refer to the CD-activating proteins as *gluten.* However, wheat products are the only foods containing the gluten protein. The proteins in barley and rye that cause an adverse reaction are hordein and secalin, respectively. For simplicity, we will refer to all dietary proteins involved in the disease pathogenesis as *gluten* in this text in keeping with the public's understanding. Oat products are not problematic for all individuals with CD. However, food manufacturers often process oats in facilities that also process wheat products, which can result in cross-contamination.

The autoimmune reaction to gluten exposure damages the mucosal surface of the small intestine; this leaves villi that are malformed and with few remaining functional microvilli (Figure 18.9). This injured mucosa effectively reduces the surface area for micronutrient and macronutrient absorption.

Symptoms can vary depending on the extent of the intestinal damage. The major symptoms of diarrhea, steatorrhea, unintended weight loss, and progressive malnutrition are secondary effects of the immunologic response to gluten.

Diagnostics. Clinical diagnosis of celiac disease requires that the individual is still consuming gluten-containing foods at the time of testing. Once on a gluten-free diet, biochemical testing is not accurate. A physician can make a clinical diagnosis with serologic testing alone or with serologic testing combined with a biopsy. Testing for the presence of tissue transglutaminase–immunoglobulin A (TG2-IgA) is the recommended first assessment in symptomatic patients. If the results show TG2-IgA levels more than 10-fold higher than the upper normal limit, then patients will undergo a second serologic test for the presence of IgA endomysial antibody. If they also test positive for that antibody, the physician can make a definitive diagnosis for CD. For those that tested positive for TG2-IgA but in lower levels, the physician will confirm the diagnosis by duodenal mucosal biopsy.[73]

Medical nutrition therapy for celiac disease. The goal of nutrition management is to avoid all dietary sources of gluten and to prevent malnutrition through healthy meal alternatives. Wheat, rye, and barley are eliminated from the diet, and a variety of other grains are used instead (Table 18.4). Some individuals with CD are sensitive to oats and must eliminate oat-containing products as well. Careful label reading is important for parents and children, because many commercial products use gluten-containing grains as thickeners or fillers. Some commercial products have a gluten-free symbol on their labels to assist with the identification

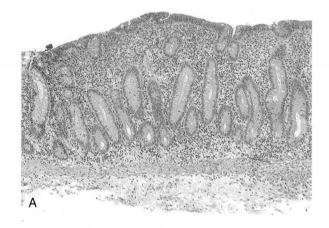

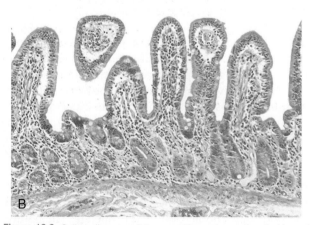

Figure 18.9 Celiac disease, gluten-sensitive enteropathy. A, Normal mucosal biopsy. B, A peroral jejunal biopsy specimen of diseased mucosa shows severe atrophy and the blunting of villi with a chronic inflammatory infiltrate of the lamina propria. (Reprinted from Kumar, V., Fausto, N., & Abbas, A. [2005]. *Robbins & Cotran pathologic basis of disease* [7th ed.]. Philadelphia: Saunders.)

Table 18.4	Gluten-Free Diet for Individuals With Celiac Disease[a]

ACCEPTABLE GRAINS AND GRAIN-SUBSTITUTE PLANT FOODS[b]	GRAINS NOT TOLERATED
Amaranth	Wheat
Arrowroot	Barley
Buckwheat	Rye
Cassava	Malt
Corn	Oats[c] (unless they are
Flax	packaged in a gluten-free
Legumes	environment)
Millet	
Nuts	
Potatoes	
Quinoa	
Rice	
Seeds	
Sorghum	
Soy	
Tapioca	
Wild rice	
Yucca	

[a]Dietary principles to address: (1) choose whole-grain, gluten-free products; (2) choose enriched, gluten-free products instead of refined, unenriched products; (3) eat more foods made with alternative plant foods, such as amaranth, quinoa, and buckwheat for good sources of fiber, iron, and B vitamins; (4) eat plenty of non-grain sources of food to meet all of the body's nutrient needs (e.g., lean meats, poultry, pork, fish, dairy products, legumes, seeds, nuts, vegetables, fruits); (5) consider taking a gluten-free multivitamin and mineral supplement.
[b]Not an exhaustive list of grain substitutes that individuals may tolerate.
[c]Individuals that tolerate oats and oat products do not need to avoid them.
Reference: Academy of Nutrition and Dietetics. (2019). *Nutrition care manual.* Chicago.

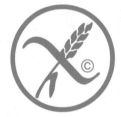

Figure 18.10 Gluten-free symbol. (Copyright Coeliac UK, Bucks, UK, 2004.)

of acceptable foods (Figure 18.10). With the increasing number of processed foods and ethnic dishes available in the marketplace, detecting all food sources of gluten is difficult. Home test kits for gluten are available and may be beneficial for individuals who consume foods without standard ingredient lists.

Adhering to a gluten-free diet is the only effective treatment for maintaining a healthy mucosa, and affected individuals must follow it for life. However, there are nutrition concerns associated with a gluten-free diet; it is generally lower in mineral (particularly calcium and iron), fiber, and B vitamin content.[14,74] Additionally, because of the nature of the malabsorption disorder, clients with CD are at risk for nutrient deficiencies and overall malnutrition during flare-ups. The health care team must consider the potential for drug-nutrient interactions and nutrient absorption interference, as with

any form of malabsorption disorder. Thus, all individuals with CD should work with a health care team that includes an RDN to ensure nutritional adequacy of their diet and address quality-of-life issues related to the restrictive nature of the diet prescription.

GASTROINTESTINAL ACCESSORY ORGANS

Three major accessory organs—the liver, the gallbladder, and the pancreas—produce important digestive agents that enter the intestine and help with the digestion and absorption of food (see Figure 5.3). A good understanding of the anatomy and physiology of the accessory organs is paramount to understanding how various diseases of these organs will subsequently affect the GI tract and nutrient metabolism.

LIVER DISEASE

The liver plays several critical roles in basic metabolism and the regulation of body functions (see Box 5.1). Diseases of the liver have the potential to disrupt any of these functions. Fortunately, the liver is an incredibly regenerative organ. In the event that a doctor diagnoses a patient with liver disease in the early stages, and the patient can remove the causative factor, the liver is capable of regenerating itself. This regenerative capacity is what allows live-donor liver transplants. After **lobectomy** for liver donation in healthy live donors, their remaining liver is capable of regenerating most of its volume within a week post-surgery.[75,76] Adequate nutrition is essential to supply the body with the necessary building blocks for this amount of successful organ regeneration.

Fatty Liver Disease

Fatty liver disease, or **steatosis**, is the excess accumulation of fat in the liver (i.e., lipotoxicity). If the disease results from alcohol abuse, we refer to it as alcoholic liver disease (ALD). If alcohol is not the cause, we refer to it as nonalcoholic fatty liver disease (NAFLD). As the condition progresses, inflammation within the liver ensues. *Steatohepatitis* is the accumulation of fat ("steato") and inflammation in the liver ("hepatitis"). There are two primary types of steatohepatitis: alcoholic steatohepatitis (ASH) and nonalcoholic steatohepatitis (NASH).

Fat accumulates in the liver in response to high levels of fatty acids in circulation, exaggerated lipogenesis, and impaired lipolysis. In other words, the liver stores more fat than it oxidizes. Alcohol-induced disturbances in the liver are multifactorial and progress from toxicity, steatosis, and mass inflammation to ultimately resulting in organ failure. Disease progression of steatohepatitis may advance to cirrhosis if the individual is not treated. Genetic and environmental factors such as obesity, metabolic syndrome, diabetes,

lobectomy surgical removal of a lobe of an organ.
steatosis accumulation of fat in the liver cells.

insulin-resistance, dyslipidemia, and dysbiosis increase the risk for the developing NASH.[77,78] Some researchers argue that nonalcoholic fatty liver disease is a direct result of insulin resistance.[79]

Basic nutrition guidelines for fatty liver disease and steatohepatitis include a balanced diet, avoidance of alcohol (if indicated), weight loss (if indicated), and tight blood glucose level control. Health care providers should evaluate patients with ASH for evidence of malnutrition and refer patients to a dietitian to establish adequate nutrient intake.

Hepatitis

Bacteria, viruses, parasites, or toxins (e.g., chloroform, alcohol, drugs, lipotoxicity) may cause the inflammatory condition of acute hepatitis. Viral infections and alcohol abuse are the most common forms of hepatitis. Viral infections are often transmitted via the oral-fecal route (e.g., hepatitis A), which is common for many epidemic diseases that involve contaminated food or water. In other cases, transfusions of infected blood or contaminated syringes or needles may transmit the virus (e.g., hepatitis B). Symptoms of hepatitis include anorexia and jaundice with underlying malnutrition.

Treatment focuses on bed rest and nutrition therapy to reduce the inflammation and support the healing and regeneration of the liver tissue (see the Case Study box, "Hepatitis"). Dietary restrictions are not usually necessary during acute hepatitis, but they may be required for chronic cases. The following requirements govern the goals of nutrition therapy[14]:

- Avoid hepatotoxic substances (e.g., alcohol, drugs, toxins).
- Consume 4 to 6 small meals per day. Most clients will tolerate oral feedings, but some will require enteral nutrition support.
- *Energy:* Consume a diet that is adequate in energy, macronutrients, and micronutrients.
- *Protein:* Protein is essential for regenerating new liver cells and preventing damage from fatty infiltration in liver tissue. The diet should supply 1.0 to 1.2 g/kg of body weight of high-quality protein daily if no complications are present.
- *Carbohydrates:* Available glucose restores protective glycogen reserves in the liver. It also helps to meet the energy demands of the disease process and prevents the breakdown of protein for energy, thus ensuring its use for tissue regeneration. The diet should supply about half of the total kilocalories as carbohydrates. Glucose intolerance and hypoglycemia are sometimes problematic in clients with liver disease. Therefore, the amount of carbohydrates in the diet depends on individual needs and any co-morbidity (e.g., diabetes).
- *Fat:* In cases of steatorrhea, the diet should not exceed 30% of total kilocalories from fat.
- Sodium is limited to 2000 mg per day to avoid fluid retention (if indicated).

- As a client's appetite and food tolerance improve, a full diet is acceptable while observing his or her likes and dislikes and planning ways to encourage optimal food intake.

Cirrhosis

Cirrhosis is a chronic state of liver disease in which damage to the liver is beyond repair with scar tissue and fatty infiltration (Figure 18.11). The nonfunctional scar tissue prevents blood flow to and through the liver and prevents the liver from performing its essential metabolic functions. Progressive cirrhosis to the point of end-stage liver disease is the ninth leading cause of death from chronic disease in the United States, and about half of all cases are the result of alcoholism.[2] Other causes include chronic hepatitis type B; autoimmune hepatitis; NASH; and genetic diseases such as Wilson disease, hemochromatosis (see Chapter 8), and galactosemia (see Chapter 5). Any form of unchecked hepatitis can progress to cirrhosis.

One of the main functions of the liver is to remove ammonia—and hence nitrogen—from the blood by converting it to urea (via the urea cycle) for urinary excretion. However, with steatohepatitis, the accompanying fatty infiltration kills liver cells and leaves only nonfunctioning fibrous scar tissue. When fibrous scar tissue replaces functional liver tissue, the blood can no longer circulate throughout the liver, which leads to **portal hypertension**. The blood, which is carrying its ammonia load, cannot get to the liver for the normal

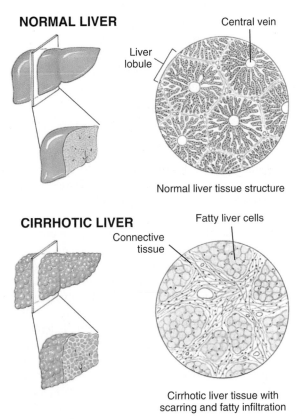

Figure 18.11 Liver disease progression from steatosis to cirrhosis.

NEXT-GENERATION NCLEX® EXAMINATION-STYLE UNFOLDING CASE STUDY
Hepatitis

See answers in Appendix A.

A 20-year-old male (Ht.: 5'10" Wt.: 165 lbs.) is a college student who spent part of his summer semester in South America. He was volunteering with an organization that was helping to establish safe drinking water in an area of very poor resources. Residents in the area previously used the local river for all of their water needs (e.g., drinking, cooking, bathing, and washing clothes). During his journey home, he began to feel ill. He had little energy, no appetite, and severe headaches, and nothing he ate seemed to agree with him. He felt nauseated, he began to have diarrhea, and he soon developed a fever. He began to show evidence of jaundice.

1. From the list provided, select all of the signs and symptoms related to hepatitis.

    a. Anorexia
    b. Constipation
    c. Jaundice
    d. Malnutrition
    e. Edema
    f. Weight gain

2. Choose the *most likely* options for the information missing from the statements below by selecting from the list of options provided.

    The patient most likely has ____1____, which is a ____2____ infection related to ____3____.

OPTION 1	OPTION 2	OPTION 3
hepatitis A	bacterial	contaminated food or water
hepatitis C	viral	blood transfusions
hepatitis B	fungal	infected syringes
hepatitis K	parasitic	infected needles

The patient was admitted to the hospital for diagnosis and treatment of hepatitis. His physical examination and lab work indicated impaired liver function. His liver and spleen were enlarged and tender upon physical examination. The physician's diagnosis was infectious hepatitis. He continues to struggle with eating and has no appetite.

3. Choose the *most likely* options for the information missing from the statements below by selecting from the list of options provided.

    The patient's lack of appetite puts him at risk for _____. It is important for him to consume adequate amounts of energy and protein to encourage liver _____.

OPTIONS	
malnutrition	degradation
anorexia	regeneration
dysbiosis	metabolism

4. From the list provided, select all the appropriate interventions related to hepatitis.

    a. Strict diet restrictions
    b. Four to six small meals per day
    c. Low protein
    d. High fat diet (i.e., >30% TEE in fat)
    e. Sodium restriction of <2000 mg
    f. Adequate calories and carbohydrate
    g. Avoid drugs and alcohol
    h. Bed rest

The patient has impaired liver function and hepatitis and is in the hospital for treatment. After a week, his symptoms of diarrhea, vomiting, and fever have improved, but he has lost weight. A registered dietitian nutritionist meets with him to discuss his diet. His estimated needs are ~2250 kcals/day.

5. Calculate the patient's carbohydrate, protein, and fat recommendations based on the medical nutrition therapy guidelines for hepatitis. Match each recommendation to the proper macronutrient. Not all recommendations will be used.

OPTIONS	MACRONUTRIENTS	ANSWER
a. 165 g/day	Carbohydrates	
b. 281 g/day	Protein	
c. 1,125 g/day	Fat	
d. 50 g/day		
e. <75 g/day		
f. 75-90 g/day		
g. <96 g/day		

6. For each assessment finding, use an X to indicate whether nutrition and nursing interventions were <u>effective</u> (helped to meet expected outcomes) or <u>ineffective</u> (did not help to meet expected outcomes).

ASSESSMENT	EFFECTIVE	INEFFECTIVE
Increased appetite		
Weight loss		
Slight yellowing of the skin		
Increased calorie intake		
Solid bowel movements		
No feelings of nausea		
Body temperature 98.6F		

removal of ammonia and nitrogen. Instead, it must follow the vessels that bypass the liver and proceed to the brain, thereby producing ammonia intoxication and **hepatic encephalopathy.** Portal hypertension causes the small blood vessels that surround the esophagus to distend, which eventually leads to the development of **esophageal varices.** The rupture of these enlarged veins with massive hemorrhage can result in death.

The liver is responsible for processing and metabolizing nutrients and medications. Thus, in the case of cirrhosis, medical treatment is limited to nutrition therapy and to removing excess sources of ammonia within the GI tract. The most common medications used are lactulose and antibiotics such as neomycin. Lactulose is an unabsorbable sugar that pulls water and ammonia into the colon for elimination. Neomycin works by destroying ammonia-producing bacteria in the gut.

Protein-energy malnutrition and vitamin/mineral deficiencies are significant issues for patients with cirrhosis. Such deficiencies exacerbate poor health-related quality of life and contribute to **ascites.**[80,81] MNT focuses on as much healing support as possible, as follows[14]:

- Avoid hepatotoxic substances (e.g., alcohol, drugs, toxins).
- Consume 4 to 6 small meals per day, including nutrient supplementation products, if indicated.
- Consume a diet that is adequate in energy, macronutrients, and micronutrients. Vitamin and mineral supplementation and/or enteral or parenteral nutrition support may be necessary to meet these needs. The health care team should monitor any supplementation of the fat-soluble vitamins to avoid toxicity.
- *Energy:* Total energy intake should equal basal energy needs plus approximately 20%. Practitioners must carefully distinguish fluid weight from actual body weight, because needs are based on dry weight. The dietitian will make adjustments for cases of hypermetabolism or if weight loss is part of the nutrition care plan.
- *Protein:* Dietary protein should equal 0.8 to 1.2 g/kg of dry or appropriate body weight in the absence of impending protein-sensitive hepatic encephalopathy. Sufficient dietary protein helps correct severe malnutrition, heal liver tissue, and restore plasma proteins.
- *Carbohydrates:* Approximately half of the total kilocalories in the diet should come from carbohydrates. The total energy provided by carbohydrates depends on individual needs and any comorbidity (e.g., diabetes, obesity).
- *Fat:* In the presence of steatorrhea, the dietary intake of fat should not exceed 30% of total kilocalories.
- Sodium is limited to 2000 mg per day to reduce the severity of ascites.

- Hyponatremia or ascites necessitates fluid restrictions.
- Reinforce the benefits of daily physical activity.

GALLBLADDER DISEASE

The basic function of the gallbladder is to concentrate and store bile and then release the concentrated bile into the small intestine when fat is present there. Bile emulsifies fat in the intestine to prepare it for digestion and then helps carry it into the mucosal cells of the intestinal wall for preparation to enter the lymphatic circulation (see Chapter 3).

Cholecystitis and Cholelithiasis

Disease process. Inflammation of the gallbladder (cholecystitis) frequently results from a low-grade chronic infection or obstruction. The impaired metabolism and supersaturation of cholesterol contributes to the formation of gallstone (cholelithiasis). Several known genetic variants contribute to the pathology of gallstone formation.[82] Exogenous risk factors for cholelithiasis include obesity, physical inactivity, hormone replacement therapy, and dietary factors such as the high intake of simple carbohydrate and saturated fatty acids.[83-85] The risk for gallbladder disease also increases in the presence of diabetes, metabolic syndrome, dyslipidemia, and liver disease. As the incidence of obesity and type 2 diabetes increases in "western societies," so does the occurrence of cholelithiasis, even in young children.[86-90]

Gallstones are composed primarily of cholesterol, bilirubin, and fatty acids; and we classify them as cholesterol stones, pigment stones, or primary bile duct stones. The majority of gallstones are cholesterol-containing gallstones. Normally, the non–water-soluble cholesterol in bile remains in solution. If the amount of cholesterol is too concentrated, cholesterol may separate out and crystallize to form gallstones. Most gallstones are asymptomatic, but some gallstone carriers experience episodes of intense pain. The typical treatment in such painful and chronic cases is cholecystectomy, which is the surgical removal of the gallbladder. Other medical treatments include litholytic therapy to dissolve the stone and shock wave lithotripsy to shatter the stone.

---

portal hypertension high blood pressure in the portal vein.
hepatic encephalopathy a condition in which toxins in the blood lead to alterations in brain homeostasis as a result of liver disease; this results in apathy, confusion, inappropriate behavior, altered consciousness, and eventually coma.
esophageal varices the pathologic dilation of the blood vessels within the wall of the esophagus as a result of liver cirrhosis; these vessels can continue to expand to the point of rupturing.
ascites the accumulation of serous fluid in the abdominal cavity.

Medical nutrition therapy for gallbladder disease. As fat enters the intestine, the hormone cholecystokinin triggers gallbladder contractions to release bile. In clients with cholecystitis or cholelithiasis, the normal contraction of the gallbladder often causes pain. MNT centers on controlling fat intake (i.e., less than 30% of calories from fat) and eating small, frequent meals.[14] Table 18.5 outlines a general low-fat diet guide, but the degree of its application depends on individual needs, acuity, and treatment plan.

After cholecystectomy, the liver continues to produce bile and release it directly into the duodenum to assist with fat digestion. Therefore, most clients will adjust to a normal diet within a few months after surgery. Without a reservoir of stored bile in the gallbladder, meals that are exceptionally heavy in fat may be uncomfortable for individuals after cholecystectomy.

PANCREATIC DISEASE

The pancreas is a key organ in normal digestion and metabolism, and it acts as both an exocrine gland and an endocrine gland. In response to hormones, the pancreas excretes digestive enzymes and bicarbonate, which are necessary for the breakdown of the macronutrients during digestion. The endocrine functions of the pancreas include the regulation of blood glucose concentrations by glucagon and insulin. Chapter 20 covers the endocrine functions of the pancreas.

Pancreatitis

Disease process. Premature trypsin activation within the pancreas causes autodigestion of pancreatic tissue and inflammation.[91] Pancreatitis (i.e., inflammation of the pancreas) inhibits normal endocrine and exocrine pancreatic function, including the secretion of digestive enzymes. Subsequently, severely altered digestion and absorption ensue, as does altered glucose control in chronic forms of pancreatitis. Mild or moderate episodes may completely subside, but the condition tends to recur, which can lead to chronic pancreatitis. Patients with pancreatitis experience severe abdominal pain and may experience nausea, vomiting, and steatorrhea.

Excessive alcohol consumption is the major causative factor of pancreatitis. Other causes of chronic pancreatitis include heredity, pancreatic duct obstruction, hypertriglyceridemia, CF, renal failure, and infectious disease.

Medical nutrition therapy for pancreatitis. Without adequate pancreatic enzymes, individuals with pancreatitis are unable to digest food properly, which eventually leads to malnutrition. Thus, supplementing with pancreatic enzyme replacement therapy is a cornerstone of treatment for chronic pancreatitis. Nutrition therapy will vary depending on the severity of symptoms and the duration of the disease. For cases of mild to moderate pancreatitis, MNT includes the following measures[14,92]:

Table 18.5	Low-Fat Diet[a]	
FOODS	**FOODS ALLOWED**	**FOODS LIMITED OR AVOIDED**
Beverages	Skim milk, coffee, tea, carbonated beverages, and fruit juices	Whole milk, cream, and evaporated and condensed milk
Bread and cereals	Most all	Rich rolls or breads, waffles, and pancakes
Desserts	Gelatin, sherbet, water ices, fruit whips made without cream, angel food cake, and rice and tapioca puddings made with skim milk	Pastries, pies, rich cakes and cookies, and ice cream
Fruits	All fresh fruits as tolerated	Fried fruits or fruit served with fat (e.g., cream, ice cream)
Eggs	Egg whites or egg substitutes	Egg yolks, fried eggs
Fats	Unsaturated fat oils, vegetable oil spreads, avocados (sparingly)	Saturated fats, shortening, mayonnaise
Meats	Lean meat such as beef, veal, lamb, liver, lean fish, and fowl that has been baked, broiled, or roasted without added fat	Fried meats, bacon, ham, pork, goose, duck, fatty fish, fish canned in oil, and cold cuts
Cheese	Low-fat or fat-free cottage cheese	All other cheeses
Potato or substitute	Potatoes, rice, macaroni, noodles, and spaghetti prepared without added fat	Fried potatoes and potato chips
Soups	Bouillon or broth without fat and soups made with skim milk	Cream soups
Sweets	Jam, jelly, and sugar candies without nuts or chocolate	Chocolate, nuts, and peanut butter
Vegetables	All vegetables as tolerated	Fried vegetables or vegetables prepared with fat (e.g., butter, cream)

[a]Such dietary restraints on fat are usually only needed during acute or unresolved cases.

- Hydration support during acute phases as determined on an individual basis. Some patients benefit from pancreatic rest while receiving fluids and corrections for electrolyte and acid-base disturbances.
- Advance to oral feedings as early as tolerated (e.g., within 24 hours). Clients with severe pancreatitis may require a continuous infusion of enteral nutrition. The health care team will consider parenteral nutrition in severe cases for patients who cannot tolerate oral or enteral feedings (see Chapter 22).

- Adequate energy and protein to prevent nutrient deficiencies and weight loss. Assess the need for vitamin and mineral supplementation, especially during periods when oral intake is insufficient to meet basic needs.
- The therapeutic diet is relatively high in protein and low in fat. The presence of fat maldigestion (e.g., steatorrhea) will determine the appropriate fat content on an individual basis.
- Strict avoidance of alcohol and smoking.

Putting It All Together

Summary

- The medical nutrition therapy for various GI diseases is specific to the degree of interference in the normal processes of ingestion, digestion, absorption, and metabolism that the disease causes.
- Problems in the upper GI tract relate to conditions that hinder chewing, swallowing, or transporting the food mass down the esophagus into the stomach. Esophageal problems interfere with the passage of food into the stomach. PUD involves the acidic erosion of the mucosal lining of the stomach or the duodenal bulb. Nutrition therapy is liberal and individual, with the goal of correcting malnutrition and supporting the healing process.
- Problems of the lower GI tract include common functional disorders such as malabsorption and diarrhea, for which the client needs symptomatic and personalized treatment. CD and CF require extensive individualized nutrition support. The inflammatory bowel diseases involve widespread tissue damage that occasionally requires surgical resection and that results in decreased absorbing surface area. Large intestine problems are often multifactorial and may be difficult to resolve. MNT is specific to each condition and generally warrants the assistance of an RDN.
- Diseases of the GI accessory organs also contribute to nutrition problems. Common liver disorders include hepatitis and cirrhosis. Nutrient and energy levels of the necessary diet therapy vary with the progression of the disease process. Gallbladder disease, infection, and stones involve some acute limitation to fat tolerance. Pancreatitis is a serious condition that requires immediate measures to counter the symptoms of severe pain followed by restorative nutrition support.

Chapter Review Questions

See answers in Appendix A.

1. The best way to prevent constipation is to _____.

   a. use stool softeners twice daily
   b. consume plenty of soluble fiber and fluids
   c. use a laxative once a week
   d. use a daily multivitamin/multimineral supplement

2. Of the options provided, the meal that is most appropriate for a client with GERD is _____.

   a. coffee, orange juice, sausage patty, and biscuit
   b. skim milk, scrambled egg, and whole-wheat toast
   c. tomato juice, country fried steak, and hash brown casserole
   d. skim milk, peppermint tea, fried chicken, and fried potatoes

3. A client with cirrhosis of the liver can help avoid progression to hepatic encephalopathy by avoiding excessive intake of

   _____.

   a. fat
   b. calories
   c. protein
   d. thiamin

4. Pancreatitis is most frequently caused by _____.

   a. excessive protein intake
   b. protein-energy malnutrition
   c. chronic food allergies
   d. excessive alcohol intake

5. A person with celiac disease should avoid _____.

   a. barley and vegetable soup
   b. grilled chicken and rice
   c. rice cakes with strawberries
   d. fresh grilled shrimp and baked potato

Next-Generation NCLEX® Examination-style Case Study

See answers in Appendix A.

A 56-year-old man (height, 5'5"; weight, 200 lbs.) experiences chest pain and frequent belching about 1 hour after eating. Currently, he is not on any medications but does take a multivitamin daily. His work and commute schedule only permit him time enough to exercise about once or twice per week. He mentions that he has been working long hours at work, which has been causing him extra stress. The dietitian collected the following 24-hour dietary recall:

Breakfast: coffee (1 c.), orange juice (1 c.), fried hash browns (½ c.), sausage links (2), and pancakes (2) with butter (1 Tbsp.)

Lunch: spaghetti and meatballs (4 c.) with pieces of garlic bread (2), soda (2 c.), and candy bar (1)

Dinner: chicken fried steak (6 oz.), mashed potatoes (1 c.), macaroni and cheese (1 c.), and alcohol (12 oz.)

1. **From the list below, select all factors from the client's history that are of nutrition-related concern.**

   a. BMI
   b. Medications
   c. Dietary supplements
   d. Physical inactivity
   e. Stress level
   f. Food choices

2. **Choose the *most likely* options for the information missing from the statements below by selecting from the list of options provided.**

   The client's nutrition assessment indicates that his weight places him in the ____1____ category. His diet is high in ____2____ and ____2____.

OPTION 1	OPTION 2
normal weight	fiber
overweight	fat
underweight	sodium
obese	fluids

3. **From the list below, identify the client's condition based on his signs, symptoms, and history.**

   a. *Helicobacter pylori* infection
   b. Gastroesophageal reflux disease
   c. Crohn's disease
   d. Ulcerative colitis
   e. Irritable bowel syndrome
   f. Diverticulitis

4. **Place the correct letter from the nursing responses below in the right column as appropriate for each client question.**

CLIENT QUESTIONS	APPROPRIATE NURSE'S RESPONSE FOR EACH CLIENT QUESTION
"Are there medications that I can take to help my condition?"	
"Can I still drink alcohol?"	
"Should I lose weight?"	
"How much physical activity should I be getting?"	

Nurse's Response Options

   a. "Medications to increase lower esophageal sphincter pressure might help, such as anticholinergics and calcium-channel blockers."
   b. "Losing weight will be helpful to reduce abdominal pressure."
   c. "Antacids and proton pump inhibitors are often used to reduce the acidity and production of stomach acid."
   d. "You can still keep your normal drinking habits without any modifications."
   e. "It might be best for you to avoid or limit alcohol as much as possible to reduce irritation."
   f. "Losing weight might be helpful to increase the abdominal pressure."
   g. "Getting at least 30 minutes of physical activity on most days of the week will be beneficial."
   h. "You should avoid physical activity with this condition."

5. For each health teaching below, use an X to identify which are indicated (appropriate or necessary) or contraindicated (could be harmful) for the client.

HEALTH TEACHING	INDICATED	CONTRAINDICATED
Consume meals in an upright position.		
After eating, it might help to lie down while your food is digesting.		
Wear tight clothing, especially after consuming meals.		
Consume small frequent meals instead of large meals.		
Drink large amounts of fluids with meals.		
Avoid irritants, such as alcohol, caffeine, chocolate, carbonated beverages, tomatoes, and spicy foods.		
Consume foods that are lower in fat and high in fiber.		

6. For each assessment finding, use an X to indicate whether nursing and collaborative interventions were effective (helped to meet expected outcomes) or ineffective (did not help to meet expected outcomes.

ASSESSMENT FINDING	EFFECTIVE	INEFFECTIVE
Lost 8 lbs. in 1 month		
Consumes fruits and vegetables throughout the day		
Replaced alcoholic beverages with soda		
Has less chest pain after consuming meals		
Skips breakfast to lower calorie intake		

Additional Learning Resources

Please refer to this text's Evolve website for answers to the Case Study questions:
http://evolve.elsevier.com/Williams/basic/.
References and **Further Reading and Resources** in the back of the book provide additional resources for enhancing knowledge.

Coronary Heart Disease and Hypertension

Key Concepts

- Cardiovascular disease is the leading cause of death in the United States.
- Several risk factors contribute to the development of coronary heart disease and hypertension, many of which are preventable by improved diet and lifestyle behaviors.
- Other risk factors for cardiovascular disease are nonmodifiable, such as age, sex, family history, and race.

- Hypertension (i.e., chronically elevated blood pressure) may be classified as primary or secondary hypertension.
- Hypertension damages the endothelium of the blood vessels.
- Early education is critical for the prevention of cardiovascular disease.

Cardiovascular disease (CVD) is the leading cause of death in the United States, and it accounts for more than 635,000 deaths annually (Figure 19.1).[1] A similar situation exists in most other industrialized societies. Every day thousands of people have heart attacks and strokes, and millions of others continue to live with various forms of rheumatic and congestive heart disease.

This chapter discusses the primary underlying disease processes of atherosclerosis and hypertension as well as the various risk factors involved. In addition, we will explore ways to use nutrition and lifestyle modifications to reduce risk factors and to help prevent disease.

CORONARY HEART DISEASE

The *coronary arteries* are the major arteries and branches that serve the heart. The arteries lie across the brow of the heart and resemble a crown. Coronary heart disease is the term we use to describe disease affecting these vessels.

ATHEROSCLEROSIS

Disease Process

Atherosclerosis is the major cause of CVD and the underlying pathologic process in coronary heart disease. The disease process is characterized by the presence of fatty plaque on the inside lining of the major blood vessels. Atherosclerotic plague is largely composed of cholesterol. Although we do not currently know all of the contributing factors involved in atherosclerosis development, scientists believe that the plaque forms in response to an endothelial injury within the artery and inflammation ensues.

Atherosclerotic plaque may begin as early as childhood in susceptible individuals. Upon examination, one can see cholesterol with the unaided eye in the debris of advanced lesions. This fatty plaque gradually thickens over time to a fibrous plaque that narrows the interior of the vessel. The thickening of the artery or the development of a blood clot may eventually cut off blood flow (Figure 19.2).

When deprived of their normal blood supply, cells die. We call the local area of dying or dead tissue an *infarct*. A myocardial infarction (MI) or *heart attack* results if the affected blood vessel is a major artery that supplies vital nutrients and oxygen to the heart muscle (i.e., the myocardium). Angina pectoris, or chest pain radiating down the left arm, is a common symptom of an MI. If the affected vessel is a major artery that supplies the brain, then the blockage causes a cerebrovascular accident or *stroke*.

---

atherosclerosis the underlying pathology of coronary heart disease; a common form of arteriosclerosis that is characterized by the formation of fatty streaks that contain cholesterol and that develop into hardened plaques in the inner lining of major blood vessels such as the coronary arteries.

coronary heart disease the overall medical problem that results from the underlying disease of atherosclerosis in the coronary arteries, which serve the heart muscle with blood, oxygen, and nutrients.

plaque thick, wax-like coating forming inside artery walls; primarily composed of cholesterol, fatty substances, cellular debris, calcium, and fibrin.

myocardial infarction (MI) a heart attack; a myocardial infarction is caused by the failure of the heart muscle to maintain normal blood circulation as a result of the blockage of the coronary arteries with fatty cholesterol plaques that cut off the delivery of oxygen to the affected part of the heart muscle.

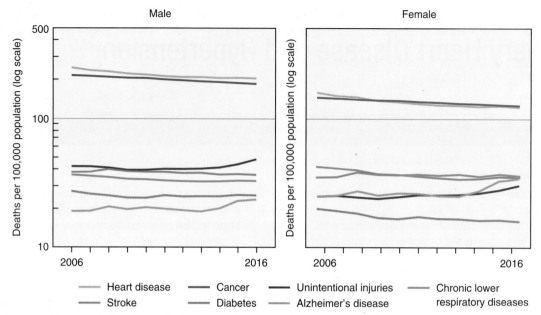

Figure 19.1 Age-adjusted death rates for selected causes of death for all ages, by sex: United States, 2006–2016. (National Center for Health Statistics. [2018]. *Health, United States, 2017: With special feature on mortality*. Hyattsville, MD: National Center for Health Statistics [U.S.].)

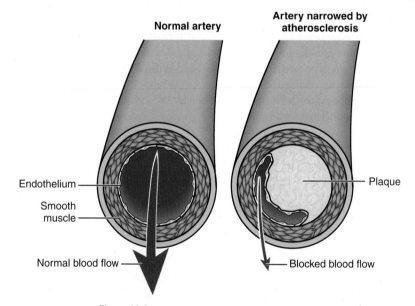

Figure 19.2 An atherosclerotic plaque in an artery.

Relation to Fat Metabolism

See Chapter 3 for details on the dietary lipids involved in the atherogenic disease process. We will briefly cover three of the substances that are specifically relevant to CVD again here.

Total cholesterol. Although cholesterol is an essential compound in the body, excess total blood levels increase the risk of heart disease in predisposed individuals. High blood cholesterol levels increase the risk for the deposition of cholesterol, fats, fibrous tissue, and macrophages in arteries throughout the body, which is the beginning of atherosclerosis. The Centers for Disease Control and Prevention reports that 27.1% of American adults ≥20 years of age have high total blood cholesterol levels exceeding 240 mg/dL, or are taking

cholesterol-lowering medications.[1] The prevalence rises precipitously along with age. Many individuals with **hypercholesterolemia** also suffer from obesity and hypertension. Such co-morbidities usually require medical intervention, and nutrition therapy is the primary focus.

---

angina pectoris a spasmodic, choking chest pain caused by a lack of oxygen to the heart; this is a symptom of a heart attack, and it also may be caused by severe effort or excitement.

cerebrovascular accident a stroke; a stroke is caused by arteriosclerosis within the blood vessels of the brain that cuts off oxygen supply to the affected portion of brain tissue, thereby paralyzing the actions that are controlled by the affected area.

hypercholesterolemia high cholesterol levels in the blood.

Lipoproteins. Fat is not soluble in water; therefore, it is carried in the bloodstream in small packages wrapped with protein called *lipoproteins.* We produce lipoproteins endogenously in the intestinal mucosal cells after consuming a meal that contains fat and in the liver as part of the ongoing process of fat metabolism. Lipoproteins carry fat and cholesterol to tissues for cell metabolism and then back to the liver for processing as needed. The percentage of protein, fat, and cholesterol content within a lipoprotein determines its density. We then categorize lipoproteins according to that density. Because protein is denser than fat and cholesterol, those lipoproteins with the highest protein content have the highest density and vice versa. The following lipoproteins are significant in relation to heart disease risk as follows:

1. *Chylomicrons:* These are predominantly composed of dietary triglycerides after digestion and absorption from the gastrointestinal tract. Chylomicrons are lipoprotein particles that transport absorbed dietary (i.e., exogenous) fat to plasma and tissues (primarily the liver) (Figure 19.3A).

2. *Very low–density lipoproteins (VLDLs):* The liver forms VLDLs from fat. VLDLs carry a relatively large load of triglycerides to cells throughout the body, and they contain approximately 12% cholesterol (Figure 19.3B). They have a very low density of protein.

3. *Intermediate-density lipoproteins (IDLs):* Degradation of VLDLs leaves IDLs in circulation. Similar to VLDLs, IDLs continue delivering triglycerides to cells and tissue throughout the body.

4. *Low-density lipoproteins (LDLs):* LDL cholesterol carries, in addition to other lipids, at least two-thirds of the total plasma cholesterol to body tissues (Figure 19.3C). The liver forms LDLs endogenously. LDLs in the serum are also a product of VLDL and IDL catabolism. Because LDLs deliver cholesterol to the tissue, we consider them "bad cholesterol." With regard to cardiovascular health, LDL cholesterol is the major lipoprotein of concern and the predominant focus of drug therapy.[2-4] Sometimes we group all of the non–high-density lipoprotein fractions (i.e., VLDLs and LDLs) together as a marker for CVD risk. LDLs have a low density of protein. Apolipoprotein B (apoB) is the primary protein found in LDL and VLDL cholesterol. ApoB is also an independent marker for atherogenic risk.

5. *High-density lipoproteins (HDLs):* HDL cholesterol carries less total fat and has a substantially higher density of protein than the other lipoproteins (Figure 19.3D). They transport cholesterol from the tissues and arteries back to the liver for catabolism. The liver endogenously produces HDLs.

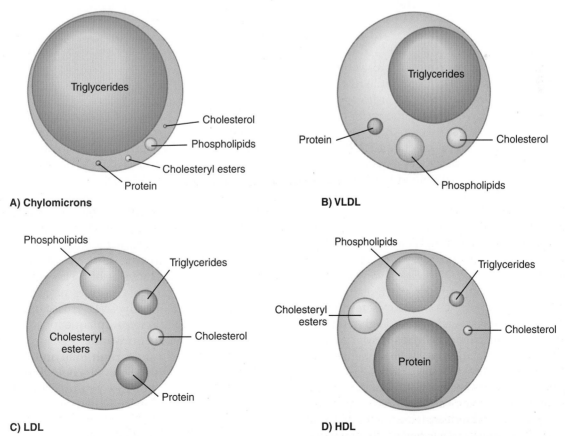

A) Chylomicrons

B) VLDL

C) LDL

D) HDL

Figure 19.3 Serum lipoprotein factions showing relative lipid composition within each lipoprotein. (A) Chylomicron. (B) Very low–density lipoprotein. (C) Low-density lipoprotein. (D) High-density lipoprotein.

Compared with LDL cholesterol, HDL is the "good cholesterol," and higher serum levels are a marker for reduce CVD risk. Genetics play a major role in a person's HDL cholesterol production. However, there are both pharmacologic interventions and lifestyle modifications that influence HDL metabolism. Individuals with a normal waist-to-hip ratio, with a non-obese BMI, and who participate in regular exercise have higher HDL cholesterol levels relative to their counterparts.[5]

We do not consume VLDL, IDL, LDL, or HDL cholesterol in our food. Thus, "eating less LDL cholesterol" or "eating more HDL cholesterol" does not address **dyslipidemia**. Other dietary modifications can improve lipid profiles, but it is not via a direct consumption or avoidance of these lipoprotein fractions in food.

Triglycerides. Simple fats, whether in the body or in food, are triglycerides. CVD screenings will test for the levels of total triglycerides circulating in the blood. **Hypertriglyceridemia** is commonly associated with low HDL cholesterol, both of which are independent risk factors for CVD.[3,4,6]

Physicians do not use blood lipid levels as the exclusive criteria for starting cholesterol-lowering medications. The algorithm for determining drug therapy takes into account many factors, including age, race/ethnicity, sex, family history, blood pressure measurements, co-morbidities (e.g., diabetes, **metabolic syndrome** [Table 19.1], chronic kidney disease, polycystic ovary syndrome), and lifestyle factors (e.g., smoking, exercise habits).

Risk Factors

The underlying disease process of atherosclerotic cardiovascular disease (ASCVD) has multiple risk factors (Box 19.1). The American College of Cardiology offers a 10-year atherosclerotic CVD Risk Estimator on their website (go to acc.org and search for "ASCVD Risk Estimator"). The current clinical practice guidelines recommend that health care providers regularly use this risk estimator tool, along with blood lipid levels, as a means of evaluating a client's risk level for CVD.[6] As you consider the risk factors for CVD, note the modifiable factors over which people have some control compared with those that individuals cannot control (i.e., nonmodifiable).

- *Age:* General risk for CVD increases with age.
- *Family history:* A family history of premature CVD increases one's risk for CVD. Early screening for children and adolescents with a high-risk family history is important so that appropriate diet and lifestyle modifications may begin before fatty streaks develop in the coronary arteries.
- *Heredity:* Certain groups (e.g., African Americans, Hispanic/Latino Americans, Native Americans, and South Asian Americans) have a higher incidence of CVD than other race/ethnicities in the

Table **19.1**	Diagnostic Criteria for Metabolic Syndrome
MEASURE[a]	**CATEGORIC CUT POINTS**
Increased waist circumference[b,c]	≥102 cm (≥40.1 inches) in men, ≥88 cm (≥34.6 inches) in women
Elevated level of triglycerides	≥175 mg/dL (2.0 mmol/L) or drug treatment for elevated triglycerides[d]
Reduced HDL-cholesterol level	<40 mg/dL (1.0 mmol/L) in men <50 mg/dL (1.3 mmol/L) in women or drug treatment for reduced HDL-cholesterol[d]
Hypertension	≥130 mm Hg systolic or ≥85 mm Hg diastolic or drug treatment for hypertension
Elevated fasting glucose level	≥100 mg/dL or drug treatment for elevated glucose

[a]Any three of these five criteria constitute a diagnosis of metabolic syndrome.
[b]To measure waist circumference, locate the top of the right iliac crest. Place a measuring tape in a horizontal plane around the abdomen at the level of the iliac crest. Before reading the tape measure, ensure that the tape is snug but that it does not compress the skin, and be sure that it is parallel to the floor. Make the measurement at the end of a normal expiration.
[c]Some U.S. adults of non-Asian origin (e.g., Caucasian, African American, Hispanic) with marginally increased waist circumferences (e.g., 94 to 101 cm [37 to 39 inches] in men and 80 to 87 cm [31 to 34 inches] in women) may have a strong genetic contribution to insulin resistance and should benefit from changes in lifestyle habits; this is similar for men with categoric increases in waist circumference. A lower waist circumference cut point (e.g., 90 cm [35 inches] in men and 80 cm [31 inches] in women) appears to be appropriate for Asian Americans.
[d]Fibrates and nicotinic acid are the most commonly used drugs for elevated triglycerides and reduced HDL-cholesterol. We can presume that clients who are taking one of these drugs have a high triglyceride level and a low HDL-cholesterol level.
From Grundy, S. M., et al. (2019). 2018 AHA/ACC/AACVPR/AAPA/ABC/ACPM/ADA/AGS/APhA/ASPC/NLA/PCNA guideline on the management of blood cholesterol: A report of the American College of Cardiology/American Heart Association Task Force on Clinical Practice Guidelines. *J Am Coll Cardiol, 73*(24), e285–e350.

United States.[4] Some of this heightened incidence rate may be related to ethnicity-associated lifestyles, acculturation, and socioeconomic status that increase the CVD risk in certain groups; there may not be solely genetic factors at play. Genetic anomalies that result in abnormally high serum lipid levels include **familial hypercholesterolemia** and **familial hypertriglyceridemia**. Both conditions require diet and drug therapy beginning in the first couple of decades of life. This is why it is important to screen lipid profiles of children with a family history of early CVD. It is more successful to prevent atherosclerotic plaque formation than to initiate treatment afterwards.

- *Blood cholesterol profile:* High total and LDL cholesterol coupled with low HDL cholesterol are major risk factors for the disease process. Physicians commonly order labs for non-HDL cholesterol (all cholesterol values with exception of HDL) because this marker is symbolic of atherogenesis.

- *Poor diet quality*: The most common dietary problems contributing to CVD are excess sodium, low nuts/seeds, high processed meats, low seafood-derived omega-3 fatty acids, excess sugar-sweetened beverages, and inadequate fruit, vegetables, and whole grains.[7]
- *Physical inactivity*: Sedentary behavior is a major risk factor for all-cause mortality and CVD in particular. Less than 22% of adults in the United States meet the national recommendations for physical activity on a regular basis.[8] See Chapter 16 for additional information on physical activity and exercise.
- *Smoking*: Smoking and exposure to secondhand smoke are major risk factors for atherosclerotic plaque formation and CVD.[9]
- *Compounding conditions*: Co-morbidities associated with obesity such as type 2 diabetes, hypertension, metabolic syndrome, premature menopause, and inflammatory diseases (e.g., rheumatoid arthritis, psoriasis, HIV) increase the risk for the development of CVD.

Box 19.1 Risk Factors for Cardiovascular Disease and Future Atherosclerotic Cardiovascular Disease Events[a,b]

MAJOR RISK FACTORS

- Dyslipidemia:
  - Elevated LDL cholesterol (≥160 mg/dL)
  - Elevated non-HDL cholesterol (≥190mg/dL)
  - Elevated triglycerides (≥175 mg/dL)
  - Elevated total cholesterol in combination with high triglycerides, non-HDL–cholesterol, or LDL cholesterol
  - Low levels of HDL cholesterol (<40 mg/dL for men; <50 mg/dL for women); >60 mg/dL is cardioprotective
- Presence of specific co-morbidities such as hypertension, diabetes, metabolic syndrome, inflammatory diseases (e.g., rheumatoid arthritis, psoriasis, HIV), premature menopause (before age 40), chronic kidney disease, congestive heart failure
- Family history of:
  - Premature atherosclerotic CVD (<55 years in men; <65 years in women)
  - Familial hypercholesterolemia
  - Family history of genetic hyperlipidemia
- High-risk race/ethnicity (e.g., South Asian ancestry)
- Advancing age (≥65 years)
- Cigarette smoking

ADDITIONAL RISK FACTORS

- Poor dietary habits such as a high intake of animal protein, sugar-sweetened beverages, saturated fat, trans fat, and sodium; or a low intake of fruits, vegetables, whole grains, unsaturated fats, nuts, and seeds
- Sedentary lifestyle
- Overweight/obesity, especially abdominal obesity
- Elevated levels of Lipoprotein (a) (≥50 mg/dL)
- Elevated levels of Apolipoprotein B (≥130 mg/dL)
- Elevated inflammatory markers such as high-sensitivity C-reactive protein (≥2.0 mg/L)
- Ankle-brachial index (<0.9)

HDL, High-density lipoprotein; *LDL*, low-density lipoprotein.
[a]Examples of atherosclerotic CVD events include acute coronary syndrome, myocardial infarction, stroke, transient ischemic attack (TIA), angina, and peripheral artery disease.
[b]The 2019 guidelines for treating high cholesterol take into account all risk factors. Physicians do not exclusively base treatment initiation on a single parameter.
Data from Arnett, D. K., et al. (2019). 2019 ACC/AHA guideline on the primary prevention of cardiovascular disease. *Circulation*, Cir0000000000000678; Grundy, S. M., et al. (2019). 2018 AHA/ACC/AACVPR/AAPA/ABC/ACPM/ADA/AGS/APhA/ASPC/NLA/PCNA guideline on the management of blood cholesterol: A report of the American College of Cardiology/American Heart Association Task Force on Clinical Practice Guidelines. *J Am Coll Cardiol*, 73(24), e285–e350; and Jellinger, P. S., et al. (2017). American Association of Clinical Endocrinologists and American College of Endocrinology guidelines for management of dyslipidemia and prevention of cardiovascular disease. *Endocr Pract*, 23(Suppl. 2), 1–87.

Recommendations to Reduce Risk

The number-one take-home message from the *2019 American College of Cardiology (ACC) and the American Heart Association (AHA) Clinical Practice Guidelines on the Primary Prevention of Cardiovascular Disease* states, "The most important way to prevent atherosclerotic vascular disease, heart failure, and atrial fibrillation is to promote a healthy lifestyle throughout life."[6] This statement symbolizes the sheer magnitude of modifiable lifestyle choices on CVD risk and the importance of lifelong healthy habits.

Poor diet quality is one of the most significant risk factors for death and disability from CVD in the United States; and poor diet quality seems to be more the rule than the exception in all age groups.[8,10] Almost half (45.4%) of all deaths from CVD are a result of modifiable diet-related inadequacies.[7] Only 0.6% of children and 1.5% of adults regularly consume a diet that meets at least 80% of the dietary recommendations for a healthy diet (defined as ≥4.5 cups/day of fruits and vegetables, ≥2 servings/week of fish, ≥3 servings/day of whole grains, <36 oz/week of sugar-sweetened beverages, and ≤1500 mg/day of sodium).[8] See the For Further Focus box "Modifiable Risk Factors for Heart Disease" for additional details on dietary behaviors in the United States.

---

dyslipidemia abnormal lipid profile (high total cholesterol, LDL, or TG; and/or low HDL).
hypertriglyceridemia high triglycerides in the blood.
metabolic syndrome a combination of disorders that, when they occur together, increases the risk of cardiovascular disease and diabetes; it is also known as syndrome X.
familial hypercholesterolemia a genetic disorder that results in elevated blood cholesterol levels despite lifestyle modifications; this condition is caused by absent or nonfunctional low-density lipoprotein receptors, and it requires drug therapy.
familial hypertriglyceridemia a genetic disorder that results in elevated blood triglyceride levels despite lifestyle modifications; it requires drug therapy.

For Further Focus

Modifiable Risk Factors for Heart Disease

The American Heart Association uses a seven-metric system for evaluating overall cardiovascular health, which includes smoking status, weight status, physical activity, diet, total blood cholesterol level, blood pressure, and fasting blood glucose level. Diet and lifestyle adjustments can address each of the modifiable risk factors. Of all of the health behaviors, poor dietary habits of American adults are the single largest modifiable risk factor contributing to preventable cardiovascular disease.[1,2] Not incidentally,

poor dietary habits negatively influence most of the other measurements in turn (e.g., body mass index, total blood cholesterol, blood pressure, and fasting blood glucose). When asked, many people overestimate the quality of their dietary patterns. However, when analyzing actual intake relative to evidence-based dietary recommendations of food group servings, 99.4% of children and 98.5% of adults *fail* to meet the recommendations (see image below for data on adults).[2]

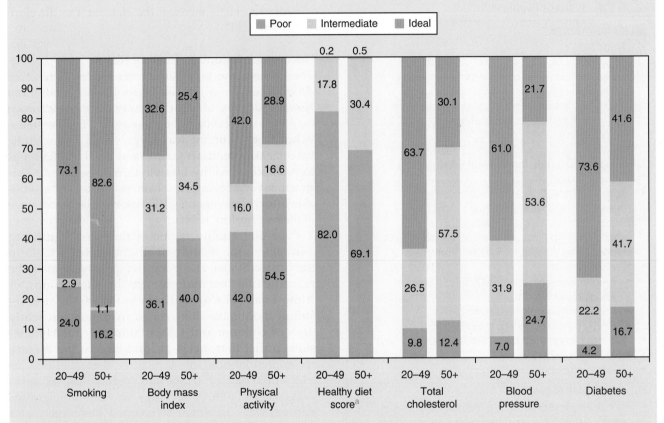

Prevalence (unadjusted) estimates of poor, intermediate, and ideal cardiovascular health for each of the 7 metrics of cardiovascular health in the American Heart Association 2020 goals among US adults aged 20 to 49 years and ≥50 years, National Center for Health Statistics, National Health and Nutrition Examination Survey (NHANES) 2013 to 2014.
[a]Healthy diet score reflects 2011 to 2012 NHANES data.

Given the pervasive nature of poor dietary habits and the impact on mortality and morbidity, there are huge implications for improvements in healthy eating patterns. See the American Heart Association diet and lifestyle recommendations for cardiovascular disease prevention in Box 19.2 for ideal lifestyle goals for adults.

REFERENCES

1   Micha, R., et al. (2017). Association between dietary factors and mortality from heart disease, stroke, and type 2 diabetes in the United States. *Journal of the American Medical Association, 317*(9), 912–924.
2   Benjamin, E. J., et al. (2018). Heart disease and stroke statistics-2018 update: A report from the American Heart Association. *Circulation, 137*(12), e67–e492.

Dietary recommendations. The *Dietary Guidelines for Americans, 2020-2025* (see Chapter 1) and the American Heart Association recommend the dietary restriction of certain types of fat and cholesterol to reduce the risk for heart disease. However, more important is the consideration of the whole diet. Changing one nutrient within an otherwise unhealthy diet will not likely make a significant difference in overall health

risk. On the other hand, a shift to a more balanced, well-rounded diet and lifestyle is the primary focus of the current clinical practice guidelines for the prevention of CVD (see Box 19.2).[6]

Clients can adapt the dietary pattern outlined in Box 19.2 to appropriate calorie requirements, personal and cultural food preferences, and nutrition therapy needs for other co-morbidities (e.g., diabetes mellitus, obesity, kidney disease). This healthy eating pattern should allow for the attainment and maintenance of a healthy weight. Clients may choose to achieve this pattern by following plans such as the *Dietary Approaches to Stop Hypertension (DASH)* (discussed later in this chapter), the *MyPlate guidelines* (see Chapter 1), or the *Mediterranean Diet* pattern (see Figure 14.5, Table 14.4, and the Clinical Applications box, "Mediterranean Diet and Heart Disease" within Chapter 14). Such dietary patterns are beneficial for CVD risk reduction and protective against other obesity-related and metabolic diseases.

Box 19.2	**American Heart Association Diet and Lifestyle Recommendations for Cardiovascular Disease Prevention**

WEIGHT AND PHYSICAL ACTIVITY
- Burn at least as many calories as consumed.
- Aim for *at least* 150 minutes of moderate physical activity or 75 minutes of vigorous physical activity (or an equal combination of both) weekly.
- To lose weight, increase the duration or intensity of physical activity to burn more calories than eaten every day.

FOODS TO FOCUS ON
- Eat a variety of nutritious foods from all food groups.
- Choose fresh vegetables and fruits, fiber-rich whole-grains, nuts, legumes, and fat-free or low-fat dairy products most often.
- Choose lean meats such as skinless poultry prepared without added saturated or trans fats.
- Eat a variety of fish, at least twice a week.
- Use monounsaturated and polyunsaturated fats instead of tropical oils and other forms of saturated fat.

FOODS TO LIMIT OR CONSUME IN MODERATION
- Limit the amount of saturated fat. For those with elevated blood cholesterol levels, limit to a maximum of 5% to 6% of total kcal/d.
- Avoid trans fat.
- Limit sodium intake. For those with elevated blood pressure, limit to a maximum of 2300 mg/day with a goal reduction to 1500 mg/d.
- Limit red meat, processed meat, and refined carbohydrates.
- Consume less of the nutrient-poor foods, such as sugar-sweetened beverages.

GENERAL RECOMMENDATIONS
- Drink alcohol in moderation, if at all (e.g., one drink per day for women and two drinks per day for men).
- Follow the American Heart Association recommendations when eating out, and uphold appropriate portion sizes.
- Do not smoke tobacco, and avoid exposure to tobacco smoke.

Modified from the American Heart Association. (n.d.). *Diet and lifestyle recommendations*. Retrieved July 24, 2019, from www.heart.org/en/healthy-living/healthy-eating/eat-smart/nutrition-basics/aha-diet-and-lifestyle-recommendations.

Lifestyle recommendations. In addition to the recommendations for a healthy eating pattern, the expert committee also recommends that adults participate in regular physical activity, minimize sedentary behaviors, abstain from tobacco, and avoid exposure to second-hand smoke as essential components of CVD risk reduction.[6] Tobacco cessation strategies for individuals who smoke should include both behavioral interventions and pharmacotherapy to aid in the process of quitting.

Health care providers should encourage weight loss for overweight or obese individuals and refer their patients to a registered dietitian nutritionist for patient-centered lifestyle intervention counseling. Clients may achieve negative energy balance through a combination of reduced energy intake and increased energy expenditure from physical activity (see Chapter 15 for healthy weight-loss approaches). An exercise tolerance test is ideal to determine the exercise limit for individuals who are older, who are obese, or who have a history of CVD or hypertension before they start an exercise program (Figure 19.4).

Social determinants of health contribute to a person's CVD risk. A successful **team-based care approach** will tailor the advice and treatment plan to the patient's socioeconomic status, education level, health literacy, and cultural, work, and home environments.[6] Health care plans must consider a person's access to adequate housing, food, transportation, financial means, social support, and safety to optimize treatment efficacy and adherence. Furthermore, providing specific food examples and healthy eating pattern details is necessary for clients to translate the advice into meaningful actions (see the Clinical Applications box, "Translating Broad Terms of Advice").

team-based care approach a multidisciplinary group of health care professionals working collaboratively.

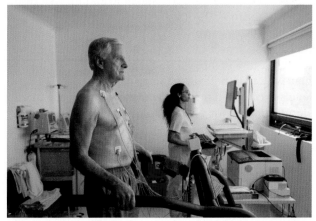

Figure 19.4 A client with a history of cardiac disease undergoing evaluation for exercise tolerance with a treadmill stress test. (Copyright iStock Photos.)

Clinical Applications

Translating Broad Terms of Advice

When health care providers recommend that their clients follow a "healthy eating pattern" (such as that outlined in Box 19.2, the Mediterranean diet, or the DASH diet) they must provide specific examples and details for their clients to translate the advice into meaningful actions. Telling a person to "eat more fruits and vegetables and replace saturated fat with monounsaturated fat" is often not definitive enough to invoke measurable changes in an otherwise typical Western diet. For example, "more" is a relative term; what would your client do with that information if he or she does not eat any plant foods? Would the addition of one serving of either fruit or vegetable make a meaningful improvement to the client's dietary risk factors? What is the health benefit if the addition of plant foods to the client's diet is French fries? Likewise, the advice to replace saturated fat with unsaturated fats may be difficult to interpret into action. What foods are your clients likely to choose if they do not know what items contain saturated fat or monounsaturated fats?

Precise and measurable healthy lifestyle recommendations that are culturally and socioeconomically sensitive are important to support change and maintain healthy behaviors. Many clients will benefit from a very specific daily menu guide to get them started on a healthier eating plan—particularly if their normal eating plan is substantially different from that of the evidence-based recommendations. The MyPlate.gov website is a great resource for menu examples and suggestions that clients can adapt to their individual needs to meet the dietary recommendations for CVD risk reduction. See Chapter 1 for additional information on MyPlate. Health care providers should refer all CVD patients to a registered dietitian nutritionist for patient-centered dietary guidance.

Drug Therapy

In the event that the LDL cholesterol level is above the goal range or an individual has multiple risk factors for CVD, the AHA/ACC *Guidelines on the Management of Blood Cholesterol* provide an algorithm for determining the appropriate lipid-lowering regimen.[4] As the number and severity of risk factors increase, so does the aggressiveness of drug therapy. For example, a person with few or no risk factors associated with CVD may wait to initiate drug therapy until LDL cholesterol levels exceed 190 mg/dL, whereas an individual with significant risk for CVD should consider drug therapy when LDL cholesterol levels rise to more than 100 mg/dL. The guidelines recommend drug therapy for the following individuals[4]:

- People with CVD or multiple risk factors who are ≤ 75 years old
- People with CVD who are >75 years old and the following contingencies are met: the patient wants treatment, there is a potential for risk reduction, and there are no significant risks for adverse events or drug-drug interactions

- People with heart failure with reduced ejection fraction resulting from ischemic heart disease and have a reasonable life expectancy

At all levels of drug therapy, the clinical practice guidelines for CVD treatment recommend the continuation of a healthy eating pattern and regular physical activity as adjunct therapy.[6]

ACUTE CARDIOVASCULAR DISEASE

When CVD progresses to the point of cutting off the blood supply to major coronary arteries, a critical vascular event (i.e., MI) may occur. It may be necessary to modify the diet during the initial acute phase of the attack to allow for healing.

Cardiac Rest

The term *infarction* means tissue death from a lack of oxygen. After infarction, the damaged heart muscle releases enzymes and proteins. These enzymes and proteins serve as cardiac markers and are one of the assessments used for diagnosis. Immediately after an MI, the health care team may treat the client with the MONA protocol (e.g., *M*orphine, supplemental *O*xygen, intravenous *N*itroglycerin, and *A*spirin). They will administer individual aspects of the MONA protocol only when indicated, with the exception of aspirin, which the patient usually receives. For example, if clients are not in pain or if their oxygen levels are normal, then morphine and/or supplemental oxygen are not necessary. The physician may prescribe other medications at this time as well such as a statin or beta-blocker. The health care team will direct all care, including the diet, toward ensuring cardiac rest to promote the return of normal functioning to the damaged heart.

Medical Nutrition Therapy for Acute Cardiovascular Disease

Medical nutrition therapy (MNT) goals for patients after MI are as follows: (1) promote recovery and strength; and (2) provide support in lowering LDL cholesterol and other known risk factors to prevent additional CVD events.[11] Initially, the dietitian may recommend diet modifications specific to energy value and texture. After the initial acute phase, dietary modifications depend on the underlying cause and other co-morbidities.

Energy. Patients experiencing a loss of appetite because of pain, medication side effects, or other complications may benefit from a brief period of reduced energy intake to reduce the metabolic workload on the damaged heart. Spreading small feedings out over the course of a day helps to decrease the level of metabolic activity that the weakened heart must perform. The client progresses to eating more as healing occurs and appetite returns to normal. During the recovery period, the dietitian will adjust the caloric intake to meet the energy needs of the client's ideal body weight.

Texture. Early feedings may include foods that are relatively soft in texture or easily digested to avoid excess effort during eating or the discomfort of gas formation. Some individuals, particularly those with poor appetite or who become short of breath from the exertion of eating, may benefit from assistance during the feeding process for a short period. Smaller and more frequent meals may provide needed nourishment without undue strain or pressure. Depending on the client's condition, he or she may benefit from avoiding gas-forming foods, caffeine-containing beverages, and hot or cold temperature extremes in both solid and liquid foods.

Long-Term Dietary Modifications

To reduce the risk for additional cardiovascular events and CVD progression, health care providers should encourage all clients who have experienced an MI to follow the dietary and lifestyle guidelines for the prevention of CVD (see Box 19.2). The Mediterranean diet and DASH diet (covered later in this chapter) are also appropriate long-term eating plans for clients with CVD who have suffered an MI.

Mediterranean diet. The basic components of a Mediterranean diet are plant-based foods; nuts; whole grains; fish and poultry, limited red meat; moderate amounts of dairy products and eggs; olive oil as the primary source of fat; the use of herbs and spices in place of salt; moderate red wine intake with meals; fresh fruit as dessert; and minimal intake of processed foods. Mediterranean lifestyles also include regular leisure time activity, physical activity, and structured exercise (see Figure 14.5). Chapter 14 provides additional details about the Mediterranean eating pattern.

Scientific studies evaluating the benefits of the Mediterranean diet are difficult to carry out and interpret because the definition of the Mediterranean diet is subjective. However, studies in areas of the world where the Mediterranean diet is the standard fare (e.g., Spain, Italy), or in studies in which participants were specifically given meal plans or provided with food, research findings are more definitive. A recent review including data from 12.8 million people found that individuals following a Mediterranean food pattern have a lower risk of mortality, neurodegenerative diseases, cancer, diabetes, cognitive impairment, and CVD.[12] Furthermore, adherence to a well-defined Mediterranean diet is associated with reduced inflammatory markers after an MI and improved endothelial function.[13,14]

Sodium. General attention to reduced sodium content in food selection is important as well (Box 19.3). Clients with hypertension may benefit from sodium restriction of 2300 mg/day or less to control edema. Using little or no salt in cooking, adding no salt when eating, and avoiding salty processed foods will help the client achieve this restriction. Nutrition Facts labels provide

---

Box 19.3	Sodium-Restricted Diet Recommendations[a]

- Choose fresh, frozen, or canned low-sodium or no-salt-added vegetables.
- Cook without salt, and avoid adding salt to prepared meals.
- Avoid salt-preserved foods such as salted or smoked meat (e.g., bacon, bacon fat, bologna, dried or chipped beef, corned beef, frankfurters, ham, kosher meats, luncheon meats, salt pork, sausage), salted or smoked fish (e.g., anchovies, caviar, salted and dried cod, herring, sardines, canned fish products), sauerkraut, and olives.[b] Use fresh poultry, fish, and lean meats instead.
- Avoid highly salted foods (e.g., crackers, pretzels, potato chips, corn chips, salted nuts, and salted popcorn). Choose foods that are lower in sodium.
- Limit processed foods and convenience foods (e.g., cheese, peanut butter, flavored rice and pasta, frozen dinners, canned soups) that are usually high in salt, or choose reduced-sodium versions.
- Limit spices and condiments such as bouillon cubes, ketchup, chili sauce, celery salt, garlic salt, onion salt, monosodium glutamate, meat sauces, meat tenderizers, pickles, prepared mustard, relishes, Worcestershire sauce, and soy sauce.[b] Choose low- or reduced-sodium or no-salt-added versions of foods and condiments, when available.

[a]These restrictions are for a mild, low-sodium diet (i.e., 2 to 4 g/day). Many clients need to reduce sodium intake further (e.g., 1.5 to 2.3 g/day).
[b]Low-sodium brands may be used.

---

specific information about the sodium content per serving of any food, and clients may use them as a tool for selectively choosing appropriate foods to include in the diet on an individual basis (see Chapter 13). Apply the MNT guidelines for acute cardiovascular disease to the Case Study box, "Myocardial Infarction."

HEART FAILURE

Congestive heart failure is a form of chronic heart disease. The progressively weakened heart muscle is unable to maintain an adequate cardiac output to sustain normal blood circulation. The resulting fluid imbalances make basic functions of living (e.g., breathing, eating, walking, sleeping) difficult to perform. The most significant risk factors for heart failure are coronary artery disease, obesity, cigarette smoking, hypertension, and diabetes.

Control of Pulmonary Edema

The goals of diet therapy for a client with congestive heart failure are to manage shortness of breath and fatigue and to control the fluid imbalance that results in **pulmonary edema**. The primary causes of fluid accumulation are altered fluid shift mechanisms and inappropriate hormonal responses.

Fluid shift mechanism. With decreased heart function, blood accumulates in the vascular system. This

See answers in Appendix A.

A 46-year-old male executive works long hours and carries the major responsibilities of his struggling small business. At his last physical checkup, the physician cautioned him about his pace because he was already exhibiting mild hypertension. In addition, his blood cholesterol level was elevated and he was overweight, with a body mass index of 28.5 kg/m². There is no history of heart disease in his family and he denies any alcohol use. At his desk job, he gets little exercise, and he finds himself smoking more and eating irregularly because of the stress of his increasing financial pressures.

1. **From the list provided, select all of the factors in the patient's history that puts him at risk for coronary heart disease.**

   a. Age
   b. Family history
   c. Elevated blood cholesterol
   d. BMI 28.5 kg/m²
   e. Desk job
   f. Smoking
   g. Working long hours with financial pressures
   h. Sex
   i. Hypertension
   j. Alcohol use
   k. Heredity
   l. Irregular diet

2. **Match each risk factor below with the correct choice describing how it increases the risk for coronary heart disease.**

RISK FACTORS	ANSWERS	RATIONALE
Increasing age		a. Diets high in saturated fat and sodium increase the risk for coronary heart disease
Elevated blood cholesterol		b. Atherosclerosis is a progressive disease that worsens over time
Poor diet quality		c. Main component of atherosclerotic plaque
Physical inactivity		d. Increases blood pressure and leads to plaque development
Smoking		e. Weight gain, hypertension, and increased cholesterol levels may come of this and lead to plaque development
Hypertension/Obesity		f. Comorbidities can contribute to further plaque development

The patient was commuting in traffic when he felt a pain in his chest and he became increasingly apprehensive. When he arrived home, the pain increased. He broke out into a cold sweat and he felt nauseated. When he became more ill after trying to eat dinner, his housemate called his physician and he was admitted into the hospital.

Test results showed elevated non-HDL-cholesterol and triglyceride levels and a low HDL cholesterol level. The electrocardiogram revealed an infarction of the posterior myocardium wall.

When the patient started eating, he could only manage consuming liquids. As his condition stabilized, the dietitian increased his diet to 1500 kcal with low saturated fat and low sodium. By the end of the first week, the dietitian increased his diet to 2000 kcal (full diet), with ≤25% of the kilocalories from fat, and replaced his dietary sources of saturated fat with monounsaturated and polyunsaturated fats.

3. **Choose the *most likely* options for the information missing from the statements below by selecting from the list of options provided.**

   Excess consumption of _____1_____ fat can lead to _____2_____ , where plaque causes narrowing of the arteries. This plaque is mostly composed of _____3_____ .

OPTION 1	OPTION 2	OPTION 3
unsaturated	atherosclerosis	triglycerides
saturated	multiple Sclerosis	cholesterol
monosaturated	osteoporosis	proteins

4. **From the list below, select all of the correct rationales for the patient's diet modification.**

   a. Excess fat may lead to atherosclerosis
   b. Saturated fat is beneficial in preventing cardiovascular disease
   c. Unsaturated fat is anti-inflammatory and protective
   d. Unsaturated fats are more shelf-stable
   e. Saturated fats increase LDL levels
   f. Unsaturated fats reduce HDL levels

After his recent myocardial infarction, the man gradually improved over the next few days and was able to go home from the hospital. The physician, the nurse, and the dietitian discussed with the patient and his housemate the need for care at home during a period of convalescence. They explained that he has dyslipidemia and that he needs to make lifestyle changes in accordance with the *ACC/AHA Guidelines on the Primary Prevention of Cardiovascular Disease* to improve his cardiometabolic health.

5. **Use an X to identify effective (helped to meet expected outcomes), or ineffective (did not help to meet expected outcomes) interventions based on the patient's condition.**

INTERVENTIONS	EFFECTIVE	INEFFECTIVE
Follow the Mediterranean Diet eating pattern		
Follow the Dietary Approach to Stop Hypertension eating pattern		
Follow a ketogenic diet		
Limit sodium to 2400 mg per day		
Consume fish twice per week		
Increase intake of refined grains		
Increase fruit and vegetable intake		
Weight gain		
Increase physical activity		

6. **From the list below, identify assessment measures that would indicate that lifestyle changes and interventions were effective for the patient.**

   a. BMI: 24 kg/m²
   b. Blood pressure: 120/80 mmHg
   c. HDL: 45 mmol/L
   d. Total cholesterol: 250 mg/dL
   e. Waist circumference: 45″
   f. Triglycerides: 175 mmol/L

buildup offsets the delicate balance of filtration pressures and causes fluid to collect within intracellular spaces instead of flowing among fluid compartments.

Hormonal alterations. Kidney nephrons sense decreased renal blood flow, which is normally an indication of dehydration and hypovolemia, and they respond by triggering the vasopressin and renin-angiotensin-aldosterone systems to increase blood pressure (see Chapter 9). Unlike dehydration, inadequate pumping of the heart causes reduced blood flow but not hypovolemia. Vasopressin from the pituitary gland, which we also know as *antidiuretic hormone,* stimulates the resorption of water in the kidneys. In addition, the adrenal glands secrete aldosterone, which causes the resorption of sodium (and thus water) in the kidneys. Consequently, an increase in fluid retention exacerbates edema by inducing hypervolemia.

Medical Nutrition Therapy for Heart Failure

MNT guidelines for patients suffering from heart failure focus on achieving nutritional adequacy of the diet while limiting sodium and fluid intake to control edema.[11]

The main source of dietary sodium is common table salt or sodium chloride. Humans acquire the taste for salt. Some people heavily salt their food out of habit without tasting it first, thereby habituating their taste to high salt levels. Others acquire a taste for less salt by gradually using smaller and smaller amounts. The Adequate Intake for sodium is 1500 mg/d for adults. In 2019 the DRI committees established 2300 mg/d as the maximum intake for **chronic disease risk reduction** (i.e., adults should not consume more than 2300 mg/d of sodium to reduce their risk for chronic disease).[15] Daily adult intakes of sodium range widely in the typical American diet; men consume an average of 4107 mg/day, and women consume an average of 3007 mg/day.[16] Other than the individual use of salt while cooking or adding it to food while eating, food manufacturers extensively use sodium as a preservative in processed food. Remaining sources of sodium include that found as a naturally occurring mineral in certain foods.

MNT guidelines focus on the following[11]:

- *Sodium restriction (2 g per day):* For those with moderate to severe heart failure. Fresh foods are encouraged and should include sodium-free flavorings such as herbs. Patients should avoid salty processed foods (e.g., pickles, olives, bacon, ham, corn chips, potato chips) and added salt at mealtime. Box 19.4 provides options for no/low-sodium seasoning that clients may find helpful for flavoring their food.
- *Fluid restriction:* Fluid is limited to 2 L per day for individuals with serum sodium levels less than 130 mEq/L.
- *Dietary supplements:* Clients may need thiamin and/or potassium supplements to overcome losses from diuretic medications. The dietitian should evaluate

the diet to ensure clients are meeting their DRIs for folate, vitamin B_{12}, and magnesium through food and/or dietary supplements.

- *Alcohol:* Alcohol intake is limited to one drink per day for women and two drinks per day for men in adults who regularly consume alcohol. The patient must completely avoid alcohol if alcohol contributed to their heart disease.

Clients may tolerate soft foods better if eating is laborious or uncomfortable. Frequent small meals (e.g., five to six per day) are better suited than large meals to prevent fatigue from eating. The dietitian should evaluate the diet to ensure that restrictions do not result in nutrient inadequacies in the diet.

HYPERTENSION

INCIDENCE AND NATURE

Hypertension is one of the most common vascular diseases worldwide, and experts estimate that the majority of people will develop hypertension during their advanced years. We frequently refer to hypertension as "the silent killer," because no signs indicate its presence. Without detection, treatment, and control, hypertension can have deleterious and lethal health effects. Using the diagnostic standards for hypertension established in 2017, 46% of American adults (≥20 years old) have hypertension (Figure 19.5), and many of them are unaware of their condition.[17] Of the adults with hypertension, about half of them do not yet have their blood pressure under control. The incidence of hypertension is higher among black or African-Americans than in whites, Hispanics, or Asian-Americans.[1]

When speaking of the chronic condition of elevated blood pressure, the term *hypertension* is more appropriate than *high blood pressure,* because blood pressure may occasionally be elevated during situations that involve overexertion, anxiety, or stress. Box 19.5 provides common modifiable and nonmodifiable risk factors for **essential (or primary) hypertension**, the predominant form of hypertension. **Secondary hypertension** is a symptom or a side effect of another primary condition. For example, individuals with kidney disease often have secondary hypertension. Approximately 10% of hypertensive

---

congestive heart failure a chronic condition of gradually weakening heart muscle; the muscle is unable to pump normal blood through the heart-lung circulation, which results in the congestion of fluids in the lungs.

pulmonary edema an accumulation of fluid in the lung tissues.

chronic disease risk reduction (CDRR) a new category within the Dietary Reference Intakes that identifies the level of intake for which there is sufficient evidence to characterize a reduced risk for chronic disease. Sodium is the first nutrient to have an established CDRR.

| Box **19.4** | **Suggestions for No/Low-Sodium Seasoning** |

FISH

Breaded, battered fillets
  Dry mustard, onion, oregano, basil, garlic, thyme
Broiled steaks or fillets
  Chili or curry powder, tarragon
Fish cakes
  Tarragon, savory, dry mustard, white pepper, red pepper, oregano

BEEF

Swiss steak
  Rosemary, black pepper, bay leaf, thyme, clove
Roast beef
  Basil, oregano, bay leaf, nutmeg, tarragon, marjoram
Beef stew
  Chili powder, bay leaf, tarragon, caraway, marjoram
Beef stroganoff
  Red pepper, onion, garlic, nutmeg, curry powder

POULTRY AND VEAL

Roast chicken or turkey
  Ginger, garlic, onion, thyme, tarragon
Chicken croquettes
  Dill, curry, chili, cumin, tarragon, oregano
Veal patties
  Italian seasoning, tarragon, dill, onion, sesame seeds
Barbecue chicken
  Garlic, dry mustard, clove, allspice, basil, oregano

GRAVIES AND SAUCES

Barbecue
  Bay leaf, thyme, red pepper, cinnamon, ginger, allspice, dry mustard, chili powder
Brown
  Chervil, onion, bay leaf, thyme, nutmeg, tarragon
Chicken
  Dry mustard, ginger, garlic, marjoram, thyme, bay leaf

SOUPS

Chicken
  Thyme, savory, ginger, clove, white pepper, allspice
Clam chowder
  Basil, oregano, nutmeg, white pepper, thyme, garlic powder
Mushroom
  Ginger, oregano, thyme, tarragon, bay leaf, black pepper, chili powder
Onion
  Curry, caraway, marjoram, garlic, cloves

Tomato
  Bay leaf, thyme, Italian seasoning, oregano, onion, nutmeg
Vegetable
  Italian seasoning, paprika, caraway, rosemary, thyme, fennel

SALADS

Chicken
  Curry or chili powder, Italian seasoning, thyme, tarragon
Coleslaw
  Dill, caraway, poppy seeds, dry mustard, ginger
Fish or seafood
  Dill, tarragon, ginger, dry mustard, red pepper, onion, garlic
Macaroni
  Dill, basil, thyme, oregano, dry mustard, garlic
Potato
  Chili powder, curry, dry mustard, onion

PASTA, BEANS, AND RICE

Baked beans
  Dry mustard, chili powder, clove, onion, ginger
Rice and vegetables
  Curry, thyme, onion, paprika, rosemary, garlic, ginger
Spanish rice
  Cumin, oregano, basil, Italian seasoning
Spaghetti
  Italian seasoning, nutmeg, oregano, basil, red pepper, tarragon
Rice pilaf
  Dill, thyme, savory, black pepper

VEGETABLES

Asparagus
  Ginger, sesame seeds, basil, onion
Broccoli
  Italian seasoning, marjoram, basil, nutmeg, onion, sesame seeds
Cabbage
  Caraway, onion, nutmeg, allspice, clove
Carrots
  Ginger, nutmeg, onion, dill
Cauliflower
  Dry mustard, basil, paprika, onion
Tomatoes
  Oregano, chili powder, dill, onion
Spinach
  Savory, thyme, nutmeg, garlic, onion

---

cases are due to secondary hypertension, and a small number of cases result from genetic mutations.

A family history of hypertension significantly increases one's risk of developing hypertension. Children of hypertensive parents are more likely to develop hypertension as early as their first decade of life; and hypertension during childhood and adolescence is strongly associated with pervasive hypertension throughout life.[18,19] Obesity worsens the condition through a multitude of pathways, including inflammation, oxidative stress, renal damage, altered blood circulation, impaired endocrine response, endothelial injury, and sympathetic nervous system dysfunction.[20,21] Smoking also increases blood pressure

through nicotine-induced vasoconstriction and the promotion of plaque formation, which further restricts blood flow.[9] Other risk factors include excessive alcohol consumption, high sodium intake, and insufficient dietary potassium, magnesium, calcium, vegetable-derived protein, fiber, and unsaturated fat from fish.[17]

essential (or primary) hypertension an inherent form of high blood pressure with no specific identifiable cause; it is considered to be familial.

secondary hypertension an elevated blood pressure for which the cause can be identified and that is a symptom or side effect of another primary condition.

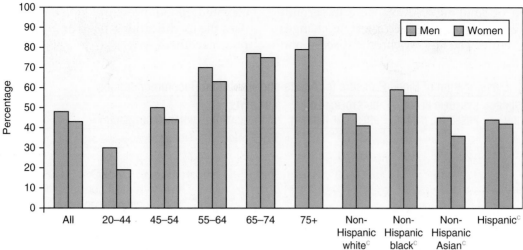

Prevalence of hypertension (SBP/DBP ≥130/80 mm Hg) or taking antihypertensive medication[a,b]

SBP: systolic blood pressure
DBP: diastolic blood pressure
[a]The prevalence estimates have been rounded to the nearest full percentage. Prevalence of hypertension based on 2 SBP/DBP thresholds.
[b]Adjusted to the 2010 age-sex distribution of the US adult population.
[c]Includes adults ≥20 years of age of specified ethnicity.

Figure 19.5 Hypertension among adults aged 20 years and older, by sex, age, and ethnicity: United States. (Source: Whelton, P. K., et al. [2018]. 2017 ACC/AHA/AAPA/ABC/ACPM/AGS/APhA/ASH/ASPC/NMA/PCNA guideline for the prevention, detection, evaluation, and management of high blood pressure in adults: A report of the American College of Cardiology/American Heart Association Task Force on Clinical Practice Guidelines. *Hypertension, 71*[6], e13–e115.)

HIGH BLOOD PRESSURE LEVELS

Blood pressure measurements indicate the pressure of the blood surge in the arteries of the upper arm with each heartbeat. Health care providers measure the power of each surge in millimeters of mercury (mm Hg). The numerator of the fraction measures the force of the blood surge when the heart contracts, which we know as the *systolic pressure*. The denominator of the fraction measures the pressure that remains in the arteries when the heart relaxes between beats; we know this as the *diastolic pressure*. A normal blood pressure for adults is less than 120/80 mm Hg. Current hypertension screening and treatment paradigms identify people with hypertension according to the degree of severity and existing co-morbidities (Table 19.2).[17] The health care team will then determine the appropriate care plan, along with the patient, after considering confounding factors.

Elevated Blood Pressure

We identify individuals with blood pressure measurements that are above normal but are not so high as to meet the diagnostic criteria for hypertension, as having *elevated blood pressure* (also known as prehypertension). It is similar in this regard to prediabetes. The assumption is that without intervention, the client will likely progress to stage 1 hypertension.

The primary focus of hypertension treatment is lifestyle modifications. Lifestyle choices that the American College of Cardiology (ACC) and the

| Box **19.5** | Risk Factors for Hypertension |

MODIFIABLE RISK FACTORS
- Smoking and exposure to secondhand smoke
- Type 2 diabetes mellitus
- Hypercholesterolemia
- Overweight/obesity
- Sedentary behaviors and physical inactivity
- Poor diet quality

RISK FACTORS THAT ARE DIFFICULT TO CHANGE
- Low socioeconomic status
- Low education
- Obstructive sleep apnea
- Chronic kidney disease
- Psychosocial stress

NONMODIFIABLE RISK FACTORS
- Family history
- Race/ethnicity
- Increasing age
- Male sex

From Whelton, P. K., et al. (2018). 2017 ACC/AHA/AAPA/ABC/ACPM/AGS/APhA/ASH/ASPC/NMA/PCNA guideline for the prevention, detection, evaluation, and management of high blood pressure in adults: A report of the American College of Cardiology/American Heart Association Task Force on Clinical Practice Guidelines. *Hypertension, 71*(6), e13–e115.

American Heart Association (AHA) *Clinical Practice Guidelines on the Detection, Evaluation and Treatment of High Blood Pressure in Adults* recommend include the following: (1) weight loss, if indicated; (2) adopting a heart-healthy diet such as the DASH diet; (3) reduced sodium intake; (4) increase potassium intake;

(5) moderation of alcohol use; (6) regular physical activity with a structured exercise program; and (7) cessation of smoking and exposure to second-hand smoke, if indicated.[17] Such lifestyle changes are able to reduce the risk of chronic disease and measurably improve blood pressure (Table 19.3). These recommendations apply to all people with elevated blood pressure, whether the individual uses the modifications alone or in combination with pharmacotherapy.

Table 19.2 Classification of Blood Pressure for Adults and Treatment Recommendations[a]

BLOOD PRESSURE CLASSIFICATION	SYSTOLIC BLOOD PRESSURE (MM HG)	DIASTOLIC BLOOD PRESSURE (MM HG)	LIFESTYLE MODIFICATION	PHARMACOTHERAPY
Normal	<120	and <80	Encourage	Not applicable
Elevated[b]	120–129	and <80	Yes	Not indicated. Reassess in 3 to 6 months.
Stage 1 Hypertension	130–139	or 80–89	Yes	If patient's 10-year CVD risk[c] is <10%, the first-line therapy is strict adherence to lifestyle modifications and reassessment in 3 to 6 months. If patient has diagnosed atherosclerotic CVD or elevated 10-year CVD risk (≥10%), health care provider will initiate hypotensive medication and reassess patient in 1 month.
Stage 2 Hypertension	≥140	or ≥90	Yes	Hypotensive medication initiated. Reassess in 1 month. If goal not achieved, health care provider will adjust dose and/or add other medications to treatment regime.

[a]Based on an average of ≥2 measurements obtained on ≥2 occasions. The highest blood pressure category determines the treatment protocol.
[b]The blood pressure is above optimal levels but not high enough for the health care provider to diagnose the client with hypertension.
[c]10-year Atherosclerotic Cardiovascular Disease Risk Estimator (tools.acc.org/ASCVD-Risk-Estimator-Plus/#!/calculate/estimate/).
Modified from Whelton, P. K., et al. (2018). 2017 ACC/AHA/AAPA/ABC/ACPM/AGS/APhA/ASH/ASPC/NMA/PCNA guideline for the prevention, detection, evaluation, and management of high blood pressure in adults: A report of the American College of Cardiology/American Heart Association Task Force on Clinical Practice Guidelines. *Hypertension, 71*(6), e13–e115.

Table 19.3 Best Proven Lifestyle Interventions for Prevention and Treatment of Hypertension[a]

LIFESTYLE INTERVENTION	GOAL	APPROXIMATE IMPACT ON SBP	
		HYPERTENSION	NORMOTENSION
Weight/body fat loss	The best goal is to achieve an ideal body weight, but aim for at least a 1-kg reduction in body weight for most adults who are overweight. Expect about 1 mm Hg for every 1-kg reduction in body weight.	–5 mm Hg	–2 to 3 mm Hg
Healthy diet (e.g., DASH dietary pattern)	Consume a diet rich in fruits, vegetables, whole grains, and low-fat dairy products, with reduced content of saturated and total fat.	–11 mm Hg	–3 mm Hg
Reduced dietary sodium intake	Optimal goal is <1500 mg/d, but aim for at least a 1000-mg/d reduction in most adults.	–5 to 6 mm Hg	–2 to 3 mm Hg
Enhanced dietary potassium intake	Aim for 3500–5000 mg/d, preferably by consumption of a diet rich in potassium.	–4 to 5 mm Hg	–2 mm Hg
Aerobic exercise	90–150 minutes per week 65%–75% heart rate reserve[b]	–5 to 8 mm Hg	–2 to 4 mm Hg
Dynamic resistance exercise	90–150 minutes per week 50%–80% 1 rep maximum 6 exercises, 3 sets/exercise, 10 repetitions/set	–4 mm Hg	–2 mm Hg
Isometric resistance exercise	4 × 2 min (hand grip), 1 min rest between exercises, 30%–40% maximum voluntary contraction, 3 session per week 8–10 weeks	–5 mm Hg	–4 mm Hg
Moderation in alcohol intake	In individuals who drink alcohol, reduce alcohol[c] to: Men ≤2 drinks daily, women ≤1 drink daily	–4 mm Hg	–3 mm Hg

[a]Type, dose, and expected impact on BP in adults with a normal BP and with hypertension.
[b]Heart rate reserve is the difference between resting heart rate and maximum heart rate.
[c]In the United States, one "standard" drink contains roughly 14 g of pure alcohol, which is typically found in 12 oz of regular beer (usually about 5% alcohol), 5 oz of wine (usually about 12% alcohol), and 1.5 oz of distilled spirits (usually about 40% alcohol).
DASH, Dietary Approaches to Stop Hypertension; *SBP,* systolic blood pressure.
Modified from Whelton, P. K., et al. (2018). 2017 ACC/AHA/AAPA/ABC/ACPM/AGS/APhA/ASH/ASPC/NMA/PCNA guideline for the prevention, detection, evaluation, and management of high blood pressure in adults: A report of the American College of Cardiology/American Heart Association Task Force on Clinical Practice Guidelines. *Hypertension, 71*(6), e13–e115.

Stage 1 Hypertension

In addition to the healthy lifestyle modifications prescribed for individuals with elevated blood pressure, the health care team may include blood pressure–lowering medications (i.e., hypotensive or antihypertensive medications) as part of the treatment plan, depending on co-morbidities. Table 19.2 provides the ACC/AHA guidelines' summary for initiating drug therapy in response to hypertensive stage.

Diuretics are one of the first-line medications used to lower blood pressure. The continuous use of some diuretic drugs may cause a loss of potassium along with the increased loss of water from the body. Because potassium is necessary for maintaining normal heart muscle action, depletion could become dangerous. Potassium replacement is sometimes necessary. Dietary replacement with the increased use of potassium-rich foods (e.g., fruits, especially bananas and orange juice; vegetables; legumes; nuts; whole grains) is an important part of therapy. Appendix C provides the sodium and potassium values of various foods. Dietary supplements may be necessary for individuals unable to meet potassium needs through foods alone. However, the decision to use potassium supplements should be part of the overall treatment plan approved by the health care team because hyperkalemia is a concern for some patients (see Chapter 8).

Stage 2 Hypertension

In addition to the lifestyle modifications for stage 1 hypertension, vigorous drug therapy is necessary for stage 2 hypertension treatment. The ACC/AHA guidelines provide practitioners with a detailed algorithm for initiating and evaluating drug therapy efficacy for hypertension management.[17] See the Drug-Nutrient Interaction box titled "Grapefruit Juice and Drug Metabolism" for more information about potential interactions with the medications that are often used for hypertension and CVD. Nutrition therapy is important for all levels of hypertension, along with other nondrug therapies such as physical activity, smoking cessation, and moderating alcohol use.

MEDICAL NUTRITION THERAPY FOR HYPERTENSION

Regardless of hypertensive stage, all patients should receive patient-centered, culturally sensitive guidance on achieving applicable behavioral and lifestyle

---

 Drug-Nutrient Interaction

Grapefruit Juice and Drug Metabolism

KELLI BOI

A common pathway for drug metabolism makes use of the enzyme CYP3A. This enzyme oxidizes lipid-soluble drugs, thereby making them more water soluble in preparation for urinary excretion. As the enzyme oxidizes more of the drug, less of the medication is bioavailable for its intended action. Scientists anticipate the enzyme action when calculating the necessary drug dosage and know that only a percentage of the therapeutic agent will actually reach the circulation.

Compounds in grapefruit juice known as *furanocoumarins* inhibit CYP3A, thereby increasing the amount of the associated drug that enters the circulation. As little as 8 oz of grapefruit juice can increase the absorption of certain drugs for up to 72 hours after consumption. The increased absorption of these medications may cause adverse events and can be fatal. Clients essentially experience drug toxicity from their prescribed dose because of the drastic increase in absorption of the active ingredient.

Several cardiovascular drugs make use of the CYP3A pathway for metabolism. The table below shows some of the cardiovascular agents susceptible to grapefruit's inhibition of CYP3A and the associated side effect. Hospitals and inpatient facilities do not serve grapefruit juice, and clients who are taking drugs that use the CYP3A pathway for metabolism should avoid drinking grapefruit juice at home.

DRUG NAME	DRUG CLASS AND ACTION	SIDE EFFECTS	ADDITIONAL COMMENTS
Amiodarone (Cordarone)	Antiarrhythmic; broad-spectrum antiarrhythmic, vasodilator	Anorexia, nausea, vomiting, constipation	High levels may cause fatal pulmonary toxicity
Amlodipine (Norvasc) Nifedipine (Procardia) Nisoldipine	Calcium channel blockers; antihypertensive	Nausea, dyspepsia, constipation, peripheral edema, muscle cramps, flushing	Alternative calcium channel blockers (e.g., verapamil) are available that do not interact with grapefruit juice
Atorvastatin (Lipitor) Lovastatin (Mevacor) Simvastatin (Zocor)	3-hydroxy-3-methylglutaryl coenzyme A inhibitors/statins; antihyperlipidemic	Nausea, dyspepsia, abdominal pain, constipation, diarrhea, possible myopathy	Alternative medications in this class are available that do not have significant interactions with grapefruit juice (e.g., fluvastatin, pravastatin, rosuvastatin)

modifications such as those provided on pages 357-358. These lifestyle interventions are the foundation for treatment. Hypertension is one of the most critical risk factors for CVD and stroke. Thus, the American Heart Association's dietary and lifestyle recommendations to reduce the risk for CVD (see Box 19.2) serve as the standard recommendations for all adults. In addition, the following recommendations are specifically encouraged for adults who would benefit from lowering their blood pressure.

Weight Management

In accordance with individual need, weight management requires losing excess body fat and maintaining a healthy weight for one's stature. Chapter 15 discusses sound approaches to managing weight loss, and Chapter 16 provides guidance for increasing physical activity. Because excess weight is closely associated with hypertension risk factors, a wisely planned personal program of weight reduction and physical activity is the cornerstone of therapy. The ACC/AHA guidelines note that weight loss (when applicable) is *the* most important intervention for treating hypertension.[17] Drastic weight loss is not necessary to realize the benefits. Overweight clients can expect their systolic blood pressure to decrease by 1 mm Hg, on average, for every 1 kg of weight loss.[17] For example, an overweight/obese person with a systolic blood pressure measurement of 130 mm Hg (stage 1 hypertension) would need to lose approximately 10 kg to achieve a blood pressure within normal range.

Physical Activity

Participating in regular physical activity is important throughout all life-cycle stages for general health and fitness. Participating in at least 30 minutes of aerobic physical activity on most days of the week can lower systolic blood pressure by 5 to 8 mm Hg in hypertensive individuals. The ACC/AHA treatment guidelines recommend that clients engage in a combination of moderate- to vigorous-intensity aerobic activity, dynamic resistance exercises, and isometric resistance exercises to lower blood pressure (see Table 19.3).[17] For some clients, the combined benefits of weight loss and physical activity are enough to correct for chronically elevated blood pressure and allow them to discontinue pharmacotherapy.

The DASH Diet

The DASH diet is the result of the successful Dietary Approaches to Stop Hypertension landmark study, which was able to lower blood pressure significantly by diet alone within a 2-week period.[22] The diet recommends eating 4 to 6 servings of fruits, 4 to 6 servings of vegetables, and 2 to 3 servings of low-fat dairy foods per day in addition to lean meats, nuts, seeds, dried beans, and high-fiber grains.

Individuals who follow the diet have an overall decreased incidence of CVD, coronary heart disease, and stroke and significantly lower blood pressure, total cholesterol, LDL cholesterol, fasting blood insulin, HbA1c (a marker of glucose levels), and body weight.[22-24] When the DASH diet is combined with a low-sodium diet, the blood–pressure-lowering effects are substantially greater.[25] Thus, the DASH diet has many benefits beyond just blood pressure control.

The ACC/AHA guidelines endorse the DASH diet as one method to achieve the lifestyle modifications to manage blood pressure nonpharmacologically. Experts recommend the DASH diet for individuals with high blood pressure, blood pressure in the elevated range, and a family history of high blood pressure; they also recommend it for those who are trying to eliminate the use of blood-pressure–lowering medications.[17] The first step in following the DASH diet is to determine the appropriate energy level (in kilocalories) based on the desired weight and activity level (see Chapter 6). The total energy needs determine the appropriate number of servings per day of each food group. Table 19.4 outlines the DASH diet and its associated serving sizes; Box 19.6 provides a 1-day sample menu for a 2000-calorie diet.

Sodium Restriction

There is a direct correlation between sodium intake and blood pressure (i.e., a low sodium intake lowers blood pressure), even in children and adults with **resistant hypertension**.[26-30] Although scientists do not yet clearly understand the mechanisms involved, experts believe that about half of the population with hypertension and a quarter of normotensive individuals are *salt-sensitive*, which means that their dietary sodium intake significantly and rapidly affects their blood pressure.[31-33] Subsequently, all dietary guidelines include the ubiquitous recommendation to restrict dietary sodium intake to 1500 to 2300 mg/day for blood pressure control.[6,11,15,17,34] However, achieving a palatable diet with sodium restrictions set at less than 2 g/day may be difficult for clients who rely heavily on processed foods. Keep in mind that 2.3 g of sodium is equivalent to approximately 5.75 g of sodium chloride (i.e., table salt). See Box 19.3 for ideas on ways to limit sodium intake.

Potassium

There is an inverse association between potassium intake and blood pressure (i.e., high potassium intake lowers

---

resistant hypertension the presence of high blood pressure despite treatment with three antihypertensive medications.

Table 19.4   The DASH Eating Plan

CALORIES PER DAY	GRAINS[a]	VEGETABLES	FRUITS	FAT-FREE OR LOW-FAT MILK AND MILK PRODUCTS	LEAN MEATS, POULTRY, AND FISH	NUTS, SEEDS, AND LEGUMES	FATS AND OILS[b]	SWEETS AND ADDED SUGARS
				SERVINGS PER DAY (UNLESS OTHERWISE SPECIFIED)				
1600	6	3 to 4	4	2 to 3	3 to 6	3 per week	2	0
2000	6 to 8	4 to 5	4 to 5	2 to 3	≤6	4 to 5 per week	2 to 3	≤5 per week
2600	10 to 11	5 to 6	5 to 6	3	6	1	3	≤2
3100	12 to 13	6	6	3 to 4	6 to 9	1	4	≤2
Serving sizes	1 slice bread; 1 oz dry cereal[c]; ½ cup cooked rice, pasta, or cereal	1 cup raw leafy vegetables, ½ cup cut-up raw or cooked vegetables, ½ cup vegetable juice	1 medium fruit; ¼ cup dried fruit; ½ cup fresh, frozen, or canned fruit; ½ cup fruit juice	1 cup milk or yogurt, 1½ oz cheese	1 oz cooked meat, poultry, or fish; 1 egg[d]	⅓ cup or 1½ oz nuts, 2 Tbsp peanut butter, 2 Tbsp or ½ oz seeds, ½ cup cooked legumes (dry beans and peas)	1 tsp soft margarine, 1 tsp vegetable oil, 1 Tbsp mayonnaise, 2 Tbsp salad dressing	1 Tbsp sugar, 1 Tbsp jelly or jam, ½ cup sorbet, gelatin; 1 cup lemonade

[a]Experts recommend whole grains for most grain servings as a good source of fiber and nutrients.
[b]Fat content changes the serving amount for fats and oils. For example, 1 Tbsp of regular salad dressing equals one serving, whereas 1 Tbsp of a low-fat dressing equals a half serving and 1 Tbsp of a fat-free dressing equals zero servings.
[c]Serving sizes vary between ½ cup and 1¼ cups, depending on the cereal type. Check the product's Nutrition Facts label.
[d]Because eggs are high in cholesterol, limit egg yolk intake to no more than four per week; two egg whites have the same protein content as 1 oz of meat.
Modified from National Heart, Lung, and Blood Institute. (2006). *Your guide to lowering your blood pressure with DASH* (NIH Publication No. 06-4082). Washington, DC: U.S. Department of Health and Human Services, National Institutes of Health.

| Box 19.6 | Sample 1-Day Menu on the Dash Diet, 2000 Calories |

BREAKFAST
- ¾ cup bran flakes cereal
- 1 medium banana
- 1 cup low-fat milk
- 1 slice whole-wheat bread
- 1 tsp unsalted soft margarine
- 1 cup orange juice

LUNCH
- ¾ cup chicken salad
- 2 slices whole-wheat bread
- 1 Tbsp Dijon mustard
- Salad with the following:
  - ½ cup fresh cucumber slices
  - ½ cup tomato wedges
  - 1 Tbsp sunflower seeds
  - 1 tsp Italian dressing, low calorie
- ½ cup fruit cocktail, juice packed

DINNER
- 3 oz beef, eye of round
- 2 Tbsp beef gravy, fat free
- 1 cup green beans, sautéed with ½ tsp canola oil
- 1 small baked potato with the following:
  - 1 Tbsp sour cream, fat free
  - 1 Tbsp grated natural cheddar cheese, reduced fat
  - 1 Tbsp chopped scallions
- 1 small whole-wheat roll
- 1 tsp unsalted soft margarine
- 1 small apple
- 1 cup low-fat milk

SNACKS
- ⅓ cup almonds, unsalted
- ¼ cup raisins
- ½ cup fruit yogurt, fat free, no sugar added

Modified from National Heart, Lung, and Blood Institute. (2006). *Your guide to lowering your blood pressure with DASH* (NIH Publication No. 06-4082). Washington, DC: U.S. Department of Health and Human Services, National Institutes of Health.

blood pressure) in hypertensive individuals.[30,35] Because a diet rich in potassium-containing fruits and vegetables (e.g., DASH diet) reduces the risk for hypertension as well as other chronic disease, the current guidelines for managing blood pressure promote the use of whole foods and an overall heart-healthy diet instead of relying exclusively on dietary supplements to meet potassium needs.[17] The recommendation for a potassium-rich diet is also part of the *Dietary Guidelines for Americans, 2020-2025* and the guidelines for CVD prevention.[6,34]

Other Nutrients

The ACC/AHA Task Force concluded that there is insufficient evidence available at this time to determine a specific and independent relationship between hypertension and dietary intake of nutrients such as magnesium and calcium.[17]

ADDITIONAL LIFESTYLE MODIFICATIONS

The ACC/AHA guidelines recommend limiting alcohol intake to no more than two drinks per day for men and one drink per day for most women and smaller men. One alcoholic drink is equal to 12 oz of regular beer, 5 oz of wine, or 1.5 oz of 80-proof whiskey. Moderation of alcohol intake is associated with a reduction of systolic blood pressure by 4 mm Hg.[17]

Additional lifestyle factors that are associated with hypertension include smoking, exposure to second-hand smoke, and chronic psychosocial stress.[17,36,37] Smoking cessation and avoiding environmental cigarette smoke exposure are accessible lifestyle modifications that can reduce the burden of CVD considerably. Psychosocial stress, mental stress, and emotional stress are typical aspects of adult life. However, chronic stress takes a toll on the body and may lead to elevated blood pressure in susceptible people.[37] Unfortunately, stress-reducing techniques (e.g., meditation, yoga) have been unsuccessful in reducing blood pressure in clinical trials thus far.[38,39]

EDUCATION AND PREVENTION

Education and disease prevention are concepts that are extremely important in our aging population. Many diseases covered in this text are preventable through modified diet and lifestyle behaviors alone. As such, the topics covered in this section are applicable for all preventable chronic diseases, not just CVD. Because CVD is the primary cause of death in the United States, we will cover the topic in this chapter.

NUTRITION EDUCATION

Food Planning and Purchasing

The *Dietary Guidelines for Americans, 2020-2025* (see Figure 1.5) and the MyPlate Guidelines (see Figure 1.4) provides basic outlines for sound food habits.[34] The American Heart Association and the Academy of Nutrition and Dietetics also provide heart-healthy eating resources online at www.heart.org (search "healthy eating"), and www.eatright.org (search "hypertension"), respectively.

An important part of purchasing food is carefully reading food labels. The Nutrition Facts labels provide basic nutrition information in a standard format that is easily recognized and clearly expressed. All food products that make health claims must follow the strict guidelines provided by the U.S. Food and Drug Administration. A good general guide is to use fresh, whole foods primarily, with a limited selection of processed foods when necessary. See Chapter 13 for background material regarding food supply and Nutrition Facts labels.

Food Preparation

The public is more aware than ever before of the need to prepare foods with less saturated fat, trans fat, and salt. Consequently, the cookbook industry has responded by providing an abundance of guides and recipes for various age groups and customs. Many seasonings (e.g., herbs, spices, lemon, wine, onion, garlic, nonfat milk and yogurt, fat-free/low-sodium broth) can help to train taste preferences for less sodium. We can use less animal products overall, and in leaner and smaller portions, combined with complex carbohydrate foods (e.g., potatoes, winter squash, rice, bulgur, and legumes) to make more healthful main dishes. Whole-grain breads and cereals provide needed fiber, and an increased use of fish adds healthier forms of fat. Encourage the creative use of a variety of vegetables and fruits to add interest, taste appeal, and nourishment to meals. The American Heart Association publishes several cookbooks that are excellent guides to lighter, more tasteful and healthier food preparation (www.shopheart.org).

Person-Centered Approach

The individual adaptation of diet principles is important in all nutrition teaching and counseling. Health care providers must give special attention to personal desires, ethnic diets, economic restrictions, food availability, and dietary habits (see Chapter 14). Effective diet planning must meet both personal and health needs. The most effective lifestyle changes are the ones that are reasonable, sustainable, and include the whole family.

PRINCIPLES OF EDUCATION

Starting Early

The prevention of hypertension and heart disease begins during childhood, especially with children from high-risk families. National data indicate that 20% of youths aged 6 to 19 years have at least one adverse lipid level.[40,41] Furthermore, total cholesterol, LDL cholesterol, and triglyceride levels are substantially higher in overweight and obese children than in non-overweight children.[42] Preventive measures in family food habits relate to healthy weight maintenance, regular physical activity, and the limited use of foods that are high in salt, saturated fats, and trans fats. For children and adults with poor CVD indicators (e.g., lipid levels, blood pressure) or diagnosed heart disease, learning should be an integral part of all therapy.

If a CVD-related event occurs, such as a heart attack or stroke, nutrition and lifestyle education should begin early during convalescence rather than at hospital discharge. This practice helps clients and their families establish clear and practical knowledge regarding positive lifestyle necessities and allows time for questions and guidance on additional outpatient resources.

Focusing on High-Risk Groups

Health care providers should especially direct education about heart disease and hypertension toward individuals with one or more high-risk factor (see Box 19.1). For example, the prevalence of premature cardiovascular mortality is significantly higher in certain high-risk populations, including Native American and South Asian Americans, individuals with low education, those with low socioeconomic resources, and overweight/obese individuals.[1] See the Cultural Considerations box, "Influence of Sociodemographics on Prevalence of Heart Disease," for more information on high-risk groups.

Using a Variety of Resources

As researchers learn more about heart disease and hypertension, the American Heart Association and other health agencies are able to provide many excellent resources. The Academy of Nutrition and Dietetics provides a website (www.eatright.org) for the public as well as for health professionals with helpful client education tools, several of which are applicable to heart disease. As professionals and the public have become more aware of health needs and disease prevention, an increasing number of resources and programs are available in most communities. These include various weight-management programs, registered dietitian nutritionists in private practice or in health care centers that provide nutrition counseling, and practical food-preparation materials found in a number of "light cuisine" cooking classes and cookbooks. Bookstores and public libraries as well as health education libraries in health centers and clinics provide an abundance of materials that address health promotion and self-care.

🌐 Cultural Considerations

Influence of Sociodemographics on Prevalence of Heart Disease

Although the death rate from heart disease has declined substantially since the 1960s, it is still the leading cause of death in the United States. The major conditions of heart disease, hypertension, and high blood cholesterol are more prevalent among individuals within certain sociodemographic categories in the United States. Some CVD risk factors are nonmodifiable (e.g., race, sex), some are modifiable but difficult to change (e.g., education and poverty level), and others are readily changeable with support and access to heathier options (e.g., dietary and physical activity habits). Note the correlation for CVD prevalence between education level and poverty level in the figure below.

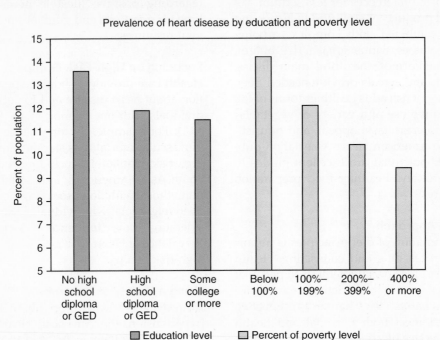

(From National Center for Health Statistics. [2018]. *Health, United States, 2017: With special feature on mortality*. Hyattsville, MD: National Center for Health Statistics [U.S.].)

Recognizing environmental and genetic factors associated with disease risk is important to help identify the modifiable contributors to disease etiology. Only after recognizing those factors can health care providers direct prevention and treatment programs on an individual basis. A complex combination of sociodemographic risk factors such as education level, annual household income, and employment status contribute to an individual's risk for death from CVD. By acknowledging the risks associated with such factors and directing education and resources toward high-risk populations, health care providers may detect warning signs earlier.

Putting It All Together

Summary

- Coronary heart disease is the leading cause of death in the United States. Atherosclerosis is the underlying blood vessel disease. If fatty buildup on the interior surfaces of the blood vessels becomes severe, it cuts off the supply of oxygen and nutrients to the cells, which in turn die. When this occurs in a major coronary artery, the result is an MI.
- The risk for atherosclerosis increases with the amount and type of blood lipids and lipoproteins in circulation.
- Current recommendations to help prevent coronary heart disease involve inclusion of a healthy and balanced diet, weight management, and increased physical activity.
- Dietary recommendations for acute CVD include measures to ensure cardiac rest. People with chronic heart disease involving congestive heart failure benefit from a low-sodium diet to control pulmonary edema.
- People with hypertension may improve their condition with weight control, exercise, sodium restriction, and a diet that is rich in fruits, vegetables, whole grains, lean meats, and low-fat dairy products.

Chapter Review Questions

See answers in Appendix A.

1. High serum level of which of the following lipoproteins is protective against CVD?

   a. HDL cholesterol
   b. LDL cholesterol
   c. Triglycerides
   d. VLDL cholesterol

2. The best sandwich choice for a client on a diet with sodium restriction would most likely be _____.

   a. grilled chicken
   b. hard salami
   c. packaged ham slices
   d. pastrami

3. Combining the _____ with a low-sodium diet significantly reduces blood pressure.

   a. DASH diet
   b. Atkins diet
   c. Paleo diet
   d. Whole 30 diet

4. An example of a profile consistent with metabolic syndrome is _____.

   a. a 19-year-old male with a waist circumference of 42 inches, triglyceride level of 225 mg/dL, and a blood pressure of 166/84 mm Hg
   b. a 20-year-old male with a waist circumference of 34 inches, triglyceride level of 134 mg/dL, and a blood pressure of 123/68 mm Hg
   c. a 28-year-old woman with a fasting glucose level of 83 mg/dL, HDL cholesterol level of 58 mg/dL, and a blood pressure of 124/76 mm Hg
   d. a 32-year-old woman with a waist circumference of 24 inches, fasting glucose level of 110 mg/dL, and HDL cholesterol level of 63 mg/dL

5. Specific recommendations to decrease high blood pressure include _____.

   a. decreasing intake of potassium
   b. increasing intake of potassium
   c. decreasing intake of magnesium
   d. increasing intake of magnesium

Next-Generation NCLEX® Examination-style Case Study

See answers in Appendix A.

A 45-year-old female (Ht.: 6'0" Wt.: 230 lbs.) was diagnosed with congestive heart failure. She has a history of coronary heart disease, hypertension, and used to smoke 2 packs of cigarettes daily. She experiences shortness of breath, making it difficult for her to eat. She consumes approximately 50% of her estimated needs and has significant edema in her lower extremities.

1. Choose the *most likely* options for the information missing from the statements below by selecting from the list of options provided.

   The client's reduced renal blood flow can causes her adrenal glands to secrete ___1___. This can cause retention of ___2___ and ___2___, which is most likely contributing to her edema.

OPTION 1	OPTION 2
renin	water
aldosterone	calcium
angiotensin	sodium
angiotensinogen	phosphorous
cortisone	potassium

2. From the list below, select all of the recommended dietary intervention strategies for this client.

   a. Limit fluid
   b. Limit sodium
   c. Utilize diuretics
   d. Supplement folate, vitamin B_{12}, and magnesium
   e. Increase sodium intake
   f. Limit potassium intake
   g. Consume large frequent meals
   h. Incorporate soft foods if eating is exhaustive

3. For each health teaching below, use an X to identify which are indicated (appropriate or necessary) or contraindicated (could be harmful) for the client.

HEALTH TEACHING	INDICATED	CONTRAINDICATED
Use herbs to season foods.		
Avoid salty processed foods such as chips, pickles, olives, and ham.		
Supplement thiamin and potassium if taking a diuretic.		
You do not have to limit alcohol consumption.		
Limit meals to 2 or 3 per day if having difficulty eating enough calories.		

4. For each assessment finding, use an X to indicate whether nursing and collaborative interventions were effective (helped to meet expected outcomes), or ineffective (did not help to meet expected outcomes).

ASSESSMENT FINDING	EFFECTIVE	INEFFECTIVE
Reduced edema in the lower extremities.		
Consumes 2300 mg of sodium per day.		
Limits fluid to 2 L per day.		
Eats foods such as mashed potatoes, applesauce, and pureed peas when eating is difficult.		
Has low potassium levels.		
Seasons chicken with sodium-free spices such as pepper and garlic powder.		

Additional Learning Resources

Please refer to this text's Evolve website for answers to the Case Study questions:
http://evolve.elsevier.com/Williams/basic/.

References and **Further Reading and Resources** in the back of the book provide additional resources for enhancing knowledge.

Diabetes Mellitus

Dana Gershenoff MS, RDN, CDCES

Key Concepts

- Diabetes mellitus is a metabolic disorder of glucose metabolism that has many causes and forms.
- A consistent and healthy eating pattern is a major component of diabetes care and management.
- Daily self-management tools enable a person with diabetes to maintain health and reduce risks for complications.

- Blood glucose monitoring is a critical practice for effective glycemic control for individuals using exogenous insulin.
- A personalized care plan that balances food intake, exercise, and insulin regulation is essential to successful diabetes management.

Approximately 30.3 million people in the United States, which is 9.4% of the population, are living with diabetes. The rate is higher in adults than in children, accounting for roughly 30.2 million cases with a staggering 7.3 million of these cases undiagnosed. The prevalence of diabetes increases with age. Currently, about 25% of adults aged 65 years or older have diabetes.[1]

Before the discovery of **insulin** in 1922, diabetes resulted in death at a young age for many people. Greater knowledge of the disease and increased diabetes self-management education now enables people with diabetes to live long and fulfilling lives. However, there is not yet a cure for diabetes, and individuals without health care and access to proper medication continue to experience significant complications and a shortened life span. Professional guidance, support, and education help those with diabetes minimize long-term complications. Some of these practices include seeing the health care team consistently, taking medication routinely, and sustaining lifestyle habits such as healthy eating, physical activity, and weight management.

This chapter examines the nature of diabetes and explains why daily self-care is essential for optimal health.

THE NATURE OF DIABETES

DEFINING FACTOR

Glucose is the primary and preferred source of energy for the body. As discussed in Chapter 2, carbohydrate foods break down during digestion in the gastrointestinal tract and they are absorbed into the bloodstream mainly as glucose. Glucose then circulates throughout the body. For cells to use glucose as energy, glucose must first leave the blood and enter into the cell. For this process to happen in most cells, the hormone insulin must be present and insulin receptors must function properly. The β cells of the pancreas produce insulin (see the For Further Focus box, "The History and Discovery of Insulin"). People with diabetes produce very little to no insulin (insulin deficiency), ineffectively use insulin (insulin resistance), or produce inadequate amounts of insulin (insulin insufficiency). Without adequate insulin, glucose accumulates in the bloodstream at abnormally high levels. The American Diabetes Association (ADA) defines diabetes as a group of metabolic diseases causing **hyperglycemia** resulting from defects in insulin secretion, insulin action, or both.[2]

CLASSIFICATION OF DIABETES MELLITUS AND GLUCOSE INTOLERANCE

The pathogenic process of the various forms of diabetes mellitus determines its classification. Classification is a critical step in matching therapy to the type of diabetes, but it is not always possible to identify the classification at the initial diagnosis.[2] As the disease progresses, the true diagnosis becomes more readily apparent. Both type 1 and type 2 diabetes occur at all ages.

Type 1 Diabetes Mellitus

An autoimmune destruction of the pancreatic β cells causes type 1 diabetes mellitus. This form of diabetes accounts for 5% to 10% of all diabetes cases. Scientists have identified at least five autoantibodies causing the destruction in the majority of this population: islet cell autoantibodies, autoantibodies to insulin, autoantibodies to glutamic acid decarboxylase (GAD65), autoantibodies to the tyrosine phosphatases (IA-2 and IA-2β), and autoantibodies to the zinc transporter protein (ZnT8).[2,3] People with type 1 diabetes are also at risk for other forms of autoimmune diseases, such as Graves' disease, Hashimoto's thyroiditis, Addison's disease,

For Further Focus

The History and Discovery of Insulin

EARLY HISTORY AND NAME

During the first century, the Greek physician Areatus wrote of a malady in which the body "ate its own flesh" and gave off large quantities of urine. He named it *diabetes,* from the Greek word meaning "to siphon" or "to pass through." During the 17th century, the word *mellitus* from the Latin word meaning "honey" was added because of the sweetness of the urine. The addition of *mellitus* distinguished the disorder from another disorder, *diabetes insipidus,* in which the patient produced excessive urine but did not experience disordered glucose metabolism. Diabetes insipidus, caused by a deficiency of antidiuretic hormone, is a rare and different disease than diabetes mellitus. Today, the term *diabetes* is usually in reference to diabetes mellitus.

DIABETIC DARK AGES

Throughout the dawning of the scientific era, many early scientists and physicians continued to puzzle over the mystery of diabetes, but the cause remained obscure. For physicians and their patients, these years were the "Diabetic Dark Ages." Individuals with diabetes had short life spans and survived on a variety of semistarvation and high-fat diets.

DISCOVERY OF INSULIN

The first breakthrough came from a clue that pointed to the involvement of the pancreas in the disease process. A young German medical student, Paul Langerhans (1847-1888), provided a clue when he found special clusters of cells scattered throughout the pancreas forming little islands of cells. Although he did not yet understand their function,

Langerhans could see that these cells were different from the rest of the tissue and assumed that they must be important. When his suspicions later proved true, scientists named these clusters of cells the *islets of Langerhans* for their young discoverer. In 1922, with the use of this important clue, Canadian scientists extracted the first insulin from animals. It proved to be a hormone that regulates the oxidation of blood glucose and that helps to convert it to heat and energy. They called the hormone *insulin* from the Latin word *insula,* meaning "island." Insulin did prove to be the effective agent for the treatment of diabetes. The first child treated with insulin was Leonard Thompson, in 1922. He lived to adulthood, but he died at the age of 27 years—not from his diabetes but from coronary heart disease caused by the diabetic diet of the day, which obtained 70% of its total kilocalories from fat. Unsurprisingly, his autopsy showed marked atherosclerosis.

SUCCESSFUL USE OF DIET AND INSULIN

The insulin discovery team was more successful with treatment on their third try with an 11-year-old girl. Initially, her health care provider prescribed a starvation diet, and her weight fell from 75 to 45 pounds (34 to 21 kg) over a 3-year period. However, the medical research team fortunately had learned the importance of a well-balanced diet for normal growth and health. Thus, with a good diet and the new insulin therapy, this child, Elizabeth Hughes, gained weight and vigor and lived a normal life. She married, had three children, took insulin for 58 years, and died of heart failure at the age of 73 years.

---

celiac disease, vitiligo, autoimmune hepatitis, myasthenia gravis, and pernicious anemia.[2] Several genetic factors are involved in the complex etiology of type 1 diabetes, the exact mechanisms of which are still under investigation.[2,3] The possible impact of environmental factors is also under investigation. The rate of β cell destruction determines the onset of diabetes. The initial onset of type 1 diabetes occurs rapidly among children and adolescents (hence its former name *juvenile-onset diabetes*) but may occur at any age, sometimes well into the eighth and ninth decade of life.[2] In infants and children, the classic symptoms that are typically present include polyuria and polydipsia with almost a third experiencing **diabetic ketoacidosis (DKA)** at diagnosis. For most adults, the rate of β cell destruction is slower, and symptoms appear less rapidly. Individuals with type 1 diabetes rely on **exogenous** insulin for survival (hence its other former name, *insulin-dependent diabetes*). At the time of diagnosis, the presence of obesity should not preclude a diagnosis of type 1 diabetes.[2]

Type 2 Diabetes Mellitus

Approximately 90% to 95% of individuals with diabetes have type 2 diabetes. This form is most closely associated with lifestyle and environmental factors that lead to excess body fat, particularly in the abdominal region, and lack of physical activity.[2] Genome-wide

association studies have identified several genetic risk factors for the development of both obesity and type 2 diabetes. Although scientists have definitively linked many specific genetic variants (130 to date) to type 2 diabetes risk, they do not account for all cases.[3] Box 20.1 provides the risk factors for the development of type 2 diabetes. The ADA recommends that health care providers consider testing individuals for diabetes who have a body mass index (BMI) ≥25 kg/m² (or ≥23 kg/m² in Asian Americans) and one or more of the risk factors listed in Box 20.1. Once individuals are 45 years or older, their health care providers should consider testing for diabetes routinely.

Unlike type 1 diabetes, an autoimmune response does not cause type 2 diabetes. This form of diabetes results from insulin resistance and, in some cases,

---

insulin a hormone produced by the β cell in the pancreas, attaches to insulin receptors on cell membranes, and allows the absorption of glucose into the cell.

hyperglycemia an elevated blood glucose level.

diabetic ketoacidosis (DKA) also known as ketoacidosis, the excess production of ketones; a form of metabolic acidosis that occurs with unmanaged diabetes or starvation from burning body fat for energy fuel; a continuing uncontrolled state can result in coma and death.

exogenous originating from outside the body.

leads to insulin insufficiency. Either the body is unable to use the insulin produced effectively or the pancreas produces inadequate insulin to cover the glucose load. Some people with type 2 diabetes experience both insulin resistance and insufficiency. Initially, these individuals do not need exogenous insulin for survival; rather, they rely on healthy eating, exercise, and oral medications for disease management. Type 2 diabetes is a progressive disease, and many clients eventually need insulin to manage their glucose levels. Previously, we called type 2 diabetes *adult-onset diabetes* or *non–insulin-dependent diabetes*

because the onset was primarily in adults that were at least 40 years old. However, between 2002 and 2012, the relative annual increase in the incidence of type 2 diabetes in youth ages 10 to 19 was almost 5%, with significant increases in all minority racial and ethnic groups.[4] Thus, the disease is increasingly becoming a cause for morbidity in children and no longer considered an *adult-onset disease* (see the Cultural Considerations box entitled "Prevalence of Type 2 Diabetes").

Many adults and children with type 2 diabetes can improve their symptoms with weight loss, healthy eating, and increased physical activity. There are several tools available for health care providers and the public to determine an individual's risk of developing prediabetes or type 2 diabetes. Individuals who meet certain criteria may consider reviewing their diabetes risk with their health care team and taking specified diagnostic tests. Table 20.1 summarizes the chief differences between type 1 and type 2 diabetes mellitus.

Gestational Diabetes

Gestational diabetes mellitus (GDM) is a form of diabetes that occurs during the second or third trimester of pregnancy, with normal blood glucose control usually recovered after delivery. Pregnant women who have preexisting type 1 or type 2 diabetes before conception do not fall into this category. GDM presents complications for both mother and fetus if the pregnant woman does not carefully monitor and manage her glucose levels. Persistent hyperglycemia is associated with an increased risk of intrauterine fetal death and macrosomia.

GDM develops in approximately 7.6% of all pregnant women.[5] Risk factors for GDM are similar to those for type 2 diabetes (see Box 20.1). Health care providers should screen pregnant women who are at

---

Box 20.1   Risk Factors for Type 2 Diabetes

NONMODIFIABLE RISK FACTORS
- First-degree relative with diabetes (e.g., mother, father, brother, sister)
- Age 45 or older
- African American, Hispanic/Latino, American Indian, Alaska Native, Asian American, Native Hawaiian, or Pacific Islander
- History of polycystic ovary syndrome or gestational diabetes

MODIFIABLE RISK FACTORS
- BMI ≥25 kg/m^2 (or ≥23 kg/m^2 for some Asian Americans)
- Sedentary lifestyle or physically inactive
- High blood pressure
- History of heart disease or stroke
- Low HDL cholesterol
- High triglycerides

Data from Centers for Disease Control and Prevention (CDC). (2019). *Who's at risk*. Retrieved June 18, 2019, from www.cdc.gov/diabetes/basics/risk-factors.html; and National Institute of Diabetes and Digestive and Kidney Disease (NIDDK). (2016). *Risk factors for type 2 diabetes*. Retrieved June 18, 2019, from www.niddk.nih.gov/health-information/diabetes/overview/risk-factorstype-2-diabetes.

Table 20.1   Differentiating Type 1 and Type 2 Diabetes Mellitus

FACTOR	TYPE 1	TYPE 2
Ethnicity	Increased rates among persons with Northern European heritage	Highest rates are found in those with Native American, Hispanic, African-American, Asian American, Pacific Islander
Age of onset	Generally younger than 30 years of age, with the peak onset before puberty; can occur in adulthood	Generally older than 40 years of age, although increased incidence at younger ages; including youth
Weight	Usually normal or underweight; unintentional weight loss often precedes diagnosis; obesity should not exclude possible diagnosis	Obesity is a risk factor; although occurs in lean individuals
Treatment	Insulin required; long-term goals include consistent activity, healthy eating, and weight management to prevent or delay complications; can still develop insulin resistance	Modest weight loss goal of 5% to 10%, healthy eating and increased physical activity; typically start with oral hypoglycemic agents and then may need insulin for glucose management
β-cell functioning	Insulin deficient and may develop insulin resistance based on lifestyle choices; very little or no insulin produced after the "honeymoon period" (a period of about 1 year after diagnosis in which residual insulin is produced)	Insulin resistance that may lead to insulin insufficiency; type 2 diabetes is a progressive disease and insulin production generally decreases over disease duration

American Diabetes Association. (2019). Standards of medical care in diabetes–classification and diagnosis of diabetes. *Diabetes Care, 42*(Suppl. 1), S13–S28. Skyler, J. S., et al. (2017). Differentiation of diabetes by pathophysiology, natural history, and prognosis. *Diabetes, 66*, 241–255.

Cultural Considerations

Prevalence of Type 2 Diabetes

Diabetes, impaired glucose tolerance, obesity, and even cardiovascular disease (CVD) are beginning to plague the children of America in a similar fashion as they do adults.

CHILDREN

Researchers concluded in 2008 that fetal exposure to maternal diabetes is a contributing factor responsible for the increased prevalence of type 2 diabetes in children, especially among diverse ethnic groups.[1] As scientists continue to follow this study population, the amount of television and computer screen time is emerging as an additional factor that is highly correlated to elevated HbA_{1c} levels.[2] Racial and ethnic groups with pronounced risks for type 2 diabetes include African Americans, Hispanic and Latino Americans, and American Indians/Alaska Natives. The estimated number

of new cases of type 2 diabetes in children younger than 20 years old is more than 5300 annually.[3]

ADULTS

The Centers for Disease Control and Prevention monitors the prevalence of prediabetes, type 1, and type 2 diabetes among racial and ethnic groups in the United States. In addition, they compare the diagnosis relative to age, sex, education, and socioeconomic levels. The most recent data reported the prevalence of diagnosed diabetes from 2013 to 2015 in adults ≥18 years old by race and ethnicity. Similar to the younger generation, adults in some racial and ethnic groups have a higher prevalence of type 2 diabetes than the white, non-Hispanic population.[3] The image below illustrates this increased risk.

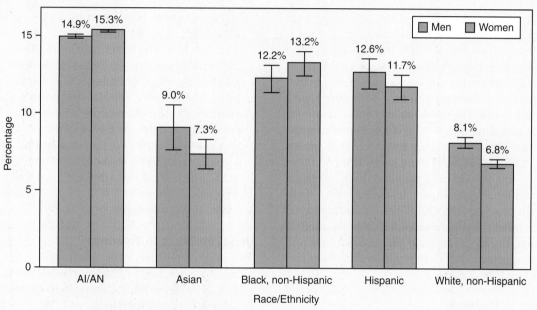

AI/AN = American Indian/Alaska Native.
Note: Error bars represent upper and lower bounds of the 95% confidence interval.

(From Centers for Disease Control and Prevention. [2017]. *National diabetes statistics report: Estimates of diabetes and its burden in the United States*. Atlanta: U.S. Department of Health and Human Services, CDC.)

REFERENCES

1. Dabelea, D., et al. (2008). Association of intrauterine exposure to maternal diabetes and obesity with type 2 diabetes in youth: The SEARCH Case-control study. *Diabetes Care, 31*(7), 1422–1426.
2. Li, C., et al. (2015). Longitudinal association between television watching and computer use and risk markers in diabetes in the

SEARCH for Diabetes in Youth study. *Pediatric Diabetes, 16,* 38s–91.
3. Centers for Disease Control and Prevention. (2017). *National diabetes statistics report: Estimates of diabetes and its burden in the United States, 2017.* Atlanta: U.S. Department of Health and Human Services, CDC.

high risk for diabetes with a fasting plasma glucose and glycosylated hemoglobin A_{1c} (HbA_{1c}) test during the first prenatal visit. The health care provider will diagnose women who meet the diagnostic criteria for diabetes at this time with diabetes (usually type 2) rather than gestational diabetes. All women who are not otherwise known to have diabetes, or who are at high risk, should be screened with a glucose tolerance test between 24 and 28 weeks' gestation.[2,6] The screening protocol for GDM is provided in the section "Gestational Diabetes" in Chapter 10.

The first-line therapy to manage blood glucose levels for women with GDM includes medical nutrition therapy (MNT), physical activity, and self-monitoring of blood glucose. Recommendations include frequent testing and the following goals: fasting glucose results less than 95 mg/dL; 1-hour **postprandial** less than 140 mg/dL and 2-hour postprandial less than 120 mg/dL.[6,7] The health care team reviews the results weekly and if blood glucose levels consistently exceed the goal level, then first-line treatment starts with insulin therapy. In the past, health care providers avoided prescribing oral hypoglycemic agents for women with GDM for fear of teratogenic effects. However, if the individual with GDM declines insulin use or cannot afford insulin, or if the team is concerned with the client's ability to safely use insulin, then they may consider oral medications.[6] Studies indicate that the maternal and fetal outcomes of diabetes management with oral medications are inferior to those of insulin treatment but that these medications may be an appropriate alternative when insulin therapy is not an option.[6,8,9] It is important that the health care provider discusses the risk with the client, such as oral medications' decreased efficacy, the medication crossing the placenta, and the unknown long-term effects for the offspring.[6]

Women can greatly reduce the risk for complications of GDM for themselves and their babies by managing blood glucose levels within recommended ranges. Diabetes management guidelines also advise women with GDM to maintain a healthy body weight or weight gain pattern and to attend all follow-up visits with their health care providers. Women with GDM are at significant risk for having subsequent pregnancies that are complicated by diabetes and for developing type 2 diabetes later in life. The ADA recommends follow-up blood glucose testing at 4 to 13 weeks postpartum using a 75-g oral glucose tolerance test (OGTT); if results are within normal parameters and depending on other risk factors, the health care provider may continue evaluation using any diagnostic test (e.g., HbA$_{1c}$, fasting blood glucose, or 75-g OGTT test).[6,7] Women who continue to follow the recommended lifestyle modifications of healthy eating, regular physical activity, and weight management after delivery minimize their risk for developing type 2 diabetes.[10]

Other Types of Diabetes

A number of conditions or agents that affect the pancreas, including the following, may produce *secondary* diabetes:

- *Monogenic diabetes syndromes:* Defects in the β cells or insulin action may bring about several forms of diabetes. These forms are not characteristic of the autoimmune destruction found in individuals with type 1 diabetes. Scientists have identified mutations on at least 11 genetic loci that impair insulin secretion (although not the action of the insulin). Other less common defects in the action of insulin (but not in the amount secreted) also lead to hyperglycemia and diabetes. Two such groupings include neonatal diabetes, diagnosed under 6 months, and maturity-onset diabetes of the young (MODY). This population makes up less than 5% of those with diabetes, yet correct diagnosis with genetic testing is critical for the appropriate treatment therapy and to minimize complications.[2]
- *Pancreatic conditions or diseases:* Any condition that causes damage to the pancreatic cells can result in

diabetes. Such conditions include tumors that affect the islet cells; acute viral infection by a number of agents, such as the mumps virus; acute pancreatitis from biliary disease, gallstones, or alcoholism; chronic pancreatic insufficiency, such as that which occurs with cystic fibrosis; pancreatic surgery; and severe traumatic abdominal injury.

- *Endocrinopathies:* Insulin works in conjunction with several other hormones in the body. Hormones such as growth hormone, cortisol, glucagon, and epinephrine are all antagonistic to the functions of insulin. Therefore, individuals with disorders such as **Cushing's syndrome**, **glucagonoma**, **pheochromocytoma**, and hyperthyroidism may suffer from hyperglycemia resulting from excess production of insulin-antagonistic hormones.
- *Drug- or chemical-induced diabetes:* This form includes the use of steroids and immunosuppressive regimes after organ transplantation surgeries to prevent organ rejection. The benefits of taking these drugs and preventing organ rejection far outweigh the possible risks of developing diabetes and requiring medication. Additionally, certain drugs and toxins can impair insulin secretion or insulin action. The following drugs and toxins have been linked to impaired glucose tolerance and diabetes in susceptible individuals: Vacor (rat poison), pentamidine, nicotinic acid, glucocorticoids, thyroid hormone, thiazides, diazoxide, phenytoin (Dilantin), β-adrenergic agonists, and α-interferon.[2]

Impaired Glucose Tolerance

The ADA identifies individuals whose fasting blood glucose level is higher than normal (≥100 mg/dL) but less than the level for the clinical diagnosis of diabetes (≥126 mg/dL and/or HbA$_{1c}$ of 5.7% to 6.4%) as impaired glucose tolerance (IGT), which is also known as *prediabetes*.[2] Risk factors for IGT are similar to those for type 2 diabetes. There are several self-administered screening tools for IGT and/or type 2 diabetes available

---

postprandial after eating; normally 1 to 2 hours after a meal.

Cushing's syndrome the excess secretion of glucocorticoids from the adrenal cortex; symptoms and complications include protein loss, obesity, fatigue, osteoporosis, edema, excess hair growth, diabetes, and skin discoloration.

glucagonoma a very rare neuroendocrine tumor found in the α cells of the pancreas that leads to an overproduction of glucagon; may be characterized by diabetes, weight loss, high levels of glucagon, and hypoaminoacidemia.

pheochromocytoma a tumor of the adrenal medulla or the sympathetic nervous system in which the affected cells secrete excess epinephrine or norepinephrine and cause headache, hypertension, and nausea.

from ADA and the Centers for Disease Control and Prevention (CDC); search "prediabetes screening test" at www.cdc.gov. ADA recommends testing for IGT beginning at 45 years old for all individuals, and earlier if individuals have a BMI ≥25 kg/m^2 (or BMI ≥23 kg/m^2 in Asian Americans) with one or more risk factors for type 2 diabetes. If the glucose test results are within normal recommended values, the ADA recommends testing the client every 3 years, unless risk status or other conditions change. If results fall within the IGT range (i.e., fasting blood glucose of 100 to 125 mg/dL), the health care provider should screen clients annually.[2] IGT is a strong risk factor for the future development of type 2 diabetes and cardiovascular disease (CVD). The Diabetes Prevention Program (DPP) demonstrated that overweight adults with IGT could reduce the risk for developing type 2 diabetes by 58% with modest weight loss (5% to 10% of body weight) and regular physical activity (at least 150 minutes per week).[11] This risk reduction persisted for many years. The researchers found that at 10 years postintervention, participants had a 34% reduction in risk and at 15 years, they experienced a 27% risk reduction.[12,13] Aerobic exercise and resistance training are particularly important aspects of treatment because they increase insulin sensitivity and glucose utilization in skeletal muscles.[14,15]

Individuals with IGT often have a complicated assortment of underlying conditions (e.g., dyslipidemia, obesity, hypertension, chronic inflammation) that build on one another to create the condition known as *metabolic syndrome* (see Table 19.1 for the diagnostic criteria of metabolic syndrome). In a 10-year follow-up of the DPP study, the participants recorded higher levels of moderate physical activity and less sedentary time when compared with a similar population that did not participant in the DPP.[16] These results highlight the efficacy of a lifestyle intervention program on long-term behavior changes. This is particularly important for individuals with metabolic syndrome and indicates that slow and modest improvements over time (e.g., more physical activity and less sedentary behavior) can help reduce risk factors for many chronic diseases of adulthood, including diabetes, CVD, hypertension, and metabolic syndrome.

Several lifestyle intervention programs (based on the original DPP[11]) are available to help individuals implement and sustain modest weight loss and prevent or delay the onset of type 2 diabetes. The CDC manages the National Diabetes Prevention Program curriculum and provides a program locator, with both in-person and virtual programs available to meet individual preferences.

SYMPTOMS OF DIABETES

Initial Signs

Early signs of diabetes include three primary symptoms: (1) increased thirst (polydipsia); (2) increased urination (polyuria); and (3) increased hunger (polyphagia). Unintentional weight loss often occurs with type 1 diabetes and sometimes with advanced undiagnosed type 2 diabetes. Additional signs include blurred vision, fatigue, dehydration, skin irritation or infection, and general weakness and loss of strength. Individuals with type 2 diabetes often do not recognize the signs because the symptoms develop gradually over many years. Commonly, patients with type 2 diabetes are already exhibiting some of the long-term complications associated with diabetes at diagnosis.

Laboratory Tests

Laboratory tests show hyperglycemia, abnormal glucose tolerance tests, elevated glycosylated hemoglobin A_{1c}, and glucosuria (i.e., glucose in the urine). Although the urinary excretion of glucose is correlated with increasing levels of blood glucose, it is not as sensitive in individuals with type 2 diabetes as it is with type 1 diabetes.[17] Glycosylated hemoglobin A_{1c}, which is usually abbreviated as HbA_{1c} or A_{1c}, represents blood glucose levels over a 3-month period. Individuals with an HbA_{1c} test within the range of 5.7% to 6.4% have IGT and are at very high risk for progressing to diabetes.[2] HbA_{1c} levels of 6.5% or more are indicative of diabetes mellitus. Box 20.2 outlines the criteria for the diagnosis of diabetes mellitus, and Table 20.2 provides the correlation between HbA_{1c} values and plasma glucose levels. Table 20.3 provides a summary of glycemic recommendations for most adults with diabetes.

Box 20.2	Criteria for the Diagnosis of Diabetes Mellitus

CRITERIA FOR THE DIAGNOSIS OF DIABETES

FPG ≥126 mg/dL (7.0 mmol/L). Fasting is defined as no caloric intake for at least 8 h.[a]

   OR

   2-h PG ≥200 mg/dL (11.1 mmol/L) during OGTT. The test should be performed as described by the WHO, using a glucose load containing the equivalent of 75-g anhydrous glucose dissolved in water.[a]

   OR

   HbA_{1c} ≥6.5% (48 mmol/mol). The test should be performed in a laboratory using a method that is NGSP certified and standardized to the DCCT assay.[a]

   OR

   In a patient with classic symptoms of hyperglycemia or hyperglycemic crisis, a random plasma glucose ≥200 mg/dL (11.1 mmol/L).

DCCT, Diabetes Control and Complications Trial; *FPG*, fasting plasma glucose; *OGTT*, oral glucose tolerance test; *WHO*, World Health Organization; *2-h PG*, 2-h plasma glucose.
[a]In the absence of unequivocal hyperglycemia, diagnosis requires two abnormal test results from the same sample or in two separate test samples.
From American Diabetes Association. (2019). Standards of medical care in diabetes–2019: Classification and diagnosis of diabetes. *Diabetes Care, 42*(Suppl.1), S13–S28.

Table 20.2	Correlation Between Glycosylated Hemoglobin A$_{1c}$ and Estimated Average Glucose Levels	
	ESTIMATED AVERAGE GLUCOSE LEVEL	
HBA$_{1c}$	**MG/DL**	**MMOL/L**
6	126	7.0
7	154	8.6
8	183	10.2
9	212	11.8
10	240	13.4
11	269	14.9
12	298	16.5

Mayo Clinic. (Reviewed 2018, December 18). *HbA1c test*. Retrieved June 1, 2019, from www.mayoclinic.org/tests-procedures/a1c-test/about/pac-20384643.

Table 20.3	Summary of Glycemic Recommendations for Most Adults With Diabetes
PARAMETER	**RECOMMENDATION**
Glycosylated hemoglobin A$_{1c}$ level	<7.0%[a]
Preprandial capillary plasma glucose level	80 to 130[a] mg/dL (3.9 to 7.2 mmol/L)
Peak postprandial capillary plasma glucose level (1 to 2 hrs from start of meal)	<180[a] mg/dL (<10.0 mmol/L)

[a]More or less stringent glycemic goals may be appropriate for some individuals. Goals are adjusted based on the following:
- Duration of diabetes
- Patient's age and life expectancy
- Comorbid conditions
- Known cardiovascular disease or advanced microvascular complications
- Hypoglycemia unawareness
- Individual patient considerations

From American Diabetes Association. (2019). Standards of medical care in diabetes—2019: Glycemic targets. *Diabetes Care, 42*(Suppl. 1), S61–S70.

THE METABOLIC PATTERN OF DIABETES

ENERGY SUPPLY AND CONTROL OF BLOOD GLUCOSE

Energy Supply

The primary source of cellular energy is glucose, and diabetes most prominently alters glucose metabolism. However, in doing so, it also alters the overall energy system, including each of the energy-yielding nutrients (i.e., carbohydrate, fat, and protein). The three basic stages of normal glucose metabolism are as follows:

1. Initial interchange with glycogen (glycogenolysis) and reduction to a smaller central compound (glycolysis pathway)
2. Joining with the other two energy-yielding nutrients, fat and protein (pyruvate link)
3. Final common energy production (citric acid cycle and electron transport chain)

Blood Glucose Management

Optimal health depends on managing blood glucose levels within recommended ranges. Normal control mechanisms ensure sufficient circulating blood glucose to meet the constant energy needs (even the basal metabolic energy needs during sleep), because glucose is the body's preferred fuel, especially for the brain and red blood cells. Figure 20.1 shows the balanced sources and uses of glucose at various levels of blood glucose concentrations.

Sources of blood glucose. To ensure a constant supply of the body's main fuel, the following two sources provide the body with glucose:

- *Dietary intake:* The energy-yielding nutrients in food (i.e., carbohydrates and the carbon backbones of fat and protein, as needed; see Chapter 2 through Chapter 6)
- *Glycogen:* The backup source from the constant turnover of stored glycogen in the liver and muscles (i.e., glycogenolysis; see Chapters 2, 5, and 6)

Uses of blood glucose. The body uses glucose as needed in the following actions:

- Burning it during cell oxidation for immediate energy needs (i.e., glycolysis)
- Changing it to glycogen (i.e., glycogenesis), which is briefly stored in the muscles and liver and then withdrawn and changed back to glucose for short-term energy needs
- Converting it to fat, which is stored for longer periods in adipose tissue (i.e., lipogenesis)

Figure 20.2 summarizes the pathways that are involved in glucose metabolism.

Pancreatic Hormonal Control

The specialized cells of the islets of Langerhans in the pancreas provide three hormones that work together to regulate blood glucose levels: insulin, glucagon, and somatostatin. The β cells of the islets produce insulin and make up about 60% of each islet gland. Figure 20.3 illustrates the specific arrangement of human islet cells.

Insulin. Insulin is the major hormone that controls the level of blood glucose. It accomplishes this through the following metabolic actions:

- Helping to transport circulating glucose into cells
- Stimulating glycogenesis
- Stimulating lipogenesis
- Inhibiting lipolysis and protein degradation
- Promoting the uptake of amino acids by skeletal muscles, thereby increasing protein synthesis
- Permitting cells to burn glucose for constant energy as needed

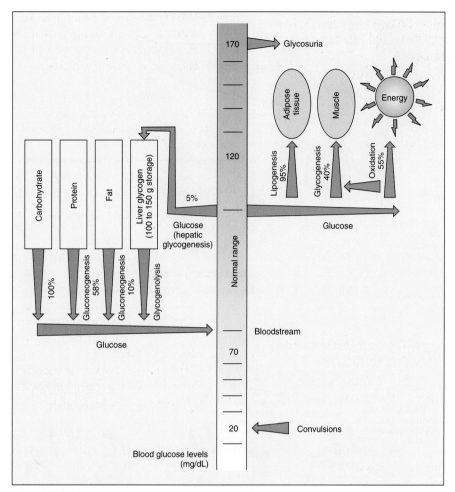

Figure 20.1 Sources of blood glucose (e.g., food, stored glycogen) and normal routes of control.

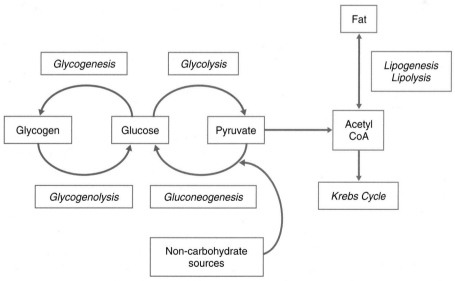

Figure 20.2 Glucose metabolism.

Glucagon. Glucagon is a hormone that acts in an opposite manner to that of insulin to balance the overall blood glucose control. **Hypoglycemia** triggers a rapid breakdown of glycogen in the liver (i.e., glycogenolysis). This action raises blood glucose concentrations as needed to protect the brain and other tissues during sleep or fasting. Glucagon is produced in the α cells of the pancreatic islets, which are arranged around the outer rim of each of these glands and make up about 30% of the gland's total cell mass. Care providers may use glucagon injections as a quick-acting antidote for a severe low blood glucose, especially if the affected individual is unresponsive.

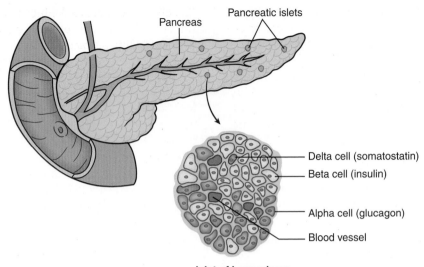

Islet of Langerhans

Figure 20.3 The islets of Langerhans, which are located in the pancreas.

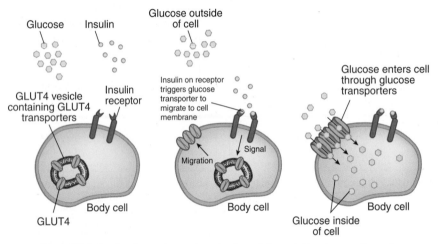

Figure 20.4 Insulin allows glucose to enter the cell through the glucose channel.

Somatostatin. Somatostatin is the pancreatic hormone that acts as a referee for several other hormones that affect blood glucose levels. Somatostatin is produced in the δ cells of the pancreatic islets, which are scattered between the α and β cells and make up approximately 10% of each islet's cells. Somatostatin inhibits the secretion of insulin, glucagon, and other gastrointestinal hormones (e.g., gastrin, cholecystokinin). Because it has more generalized functions in the regulation of circulating blood glucose levels, other parts of the body (e.g., the hypothalamus) also produce somatostatin.

ABNORMAL METABOLISM IN DIABETES WITH HYPERGLYCEMIA

When insulin action is insufficient or deficient, abnormal metabolic changes and imbalances occur among the three macronutrients.

Glucose

Unlike other areas of the body, the pancreatic cells do not need insulin for glucose transport. Normally what happens after a meal or snack is that glucose is absorbed into the pancreatic cells and triggers the secretion of insulin into the bloodstream. The blood then circulates insulin throughout the body, attaching to insulin receptor sites on cell membranes throughout. Once bound, a signaling cascade begins that phosphorylates **GLUT4** vesicles (within the cell) and results in the migration of GLUT4 vesicles to the cell membrane. Ultimately, GLUT4 transporters allow for the uptake of glucose into the cell (Figure 20.4). Without adequate insulin, this process cannot happen; or if insulin resistance is present, this process occurs in a less efficient manner. Therefore, cells are essentially starving for glucose as glucose concentrations increase in the blood, resulting in hyperglycemia.

Fat

Insulin promotes lipogenesis and inhibits lipolysis. In essence, when adequate blood glucose is available and insulin is functioning properly, the body uses its preferred energy source (glucose) and stores extra energy for later use as triglycerides in adipose tissue. In the absence of functioning insulin, lipolysis in the adipose tissue increases in an effort to burn fatty acids for energy. This release of fatty acids into the blood results in elevated triglyceride levels. In addition, **ketogenesis** ensues in the liver. The intermediate products of fat metabolism, called **ketones**, accumulate in the body. Ketones are acids, and their excess accumulation leads to DKA. DKA is a risk for individuals with type 1 diabetes, but this rarely occurs in those with type 2 diabetes. The appearance of the ketone **acetone** in the urine is one indicator of unmanaged hyperglycemia as well as of the adverse development of ketoacidosis. DKA may result in a coma and, in some instances, death.

Protein

In the absence of insulin, protein tissues are also broken down in the body's effort to secure energy sources, thereby causing weight loss, muscle weakness, and urinary nitrogen loss.

LONG-TERM COMPLICATIONS

Chronic hyperglycemia causes the long-term complications associated with diabetes. These health problems mainly relate to microvascular and macrovascular dysfunction in the vital organs. Managing glucose levels helps to minimize the risk, or delays the onset, of such complications. See Table 20.3 for a summary of glycemic recommendations for most adults with diabetes.

Retinopathy

Retinopathy involves damage to the small blood vessels in the retina. It often leads to small hemorrhages in the retina that involve yellow, waxy discharge or retinal detachment. Diabetic retinopathy is the leading cause of blindness in adults but has few warning signs. The risk for retinopathy significantly increases with incessant hyperglycemia. The number of individuals suffering from diabetic retinopathy is expected to almost double from 7.7 million people in 2010 to 14.6 million by 2050.[18] Some treatment modalities (e.g., laser photocoagulation therapy) can delay or prevent the onset of this condition; thus, ongoing eye evaluations are an important part of the care plan. The ADA recommends that individuals with type 1 diabetes have their first-time eye examination within 5 years after diagnosis and that those with type 2 diabetes have their first eye examination shortly after diagnosis. Examinations with dilation should continue from that point forward every 1 to 2 years for individuals who have had no evidence of retinopathy and annually for individuals with retinopathy.[19] Tight glucose management during the early stages of diabetes is critical for long-term health. Participants in a study that focused on early and intensive glucose management experienced lasting benefits with increased quality of life while maintaining visual acuity, reduced retinopathy progression, and decreased development of severe diabetic retinopathy.[19,20]

Do not confuse retinopathy with the blurry vision that sometimes occurs as one of the first signs of diabetes. The increased glucose concentration in the fluids of the eye causes brief changes in the curved, light-refracting surface of the eye; thus, blurry vision. Glycemic management usually improves this form of temporarily impaired vision.

Nephropathy

As with retinopathy, hyperglycemia also damages the small vessels within the kidneys. Diabetes is one of the leading causes of end-stage renal disease in the United States. Approximately 36% of individuals with diabetes also developed chronic kidney disease (CKD), stages 1 to 4.[1] The presence of either **albuminuria** or decreased **estimated glomerular filtration rate (eGFR)** is diagnostic for diabetic kidney disease.[19] Nephropathy and end-stage renal disease are incurable; however, with improved glucose management and antihypertensive therapy, disease progression can be slowed.[21,22] Recommendations for screening are similar to those for retinopathy: within 5 years of diagnosis in type 1 diabetes and at diagnosis in type 2 diabetes, with annual follow-up in both groups.[19]

Neuropathy

Diabetes is one of the most common causes of neuropathy. There is also evidence that neuropathy occurs in many individuals with IGT before blood glucose levels are high enough for a diabetes diagnosis.[23,24] This indicates the highly sensitive nature of the small nerves throughout the body to chronic hyperglycemia.

Damage to the nerves most commonly involves injury in the peripheral nervous system, especially in the legs and feet. For some individuals this causes prickly sensations, increasing pain, and the eventual loss of sensation from damaged nerves. Up to half of the cases of diabetic neuropathy have no symptoms. The loss of nerve sensation can lead to further tissue damage and infection from unfelt foot injuries such as bruises, burns, and deeper **cellulitis**. Asymptomatic individuals are at a particularly high risk for complications. Amputations and foot ulcerations are the most common results of severe neuropathy. More than 100,000 people with diabetes have lower-limb amputations annually, amounting to 5 out of every 1000 individuals with diabetes.[21] Autonomic neuropathy also results in significant clinical concerns such as hypoglycemia unawareness, gastroparesis, orthostatic hypotension, erectile dysfunction, constipation or diarrhea, and bladder dysfunction.[25] The most important form of treatment for neuropathy is prevention with intensive glucose management and maintaining a healthy lifestyle. Recommendations for screening are the same as those for other microvascular diseases: within 5 years of diagnosis for type 1 and at diagnosis for type 2, with annual follow-up for both groups.[19]

Heart Disease

CVD is a major cause of death for people with diabetes, and their risk of death from heart attack or stroke is almost double that of their counterparts without diabetes.[26,27] The standards of medical care for individuals with diabetes include recommendations for the prevention and management of CVD that are specifically aimed at blood lipid levels, blood pressure control, aspirin use, lifestyle changes incorporating weight loss, and smoking cessation.[26] **Glycemic control** is not as strongly related to *macro*vascular complications (i.e., dyslipidemia and hypertension) as it is to other long-term *micro*vascular complications of diabetes (i.e., retinopathy, nephropathy, and neuropathy). However, the co-morbid conditions of hyperglycemia and dyslipidemia greatly increase the risk of CVD; thus, evaluation and treatment for CVD must be part of the overall health care plan for individuals with diabetes.

Dyslipidemia. Elevated triglyceride levels and decreased high-density lipoprotein (HDL) cholesterol levels are characteristic of dyslipidemia in individuals with type 2 diabetes. The management of dyslipidemia is prioritized as follows: (1) incorporating lifestyle modifications that focus on the reduction of saturated fats and avoidance of trans fats; increased intake of omega-3 fatty acids, viscous fiber, and plant stanols/sterols; weight loss, if indicated; and increased physical activity; (2) lowering low-density lipoprotein cholesterol levels; and (3) lowering triglyceride levels.[26] Chapter 19 discusses dietary and lifestyle recommendations to improve lipid profiles for adults; depending on other health factors, a person with diabetes may have more stringent recommendations.

Hypertension. Hypertension affects 73.6% of adults with diabetes, and it is a major risk factor for microvascular complications.[21] CVD mortality is significantly higher for people with both diabetes and hypertension, thereby making blood pressure evaluation and treatment an important part of the health care plan. In adults with an elevated risk for CVD and diabetes, the goal blood pressure is below 130/80 mm Hg (if safely achievable).[26] The health care team should encourage individuals with diabetes to lower their blood pressure by adopting lifestyle modifications such as reducing sodium intake; losing weight (if indicated); increasing the consumption of fruits, vegetables, and low-fat dairy products (i.e., following the DASH diet; see Chapter 19); moderating alcohol intake; and increasing physical activity levels.[26]

GENERAL MANAGEMENT OF DIABETES

EARLY DETECTION AND MONITORING

The guiding principles for the management of diabetes are early detection and the prevention of complications. Community screening programs and annual physical examinations help identify people with elevated blood glucose levels who may benefit from a fasting blood glucose or HbA_{1c} test and medical evaluation. The HbA_{1c} assay (normal value <5.7%) provides an effective tool for evaluating the long-term management of diabetes and the degree of control. Because glucose attaches itself to the hemoglobin molecule over the life of the red blood cell, this test reflects the average level of blood glucose over the preceding 3 months. Other tests such as measurement of fructosamine and glycated albumin levels are sometimes used for diagnostic purposes.[28] However, HbA_{1c} is the most commonly used assessment tool for monitoring ongoing blood glucose management and the risk for complications.

BASIC GOALS OF CARE

The health care team includes physicians, nurse practitioners, physician assistants, nurses, dietitians, pharmacists, and mental health professionals with expertise in diabetes. Many of these practices use a diabetes self-management education (DSME) program described later in this chapter. The team focuses on several objectives when caring for individuals with diabetes, as follows.

Glycemic Management and Medication

This objective seeks to keep a person relatively free from symptoms of hyperglycemia, hypoglycemia,

---

hypoglycemia a low blood glucose level; a serious condition in diabetes management that requires immediate fast-acting glucose intake to increase blood glucose to safe levels.

GLUT4 an insulin-regulated protein that is responsible for glucose transport into cells.

ketogenesis a metabolic pathway that produces ketones bodies as an alternative source of energy for the body; manifests when carbohydrate stores are significantly reduced, and the body breaks down fatty acids that are converted into acetone, acetoacetate, and beta-hydroxybutyrate.

ketones the chemical name for a class of organic compounds that includes three keto acid bases that occur as intermediate products of fat metabolism.

acetone a major ketone compound that results from fat breakdown for energy in individuals with unmanaged diabetes; persons with diabetes periodically take urinary acetone tests to monitor the status of ketone production.

albuminuria higher than normal levels of albumin in the urine; the health care team uses as a clinical tool to diagnosis and monitor kidney disease.

estimated glomerular filtration rate (eGFR) estimated glomerular filtration rate is an equation used to measure kidney function.

cellulitis the diffuse inflammation of soft or connective tissues from injury, bruises, or pressure sores that leads to infection; poor care may result in ulceration and abscess or gangrene.

glycemic control management of blood glucose levels within individualized targets.

and glycosuria, which indicate poor glycemic management. A number of factors are involved in supporting this goal, such as pharmacology (e.g., insulin injections, oral medications), healthy eating, regular physical activity, and glucose monitoring. Consistently managing blood glucose levels within the target range helps to reduce the risks of chronic complications. Although it is not within the scope of this textbook to extensively cover medications, a brief summary follows.

Exogenous insulin. Current medication options include several types of insulin with different durations of action (Table 20.4). When choosing a type of insulin regime, the health care team considers the person's lifestyle, routine, and financial budget (see the For Further Focus box, "Comparative Types of Insulin"). The health care team also provides education on how exogenous insulin works in the body and how its action correlates to food intake and physical activity. It is also important to include training on proper insulin injection technique, storage, and timing. In addition to standard injections with needle and syringe or insulin pen, insulin pumps can administer insulin (Figure 20.5). Insulin-pump therapy continuously delivers rapid-acting insulin to the body at preprogrammed basal rates that more closely mimic natural insulin secretion. For mealtimes, the individual uses the pump to administer small amounts of insulin specific to the individual's carbohydrate intake.

Oral and noninsulin injectable medications. Several noninsulin medications provide varying mechanisms to manage blood glucose levels for individuals with type 2 diabetes (Table 20.5). Several organizations (e.g., ADA, American Association of Clinical Endocrinologists) provide an algorithm that assists providers in deciding which medication to use, when to add another medication, and when to start insulin. The individual's routine, lifestyle, and other personal preferences are important factors for the health care team to consider when prescribing medications to manage diabetes. Considering factors such as risk of hypoglycemia, medication cost, the number of doses required, and medication timing is important for improving medication adherence and clinical outcomes.[29] The Drug-Nutrient Interaction box, "SGLT2 Inhibitors and Glucose Management," describes the action of one such glucose-lowering medication.

Table 20.4 Types of Insulin

TYPE	EXAMPLES	ONSET OF ACTION	PEAK ACTION	DURATION OF ACTION
Rapid-acting (used as bolus insulin)	Fiasp (aspart) NovoLog (aspart) Apidra (glulisine) Humalog (lispro), u100 Humalog (lispro), u200	15 min	30 to 90 min	3 to 5 hours
Short-acting (regular) (used as bolus insulin)	Humulin R Novolin R	30 to 60 minutes	2 to 4 hours	5 to 8 hours
Intermediate-acting (used as basal insulin)	Humulin N (NPH) Novolin N (NPH)	1 to 2 hours	8 hours	12 to 16 hours
Long-acting (used as basal insulin)	Lantus (glargine) Basaglar (glargine) Levemir (detemir)	1 to 3 hours	None	20 to 26 hours
Ultra–long-acting (used as basal insulin)	Tresiba (degludec), u100 Tresiba (degludec), u200 Toujeo (glargine), u300	1 to 6 hours	None	36 to 42 hours
Premixed (intermediate-acting and regular short-acting)	Humulin 70/30 Novolin 70/30	30 to 60 minutes	Varies	10 to 16 hours
Premixed insulin lispro protamine suspension (intermediate-acting) and insulin lispro (rapid-acting)	Humalog Mix 75/25 Humalog Mix 50/50	10 to 15 minutes	Varies	10 to 16 hours
Premixed insulin aspart protamine suspension (intermediate-acting) and insulin aspart (rapid-acting)	NovoLog Mix 70/30	5 to 15 minutes	Varies	10 to 16 hours

All insulins listed are u100 unless noted otherwise.
Data from American Diabetes Association. (2019). *Insulin basics*. Retrieved May 30, 2019, from www.diabetes.org/living-with-diabetes/treatment-and-care/medication/insulin/insulin-basics.html; Cleveland Clinic. (2018). *Injectable insulin medications*. Retrieved May 30, 2019, from my.clevelandclinic.org/health/drugs/13902-injectable-insulin-medications; Novo Nordisk. (2018). *Fiasp* (PDF packet insert). Retrieved May 30, 2019, from www.novo-pi.com/fiasp.pdf; and NIDDK. (2016). *Insulin, medicines & other diabetes treatments*. Retrieved May 30, 2019, from www.niddk.nih.gov/health-information/diabetes/overview/insulin-medicines-treatments.

Comparative Types of Insulin

Flexible insulin plans allow clients to use rapid-acting or regular insulin and longer-acting types of insulin as part of their daily medication regime. Each person's specific needs determine the amount of insulin that he or she uses. With rapid-acting or regular insulin (i.e., bolus insulin), individuals count their carbohydrates and then calculate the amount of insulin needed at mealtimes. By injecting the long-acting insulin (i.e., basal insulin) once or twice daily, they cover their background insulin needs. See Table 20.4 for the various types of insulin and their onset, peak, and duration of action. See image below regarding the activity profile for rapid-acting, regular, intermediate, and long-acting insulins.

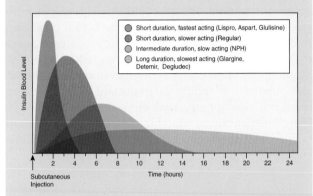

- ● Short duration, fastest acting (Lispro, Aspart, Glulisine)
- ● Short duration, slower acting (Regular)
- ● Intermediate duration, slow acting (NPH)
- ● Long duration, slowest acting (Glargine, Detemir, Degludec)

People with diabetes monitor their blood glucose levels with glucose meters and finger pricks or the use of a continuous glucose monitor that provides a glucose reading every 5 minutes. Throughout the day, individuals adjust their bolus insulin dose according to their current glucose levels, carbohydrate intake, work schedule, and activity level. Some individuals use an insulin pump (instead of the multiple daily injection regime) that continuously delivers insulin into the subcutaneous layer of skin.

Fixed insulin regimes allow people to cover their day's insulin needs using a premixed insulin dose containing both rapid-acting or regular insulin (bolus) and intermediate-acting insulin (basal) combinations. This protocol requires fewer injections per day and is a simpler regime. If cost is a concern, using a premixed insulin option is less expensive, but a routine schedule is critical to prevent hypoglycemia. Because of the insulin duration of action, once the person injects the premixed insulin, he or she must eat meals at the same time each day, eat similar carbohydrate amounts at each meal, avoid skipping meals, and inject his or her insulin at the same time each day.

Optimal Nutrition

Within the basic goals of care, the second objective is to maintain healthy eating patterns to support optimal health, adequate growth and development, and the maintenance of an appropriate body weight. MNT is an important part of diabetes management and the prevention of complications throughout the life span. We discuss it in detail later in this chapter.

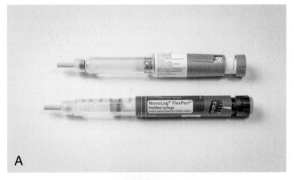

A

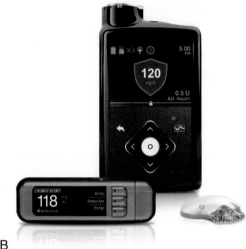

B

Figure 20.5 (A) Examples of prefilled insulin pens for insulin injections. (From Lilley, L. L., et al. [2020]. *Pharmacology and the nursing process* [9th ed.]. St. Louis: Elsevier.) (B) MiniMed 670G and Guardian3 continuous glucose monitor sensor.

Physical Activity

Current recommendations for adults with diabetes are to perform at least 150 minutes per week of moderate-intensity aerobic physical activity (i.e., 50% to 70% of maximum heart rate). Ideally, exercise bouts occur at least 3 days per week with no more than 2 consecutive days without exercise. In addition, people with diabetes are encouraged to perform resistance training at least twice per week in the absence of contraindications.[30] Regular moderate-intensity exercise programs help individuals with both type 1 or type 2 diabetes manage their blood glucose levels and reduce their risk for CVD, hyperlipidemia, hypertension, and obesity. If the individual exhibits long-term complications of diabetes such as retinopathy, neuropathy, or CVD, certain types of exercise may be contraindicated. Health care providers can help make individualized plans for optimal benefits. People with type 1 diabetes may experience high glucose variability, depending on type and duration of exercise. See additional information under the section titled "Physical Activity and Glycemic Management."

Diabetes Self-Management Education and Support

Glycemic management plays a significant role in preventing or delaying the long-term complications of

Table **20.5**	Oral and Noninsulin Injectable Medications	
CATEGORY OF MEDICATION	**EXAMPLES**	**ACTION**
α-Glucosidase inhibitor	Acarbose (Precose) Miglitol (Glyset)	Slows breakdown and absorption of starches, thereby delaying the rise in blood glucose level that occurs after a meal
Amylin agonists (injectable)	Pramlintide (Symlin)	Suppresses glucagon production and prevents hyperglycemia after meals; slows gastric emptying
Biguanide	Metformin (Glucophage) Metformin extended release (Glucophage XR)	Suppresses hepatic glucose production
Dipeptidyl peptidase-4 inhibitor (DPP-4)	Alogliptin (Nesina) Linagliptin (Tradjenta) Saxagliptin (Onglyza) Sitagliptin (Januvia)	Prevents the breakdown of GLP-1 compound that lowers glucose, increase insulin secretion and suppress glucagon production
Glucagon-like peptide-1 receptor agonists (injectable)	Exenatide (Byetta) Exenatide Extended Release (Bydureon) Dulaglutide (Trulicity) Liraglutide (Victoza) Semaglutide (Ozempic)	Improves the glucose-dependent secretion of insulin; decreases glucagon secretion after eating; slows gastric emptying and increases satiety
Meglitinide	Nateglinide (Starlix) Repaglinide (Prandin)	Increases insulin secretion from β cells
Sodium-glucose transport protein inhibitors (SGLT2)	Canagliflozin (Invokana) Dapagliflozin (Farxiga) Empagliflozin (Jardiance) Ertugliflozin (Steglatro)	Blocks and thus reduces the reabsorption of glucose in the kidneys; extra glucose released in urine
Sulfonylurea (second-generation)	Glipizide (Glucotrol, Glucotrol XL) Glyburide (Glynase PresTabs) Glimepiride (Amaryl)	Increases insulin secretion from β cells
Thiazolidinedione	Pioglitazone (Actos) Rosiglitazone (Avandia)	Increases insulin sensitivity in muscle and fat

Data from American Diabetes Association. (2018). *Oral medication: What are my options?* Retrieved May 30, 2019, from www.diabetes.org/living-with-diabetes/treatment-and-care/medication/oral-medications/what-are-my-options.html; and Davies, M. J., et al. (2018). Management of hyperglycemia in type 2 diabetes, 2018; A consensus report by the American Diabetes Association (ADA) and the European Association for the Study of Diabetes (EASD). *Diabetes Care, 41*(12), 2669–2701.

Drug-Nutrient Interaction

SGLT2 Inhibitors and Glucose Control

Oral medication options for people with type 2 diabetes have expanded rapidly in the last decade. The sodium-glucose co-transporter 2 (SGLT2) inhibitor is one of the newest classes of medications that help to lower blood glucose levels. Currently, there are four medications approved for use in the United States. These inhibitors work by blocking the kidneys from reabsorbing glucose back into the blood and excreting it via urine instead, thus lowering overall glucose levels.[1] The drug is glucose dependent and independent of insulin action. This function minimizes the risk for hypoglycemia after taking the medication.[1,2] SGLT2 inhibitors are also associated with weight loss and reduction of blood pressure. As the mechanism relies on adequate renal function, the start and continuation of the medication is dependent upon the client's renal status.[2]

SGLT2 inhibitors may provide cardiovascular benefits in addition to lowering blood glucose concentrations. In a population with both type 2 diabetes and atherosclerotic cardiovascular disease (ASCVD), the medication reduced the risk for major adverse cardiovascular events by 14%. Additionally, for people with diabetes, regardless of ASCVD or heart failure

at baseline, the SGLT2 inhibitors reduced risk of cardiovascular death or hospitalization secondary to heart failure by 23%.[3]

Common side effects for this medication include polyuria, hypotension, dizziness, genital infections, and increased risk of urinary tract infection.[2] One specific medication in this class increases the risk for lower-limb amputation and fracture.[2,4] See Table 20.5 for a list of medication options.

REFERENCES
1. Kalra, S. (2014). Sodium glucose co-transport-2 (SGLT2) inhibitors: A review of their basic and clinical pharmacology. *Diabetes Therapy, 5*(2), 355–366.
2. Davies, M. J., et al. (2018). Management of hyperglycemia in type 2 diabetes, 2018. A consensus report by the American diabetes association (ADA) and the European association for the study of diabetes (EASD). *Diabetes Care, 41*(12), 2669–2701.
3. Zelniker, T. A., et al. (2019). SGLT2 inhibitors for primary and secondary prevention of cardiovascular and renal outcomes in type 2 diabetes: A systematic review and meta-analysis of cardiovascular outcome trials. *Lancet, 393*(10166), 31–39.
4. MedlinePlus. (2019, January 15). *Canagliflozin.* Retrieved January 15, 2019, from medlineplus.gov/druginfo/meds/a613033.html.

chronic hyperglycemia with daily self-care being a critical factor. Comprehensive diabetes education programs facilitate the development of these self-care skills and empower the individual for the day-to-day management needed for healthier outcomes.[31] There are four critical timeframes when the diabetes care and education specialist should provide diabetes self-management education and support (DSME/S): (1) at diagnosis, (2) during the annual assessment of education, nutrition, and emotional needs; (3) when new complicating factors influence self-management; and (4) when transitions in care occur.[32]

The objectives of DSME are to improve clinical outcomes, health status, and quality of life by supporting informed decision making, self-care behaviors, problem solving, and active collaboration with the health care team.[33] A Certified Diabetes Care and Education Specialist (CDCES) or a health care professional with a Board Certification in Advanced Diabetes Management (BC-ADM) may provide the DSME/S services. Other professionals may assist in providing services with additional education and supervision.[33] As experts fine-tune the evidenced-based recommendations with new medications and emerging technology, continuing medical education is essential for all professionals on the health care team. Individuals and health care providers can locate trained diabetes care and education specialist at www.diabeteseducator.org.

Many medical insurance plans, Medicare, and Medicaid cover DSME/S appointments annually. The core content of the DSME/S services generally includes a comprehensive list of training topics[34] (listed later in this chapter) while also individualizing the contents to match the person's needs and levels of health literacy and numeracy.[33]

Dietary and lifestyle management. Cultivating a lifestyle that includes healthy eating patterns specific to individual nutrition needs, cultural preferences, and socioeconomic situation is an important part of management for people with diabetes. Healthy eating and consistent physical activity are vital to glycemic management, weight management, and prevention of complications. If a medication regime includes insulin or **insulin secretagogue** (one class of oral medications) that increases the risk for hypoglycemia, then the health care team will work together with the client to create a physical activity, food, and medication plan.

Monitoring. Monitoring blood glucose levels, urinary acetone levels, body weight, and blood pressure are fundamental to diabetes management and mitigating long-term complications. This includes learning accurate self-testing procedures as well as understanding the results and knowing what action to take in relation to food, medications, or physical activity. A blood glucose meter is a medical device that uses a blood sample obtained by fingerstick to measure a single point-in-time glucose reading. There are a variety of meters available, and they provide results within seconds. Additionally, there are continuous glucose monitors (CGMs) available that provide the user with real-time glucose values every 5 minutes (see Figure 20.5). These monitors also provide users with data about which direction their blood glucose levels are trending. This information assists in making treatment decisions to correct for impending hypo- or hyperglycemia.

Medications. An important role of the health care team is to help individuals understand their treatment plan, how all their medications work, when to take them, and what to do in the event of a missed or delayed medication dose. Additionally, the education encompasses details about their medication, such as side effects, toxicity, dosage, and storage. Various members of the health care team can aid in this process. The educator should use tools, such as the teach-back method, to ensure comprehension and provide an atmosphere where questions are welcome.

Problem solving. Managing blood glucose levels involves planning and preparation on a daily basis. Even the best-planned days go awry, thus helping individuals plan and problem-solve for acute complications, such as hypoglycemia, is an integral part of DSME/S. When unexpected hypoglycemia or hyperglycemia events occur, the goal is not to assign blame, rather work with the person to assess what happened and take preventative steps to minimize future events. Knowing how to address the situation in the short- and long-term is critical for success. The Association of Diabetes Care and Education Specialist curriculum includes a 4-step problem-solving cycle: (1) act, (2) analyze and evaluate, (3) discuss solutions, and (4) learn from experience.[34] Other circumstances that necessitate problem-solving skills are illness, travel, exercise, stress, healthy food options, and medication access.

Reducing risk. Another goal of DSME/S is to provide individuals with a thorough knowledge of prevention, detection, and understanding of treatment options for acute and chronic diabetes complications. Tools, skills, and checklists generally include monitoring blood glucose and blood pressure levels, smoking cessation, foot care, and knowing which annual health care visits are

---

insulin secretagogues an oral medication that stimulates the β cells to secrete insulin to help lower overall blood glucose levels. Side effects are increased risk of hypoglycemia and weight gain.

recommended and how often (e.g., primary care provider, dietitian, dentist, optometrist).

Psychosocial assessment and care. Healthy coping skills play a significant role in daily management of an individual's diabetes management and are covered in many DSME/S programs. Health care providers routinely screen for psychosocial concerns such as depression, diabetes-related stress, anxiety, eating disorders, and cognitive impairment.[30] Working with individuals to develop personal strategies around healthy behavior choices improves their long-term health status and quality of life. The health care team helps individuals identify appropriate coping mechanisms and support systems.

Resource awareness. A number of organizations furnish a wealth of evidenced-based tools for both the health care team and the person with diabetes, such as the ADA, the Academy of Nutrition and Dietetics (AND), and the Association of Diabetes Care and Education Specialist. These organizations' websites include educational handouts as well as program locators for diabetes educators, hospital and outpatient-based diabetes programs, dietitians, and local support groups. Matching resource materials to the person's cultural and socioeconomic needs are vital for long-term success. ADA materials include numerous topics (e.g., basics of diabetes, healthy eating, annual health visits) in several languages. For continual support, there are many in-person or online support groups for people with diabetes and their caregivers. A key element of the DSME/S program involves helping each person find a credible and evidenced-based material source and a long-term support system.

MEDICAL NUTRITION THERAPY

Glucose management is the primary focus of diabetes management for all individuals with diabetes. MNT contributes to improved glycemic outcomes by addressing lifestyle recommendations, energy balance, nutrient distribution, food and medication timing, healthy eating patterns, and other special concerns.

PATIENT-CENTERED APPROACH

Many people find that diabetes management is challenging because they do not fully understand what they can eat or how to create a feasible healthy eating plan. There is not a "one size fits all" diet plan. Thus, all people with diabetes should receive an MNT referral to work with a registered dietitian nutritionist (RDN) for an individualized nutrition plan.[30] When MNT is delivered by an RDN, studies have shown a significant decrease in HbA$_{1c}$ levels (up to 2% in individuals with type 2 diabetes and 1.0% to 1.9% in those with type 1 diabetes).[35] Continued care with an RDN helps maintain more

ideal HbA$_{1c}$ levels.[35] Many insurance plans, including Medicare, and frequently Medicaid, cover 2 to 3 annual visits with an RDN for MNT. Additionally, the health care team supplements nutrition therapy with evidence-based guidance that meets individuals' needs, respects their cultural preferences, and provides healthy food choices to optimize their health.[36] The following sections describe the MNT recommendations and interventions for people with prediabetes or with diabetes.

Prediabetes

Individuals with prediabetes or those at risk for type 2 diabetes can decrease their risk of diabetes and CVD by choosing healthier foods and increasing physical activity to promote and maintain modest weight loss of 5% to 10% of body weight.[11] Well-rounded dietary patterns such as the Mediterranean diet or DASH diet (see Chapter 19) support these goals. Other recommendations regarding specific nutrients (e.g., saturated fat, trans fat, and sugar-sweetened beverage intake) align with the same MNT guidelines as those provided for individuals with type 2 diabetes.

Diabetes

There are several facets for the RDN to consider when providing individualized nutrition therapy for clients with diabetes. Following is a summary of the ADA recommendations[30,36]:

1. The primary focus of the RDN is to provide evidence-based recommendations that promote and support healthy eating patterns with a focus on a varied intake of nutrient-dense foods while maintaining appropriate portion sizes. Overall goals are to improve diabetes outcomes (e.g., HbA$_{1c}$, blood pressure, and lipid levels), either maintain or achieve a healthy body weight, and prevent or delay the onset of diabetes complications.
2. The RDN considers the overall nutrient intake and balances this with the individual's cultural and personal preferences. The RDN communicates in a mode that accounts for the person's health literacy and numeracy.
3. The RDN provides practical daily tools to help with meal planning and takes into account the person's access to healthy food choices while also keeping the message positive and nonjudgmental about food choices.

Additional Considerations

The goals of MNT that apply to specific situations include the following:

- For youth with type 1 diabetes, youth with type 2 diabetes, and older adults with diabetes, meet the nutrition and psychosocial needs of these unique times of the life cycle.
- When a woman with diabetes becomes pregnant or when pregnancy induces GDM, her body

metabolism changes to meet the increased physiologic needs of the pregnancy while battling the manifestations of diabetes (see Chapter 10). Careful team monitoring of the mother's diabetes management ensures her health and the health of her baby. Her health care team calculates the energy and nutrient intake for optimal outcomes.

- Provide self-management training for safe conduct of exercise, including the prevention and treatment of hypoglycemia and diabetes treatment during acute illness.

TOTAL ENERGY BALANCE

Type 1 diabetes most commonly begins during childhood. Health care providers can use the normal growth charts for children to monitor for adequate growth and development. During adulthood, maintaining a healthy weight continues to be a basic goal. For overweight or obese individuals with prediabetes, working toward persistent and modest weight loss helps to prevent or delay the onset of type 2 diabetes.[11-13] For overweight or obese individuals with type 2 diabetes, weight loss of 5% or more produces clinically positive outcomes in glycemic control, blood pressure, and blood lipid levels.[37] Additional clinical benefits are realized with even greater weight loss (~15%), as the outcomes are progressive. Some individuals are capable of driving their diabetes (type 2) into remission through weight loss and healthy lifestyle alone.[38]

The total energy value of the diet for a person with diabetes should be sufficient to meet individual needs for normal growth and development, physical activity, and the maintenance of a healthy weight. Physical activity improves the cellular uptake of glucose and is a fundamental component of glycemic management. Energy intake should equal energy output, unless weight loss is desired, in which a negative energy balance helps achieve the goal. The Dietary Reference Intakes (DRIs) for children and adults (see Appendix B) can serve as guides for total energy needs, with appropriate reductions in kilocalories made for overweight adults (see Chapter 15).

NUTRIENT BALANCE

There is no specific macronutrient distribution recommendation for individuals with diabetes.[30,36] ADA recommendations emphasize the importance of people with diabetes meeting with an RDN who specializes in diabetes-related nutrition therapy to have their meal and macronutrient plan customized for their needs.[30,36,39] Healthy eating for any person with diabetes incorporates the normal nutrition needs for that individual, including optimal health, personal preferences, metabolic goals, meal schedule, and physical activity (see the section "Healthy Eating Patterns").[30,36,39] For individuals who are overweight or obese, the dietitian considers the overall energy intake and weight loss goals when providing MNT.[30,36] The guidelines for

macronutrient, micronutrient, and alcohol intake provided in Box 20.3 reflect the recommendations from the ADA Standards of Medical Care.

Carbohydrate

The primary focus in diabetes care is glycemic control, which involves the regulation of the body's primary fuel, which is glucose. The quantity and quality of a carbohydrate food consumed influences the postprandial glycemic response. The ADA recommends a diet that includes nutrient-dense carbohydrates from fruits, vegetables, whole grains, legumes, and dairy products for optimal health.[30] Studies indicate that most individuals with diabetes consume a moderate amount of carbohydrates at approximately 45% of total caloric intake, and when efforts were made to change an individual's dietary habits, most returned to their baseline macronutrient distribution.[39] Dietitians and diabetes educators work with clients to create sustainable and culturally appropriate food plans centered on healthy carbohydrate options and appropriate portion sizes. For additional information regarding low-carbohydrate and very low–carbohydrate eating patterns see the For Further Focus box, "Low- and Very-Low–Carbohydrate Diets."

Starch and sugar. Carbohydrate-rich foods make up a large portion of the food supply. The most obvious of these include breads, cereals, grains, and sugary sweets. Almost all of the calories provided by fruit and vegetables are carbohydrates as well. For individuals with diabetes, understanding the difference between starchy vegetables and nonstarchy vegetables is important when balancing overall carbohydrate intake. Vegetables that have a low carbohydrate concentration, such as green leafy vegetables, onions, and green beans, are nonstarchy vegetables. Vegetables that are denser in carbohydrates, such as potatoes, corn, peas, and legumes are examples of starchy vegetables. Individuals with diabetes do not need to avoid carbohydrate-rich foods because they provide an important source of energy, vitamins, minerals, and fiber. Rather, it is important for the person with diabetes to monitor portion size and balance carbohydrates with other macronutrient intake. Although the complete elimination of sucrose-containing foods is not necessary, the health care provider should emphasize the importance of small portions and infrequent consumption. ADA does recommend that clients minimize their intake of *added* sugar, refined grains, and that they avoid all sugar-sweetened beverages.[30]

Glycemic index. The use of the glycemic index for individuals with diabetes may provide a modest benefit for lowering glucose values; however, there are mixed results of its effectiveness.[30,36] Personal preference dictates the use of the glycemic index values. See the For Further Focus box in Chapter 2 titled "Carbohydrate Complications" for more details about the glycemic index.

Box 20.3 Summary of American Diabetes Association Medical Nutrition Therapy Recommendations

TOPIC	RECOMMENDATIONS	EVIDENCE RATING[a]
Eating patterns and macronutrient distribution	There is no single ideal dietary distribution of calories among carbohydrates, fats, and proteins for people with diabetes; therefore, meal plans should be individualized while keeping total calorie and metabolic goals in mind.	E
	A variety of eating patterns are acceptable for the management of type 2 diabetes and prediabetes. Reducing overall carbohydrate intake for individuals with diabetes has demonstrated the most evidence for improving glycemia and may be applied in a variety of eating patterns that meet individual needs and preferences. For select adults with type 2 diabetes not meeting glycemic targets or where reducing glucose-lowering medications is a priority, reducing overall carbohydrate intake with low- or very low carbohydrate eating plans is a viable approach.	B
Carbohydrates	Carbohydrate intake should emphasize nutrient-dense carbohydrate sources that are high in fiber, including vegetables, fruits, legumes, whole grains, as well as dairy products.	B
	People with diabetes, and those at risk, are advised to avoid sugar-sweetened beverages (including fruit juices) to control glycemia and weight and reduce their risk for cardiovascular disease and fatty liver (**B**) and should minimize the consumption of foods with added sugar that have the capacity to displace healthier, more nutrient-dense food choices (**A**).	B, A
Protein	In individuals with type 2 diabetes, ingested protein appears to increase insulin response without increasing plasma glucose concentrations. Therefore, carbohydrate sources high in protein should be avoided when trying to treat or prevent hypoglycemia.	B
Dietary fat	Data on the ideal total dietary fat content for people with diabetes are inconclusive, so an eating plan emphasizing elements of a Mediterranean-style diet rich in monounsaturated and polyunsaturated fats may be considered to improve glucose metabolism and lower cardiovascular disease risk and can be an effective alternative to a diet low in total fat but relatively high in carbohydrates.	B
	Eating foods rich in long-chain n-3 fatty acids, such as fatty fish (high in EPA and DHA) and nuts and seeds (high in ALA), is recommended to prevent or treat cardiovascular disease (**B**); however, evidence does not support a beneficial role for the routine use of n-3 dietary supplements (**A**).	B, A
Micronutrients and herbal supplements	There is no clear evidence that dietary supplementation with vitamins, minerals (such as chromium and vitamin D), herbs, or spices (such as cinnamon or aloe vera) can improve outcomes in people with diabetes who do not have underlying deficiencies and they are not generally recommended for glycemic control.	C
Alcohol	Adults with diabetes who drink alcohol should do so in moderation (e.g., no more than one drink per day for adult women and no more than two drinks per day for adult men).	C
	Alcohol consumption may place people with diabetes at increased risk for hypoglycemia, especially if taking insulin or insulin secretagogues. Education and awareness regarding the recognition and management of delayed hypoglycemia are warranted.	B
Sodium	As for the general population, people with diabetes should limit sodium consumption to <2300 mg/day.	B
Nonnutritive sweeteners	The use of nonnutritive sweeteners may have the potential to reduce overall calorie and carbohydrate intake if substituted for caloric (sugar) sweeteners and without compensation by intake of additional calories from other food sources. For those who consume sugar-sweetened beverages regularly, a low-calorie or nonnutritive-sweetened beverage may serve as a short-term replacement strategy, but overall, people are encouraged to decrease both sweetened and nonnutritive-sweetened beverages and use other alternatives, with an emphasis on water intake.	B

EPA, eicosapentaenoic acid; DHA, docosahexaenoic acid; ALA, alpha-linolenic acid

[a]The American Diabetes Association created a grading system for guidelines based on the quality of the scientific evidence. ADA classifies its recommendations with 4 levels of evidence and ratings of A, B, or C and a separate category, E for expert opinion. This last category is used if a clinical trial is impractical, there are no clinical trials, or if the evidence is conflicting. Recommendations that are based on large, well-designed clinical trials or meta-analysis receive an A rating and have the most likelihood of improving diabetes outcomes in the specified population. Recommendations with B or C ratings may still play an important role in improving diabetes outcomes but do not have the same level of scientific evidence as an A rating.

From American Diabetes Association. (2019). Standards of medical care in diabetes–2019: Lifestyle management. *Diabetes Care, 42*(Suppl. 1), S46–S60; and American Diabetes Association. (2019). Standards of medical care in diabetes–2019: Introduction. *Diabetes Care, 42*(Suppl. 1), S1–S2.

For Further Focus

Low- and Very-Low–Carbohydrate Diets

One eating pattern that has gained significant attention in recent years is the low-carbohydrate or very-low–carbohydrate diet. There are a few factors to consider as we learn more about this eating pattern. One of the challenges with evaluating this diet is that the definition used for *low-carbohydrate diet* varies widely among the available studies.[1] Some researchers define a low-carbohydrate diet as one that contains less than 50 g of carbohydrates per day, whereas others define a low-carbohydrate diet as one that contains up to 40% of total daily kilocalories coming from carbohydrates. For a person consuming 2000 kcal/day, these two definitions vary from 50 g of carbohydrates per day (10% of total kcals) to 200 g of carbohydrates per day (40% of total kcals). Additionally, adherence to a strict low-carbohydrate plan, even within a research study, is low. Wide deviations between instructed and actual intake of carbohydrates prevent definitive conclusions. One meta-analysis reviewed this variance in three studies that instructed participants on a very-low–carbohydrate intake of up to 50 g a day. Despite the instructions, the average daily carbohydrate intake of the participants following the very-low–carbohydrate diet ranged from 49 g to 154 g per day by 6 months into the study. In the studies that measured intake at 1 year, the participants were consuming between 132 g to 162 g per day (~3 times the amount instructed to consume).[2] This brings attention to the difficulty of sustaining this type of eating pattern.

The most recent consensus report on nutrition therapy for adults with prediabetes or diabetes states that low-carbohydrate and very-low-carbohydrate eating patterns reduce HgA$_{1c}$ and the need for antihyperglycemic medications (for patients with type 2 diabetes), thus this form of eating pattern may provide a viable approach for improving glycemic control.[3] Additional studies are needed for more definitive recommendations and it is not appropriate for all patients (e.g., those with chronic kidney disease, pregnant women, and individuals with disordered eating patterns).

A few long-term clinical studies are ongoing with strict adherence guidelines and clear definitions of what constitutes a low-carbohydrate diet. In these studies, the researchers are providing the participants with all of their meals to address issues of noncompliance. It will be interesting to see the results as they are published in the next few years. Any patient considering a low- or very-low-carbohydrate diet should work closely with their provider or care team before initiating the diet as their medications may need adjustment to prevent hypoglcyemia.

REFERENCES

1. Snorgaard, O., et al. (2017). Systematic review and meta-analysis of dietary carbohydrate restriction in patients with type 2 diabetes. *BMJ Open Diabetes Research & Care, 5*(1), e000354.
2. van Wyk, H. J., et al. (2016). A critical review of low-carbohydrate diets in people with type 2 diabetes. *Diabetes Medicine, 33*(2), 148–157.
3. Evert, A. B., et al. (2019). Nutrition therapy for adults with diabetes or prediabetes: A consensus report. *Diabetes Care, 42*, 731–754.

Fiber. As for all individuals, health care providers should encourage the consumption of dietary fiber for people with diabetes. There is no reason for these individuals to consume greater amounts of fiber than the general population. Current recommendations are to consume approximately 14 g of fiber per 1000 kcal (approximately 25 g/d for women and 38 g/d for men).[40]

Sugar substitutes and sweeteners. Nutritive and non-nutritive sweeteners are safe to consume in moderation and may help individuals with diabetes reduce their intake of added sugar. If an individual uses nutritive sweeteners (e.g., sucrose, fructose, sorbitol), which are not calorie free, the person needs to account for these calories as part of their overall caloric intake. The American Heart Association, with support from the ADA, recently published a science advisory encouraging the general population to decrease their intake of artificially sweetened beverages and to choose water instead.[41]

Protein

There is no evidence that a protein intake different than the DRI guidelines for the general population will improve glucose control for clients with diabetes.[30,39] Experts do not recommend excessively high protein intake for individuals with diabetic kidney disease (DKD) because of its unnecessary stress on the kidneys. Likewise, consuming less protein than the general recommendation of 0.8 g/kg/day does not provide clinical benefits on glucose levels, CVD risk, or the eGFR.[30]

Fat

There is no evidence that a fat intake different than the DRI guidelines for the general population will improve clinical outcomes for clients with diabetes. Fat quality appears to be more important than fat quantity; thus, recommendations for dietary patterns such as Mediterranean diet (which is high in monounsaturated fats) are favored over low-fat, high-carbohydrate diets.[30,36] Recommendations for omega-3 fatty acids, saturated fat, and trans fat are the same for individuals with diabetes as for the general population. With the increased risk of CVD in those with diabetes, the healthy eating plan must incorporate cardioprotective nutrition interventions.

NUTRIENT INTAKE, PHYSICAL ACTIVITY, AND MEDICATION TIMING

Individuals with diabetes balance their meal schedule and carbohydrate intake with their daily work and family schedule, physical activity, and medications—all of which are important factors in the daily challenge of managing glucose levels.

Daily Schedule

For clients taking insulin or insulin secretagogues, preplanning meals and having a backup plan help to prevent or minimize hypoglycemia. The careful distribution of food and snacks plays a particularly important role for children and adolescents with diabetes to balance insulin and glucose levels during growth spurts and the changing hormone patterns of puberty.

Practical considerations include school and work schedules, athletics, social events, and stressful situations. A high-stress event caused by any source (e.g., injury, anxiety, fear, pain) brings an adrenaline (epinephrine) rush. This fight-or-flight effect counteracts insulin function and contributes to a glucose response.

Physical Activity and Glycemic Management

People using insulin secretagogues or insulin, especially both basal and bolus insulin together, must balance their physical activity with their medication and carbohydrate intake. Despite the additional scheduling demands, physical activity remains a vital component of diabetes self-care and healthy body weight maintenance. Chapter 16 discusses the energy demands of exercise. The following guidelines provide general steps to manage blood glucose levels with physical activity:

1. Aim for normal glucose levels before physical activity:
   - If glucose levels are less than 100 mg/dL, ingest 10 g to 20 g of carbohydrates before exercise.
   - In the presence of hyperglycemia ≥250 mg/dL:
     - People with type 1 diabetes need to check for ketones; avoid moderate to vigorous activity with high levels of ketones.[42]
     - Use caution with elevated glucose levels, even in the absence of ketones.
2. Monitor glucose levels before, during, and after physical activity.
   - Identify when changes in insulin or food intake are necessary.
   - CGMs are a useful tool for clients to understand the impact of activity and when they need to make adjustments.
   - Work with the health care team to learn and understand the glucose response to different physical activity types.
3. Monitor food and fluid intake.
   - Consume added carbohydrate as needed to minimize or prevent hypoglycemia (Table 20.6).
   - Carry fast-acting carbohydrate sources that are easily available during and after physical activity.
   - Ensure adequate fluid intake.

Medications and Meal Timing

Depending on the type of insulin or noninsulin medication prescribed, the medication regimen may influence the timing of meals. Individuals using basal and bolus insulin have two options (see Table 20.4 for insulin types and examples). The first option provides the most flexibility and uses different types of insulin: long-acting insulin for their background (basal) needs and rapid-acting or regular insulin for their meal (bolus) needs. If the person is using rapid-acting insulin, taking it 10 to 15 minutes before eating a meal matches the insulin action to the timing of carbohydrate absorption. Individuals using regular insulin need to inject the medication 30 minutes before eating a meal for the best results. With both rapid and regular insulin,

Table 20.6	Type 1 Diabetes and Carbohydrate Requirements for Endurance (Aerobic) Exercise Performance	
ACTIVITY LEVEL	**CARBOHYDRATE NEEDS**	**EXAMPLES**
Moderate		
30 minutes	Usually not necessary unless blood glucose is <100 mg/dL	
1 hour	15 g carbohydrates per hour	1 small apple, ½ medium banana, ½ peanut butter sandwich, 2 tablespoons raisins, or 1 energy gel
Strenuous		
1 to 2 hours	30–60 g carbohydrates per hour	Peanut butter and jelly sandwich; 1 large banana; granola or energy bar (check label); sports drink 8–12 oz (check label)
>150 min (2.5 hours)	30–90 g carbohydrates per hour; spread over the activity; for example, 20 g every 20 min	Use carbohydrate sources that use different gut transporters (e.g., glucose and fructose)

Modified from Riddell, M., et al. (2017). Exercise management in type 1 diabetes: A consensus statement. *Lancet Diabetes Endocrinol, 5*(5), 377–390.

they match the bolus insulin to the amount of carbohydrates consumed, also known as an insulin-to-carbohydrate ratio. The specific needs of each person dictate his or her ratio (see the next section on carbohydrate counting). For individuals using a premixed insulin, rapid-acting, or regular insulin mixed with an intermediate insulin, the timing of meals is critical to prevent hypoglycemia. Individuals using premixed insulin need to eat meals at similar times each day and similar carbohydrate intake at each meal. Skipping, delaying, or eating fewer carbohydrates than normal increases the risk for hypoglycemia.

Individuals taking noninsulin medications do not adjust their dose to their carbohydrate intake, but meal timing continues to play a role. An ideal eating pattern allows for a moderate and relatively consistent amount of carbohydrates throughout the day. Dietitians and diabetes educators should consider the following guidelines when working with clients who use noninsulin medications: those using insulin secretagogues need to include a source of carbohydrates at each meal; those using biguanides must take their medication with meals to minimize gastric intestinal side effects; those using alpha-glucosidase inhibitors must take their medications at the very beginning of a meal; and the meal timing will vary depending on the specific medication for those taking incretin mimetics. Successful self-care and management of diabetes means matching the medication to the individual's medical needs, personal preferences, budget, and schedule.

Carbohydrate Counting

For clients using rapid-acting or regular insulin at mealtimes, carbohydrate counting provides an option to balance carbohydrate intake with insulin needs for a particular meal. It also provides flexibility in carbohydrate intake because individuals match the insulin to the specific amount of carbohydrates they choose for that meal. After summing up the total carbohydrates planned for the meal, individuals then calculate insulin needs based on their insulin-to-carbohydrate ratio. The Nutrition Facts Label assists greatly with carbohydrate counting, although the client needs to consider their portion size compared with the size specified on the label. Many fresh foods do not have a Nutrition Facts Label, but there are several tools to help count carbohydrates and are available through various means (e.g., smartphone apps, online programs, and books).

Using an insulin-to-carbohydrate ratio is a complex process that requires the client to have advanced health literacy and numeracy to use successfully. The ADA (www.diabetes.org) and the AND (www.eatright.org) provide additional information and tool kits for meal planning based on carbohydrate counting techniques.

The Exchange System is another method used (although infrequently) to help individuals match their insulin dose to their carbohydrate intake. The dietitian typically calculates the person's energy and nutrients needs and creates a customized meal plan. Commonly used foods are grouped into exchange lists based on roughly equal macronutrient values. The exchange list includes defined portions based on macronutrient content for carbohydrates, meat, fats, and alcohol. The individual then chooses a specific number of "exchanges" at each meal. The use of carbohydrate counting has mostly replaced this method of meal planning for those with diabetes.

Healthy Eating Patterns

One of the main concerns for many people with diabetes is to understand what they "can and cannot eat." Dietary recommendations for diabetes management have changed, along with scientific advancement and discovery, over the years. The concept of prescribing a specific diet plan for people with diabetes no longer exists. The patient-centered care approach emphasizes education and overall healthy eating patterns. In today's society, there are many sources, regardless of evidence, telling individuals what to eat. Most clients seek and appreciate dietary guidance. The health care team plays a vital role in helping the individual sort sound evidence from myth.

There are several acceptable eating patterns for individuals managing prediabetes and type 2 diabetes.[30,36]

The Mediterranean diet, DASH diet, and plant-based eating patterns are a few long-standing examples that produce positive results in research. These options can serve as a baseline plan and then the RDN customizes them to the individual's health status, preferences, and long-term goals.[30,36] Emerging evidence indicates that following a low-carbohydrate or very low–carbohydrate eating pattern may improve HbA$_{1c}$ levels in individuals with type 2 diabetes over a 3- to 6-month timeframe. However, this benefit is attenuated at 12 and 24 months.[43-45] See the For Further Focus box titled "Low- and Very-Low–Carbohydrate Diets" for additional information. The low-carbohydrate plan is not recommended for those individuals who are pregnant, lactating, or at risk of disordered eating or for those with renal disease.[30,36]

As current evidence does not indicate that one eating pattern is preferred over another, there are a few key messages the health care team can relay to their clients, as follows: (1) include nonstarchy vegetables at most meals, (2) minimize the intake of refined grains and added sugars, and (3) avoid highly processed foods by choosing whole foods instead.[30,36] Additionally, Box 20.3 summarizes the nutrition recommendations from ADA. Box 20.4 outlines a sample menu based on these principles.

Additional Concerns

Additional concerns arise in daily living and become an important part of ongoing MNT. The following sections provide some suggestions for these concerns.

Special diet food items. Little need exists for special "diabetic" foods. Similar to the general population, people with diabetes following a healthy eating plan that promotes well-balanced meals and a regular meal schedule optimize their overall health and minimize (or prevent) chronic disease. Healthy eating patterns primarily include fresh foods, whole foods, and limits processed foods. The simple principles of moderation and variety guide food choices and amounts.

Alcohol. The guidelines for alcohol use for people with diabetes or prediabetes follow those for the general population: one drink or less per day for adult women and two drinks or less for adult men. Individuals using either insulin or insulin secretagogues must monitor their blood glucose carefully because alcohol increases the risk for delayed hypoglycemia. Education regarding the signs, symptoms, and treatment of hypoglycemia is an important part of diabetes education and lifestyle management.[30] Equivalent portions of a single alcohol serving are 12 oz of beer, 5 oz of wine, 1.5 oz of 80-proof whiskey.

A person with type 1 diabetes should not substitute alcohol for carbohydrate options in meal planning. When a person's blood glucose levels begin to drop, the liver typically responds to the hormone glucagon and releases glucose into the blood to reestablish normal blood glucose levels. However, with the consumption of alcohol, the liver detoxifies the blood of alcohol and suspends the normal response to impending hypoglycemia until it has cleared the alcohol. Thus, when alcohol consumption occurs slowly, in moderation, and with food, it minimizes the risk of hypoglycemia. Using alcohol in cooking poses less concern because the alcohol vaporizes in the cooking process and contributes only its flavor to the finished product.

Hypoglycemia. The brain depends on a constant supply of glucose for metabolism and proper function; a prolonged lack of glucose can lead to brain damage. When adjusting medication options, it is important to consider the risk for hypoglycemia.[46] The three classifications for hypoglycemia are defined as follows: level 1 is a blood glucose level between 54 mg/dL and 70 mg/dL; level 2 is less than 54 mg/dL; and level 3 is a severe event characterized by needing assistance from another person, regardless of blood glucose level.[46]

Hypoglycemic events occur because there is too much insulin or oral hypoglycemic medication in the body relative to the blood glucose level. Factors precipitating hypoglycemia include incorrect insulin dose based on food intake, increased physical activity, and delayed or skipped meal. Table 20.7 provides some symptoms of hyperglycemia and hypoglycemia. Individuals suffering from hypoglycemia may be mistaken as intoxicated because their behavior can appear irrational or uncoordinated. Thus, any form of diabetes identification (e.g., bracelet, pendant, or other item) helps prevent this mistake and helps with proper treatment of hypoglycemia, either in the form of a fast-acting glucose source or injection of glucagon.

People with diabetes and using insulin or insulin secretagogues need to plan for unexpected hypoglycemia events and carry a convenient source of fast-acting glucose. If an event occurs, the "rule of 15" serves as a reminder for appropriate treatment. The "rule of 15" states to provide 15 to 20 g of fast-acting glucose, checking glucose levels 15 minutes later, and if blood glucose is less than 70 mg/dL, repeat as needed. During a hypoglycemic event, people with diabetes should not use food sources containing dietary fat as it slows down absorption of glucose into the bloodstream. Similarly, protein is also avoided because protein increases insulin response without increasing glucose levels in some individuals. Thus, we use neither fat nor protein to treat hypoglycemia (see the Case Study box, "Type 1 Diabetes").[46] Once blood glucose levels return to normal, the individual should consume a small snack of mixed macronutrients and closely monitor

---

Box 20.4	**Sample Healthy Eating Pattern: ~2250 Kilocalories**

- 255 g of carbohydrate (45% kcal)
- 110 g of protein (20% kcal)
- 88 g of fat (35% kcal)

BREAKFAST
- 1 cup whole strawberries
- 2 slices of whole wheat toast (2 oz)
- 2 scrambled eggs with spinach and tomatoes
- ¼ avocado
- Coffee or tea without sweetener

LUNCH
- Green salad with cucumbers, baby carrots, cherry tomatoes, 1 Tbsp parmesan cheese, and 1.5 tbsp of balsamic dressing
- Tuna sandwich on 2 slices of whole-wheat bread
  - Tuna (½ cup, drained)
  - Mayonnaise (1 Tbsp)
  - Chopped dill pickle
  - Chopped celery
- 1 medium fresh pear

DINNER
- Pan-broiled pork chop (well-trimmed)
- 1 cup of oven roasted potatoes
- 1 cup of grilled mushrooms, bell peppers, and tomatoes
- 1 cup of tossed spinach and romaine salad, tomatoes, bell peppers, onions
- Balsamic salad dressing (1½ Tbsp)
- Large glass of water

AFTERNOON SNACK
- 1 small whole wheat pita pocket with 1 Tbsp of peanut butter
- 2 clementine oranges

EVENING SNACK
- 1 cup Greek plain yogurt
- 1 tbsp sliced almonds
- 1 cup of raspberries

Table 20.7	**Symptoms of Hyperglycemia and Hypoglycemia**	
FACTOR	**HYPERGLYCEMIA**	**HYPOGLYCEMIA**
Cause(s)	Too much food, not enough insulin, illness, some medications, or stress	Not enough food, too much insulin, too much exercise, or alcohol intake without food
Symptoms	Polydipsia Polyuria Polyphagia Dry or itchy skin Blurred vision Drowsiness Nausea Fatigue Shortness of breath Weakness Confusion Coma	Sudden shaking Nervousness Sweating Anxiety and irritability Dizziness Impaired vision Weakness Headache Hunger Confusion Tingling sensations around the mouth Seizure

NEXT-GENERATION NCLEX® EXAMINATION-STYLE UNFOLDING CASE STUDY
Type 1 Diabetes

See answers in Appendix A.

A 21-year-old male has type 1 diabetes mellitus. He gives himself four injections daily; 1 injection for his long acting (basal) insulin and then 3 injections with rapid-acting insulin at mealtimes (bolus). He checks his blood glucose levels 4 to 5 times per day: when he wakes up, before each meal, and at bedtime. He studies architecture and generally plays basketball several days a week to decrease stress and spend time with friends.

However, this is final examination week, and his schedule is irregular. He is putting in long hours of study, and he is under considerable stress with less time for activity. On the day before a particularly difficult examination, he is reviewing his study materials at home, and although he checks his glucose level before lunch and takes his mealtime insulin before eating lunch, he doesn't finish all his meal (including some potatoes) as he heads to the university early to find a parking spot before the exam.

Unfortunately, he has to park further away than normal and runs to his class for his final exam. During the middle of the exam, he begins to feel faint and sweaty. He realizes that without eating all of his lunch and with the unplanned activity, his glucose level is too low.

1. **Select all the situations that put the patient at risk for irregular blood glucose levels.**

   a. Mixing two different types of insulin
   b. Irregular carbohydrate intake
   c. Taking insulin before meal
   d. Irregular physical activity
   e. Irregular schedule
   f. Elevated stress levels

2. **Choose the *most likely* option for the information missing from the statements below by selecting from the list of options provided.**

   Irregularities in diet and physical activity can result in _____ (i.e., high levels of glucose in the blood) and _____ (i.e., low levels of glucose in the blood).

OPTIONS	
hyponatremia	hypernatremia
macrosomia	hypoglycemia
microsomia	hypovolemia
hyperglycemia	

3. **Select all of the following explanations that are related to the patient's given signs and symptoms.**

   a. Administered too much insulin for amount of carbohydrates ingested leading to hyperglycemia
   b. Administered too much insulin for amount of carbohydrates ingested leading to hypoglycemia
   c. Unplanned activity leading to hypoglycemia
   d. Unplanned activity leading to hyperglycemia
   e. Eating a meal rich in carbohydrates leading to hypovolemia
   f. Checking blood glucose before eating a meal
   g. Unplanned activity leading to hypernatremia

4. **For each intervention option, use an X to identify <u>effective</u> (will help to meet expected outcomes), or <u>ineffective</u> (will not help to meet expected outcomes) strategies for immediate treatment of hypoglycemia in the patient**

INTERVENTION	EFFECTIVE	INEFFECTIVE
Administer more insulin		
Exercise		
Consume rapid acting carbohydrates		
Consume a mixture of rapid and slow acting carbohydrates with protein		
Consume protein		
Consume fat		

He remembers that he keeps snacks in his backpack. After eating, he checks his blood glucose.

5. **From the options provided, select the best food choices for the patient to eat in the given situation to bring his blood glucose back into normal range most rapidly.**

   a. Beef jerky
   b. Almonds
   c. Baby carrots
   d. Jellybeans
   e. Apple juice
   f. String cheese

6. **Select all of the client's blood glucose measurements that were within normal limits.**

   a. 65 mg/dL
   b. 79 mg/dL
   c. 50 mg/dL
   d. 55 mg/dL
   e. 90 mg/dL
   f. 95 mg/dL

for recurrent hypoglycemia over the next 24 hours. Individuals experiencing a level 3 hypoglycemic event may need assistance in the form of a glucagon injection. It is imperative to train friends and family members (who are close to an individual prone to hypoglycemia events) on proper glucagon kit use.[46]

Illness. Illness complicates healthy eating patterns and blood glucose levels. As such, recommendations include that individuals with diabetes receive an annual influenza vaccination plus other preventative vaccines as indicated (e.g., pneumococcal polysaccharide vaccine, hepatitis B vaccines).[47] When general illness occurs, the person with diabetes adjusts food and insulin accordingly. Modifying the texture of food or using liquid forms may help with the continual intake of carbohydrates during illness. In general, people with diabetes experiencing short-term illness (e.g. cold, flu, vomiting, diarrhea) should do the following[47]:

- Monitor glucose levels more frequently. Fever, infection, or stress hormones can raise glucose levels.
- Possibly adjust their insulin dose according to what their health care team recommends.
- Monitor urine for ketones, a sign of DKA.
- Maintain food and fluid intake. Replace lost fluids, carbohydrates, and electrolytes. Liquid or soft foods may replace solid carbohydrates foods if necessary.
- Contact a health care provider if illness lasts for more than 24 hours, if fever remains high, or if glucose levels are 250 mg/dL or more and moderate to large ketone levels are present.

Travel. When planning for a trip, individuals may benefit from consulting with the dietitian or diabetes educator to help with healthy eating plans in new environments. In general, preparation activities include the following:

- Review how to choose healthier options when eating out, estimating portion sizes; match carbohydrate intake with insulin; and budget their favorite treat size and frequency.
- Carry healthier snack options and items that travel well; e.g., 1 oz nuts, small piece of fruit, 1 oz cheese, 8 to 10 whole-grain crackers, ¼ cup hummus and vegetables.
- Bring fast-acting glucose options in case of hypoglycemia and educate traveling partners on signs, symptoms, and treatment of hypoglycemia.
- Plan for time-zone changes regarding medications, activity, and meals.
- Wear identification bracelet, necklace, or another item.
- Obtain health care provider letter that addresses medications and other medical devices needed.

Eating out. Similar to the general population, a small amount of pre-planning will help the person with diabetes to identify healthier choices when eating out. Selecting restaurants with fresh, less processed options and appropriate portions sizes assists in following a healthy eating pattern. For individuals using mealtime insulin, understanding carbohydrate content of various foods helps to match their insulin dose correctly. Another important consideration is the timing of the meal and insulin dose to avoid either hypoglycemia or hyperglycemia.

Stress. Physiologic or psychosocial stress affects glycemic management in individuals with diabetes due to the hormone responses that are antagonistic to insulin. Additionally, diabetes distress is common, and addressing its potential in each health care visit is recommended, especially if the individual's glycemic targets are not met or with the onset of a new diabetes complication.[30] Diabetes-specific emotional stress correlates with higher HbA$_{1c}$ values and less healthy lifestyle choices.[30] Stress-reduction exercises help people with diabetes manage their self-care and glucose levels. Preferred stress-reducing activities vary greatly from one person to the next (e.g., medication, running, yoga, journaling, playing music). The health care team supports individuals in finding their best coping mechanisms.

---

diabetes distress psychological reaction to the intense emotional burden and negative impact of daily concerns when managing the serious and complex lifelong disease of diabetes.

Putting It All Together

Summary

- Diabetes mellitus is a syndrome with varying forms and degrees with the common characteristic of hyperglycemia. The underlying metabolic disorder involves all three of the energy-yielding nutrients and influences energy balance. The most influential hormone is insulin and people with diabetes experience insulin deficiency, resistance, or insufficiency.

- Type 1 diabetes affects approximately 5% to 10% of all people with diabetes, although it typically occurs in childhood or adolescent, it can occur at any age. Treatment includes exogenous insulin (either by injection or via insulin pump), healthy eating patterns, and physical activity.

- Type 2 diabetes occurs mostly in adults; however, the incidence in childhood is increasing. There is a high correlation between high body weight and type 2 diabetes. Treatment includes modest weight loss, healthy eating, and physical activity. Individuals may need oral medications and/or exogenous insulin.

- Diabetes self-management education is a cornerstone of the overall success of diabetes management.

- MNT plays a significant role in overall glucose management. Basic healthy eating pattern includes foods rich in complex carbohydrates and dietary fiber, low in added sugars, saturated fats, and moderate in protein. Other important factors for healthy meal planning include cultural preferences, meal schedules, food accessibility, and client health and numeral literacy.

Chapter Review Questions

See answers in Appendix A.

1. A risk factor for type 2 diabetes is _____.
   a. a BMI of 20 kg/m^2
   b. a BMI of 28 kg/m^2
   c. exercising 60 minutes a day
   d. a blood pressure of 125/85 mm Hg

2. A form of metabolic acidosis that occurs in unmanaged type 1 diabetes is called _____.

   a. metabolic syndrome
   b. ketoacidosis
   c. ketoalkalosis
   d. hypoglycemia

3. The hormone responsible for promoting the uptake of amino acids by skeletal muscle is _____.

   a. insulin
   b. somatostatin
   c. glucagon
   d. leptin

4. A healthy eating plan that can assist an individual with type 2 diabetes includes _____.

   a. replacing all sugar with noncaloric sweeteners
   b. restricting carbohydrate intake to 20 g or less per day
   c. focusing on healthy portions sizes, increasing nonstarchy vegetables, and minimizing processed foods
   d. choosing foods with a high glycemic index

5. Factors to consider when helping clients with diabetes and their healthy eating pattern include _____.

   a. telling the clients what foods they can and cannot have
   b. limiting their intake of all sucrose-containing foods
   c. understanding their personal preferences, cultural needs, and budget
   d. recommending that they never eat out because the food choices are always unhealthy

Next-Generation NCLEX® Examination-style Case Study

See answers in Appendix A.

A 35-year-old male (Ht.: 6'3" Wt.: 280 lbs.) has been diagnosed with type 2 diabetes mellitus. Before he came into the clinic, he was feeling thirsty and noticed that he was urinating more than normal. His previous medical history indicates hypertension and atherosclerosis. He reports getting about one hour of exercise per week. His clinical and biochemical findings are as follows:

Blood pressure: 127/90 mmHg
Triglycerides: 165 mmol/L
HDL-cholesterol: 45
LDL-cholesterol: 190

1. From the list below, select all of the client's risk factors that relate to type 2 diabetes.

   a. BMI
   b. 1 hour of exercise per week
   c. Blood pressure
   d. Medical history
   e. HDL and LDL cholesterol levels
   f. Triglyceride levels

2. Choose the *most likely* option for the information missing from the statements below by selecting from the list of options provided.

   The client is experiencing ____1____ (increased thirst), and ____1____ (increased urination). This is the body's attempt to remove excess ____2____ in the blood caused by insulin resistance.

OPTION 1	OPTION 2
polydipsia	sodium
dysphagia	glucose
polyuria	phosphorous
polyphagia	calcium
oliguria	cholesterol

3. From the list below, select all the appropriate nutrition interventions related to a new diagnosis of type 2 diabetes.

   a. Diuretics
   b. Weight loss
   c. Healthy eating
   d. Surgery
   e. Statins
   f. Fasting
   g. Physical activity
   h. Exogenous insulin

4. For each assessment finding, use an X to indicate whether nursing and collaborative interventions were <u>effective</u> (helped to meet expected outcomes), or <u>ineffective</u> (did not help to meet expected outcomes).

ASSESSMENT FINDING	EFFECTIVE	INEFFECTIVE
Client weighs 250 lbs. after 1 month		
Blood pressure: 120/85 mmHg		
Triglycerides: 145 mmol/L		
Participates in 150 minutes of moderate intensity physical activity per week		
Avoids eating dinner with family and friends at restaurants		
Replaced soda with diet soda		

Additional Learning Resources

Please refer to this text's Evolve website for answers to the Case Study Questions:
http://evolve.elsevier.com/Williams/basic/.
References and **Further Reading and Resources** in the back of the book provide additional resources for enhancing knowledge.

Kidney Disease

Melody Kienholz BS, RDN, CSR

Key Concepts

- Kidney disease interferes with the normal capacity of nephrons to filter the waste products of metabolism.
- Short-term kidney disease requires basic nutrition support for healing.
- The progressive degeneration of chronic kidney disease requires dialysis treatment and nutrient

modification in accordance with the individual's disease status.
- Current therapy for kidney stones depends more on basic nutrition and health support for medical treatment than on major food and nutrient restrictions.

There are more than 120,000 Americans diagnosed with end-stage renal disease (ESRD) annually.[1] There are many more with compromised kidney function who remain undiagnosed and untreated. The National Health and Nutrition Examination Survey found that less than 15% of individuals with chronic kidney disease (CKD) stage 3 or 4 are aware of their condition.[2] Kidney diseases are costly to both the individual and society because they result in a loss of productivity, income, leisure time, and overall quality of life.

This chapter reviews the medical nutrition therapy (MNT) for people with various forms of kidney disease. Dialysis extends the lives of individuals with CKD; however, it does so at an emotional, physical, and financial cost.

BASIC STRUCTURE AND FUNCTION OF THE KIDNEY

The kidneys filter tremendous quantities of fluid (approximately 1.2 L) every minute. The kidneys reabsorb and return most of this fluid to the vascular system to maintain circulating blood volume. As the blood circulates through the kidneys, these twin organs repeatedly "launder" it to monitor and maintain its quantity and quality. Indeed, the composition of various body fluids is determined not as much by what the mouth takes in as by what the kidneys keep; they are the master chemists of the internal environment.

STRUCTURE

The basic functional unit of the kidney is the nephron. Each kidney contains approximately 1 million nephrons, all of which are independently capable of forming urine. Each nephron has two components: (1) a vascular component and (2) a tubular component (Figure 21.1).

Vascular Components

The glomerulus is a cluster of capillaries, surrounded by Bowman's capsule, that branch from the afferent

arteriole and then rejoin into the efferent arteriole (see Figure 21.1). Only the larger blood proteins and cells remain behind in the circulating blood as it leaves the glomerulus via the efferent arteriole. The glomerular filtration rate (GFR) is the rate at which the glomerulus filters blood. This is the current method for monitoring kidney function and for defining stages of kidney disease. The current standards of care define chronic kidney disease as a GFR of less than 60 mL/min (adjusted to a standard body surface area of 1.73 m^2) for 3 or more months or a urinary albumin-to-creatinine ratio of more than 30 mg/g.[3]

---

dialysis the process of separating crystalloids (i.e., crystal-forming substances) and colloids (i.e., glue-like substances) in solution by the difference in their rates of diffusion through a semipermeable membrane; crystalloids (e.g., blood glucose, other simple metabolites) pass through readily, and colloids (e.g., plasma proteins) pass through slowly or not at all. Dialysis is the process of removing waste and excess fluid from the blood when one's kidneys are not functioning.

nephron the functional unit of the kidney that filters and reabsorbs essential blood constituents, secretes hydrogen ions as needed to maintain the acid-base balance, reabsorbs water, and forms and excretes a concentrated urine for the elimination of wastes.

glomerulus the first section of the nephron; a cluster of capillary loops that are cupped in the nephron head that serves as an initial filter.

Bowman's capsule the membrane at the head of each nephron; this capsule is named for the English physician Sir William Bowman, who in 1843 first established the basis of plasma filtration and consequent urine secretion in the relationship of the blood-filled glomeruli and the filtration across the enveloping membrane.

glomerular filtration rate (GFR) the volume of fluid filtered from the renal glomerular capillaries into Bowman's capsule per unit of time; this term is used clinically as a measure of kidney function.

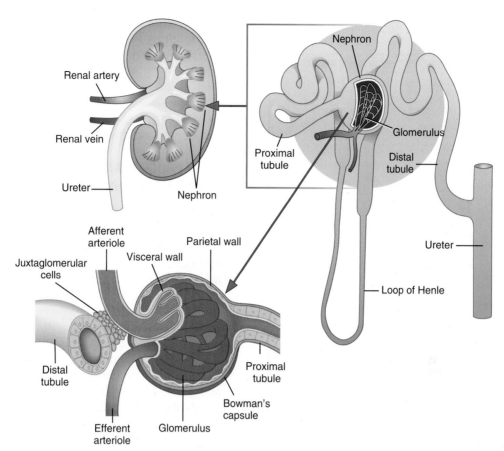

Figure 21.1 Anatomy of the kidney. (*Top*, Reprinted from Peckenpaugh, N. J. [2010]. *Nutrition essentials and diet therapy* [11th ed.]. St. Louis: Saunders. *Bottom*, Reprinted from Thibodeau, G. A., & Patton, K. T. [2007]. *Anatomy & physiology* [6th ed.]. St. Louis: Mosby.)

Tubular Component

A small tubule carries the filtered fluid from Bowman's capsule through its winding pathway and empties into the central area of the kidney medulla. The four sections of the tubular component reabsorb and secrete specific substances throughout, as follows:

- A brush border membrane containing thousands of microvilli greatly increase the surface area of the first section, called the proximal tubule. This section usually reabsorbs glucose and amino acids as well as approximately 80% of the water.
- The remaining 20% of the filtered fluid then enters the loop of Henle. Here, the important exchange of sodium, chloride, and water occurs. This fluid environment maintains the necessary osmotic pressure to concentrate the urine as it passes through the distal tubule and ureter on its way to the bladder for elimination.
- In the distal tubule, the secretion of hydrogen ions occurs as needed to control the acid-base balance. Reabsorption of additional sodium, as needed, under the influence of the adrenal hormone aldosterone occurs here (see Chapter 9).
- Concentrated urine is produced in the collecting tubule section by the following water-reabsorbing actions: (1) the influence of antidiuretic hormone (see Chapter 9); and (2) the osmotic pressure from the dense surrounding fluid in the central area of the

kidney. The concentrated urine, ready for excretion, only amounts to 0.5% to 1% of the original fluid and materials filtered through the glomerulus.

See Table 21.1 for additional details of the resorption and secretion functions of the tubules.

FUNCTION

Nephron structure is adapted in fine detail to balance the internal fluids that are necessary for life. At birth, most people have far more nephrons than needed, but the number decreases with advancing age. Chronic hyperglycemia (see Chapter 20) and hypertension (see Chapter 19) exacerbate damage to the glomerulus and increase the rate of lost functioning nephrons.

Excretory and Regulatory Functions

The kidneys perform the following excretory and regulatory tasks while blood flows through the nephron:

- *Filtration:* The kidneys filter most particles in blood except for the larger components of red blood cells and proteins.
- *Reabsorption:* The winding tubules selectively reabsorb and return to the blood substances within the filtrate that the body needs. This process helps maintain the electrolyte, acid-base, and fluid balances.
- *Secretion:* Along the tubules, secretion of additional hydrogen ions occurs as needed to maintain the acid-base balance.

Table **21.1**	Reabsorption and Secretion in Parts of the Nephron	
PART	**FUNCTION**	**SUBSTANCE MOVED**
Proximal tubule	Reabsorption (active)	Sodium, glucose, amino acids
	Reabsorption (passive)	Chloride, phosphate, urea, water, other solutes
Loop of Henle		
Descending limb	Reabsorption (passive)	Water
	Secretion (passive)	Urea
Ascending limb	Reabsorption (active)	Sodium
	Reabsorption (passive)	Chloride
Distal tubule	Reabsorption (active)	Sodium
	Reabsorption (passive)	Chloride, other anions, water (in the presence of antidiuretic hormone)
	Secretion (passive)	Ammonia
	Secretion (active)	Potassium, hydrogen, some drugs
Collecting duct	Reabsorption (active)	Sodium
	Reabsorption (passive)	Urea, water (in the presence of antidiuretic hormone)
	Secretion (passive)	Ammonia
	Secretion (active)	Potassium, hydrogen, some drugs

From Thibodeau, G. A., & Patton, K. T. (2010). *Anatomy & physiology* (7th ed.). St. Louis: Mosby.

- *Excretion:* The now-concentrated urine contains waste materials ready for excretion.

Endocrine Functions

In addition to the regulatory and excretory functions, the kidneys perform several endocrine functions. The endocrine system is composed of glands that secrete hormones directly into the circulatory system. Many of these hormones have a response within the kidney, as follows:

- *Renin secretion:* When the **arteriole** pressure falls, the kidneys activate and secrete renin, which is an enzyme that initiates the renin-angiotensin-aldosterone mechanism to reabsorb sodium and to maintain hormonal control of the body water balance (see Chapter 9).

- *Erythropoietin secretion:* The kidneys are responsible for producing the body's major supply (80% to 90%) of **erythropoietin**.
- *Vitamin D activation:* The kidneys convert an intermediate inactive form of vitamin D into the final active vitamin D hormone in the proximal tubules of the nephrons (see Chapter 7). The parathyroid hormone stimulates this action.

DISEASE PROCESS AND DIETARY CONSIDERATIONS

GENERAL CAUSES OF KIDNEY DISEASE

Several disease conditions may interfere with the normal functioning of nephrons and eventually result in kidney disease.

- Infections (including urinary tract infections) can lead to chronic disease and obstruction from kidney stones.
- Other causes of obstruction, such as prostatic hypertrophy, which blocks urinary tract drainage, may lead to general tissue damage and kidney disease.
- Various environmental agents, animal venom, certain plants, heavy metals, and some drugs (e.g., nonsteroidal anti-inflammatory drugs, aminoglycoside antibiotics, and radiographic contrast dye) are **nephrotoxic** and can cause kidney damage.

Damage From Other Diseases

Diabetes mellitus is the leading reported cause of ESRD in the United States.[1] Hyperglycemia and hypertension associated with diabetes causes damage to the small renal arteries, thereby leading to glomerulosclerosis (i.e., the loss of functioning nephrons) and eventual CKD. Circulatory disorders such as prolonged and poorly controlled hypertension can cause the degeneration of the small arteries within the kidney and ultimately interfere with normal nephron function. Increased demands on the remaining nephrons may in turn exacerbate hypertension and cause additional damage. Although diabetes and hypertension are common causes of CKD, reported awareness of CKD diagnosis in this population is alarmingly low at approximately 15% (Figure 21.2).[2] Other chief causes are glomerulonephritis and cystic kidney disease. Autoimmune diseases such as systemic lupus erythematosus may also lead to compromised kidney function or disease.

Genetic or Congenital Defects

Cystic diseases (e.g., polycystic kidney disease, medullary cystic disease) are genetically linked kidney

---

arteriole the smallest branch of an artery that connects with the capillaries.
erythropoietin hormone that stimulates the production of red blood cells in the bone marrow.
nephrotoxic toxic to the kidney.

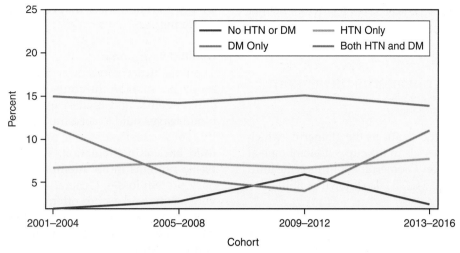

Figure 21.2 Percentage of people with diabetes and/or hypertension who are aware they have CKD. *HTN*, Hypertension; *DM*, diabetes mellitus. (U.S. Renal Data System. [2018]. *2018 Annual data report: CKD in the general population.* Bethesda, MD: National Institutes of Health, National Institute of Diabetes and Digestive and Kidney Diseases.)

diseases that may lead to ESRD later in life. Congenital abnormalities of both kidneys can contribute to kidney disease with extensive distortion of kidney structure. Individuals missing one kidney do not necessarily have kidney disease or even impaired function as long as the remaining kidney functions properly.

Risk Factors

Risks for CKD are higher among individuals who have diabetes, hypertension, or cardiovascular disease (CVD); are older than 60 years; are obese; and have a family history of kidney disease.[1] Malnutrition can intensify the rate of renal tissue destruction and increase susceptibility to infection. The prevalence of CKD is higher in racial and ethnic minority populations and among individuals with low-socioeconomic status. This increased prevalence is due in part to modifiable contributing factors such as smoking, alcohol intake, and limited access to health care.[4] Box 21.1 summarizes risk factors and common causes of kidney disease.

MEDICAL NUTRITION THERAPY IN KIDNEY DISEASE

During the treatment of kidney disease, the dietitian will determine the appropriate MNT based on the severity of the disease, the presence of metabolic abnormalities, and the treatment modality in use (e.g., renal replacement therapy, medications).

Length of Disease

Drug therapy with antibiotics usually controls short-term acute disease resulting from bacterial infection. The goal of nutrition therapy is to provide optimal nutrition support for healing and normal growth. The dietitian may deem that specific nutrient modifications are necessary if the patient is a child or if the disease progresses to a chronic state.

Box 21.1	Risk Factors and Common Causes of Kidney Disease

SOCIODEMOGRAPHIC FACTORS
- Older age
- Family history of chronic kidney disease
- Hereditary diseases affecting the kidneys (e.g., polycystic kidney disease)

CLINICAL FACTORS
- Chronic hyperglycemia
- Hypertension
- Obesity
- Autoimmune disease
- Glomerulonephritis
- Systemic infection
- Repetitive urinary tract infection or kidney stones
- Lower urinary tract obstruction
- History of acute kidney injury
- Reduction in kidney mass or congenital malformations
- Exposure to certain nephrotoxic drugs or environmental conditions

Degree of Impaired Kidney Function and Clinical Symptoms

When there are only a few nephrons involved in a case of mild acute kidney disease, there is less interference with overall kidney function. Because there are so many nephrons in the kidney, the unaffected nephrons can usually meet basic needs. However, in cases of progressive chronic disease, more and more nephrons become involved, which eventually results in CKD. Such cases require extensive MNT to help maintain kidney function as long as possible. Intentional nutrient modifications help to meet individual needs and address clinical symptoms as the disease progresses. Working closely with a dietitian that is board certified as a specialist in renal nutrition for personalized MNT is especially important for those with advanced kidney disease.

This chapter's discussion focuses primarily on the serious degenerative process of CKD. The following sections cover the MNT and clinical practice guidelines for each type of kidney disease.

NEPHRON DISEASES

ACUTE GLOMERULONEPHRITIS OR NEPHRITIC SYNDROME

Disease Process

This inflammatory process affects the glomeruli, which are the small blood vessels in the cupped membrane at the head of the nephron. Glomerulonephritis is the third leading cause of stage 5 CKD (also known as ESRD).[1]

Clinical Symptoms

Classic symptoms include **hematuria** and **proteinuria**, although edema and hypertension also may occur. These individuals may experience anorexia in advanced stages, which contributes to feeding problems and malnutrition. If the disease progresses to more kidney involvement, signs of **oliguria** or **anuria** may develop. Table 21.2 outlines the five glomerular syndromes and their respective clinical manifestations.

Medical Nutrition Therapy for Glomerulonephritis

Nephrologists and dietitians favor overall optimal nutrition support for growth with adequate protein. Diet modifications are not crucial in most clients with acute short-term disease. Output and insensible losses determine fluid intake recommendations.

NEPHROTIC SYNDROME

Disease Process

Nephrotic syndrome or **nephrosis** results from nephron tissue damage to the major filtering membrane of the glomerulus, thereby allowing protein to pass into the tubule. This high protein concentration may cause further damage to the tubule. Disruption of both filtration and reabsorption functions of the nephron ensues. Common causes of nephrosis include infection, medications, neoplasms, preeclampsia, progressive glomerulonephritis, or diseases such as poorly controlled diabetes and systemic lupus erythematosus.

Clinical Symptoms

The large urinary loss of protein from nephrosis (e.g., ≥3 g/day or more in adults) leads to hypoalbuminemia, edema, and ascites. Inadequate protein in the blood leaves fluid to accumulate in the abdominal cavity (i.e., ascites) as osmotic pressure is too low to pull fluid back into circulation. The body will catabolize tissue proteins in an attempt to compensate for urinary protein losses. General malnutrition follows. Severe edema and ascites often mask the extent of body tissue wasting. Other clinical manifestations include hyperlipidemia, **lipiduria**, blood clotting abnormalities, and imbalances in several minerals (e.g., iron, copper, zinc, calcium) resulting from the loss of key proteins that are necessary for their transport or metabolism.

Medical Nutrition Therapy for Nephrotic Syndrome

The goals of MNT are to control major symptoms, replace nutrients lost in the urine, reduce the progression to CKD, and to decrease the risk of atherosclerosis. The Academy of Nutrition and Dietetics (AND) recommends the following standards of care[5]:

- *Protein:* A diet containing moderate amounts of protein (0.8 to 1.0 g/kg of body weight/day), with an emphasis on protein from high biologic value sources, including soy protein. **Blood urea nitrogen** and GFR levels help the dietitian fine-tune the ideal total protein intake. When patients experience an elevated blood urea nitrogen level and decreased urine output, they may need to restrict their dietary protein intake.
- *Energy:* Total energy intake should be adequate to support nutrition status. Needs may be as high as 35 kcal/kg/day. Liberal complex carbohydrates provide sufficient energy in kilocalories and help to combat the catabolism of tissue protein and to prevent starvation **ketosis.**

Table **21.2** Glomerular Syndromes	
SYNDROME	**CLINICAL MANIFESTATIONS**
Acute nephritic syndrome	Hematuria, azotemia, variable proteinuria, oliguria, edema, and hypertension
Rapidly progressive glomerulonephritis	Acute nephritis, proteinuria, and acute kidney failure
Nephrotic syndrome	>3.5 g of proteinuria, hypoalbuminemia, hyperlipidemia, and lipiduria
Chronic kidney failure	Azotemia and uremia that progress for years
Asymptomatic hematuria or proteinuria	Glomerular hematuria and subnephrotic proteinuria

From Kumar, V., Fausto, N., & Abbas, A. *Robbins and Cotran pathologic basis of disease* (7th ed.). Philadelphia: Saunders.

hematuria the abnormal presence of blood in the urine.
proteinuria an abnormal excess of serum proteins (e.g., albumin) in the urine.
oliguria the secretion of small amounts of urine in relation to fluid intake (i.e., 0.5 mL/kg per hour or less).
anuria the absence of urine production; anuria indicates kidney failure.
nephrosis degenerative lesions of the renal tubules of the nephrons and especially of the thin basement membrane of the glomerulus that helps to support the capillary loops; marked by edema, albuminuria, and a decreased serum albumin level.
lipiduria lipid droplets found in the urine that are composed mostly of cholesterol esters.
blood urea nitrogen a test of nephron function that measures the ability to filter urea nitrogen, which is a product of protein metabolism, from the blood.
ketosis the accumulation of ketones, which are intermediate products of fat metabolism, in the blood.

- *Fat:* Total fat intake should not exceed 30% of total kcal/day, and cholesterol intake should not exceed 200 mg/day. Controlling the dietary intake of fat and cholesterol may help to alleviate dyslipidemia and the resulting risk for atherosclerosis. Patients should include dietary sources of polyunsaturated fats (e.g., fish) to account for up to 10% of their total kilocalories.
- *Sodium and potassium:* To reduce symptoms of edema, patients should limit sodium intake to 1 to 2 g/day. Sodium overload is difficult to treat because of the characteristic hypoalbuminuria and **hypotension**; therefore, the health care team must monitor patients carefully. Oliguria impairs the renal clearance of potassium. The provider will monitor potassium intake and labs, making adjustments in accordance with individual needs.
- *Calcium and phosphorus:* Some calcium is bound to albumin in the blood. As albumin is lost through the damaged tubule, bound calcium is also lost. In addition, low serum levels of active vitamin D decrease calcium absorption. Thus, AND recommends that individuals consume 1 to 1.5 g of calcium per day but not to exceed 2 g of calcium (including supplements and/or calcium-based phosphorus binders). Patients should limit phosphorus intake to 12 mg/kg/day.
- *Fluid:* The health care team may restrict fluid intake in response to urine output and insensible losses. If not, then the patient may consume fluids as desired.

KIDNEY FAILURE

The two types of kidney failure—acute and chronic—have a number of symptoms that reflect interference with normal nephron functions and nutrient metabolism. The MNT is similar for both forms, depending on the extent of renal tissue damage and the treatment method used.

ACUTE KIDNEY INJURY

Disease Process

Healthy kidneys may suddenly shut down after metabolic insult or traumatic injury, thereby causing a life-threatening situation. Primary risk factors for the development of acute kidney injury (also known as *acute renal failure*) include older age, diabetes, and hypertension.[6] This is a medical emergency in which the dietitian and the nurse play important supportive roles. There are three categories of AKI depending on the underlying cause[7]:

1. *Prerenal:* Prerenal injury is the most common form of AKI, accounting for 60% to 70% of cases. It involves inadequate blood flow to the kidneys and a subsequent reduction in GFR. Common causes include renal vasoconstriction or occlusion, nephrotoxic medications (e.g., nonsteroidal antiinflammatory drugs, angiotensin-converting enzyme inhibitors, angiotensin receptor blockers), systemic vasodilation (e.g., sepsis, shock), and severe dehydration and hypotension.
2. *Intrinsic:* Intrinsic AKI results from damage to a specific part of the kidney. Common causes include glomerulonephritis, acute tubular necrosis, acute interstitial nephritis, vascular obstruction, infection, or nephrotoxicity from antibiotics, antimicrobial agents, radiographic contrast agents, chemotherapeutic agents, or other nephrotoxic drugs.
3. *Postrenal obstruction:* Postrenal obstruction involves the obstruction of urine flow. Common causes include prostatic hypertrophy with urinary retention, ureteral stones, and other obstructions (e.g., tumors, blood clots).

AKI occurs in as many as one in six hospitalizations and significantly increases the length of stay in the hospital, hospital costs, and mortality.[8] For those who do recover, the episode of AKI may last from days to weeks, with normal function returning once there is a resolution of the etiology. Depending on the extent of renal tissue damage, regaining full function may take months. However, some individuals do not regain normal kidney function, and the disease then progresses to CKD. Individuals suffering an AKI and who have a high risk for advancing to chronic kidney disease are those with significantly reduced GFR (measurement of severity), repetitive and/or long episodes of AKI, endothelial damage, and persistent fibrosis.[9,10]

Clinical Symptoms

The RIFLE classification system, which assesses the severity of *risk, injury, failure,* and the outcomes of either *loss* or ESRD and the Acute Kidney Injury Network (AKIN) criteria classify the degree of AKI.[7] The diagnostic criteria for AKI are an increase in serum **creatinine** levels and oliguria, which occurs when cellular debris from the tissue damage blocks the tubules. Proteinuria or hematuria may accompany diminished urine output. Other symptoms include nausea, vomiting, fatigue, muscle weakness, swelling in the lower extremities, itchy skin, confusion, uremia, and malnutrition. Fluid balance also becomes a crucial factor. **Continuous renal replacement therapy**, which is a type of dialysis, supports kidney function for some critically ill patients.

Medical Nutrition Therapy for Acute Kidney Injury

Basic objectives. The major challenge during AKI is to improve or maintain nutrition status while the patient experiences marked catabolism. Current standards indicate the need for highly individualized therapy focusing on the following: (1) treating the underlying cause; (2) preventing further kidney damage and complications from nutrient deficiencies; and (3) correcting any fluid, electrolyte, or uremic abnormalities.[5] Loss of appetite is common, often requiring enteral nutrition support. Parenteral nutrition support may be necessary (see Chapter 22) if enteral nutrition is contraindicated.

Principles. Nutrition support in acutely ill patients helps reduce the risks for energy and protein malnutrition. This section presents general recommendations for AKI. Keep in mind that kidney function and treatment modality may vary greatly; accordingly, the dietitian will make adjustments in MNT to meet the patient's needs. AND recommends the following standards of care for individuals with AKI[5]:

- *Protein:* Adequate protein is important for supporting kidney function and for preserving lean tissue. Therefore, AND recommends a protein intake of 0.8 to 1.2 g/kg for patients who are not receiving dialysis and who are not experiencing catabolism. Individuals who are experiencing catabolism or who are on dialysis may need 1.2 to 1.5 g/kg of daily protein. This allows for nutrient replenishment and accounts for losses.
- *Energy:* AND suggests an energy intake in the range of 25 to 35 kcal/kg. The dietitian will adjust this amount on an individual basis, depending on metabolic stress and the nutrition status of the individual. If the patient is on **peritoneal dialysis**, the total energy intake should include energy obtained from the **dialysate**.
- *Sodium and potassium:* During a diuretic phase, patients may lose excessive electrolytes. The diet should replace losses of both sodium and potassium (2 to 3 g/day each) during this phase. Blood pressure trends and the presence of edema will determine any necessary adjustments to these levels. During oliguria or anuria phases, the health care team may place the patient on electrolyte restrictions because of their accumulation in the blood and increased risk for hyperkalemia, a potentially fatal condition (see Chapter 8).
- *Phosphorus and calcium:* The dietitian will determine the appropriate dietary phosphorus intake based on body weight, with a range of 8 to 15 mg of phosphorus per kg of body weight. Hyperphosphatemia during anuria phases results in calcium resorption from bones. Phosphorus binders help prevent phosphorus absorption when taken with meals. The MNT goal for calcium is to maintain serum value levels within normal limits and to adjust dietary intake accordingly.
- *Vitamins and minerals*: A balanced diet will help prevent nutrient deficiencies by meeting the Dietary Reference Intakes (DRIs) for all other vitamins and minerals. If the patient is experiencing catabolism or other complications, the dietitian must make modifications to his or her nutrient intakes to meet specific needs.
- *Fluid:* Fluid needs are highly variable with AKI. The health care team must consider the treatment modality, hydration status, and fluid loss on an individual basis when setting fluid intake guidelines. Insensible fluid loss may increase because of fever, and sensible fluid loss (e.g., urine output, vomitus, diarrhea) will vary considerably among patients. A starting point recommendation is 500 mL of fluid plus urine output daily.

CHRONIC KIDNEY DISEASE

Disease Process

CKD is a progressive breakdown of kidney tissue, which impairs all kidney functions. Few functioning nephrons remain, and they gradually deteriorate. CKD develops slowly, and no cure exists. Approximately 15% of the U.S. population has CKD; individuals more than 60 years of age have the highest prevalence.[1]

CKD is most commonly a result of the following:

- Metabolic diseases with kidney involvement (e.g., diabetes, hypertension, CVD, metabolic syndrome, obesity)
- Primary glomerular disease
- Inherited diseases (e.g., polycystic kidney disease) or congenital abnormality
- Other causes: immune disease such as lupus, obstructions such as kidney stones, chronic urinary tract infections, and long-term use of nephrotoxic medications

hypotension low blood pressure.
creatinine a nitrogen-carrying product of normal tissue protein breakdown; excreted in the urine; serum creatinine levels are an indicator of renal function.
continuous renal replacement therapy (CRRT) a method of blood purification that is continuous (i.e., 24 h/day) for critically ill patients in intensive care settings. There are several forms of CRRT that vary according to the vascular access route, presence or absence of dialysate, type of semipermeable membrane used, and the mechanism of solute removal.
peritoneal dialysis a form of dialysis in which the waste/excess fluid is filtered using the individual's peritoneal membrane. There are three basic steps: (1) fill the peritoneal membrane with dialysate, (2) allow the dialysate to dwell, (3) drain the dialysate, which now contains waste and excess fluid.
dialysate the cleansing solution used in dialysis; contains dextrose and other chemicals similar to those in the body.

Modifiable risk factors include blood pressure, glycemic control, and addressing dyslipidemia; reducing sodium intake; making necessary dietary adjustments to potassium, phosphorus, and protein intake; increasing physical activity; achieving a healthy body weight; and quitting smoking.[3] There are five stages of chronic kidney disease based on the GFR (Table 21.3). This section focuses on stages 1 through 4, and the following section covers stage 5.

Clinical Symptoms

Depending on the nature of the underlying kidney disease, chronic kidney changes may involve extensive scarring of renal tissue, which distorts the kidney structure and causes vascular damage. The kidneys gradually lose their ability to sustain metabolic balance as functioning nephrons decrease. Long-term complications most commonly include malnutrition, bone and mineral disorders, anemia, and CVD.

Water balance. During the early stages of chronic kidney failure, the kidneys are unable to reabsorb water or to concentrate urine properly. Therefore, the afflicted individual produces a large amount of dilute urine (i.e., polyuria). Dehydration is a risk factor at this point, and it may become critical. As the disease progresses, the patient's urine production will decline to a point of oliguria and then finally to a point of anuria. Without the urinary excretion of waste products, dangerous levels of urea accumulate in the blood.

Nitrogen retention. An increasing loss of nephron function results in elevated levels of nitrogenous metabolites such as **urea**. Elevated blood urea nitrogen, serum creatinine, and serum uric acid levels reflect the characteristic laboratory finding of **azotemia**. Protein-energy malnutrition is a common complication of protein catabolism.

Electrolyte and mineral balance. Decreasing nephron function causes several imbalances among electrolytes. The failing kidney cannot appropriately maintain the vital sodium and potassium balance that guards body water (see Chapter 9). The metabolism of nutrients produces a concentration of materials (e.g., phosphate, sulfate, organic acids). Without appropriate filtering, these materials accumulate in the blood, thereby causing metabolic acidosis. The disturbed metabolism of calcium and phosphorus, the abnormal levels of parathyroid hormone, and the lack of activated vitamin D (a process that occurs in the kidneys) lead to bone pain, abnormal bone metabolism, and **chronic kidney disease-mineral and bone disorder** (CKD-MBD) or **osteodystrophy**.

Anemia. The damaged kidney cannot produce enough erythropoietin to accomplish its normal initiation of red blood cell production. Therefore, there are fewer red blood cells produced, and those that are have a decreased survival time. The Kidney Disease–Improving Global Outcomes Work Group maintains the clinical practice guidelines for the monitoring and treatment of anemia in individuals with CKD.[11]

Hypertension. When blood flow to the kidney tissues is increasingly impaired, renal hypertension develops. In turn, hypertension causes cardiovascular damage and the further deterioration of the nephrons. The Kidney Disease–Improving Global Outcomes Work Group also maintains specific clinical practice guidelines for the monitoring and treatment of hypertension in individuals with CKD.[12]

Table 21.3 Stages of Chronic Kidney Disease[a]

STAGE	DESCRIPTION	GLOMERULAR FILTRATION RATE (ML/MIN/1.73 M²)
1	Kidney damage with normal or elevated GFR	≥90
2	Kidney damage with mild decrease in GFR	60 to 89
3	Mild to moderate decrease in GFR	30 to 59
4	Severely decreased GFR	15 to 29
5	Kidney failure or end-stage renal disease	<15 (or dialysis)

GFR, Glomerular filtration rate.
[a]Chronic kidney disease is defined as either kidney damage or a glomerular filtration rate of less than 60 mL/min per 1.73 m² for 3 or more months. Kidney damage is defined as pathologic abnormalities or markers of damage, including abnormalities in blood or urine tests or imaging studies.
Data from Kidney Disease: Improving Global Outcomes (KDIGO) CKD Work Group. (2013). KDIGO 2012 clinical practice guideline for the evaluation and management of chronic kidney disease. *Kidney Int*, 3(Suppl.), 1–150.

urea the chief nitrogen-carrying product of dietary protein metabolism; urea appears in the blood, lymph, and urine.
azotemia an excess of urea and other nitrogenous substances in the blood.
chronic kidney disease-mineral and bone disorder a clinical syndrome that develops as a systemic disorder of mineral and bone metabolism in patients with chronic kidney disease; results from abnormalities of calcium, phosphorus, parathyroid hormone, or vitamin D metabolism; causes abnormalities in bone turnover, mineralization, volume, linear growth, strength, and soft-tissue calcification.
osteodystrophy an alteration of bone morphology found in patients with chronic kidney disease.

General Signs and Symptoms

Increasing loss of kidney function causes progressive weakness, shortness of breath, fatigue, anemia, swelling in the extremities, and itchy skin rashes. Anorexia, nausea, and vomiting are common, thus worsening malnutrition and weight loss. Protein-energy wasting (PEW) syndrome is a common occurrence in patients with CKD. PEW is multifactorial, results in a loss of muscle and visceral protein stores, and is associated with high morbidity and mortality.[13,14] Malnutrition lowers resistance to infection, and some individuals may experience bone and joint pain. In advanced stages, irregular cyclic breathing (i.e., Kussmaul breathing) indicates acidosis. Acidosis may cause mouth ulcers, a foul taste, and bad breath. Nervous system involvement may involve muscular twitching and peripheral neuropathy.

Medical Nutrition Therapy for Chronic Kidney Disease

Basic objectives. Treatment must always be individualized and adjusted according to the progression of the illness, the type of treatment, and the patient's response. The dietitian will monitor the patient's nutrition status at regular intervals to identify dietary risk factors and to help prevent malnutrition.[15]

Principles. Nutrition therapy for individuals with CKD who are not on dialysis involves several nutrient adjustments based on individual needs. The MNT recommendations for individuals with CKD are as follows[5]:

- *Protein:* The goal is to provide adequate protein to maintain tissue integrity while avoiding excess. Limit dietary protein intake to 0.6 to 0.8 g/kg/day for those without diabetes, not on dialysis, and who have a GFR of <30 mL/min per 1.73 m^2. AND recommends a protein intake of 0.8 to 0.9 g/kg/day when diabetic nephropathy coexists with CKD (a protein intake of less than 0.8 g/kg/day may result in hypoalbuminemia for these individuals). To encourage the use of plant-based protein, AND recommends that at least two-thirds of the individual's protein intake come from high-quality plant protein sources and/or plant and animal combinations.[3] Ensuring that the combinations provide complete, essential amino acid profiles is crucial to avoid deficiencies.
- *Energy:* Carbohydrate and fat must provide sufficient nonprotein kilocalories to supply energy and spare protein for tissue synthesis. The recommended energy intake is 23 to 35 kcal/kg/day. Energy needs are lower for overweight individuals with both CKD and diabetes to allow for weight loss. Remaining calories should support cardiovascular health principles (e.g., substitute monounsaturated and polyunsaturated fats for saturated and trans fats, reduce total cholesterol intake; see Chapter 19) as patients with CKD have accelerated cardiovascular disease. For individuals with diabetes, glycemic control is an important part of their nutrition intervention (see Chapter 20). The recommendation is to achieve an HbA$_{1c}$ value of approximately 7%.[3]

- *Sodium and potassium:* The general population recommendations for sodium (<2.3 g/day) and potassium are applicable until complications are present. If hypertension and edema are present, limit sodium intake to 2 g/day.[3] Less potassium is cleared from the blood as CKD advances to stages 3 and 4. Dietary intake is determined by assessing laboratory values. If there are elevated blood levels of potassium and other non-dietary causes are eliminated, the dietitian will place the patient on a potassium-restricted diet (<2.4 g/day).

- *Phosphorus and calcium:* Inappropriate blood phosphorus and calcium levels negatively affect bone composition. As the kidneys lose function, they are no longer capable of activating vitamin D or controlling blood calcium levels. Excess blood phosphorus levels worsen this problem, resulting in calcium resorption from the bone to establish a calcium/phosphorus equilibrium in the blood. Thus, moderate dietary phosphorus restriction depends on laboratory values, and it is generally limited to 800 to 1000 mg/day when the serum phosphorus level is ≥4.6 mg/dL or with an elevated parathyroid hormone level. Restriction of total elemental calcium intake (to include dietary, supplementation, and calcium-based phosphorus binders) is to no more than 2 g/day in CKD stages 3 and 4.

- *Vitamins and minerals:* An individualized CKD diet makes it challenging to meet the daily requirement of all essential nutrients (review the Case Study box, "Chronic Kidney Disease"). AND recommends avoiding supplemental fat-soluble vitamins A and E because they may accumulate to toxic levels in those with kidney failure. Likewise, patients should avoid excess vitamins D and K, because the kidney cannot convert vitamin D to its active form, and surplus vitamin K can adversely affect clotting time. The specific MNT recommendations are to help individuals meet their DRIs for the B-complex vitamins and vitamin C and to determine the patient-specific needs for vitamin D and iron.

- *Fluid:* Fluid intake should be sufficient to maintain adequate urine volume in patients who are not undergoing dialysis. The health care team will determine fluid restrictions based on medical factors such as edema, blood pressure control, and changes in urine output.

NEXT-GENERATION NCLEX® EXAMINATION-STYLE UNFOLDING CASE STUDY
Chronic Kidney Disease

See answers in Appendix A.

A 49-year-old active male works at a large manufacturing plant. Recently he has begun to tire more easily, has little appetite, has unintentionally lost 5% of his normal body weight, and generally feels ill most of the time. He recently noticed some ankle swelling and blood in his urine. At his partner's insistence, he finally decided to see his physician.

After a complete workup, the physician's findings included the following:

- No prior illness except a case of the flu with a throat infection during his overseas service in the Army
- Laboratory tests: Presence of albumin, red blood cells, and white blood cells in the urine; high blood potassium, phosphorus, creatinine, and urea levels; and severely decreased glomerular filtration rate of 20 mL/min per 1.73 m^2
- Other symptoms: Hypertension, edema in the lower legs, headache, occasional blurry vision, and low-grade fever

1. Select all clinical symptoms assessed in the patient that are most indicative of chronic kidney disease.

   a. Dysphagia
   b. Proteinuria
   c. Hematuria
   d. Dyspnea
   e. Azotemia
   f. Low GFR
   g. Analgesia
   h. Electrolyte imbalances

2. Choose the *most likely* options for the information missing from the statements below by selecting from the list of options provided.

   The nurse recognizes that the patient's ___1___ imbalance is causing ___2___. The health care team needs to account for this when analyzing the patient's ___3___.

OPTION 1	OPTION 2	OPTION 3
acid-base	hyponatremia	weight
hormone	anorexia	height
electrolyte	hematuria	GFR
enzyme	edema	BUN

The physician discussed the findings and the serious prognosis of stage 4 chronic kidney disease with the patient and his partner. Together with the renal dietitian, they explored his immediate medical and nutrition needs. They also discussed the ultimate need for medical management with dialysis or transplantation. The physician prescribed medications to control the patient's growing symptoms and discomfort.

3. Choose the *most likely* options for the information missing from the statements below by selecting from the list of options provided.

   An increasing loss of ___1___ function requires external modifications to regulate ___2___ imbalances. This ensures that the body is in ___3___.

OPTION 1	OPTION 2	OPTION 3
cortex	musculoskeletal	homeostasis
medulla	chemical	homogenous
nephron	physical	heterogenous
glomerular	congenital	osmosis

4. Use an X to indicate intervention strategies that are indicated (appropriate or necessary) or contraindicated (could be harmful) for the patient.

INTERVENTION	INDICATED	CONTRAINDICATED
Maintain lean body mass with adequate protein intake		
Restrict carbohydrates and fat		
Restrict sodium intake to reduce fluid retention		
Restrict potassium		
Restrict phosphorous		
Encourage high intakes of calcium		
Supplement Vitamins A and E		
Supplement Vitamins D and K		
Provide adequate fluid to meet patient's individualized needs		

Over the next 10 months, his symptoms worsened. He lost more weight, became anemic, and had increased bone and joint pain. Nausea and fatigue increased, and he had occasional muscle twitching and spasms. Small mouth ulcers made eating a painful effort. He made an appointment with his dietitian to learn how to increase his food intake at home.

5. Select all food choices that would be appropriate for the patient to eat in the given situation.

   a. Scrambled eggs
   b. Whole wheat toast
   c. Apple sauce
   d. Cauliflower rice
   e. Baked salmon
   f. Canned green beans

6. Identify assessment measures that would indicate the nursing and collaborative interventions were effective (helped to meet expected outcomes) for the patient.

   a. GFR 35 mL/min
   b. GFR 15 mL/min
   c. Edema in proximal extremities
   d. Decrease in blood pressure
   e. Reduced albuminuria
   f. Weight loss
   g. Lean body mass accrual

END-STAGE RENAL DISEASE

Disease Process

When CKD advances to its end stage, life-support decisions face the patient, the family, and the physician. To make the diagnosis of ESRD the patient's GFR must decrease to less than 15 mL/min per 1.73 m² body surface area. This decrease in GFR indicates irreversible damage to a majority of the kidneys' nephrons. At this point, the patient has three options: long-term kidney dialysis, kidney transplant, or conservative care (such as hospice). Dialysis and kidney transplants prolong the lives of an estimated 720,000 people in the United States annually.[1] Dialysis is the principal treatment for ESRD.

There are two forms of dialysis: hemodialysis and peritoneal dialysis. For a thorough understanding of the treatment options that are available for ESRD, please see the National Kidney Foundation's website at www.kidney.org. A site search for "Understanding kidney disease and treatment options" will provide the viewer with an excellent series of short videos on kidney function, disease, and treatment modalities.

Treatment Options and Medical Nutrition Therapy for End-Stage Renal Disease

Hemodialysis. Hemodialysis is the use of an "artificial kidney machine" to remove toxic substances from the blood and to restore nutrients and metabolites to normal blood levels (Figure 21.3). Before beginning hemodialysis, the surgeon must establish a vascular access in the patient. This procedure ideally takes place 4 to 16 weeks before treatments begin to allow for adequate healing. The three basic kinds of vascular access for hemodialysis are arteriovenous fistula, arteriovenous graft, and a central venous catheter (Figure 21.4). An arteriovenous fistula is the most commonly used and preferred access for long-term dialysis.[1] To create an arteriovenous fistula, a surgeon joins an artery and a vein just beneath the skin, typically on the arm. Once healed, the dialysis technician will insert two cannulas (i.e., a large-bore needle) through the tissue and into the bloodstream to allow the blood to flow through tubes to the dialysis machine.

Patients on in-center hemodialysis usually receive three treatments per week, each of which lasts 3 to 4 hours. During each treatment, their blood cycles through the dialyzer, which removes excess waste

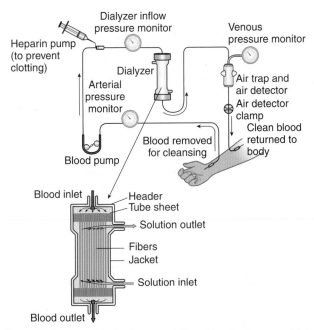

Figure 21.3 Hemodialysis cleans and filters blood with a special filter called a *dialyzer* that functions as an artificial kidney. Blood travels through tubes into the dialyzer, which filters wastes and extra water, and then the cleaned blood flows through another set of tubes and back into the body. (From National Institute of Diabetes and Digestive and Kidney Diseases. [2006]. *Treatment methods for hemodialysis* [NIH Publication No. 07-4666]. Bethesda, MD: National Institutes of Health.)

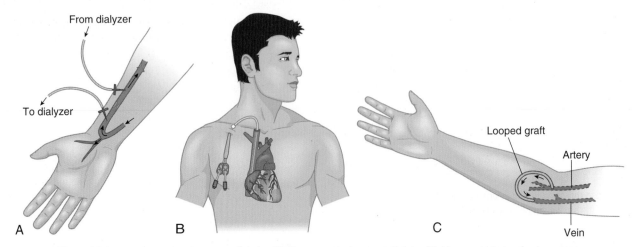

Figure 21.4 Types of access for hemodialysis. (A) Forearm arteriovenous fistula. (B) Venous catheter for temporary hemodialysis access. (C) Artificial loop graft. (From National Institute of Diabetes and Digestive and Kidney Diseases. [2007]. *Kidney failure: Choosing a treatment that's right for you* [NIH Publication No. 00-2412]. Bethesda, MD: National Institutes of Health.)

to maintain normal blood levels of life-sustaining substances, a function that the patient's own kidneys can no longer accomplish. A selective semipermeable membrane separates two compartments in the machine: one compartment contains blood from the patient with all of the excess fluids and waste; the other contains the dialysate, which is a type of "cleaning fluid." As during normal capillary filtration, the blood cells are too large to pass through the pores in the membrane. However, the remaining smaller molecules in the blood pass through the membrane and the dialysate carries them away as waste. The dialysate is individualized to the patient's needs. If a patient is deficient in a specific nutrient, the health care team can specify that those nutrients be added to the dialysate. These nutrients will cross the membrane via osmosis or diffusion to establish equilibrium between the dialysate and the blood and help meet the patient's nutrient needs.

Studies indicate that individuals receiving hemodialysis up to six times per week with shorter sessions experience health benefits such as improved general health and mental health with no reported loss in quality of life.[16] For this reason, some clients opt to do home hemodialysis, during which they perform their own dialysis treatment with the care of a partner or care provider; this is typically five to six treatments per week, ranging from about 2 to 4 hours per treatment. Some dialysis centers offer nocturnal hemodialysis and/or nocturnal home hemodialysis, which typically last 6 to 8 hours on 3 or more nights per week.

Medical nutrition therapy for hemodialysis. The diet of a person who is undergoing hemodialysis is an important aspect of maintaining biochemical balance. PEW syndrome remains a significant concern for patients on hemodialysis. The loss of muscle mass through progressive protein catabolism is associated with mortality.[14] Registered dietitian nutritionists who specialize in renal care are responsible for meal planning and diet education. The goal of the MNT during hemodialysis is to maintain optimal nutrition while preventing the accumulation of excess waste products between treatments. In most cases, MNT can allow for more liberal nutrient allowances than for nondialysis patients, as follows[5]:

- *Protein:* Protein-energy malnutrition, as indicated by dietary intake and the biomarkers of protein status, is a major concern for patients on dialysis and is one of the most significant predictors of overall malnutrition and adverse outcomes.[17-19] For most individuals on dialysis, a protein allowance of 1.2 g/kg or greater is ideal to prevent protein malnutrition. This amount provides nutrition needs, maintains positive nitrogen balance, does not produce excessive nitrogenous waste, and replaces the amino

acids lost during each dialysis treatment. At least 50% of this daily allowance should consist of protein foods of high biologic value (e.g., eggs, meat, fish, poultry).

- *Energy:* MNT recommendations for energy intake are 30 to 35 kcal/kg/day to achieve and maintain goal body weight for individuals older than 60 years of age. For those individuals under 60 years of age, recommendations are 35 kcal/kg/day. Interestingly, the death rate decreases as the body mass index increases above normal ranges (i.e., ≥ 25 kg/m^2), purportedly as the result of a complex association between malnutrition and clinical outcomes.[20,21] The unfortunate combination is that decreased appetite is common in ESRD when the GFR falls below 60 mL/min per 1.73 m^2. A generous amount of carbohydrates with some fat continues to supply needed kilocalories for energy and protein sparing.
- *Sodium and potassium:* Recommendations are to limit sodium to less than 2.4 g/day to control body fluid retention and hypertension. Reducing sodium restrictions further may help manage thirst and help patients conform to fluid restrictions. To prevent potassium accumulation, which can cause cardiac problems, limit intake to less than 2.4 g/day, with adjustments based on serum potassium levels as indicated.
- *Phosphorus and calcium:* With careful monitoring to control for co-morbid bone conditions, the dietary intake of phosphorus recommendations is less than 800 to 1000 mg/day or 10 to 12 mg of phosphorus per gram of protein when serum phosphorus levels exceed 5.5 mg/dL or with elevated parathyroid hormone levels. Calcium intake should not exceed 2 g/day, including the amount received through food, dietary supplements, and medications such as calcium-based phosphorus binders.
- *Vitamins and minerals:* The general recommendation for all water-soluble vitamins is to achieve the DRIs. Biochemical markers allow for individualization of iron and vitamin D intake recommendations. Other micronutrients of special interest are as follows:
  - Vitamin C: 60 to 100 mg/day
  - Vitamin B$_6$: 2 mg/day
  - Folate: 1 to 5 mg/day
  - Vitamin B$_{12}$: 3 mcg/day
  - Vitamin E: 15 IU/day
  - Zinc: 15 mg/day
- *Fluid:* The MNT recommendations for patients with ESRD on hemodialysis are to limit their fluid intake to 1000 mL/day plus an amount equal to any urine output.

Peritoneal dialysis. An alternate form of treatment is peritoneal dialysis, which has the convenience of mobility. Approximately 10% of patients with ESRD who are on dialysis use this form of dialysis.[1] During this process, the patient introduces the dialysate solution directly into the **peritoneal cavity**, where the peritoneal membrane serves as the filter in which metabolic waste products can pass into the dialysate for removal from the body. *Continuous ambulatory peritoneal dialysis* is a form of continuous dialysis within the body. *Continuous cycling peritoneal dialysis* is a form of dialysis, using an automated device, providing several solution exchanges during sleep hours and one continuous exchange during the day.

First, the surgeon prepares the patient by placing a permanent catheter into the peritoneal cavity. Treatments are then carried out by doing the following: (1) attaching a disposable bag that contains the dialysate solution to the abdominal catheter, which leads into the peritoneal cavity; (2) emptying the dialysate into the peritoneal cavity and allowing 4 to 6 hours for the

solution exchange, known as dwell time; (3) allowing gravity to pull the waste-containing fluid back out of the peritoneal cavity into an empty bag; and (4) repeating the procedure (Figure 21.5). Individuals on peritoneal dialysis can move about in their normal daily activities throughout the dwell times but must remain stationary during the exchange of the dialysate and waste solution into and out of the bags (typically 20 to 30 minutes). The use of peritoneal dialysis at home gives the patient a sense of control, independence, and improved satisfaction with care.

peritoneal cavity a serous membrane that lines the abdominal and pelvic walls and the undersurface of the diaphragm to form a sac that encloses the body's vital visceral organs.

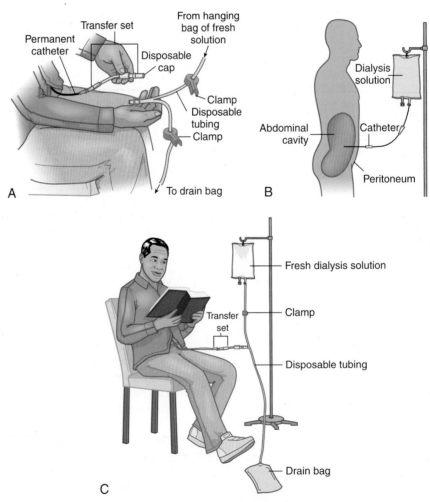

Figure 21.5 Continuous ambulatory peritoneal dialysis. (A) A soft tube catheter fills the abdomen with a cleansing dialysis solution. (B) A peritoneal membrane lines the walls of the abdominal cavity and allows waste products and extra fluid to pass from the blood into the dialysis solution. (C) Waste and fluid then leave the body during draining of the dialysis solution. The time during which the dialysis solution remains in the abdominal cavity (i.e., dwell time) ranges from 4 to 6 hours, and the patient can be mobile during this time. An exchange takes approximately 30 to 40 minutes, and a typical schedule requires four to five exchanges every day. (From National Institute of Diabetes and Digestive and Kidney Diseases. [2006]. *Treatment methods for kidney failure: Peritoneal dialysis* [NIH Publication No. 06-4688]. Bethesda, MD: National Institutes of Health.)

Medical nutrition therapy for peritoneal dialysis. Peritoneal dialysis allows for a slightly more liberal diet, as follows[5]:

- *Protein and energy:* AND recommends a protein intake of 1.2 to 1.3 g/kg of body weight for patients on peritoneal dialysis. Energy intake recommendations are the same as those for hemodialysis.
- *Sodium and potassium:* Depending on their fluid balance status, patients will limit sodium intake to 2 g/day. Potassium intake recommendations are 3 to 4 g/day, depending on serum levels.
- *Phosphorus, calcium, and fluid intake:* Recommendations for phosphorus, calcium, and fluid intake remain the same as those for hemodialysis.
- *Vitamins and minerals:* All recommendations are the same as those for hemodialysis, as described previously, with the following exception: individuals may need 1.5 to 2 mg/day of thiamin (vitamin B_1) because of losses that occur during

dialysis. Increased mean corpuscular volume (MCV) of greater than 100 ng/mL, low serum B_{12}, or folate levels indicate the need for additional supplementation.

Transplantation. Kidney transplantation, which is another treatment modality, improves quality of life and survival rates, and it is more cost effective than maintenance dialysis.[1,22] Current advances in surgical techniques, immunosuppressive drugs to prevent rejection, and antibiotics to control infection have helped to ensure successful outcomes (see the Drug-Nutrient Interaction box, "Immunosuppressive Therapies after Kidney Transplantation"). Clients who have undergone kidney transplantation have significantly lower rates of CVD progression and CVD mortality than those who remain on dialysis, despite the continuous use of immunosuppressive therapy.[1]

 Drug-Nutrient Interaction

Immunosuppressive Therapies After Kidney Transplantation

The kidney is the most commonly transplanted solid organ worldwide, and the need for kidney transplantation has grown over the past decade. Survival after kidney transplant is largely dependent on a successful immunosuppressive regimen with several antirejection medications. Most kidney transplant recipients undergo multidrug immunosuppressive therapy that includes corticosteroids to reduce the risk of acute rejection.[1] Over time, the patient may wean from steroid use but will continue on long-term maintenance regimens that include other antirejection medications. The use of corticosteroids is associated with a number of adverse side effects that specifically alter overall nutrition status, such as the following:

- Gastrointestinal irritation: esophagitis, dyspepsia, peptic ulcer disease
- Increased appetite and unintentional weight gain
- Hyperglycemia
- Protein catabolism and negative nitrogen balance
- Fluid retention
- Growth retardation (in children)
- Bone disease
- Cardiovascular disease and mortality

Corticosteroids also increase the excretion of several nutrients. Subsequently, individuals may need additional sources (from either the diet or dietary supplements) of folate, potassium, phosphorus, magnesium, zinc, protein, and vitamins A, B_6, B_{12}, and C. MNT recommendations include supplemental calcium and vitamin D for patients on

long-term corticosteroid treatment plans. If a patient is taking other antirejection medications concomitantly with corticosteroids, these medications may interact with nutrient bioavailability. For example, cyclosporine and tacrolimus (Prograf) are calcineurin inhibitors. These immunosuppressants may cause hyperkalemia; thus, patients must limit their intake of high-potassium foods or supplements when these drugs are part of the drug regimen. The health care team can monitor the patient's serum drug levels and electrolyte levels to adjust the medication dosage for optimal therapeutic benefit. Azathioprine (Imuran) and mycophenolate (CellCept) are other antirejection medications that do not have significant nutrient interactions, but they can cause nausea, vomiting, abdominal pain, and diarrhea in some individuals. This is especially a concern for patients who are unable to consume adequate nutrition and are at risk for malnutrition.

Research continues to explore alternative immunosuppressive regimens that avoid or reduce long-term steroid use. In the last two decades, the prevalence of steroid-free transplant regimens has increased but long-term survival rates have not improved. Experts need additional evidence-based research before they can explore new protocols.

REFERENCE

1. Axelrod, D., Naik, A. S., Schnitzler, M. A., et al. (2016). National variation in use of immunosuppression for kidney transplantation: A call for evidence-based regimen selection. *American Journal of Transplantation*, 16(8), 2453–2462.

The difficulty with transplantation is that waiting times can be long and donor matches difficult to find. See the Cultural Considerations box entitled "Cultural Disparities in Kidney Transplant Availability and

Success in Certain Ethnic and Racial Groups" for more details. Recipients of living donor transplants experience improved survival rates over those of deceased donors.[1]

Cultural Considerations

Cultural Disparities in Kidney Transplant Availability and Success in Certain Ethnic and Racial Groups

Kidney transplantation is the optimal treatment for individuals with end-stage renal disease. Surgeons performed more than 21,000 kidney transplants in the United States in 2018, of which approximately 14,500 of the donated kidneys were from deceased donors, and 6000 were from living donors.[1] Historically, white individuals had higher rates of receiving deceased-donor kidneys than minority individuals. Since 2016, the rates of deceased-donor transplants for African Americans and American Indians/Alaska Natives were similar to that of whites.[1] This improvement in kidney transplantation distribution is in part due to the recent changes in kidney allocation system (KAS) (activated in 2014). Another noted change is the increase in deceased-donation by African-American and Hispanic individuals, which may help match donors to recipients who are more immunologically compatible.[2] Advances in both medical technology and immunosuppressive therapies have led to longer lives for transplant recipients among all racial groups over the past several decades. Despite this increase in survival rates, African-American kidney transplant recipients continue to have lower 5-year survival rates among transplant recipients compared with their white counterparts. Hispanic and Asian transplant recipients have the best outcomes.[1]

Racial variation with regard to transplant success is related in part to differences in immunologic function among different racial groups. There are also social factors that affect the disparities in kidney transplantation survival rates. Researchers reported a correlation between transplant failure in African Americans and social factors such as a young age, lower education level, above-normal BMI, and lack of medical insurance.[3] To compound this issue, African-American individuals are more likely to have been on dialysis for a longer period and suffer comorbidities such as hypertension and diabetes. The longer that a recipient is on dialysis while waiting for a transplant, the lower the success rate of the transplant.[3]

The disparities in kidney transplant success rates are likely multifactorial and involve many of the above factors known to influence success rates. However, to decrease these disparities, researchers offer several suggestions for improvement. Effective education methods and materials must be culturally sensitive and consider the patients' beliefs, values, language, socioeconomic status, and social context. In addition, health care providers managing dialysis should receive education regarding kidney transplantation. This will allow them to supply quality education to both potential transplant patients and potential live donors during dialysis treatment sessions with patients. Likewise, offering education about live donor kidney transplant to families of patients with end-stage renal disease may improve the donor pool and thus ease the matching process for donors and recipients awaiting transplant. Research indicates that including education early during the course of treatment and frequently throughout treatment leads to an increase across all ethnic groups with regard to the patients' pursuit of transplantation.[4]

REFERENCES

1. Hart, A., et al. (2019). OPTN/SRTR 2017 Annual data report: Kidney. *American Journal of Transplantation*, 19(2), 19–123.
2. United States Renal Data System (2018). *2018 USRDS annual data report: Epidemiology of kidney disease in the United States.* Bethesda, MD: National Institutes of Health, National Institute of Diabetes and Digestive and Kidney Diseases.
3. Taber, D. J., Egede, L. E., & Baliga, P. K. (2017). Outcome disparities between African Americans and Caucasians in contemporary kidney transplant recipients. *The American Journal of Surgery*, 213(4), 666–672.
4. Jones, D., You, Z., & Kendrick, J. (2018). Racial/ethnic differences in barriers to kidney transplant evaluation among hemodialysis patients. *American Journal of Nephrology*, 47(1), 1–7.

The dietitian works with individuals who have undergone a kidney transplant to ensure highly individualized MNT that takes into consideration any co-morbidities and level of kidney function after surgery. Table 21.4 summarizes the nutrition guidelines for various levels of kidney disease and treatments.

Complications

Long-term complications of ESRD and dialysis include bone disorders, malnutrition, anemia, hormonal and blood pressure imbalances, depression, and diminished quality of life because of constant dependence on treatments. We addressed several of these conditions earlier in this chapter. Additional complications of CKD found in patients with ESRD include the following.

Enteral or parenteral nutrition support. There are special considerations for patients on dialysis who are in medical need of nutrition support via enteral or parenteral feedings. A medical necessity of nutrition support usually means that the patient is experiencing severe malnutrition, inflammation, and anorexia. The type and tolerance of dialysis is a consideration when choosing an appropriate nutrition support modality, as well as the current GFR, metabolic state, stress, and nitrogen balance. The American Society for Parenteral and Enteral Nutrition has published clinical guidelines for administering and evaluating nutrition support specifically for patients with CKD.[23]

Osteodystrophy. Bone disease and disorders are prevalent in cases of CKD, and they are a leading cause of morbidity. Several factors contribute to renal osteodystrophy and CKD-MBD. The decreased activation of vitamin D has a cascading effect that results in elevated levels of parathyroid hormone, reduced calcium absorption from the gastrointestinal tract, and low serum calcium levels. Patients also have elevated serum phosphorus levels because of the inability of the kidney to excrete phosphorus. This combination

Table **21.4**   **Recommended Nutrition Guidelines for Adults With Chronic Kidney Disease**

NUTRIENT	CKD STAGES 3 TO 5 WITHOUT RRT (GFR CATEGORIES 3 TO 5)	CKD STAGE 5 WITH RRT (KIDNEY FAILURE)	POST-TRANSPLANTATION (GUIDED BY CKD STAGE/CATEGORY OF KIDNEY FUNCTION)
Protein	0.6 to 0.8 g/kg of BW/day with at least 50% HBV to potentially slow disease progression (particularly in patients with diabetes) and achieve/maintain adequate serum albumin	1.1 to 1.5 g/kg of BW/day (HD with at least 50% HBV to achieve/maintain adequate serum albumin levels in conjunction with sufficient protein-sparing caloric intake)	0.8 to 1.0 g/kg of BW/day with 50% coming from HBV sources
Energy	25 to 35 kcal/kg of BW/day to achieve or maintain goal body weight	25 to 35 kcal/kg of BW/day to achieve or maintain goal body weight; include estimated caloric absorption from PD fluid as applicable	25 to 35 kcal/kg of BW/day to achieve or maintain goal body weight
Fat	General population recommendation of <30% of total calories from fat; emphasis on healthy fat sources	Focus on type of fat and carbohydrate to manage dyslipidemia, if present	Focus on type of fat and carbohydrate to reduce cardiovascular risk or manage immunosuppressant medication adverse effect (e.g., dyslipidemia, glucose intolerance)
Saturated fat	Same as for general population; <7% of total fat	Reduce and substitute saturated fat sources with healthier fat sources	Reduce and substitute saturated fat sources with healthier fat sources
Sodium	General population recommendation of ≤2.3 g/day	2.0 to 3.0 g/day (HD) to control interdialytic fluid gain; 2.0 to 4.0 g/day (PD) to control hydration status	General population recommendation of ≤2.3 g/day
Potassium	Typically not restricted until hyperkalemia is present, then individualized	2.0 to 4.0 g/day or 40 mg/kg of BW/day in HD or individualized in PD to achieve normal serum levels	No restriction unless hyperkalemia is present, then individualized
Calcium	No restriction	2 g elemental/day from dietary and medication sources	Individualized to kidney function
Phosphorus	Typically not restricted until hyperphosphatemia is present, then individualized to maintain normal serum levels by diet and/or phosphate binders	800 to 1000 mg/day to achieve goal serum level of 3.5 to 5.5 mg/dL or below; coordinate with oral phosphate binder prescription	Individualized to stage of kidney function
Fiber	Same as general population; 25 to 38 g/day	Same as general population; 25 to 38 g/day	Same as general population; 25 to 38 g/day
Fluid	No restriction	1000 mL/day (+ urine output if present) in HD; greater in PD; individualized to fluid status	No restriction; matched to urine output if appropriate

BW, Body weight; *CKD,* chronic kidney disease; *GFR,* glomerular filtration rate; *HBV,* high biologic value; *HD,* hemodialysis; *PD,* peritoneal dialysis; *RRT,* renal replacement therapy (i.e., hemodialysis, peritoneal dialysis).
From Beto, J. A., Ramirez, W. E., & Bansal, V. K. (2014). Medical nutrition therapy in adults with chronic kidney disease: Integrating evidence and consensus into practice for the generalist registered dietitian nutritionist. *J Acad Nutr Diet, 114*(7), 1077–1087.

causes abnormal changes in bone structure and function. Hyperphosphatemia is associated with increased mortality risk; thus, phosphate binders are an important management aspect of CKD. The health care team will evaluate patients with a GFR less than 45 mL/min per 1.73 m^2 for bone disease and disorders of calcium and phosphorus metabolism. Treatment strategies for bone disorders require a highly individualized management plan and continue to evolve in the light of new research.[24]

Neuropathy. In the absence of functioning kidneys, toxic substances accumulate in the blood, resulting in a uremic state. These toxic substances damage nerve tissues and lead to painful neuropathies in the majority of individuals with ESRD. Central and peripheral neurologic disturbances may be present at the initiation of dialysis, particularly for patients with diabetes. Symptoms of neuropathy are more common when the GFR falls below 20 mL/min per 1.73 m^2 and when serum creatinine levels rise. The health care team will periodically assess patients for neuropathy irrespective of symptoms because some cases are asymptomatic. Addressing and managing pain are important aspects of health care to maintain quality of life in patients with ESRD.

KIDNEY STONE DISEASE

In the United States, approximately 9.4% of women and 10.9% of men form kidney stones at some point during their lives.[25] The etiology of **nephrolithiasis** is unknown, but many factors that relate to the nature of the urine itself (e.g., pH, concentration) or to conditions of the urinary tract environment contribute to **supersaturation** and stone formation. Co-morbidities such as obesity, diabetes, gout, and hyperparathyroidism increase the risk for stone formation.[26-28] The most common types of kidney stones are calcium, struvite, and uric acid. Figure 21.6 illustrates various types of stones. Box 21.2 lists additional risk factors that are associated with kidney stone development.

DISEASE PROCESS

Calcium Stones

Calcium oxalate and calcium phosphate stones are the most common types, and they account for approximately 80% of all kidney stones. The supersaturation of kidney stone materials in the urine may result from the following[28]:

- Excess calcium in the blood (hypercalcemia) or urine (hypercalciuria)
- Excess oxalate (hyperoxaluria) or uric acid in the urine (hyperuricosuria)
- Low levels of citrate in the urine (hypocitraturia)

High levels of urinary oxalate increase the risk of an individual forming a calcium oxalate stone. We synthesize oxalates endogenously (relative to lean body mass) and consume oxalates in the diet. High-oxalate food sources include dark green leafy vegetables (e.g., spinach, kale, collard greens), beans (e.g., wax, dried), beets, potatoes, bran products, cocoa, tea, and some nuts. Small percentages of the population are "hyperabsorbers" of dietary oxalate and thus are at higher risk of forming stones. Oxalic acid is a metabolite of ascorbic acid. Therefore, the long-term supplementation of vitamin C in excess of the tolerable upper intake (2000 mg/day) may pose a potential health risk for kidney stone formation, especially for women.[29,30]

Adequate dietary calcium intake helps to prevent calcium oxalate stone formation.[28,31] Individuals with a low dietary intake of calcium are at a *higher* risk for calcium oxalate stone formation than those who consume the DRI for calcium. Dietary calcium binds oxalates in the intestines, which prevents oxalate absorption and concentration in the urine. It was common to restrict the dietary intake of calcium in patients who formed calcium oxalate stones in the past. We now know that this practice exacerbates the risk for stone formation.

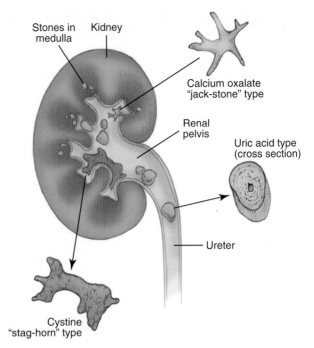

Figure 21.6 Renal calculi: stones in the kidney, renal pelvis, and ureter.

Box 21.2	Risk Factors for the Development of Kidney Stones

DIETARY
- Inadequate fluid intake
- Low calcium intake
- High animal protein intake
- High sodium intake
- Frequent sugar-sweetened beverage consumption

DISEASES OR DISORDERS
- Eating disorders, multiple food restrictions, or food intolerances or allergies
- Chronic diarrhea from malabsorption disorders or bowel disease
- Obesity, type 2 diabetes, gout, hyperparathyroidism, metabolic syndrome
- Chronic urinary tract infections

FAMILIAL
- Personal history or family history of urolithiasis
- Genetic predisposition for stone formation
- Congenital disorders of the kidneys

Struvite Stones

Struvite stones, which account for approximately 10% of all kidney stones, are composed of magnesium ammonium phosphate and carbonate apatite. We frequently refer to them as *infection stones* because they are primarily caused by urinary tract infections and not associated with any specific nutrient. Thus, there is not a particular MNT recommended for individuals

---

nephrolithiasis the formation of a kidney stone.
supersaturation (pertaining to urine) excess concentration of solutes

with struvite stones. Struvite stones are usually large "staghorn" stones that require surgical intervention.

Uric Acid Stones

Approximately 10% to 20% of kidney stones are uric acid stones. The primary risk factors for uric acid stone formation are overly acidic urine, excess urinary excretion of uric acid, and low urine volume.[28] Hyperuricosuria may result from an impairment of purine metabolism. Purine is a nitrogen product of protein metabolism and forms uric acid. This impairment occurs with diseases such as gout, and it can occur with rapid tissue breakdown during wasting disease. Other conditions that are associated with persistently acidic urine and uric acid stone formation are diarrheal illness (e.g., short-gut syndrome, inflammatory bowel disease), type 2 diabetes, obesity, and metabolic syndrome.[32,33]

Other Stones

Other rare forms of kidney stones are often reflective of hereditary disorders or complications of medications. For example, cystine stones are the result of a genetic defect in the renal reabsorption process of the amino acid cystine (the oxidized dimer form of the amino acid cysteine). Without reabsorption, cystine accumulates in the urine (cystinuria). Cystine is not soluble, and thus a high concentration may result in stone formation.

Clinical Symptoms

The main symptom of kidney stones is severe pain. Many other urinary symptoms may result from the presence of the stones, and general weakness and sometimes fever are present. Laboratory examination of the urine and of any passed stones helps to determine treatment.

MEDICAL NUTRITION THERAPY FOR NEPHROLITHIASIS

General Objectives

MNT may include several aspects, and it will vary depending on the type of stone. General MNT recommendations are as follows[5]:

- *Energy:* Overweight and obesity increase the risk for several chronic diseases as well as for kidney stone formation. The dietitian will customize the patient's total energy intake to achieve an ideal body weight. Healthy eating patterns such as the DASH diet or Mediterranean diet are ideal (see Chapter 19). Health care providers should discourage high-protein, low-potassium diets for individuals at risk for stone formation.[34]
- *Protein:* Excessive protein intake from animal sources is a risk factor for kidney stone formation. Thus, individuals should normalize their intake to healthy population standard recommendations of 0.8 to 1.0 g/kg/day.
- *Calcium:* Low dietary calcium intake is a risk for calcium oxalate stone formation. Thus, the dietitian or health care provider should encourage the patient

to meet the DRI for calcium (1000 to 1200 mg/day) and balance intake throughout the day.

- *Phosphorus:* If patients are consuming phosphorus in amounts higher than the DRI (i.e., >700 mg/day), then the dietitian will encourage them to limit their intake to the DRI amount and no more. Many convenience food items use phosphorus as an additive or preservative and are therefore high in phosphorus.
- *Sodium and potassium:* High sodium intake increases the amount of calcium excretion in the urine, thereby precipitating hypercalciuria, and it is associated with an increased risk of stone formation. All stone formers should observe a low-sodium diet (<2300 mg/day). Citrate and potassium are helpful in solubilizing calcium salts and preventing calcium oxalate stone formation. Consuming a diet that is rich in fruits (particularly citrus fruits) and vegetables helps provide a potassium intake of more than 4.7 g/day.
- *Oxalates:* Limiting dietary oxalates reduces urinary oxalate excretion and the risk of calcium oxalate stone formation.[28] Individuals prone to calcium oxalate stones should avoid unnecessary intake of high-oxalate foods.
- *Vitamins and minerals:* Vitamin C should not exceed the DRI, and all other vitamin and mineral intakes should meet the DRI standards.
- *Fluid:* A large fluid intake of at least 2 to 3 L/day helps to produce more dilute urine and thus to prevent the accumulation of materials that concentrate into stones. Exact fluid intake needs vary by individual, but health care providers should encourage enough fluids—preferably water—to produce at least 2 to 2.5 L of clear urine daily. For individuals who consume soft drinks, reducing sugar-sweetened beverage intake may lower the risk of recurrent stone formation.[35]

Objectives Specific to Type of Stone

The dietitian may further individualize the nutrition care plan specific to the nature of the stone formed. Varieties of medications are useful for the treatment of kidney stones in combination with MNT. Identifying the specific type of stone formed allows the physician to prescribe the most effective medication. However, collecting and analyzing a kidney stone is not always possible and subsequently limits drug therapy in some individuals.

Table 21.5 is a summary of dietary recommendations relative to specific type of stone formation.

Calcium stones. In some cases, dietary control of the stone constituents may help to reduce the recurrence of such stone formation. If a stone consists of calcium oxalate, then avoiding foods that are high in oxalate may be beneficial. If a stone consists of calcium phosphate, the client can minimize unnecessary dietary sources of phosphorus (e.g., foods containing phosphorus as an additive, meat, legumes).

Table **21.5**   Summary of Dietary Principles in Kidney Stone Disease

	NUTRIENT INTAKE RECOMMENDATION							
STONE TYPE	CALCIUM	OXALATE	SODIUM[a]	POTASSIUM[b]	ANIMAL PROTEIN	CITRATE	FRUCTOSE	FLUIDS
Calcium								
• Idiopathic calcium oxalate	1000–1200 mg	Avoid oxalate-rich foods	Reduce to <2000 mg	Increase to >120 mEq	Reduce to <0.8 g/kg	Increase	Reduce	Increase
• Calcium phosphate	800–1200 mg		Reduce to <2300 mg	?	Reduce to <1.2 g/kg	?		Increase
Uric acid				Increase	Reduce (also purines)	Increase		Increase
Cystine			Reduce to <2300 mg	Increase	Reduce to <1.2 g/kg	Increase		Increase
Struvite	1000–1200 mg		Reduce to <2300 mg					Increase

Empty box indicate that nutrient intake is not relevant; question marks indicate that it is currently unclear if dietary modification is beneficial or adverse.
[a]2300 mg Na corresponds to about 6 g of NaCl.
[b]120 mEq K corresponds to 4.7 g of K.
Data from Morgan, M. S. C., & Pearle, M. S. (2016). Medical management of renal stones. *Br Med J, 352,* i52; and Khan, S. R., Pearle, M. S., Robertson, W. G., et al. (2017). Kidney stones. *Nat Rev Dis Primers, 2,* 16008.

In addition to the recommendations listed previously, some calcium stone formers may also benefit from added sources of specific types of dietary fiber. Materials that bind potential stone elements in the intestine can prevent their absorption and remove these elements from the body through defecation. For example, phytate can bind calcium in the intestine and thus it helps to prevent the crystallization of oxalate calcium salts. Phytates are commonly in high-fiber plant foods such as whole wheat, bran, and soybeans.

Uric acid stones. Dietary attempts to alter urinary pH with **alkaline diets** that are low in purines may help to prevent uric acid concentration and stone formation within the kidneys. Acidic urine favors the kidneys' reuptake of uric acid, whereas alkaline urine favors the excretion of uric acid.[27] Potassium citrate treatments raise the urinary pH, which decreases the potential for uric acid supersaturation by favoring its excretion.[36] The primary goals of therapy are to establish and maintain a healthy weight and alkalization of the urine through a vegetarian-type diet with limited animal protein (including red meat, fish, and poultry).[31,34]

Cystine stones. The following dietary modifications help reduce cystine stone formation: reduce urinary cystine concentrations by decreasing intake of animal foods high in cystine and methionine; reduce sodium intake; increase intake of vegetables that are high in organic anions; and dilute the urine.[37] Diluting the urine requires the intake of copious amounts of water daily to void 3 to 4 L of urine per day.[37]

---

alkaline diet diet that is low in animal protein and high in fruits and vegetables.

Putting It All Together

Summary

- The nephrons are the functional units of the kidneys. Through these unique structures, the kidney maintains homeostasis of the materials required for life and health. The nephrons accomplish their tremendous task by constantly cleaning the blood, returning necessary elements to the blood, and eliminating the remainder in concentrated urine.

- Various diseases that interfere with the vital functions of nephrons can cause kidney disease. Kidney diseases have predisposing factors, such as diabetes, recurrent urinary tract infections that may lead to renal calculi, and progressive glomerulonephritis that may lead to chronic nephrotic syndrome and kidney failure.

- Dialysis or kidney transplantation are the two treatment options available for CKD at its end stage. Individuals who are undergoing dialysis require close monitoring for protein, water, nutrient, and electrolyte balance.

- Varieties of substances form kidney stones. For some individuals, a change in the dietary intake of the identified substance (e.g., sodium, oxalate, purine) and an increase in fluid intake may decrease stone formation.

Chapter Review Questions

See answers in Appendix A.

1. The hormone that acts on the distal nephron tubule to stimulate reabsorption of sodium is _____.

   a. aldosterone
   b. antidiuretic hormone
   c. insulin
   d. erythropoietin

2. Which of the following do the kidneys convert from an intermediate inactive form to its active form?

   a. Hemoglobin
   b. Nitrogen
   c. Vitamin D
   d. Vitamin E

3. A woman with nephrotic syndrome is likely to have _____.

   a. low serum albumin levels
   b. high serum albumin levels
   c. low plasma glucose levels
   d. high plasma glucose levels

4. Medical nutrition therapy for a man with stage 3 CKD, not treated with dialysis, who does not have diabetes includes _____.

   a. energy intake limited to 20 kcal/kg body weight
   b. fluid intake limited to 500 mL per day
   c. protein intake limited to 0.6 to 0.8 g/kg body weight
   d. sodium intake limited to 4 g per day

5. A protein source that is of high biologic value is _____.

   a. baked beans
   b. grilled chicken
   c. oatmeal
   d. spinach

Next-Generation NCLEX® Examination-style Case Study

See answers in Appendix A.

A 28-year-old female (Ht.: 5'6 Wt.: 132 lbs.) has been having severe side pain, nausea, and blood in her urine caused by a kidney stone. She has no previous medical history and does not take any medications. She mentions that she has been taking 3000 mg of vitamin C every day to avoid getting COVID-19. A diet analysis indicated that her intake of calcium was ~600 mg/day and phosphorous was ~3 mg/day. Her blood pressure was 127/85 mmHg and her fasting glucose levels were 90 mg/dL. She stated that she usually drinks about 30 oz. of fluid each day.

1. From the list below, select all factors from the client's history that are concerning.

   a. BMI
   b. Vitamin C intake
   c. Calcium intake
   d. Phosphorous intake
   e. Blood pressure
   f. Fasting glucose level
   g. Fluid intake

2. Choose the *most likely* options for the information missing from the statements below by selecting from the list of options provided.

   After a dietary recall was collected from the client, the dietitian identified large amounts of foods high in oxalate such as _____ and _____, which can increase the risk of kidney stone development.

OPTIONS	
spinach	collard greens
pasta	chicken
rice	beef

3. From the list below, select all the appropriate nutrition interventions related to the client's diagnosis of kidney stones.

   a. Maintain healthy weight
   b. Reduced protein needs
   c. Reduced calcium intake
   d. Phosphorous intake ≤DRI
   e. Reduced sodium intake
   f. Increased oxalate intake
   g. Reduced vitamin C intake
   h. Increased fluid intake

4. For each assessment finding, use an X to indicate whether nursing and collaborative interventions were <u>effective</u> (helped to meet expected outcomes), or <u>ineffective</u> (did not help to meet expected outcomes).

ASSESSMENT FINDING	EFFECTIVE	INEFFECTIVE
Client carries water bottle throughout the day to consume 2-3 L of fluid per day.		
Blood pressure: 119/79 mmHg		
Client focuses on consuming more fruits and vegetables such as oranges, grapefruits, and berries.		
Increased consumption of lean meats from animal sources.		
Client consumes low sodium dairy foods.		
Client reduces vitamin C supplementation to 60 mg of vitamin C per day.		
Client has resolution of hematuria.		

Additional Learning Resources

Please refer to this text's Evolve website for answers to the Case Study questions:
http://evolve.elsevier.com/Williams/basic/.
References and **Further Reading and Resources** in the back of the book provide additional resources for enhancing knowledge.

Surgery and Nutrition Support

Jean Zancanella MS, RDN

Key Concepts

- Surgical procedures may require nutrition support for tissue healing and recovery.
- Gastrointestinal (GI) surgery may necessitate diet modifications if the surgery alters the normal digestion or passage of food.
- To ensure optimal nutrition for postsurgical or critically ill patients, diet management may involve enteral or parenteral nutrition support.

Malnutrition is a significant risk for patients because it contributes to morbidity, mortality, extended length of stay in the hospital, and significant additional treatment costs.[1-3] Effective nutrition support should reverse malnutrition, improve prognosis, and speed recovery in a cost-effective manner.[4] The surgical process also places physiologic and psychologic stress on the client, which may lead to additional nutrition demands and elevates the risk for clinical complications.[5]

This chapter looks at the nutrition needs of surgical clients, burn patients, and the enteral and parenteral feeding methods for providing nutrition support. Careful attention to both preoperative and postoperative nutrition support can reduce complications and supply essential nutrient resources necessary for healing and health.

NUTRITION NEEDS OF GENERAL SURGERY PATIENTS

A client undergoing surgery often faces significant physical and psychologic stress. As a result, the body requires more nutrients during this period, and deficiencies can develop that manifest as malnutrition with subsequent clinical complications. Therefore, caregivers must pay careful attention to nutrition status in preparation for surgery as well as to the individual nutrition needs that follow surgery to address wound healing and recovery. Poor nutrition status and the following clinical problems are well documented[2,6-8]:

- Impaired wound healing and increased risk of infection
- Increased necessity of **enteral** or **parenteral** nutrition support
- Longer hospital stays and increased medical cost
- Increased morbidity and mortality rate
- Reduced quality of life

The diagnosis of malnutrition includes the following general characteristics: insufficient energy intake; weight loss; loss of muscle mass; loss of subcutaneous fat; localized or generalized fluid accumulation; and diminished functional status as measured by strength of handgrip.[9] A diagnosis requires that a patient meet two or more of these criteria. Table 22.1 provides the clinical diagnostic criteria for malnutrition.

PREOPERATIVE NUTRITION CARE: NUTRIENT RESERVES

When clients have elective surgery (i.e., not emergent), they have time to prepare beforehand for the nutrient demands of surgery and the period of limited food intake that often follows.

Protein

Protein deficiency among pediatric and geriatric hospital patients is common, particularly among critically ill patients.[10] Every surgical patient should be equipped with adequate body protein to counteract blood that is lost during surgery and prevent tissue catabolism during the immediate postoperative period (see the Clinical Applications box, "Protein-Energy Malnutrition after Surgery"). The adequate dietary consumption of high-quality complete proteins (i.e., those that have all of the essential amino acids) improves the body's ability to maintain lean tissue.[11]

---

enteral a mode of feeding that makes use of the gastrointestinal tract through oral or tube feedings.

parenteral a mode of feeding that does not involve the gastrointestinal tract but that instead provides nutrition support via the intravenous delivery of nutrient solutions.

| Table 22.1 | Clinical Diagnostic Criteria for Malnutrition |

CHARACTERISTICS TO DIAGNOSE SEVERE MALNUTRITION		
CHARACTERISTIC	**ACUTE ILLNESS OR INJURY RELATED MALNUTRITION**	**CHRONIC DISEASE RELATED MALNUTRITION**	**SOCIAL OR ENVIRONMENTAL RELATED MALNUTRITION**
Weight loss	>2%/1 week >5%/1 month >7.5%/3 months	>5%/1 month >7.5%/3 months >10%/6 months >20%/1 year	>5%/1 month >7.5%/3 months >10%/6 months >20%/1 year
Energy intake	≤50% for ≥5 days	≤75% for ≥1 month	≤50% for ≥1 month
Body fat	Moderate depletion	Severe depletion	Severe depletion
Muscle mass	Moderate depletion	Severe depletion	Severe depletion
Fluid accumulation	Moderate —> severe	Severe	Severe
Grip strength	Not recommended in intensive care unit	Reduced for age/sex	Reduced for age/sex

CHARACTERISTICS TO DIAGNOSE MODERATE MALNUTRITION		
CHARACTERISTIC	**ACUTE ILLNESS OR INJURY RELATED MALNUTRITION**	**CHRONIC DISEASE RELATED MALNUTRITION**	**SOCIAL OR ENVIRONMENTAL RELATED MALNUTRITION**
Weight loss	1%–2%/1 week 5%/1 month 7.5%/3 months	5%/1 month 7.5%/3 months 10%/6 months 20%/1 year	5%/1 month 7.5%/3 months 10%/6 months 20%/1 year
Energy intake	<75% for >7 days	<75% for ≥1 month	<75% for ≥3 months
Body fat	Mild depletion	Mild depletion	Mild depletion
Muscle mass	Mild depletion	Mild depletion	Mild depletion
Fluid accumulation	Mild	Mild	Mild
Grip strength	Not applicable	Not applicable	Not applicable

From Malone, A., & Hamilton, C. (2013). The Academy of Nutrition and Dietetics/the American Society for Parenteral and Enteral Nutrition consensus malnutrition characteristics: Application in practice. *Nutr Clin Pract, 28*(6), 639–650.

⬆ Clinical Applications

Protein-Energy Malnutrition After Surgery

Malnutrition compromises quality of life and the ability to recover from surgery and injury. As general health declines with age and the risk for unplanned surgery increases, so does the prevalence of malnutrition. Evaluating the nutrition status of older people in the home, the hospital, or a long-term care facility can help to identify clients who may benefit from improved nutrient intake before surgery. Using oral supplements or enteral feedings for malnourished patients before surgery improves clinical outcomes such as reducing infection and preventing unintentional weight loss.

The medical team should identify and monitor patients for malnutrition to prevent unintended weight loss associated with protein-energy malnutrition. Unplanned weight loss is indicative of malnutrition as well as of the inability to deal with physiologic stress. The Academy of Nutrition and Dietetics defines *moderate malnutrition* as an unintentional weight loss of up to 5% over a 1-month period or of 10% over a 6-month period. Unintentional weight loss beyond these amounts is diagnostic for *severe malnutrition*.[1] Identifying and treating those individuals who are at risk for malnutrition may also prevent poor outcomes in the event of injury or emergency surgery.

REFERENCE
1. Malone, A., & Hamilton, C. (2013). The Academy of Nutrition and Dietetics/the American Society for Parenteral and Enteral Nutrition consensus malnutrition characteristics: Application in practice. *Nutrition in Clinical Practice, 28*(6), 639–650.

Energy

Sufficient energy intake spares protein for its tissue-building function. When energy is not readily available, the body sacrifices protein for its kilocalories. Thus, providing adequate energy from carbohydrates and fats is necessary when clients need protein to build and repair tissue. Before surgery, underweight clients may benefit from extra energy to increase weight to a desired maintenance level. For overweight or obese individuals, reasonable weight reduction before elective surgery may help reduce surgical complications.

Micronutrients

When a client needs extra protein and energy, it is also important to supply the body with the necessary vitamins and minerals required for protein and energy metabolism (e.g., B-complex vitamins). The health care team must identify and correct any nutrient deficiencies (e.g., iron-deficiency anemia) or electrolyte and water imbalances before surgery.

Immediate Preoperative Period

The usual preparation for surgery requires that nothing is taken orally for at least 8 hours before the procedure.[12] This protocol ensures that the stomach does not retain food during surgery. The presence of food may cause complications, such as aspirating food particles during anesthesia or vomiting in the course of recovery from anesthesia. In addition, any food present in the stomach may interfere with the surgical procedure or increase the risk for postoperative gastric retention and expansion. The health care team often recommends fiber-restricted diets for several days before GI surgery to clear the surgical site of any food residue (Table 22.2). Commercial elemental formulas that are free of residue can supply a complete diet in liquid form. Clients can drink these formulas or take them through an enteral feeding tube. Adding flavoring to formulas or drinking them through a straw improves palatability.

Emergency Surgery

When surgery is urgent, there is no time to maximize nutrition reserves. Clients who are well nourished have fewer risks associated with surgery because their reserves are available to meet their needs during times of stress.[13]

POSTOPERATIVE NUTRITION CARE: NUTRIENT NEEDS FOR HEALING

To help with recovery from surgery, patients need nutrition support to replenish nutrient stores. Clients may experience diminished or a complete lack of food intake for a period after surgery. If clients are not able to resume adequate oral intake within a few days, the health care team may consider an alternative form of nutrition support. Several nutrients require attention during this time, as discussed in the following sections.

Protein

As with the preoperative period, it is important for clients to consume optimal amounts of protein during the postoperative recovery period. Immediately after major surgery, the body tissues may undergo considerable catabolism, which means that the process of tissue breakdown and loss exceeds the process of tissue buildup (i.e., anabolism). Weight loss and malnutrition are common among patients who are experiencing catabolic stress. The maintenance of lean body mass improves the outcomes for some catabolic patients.[14]

In addition to protein losses from the breakdown of tissue, other losses of protein from the body may occur. These losses include plasma protein from hemorrhage, blood loss, and various body fluids or exudates. The health care team should monitor patients for increased

---

residue any undigested or unabsorbed food remaining in the colon after digestion has taken place; includes fiber and substances that stimulate contractions of the GI tract.

elemental formula a nutrition support formula composed of simple elemental nutrient components that require no further digestive breakdown and are thus readily absorbed (e.g., glucose, amino acids, medium-chain triglycerides).

exudate a fluid with a high content of protein and cellular debris, which has escaped from blood vessels and deposited in tissues or on tissue surfaces, usually a result of inflammation.

Table 22.2	Fiber-Restricted Diet[a]	
FOOD TYPE	**FOODS ALLOWED**	**FOODS NOT ALLOWED**
Dairy	Buttermilk and kefir Fat-free and low-fat milk and milk-substitute products (e.g., soy, rice, almond milk) Yogurt and mild cheese Lactose-free dairy products	Whole milk Half-and-half Cream and sour cream Dairy products with nuts or fruit
Grains	Grains with <2 g of fiber per serving Grain products made with white or refined flour	Grains made with whole wheat or whole grains Grains made with seeds or nuts Popcorn
Fruit	Canned, soft, or well-cooked fruit without skin, seeds, or membranes Fruit juice without pulp	Raw fruits Fruit with skin Dried fruit Fruit juice with pulp Prune juice
Vegetables	Canned, soft, or well-cooked vegetables without skin, seeds, or hulls Mashed potatoes Vegetable juice without skin	Raw or undercooked vegetables High-fiber vegetables Gas-forming vegetables
Fats and oils	Limit to less than 8 tsp daily	Coconut Avocado

[a]Fiber-restricted diet: This diet contains less than 13 grams of fiber and includes foods that are low in fiber, seeds, and skins and with a minimal amount of residue. The diet should be adequate in protein and energy but may be inadequate in micronutrients. Consider supplementary vitamins and minerals if clients are to continue this diet for a long period.
Reference: Academy of Nutrition and Dietetics. (2019). *Nutrition care manual.* Chicago: Academy of Nutrition and Dietetics.

loss of plasma protein from extensive tissue destruction, inflammation, infection, and trauma. If any degree of prior malnutrition or chronic infection exists, a state of protein deficiency may contribute to significant clinical complications. Such problems include poor wound healing, the rupture of the suture lines (i.e., **dehiscence**), the delayed healing of fractures, depressed heart and lung function, anemia, the failure of GI **stomas**, a reduced resistance to infection, liver damage, extensive weight loss, muscle wasting, and an increased mortality risk.

Building tissue. The process of wound healing requires building new body tissue, which depends on adequate amounts of essential amino acids. During wound healing, a client's dietary protein needs increase beyond normal to restore lost protein and to build new tissues at the wound site.

Protein and minerals are essential to the foundation of bone tissue and for proper bone formation and healing. Protein supplies the matrix for calcium and phosphorus, which strong bones require.

Controlling edema and shock. An adequate supply of the plasma protein albumin is necessary to maintain blood volume. When a client's albumin level drops, pressure to keep tissue fluid circulating between the capillaries and cells is insufficient. Without adequate pressure, capillaries lose water, which results in edema (see Chapter 9). Edema is the swelling of tissue from excess fluid that that does not return to circulation. Generalized edema may adversely affect heart and lung function. Local edema at the wound site interferes with the closure of the wound and hinders the healing process.

Excessive loss of blood from circulation (because of low albumin level and subsequent edema) may lead to symptoms of shock as the body attempts to restore **euvolemia**.

Resisting infection. Protein is the major component of the body's immune system. The immune system's defensive agents include specialized white cells called *lymphocytes* as well as antibodies and various other blood cells, hormones, and enzymes. Strong body tissue provides a major defense barrier against infection.

Transporting lipids. Fat is another vital component of tissue structure. It forms the lipid bilayer of cell membranes, and it takes part in many other metabolic activities. Protein is necessary to transport fat through circulation to all tissues and to the liver for metabolism (e.g., lipoproteins).

Energy

When the body needs to build tissue, we must supply it with adequate amounts of kilocalories from carbohydrates and fat in order to spare protein for this vital function. In situations of acute metabolic stress (e.g., with extensive surgery or burns), energy needs may increase to as much as 1.2 to 2 kcal/kg of body weight/day over basal energy requirements. We estimate energy requirements by first calculating the individual's basal metabolic rate (BMR) with the Mifflin-St. Jeor equation (see Chapter 6) and then multiplying by an injury factor (1 to 2, depending on the client's status) to meet the added energy needs of metabolic stress and **sepsis**:

$$\text{Male} = [(10 \times \text{Weight in kg}) + (6.25 \times \text{Height in cm}) - (5 \times \text{Age in years}) + 5] \times \text{injury factor}$$

$$\text{Female} = [(10 \times \text{Weight in kg}) + (6.25 \times \text{Height in cm}) - (5 \times \text{Age in years}) - 161] \times \text{injury factor}$$

The clinical dietitian carefully estimates energy requirements in surgical patients to prevent overfeeding, which is associated with several complications.

Water

Surgery may cause altered fluid distribution in the body. Fluid replacement is necessary to prevent dehydration, maintain circulation, and reduce complications. Each client requires an individualized plan for meeting fluid therapy goals during and after surgery.[15] Elderly clients, whose thirst mechanisms may be depressed, call for special attention to total fluid intake and hydration status. During the postoperative period, large water losses may occur from vomiting, hemorrhage, fever, infection, or **diuresis**. An assortment of solutions is available for intravenous (IV) administration, depending on the client's needs. IV fluids after surgery supply initial hydration needs, but clients should transition to oral intake as soon as possible

Vitamins

Some vitamins play a vital role in wound healing. For example, vitamin C is vital for building connective tissue and capillary walls during the healing process, yet vitamin C levels may be low, particularly in critically ill malnourished individuals. In some post–cardiac

---

dehiscence a splitting open; the separation of the layers of a surgical wound that may be partial, superficial, or complete and that involves total disruption and re-suturing.

stoma an opening that is established in the abdominal wall that connects with the ileum or the colon for the elimination of intestinal wastes after the surgical removal of nonfunctional portions of the intestines.

euvolemia normal blood volume.

sepsis a life-threatening immune response to a bacterial infection.

diuresis the increased excretion of urine.

surgery patients, vitamin C protects the microvascular function and helps to decrease the length of hospital stay; additionally, vitamin C and thiamin combined with certain medications may be particularly beneficial for critically ill patients with sepsis.[16-18]

Supplementation with various combinations of antioxidants and polyunsaturated fatty acids shows promise in preventing postsurgical complications such as arrhythmias, oxidative stress, and inflammation.[19,20] Among malnourished individuals with pressure ulcers, supplementation with antioxidants, arginine, and zinc specifically improves the healing of wounds.[21]

When energy and protein needs increase, the B vitamins that have important coenzyme roles in protein and energy metabolism (e.g., thiamin, riboflavin, niacin) should increase as well. Other B vitamins (e.g., folate, B₁₂, pyridoxine, pantothenic acid) play important roles in building hemoglobin, and thus adequate amounts must be present to meet the demands of an increased blood supply and general metabolic stress.

Minerals

Attention to mineral deficiencies is important, and supplementation may prove helpful in recovery from surgery. However, there is no universally accepted list of minerals or dosing recommendations required for postsurgical or critically ill individuals.[18,22] Tissue catabolism results in the loss of potassium and phosphorus from cells. Electrolyte imbalances of sodium and chloride also result from fluid imbalances. Iron-deficiency anemia may develop from blood loss or inadequate iron absorption. Individuals with critical illness or sepsis, who have low levels of zinc and selenium in reaction to the inflammatory response, have elevated risk for added oxidative stress and inflammation.[23,24] Furthermore, mortality rates are significantly lower in critically ill patients who have adequate serum levels of zinc and copper.[25] Zinc is also important for wound healing; however, even if clients have adequate zinc intake, surgical trauma and infection may lead to reduced serum zinc status and elevated needs.

GENERAL DIETARY MANAGEMENT

The nutrition support needed for hospitalized individuals varies. Patients' medical nutrition therapy (MNT) plan depends on their nutrition status upon arrival, the metabolic results of their condition, their ability to consume food, and their advance directive, or living will.

INITIAL INTRAVENOUS FLUID AND ELECTROLYTES

Routine IV fluids supply hydration and electrolytes; they cannot sustain energy and nutrient balance. For example, a 5% dextrose solution with normal saline (i.e., 0.9% sodium chloride solution) contains only 5 g of dextrose/dL. This equals approximately 170 kcal/L

because dextrose provides only 3.4 kcal/g. Meanwhile, the person's total energy need is typically more than 10 times that amount. For clients receiving only IV fluids, the return to regular food should occur as soon as possible. Methods of preparing people for surgery and the recovery that follows is undergoing a paradigm shift and hospitals are looking at ways to enhance the pre and postsurgical experience (see the For Further Focus box: Enhanced Recovery After Surgery Protocol).

🔍 **For Further Focus**

Enhanced Recovery After Surgery Protocol

The Enhanced Recovery After Surgery (ERAS) protocol questions many long-held beliefs and surgical practices. The ERAS protocol decreases the physiologic stress of surgery and promotes a faster and easier recovery. ERAS considers many aspects of treating patients before and after surgery, of which nutrition is just one of the important components. These protocols appear to be highly effective[1]; however, hospitals have been slow to adopt them.

Requiring clients to fast after midnight on the night before an elective surgical procedure is a tradition. However, support in the literature for this practice is lacking. ERAS eliminates the midnight fast and even recommends drinking high-carbohydrate beverages before surgery. Clients drink a clear, carbohydrate-rich beverage on the night before surgery and another high-carbohydrate beverage 2 hours before surgery on the day of the procedure. These carbohydrate-containing beverages reduce thirst and hunger and appear to have other metabolic benefits. Allowing people to eat (and drink) puts them in an anabolic, rather than catabolic, state before surgery. After surgery, caregivers may begin feeding patients within 12 hours, and most people tolerate feedings well.[2]

ERAS protocols involve many aspects of patient care. By adopting these protocols, some hospitals have been able to reduce postop infection occurrence, hospital length of stay, client satisfaction, and even hospital costs.[2,3]

REFERENCES
1. Horosz, B. K., Nawrocka, K., & Malec-Milewska, M. (2016). Anaesthetic perioperative management according to the ERAS protocol. *Anaesthesiology Intensive Therapy, 48*(1), 49–54.
2. Liu, V. X., et al. (2017). Enhanced recovery after surgery program implementation in 2 surgical populations in an integrated health care delivery system. *JAMA Surgery, 152*(7), e171032.
3. Stone, A. B., et al. (2016). Implementation costs of an enhanced recovery after surgery program in the United States: A financial model and sensitivity analysis based on experiences at a quaternary academic medical center. *Journal of the American College of Surgeons, 222*(3), 219–225.

METHODS OF NUTRITION SUPPORT

Malnutrition during hospital stays is a common occurrence, and the risk for malnutrition increases with advanced age, disease status, and the length of the hospital stay.[1,2,26] The physician, the dietitian, and the nurse work together to manage the diet with oral, enteral, or parenteral feeding as necessary:

- *Oral:* Nourishment through the regular GI route by oral feedings; may include a variety of diet plans, textures, and meal replacement liquid supplements

- *Enteral:* Technically refers to nourishment through the regular GI route either by regular oral feedings or by tube feedings; however, in medical nutrition therapy, enteral feedings imply *tube feedings*
- *Parenteral:* Nourishment through the veins (either small peripheral veins or a large central vein) bypassing the GI tract

Nutrition support provides nutrition when individuals cannot meet their needs with oral feedings. Table 22.3 provides a list of conditions that may require nutrition support by tube feeding or parenteral nutrition. Box 22.1 lists the general criteria for selecting the most appropriate nutrition support method. In addition, Figure 22.1 provides the algorithm for determining the route for nutrition support administration.

Oral Feedings

When the GI tract is functional, it is the preferred route of feeding: orally if possible and by feeding tube if not. Most general surgical patients can and should receive

Table 22.3	Conditions That Often Require Nutrition Support	
RECOMMENDED ROUTE OF FEEDING	**CONDITION**	**EXAMPLES**
Enteral nutrition	Impaired nutrient ingestion	Neurologic disorders Facial, oral, or esophageal trauma or surgery Congenital anomalies Respiratory failure Cystic fibrosis Traumatic brain injury Anorexia and wasting with severe eating disorders
	Inability to consume adequate nutrition orally	Hyperemesis gravidarum Hypermetabolic states (e.g., burns) Comatose states Anorexia with congestive heart failure, cancer, chronic obstructive pulmonary disease, and eating disorders Congenital heart disease Severe dysphagia Premature birth without suck reflex Spinal cord injury
	Impaired digestion, absorption, and metabolism	Severe gastroparesis Inborn errors of metabolism Crohn's disease Obstruction in the upper gastrointestinal tract Short-bowel syndrome with minimal resection
	Severe wasting or depressed growth	Cystic fibrosis Failure to thrive Cancer, HIV/AIDS Sepsis Cerebral palsy Myasthenia gravis
Parenteral nutrition	Gastrointestinal incompetence	Nothing by mouth before surgery for more than 7 days Obstruction in the lower gastrointestinal tract Intestinal infarction Short-bowel syndrome or major resection Severe acute pancreatitis Severe inflammatory bowel disease Small-bowel ischemia Intestinal atresia Severe liver failure Major gastrointestinal surgery
	Critical illness with poor enteral tolerance or accessibility	Multiorgan system failure Major trauma or burns Bone marrow transplantation Acute respiratory failure with ventilator dependency and gastrointestinal malfunction Severe wasting with renal failure and dialysis Small-bowel transplantation, immediately after surgery

Modified from Mahan, L. K., & Escott-Stump, S. (2012). *Krause's food & nutrition therapy* (13th ed.). St. Louis: Saunders.

Criteria for Selecting a Nutrition Support Method

The physician and registered dietitian nutritionist (RDN) will decide the most appropriate method of medical nutrition therapy for the patient with the use of the following criteria. Either the pharmacist or the RDN will make the calculations for the enteral formula or parenteral nutrition solution. There is typically no indication for nutrition support when prognosis does not warrant continued aggressive therapies or if the patient/caregivers refuse nutrition support.

ENTERAL NUTRITION SUPPORT
Indicated for patients with the following characteristics:
- They have enough functional gastrointestinal tract to allow adequate digestion and absorption.
- They cannot eat enough to meet their nutrient needs orally.
- They are at risk for malnutrition without nutrition support.

PARENTERAL NUTRITION SUPPORT
Indicated for patients with the following characteristics:
- They do not have sufficient gastrointestinal tract function, and they need long-term nutrition support.
- They are unable to meet nutrient needs after 7 to 10 days of enteral nutrition.
- There is a need for bowel rest (e.g., enteral fistulas, acute inflammatory bowel disease).
- They do not have access for feeding tube placement and need nutrition support.
- They repeatedly pull out their feeding tubes.

If parenteral nutrition support is necessary, the health care team must then decide on the specific location to administer the nutrition support:

Peripheral Parenteral Nutrition
- Length of therapy of ≤10 to 14 days
- Not hypermetabolic
- No fluid restriction

Central Parenteral Nutrition
- Long-term therapy needed
- Hypermetabolic
- Poor peripheral access or central access already in place

"house" diets. House diets offer texture modifications ranging from clear liquid (liquids you can see through) to full liquid (including milk, strained cream soups, etc.) and from soft food to a full regular diet. Clients with chewing or swallowing problems benefit from mechanically altered, soft diets. Caregivers may add small amounts of liquid to regular foods to achieve an appropriate pureed consistency. Mechanically altered diets can range from low sodium, low fat, to high fat, or high protein depending on the client's needs. Therapeutic soft diets help clients to transition from liquid to regular diets. Table 22.4 summarizes the basic details of routine hospital diets.

Assisted oral feeding. Clients may need help with eating, depending on their condition. Health care providers should encourage clients to remain independent and help them to do so with whatever degree of assistance that is necessary. Caregivers can provide plate guards or special utensils to facilitate independence. The staff should try to learn each client's needs and limitations because small actions such as cutting meat or buttering bread before bringing the tray to the bedside promote feelings of independence. Box 22.2 provides guidelines for personnel for assisting clients at mealtimes.

Providing a client with assistance at mealtime is an opportunity for nutrition counseling and support. Attentive caregivers make important observations during this time. For example, the assistant can closely observe the client's appetite, physical appearance, and tolerance to the foods served. These observations help the nurse and the dietitian adapt the client's diet to meet individual needs. Helping clients learn more about their own nutrition needs is an important part of personal care. It may encourage clients to maintain sound eating habits after discharge from the hospital as well as to improve their eating habits in general.

oral feedings as soon as possible to provide adequate nutrition. Early initiation of oral feedings (i.e., within 24 hours after injury, surgery, or hospital admission) is associated with reduced complications and infections, and, in some cases, reduced hospital stays.[27] When oral feedings begin, the client may begin to consume clear or full liquids and then progress to a soft or regular diet as indicated. If inadequate caloric intake is a concern, the dietitian may increase the energy value of foods in the regular diet with added sauces, dried protein powder, or dressings. Caregivers may add supplemental nutrition drinks such as Boost or Ensure with or between meals to improve oral intake. Some clients benefit from small, frequent, energy-dense meals or snacks to help make every bite count.

Routine house diets. Most hospital food service departments follow a cycle menu consisting of routine

Enteral Feedings
When a client cannot eat or drink, but the remaining portions of the GI tract are functioning, an alternate form of enteral nutrition (EN), delivered to the GI tract by tube, provides nutrition support. Enteral tube feedings preserve gut function and are less invasive and less expensive than parenteral nutrition. Even when clients can only tolerate small amounts of enteral feedings, providing some portion of the day's nutrient needs through the GI tract is helpful. Maintaining some level of gut function helps to prevent atrophy of the GI tract.

If a client requires enteral tube feeding for a short time (less than 4 weeks), a feeding tube is usually inserted into the stomach through the nose (nasogastric). For clients who are at risk for aspiration, reflux, or continual vomiting, a nasoduodenal or nasojejunal tube may be more appropriate (Figure 22.2A).[28] In both cases, a practitioner passes a tube through the nose and then down

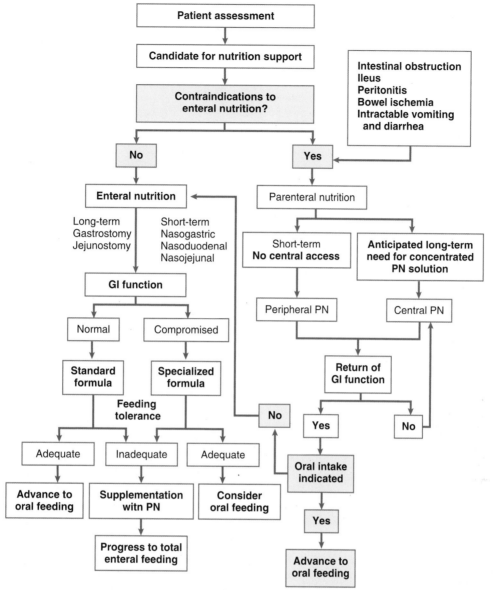

Figure 22.1 Route of administration algorithm for nutrition support. *PN*, Parenteral nutrition. (Reprinted from Ukleja, A., et al. [2010]. Standards for nutrition support: Adult hospitalized patients. *Nutr Clin Pract*, 25[4], 403–414.)

the esophagus and into the stomach. The tube passes through the stomach and into the proper location of the small intestine by peristaltic activity, endoscopic, or fluoroscopic guidance. To verify the correct placement of the tube, a health care provider will use one of the following methods: radiography, **auscultation**, or gastric content aspiration.[28] Modern small-bore nasoenteric feeding tubes are made of soft and flexible polyurethane and silicone materials. These feeding tubes are relatively comfortable for the client, and deliver the nutrients provided by EN formulas easily.

Routes. The patient's disease state, estimated length for enteral therapy, GI anatomy and function, and ability to access the GI tract safely are important aspects to consider when determining the most appropriate access point for EN. In many clinical situations, using the nasoenteric route for short-term therapy of 4 to 6 weeks

or less is beneficial. For long-term feedings, however, an enterostomy (i.e., the surgical placement of the tube at progressive points along the GI tract) provides a more comfortable route, as follows (Figure 22.2B):

- *Esophagostomy:* The surgeon places a cervical esophagostomy at the level of the cervical spine to the side of the neck after head and neck surgeries or traumatic injury. This placement removes the discomfort of the nasal route and enables concealment of the entry point under clothing.
- *Percutaneous endoscopic gastrostomy:* If the client is not at risk for aspiration, the surgeon will place a gastrostomy tube through the abdominal wall into the stomach.

auscultation listening to the sounds of the gastrointestinal tract with a stethoscope.

Table 22.4 Routine Hospital Diets

FOOD	CLEAR LIQUID[a]	FULL LIQUID[b]	MECHANICAL SOFT[c]	REGULAR HOUSE DIET
Soup	Clear, fat-free broth; bouillon	Same as clear, plus strained, or blended cream soups	Same as clear and full, plus all cream soups	All
Cereal	Not included	Cooked, very-thin, refined cereal	Cooked cereal, corn flakes, rice, noodles, macaroni, and spaghetti	All
Bread	Not included	Not included	White bread, crackers, Melba toast, and Zwieback	All
Protein foods	Not included	Milk, cream, milk drinks, and yogurt	Same as full, plus eggs (not fried), mild cheeses, cottage and cream cheeses, poultry, fish, tender beef, veal, lamb, and liver	All
Vegetables	Not included	Vegetable juices or puréed vegetables	Potatoes: baked, mashed, creamed, steamed, or scalloped; tender, cooked, whole, bland vegetables; fresh lettuce, and tomatoes	All
Fruit and fruit juices	Strained fruit juices as tolerated and flavored fruit drinks	Fruit juices	Same as full, plus cooked fruit: peaches, pears, applesauce, peeled apricots, and white cherries; ripe peaches, pears, and bananas; orange and grapefruit sections without membrane	All
Desserts and gelatin	Fruit-flavored gelatin, fruit ices, and popsicles	Same as clear, plus sherbet, ice cream, puddings, custard, and frozen yogurt	Same as full, plus plain sponge cakes, plain cookies, plain cake, puddings, and pies made with allowed foods	All
Miscellaneous	Soft drinks as tolerated, coffee, tea, sugar, honey, salt, hard candy, Polycose (Abbott Nutrition, Columbus, OH), and residue-free supplements	Same as clear, plus margarine and all supplements	Same as full, plus mild salad dressings	All

[a]Clear liquids consist of foods that are transparent liquid at body temperature and require minimal digestion. Limited to 24 to 48 hours.
[b]Full-liquid diets contain anything that would melt at room temperature. Use only temporarily during recovery.
[c]Mechanically altered diets can vary depending on the condition of the client. This diet consists of foods that are easy to swallow because they are blended, chopped, grinded, or mashed so that they are easy to chew and swallow.

Box 22.2 Assisted Oral Feeding Guidelines

- Have the tray securely placed within the client's sight.
- Sit down beside the bed if this is more comfortable and make simple conversation or remain silent as the client's condition indicates. Do not exclude the client by carrying on a conversation with another client or co-worker or engaging in any form of mobile phone/device use.
- Offer small amounts, and do not rush the feeding.
- Allow ample time for a client to chew and swallow or to rest between mouthfuls.
- Offer liquids between the solids, with a drinking straw if necessary.
- Wipe the client's mouth with a napkin during and after each meal, or offer a napkin if he or she can do this independently.

- Let the client hold his or her bread if desired and able to do so.
- When feeding a client who is sight-impaired, describe the food on the tray so that a mental image helps create a desire to eat. Sometimes the analogy of the face of a clock helps a client to visualize the position of certain foods on the plate (e.g., indicate that the meat is at 12 o'clock, the potatoes are at 3 o'clock, and so on).
- Warn the client that sipping soup through a straw feels particularly hot.
- Ask if clients are ready for more food before you feed it to them.
- Stop feeding clients if they tell or show you that they have had enough.

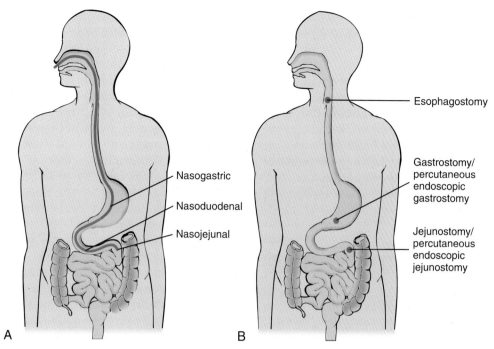

Figure 22.2 Types of enteral feeding. (A) Nonsurgical routes accessed through the nasal cavity. (B) Surgically placed feeding routes. (Copyright Rolin Graphics.)

Labels in figure A: Nasogastric, Nasoduodenal, Nasojejunal

Labels in figure B: Esophagostomy, Gastrostomy/percutaneous endoscopic gastrostomy, Jejunostomy/percutaneous endoscopic jejunostomy

- *Percutaneous endoscopic jejunostomy:* The surgeon will place a jejunostomy tube through the abdominal wall and pass it through the duodenum into the jejunum.

Enterostomy procedures may be good options for clients with gastroparesis, gastric obstructions, or a history of reflux or aspiration or for those who otherwise cannot tolerate gastric feedings.

Formula. The physician and the clinical dietitian, in accordance with the client's nutrition needs and tolerance, usually prescribe the EN formula. In addition to the specific and immediate needs of the client, other considerations include preexisting conditions, co-morbidities, food allergies, and food intolerances. Several varieties of commercial formulas are available and designed to meet individual needs. Polymeric formulas, which are composed of intact nutrients, are appropriate for use in clients with a fully functioning GI system that is capable of digestion and absorption. Other formulas use readily absorbable hydrolyzed elemental or semielemental nutrients with minimal amounts of residue. Still others are a mixture of single-nutrient modules of protein, carbohydrate, and fat combined (as calculated by the dietitian) to meet a client's specific needs.

Commercial formulas provide a nutritionally adequate, sterile, homogenized solution suitable for small-bore feeding tubes. With the development of improved formulas and feeding equipment, the need for blender-mixed formulas of regular foods seldom arises. However, an increasing number of clients would like the option of formulas made from whole foods that are plant-based and organically grown. Formulas

such as this are commercially available and are safe for enteral use.[29] Clients and caregivers may prefer the use of homemade puréed table food for tube feedings; however, puréed food may present the following problems[30]:

- *Physical form:* Foods do not pass through the small feeding tubes easily and thus require the use of the uncomfortable large-bore tubing.
- *Safety:* Blender-mixed formulas carry problems of bacterial growth and infection as well as inconsistent nutrient composition because the solid components settle out.
- *Digestion and absorption:* Puréed food requires a fully functioning GI system to digest the food and absorb its released nutrients. Many clients have GI deficits that require nutrients with varying degrees of hydrolysis or smaller molecular structure.

Enteral feeding formulas are available in varying caloric densities (e.g., 1 kcal/mL, 1.5 kcal/mL, 2 kcal/mL) to meet the individual's energy needs in a given volume of fluid. The formulas provide carbohydrates in the form of sucrose, maltodextrins, or corn syrup; protein is derived from soy, casein, or whey protein; and fat is usually from soy, canola, corn, or safflower oil, or medium-chain triglycerides as indicated. Some formulas also have added fiber. All formulas are fortified with essential vitamins and minerals that will meet the daily recommended intake in amounts commonly prescribed.[31] In addition to the standard formulas, there are also "specialty formulas" that are marketed to meet the needs of clients with unique requirements. Some examples of specialty formulas include those that are designed for patients with diabetes, trauma, cancer, renal conditions, and pediatric conditions.[31,32]

Methods of administration. Nurses work with dietitians to monitor and regulate the amount of formula and the administration rate for any form of EN. There are several methods of administration, including continuous, cyclic, intermittent, and bolus feedings. The health care team can use either feeding method alone or in combination to meet the client's nutrition needs.[33] See the Clinical Applications box entitled "Calculating a Tube Feeding" for details about setting the rate of administration for a tube feeding.

🔱 Clinical Applications

Calculating a Tube Feeding[a]

Calculating the nutrient needs and feeding schedule of a person receiving enteral nutrition requires the following information:

1. Energy needs:
   - Basal metabolic rate[b] × Injury factor (which depends on the condition of the person)
2. The type of formula that will meet the needs of the individual
3. Total volume of formula needed for the day to meet energy requirements (energy needs [kcal/day] ÷ formula [kcal/mL])
4. Volume of formula to be provided at each feeding based on the prescribed feeding schedule (total formula for the day ÷ number of feedings or hours for continuous feedings)

CRITICAL THINKING

How many milliliters of formula does the following woman need at each feeding?

- She is 37 years old, 5 feet and 7 inches tall, and weighs 140 pounds (63.6 kg).
- She is under considerable catabolic stress, with an injury factor of 1.5.
- The energy value of formula that she will receive is 1.5 kcal/mL.
- She is to receive 6 equal feedings per day.

Steps

1. Calculate her energy needs:
   - BMR: $(10 \times 63.6 \text{ kg}) + (6.25 \times 170.2 \text{ cm}) - (5 \times 37) - 161 = 1353$ kcal/day
   - Total energy needs (BMR × injury factor): 1353 kcal/day × 1.5 (injury factor) = 2029 kcal/day
2. We will use a formula that provides 1.5 kcal/mL in this case. Therefore, we need to calculate the total formula needed to meet her energy needs:
   2029 kcal/day ÷ 1.5 kcal/mL = 1352mL/day
3. Feeding schedule: 1352mL/day ÷ 6 feedings/day = 225.4 mL/feeding

[a]These equations require the weight in kilograms, the height in centimeters, and the age in years.
[b]As calculated by the Mifflin-St. Jeor equation: Female basal metabolic rate = (10 × Weight) + (6.25 × Height) − (5 × Age) − 161; Male basal metabolic rate = (10 × Weight) + (6.25 × Height) − (5 × Age) + 5.

Continuous feedings provide EN over a 24-hour period with assistance of a feeding pump. The pump is set to administer the formula at an hourly rate. Pump-assisted feedings are appropriate for critically ill patients to allow for the slower administration of continuous feedings into the small bowel. Critically ill patients or those who have not been fed enterally for some time may not be able to tolerate large feedings at initiation and should start with slow rates (e.g., 10 to 40 mL/h), increasing gradually to the goal rate (e.g., increase by 10 to 20 mL/h every 8 to 12 hours).[32]

Nurses administer cyclic feedings using a feeding pump over a period that is less than 24 hours. For example, the health care team may set the feeding rate to administer the formula over a shorter continuous period of time (e.g., 12-hour infusion or 8-hour nocturnal infusion). To determine the goal infusion rate, divide the desired formula volume by the number of hours of administration. One advantage of cyclic feedings is that it enables clients to be free from a feeding pump for a period of time.

An intermittent feeding is the administration of EN over 20 to 60 minutes every 4 to 6 hours using a pump or gravity. Typically, intermittent feedings supply 240 to 720 mL of formula depending on the client's needs. Intermittent feedings also allow clients to be mobile between feeding times.

Bolus feedings are the administration of EN over a few minutes using a syringe or gravity drip. Care providers, or the client themselves, give a bolus of approximately 240 mL of feeding 3 to 6 times daily. Before introducing bolus feedings, clients have usually demonstrated the ability to tolerate a continuous feeding into the stomach. Bolus feedings are easy to administer but may increase the client's risk for aspiration.[34]

Many hospitals have implemented volume-based tube feeding polices, which increase success in reaching enteral formula infusion goals. These protocols empower nurses to increase feeding rates to make up for volume lost while EN is interrupted (see the For Further Focus box titled "Volume-Based Enteral Feeding").[34]

Monitoring for complications. Nurses monitor clients who are receiving EN for appropriate feeding schedules, tolerance, and potential complications.

---

continuous feeding an enteral feeding schedule with which formula is infused via a pump over a 24-hour period.

bolus feeding a volume of feeding administered by a syringe over a short period of time (usually 10 to 15 minutes) that is given in several feedings per day.

Diarrhea is a frequently reported GI complication in individuals receiving nutrition via tube feeding. A number of factors may contribute to diarrhea in tube-fed clients, including medications, bacterial overgrowth, infections, or conditions that predispose the client to diarrhea.[32] Before making changes to the enteral feeding protocol, the health care team should rule out the common culprits such as medications and *Clostridium difficile* enterocolitis. If there is evidence of persistent diarrhea, commercially prepared, fiber-containing formulas may help promote bowel regularity.[34] If clients do not respond to fiber, then small peptide-based formulas may be an effective alternative.[34]

Despite meeting a client's physiologic needs through any number of feeding tube and formula options, this feeding method may contribute to psychologic stress.[35] Providing support to maintain quality of life is an important part of care planning.[35] Box 22.3 provides guidelines for an ideal monitoring schedule, and Table 22.5 provides problem-solving suggestions for common issues encountered with EN.

For Further Focus

Volume-Based Enteral Feeding

Hospitalized patients often do not receive the full volume of enteral feeding ordered by the physician because of interruptions from tests and procedures that are part of their care.[1] The tradition of giving enteral nutrition using a continuous rate-based method contributes to this problem.

Volume-based enteral feeding allows the nurse to adjust the hourly rate of the feeding to achieve the desired daily volume. When using volume-based enteral feeding, nurses 1) calculate the amount of formula that the patient missed during interruptions; 2) recalculate the volume needed to meet the patient's nutrient needs for the day, and 3) give it over the remaining hours of the day. For example, if a client requires 1200 mL of formula over a 24-hour period, delivered at 50 mL per hour, and the health care team has to discontinue the feeding for 4 hours, the client only receives 20 hours' worth (or 1000 mL) of the formula. Volume-based enteral feeding would allow the nurse to add the 200 mL that the client missed over the remaining hours of the nurse's shift. Hospitals that adopt volume-based enteral feeding protocols place the emphasis on meeting the clients' nutrient needs regardless of interruptions.

Ongoing research will help determine if this method of volume-based tube feeding improves patient outcomes for all patients or if there are certain conditions that preclude benefits.[2,3] One potential concern for clients receiving volume-based tube feeding is that it may be difficult to account for the carbohydrates that individuals with diabetes receive, which may affect their insulin requirements.

REFERENCES

1. McClave, S. A., et al. (2015). Volume-based feeding in the critically ill patient. *JPEN Journal of Parenteral and Enteral Nutrition*, *39*(6), 707–712.
2. Kinikin, J., Phillipp, R., & Altamirano, C. (2020). Using volume-based tube feeding to increase nutrient delivery in patients on a rehabilitation unit. *Rehabilitation Nursing*, *45*(4), 186–194.
3. Krebs, E. D., et al. (2018). Volume-based feeding improves nutritional adequacy in surgical patients. *American Journal of Surgery*, *216*(6), 1155–1159.

Box 22.3 Monitoring the Patient Who Is Receiving Enteral Nutrition

NUTRITION-RELATED HISTORY
- Energy intake
- Diet order
- Macro- and micronutrient intake
- Enteral and parenteral nutrition administration
- Medications

ANTHROPOMETRICS
- Weight (daily for 3 to 4 days until stable and then at least three times per week)
- Length or height in pediatric patients (monthly)
- Weight change

PHYSICAL ASSESSMENT
- Signs and symptoms of edema (daily)
- Fluid balance (daily)
- Adequacy of enteral intake (several times per week)
- GI motility (every 2 to 4 hours during initiation of feedings, every 8 hours when stable) such as the following:
  - Abdominal distention and discomfort

- Nausea and vomiting; risk for aspiration
- Gastric residuals
- Stool output and consistency
- Tube placement: make sure that the tube is in the desired location (daily for the short term or as needed if there are indications of migration)

BIOCHEMICAL MEASURES
- Glucose (three times daily until stable, then two to three times per week)
- Serum electrolytes (daily until stable, then two to three times per week)
- Blood urea nitrogen (one to two times per week)
- Serum calcium, magnesium, and phosphorus (one to two times per week)
- Complete blood count and transferrin or prealbumin (once a week)

Modified from Academy of Nutrition and Dietetics. (2019). *Nutrition care manual.* Retrieved May 21, 2019, from nutritioncaremanual.org; Bankhead, R., Boullata, J., Brantley, S., et al. (2009). A.S.P.E.N. Board of Directors. Enteral nutrition practice recommendations. *JPEN J Parenter Enteral Nutr, 33*(2), 122–167; and Moore, M. C. (2009). *Nutrition assessment and care* (6th ed.). St. Louis: Mosby.

Table 22.5	Problem-Solving Tips for Individuals Receiving Enteral Nutrition
PROBLEM	**SUGGESTED SOLUTIONS**
Thirst and oral dryness	Lubricate the lips Chew sugarless gum Brush the teeth Rinse the mouth frequently
Tube discomfort	Gargle with a mixture of warm water and mouthwash Gently blow the nose Clean the tube regularly with water or a water-soluble lubricant If persistent, gently pull out the tube, clean it, and reinsert it Request a smaller tube
Tension and fullness	Relax and breathe deeply after each feeding
Reflux or aspiration	Lift the head of the bed to 30 to 45 degrees Reduce infusion rate
Constipation	Use a fiber-containing formula Assess for adequate fluid intake
Diarrhea	Take antidiarrheal medications if there are no bacterial infections Avoid excess sorbitol and hypertonic solutions Use continuous feedings instead of bolus feedings Evaluate for lactose intolerance and intestinal mucosal atrophy Consider probiotics Consider formula that is low in fat or contains MCT oil
Gustatory Distress[a]	
General dissatisfaction with feeding	Warm or chill feedings *Caution:* Feedings that are too cold may cause diarrhea Serve favorite foods in liquefied form
Persistent hunger	Chew gum Suck hard candy
Inability to drink	Rinse the mouth frequently with water and other liquids

MCT, Medium-chain triglycerides.
[a]This refers to the frustration clients experience when the sense of taste is not satisfied.

Parenteral Feedings

If a client cannot tolerate or absorb food or formula in the GI tract, alternative methods of nutrition support are necessary. The term *parenteral nutrition* refers to any feeding method not involving the GI route. In current medical terminology, parenteral nutrition (PN) specifically refers to the feeding of nutrients directly into the blood circulation through certain veins

(e.g., a peripheral vein in the arm or the subclavian vein). Compared with EN, parenteral feedings are more invasive and expensive, and they introduce more risk. However, for individuals without a functioning lower GI system, it is necessary. Table 22.3 summarizes common indications for PN. Depending on the nutrition support necessary, the following two routes are available:

- *Peripheral PN:* Appropriate for use when a solution of 900 mOsm/L or less is enough to provide nutrient needs and when feeding is necessary for only a brief period (e.g., no more than 10 to 14 days) or as a supplement to enteral feedings. The osmolality (i.e., mOsm/L) of a solution depends on the concentration of its total particles, including dextrose, protein, and electrolytes. Small peripheral veins, usually in the arm, deliver the less-concentrated solutions (Figure 22.3).
- *Central PN:* Appropriate for use when the energy and nutrient requirement is large or when the client needs full nutrition support for longer periods. The surgeon will place the catheter into a large central vein (usually the subclavian vein that leads directly into the rapid flow of the superior vena cava to the heart). The catheter may access the superior vena cava directly (Figure 22.4A); a peripherally inserted central catheter (Figure 22.4B); or a tunneled catheter (Figure 22.4C). The central veins tolerate nutrition support solutions of high osmolality.

We use PN in cases of major surgery or complications, especially those that involve the GI tract or when the client is unable to obtain enough nourishment enterally. PN provides crucial nutrition support from solutions that contain glucose, amino acids, electrolytes, vitamins, and minerals. Fat in the form of lipid emulsions supplies needed energy and essential fatty acids. Oils used in lipid emulsions come from a variety of sources, including soybean, safflower, olive, fish, and coconut oils. A basic PN solution may contain between 3% and 20% crystalline amino acids, 2.5% to 70% dextrose, and 10% to

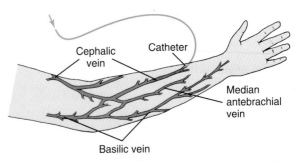

Figure 22.3 Peripheral parenteral nutrition feeding into the small veins of the arm.

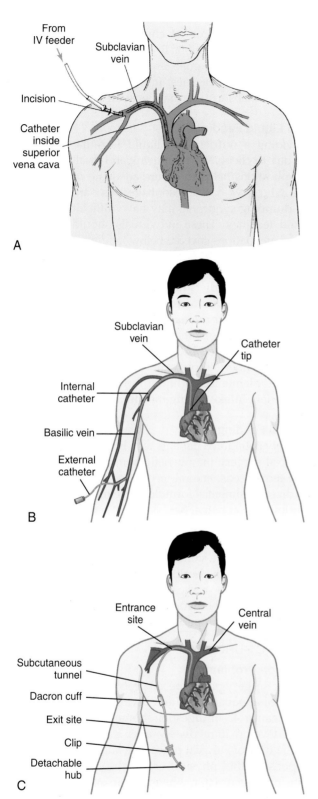

Figure 22.4 Catheter placement for parenteral nutrition. (A) A direct line via the subclavian vein to the superior vena cava. (B) A peripherally inserted central catheter line. (C) A tunneled catheter.

30% fat emulsions, with added micronutrients that are specific to the client's needs. Each constituent of the parenteral solution contributes to the overall osmolality. The health care team must consider that the peripheral veins have a limited capacity for high-osmolality solutions when choosing which infusion site to use.

A team of specialists including physicians, dietitians, pharmacists, and nurses works closely together during the administration of PN. The physician, pharmacist, and the clinical dietitian will design the most appropriate formula based on a detailed individual nutrition assessment and concurrent medication use (see the Drug-Nutrient Interaction box, "Propofol and Lipids in Nutrition Support"). The pharmacist on the nutrition support team mixes the PN solutions by following the prescription. The administration of the solution is an important nursing responsibility.

Drug-Nutrient Interaction

Propofol and Lipids in Nutrition Support

KELLI BOI

Medical providers use the drug propofol for sedation and anesthesia during surgery, and in the intensive care unit to maintain sedation in mechanically ventilated patients. Propofol is a fat-soluble drug that is emulsified in an oil and water solution for IV administration. During long-term sedation, patients often receive nutrition support in the form of EN or PN. One important consideration for the nutrition support team is the concurrent administration of propofol because the lipid emulsion contributes 1.1 kcal/mL. Therefore, the RDN will reduce the calories from EN or PN solutions to compensate for the calories provided in propofol.

Elevated serum triglyceride levels may result if the infusion rate of propofol exceeds the body's ability to clear it. This is more likely to occur with long-term use of propofol when other risk factors are present (e.g., advanced age, cardiovascular disease, renal failure) or when the overall amount of lipids provided exceeds the patient's needs. The health care team will monitor serum triglyceride levels during propofol infusion to prevent hypertriglyceridemia.

The health care team will discuss the use of either PN or EN with the patient or their designated care providers (e.g., family, friends). Some clients and/or families do not welcome the use of assisted medical technology in feeding. It may be against their will for ethical, cultural, religious, or personal reasons. See the Cultural Considerations box entitled "Cultural Differences in Advanced Care Planning" for more information.

Cultural Considerations

Cultural Differences in Advanced Care Planning

JENNIFER E. SCHMIDT

Advanced care planning spells out the type of treatment a person wants at the end of his or her life. In the United States, health care institutions recognize advanced directives and living wills as legal documents. The Patient Self-Determination Act of 1991 promotes the use of advanced care procedures and strengthens the rights of individuals making end-of-life medical decisions. For example, if a person is unconscious or unresponsive, advanced care planning ensures that the health care team knows the patient's treatment preferences.

People sometimes refer to EN and PN support as *artificial nutrition and hydration*. Patients do not always welcome these potentially life-sustaining interventions. For individuals nearing the end of life, artificial nutrition is unlikely to prolong life and may even lead to medical complications and increase suffering.

Studies suggest that significant differences exist among various racial and ethnic groups and their caregivers about advanced care planning and end-of-life decisions. When demographic values are examined, several factors influence the completion of a living will, a do-not-resuscitate order, or orders that address the removal of life support. These values include the following[1]:

- *Sex:* Females are more likely than males to complete advance directives.
- *Education:* Individuals with at least a high school education are more likely to have completed an advance directive.
- *Religion:* Individuals with a religious affiliation are more likely to have end-of-life preferences or a living will.
- *Age:* Individuals who have completed advance directives are more likely to be older and have had some personal experience with end-of-life decision making in the past.
- *Ethnicity:* Researchers have also found that Caucasians are less likely to request life-supportive treatments than African-Americans are.

By recognizing cultural differences and the likelihood of patients having advanced care planning, health care professionals can assist individuals with greater awareness and sensitivity and provide culturally appropriate education to them and their families about advance directives, living wills, and appropriate end-of-life care. Even when patients have verbally expressed their wishes to the family, family members may find it difficult to follow through. Advanced care planning ensures that caregivers and the medical team know and honor the patient's wishes.

REFERENCE

1. Hart, J. L., et al. (2018). Are demographic characteristics associated with advance directive completion? A secondary analysis of two randomized trials. *Journal of General Internal Medicine, 33*(2), 145–147.

SPECIAL NUTRITION NEEDS AFTER GASTROINTESTINAL SURGERY

A surgical procedure on any part of the GI system requires special dietary attention and potentially nutrient modification.

MOUTH, THROAT, AND NECK SURGERY

Surgery that involves the mouth, jaw, throat, or neck may require modification regarding the mode of eating. Clients who cannot chew or swallow normally require accommodations to address individual limitations. The ultimate goals are to promote healing, prevent nutrient deficiencies, and minimize complications such as malabsorption, maldigestion, and dysphagia.[32]

Oral Liquid Feedings

Providing a nutrient-rich liquid formula throughout the day to clients who can drink and swallow without complications helps to ensure adequate nutrition. Clients who have had an esophagectomy and are at risk for dumping syndrome may have difficulty tolerating liquid feedings. These individuals should follow the recommendations covered below for *dumping syndrome*.

Mechanical Soft Diets

Mechanical soft diets help to transition between full-liquid and regular diets. These diets may include whole foods that are easy to chew and swallow (see Table 22.4). Because mechanical soft diets do not include high-fiber foods, it may be prudent to provide a functional fiber supplement. Multivitamins and minerals supplemented in liquid form help to ensure micronutrient intake during the initial recovery period.

Enteral Feedings

Severely debilitated patients who have had radical neck or facial surgery may benefit from tube feedings. For long-term needs, enteral feeding equipment and standardized commercial formulas have made it possible to continue EN at home. Nasogastric tubes are the tube of choice unless an obstruction of the esophagus or other complication requires the surgeon to create a gastrostomy to access the stomach. To support the integrity of the client's gut, the health care team should initiate the feeding tube at the earliest functioning point of access to the GI tract. In other words, if the esophagus and stomach are working properly, the best practice is to use it.

GASTRIC SURGERY

Nutrition Problems

Gastric surgery poses special problems for the maintenance of adequate nutrition because of the stomach's significant role in digestion. Some of these problems may develop immediately after surgery, depending on the type of surgical procedure and the individual's response. Other physical or malabsorption complications may occur later, when the person begins to eat a regular diet. Refer to Chapter 5 to review the digestive processes that take place in the stomach. The goals of nutrition therapy are to promote healing, to prevent dumping syndrome and nutrient deficiency, and to minimize complications such as malabsorption and maldigestion. To maintain nutrient balance, the health care team may consider using multivitamin/mineral supplements in liquid form, vitamin B$_{12}$ injections, or functional fiber supplements.[32]

Gastrectomy

Serious nutrient deficits sometimes occur after a gastrectomy. Increased gastric fullness and distention may result if the gastric resection also involved a **vagotomy**. Because it lacks the normal nerve stimulus, the stomach becomes **atonic** and empties poorly. Food fermentation occurs, and this produces discomfort, gas, and diarrhea. Weight loss is common after extensive gastric surgery.

To cover the immediate postoperative nutrition needs after a gastrectomy procedure, surgeons may create a jejunostomy through which the patient can ingest an enteral formula. Patients may have frequent small oral feedings as tolerated. A typical pattern of simple dietary progression may occur over several weeks. The basic principles of diet therapy for the immediate postgastrectomy period involve both the size of the meals (which should be small and frequent) and the nature of the meals (which are generally simple, easily digested, bland, and low in bulk).

Dumping Syndrome

Dumping syndrome is the most frequently encountered complication subsequent to extensive gastric resection. After the initial recovery from surgery, when the person begins to feel better and eat a regular diet, he or she may experience discomfort 10 to 20 minutes after meals. With *early onset dumping syndrome* a cramping and full feeling develops, the pulse rate becomes rapid, and a wave of weakness, cold sweating, and dizziness may follow. Abdominal pain and diarrhea terminate the event. For individuals with *intermediate dumping syndrome,* symptoms begin within 20 to 30 minutes after eating; and for those experiencing *late onset dumping syndrome,* the symptoms begin 1 to 3 hours after a meal.

This multifaceted condition is a shock syndrome that results when a meal containing a sizeable proportion of readily absorbable carbohydrates rapidly enter or "dump" into the small intestine. A stomach bypass allows food to pass quickly from the esophagus into the small intestine. This concentrated food mass draws water from the circulatory system into the GI tract to achieve osmotic balance (i.e., a state of equal concentrations of fluids within the small intestine and the surrounding blood circulation). This water shift rapidly shrinks the vascular fluid volume, thereby causing shock. Blood pressure drops, and signs of rapid heart rate to rebuild the blood volume appear; these include a rapid pulse rate, sweating, weakness, and tremors.

If a client eats a meal consisting of simple carbohydrates, late dumping may occur approximately 2 hours after eating. The quick absorption of a concentrated simple carbohydrate solution results in the rapid rise of blood glucose and an overproduction of insulin. Blood sugar level eventually drops below normal, causing symptoms of hypoglycemia (e.g., weakness, shaky,

sweating, confusion). As a result, susceptible individuals are often reluctant to eat much food, and this may lead to unintentional weight loss and general malnutrition.

Careful adherence to the postoperative diet produces dramatic relief from these distressing symptoms. Clients may find that choosing carbohydrates with a low glycemic index, eating slowly, eliminating fluids during meals, reducing dietary fat and lying down for 15 to 30 minutes after eating help to decrease the rate of gastric emptying (see the Case Study box, "Gastrectomy").[36]

BARIATRIC SURGERY

Clients undergoing bariatric surgery are often malnourished before the surgery, which may exacerbate complications. These individuals are at high risk for several micronutrient deficiencies that require special consideration (see the For Further Focus box, "Nutrient Deficiencies after Bariatric Surgery").[37] After gastric bypass, clients progress slowly from a clear liquid diet to a regular balanced solid diet over a period of approximately 2 months.[38] After bariatric surgery, the combination of severely reduced food intake and (potential) malabsorption or dumping syndrome dramatically decreases nutrient availability.

As with other forms of gastric surgeries, adherence to the postoperative diet should provide relief from difficult symptoms as well as the gradual stabilization of weight. Given the high variability among clients regarding their eating progression, experts recommend that they receive consultations with a bariatric dietitian for individualized diet plans.[38] Chapter 15 covers various forms of bariatric surgery.

GALLBLADDER SURGERY

For patients with acute gallbladder inflammation (i.e., cholecystitis) or gallstones (i.e., cholelithiasis) (Figure 22.5), the treatment is usually cholecystectomy (see Chapter 18). The modern procedure for this removal, called *laparoscopic cholecystectomy,* requires only minimal surgery that involves small skin punctures. Through these small openings, the surgeon can insert needed instruments and a laparoscope fitted with a miniature camera and bright fiberoptic lighting.

After surgery, reducing fat in the diet (e.g., less than 30% of total energy intake as fat) facilitates wound healing and comfort.[32] The hormonal stimulus for bile continues to function, thus causing pain with the high intake of fatty foods. The body needs a period to adjust to the more dilute supply of bile that is available to assist with fat digestion and absorption directly from the liver; see the low-fat diet guide given for gallbladder disease in Chapter 18, Table 18.5.

---

vagotomy the cutting of the vagus nerve, which supplies a major stimulus for gastric secretions.
atonic without normal muscle tone.

NEXT-GENERATION NCLEX® EXAMINATION-STYLE UNFOLDING CASE STUDY
Gastrectomy

See answers in Appendix A.

A 40-year-old male had a long experience with persistent peptic ulcer disease involving increasing amounts of stomach tissue. His physician decided that he would need surgery and admitted him into the hospital for a total gastrectomy. He weathered the surgery well and received some initial nutrition support from an elemental formula fed through a percutaneous endoscopic jejunostomy (PEJ) tube that the surgeon had placed into his jejunum. After a few days, the doctors removed the tube. Over the next 2 weeks, the patient was gradually able to tolerate small amounts of soft food orally. He soon recovered enough to go home and gradually felt his strength returning. The patient was relieved to be free of his ulcer pain, and he began to resume more of his usual activities, including eating a regular diet in increasing amounts and variety.

1. From the list below, select all of the *most likely* problems that the patient may experience after his procedure.

   a. Rapid weight gain
   b. Inadequate bile secretion
   c. Malabsorption
   d. Loss of pancreatic enzymes
   e. Development of type 1 diabetes
   f. Maldigestion
   g. Infection
   h. Changes in transit time
   i. Malnutrition
   j. Physical complications

2. From the list below, select appropriate nutrition needs for the patient after discharge.

   a. Three large meals per day
   b. Foods high in insoluble fiber
   c. Five to six small meals per day
   d. Avoiding spicy and heavily seasoned foods
   e. Consuming foods that are easy to digest
   f. Emphasizing high quality protein foods

A few months after his gastrectomy, the patient was recovering well. However, as time went by, he began having more discomfort after meals. He felt a cramping sensation and an increased heart rate, followed by a wave of weakness with sweating and dizziness. He would often become nauseated and have diarrhea. As his anxiety increased, he began to eat less and less, and his weight began to drop. He was soon in a state of general malnutrition.

3. Choose the *most likely* options for the information missing from the statements below by selecting from the list of options provided.

   The patient is most likely experiencing ____1____ syndrome. This can occur after consuming a meal with a large amount of readily absorbable ____2____ that rapidly enter the ____3____.

OPTION 1	OPTION 2	OPTION 3
refeeding	protein	small intestine
short bowel	carbohydrates	stomach
dumping	fats	liver
irritable bowel	fiber	large intestine

4. Use an X to identify effective nutrition and lifestyle intervention strategies that are <u>indicated</u> (appropriate or necessary) or <u>contraindicated</u> (could be harmful) for the patient.

INTERVENTION	INDICATED	CONTRAINDICATED
Consuming carbohydrates with a low glycemic index		
Drinking 16 to 20 oz. of fluids with meals		
Eating meals slowly		
Reducing dietary fat		
Participating in physical activity shortly after eating		
Laying down for 15-30 minutes after meals		

The patient met with a dietitian to discuss how to manage these symptoms with his diet. The dietitian planned a follow-up appointment 2 weeks later to see how he was doing.

5. From the list below, select the most appropriate meal to reduce the patient's symptoms.

   a. Grilled cheese on whole wheat bread with tomato soup
   b. Turkey sandwich on whole wheat bread, plain yogurt, carrots, medium apple
   c. Waffles, strawberry yogurt, scrambled eggs
   d. Brown rice, beans, chicken, canned pears in heavy syrup, creamed corn, water
   e. Chocolate milk, pretzels, string cheese, peanut butter and jelly sandwich
   f. Hamburger with fries, steamed vegetables, sweet tea

6. For each assessment finding, use an X to indicate whether nursing and collaborative interventions were <u>effective</u> (helped to meet expected outcomes), or <u>ineffective</u> (did not help to meet expected outcomes).

ASSESSMENT	EFFECTIVE	INEFFECTIVE
Weight has not returned to normal		
Muscle mass has improved		
Less discomfort after meals		
Diarrhea		
Displays feelings of fear towards foods		
Avoids protein foods		
Avoids carbohydrates with high GI index		
Consumes liquids with foods		

Nutrient Deficiencies After Bariatric Surgery

Bariatric surgery for obese individuals is becoming more common around the world. Bariatric surgery is effective for weight loss and maintenance, but it is not without drawbacks. Restrictive eating patterns, dumping syndrome, and nutrient deficiencies from malabsorption are common complications. The quality-of-life to cost-benefit ratio of surgery is difficult to assess. Although obesity increases morbidity and mortality rates, the complications of surgery can introduce a new set of risks.

The Roux-en-Y gastric bypass procedure (see Chapter 15), which reduces the amount of bowel that is capable of absorbing nutrients, is the surgery of choice for obesity in the United States. Obese clients are at risk for complications during surgery from co-morbid conditions such as diseases of the cardiovascular, endocrine, renal, pulmonary, gastrointestinal, and musculoskeletal systems. Therefore, the health care team must take special care to prepare the patient for surgery.

Bariatric surgeries that induce malabsorption (e.g., gastric bypass, biliopancreatic diversion) present nutrition problems. Protein deficiency is a significant risk for many patients and may result in hospitalization and the necessity of nutrition support in severe cases. In addition, micronutrient deficiencies from limited intake and malabsorption warrant multivitamin/mineral supplementation postoperatively for life. The nutrients at risk for deficiency are highly dependent upon the form of bariatric surgery performed.[1] Specific nutrients of concern include the following[2]:

- Vitamins: A, B_1, B_6, B_{12}, C, D, E, K, and folate
- Minerals: calcium, copper, iron, selenium, and zinc

Clients who have undergone bariatric procedures should discuss dietary adequacy with a registered dietitian nutritionist. Registered dietitian nutritionists recommend that bariatric clients take the following supplements daily after surgery: two multivitamin/mineral supplements with iron; calcium citrate (600 to 1200 mg/day); vitamin D (3000 IU/day).[3] These supplements should be in chewable or liquid form for the first couple of months after surgery. In addition, clients should take a sublingual vitamin B_{12} supplement (250 to 350 mcg/day) or receive a monthly injection of 1000 mcg.[3]

REFERENCES

1. Lupoli, R., et al. (2017). Bariatric surgery and long-term nutritional issues. *World Journal of Diabetes, 8*(11), 464–474.
2. Torres-Landa, S., et al. (2018). Surgical management of obesity. *Minerva Chirurgica, 73*(1), 41–54.
3. Sherf Dagan, S., et al. (2017). Nutritional recommendations for adult bariatric surgery patients: Clinical practice. *Advances in Nutrition, 8*(2), 382–394.

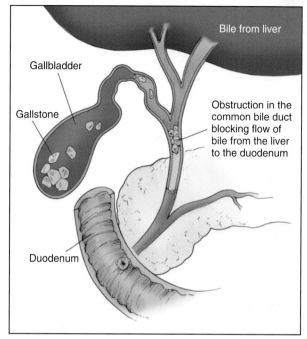

Figure 22.5 Gallbladder with stones (i.e., cholelithiasis).

INTESTINAL SURGERY

Intestinal disease that involves tumors, lesions, or obstructions may require the surgical resection of the affected intestinal area. For complicated cases that require the removal of large sections of the small intestine, the use of EN support may be difficult at first. In this case, the medical team may use PN support, with a small allowance for oral feeding. After general resection for less severe cases, a diet that is relatively low in dietary fiber may be beneficial in the beginning to allow for healing and comfort.

Intestinal surgery involving the latter portions of the GI tract sometimes requires creating a stoma (i.e., opening in the abdominal wall) to the intestine for the elimination of fecal waste. An *ileostomy* is an opening from the ileum, which is the last section of the small intestine, to the outside of the body (Figure 22.6A). At this point in the GI tract, the stool is still liquid, which may cause problems in managing the ileostomy output. A *colostomy* is an opening in the large intestine to the outside of the body (Figure 22.6B). The large intestine reabsorbs water, and the remaining feces are more solid, thereby making colostomy management less difficult. Clients with an ostomy begin a clear liquid diet during the immediate postoperative period. They then progress toward small, frequent feedings of meals that are relatively low in dietary fiber, as tolerated.[32] Encouraging clients to limit fluids with meals and instead drink adequate fluids between meals may help to reduce diarrhea. By monitoring individuals with an ileostomy for lactose intolerance and fat malabsorption, dietitians can make dietary adjustments as needed.

Clients need support and practical help with learning about self-care for an ostomy. Eliminating gas-producing foods, odor-causing foods, and foods that may cause an obstruction will help to facilitate maintenance. The goal is to advance to a customized diet that is acceptable to the client and accommodates individual food preferences as soon as tolerated. Progression to a regular diet is important for nutrition and emotional value.

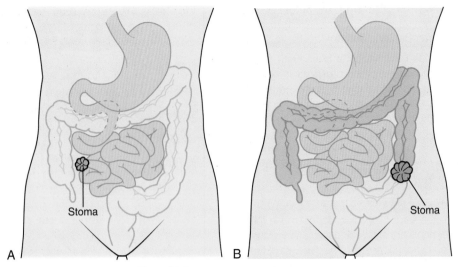

Figure 22.6 (A) Ileostomy. (B) Colostomy.

RECTAL SURGERY

For a brief period after rectal surgery or hemorrhoidectomy, clear fluid, or fiber-restricted diets (see Table 22.2) help to reduce painful elimination and to allow for healing. Nonresidue commercial elemental formulas help delay bowel movements until the surgical area has healed. Clients usually return to a regular diet rapidly.

SPECIAL NUTRITION NEEDS FOR PATIENTS WITH BURNS

In the United States, there are approximately 486,000 visits to emergency departments and 3300 deaths annually as a result of burn injuries.[39] The treatment of severe burns presents a tremendous nutrition challenge. The location and severity of the burn will greatly affect the prognosis and plan of care.

TYPE AND EXTENT OF BURNS

The depth of the burn affects its treatment and its healing process (Figure 22.7). Superficial (i.e., first-degree) burns involve cell damage to the epidermis. Second-degree burns are either superficial partial-thickness burns, which involve cell damage to the dermis, or deep partial-thickness burns, which involve both the first and second layers of skin. Full-thickness (i.e., third degree) burns result in complete skin loss, including the underlying fat layer. Subdermal (i.e., fourth degree) burns leave bone and tendon exposed. Medical teams refer patients with burn injuries involving more than 10% of the total body surface area (TBSA) to a regional burn unit facility for specialized burn team care that includes nutrition support.

STAGES OF NUTRITION CARE

The nutrition care of patients with massive burns is a considerable challenge that requires continual

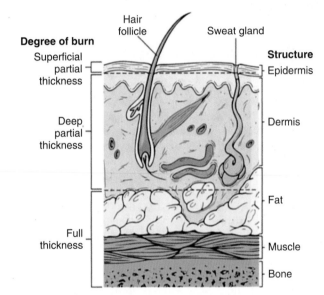

Figure 22.7 Depth of skin area involved in burns. (Reprinted from Lewis, S. M., Heitkemper, M. M., & Dirksen, S. R. [2007]. *Medical-surgical nursing: Assessment and management of clinical problems* [7th ed.]. St. Louis: Mosby.)

monitoring and adjustment. Energy expenditure in burn patients can be extremely high, and it will fluctuate depending on the stage of healing and the extent of the body surface area involved.

Burn Shock or the Ebb Phase

The ebb phase is the period immediately after a trauma such as a burn. During this time, patients experience a decrease in metabolism and tissue perfusion. Burn shock is a condition resulting from the loss of large amounts of fluid that occurs during the first hours until approximately the second day after a burn. The destruction of protective skin leads to immediate losses of heat, water, electrolytes, and protein. Blood volume and pressure drop, and urine output decreases to replace the fluid lost from the wound. Cellular dehydration occurs as intracellular water balances the loss of fluid. Potassium increases in the circulation as the body withdraws potassium from the cells. To prevent shock, physicians replenish patients with large amounts of IV fluid and electrolyte therapy given as lactated Ringer's solution. After approximately 12 hours, when vascular permeability returns to normal and fluid losses begin to decrease at the burn site, infusions of albumin solutions or plasma help restore blood volume.

After the patient receives fluid resuscitation, the dietitian establishes nutrition needs. Typically, nutrition therapy begins within 24 to 48 hours of injury. When burn patients are not able to take food orally, enteral feedings meet nutrition needs. Enteral feedings help prevent mucosal atrophy. In severe cases, introducing enteral feeding into the small intestine is indicated to help prevent complications such as intestinal permeability and infection.[34]

Acute or Flow Phase

After the ebb phase, patients experience a period of increased cardiac output and metabolism known as the flow phase. During this time, the body has added nutrient and energy demands because of metabolic stress, tissue growth, and repair. If feedings do not meet nutrient demands, patients may lose muscle mass and experience a decreased ability to heal wounds. This acute phase of hypermetabolism may last from weeks to months.

During this phase, the patient's blood flow and urine output begin to return to normal. Constant attention to fluid intake and output with evaluation for any signs of dehydration or overhydration is essential.

Medical Nutrition Therapy for Burn Patients

Most patients with burns of less than 20% of the TBSA can consume an oral meal plan that is adequate in nutrient needs, unless the burn site hinders eating. Successful nutrition therapy during this critical feeding period is based on vigorous protein and energy intake as follows[32]:

- *Adequate energy:* The dietitian will calculate energy needs with the most precise method available. If indirect calorimetry (see Chapter 6) is not available, the dietitian will calculate energy needs according to the equations provided in Table 22.6. Energy expenditure fluctuates after burn injuries, and fixed formulas often lead to underfeeding during periods of highest energy needs and to overfeeding late in the treatment course.[40] Thus, the dietitian must reassess energy needs frequently to meet the patient's changing requirements.

- Adequate energy intake spares protein for tissue rebuilding and meets the increased metabolic demands of the whole body. Approximately 55% to 60% of the total kilocalories should come from carbohydrates along with a moderate amount of fat (<35% of kcal). Overfeeding the patient is harmful as it increases metabolic stress.[40] The frequent recalculation of energy needs may be necessary if the patient is gaining or losing weight. One goal of MNT is for patients to avoid losing more than 10% of their body weight from the point of admission.[40]

- *High protein:* High-quality protein intake is crucial to promote early wound healing and to support immune function. Depending on the extent of the burn and the associated catabolic losses, individual protein needs vary from 1.5 to 2 g/kg/day in adults and from 2.5 to 4g/kg/day in children. This level of protein will equal 20% to 25% of energy intake.[40]

- *High micronutrient needs:* Increased vitamin C (500 mg/day) partners with amino acids to rebuild tissue. Supplementation of vitamin A (10,000 IU/day) and zinc is important for optimal immune function. Increased thiamin, riboflavin, and niacin are necessary for increased energy and protein metabolism. Special attention to electrolyte levels can help to prevent imbalances resulting from increased losses. Patients usually receive a daily multivitamin-mineral supplement.

> **lactated Ringer's solution** a sterile solution of calcium chloride, potassium chloride, sodium chloride, and sodium lactate in water that replenishes fluid and electrolytes; the English physiologist Sidney Ringer (1835-1910) developed this solution.

Table 22.6	Estimated Energy Needs for Burn Patients	
	EQUATION	**FORMULA**
Adults	Toronto	kcal/day = −4343 + 10.5 × %TBSA + 0.23 × previous 24 hours' caloric intake + 0.84 × Harris-Benedict equation + 114 × previous 24 hours' maximal temperature − 4.5 × days post-burn injury
Girls 3–10 yr	Shofield	kcal/day = (16.97 × weight in kg) + (1.618 × height in cm) + 371.2
Boys 3–10 yr	Shofield	kcal/day = (19.6 × weight in kg) + (1.033 × height in cm) + 414.9
Girls 10–18 yr	Shofield	kcal/day = (8.365 × weight in kg) + (4.65 × height in cm) + 200
Boys 10–18 yr	Shofield	kcal/day = (16.25 × weight in kg) + (1.372 × height in cm) + 515.5

From Rousseau, A. F., et al. (2013). ESPEN endorsed recommendations: Nutritional therapy in major burns. *Clin Nutr, 32*(4), 497–502.

Dietary management. With any method, a careful dietary intake record measures progress toward meeting the nutrition goals. Caregivers may provide nutrient-dense beverages with added protein or amino acids or commercial formulas such as Ensure, or Boost to supplement the patient's diet. Patients usually tolerate solid foods by the second week; however, hypermetabolic states, pain, and poor appetite make oral feedings difficult for individuals with major burns.

When oral intake is less than 75% of the goal for intake for more than 3 days, the health care team should implement either enteral or parenteral methods of feeding to meet crucial nutrient demands. When enteral feedings are impossible because of associated injuries or complications, parenteral feeding can supply essential nutrition support. Studies evaluating early versus delayed EN support indicate that initiating nutrition support soon after the burn injury (e.g., as early as 4 to 6 hours after injury) is effective and safe, stimulates protein retention, and reduces the hypermetabolic response, stress hormones, risk of infection, and length of hospital stay.[34]

Follow-up reconstruction. Continued nutrition support is essential to support tissue strength for successful skin grafting or reconstructive plastic surgery. Patients need the physical rebuilding of body resources that surgery requires as well as personal support to rebuild their will and spirit, because disfigurement and disability are possible. Optimal physical stamina gained through persistent and supportive medical, nutrition, and nursing care helps clients to rebuild the personal resources that they need to cope.

Putting It All Together

Summary

- Before surgery, the nutrition goals are to correct any existing deficiencies and to build nutrition reserves to meet surgical demands. After surgery, the nutrition goals are to replace losses and to support recovery. The added task of encouraging eating is often necessary during this period of healing.

- Caregivers give postsurgical feedings in a variety of ways, and patients should take food orally whenever possible. However, the inability to eat or damage to the intestinal tract may require enteral tube feedings or parenteral feedings.

- For clients who are undergoing surgery of the GI tract, the dietitian modifies their diet in accordance with the surgical procedure protocol.

- For patients with severe burns, increased nutrition support is necessary in successive stages in response to the burn injury and to the continuing requirements of tissue rebuilding.

Chapter Review Questions

See answers in Appendix A.

1. Edema may indicate inadequate intake of _____.

   a. sodium
   b. vitamin C
   c. dietary fiber
   d. protein

2. Parenteral nutrition support is most appropriate for a patient with _____.

   a. short-bowel syndrome
   b. failure to thrive
   c. facial trauma
   d. a comatose state of unknown prognosis

3. Clients receiving tube feedings who have a fully functioning GI system may have improved bowel function and less diarrhea when given an enteral formula that is _____.

   a. supplemented with fiber
   b. high in protein
   c. hydrolyzed elemental
   d. semielemental

4. After gastric resection for treatment of gastric cancer, a patient would be most likely to experience dumping syndrome if he or she ate _____.

   a. string cheese
   b. peanuts
   c. cupcakes
   d. chicken

5. Medical nutrition therapy during the acute or flow phase of recovering from a large burn consists of feedings that are _____.

   a. high in protein and high in calories
   b. high in protein and low in carbohydrates
   c. high in protein and low in calories
   d. low in protein and high in calories

Next-Generation NCLEX® Examination-style Case Study

See answers in Appendix A.

An 8-year-old male (Ht.: 120 cm Wt.: 121 kg) with a history of ulcerative colitis had a bowel resection. His ileum and colon were both removed, and he now has an ostomy. At his last appointment 30 days ago, he weighed 128 kg. He now weighs 121 kg. The nurse plots the patient's anthropometrics on the age- and sex-appropriate growth chart and notes that his weight is in the 43rd percentile and his height is in the 8th percentile. He eats food by mouth but has not eaten more than 1000 kcals total over the last three days due to a lack of appetite. He does not have any signs of dysphagia or other swallowing difficulty. He takes a multivitamin dietary supplement daily.

1. From the list below, select all factors from the patient's history that are concerning.

   a. Weight history
   b. Nutrient absorption
   c. Energy intake
   d. Height
   e. Dysphagia
   f. Supplement use

2. Choose the *most likely* options for the information missing from the statements below by selecting from the list of options provided.

   The patient's bowel resection may have resulted in ___1___. The patient's weight history indicates that this may have caused compromised ___2___ and ___2___ resulting in impaired growth.

OPTION 1	OPTION 2
refeeding syndrome	defecation
small intestinal bacterial overgrowth	digestion
short bowel syndrome	peristalsis
irritable bowel syndrome	absorption
ryes syndrome	metabolism

3. Choose the *most likely* options for the information missing from the statement below by selecting from the list of options provided.

   The patient's weight loss and oral intake indicate that he may not be getting enough _____ and _____ orally.

OPTIONS	
calcium	protein
vitamin D	fluid
calories	cholesterol

4. From the list below, select all the appropriate nutrition interventions for this patient's situation at the given time.

   a. Enteral nutrition support
   b. Peripheral parenteral nutrition support
   c. Central parenteral nutrition support
   d. Oral intake
   e. Nothing by mouth

5. Use an X to identify effective nutrition intervention strategies that are <u>indicated</u> (appropriate or necessary) or <u>contraindicated</u> (could be harmful) for the patient at this point.

INTERVENTION	INDICATED	CONTRAINDICATED
Nasogastric tube		
Gastrointestinal tube		
Standard formula		
Elemental formula		
Continuous feeds		
Bolus feeds		

6. For each assessment finding, use an X to indicate whether nursing and collaborative interventions were <u>effective</u> (helped to meet expected outcomes), or <u>ineffective</u> (did not help to meet expected outcomes).

ASSESSMENT FINDING	EFFECTIVE	INEFFECTIVE
Patient gained 200g in the last 48 hours.		
Patient experienced vomiting.		
Patient's chart shows 1 stool output over the last 46 hours.		
Abdomen is distended.		
Patient received 50% of recommended feeds.		
Patient is taking a multivitamin.		
Small snacks are eaten throughout the day.		

Additional Learning Resources

Please refer to this text's Evolve website for answers to the Case Study Questions:
http://evolve.elsevier.com/Williams/basic/.
References and **Further Reading and Resources** in the back of the book provide additional resources for enhancing knowledge.

- Environmental agents, genetic factors, and weaknesses in the body's immune system can contribute to the development of cancer.
- A person's nutrition status influences the strength of his or her body's immune system.
- Nutrition problems affect the nature of the disease process and the medical treatments for individuals with cancer or human immunodeficiency virus (HIV).

- The progressive effects of HIV to the final stage of acquired immunodeficiency syndrome (AIDS) have many nutrition implications and often require aggressive medical nutrition therapy.

Cancer is a prevalent cause for morbidity and mortality worldwide. Because cancer is generally associated with aging, increases in life expectancy contribute to this growing incidence. Although cancer and HIV/AIDS share a direct relationship with the body's immune system and basic nutrition needs, their courses and outcomes are distinct.

This chapter looks at nutrition support in relation to both cancer and HIV/AIDS. Both diseases have important nutrition connections for prevention and therapy.

SECTION 1 CANCER

PROCESS OF CANCER DEVELOPMENT

THE NATURE OF CANCER

One of the difficulties with the study and treatment of cancer is that it is not a single problem: it has a highly variable nature, and it expresses itself in multiple forms. Cancer is the second leading cause of death in the United States. It is responsible for 21% of all deaths, whereas cardiovascular disease causes 23% of all deaths.[1] We use the term *cancer* to designate a malignant tumor or **neoplasm**. The many forms of cancer vary in prevalence worldwide and change as populations migrate to different environments. The Cultural Considerations box entitled "Incidence of Cancer in American Populations" outlines the prevalence of cancer in the United States relative to race/ethnicity.

The genetic code contained in the deoxyribonucleic acid (DNA) of the cell nucleus guides the continuous process of cell division. A **mutation** may disrupt this orderly process, particularly when the mutation occurs in a regulatory gene. Growth of a mutated cell may form a malignant tumor when normal gene control is lost. Thus, the misguided cell and its tumor tissue represent normal cell growth that has gone awry. Malignancies are identified by their primary site of origin, their stage or tumor size, the presence of **metastasis**, and their grade (i.e., how aggressive the tumor growth is).

There are three phases of **carcinogenesis**: initiation, promotion, and progression. *Initiation* is the point at which a mutagen causes irreversible damage to the DNA. An agent that prompts the mutated cell to grow and reproduce initiates the *promotion* phase. *Progression* is the phase during which the cancer cells advance and become a malignant tumor that is capable of metastasizing.

CANCER CELL DEVELOPMENT

The underlying cause of cancer is the fundamental loss of cell control over normal cell reproduction. Several factors may contribute to this loss and change a normal cell into a cancer cell, including chemical carcinogens, radiation, dietary factors, oncogenic viruses, and epidemiologic factors (e.g., race, age, heredity, occupation) (Figure 23.1). As such, many aspects of cancer are outside of the scope of this text, and we will not cover them in detail. This chapter focuses on cancer development and treatment as it relates to nutrition.

Dietary Factors

The relationship between diet and cancer is complex, as are the efforts to study the associations.[2] Foods naturally contain both carcinogenic and anticarcinogenic compounds. Researchers have documented the connection between some dietary patterns and specific forms of cancer, such as diets high in processed meat or meat cooked at high temperatures and the risk for

Incidence of Cancer in American Populations

The prevalence of cancer at any given time has many variables. The image below depicts the prevalence of cancer by one such factor: race/ethnicity. The confounding dynamics associated with cancer risk are complicated and multifactorial and extend well beyond this variable. However, heritage does affect a person's dietary patterns, lifestyle behaviors, and environmental exposures. A health care trend toward the prevention of cancer is a national goal specified in the *Healthy People 2030*. With the continued efforts and advancement of research, perhaps the prevention of cancer (instead of treatment after diagnosis) will become the norm. Identifying high-risk clients and encouraging regular physical examinations are important aspects of general health care as well as valuable prevention tools.

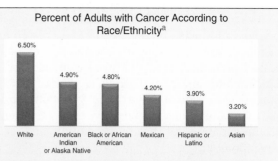

Percent of Adults with Cancer According to Race/Ethnicity[a]

6.50% White
4.90% American Indian or Alaska Native
4.80% Black or African American
4.20% Mexican
3.90% Hispanic or Latino
3.20% Asian

[a]Age 18 or older. Cancer is based on self-reported responses to a question about whether respondents had ever been told by a doctor or other health professional that they had cancer or a malignancy of any kind. Excludes squamous cell and basal cell carcinomas.

(From National Center for Health Statistics. [2019]. *Health, United States, 2018.* Hyattsville, MD: National Center for Health Statistics.)

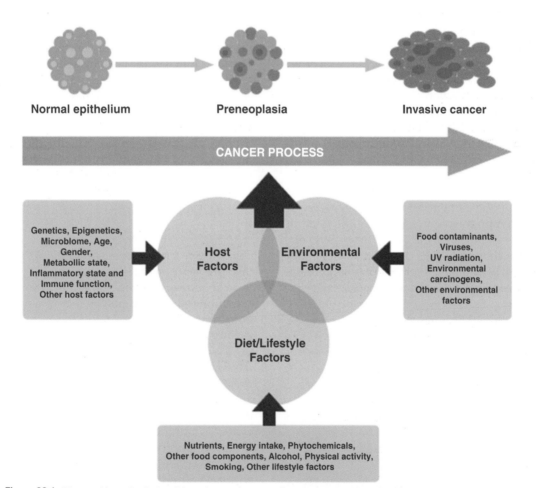

Figure 23.1 Diet, nutrition, physical activity, other environmental exposures, and host factors interact to affect the cancer process. (From World Cancer Research Fund/American Institute for Cancer Research. [2018]. *Diet, nutrition, physical activity and cancer: A global perspective, Continuous Update Project expert report.* www.wcrf.org/dietandcancer.)

colorectal and stomach cancer.[3-5] However, many other questions about diet and cancer remain unanswered. A general consensus is that obesity and a poor diet (defined as low intake of fruits, vegetables, whole grains and dairy products, and high intake of processed meat, red meat, alcohol, and sugar-sweetened beverages) increases cancer incidence.[5-11] Thus, a well-balanced diet (e.g., Mediterranean and MyPlate dietary patterns) coupled with regular physical activity that supports and maintains a healthy body weight is the general recommendation for health promotion and cancer prevention.[12,13]

THE BODY'S DEFENSE SYSTEM

The body's defense system is remarkably efficient and complex. Special cells protect the body from external invaders such as bacteria and viruses and from internal aliens such as cancer cells.

Defensive Cells

Two major cell populations provide the immune system's primary "search and destroy" defense for detecting and killing non-self substances that propagate potential disease. These two populations of lymphocytes, which are special types of white blood cells, develop early during life from a common stem cell in the bone marrow. The two types are T cells and B cells, and they originate from the thymus cells and bursal intestinal cells, respectively (Figure 23.2). A major function of T cells is to activate the phagocytes, which are the cells that destroy invaders and kill disease-carrying **antigens**. A major function of B cells is to produce **antibodies**, which also kill antigens.

Nutrition and Immunity

Immunity. Balanced nutrition is necessary to maintain the integrity of the human immune system. Severe malnutrition compromises the capacity of the immune system because of **atrophy** of the organs and tissues that are involved in immunity (e.g., liver, bowel wall, bone marrow, spleen, lymphoid tissue). Nutrition is also fundamental for combating sustained attacks of diseases

> **neoplasm** any new or abnormal cellular growth, specifically one that is uncontrolled and aggressive.
> **mutation** a permanent transmissible change in a gene.
> **metastasis** the spread to other tissue.
> **carcinogenesis** the transformation of normal cells into cancer cells.
> **antigen** any foreign or non-self substance (e.g., toxins, viruses, bacteria, foreign proteins) that triggers the production of antibodies that are specifically designed to counteract their activity.
> **antibodies** any of numerous protein molecules produced by B cells as a primary immune defense for attaching to specific related antigens.
> **atrophy** tissue wasting.

such as cancer. Internally derived antibodies constitute the core of the immune system. A direct and simple example of the important role of nutrition in immunity is the link between protein-energy malnutrition and the subsequent suppression of immune function.

Healing. The constant building and rebuilding of tissue protein maintains the strength of body tissue. Strong tissue is a front line of the body's defense. This process of tissue building and healing requires optimal nutrition intake. The diet must constantly supply specific nutrients that include protein, essential fatty acids, and key vitamins and minerals. Individuals entering cancer treatment with suboptimal nutrition status have compromised outcomes (e.g., longer hospital stay, infection, mortality).[14-16] Thus, maintaining good nutrition is a cornerstone for reducing the risk of cancer incidence and improving prognosis after treatment in the event that cancer does develop.

NUTRITION COMPLICATIONS OF CANCER TREATMENT

Oncologists use three major forms of medical treatment for cancer: surgery, radiation, and chemotherapy. Each requires nutrition support. Drug-nutrient interactions are also a complication that may happen with any form of treatment.

SURGERY

Surgery necessitates nutrition support for the healing process. This requirement is particularly true for individuals with cancer, because the disease process and its drain on the body's resources often weaken their general condition. With early diagnosis and sound nutrition support before and after surgery, surgeons may successfully remove many tumors providing patients with a good prognosis. Depending on the site of the surgery and the function of involved organs, medical nutrition therapy (MNT) may involve food texture or specific nutrient composition modifications. Chapter 22 covers various methods of nutrition support after surgery.

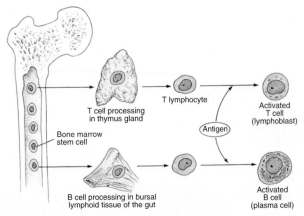

Figure 23.2 The development of the T and B cells, which are the lymphocyte components of the body's immune system. (Courtesy Eileen Draper.)

RADIATION

Oncologists may use radiation therapy by itself or in conjunction with other treatments. This type of therapy involves high-energy radiography beams converging on the cancer site to kill or shrink tumors. An external machine (Figure 23.3) or implanted radioactive materials at the cancer site administer the radiation to the body. Although the goal is for only the cancer cells to die, other cells within close proximity to the target site and rapidly growing cells often die as well.

The site and intensity of the radiation treatment determine the nature of the nutrition-related problems that the patient may encounter. For example, radiation of the head, neck, or esophagus disturbs the oral mucosa and salivary secretions, thereby affecting taste sensations and sensitivity to food texture and temperature. Resultant anorexia and nausea may exacerbate malnutrition. The registered dietitian nutritionist (RDN) can help the individual explore means of appetite improvement through food appearance and aroma as well as texture variety. Similarly, radiation to the abdominal area compromises the intestinal mucosa, causing a loss of villi and possibly nutrient malabsorption. Tissue breakdown may cause ulcers, inflammation, obstructions, or fistulas, and these conditions interfere with the normal functioning of the involved tissue.

CHEMOTHERAPY

Chemotherapeutic agents destroy rapidly growing cancer cells. Unlike radiation therapy, the health care team administers chemotherapy via general blood circulation throughout the body. Because chemotherapeutic medications are highly toxic, they also affect normal, healthy cells. This accounts for their side effects on rapidly growing tissues (e.g., bone marrow, gastrointestinal [GI] tract, hair follicles) and the complications associated with nutrition

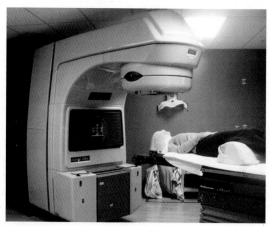

Figure 23.3 A radiation treatment machine. (Courtesy Jormain Cady, Virginia Mason Medical Center, Seattle, WA. In Lewis, S. M., Heitkemper, M. M., Dirksen, S. R., et al. [Eds.]. [2007]. *Medical-surgical nursing: Assessment and management of clinical problems* [7th ed.]. St. Louis: Mosby.)

management. General complications include the following:

- *Bone marrow:* Interference with the production of specific blood factors causes a reduced red blood cell count and anemia, a reduced white blood cell count and lowered resistance to infections, and a reduced blood platelet level that may prevent the formation of blood clots when needed to stop bleeding.
- *GI tract:* Patients may experience numerous problems that interfere with food tolerance, such as nausea and vomiting, a loss of normal taste sensations, anorexia, diarrhea, ulcers, malabsorption, and mucositis.
- *Hair follicle:* Interference with normal hair growth results in general hair loss.

DRUG-NUTRIENT INTERACTIONS

Many medications used in cancer treatment have a high potential for drug-nutrient interactions. Several antineoplastic drugs have well-documented drug-nutrient interactions that the health care team should address with patients on an individual basis. In addition, many people experiment with dietary supplements and herbs that they believe have a protective role in cancer treatment or prevention. Some of the more commonly used herbs have well-known food-drug interactions that may adversely affect patients or their treatment regimen (see the complementary and alternative medicine information at www.cancer.gov). Open dialog between a patient and the health care team helps to reveal any dietary supplement and herb use and presents an opportunity to discuss potential interactions.

MEDICAL NUTRITION THERAPY IN THE PATIENT WITH CANCER

Although the dietitian and the physician have the primary responsibility for planning and managing the MNT strategy, the nursing staff and other health care personnel make a tremendous contribution with regard to day-to-day support and counseling to help patients meet their nutrient requirements and manage complications.

NUTRITION-RELATED COMPLICATIONS OF CANCER

Individual nutrition problems throughout the continuum of care for cancer patients vary greatly. Not all individuals with cancer need MNT. For example, basal cell carcinoma is the most common type of skin cancer, and in most cases, excision of the lesion is the only intervention required. In such circumstances, nutrition intervention is rarely necessary. However, general nutrition obstacles may pose a challenge for patients with advanced stages of cancer, for those undergoing surgery or radiation therapy affecting the GI system, and for patients receiving chemotherapy. Such problems relate to the overall systemic effects of cancer as well as to the specific individual response to the treatment method.

General Systemic Effects

Cancer generally causes the following systemic effects with regard to nutrition status:

- *Anorexia,* or loss of appetite, which results in poor food intake
- *Increased metabolism,* which results in increased nutrient and energy needs
- *Negative nitrogen balance,* which results in lean tissue catabolism, fatigue, and compromised physical function

Unfortunately, this creates a snowball effect: cancer causes poor nutrition status and poor nutrition status is associated with an increased rate of hospital admission and poor overall outcome for patients with cancer.[14-16] The extent of these effects varies widely from a mild response, to malnutrition, or to an extreme form of debilitating cachexia. An inability to ingest or use nutrients causes weight loss, tissue catabolism, and weakness. Although the prevalence of cachexia varies with the type of cancer, a significant number of patients with advanced cancer experience some level of cachexia-associated weight loss, particularly older individuals.[17,18] An involuntary weight loss with ongoing loss of skeletal muscle mass (with or without loss of fat mass) is indicative of cachexia. Clinical weight loss is generally defined as >5% of body weight in 6 months or >2% of body weight for individuals with a body mass index (BMI) of $<20 \text{ kg/m}^2$. Cachexia greatly increases morbidity, mortality, length of hospital stays, and medical costs and contributes to poor quality of life and loss of function.[18-20] The best way to treat cancer-related cachexia is to alleviate the cancer and the metabolic abnormalities associated with it. However, because this is not always a possibility and there is not a standard effective treatment for cachexia, the health care team must practice aggressive MNT and medication therapy aimed at alleviating symptoms.[18,21-23]

Effects Specific to the Type or Treatment of Cancer

In addition to the primary nutrition problems that the disease process produces, secondary problems with eating or nutrient metabolism result from obstructive tumors or lesions in the GI tract, accessory organs, or the surrounding tissue. Such conditions limit food intake and digestion as well as nutrient absorption. Patients with forms of cancer that involve hormone or steroid therapy (e.g., breast and prostate cancer) are at risk for significant weight gain. Their MNT should focus on diet and lifestyle modifications that help to avoid unintentional weight gain. Dietitians must individualize each patient's MNT protocol relative to the nature and location of the cancer and the mode of treatment to help overcome cancer-specific difficulties.

Loss of appetite. Anorexia is a common problem in patients with cancer, and it curtails food intake when the individual needs it the most. Anorexia often sets up a vicious cycle that can lead to the gross malnutrition of cancer-related cachexia, as discussed previously. The dietitian, along with the patient and his or her support system, must plan a vigorous schedule for eating that does not depend on appetite for stimulus. The overall goal is to provide food with as much nutrient density as possible so that every bite counts.

Oral complications. Various problems that contribute to eating difficulties may stem from a sore mouth, mucositis, or altered taste and smell acuity. Decreased saliva and mucositis often result from radiation to the head and neck area or from chemotherapy. Spraying the mouth with artificial saliva or an oral numbing solution may be helpful. Good oral care habits are important to avoid infection and to prevent dental caries, both of which could further impede healthy eating. Basic mouth care includes regular dental cleaning and maintenance, examining the mouth daily for sores or irritation, ensuring that dentures fit correctly (if applicable), and using an alcohol-free mouthwash.

Treatments may alter the tongue's taste buds, thereby causing taste distortion, taste blindness, and the inability to distinguish sweet, sour, salt, or bitter, thereby resulting in more food aversions. Strong food seasonings (for those who can tolerate them) and high-protein liquid drinks may be helpful. Because the treatment may also alter salivary secretions, foods with a high liquid content are favored. Clients may swallow solid foods more easily with the use of sauces, gravies, broth, yogurt, or salad dressings. A food processor or blender can turn foods into semisolid or liquid forms for easier swallowing.

Gastrointestinal problems. Chemotherapy often causes nausea and vomiting, which require special individual attention. Food that is hot, sweet, fatty, or spicy sometimes exacerbates nausea. Affected individuals should avoid them in accordance with their specific tolerance. Slowly consumed small and frequent feedings of soft or liquid cold or room temperature foods may ease discomfort. The use of antinausea drugs (e.g., prochlorperazine, ondansetron) aids with food tolerances. Surgical treatment that involves the GI tract requires related dietary modifications as covered in Chapter 22. Chemotherapy and radiation treatment can affect the mucosal cells that secrete lactase and thus induce lactose intolerance. In such cases, soy-based dairy substitutes or nutrient supplements (e.g., Ensure, Boost) are appropriate alternatives. Table 23.1 provides

---

fistulas from the Latin word for "pipe," an abnormal opening or passageway within the body or to the outside.

mucositis an inflammation of the tissues around the mouth or other orifices of the body.

cachexia a specific profound syndrome that is characterized by wasting, reduced food intake, and systemic inflammation.

Table **23.1**	Dietary Modifications for Nutrition-Related Side Effects of Cancer, Human Immunodeficiency Virus, and Acquired Immunodeficiency Syndrome

SYMPTOM	SUGGESTIONS
Anorexia	Consume small, frequent, high-calorie meals and snacks (regardless of hunger) Add extra protein and calories to food to get the most out of each bite Choose foods that appeal to the sense of smell Experiment with different foods Prepare and store small portions of favorite foods for ready access Arrange for help with purchasing and preparing food and meals Perform frequent mouth care to relieve symptoms and to decrease aftertastes Participate in physical activity when possible to increase appetite
Nausea and vomiting	Avoid spicy foods, greasy foods, sweets, and foods with strong odors Have others prepare food for you if cooking causes nausea Eat dry, bland, soft, and easy-to-digest foods such as crackers, breadsticks, and toast throughout the day Cold and room temperature foods may be better tolerated Avoid heavy meals Remain upright for at least 1 hour after eating Avoid eating in areas with strong cooking odors or that are too warm Drink plenty of water throughout the day to replace lost fluids Rinse out the mouth before and after eating Suck on hard candies (e.g., peppermints, lemon drops) if there is a bad taste in the mouth Use antiemetics and electrolyte replacements as necessary
Taste and smell alterations	Try new foods when feeling best Plan meals that include favorite foods Add spices, herbs, seasonings, and sauces to foods If red meat tastes bitter, choose poultry, eggs, fish, and other high-protein foods instead; marinate meat with something sweet; or eat with a sweet sauce such as cranberry sauce, jelly, or applesauce Use plastic or wood utensils if foods taste metallic Use sugar-free lemon drops, gum, or mints when experiencing a bitter taste in the mouth Rule out zinc deficiency
Xerostomia	Drink plenty of fluids and keep a water bottle handy at all times to moisten the mouth Eat moist foods with extra sauces and gravies Perform oral hygiene at least four times per day, but avoid rinses that contain alcohol Consume tart foods and beverages to stimulate saliva production Avoid coffee, tea, and alcohol Use sugar-free chewing gum, hard candy, frozen desserts, and ice pops between meals to moisten the mouth
Mucositis and stomatitis	Eat foods that are soft and easy to chew and swallow Moisten foods with gravy, broth, or sauces Avoid alcohol and known irritants such as acidic, spicy, salty, and coarse-textured foods (e.g., crunchy foods) Cook foods until they are soft and tender, or cut foods into small bites Eat foods at room temperature Supplement meals with high-calorie, high-protein milkshakes or smoothies Maintain good oral hygiene Numb the mouth with ice chips or flavored ice pops
Dehydration	Drink 8 to 12 cups of liquids a day, regardless of thirst Add soup, flavored ice pops, and other sources of fluid to the diet Limit caffeine and alcohol Use antiemetic and antidiarrheal medications as needed for relief from vomiting and diarrhea
Diarrhea	Avoid greasy foods, hot and cold liquids, caffeine, and foods high in sugar alcohols (e.g., sorbitol) Rule out lactose intolerance Drink fluids throughout the day and at least 1 cup of liquid after each loose bowel movement Limit gas-forming foods and beverages (e.g., soda, cruciferous vegetables, legumes, lentils, chewing gum) Use antidiarrheal medications and electrolyte replacements as necessary
Constipation	Gradually increase fiber and fluid intake Maintain regular physical activity Consult the health care team following intestinal surgery or if there is an intestinal obstruction
Neutropenia[a]	Prevent food-borne illness by practicing safe food purchasing and handling guidelines (see Chapter 13) Avoid salad bars and buffets when eating out Wash fruits and vegetables well or peel and discard the outer layer Limit exposure to large groups of people and people with infections Practice good hygiene (clean hands and teeth often)

[a]Neutropenia involves a low white blood cell count and an increased risk of infection.

suggestions for dietary modifications in response to nutrition-related side effects.

Loss of lean tissue. Dietary supplements containing fish oil may be effective at preserving or improving lean body mass in adult oncology patients experiencing unintentional weight loss. Therefore, the dietitian may recommend a dietary supplement or a medical food supplement containing fish oil with 1.2 to 2.2 g of eicosapentaenoic acid daily as a nutrition intervention for individuals who continue to lose weight and lean body mass.[24]

Pain and discomfort. Patients are more able to eat if severe pain is controlled and if they are sitting in a comfortable position. The current medical consensus is to administer pain-controlling medication as needed in close consultation with the patient and their care providers or family and then to carefully monitor responses. This is especially important for children with cancer who are undergoing painful treatments. Constipation is a common side effect of several pain medications. Preventive therapy to avoid additional discomfort from constipation should focus on adequate fluids, soluble fiber, and regular physical activity (even short walks can help).

NUTRITION CARE PLAN

The fundamental principles of identifying needs and planning care based on those requirements underlie all sound patient care (see Chapter 17).

Nutrition Screening and Assessment

Assessing and monitoring the nutrition status of each client is the primary responsibility of the RDN. Various members of the health care team may take part in anthropometric measurements and the calculations of body composition, laboratory tests and the interpretation of their results, physical examination and clinical observations, and dietary analysis. Weight can change rapidly in some individuals; therefore, the health care provider must obtain accurate measurements instead of relying on self-reported or estimated values. The oncologist or dietitian should evaluate all cancer patients for malnutrition. There are validated and reliable assessment tools available to screen for malnutrition in the oncology population, such as the Malnutrition Screening Tool, Malnutrition Screening Tool for Cancer Patients, and the Malnutrition Universal Screening Tool.[24] Malnutrition or severe alterations in weight indicate complications that may change medication dosages, alter the treatment plan, or otherwise require medical intervention.

Nutrition Intervention

The basic objectives of the nutrition intervention plan for patients with cancer are as follows[25,26]:
- Prevent nutrient deficiencies and unintentional changes in body weight.

- Maintain or improve lean body mass, strength, energy, functional ability, tolerance to treatment, immune function, and quality of life.
- Identify and manage nutrition-related side effects of cancer and treatment modalities.

Based on detailed information that is gathered about each patient, including his or her living situation and other personal and social needs, the dietitian develops a personal MNT plan to meet these objectives. An oral diet is the most desired form of feeding when tolerated. However, achieving these nutrition goals in the face of frequent food intolerance, anorexia, or the inability to eat presents a great challenge for the patient and the nutrition support team. Patient-centered MNT varies, depending on the cancer site, the stage of disease, the treatment modality, and the patient's current nutrition status. The patient and dietitian work together to create a personalized food plan, including adjustments in food texture and temperature and alternative food options to account for intolerances. If normal oral intake does not meet the patient's nutrient needs, the dietitian may recommend energy-dense nutrition supplements (e.g., Ensure, Boost) in addition to meals. If nutrition status continues to decline, the health care team must consider enteral or parenteral nutrition support (see Chapter 22).[26]

Prevention of catabolism. The nutrition care plan will make every effort to meet the increased metabolic demands of the disease process in an effort to prevent extensive catabolic effects and tissue breakdown. Maintaining nutrition from the beginning is far more efficient than rebuilding the body after extensive wasting. The nutrition intervention recommendations for patients with or at risk for cancer-related cachexia are to maximize the oral intake of nutrient-dense foods while liberalizing any diet restrictions and encouraging small, frequent meals. Dietary supplements containing eicosapentaenoic acid and nutrient-dense nourishments (e.g., Ensure, Boost, Carnation Breakfast Essentials) may benefit the patient and help them to meet nutrient needs.[24]

Varieties of interventions are currently in use or under investigation to increase appetite, spare protein degradation, improve caloric intake, and decrease nausea and inflammation. Some examples include progesterone derivatives, ghrelin, antiinflammatories, anabolic agents, various nutrition supplements, and cannabinoids, all of which have limitations.[22,23] See the Clinical Applications box entitled "Cannabis as a Treatment for Anorexia" for information about the use of cannabis for combating unintended weight loss in clients who suffer from cancer-related cachexia. Table 23.1 provides strategies for improving food intake in clients with cancer or HIV.

Clinical Applications

Cannabis as a Treatment for Anorexia

Medical marijuana is currently legal in Canada, some European countries, and several states within the United States. The debate for legalization of cannabis continues in many areas with genuine concerns on both sides. Proponents argue in favor of the effectiveness that marijuana has on relieving the nausea caused by cancer treatment, the wasting effects of HIV, chronic pain, and the pain of glaucoma. Critics argue against the legalization of marijuana because there are other medications available for treating the same symptom, it carries a potential for dependency, it is associated with child development problems if used during pregnancy, and there are cardiovascular and respiratory related adverse effects associated with marijuana use. Additional clinical studies on human subjects are required to elucidate the benefits and risk related to marijuana use in individuals with various disorders.

Dronabinol (Marinol and Syndros) is a capsule form of marijuana that the U.S. Food and Drug Administration have approved for medical use. It contains synthetic delta-9-tetrahydrocannabinol, which is the active ingredient found in the marijuana plant; thus, the drug has similar side effects, such as:

Anxiety	Nightmares
Dizziness	Stomach pain
Paranoid reaction	Nausea/vomiting
Cognitive impairment	Sedation
Memory loss	Syncope
Visual disturbances	Palpitations

Providers prescribe dronabinol for the treatment of anorexia associated with unintentional weight loss in patients with HIV and for the nausea and vomiting associated with cancer chemotherapy in patients who have not adequately responded to conventional antiemetic treatments. Because this drug can be habit forming, prescribing guidelines recommend using the lowest dose needed to produce the desired result. Individuals using dronabinol should communicate clearly with their health care provider regarding any adverse reactions or concerns because the side effects are unique to each person.

Energy. An adult with good nutrition status needs approximately 25 to 30 kcal/kg of body weight for maintenance requirements. If these energy estimates are not maintaining body weight, an indirect calorimetry can determine more precise energy needs as predictive equations (e.g., Harris Benedict, Mifflin St.-Jeor equations) have significant limitations with this population.[27] Patients may need more kilocalories in accordance with the degree of metabolic stress, the amount of anabolism that is taking place, and their physical activity levels. A malnourished patient may require significantly more energy, depending on the degree of malnutrition. However,

refeeding syndrome is also a risk for these individuals. Thus, a slow increase in energy intake is crucial to avoid potentially fatal complications.[26] Symptoms and side effects of the cancer or of the cancer treatment also have significant impacts on energy needs and oral intake. Anorexia, diarrhea, cachexia, nausea, malabsorption, fever, xerostomia, pain, infection, and early satiety are all examples of complications that will alter a patient's energy needs and consumption. Some individuals are more successful in meeting nutrient needs through small-volume energy- and nutrient-dense meals instead of three large meals daily.

Protein. Adequate dietary protein is necessary for tissue building and healing and to offset the tissue breakdown that the disease or the treatment causes. Efficient protein use depends on an optimal protein-to-energy ratio to prevent catabolism. An adult nonstressed cancer patient with good nutrition status needs 1.0 to 1.5 g/kg/day of protein to meet maintenance requirements, with an emphasis on high-quality protein sources.[26] Malnourished individuals need additional protein to replenish deficits and to restore a positive nitrogen balance. Dietary protein intakes up to 2 g/kg/day are safe in patients with normal kidney function. Expert guidelines encourage patients to obtain all protein from food sources, as opposed to amino acid supplements. Currently available data do not consistently show a benefit to nutrition status or lean body mass from such supplementation.[26]

Vitamins and minerals. Key vitamins and minerals help to control protein and energy metabolism through their coenzyme roles in specific cell enzyme pathways, and they play important roles in building and maintaining strong tissue (see Chapter 7 and Chapter 8). Therefore, an optimal intake of vitamins and minerals (at least to the Dietary Reference Intake standards) is ideal. Some individuals may require vitamin and mineral supplements to ensure dietary intake. However, the efficacy and safety of using dietary supplement megadoses or intravenous administration of select vitamins (specifically those that contain antioxidants) remain controversial (see the Drug-Nutrient Interaction box, "Antioxidants and Chemotherapy").

RDNs who specialize in oncology can assist patients in sorting through the supportive data on dietary supplements for specific forms of cancer and specific forms of treatment. There are some evidence-based recommendations for supplementation in select cases.[24,25] A holistic approach to patient-centered care requires collaboration with all health care team members, and this includes the decision about dietary supplement use as part of the care plan.

Drug-Nutrient Interaction

Antioxidants and Chemotherapy

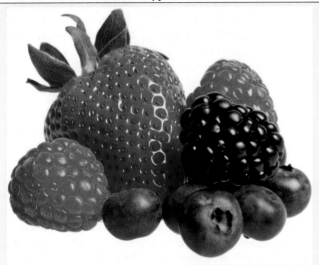

Complementary and alternative medicine (CAM) is a diverse set of health care systems, products, and practices that are not generally considered part of conventional medicine. This type of treatment includes dietary supplement use, acupuncture, massage, herbal medicines, and mind-body techniques. The use of CAM—and most notably dietary supplement use—is highly prevalent in individuals with cancer.

Oncologists characterize tumor cells by their rapid rate of division. Antineoplastic drugs work by producing free radicals that cause oxidative damage and cell death to these rapidly dividing cells. However, normal, healthy cells such as skin cells, hair follicles, and the cells that line the digestive tract divide quickly as well. This is why systemic cancer treatments, such as chemotherapy, effect these areas of healthy cells during treatment. As far back as 1969, cancer patients have used antioxidant supplements, particularly megadoses of vitamin C, in an effort to boost their immune system while undergoing cancer treatment or as the sole treatment method. Historically, this practice has been controversial, primarily because of the lack of high-quality clinical trials to support either the safety or efficacy of the practice. Because vitamin C is an antioxidant and some chemotherapeutic agents specifically use oxidative stress to target the cancer cells, health care professionals speculated that simultaneous vitamin C treatment would reduce the effectiveness of the anticancer treatment. One study found that even at typical oral supplemental doses of 500 mg per day, vitamin C prevented the cytotoxic effects of antineoplastic agents from killing tumor cells, not just healthy cells.[1] In other words, the vitamin C *protected the cancer cells.*[2] However, studies that are more recent indicate that intravenous administration of vitamin C is probably safe and may help mitigate cancer and treatment symptoms for some patients (e.g., fatigue, pain, mood).[3,4] However, high-quality clinical trials are necessary to determine the role of large-dose intravenous administration of vitamin C for cancer patients.[5]

Resveratrol is a phytochemical found in berries and other fruits with anticancer and antioxidant activity. It is also available in dietary supplement form, and individuals commonly use it as a cancer prevention prophylaxis and an adjunct to cancer treatment. In vitro studies suggest that resveratrol increases tumor cell response to the effects of chemotherapeutic agents and increases apoptosis of breast cancer cells.[6,7] This research is still in its infancy, and experts cannot yet make general recommendations regarding dietary supplements of resveratrol during cancer treatment until high-quality in vivo studies are completed.[8] To ensure safety during chemotherapy, patients should carefully discuss their use of supplemental vitamin C or other potent dietary antioxidants with their health care providers and take no more than the Upper Tolerable Intake according to the Dietary Reference Intakes unless otherwise advised.

REFERENCES

1. Heaney, M. L., et al. (2008). Vitamin C antagonizes the cytotoxic effects of antineoplastic drugs. *Cancer Research*, *68*(19), 8031–8038.
2. Subramani, T., et al. (2014). Vitamin C suppresses cell death in MCF-7 human breast cancer cells induced by tamoxifen. *Journal of Cellular and Molecular Medicine*, *18*(2), 305–313.
3. Bazzan, A. J., et al. (2018). Retrospective evaluation of clinical experience with intravenous ascorbic acid in patients with cancer. *Integrative Cancer Therapies*, *17*(3), 912–920.
4. Fritz, H., et al. (2014). Intravenous vitamin C and cancer: A systematic review. *Integrative Cancer Therapies*, *13*(4), 280–300.
5. van Gorkom, G. N. Y., et al. (2019). The effect of Vitamin C (ascorbic acid) in the treatment of patients with cancer: A systematic review. *Nutrients*, *11*(5), 977.
6. Dewangan, J., et al. (2017). Novel combination of salinomycin and resveratrol synergistically enhances the anti-proliferative and pro-apoptotic effects on human breast cancer cells. *Apoptosis*, *22*(10), 1246–1259.
7. Venkatadri, R., et al. (2017). A novel resveratrol-salinomycin combination sensitizes ER-positive breast cancer cells to apoptosis. *Pharmacological Reports*, *69*(4), 788–797.
8. Bartolacci, C., et al. (2018). Walking a tightrope: A perspective of resveratrol effects on breast cancer. *Current Protein & Peptide Science*, *19*(3), 311–322.

Fluid. Maintaining adequate fluid balance is essential to replace GI losses from fever, infection, vomiting, or diarrhea. Encourage patients to drink at least 1 cup of fluid for each incidence of diarrhea. In cases in which dehydration persists, the health care provider may order intravenous fluids. The kidneys filter the blood to dispose of metabolic waste from destroyed cancer cells and toxins from the chemotherapeutic drugs. Ample urine output is favorable for toxin clearance.

Enteral and parenteral nutrition support. Patients who have a functioning GI tract but are unable to eat may require nutrition support in the form of a tube feeding to achieve essential nutrition goals. Patients without a functioning GI tract and patients who cannot tolerate enteral feedings may require parenteral feedings for nutrition support. We sometimes refer to such forms of nutrition support as *artificial nutrition.* Guidelines recommend considering artificial nutrition when patients have not eaten in more than a week or have only been able to consume 60% or less of their nutrient needs for more than 1 to 2 weeks.[26] See Box 22.1 in Chapter 22 for indications requiring enteral and parenteral nutrition support. Chapter 22 covers the details of enteral and parenteral methods of feeding.

Nutrition Monitoring and Evaluation

As with all MNT strategies, the dietitian will evaluate the nutrition care plan for efficacy on a regular basis with the patient and care providers. Likewise, the dietitian will update the plan as needed to meet the nutrition demands of the patient's condition as well as his or her individual desires and tolerances.

CANCER PREVENTION

Experts estimate that 42% of cancer cases in adults are the result of potentially modifiable lifestyle choices (e.g., diet, physical activity, alcohol intake, smoking/ smoke exposure, UV radiation, obesity).[9] Thus, the American Cancer Society, the American Institute for Cancer Research, and the World Cancer Research Fund International highlight the significance of a healthy diet and regular physical activity in their cancer prevention guidelines.[12,13] In addition, the U.S. Food and Drug Administration (FDA) has approved specific food-labeling guidelines for associating certain foods and nutrients to the decreased risk of cancer.[28] The next section of this chapter summarizes the combined recommendations from these organizations.

GUIDELINES FOR CANCER PREVENTION

The most recent expert panel publications recommend the following lifestyle factors to reduce the risk of cancer[12,13]:

1. Be as lean as possible within the normal range of body weight throughout life.
   - Balance caloric intake with physical activity.
   - Avoid excessive weight gain at all ages. For overweight or obese individuals, losing even a small amount of weight is helpful.
2. Adopt a physically active lifestyle.
   - Children and adolescents: participate in at least 60 minutes every day of moderate to vigorous physical activity, with vigorous intensity activity included at least 3 days per week.
   - Adults: engage in at least 150 minutes of moderate intensity or 75 minutes of vigorous physical activity each week; preferably spread throughout the week.
   - Limit sedentary behaviors.
3. Consume a healthy diet that has an emphasis on plant-based food.
   - Become familiar with standard serving sizes and read food labels to become more aware of actual servings consumed. Choose foods that will help achieve and maintain a healthy body weight.

- Limit the consumption of salty foods and salt-preserved foods.
- Limit the consumption of energy-dense foods, particularly processed foods that are high in added sugar, low in fiber, or high in fat. Avoid sugar-sweetened beverages.
- Choose a variety of different fruits and vegetables. Eat at least 2.5 cups of vegetables and fruits every day.
- Choose whole grains instead of processed (refined) grains and sugars. Avoid moldy grains and legumes.
- Choose fish, poultry, and beans as alternatives to red meat. Select lean cuts and small portions, and prepare the meat by baking, broiling, or poaching rather than frying. Avoid processed meats.
4. If alcohol is consumed, limit intake to two drinks per day for men and one drink per day for women. One drink is defined as 12 oz of beer, 5 oz of wine, or 1.5 oz of 80-proof distilled spirits.
5. Meet nutrient needs through diet alone; do not rely on dietary supplements.
6. Aim to breastfeed infants exclusively for 6 months and continue to breastfeed for at least 1 year while offering complementary food after 6 months.

Dietary choices and physical activity are the most modifiable risk factors for cancer prevention. Large-scale epidemiology studies show that individuals adhering to cancer prevention guidelines (specifically diet and physical activity) have a reduced risk for all-cause and cancer-specific mortality.[29-32] One study including more than 476,000 participants followed for 10+ years reported that adherence to the preceding guidelines significantly reduced the incidence of cancer and cancer mortality for both men and women.[33] The reduction in risk varies between sex and type of cancer with risk reduction ranging from 15% (lung cancer in men) to 65% (gallbladder cancer in both sexes). Adopting a healthy lifestyle and avoiding tobacco have tremendous health benefits and reduce the risk of several other forms of chronic disease as well.

Health Claims

The FDA regulates health claims approved for use on food labels (see Chapter 13). The qualified health claims about cancer risk in the United States link the following nutrients with reduced risk[28]:

- *Dietary lipids (fat) and cancer.* An example claim approved for use: "Development of cancer depends on many factors. A diet low in total fat may reduce the risk of some cancers."
- *Fiber-containing grain products, fruits, vegetables, and cancer.* An example claim approved for use: "Low-fat diets rich in fiber-containing grain products, fruits, and vegetables may reduce the risk of some types of cancer, a disease associated with many factors."
- *Fruits and vegetables and cancer.* An example claim approved for use on oranges: "Development of cancer

depends on many factors. Eating a diet low in fat and high in fruits and vegetables, foods that are low in fat and may contain vitamin A, vitamin C, and dietary fiber, may reduce your risk of some cancers. Oranges, a food low in fat, are a good source of fiber and vitamin C."

Based on these associations, the Centers for Disease Control and Prevention (CDC) and the *Healthy People 2030* encourage Americans to eat several servings of fruits and vegetables every day.[34] Most people need at least 5 servings of fruits and vegetables daily.

Cancer Research

Research that links specific elements of the diet with the risk for cancer is difficult to do and complicated to interpret. As previously mentioned, some studies have shown that diets consistent with cancer prevention guidelines are associated with decreased incidences and mortality rates for various cancers. The exact mechanisms by which such diets are protective against cancer are still under investigation. Some examples of recent findings include the following:

- *Breast cancer:* Excess body fat (regardless of BMI) considerably increases the risk for breast cancer through several metabolic and inflammatory pathways.[35-37] Women following the World Cancer Research Fund and the American Institute for Cancer Research guidelines significantly reduce their risk for breast cancer. Meeting the following specific guidelines is protective against breast cancer development: avoiding red meat, processed meat, saturated fat, sugar-sweetened beverages, and dietary supplements (as the primary source of nutrients); consuming a plant-based diet; and getting regular physical activity.[38,39]
- *Colorectal cancer:* Over one-third of colorectal cancer incidence is attributable to dietary factors (36.7%) and physical inactivity (16.3%) alone.[9] Diets rich in whole grains, fiber, and calcium appear to be protective against colorectal cancer. Lifestyle factors that increase the risk for colorectal cancer include high intakes of red meat and processed meat, excess body fat, and alcohol consumption.[36]
- *Gastric cancer:* A diet rich in fruits and vegetables such as the Mediterranean diet appears to be protective against gastric cancer compared with the typical Western diet, which is rich in salty foods, sweets, processed meat, and fat.[40] Specifically, the intake of white vegetables, total fruit, and citrus fruits high in vitamin C are protective.[41] Excess body weight and a high intake of processed meat, salty foods, and alcohol are risk factors.[9,41]

Scientists have investigated many other associations with some controversy. The article by Islami and colleagues[9] provides detailed information about the dietary factors and lifestyle choices that are associated with a reduced risk of specific types of cancer (see the references for Chapter 23 listed at the back of this textbook).

Many programs hosted by the CDC aim to prevent and control cancer as well as research cause-and-effect relationships. Some examples of these programs include the National Comprehensive Cancer Control Program; the National Breast and Cervical Cancer Early Detection Program; the National Program of Cancer Registries; and the Colorectal Cancer Control Program. In addition to these programs, there are several initiatives that focus on education and awareness campaigns and research activities that are aimed at lung, skin, prostate, and gynecologic cancers and cancer survivorship.[42] Many of these programs have nutrition-related objectives.

DIETS AND SUPPLEMENTS

Diets and dietary supplements promoting the ability to cure cancer have been around for many decades, the vast majority of which are inconsequential, some of which are downright dangerous, and some of which are currently undergoing clinical trial. The Academy of Nutrition and Dietetics *Nutrition Care Manual* reports on the following non–evidence-based diets and supplements that are commonly associated with cancer: Gerson diet, Gonzalez diet, acid-base diets, macrobiotic diets, high-dose vitamin C supplements, hydrazine sulfate, laetrile, shark cartilage, and juice therapies.[25] Some of these purported "cancer treatments" have undergone clinical experimentation and failed to produce any positive or cancer-protective results or are not safe in patients with cancer. Despite their popularity, experts discourage the use of macrobiotic diets for cancer prevention because of the restrictive nature of the diet and the risk for multiple nutrient deficiencies.

Complementary and alternative medicine (CAM) is commonly used by individuals with cancer,[43-45] but less than half of those clients, on average, disclosed that information to their oncologist.[46,47] Health care practitioners should always be open to the needs of their clients and respectful of their desires. The most important thing to ensure is that the patient and the health care team discuss all alternative practices to determine any potential interactions, dangers, or risks. Alternative practices that may have nutrient or drug-nutrient interaction potentials include specific diets, supplements, herbs, infusions, injections, and enemas, for example. As a health care provider, be sure to ask about the use of any of these practices. Some dietary supplements can have dangerous interactions with chemotherapeutic agents or other treatment regimens (see the Drug-Nutrient Interaction box, "Antioxidants and Chemotherapy"). If clients feel uncomfortable about discussing their CAM practices with their health care provider, they are much less likely to disclose the use of CAM and serious consequences may result.

SECTION 2 HUMAN IMMUNODEFICIENCY VIRUS

PROGRESSION OF HUMAN IMMUNODEFICIENCY VIRUS

This section looks at HIV and compares its relationship to the body's immune system and course of development with that of cancer. According to the CDC, about 38,700 people are infected with HIV every year in the United States alone, approximately 81% of whom are male.[48] See the Cultural Considerations box, "Incidence of Human Immunodeficiency Virus and Acquired Immunodeficiency Syndrome in American Populations," for more information on the incidence of HIV in the United States.

EVOLUTION OF HUMAN IMMUNODEFICIENCY VIRUS

Scientists identified the earliest known case of AIDS in a blood sample collected in 1959 from a Bantu man living in what is currently the Democratic Republic of Congo, an area from which the current world epidemic is believed to have originated.[49] Early during the 1960s in the African country of Uganda, strange deaths began to occur from simple common infections such as pneumonia that did not respond to the usual antibiotic drugs. By the late 1970s and early 1980s, the same peculiar deaths were occurring in Europe and America. Similar reports of unexplained immune system failure increased rapidly in various parts of the world, and the

pandemic spread. These early cases came from people with diverse social and medical backgrounds, including heterosexual and homosexual men, intravenous drug users, and recipients of transfused blood and blood products (e.g., clients with hemophilia, medical and surgical patients). After feverish research, scientists discovered the underlying infectious agent in May 1983. The French scientist Luc Montagnier, a leading pioneer in AIDS research, reported that he and his team at the Pasteur Institute in Paris had isolated the viral cause, which we now know as *HIV*.

PARASITIC NATURE OF THE VIRUS

No virus can have a life of its own. Because of their structure and reproductive nature, viruses are the ultimate **parasites**. They are mere shreds of genetic material, a small packet of genetic information encased in a protein coat. Viruses only contain a small chromosome of nucleic acids (RNA or DNA), usually with fewer than five genes. They can live only through a host that they invade and infect, and they hijack the host's cell machinery to make a multitude of copies of themselves. Scientists agree that HIV, which is genetically similar to a virus found in African primates (simian immunodeficiency virus), was probably transmitted to human beings as hunters accidentally cut themselves while butchering their kills for food. The deadly strength of HIV results from its aggressive growth within an increasing number of hosts. Worldwide, 38 million people are living with HIV/AIDS; the majority of these individuals are in eastern and southern Africa.[50]

🌎 Cultural Considerations

Incidence of Human Immunodeficiency Virus and Acquired Immunodeficiency Syndrome in American Populations

More than 1.1 million people in the United States are currently living with HIV, and an estimated 14% of them are unaware of their infection.[1] The largest percentage of new HIV infections each year occurs because of male-to-male sexual contact.

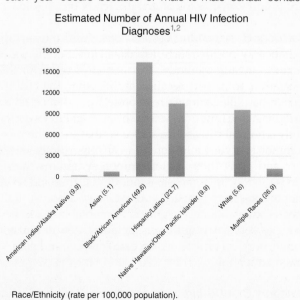

Estimated Number of Annual HIV Infection Diagnoses[1,2]

Race/Ethnicity (rate per 100,000 population).

High-risk heterosexual activity and injection drug use are the next most common causes of HIV transmission. Acquired immunodeficiency syndrome (AIDS) is the ninth leading cause of death among Americans between the ages of 25 and 44 years.[2]

The percentage of new HIV infections according to race/ethnicity is disproportionately high in some populations. For example, for every 100,000 African-American individuals, health care providers diagnose approximately 50 with HIV infection annually. Likewise, the incidence rate is high for Hispanic/Latino individuals with a rate of approximately 24 infected individuals per 100,000 people of the same race/ethnicity (compared to 5 Asian and 5.6 white individuals per 100,000, respectively).[1] Efforts to increase prevention are critically important for populations most affected.

The graph below shows the race and ethnicity of people diagnosed with HIV/AIDS in 2016.[1] Because no cures or vaccines for HIV are currently available, prevention is the only means of protection, regardless of race or sex.

REFERENCES

1. Centers for Disease Control and Prevention. (2019). Estimated HIV incidence and prevalence in the United States, 2010–2016. *HIV Surveillance Suppl Report*, 24(1).
2. National Center for Health Statistics. (2019). *Health, United States, 2018*. Hyattsville, MD: National Center for Health Statistics (U.S.).

pandemic a widespread epidemic distributed throughout a region, a continent, or the world.

parasite an organism that lives in or on an organism of another species, known as the host, from whom all nourishment is obtained.

TRANSMISSION AND STAGES OF DISEASE PROGRESSION

An infected person can transmit HIV to another person through sexual contact, through the sharing of needles or syringes, or through mother-to-child transmission. Most countries now closely screen all blood, tissue, and organ donations for HIV antibodies, thereby reducing this form of transmission. The primary mode of HIV transmission is sexual contact, which accounts for the vast majority of new cases (Figure 23.4).

The individual clinical course of HIV infection varies substantially, but the following three distinct stages mark the progression of the disease:

- Acute HIV infection
- Clinical latency (HIV inactivity or dormancy)
- AIDS

There are two classification systems for staging HIV: the CDC Classification System and the World Health Organization Clinical Staging and Disease Classification System. The CDC Classification System assesses HIV stages based on the lowest documented helper T white blood cell count (i.e., CD4 cell count stages 0, 1, 2, 3, and unknown) and the presence of specific HIV-related opportunistic illnesses.[51] Clinicians generally use the World

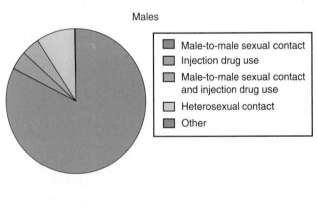

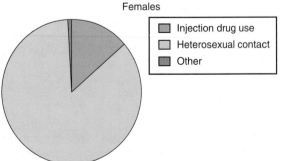

Figure 23.4 Mode of HIV transmission for males and females. (From Centers for Disease Control and Prevention. [2018]. *HIV surveillance report* [2017, vol. 29]. Retrieved August 18, 2019, from www.cdc.gov/hiv/library/reports/hiv-surveillance.html.)

Health Organization Staging System in areas where laboratory values of CD4 cell counts are unavailable. This system relies on clinical manifestations to stage the severity of HIV. The United States uses the CDC Classification System, which we will refer to in this text.

CDC Classification System for HIV

Table 23.2 provides the CDC Classification System for HIV-infected adults and adolescents 6 years of age and older. In addition to stages 1, 2, and 3, there are also *stages 0* and *unknown* as follows:

- *Stage 0:* Early HIV infection, inferred from a negative or indeterminate HIV test result within 6 months of a confirmed positive test
- *Stage unknown:* HIV test positive but no CD4+ T-lymphocyte count available

After the physician has determined the patient's stage (relative to the CD4+ T-lymphocyte count), the health care team will assess the patient's clinical category relative to his or her symptomatic conditions.

Category A: asymptomatic or acute HIV. Approximately 2 to 4 weeks after initial exposure and infection, a mild flu-like episode may occur. This brief (i.e., days to weeks) and mild response reflects the initial development of antibodies to the viral infection. Any subsequent HIV testing is positive. For a number of years, the person typically feels well. This long well period is deceptive, however, because it is a critical stage of viral incubation. The virus is hiding in lymphoid tissues (e.g., lymph nodes, spleen, adenoid glands, tonsils), where it rapidly multiplies as part of its parasite life cycle within the host, taking over more and more of the host's CD4 cells and gaining power. Researchers emphasize the crucial nature of this incubation period and the importance of early medical treatment intervention after a positive HIV test. Early treatment may slow the viral strengthening time, while scientists develop drugs and vaccines to combat its steady progression.

Category B: symptomatic conditions. After the asymptomatic HIV-positive stage, associated infectious illnesses begin to invade the body. This period of opportunistic illnesses is so named because, at this point, the HIV infection has killed enough host-protective T lymphocytes to damage the immune system severely and to lower the body's normal disease resistance so that even the most common everyday infections have an opportunity to take root and grow (Box 23.1). Common symptoms during this period include persistent fatigue, diarrhea and fever, mouth sores from thrush (i.e., oral *Candida albicans*), night sweats, unintentional weight loss, remarkable headaches, shingles, cervical dysplasia or carcinoma, new or unusual cough, unusual bruises or skin discoloration, and peripheral neuropathy.

Category C: AIDS-indicator conditions. Rapidly declining T-lymphocyte counts and the presence of opportunistic illnesses (Box 23.1) mark the terminal stage of

| Table 23.2 | CDC Classification System for HIV |

CD4+ T-LYMPHOCYTE COUNT	CLINICAL CATEGORIES		
	A ASYMPTOMATIC, ACUTE HIV, OR PGL	**B** SYMPTOMATIC CONDITIONS	**C**[a] AIDS-INDICATOR CONDITIONS
Stage 1: ≥500 cells/mcL	A1	B1	C1
Stage 2: 200-499 cells/mcL	A2	B2	C2
Stage 3: <200 cells/mcL[a]	A3	B3	C3

PGL, Persistent generalized lymphadenopathy.
[a]Clients in any stage 3 CD4+ lymphocyte count or clinical category C are considered to have AIDS (shaded in gray in the table).

| Box 23.1 | Common Types of Opportunistic Infections in Clients Infected With Human Immunodeficiency Virus |

- Candidiasis of bronchi, trachea, esophagus, or lungs[a]
- Cervical dysplasia (invasive)
- Coccidioidomycosis
- Cryptococcosis
- Cryptosporidiosis, chronic intestinal (>1 month in duration)
- Cytomegalovirus diseases (specifically retinitis)
- Encephalopathy (HIV-related)
- Herpes simplex (chronic); or bronchitis, pneumonitis, or esophagitis[a]
- Histoplasmosis
- Isoporiasis (>1 month in duration)
- Kaposi's sarcoma
- Lymphoma
- Tuberculosis
- *Mycobacterium avium* complex or *Mycobacterium kansasii*
- *Pneumocystis carinii* pneumonia
- Pneumonia, recurrent
- Progressive multifocal leukoencephalopathy
- *Salmonella* septicemia, recurrent[a]
- Toxoplasmosis of the brain[a]
- Wasting syndrome (HIV-related)

[a]Most common opportunistic infections in people with HIV in the United States.
From Centers for Disease Control and Prevention. (2019). *AIDS and opportunistic infections*. Retrieved August 18, 2019, from www.cdc.gov/hiv/basics/livingwithhiv/opportunisticinfections.html.

HIV infection, known as *AIDS*. Kaposi's sarcoma is the most common AIDS-associated cancer. Malignant and rapidly growing tumors of the skin and mucous linings of the GI and respiratory tracts characterize Kaposi's sarcoma. The health care team may use low-dose radiation therapy or anticancer drugs to slow the spread of tumors.

During severe immunodeficiency, protozoan parasites (i.e., primitive single-celled organisms) appear and infect a number of body organs. At lymphocyte counts of less than $50/mm^3$, cytomegalovirus (i.e., a herpes virus that causes lesions on the mucous linings of body organs) and lymphoma (i.e., any cancer of the lymphoid tissue) can flourish. This series of HIV effects on the body brings marked changes in body weight in both men and women (i.e., wasting syndrome), with women losing disproportionately more body fat.

If the virus kills enough white cells to overwhelm the immune system's weakened resistance to the disease complications, death follows.

MEDICAL MANAGEMENT OF THE PATIENTS WITH HIV/AIDS

The medical management of HIV infection is constantly evolving because of intensive medical research. Basic goals are to achieve the following:
- Early diagnosis and treatment initiation
- Delay the progression of the infection and support the immune system
- Prevent opportunistic illnesses

INITIAL EVALUATION AND GOALS

The initial medical evaluation of a newly diagnosed person with HIV is critical to provide guidelines for ongoing comprehensive care by the HIV/AIDS health care management team. This professional team includes medical, nutrition, nursing, psychosocial health care specialists, and others as needed on an individual basis. The current HIV screening guidelines recommend HIV testing for all individuals age 15 to 65 years, all pregnant women, and others deemed at high risk or who request testing.[52] Early detection and treatment initiation are critical to reduce the risk of transmission, HIV-related complications, and AIDS-related death.

DRUG THERAPY

Developing effective drugs is difficult because of the highly evolved nature of the virus. One of the earliest findings in the drug research for HIV has been a group of compounds called nucleoside/nucleotide reverse transcriptase inhibitors (NRTIs) that inhibit the virus's necessary enzyme for copying itself, thereby effectively preventing viral increase. Multiple toxic side effects have been reported, but some of these (e.g., nausea, diarrhea, altered taste, hyperglycemia, GI intolerance) may be helped by dietary modifications or antinausea/antidiarrheal medications. Other types of antiretroviral drugs approved by the FDA and currently in use in the United States are non-NRTIs (NNRTIs), protease inhibitors, fusion inhibitors, entry inhibitors, latency-reversing agents, attachment and post-attachment inhibitors, and HIV integrase inhibitors.[53] NNRTIs prevent the reproduction of the viral cells by inhibiting reverse transcriptase. Protease inhibitors help to stop HIV by inhibiting the basic enzyme protease, which is essential to HIV's development. Unfortunately, the virus is capable of mutation in response to some drugs (specifically protease inhibitors) and thus becomes resistant to treatment. Fusion inhibitors prevent the infection of healthy cells by binding to HIV. *Antiretroviral therapy* (ART), which is a combination of these medications, is the primary drug treatment regimen that physicians prescribe to slow the progression of HIV.

In addition to these antiretroviral drugs, the FDA has approved many other drugs to prevent or treat AIDS-related illnesses. The FDA website (www.fda.gov) and the AIDSinfo website (aidsinfo.nih.gov) provide full descriptions and current approved therapies and medications under investigation for the treatment of HIV/AIDS complications.

VACCINE DEVELOPMENT

The CDC and the National Institutes of Health are involved in coordinating vaccine research in the United States, and they are working in conjunction with other agencies worldwide to expedite the development of a more effective vaccine. A successful HIV vaccine would train the body's immune system to identify and destroy the virus. The development and testing of vaccines takes several years. After identifying a potential vaccine, it must go through the following three phases of testing and be deemed safe and effective before the FDA will approve it for public use[54]:

- *Phase I:* The vaccine is tested in small groups of healthy, low-risk participants
- *Phase II:* The vaccine is tested in hundreds of high-risk and low-risk participants
- *Phase III:* The vaccine is tested in thousands of high-risk participants for safety, efficacy, and side effects of the vaccine

A combination medication consisting of tenofovir disoproxil fumarate and emtricitabine is an effective preexposure prophylaxis that the FDA has approved for use in the United States. High-risk individuals who maintain good adherence (i.e., >70%) to the medication protocol can reduce their risk for acquiring HIV by 75%.[55] Therefore, the current U.S. Preventive Services Task Force recommends using the medication as a means of preventing HIV acquisition, specifically in high-risk populations.[56] You can find more information about preventive and therapeutic vaccines at aidsinfo.nih.gov.

MEDICAL NUTRITION THERAPY IN THE PATIENT WITH HIV

NUTRITION-RELATED COMPLICATIONS OF HIV

As they do with cancer, individual nutrition problems throughout the continuum of care for HIV patients vary greatly. HIV- and medication-induced metabolic disturbances can considerably alter the individual's nutrient requirements. In addition, co-morbidities, opportunistic illnesses, and treatment regimen further influence the degree of nutrition-related complications a person may experience. Common co-morbidities include cardiovascular disease, obesity, osteoporosis, diabetes, cancer, liver disease, and malnutrition.

Wasting Effects

Clients with advanced stages of HIV regularly have a decreased appetite and an insufficient energy intake coupled with metabolic dysregulation. Some of the energy imbalance is due to the nature of the disease, while the rest is likely attributable to medication side effects. Significant weight loss follows and eventually leads to cachexia that is similar to cancer cachexia. Malnutrition suppresses cellular immune function, thereby perpetuating the onset of opportunistic infections, which is the ultimate cause of death in persons with AIDS. This wasting process plays a major role in the individual's debilitating weakness and fatigue, decreased quality of life, and the progression of the disease.

The characteristic body wasting of HIV infection may result from any of the following processes, either alone or in combination:

- *Inadequate food intake:* An important factor in the profound weight loss seen in HIV/AIDS patients is anorexia. The patient's life-changing situation as well as the body's physiologic response to the disease and to drug-nutrient interactions may precipitate the condition. In addition to anorexia, food insecurity complicates the lives of many individuals who are living with HIV, especially in developing countries. Clinicians and researchers have recognized the importance of incorporating nutrition support and food assistance programs within the treatment regimen for individuals with HIV worldwide.[57-59]
- *Malabsorption of nutrients:* Drug-diet interactions and the progressive effects of HIV infection commonly manifest as diarrhea and malabsorption. In addition, both the virus and the ART treatments alter the gut microbiota, which further compromises gut and immune function.[60,61] During the later stages of AIDS, the damaged intestinal tissues are open to opportunistic organisms, which results in debilitating diarrhea and malabsorption. Probiotics and prebiotics may be beneficial for preserving gut function and reducing inflammation in some clients, but evidence-based recommendations require more investigation.[62,63]
- *Disordered metabolism:* Some patients with HIV experience elevated resting energy expenditure and abnormal macronutrient metabolism.[64] Despite an increase in resting energy expenditure, if the patient is no longer participating in physical activity, the total energy needs may not change as the two offset one another.
- *Lean tissue wasting:* Terminally ill patients who are undergoing extensive medical therapy with a multitude

of negative side effects are not likely to participate in regular physical activity or exercise. Disuse coupled with systemic inflammation exacerbates muscle wasting and increases mortality. Resistance training, increased protein intake, and hormone therapy may be effective for preventing lean tissue losses in some conditions of muscle wasting.[63]

Lipodystrophy

Lipodystrophy is a disproportionate gaining of fat mass in the neck and abdomen with a concurrent loss of body fat in the face, buttocks, arms, and legs. Individuals with lipodystrophy continue to lose lean tissue while unbalanced changes in fat mass are taking place. The combined effects add to the abnormal body composition seen in patients with AIDS and contribute to the development of chronic kidney disease and cardiometabolic co-morbidities (e.g., hypertension, dyslipidemia, and insulin resistance).[65-68]

The most well-understood causative factor for lipodystrophy is treatment with antiretroviral therapy (see the For Further Focus box, "Highly Active Antiretroviral Therapy and Lipodystrophy"). Other possible risk factors include age, sex, body mass index, ethnicity, genetic factors, CD4 count, viral load, ART regimen, and duration of HIV infection.[69] Scientists continue to explore effective interventions to mitigate the burden of lipodystrophy in ART-treated individuals. The dietary recommendations are to follow a well-balanced diet that is particularly heart-healthy,[63] such as those discussed in Chapter 19 (e.g., DASH diet, Mediterranean diet).

🔍 For Further Focus

Highly Active Antiretroviral Therapy and Lipodystrophy

Lipodystrophy in clients with HIV involves lipoatrophy (i.e., body fat reduction) in the limbs and face and lipohypertrophy (i.e., increased fat mass) around the abdomen and the back of the neck. This redistribution of fat is associated with metabolic abnormalities and an increased risk for chronic conditions such as dyslipidemia, cardiovascular disease, and insulin resistance.

The introduction of antiretroviral drugs was an important step in the treatment of HIV. Since that time, mortality and morbidity from HIV have significantly declined. Although the natural process of aging over time and the HIV infection can lead to lipodystrophy, antiretroviral drugs are responsible for other body fat changes. Nucleoside reverse transcriptase inhibitors and protease inhibitors are associated with lipoatrophy, and protease inhibitors may be associated with lipohypertrophy.

There is no cure for lipodystrophy; however, diet and exercise are key interventions to manage hyperlipidemia, insulin resistance, and central adiposity related to HIV-associated lipodystrophy. The dietary management is similar to that of individuals without HIV who have cardiovascular risk factors. A diet that is low in saturated and trans fats; rich in fruits, vegetables, and whole grains; and adequate in protein, in combination with daily exercise, can reduce cardiovascular risk.

NUTRITION CARE PLAN

The role of the RDN is to help maintain the health of HIV patients as it relates to nutrition through education and nutrition support, as their condition requires.

Assessment

There are specific nutrition status screening tools available for use in individuals with HIV, such as the Subjective Global Assessment-HIV.[63] Such a screening tool will identify patients at risk for malnutrition quickly and efficiently to expedite their referral to a nutrition professional. The dietitian on the multidisciplinary team will then conduct a comprehensive nutrition assessment to obtain baseline information that is necessary for starting and continuing nutrition care. The assessment should include the typical ABCD nutrition evaluations: *a*nthropometric, *b*iochemical, *c*linical, and *d*ietary parameters (see Chapter 17). HIV-infected patients may require further person-centered nutrition care, as discussed in the Clinical Applications box, "The ABCDEFs of Nutrition Assessment for Individuals with HIV/AIDS."

🏥 Clinical Applications

The ABCDEFs of Nutrition Assessment for Individuals With HIV/AIDS

The initial nutrition assessment visit with a client infected with HIV is a vital encounter serving informational and relational functions. It provides the necessary baseline information for planning practical, individual nutrition support. More importantly, however, the initial visit establishes the essential provider/patient relationship, which is the human context in which the dietitian provides nutrition care and support. The basic ABCDs of nutrition assessment (*a*nthropometry, *b*iochemical tests, *c*linical observations, and *d*ietary evaluations) provide a practical guide, with two more points added for HIV-infected individuals.

*E*nvironmental, behavioral, and psychologic assessment:
- Living situation, personal support
- Food security, access to nutritionally balanced food
- Food environment, types of meals, eating assistance needed

*F*inancial assessment:
- Medical insurance
- Income, financial support through caregivers
- Ability to afford food, enteral supplements, additional vitamins or minerals

Intervention

This portion of the nutrition care process includes planning, implementing, and documenting appropriate patient-specific interventions. The key MNT objective is to reduce or eliminate malnutrition and to correct nutrition problems that the dietitian identified in the nutrition assessment. The dietitian must address altered energy needs and micronutrient deficiencies with appropriate dietary modifications or nutrient supplementation. Additionally, the nutrition care plan must address issues related to drug-nutrient interactions, co-morbidities, food security, and strategies to support the immune system.[63] Table 23.1 provides suggestions for nutrition-related symptom management.

Dietitians can help to plan an individualized eating plan so that the patient meets his or her nutrient needs while not interfering with medication schedules. Food and water safety are important for all clients with compromised immunity, especially those with HIV. Thus, the dietitian should address the prevention of food-borne illness through appropriate cooking and storing food methods during nutrition counseling. The health care team should also discuss complications from medications, use of complementary and alternative medicine, and co-morbidities with the patient.

Nutrition Counseling, Education, and Supportive Care

Education and counseling are important factors of MNT and should focus on the following[63]:

- Adequate food intake to maintain appropriate body composition and nutrition status
- A review of nutrition strategies and additional therapies for symptom management to reduce the effects of disease progression, co-morbidities, and medication intolerance
- Food safety and food security
- Potential drug-nutrient interactions (with prescribed medications, supplements, alcohol, and other drugs)

The basic goal of nutrition counseling is to make the least amount of changes necessary in a person's lifestyle and food patterns to promote optimal nutrition status while providing maximal comfort and quality of life. In this person-centered care process, the following counseling principles are particularly important:

- *Motivation:* Changes in behavior in any area require the motivation, desire, and ability to achieve one's goals. HIV/AIDS is no exception. Until a patient is capable of prioritizing food patterns and behaviors as appropriate goals, wait for a better time, and start with establishing a general supportive climate in which to continue working together. The patient may raise specific obstacles (e.g., time, physical limitations, money, anxiety, access) that the dietitian can meet with related suggestions to consider, while also respecting the individual's apprehensions.
- *Rationale:* The dietitian must clearly explain any possible benefits or risks associated with food behavior suggestions. Those with HIV/AIDS may be particularly vulnerable to the lure of unproven therapies.
- *Manageable steps:* All information and actions should proceed in manageable steps that are as small as necessary and in order of complexity and difficulty. Tackle the simple and easy things first. Information overload can discourage anyone. Keep in mind any cognitive or central nervous system decline in the individual. Such decline may contribute to memory loss and the inability to follow nutrition advice. Include individuals from the patient's support group in consultations and provide them with written instructions.

Personal food management skills. The dietitian must consider the client's living situation and general practical skills with regard to planning, purchasing, and preparing food. It is also important to discuss the patient's need for training or guidance when developing these skills and locating educational resources. The dietitian is also responsible for establishing patient-specific dietary plans that support their medication regimens; this may include individualized plans for meal timing, macronutrient and micronutrient modulations, and symptom management.

Community programs. The patient may need information about available community food programs (e.g., Meals on Wheels for the delivery of prepared meals when the person is too ill to shop for food or prepare it). Information about food-assistance programs (e.g., the Supplemental Nutrition Assistance Program [SNAP] or food commodities [see Chapter 13]), for which lower-income clients may qualify, may be warranted. As mentioned earlier, nutrition support is a recognized important aspect of the care plan. Health care providers should ensure that patients are economically, physically, and mentally capable of meeting their daily food needs or refer them to a social worker to assist in finding available programs within their community to help secure access to food.

Psychosocial support. The health care team should provide every aspect of health care in a form and manner that provides genuine psychosocial support. All health care providers who work with HIV/AIDS populations must be particularly sensitive to the psychologic and social issues that confront their patients. Major stress areas include issues related to autonomy and dependency, a sense of uncertainty and fear of the unknown, grief, change and loss, fear of symptoms and abandonment, spirituality, and quality of life. Health care providers must always be aware of how the patient and his or her caregivers relate to the disease and use the assistance of social workers and clinical psychologists as needed. Stress-reduction groups and activities—including exercise training—are helpful, as they are for other chronic conditions.

Health care workers must also examine their own stresses, values, and fears about sexual orientation, lifestyle behaviors, intravenous drug use, and fear of HIV transmission. Clients easily sense preconceived judgments, and this can threaten the provider-patient relationship. Before they can be effective with patients, all health care workers must first deal with their own fears and prejudices and learn to let go of judgmental behavior and support the needs of the individual.

Putting It All Together

Summary

- Cancer cells are normal cells that have lost control over their own growth and reproduction. Cancer cell development occurs because of the mutation of regulatory genes. Other lifestyle factors associated with an increased risk for cancer include poor diet, excessive alcohol use, and smoking.

- The body's immune system mediates cell integrity, primarily through its two types of white blood cells: T cells that kill invading agents that cause disease and B cells that make specific antibodies to attack these agents.

- Cancer treatment primarily consists of surgery, radiation, and chemotherapy. Supportive nutrition care must be highly individualized in accordance with the client's responses to the disease and its treatment.

- The overall disease progression of HIV follows the three distinct stages: (1) HIV infection; (2) symptomatic disease with opportunistic infection and illnesses; and (3) symptomatic AIDS with complicating diseases that lead to death.

- The medical management of HIV infection involves the supportive treatment of associated illnesses and diseases. During the terminal AIDS stage, the virus eventually gains enough strength to destroy the host's immune system.

- Nutrition management centers on providing individual nutrition support to counteract the body wasting and malnutrition that are characteristic of HIV. The process of nutrition care involves a comprehensive nutrition assessment, the evaluation of personal needs, the planning of care with client and caregivers, and the meeting of food needs.

Chapter Review Questions

See answers in Appendix A.

1. Cells that activate phagocytes are called _____.

   a. antigens
   b. antibodies
   c. B cells
   d. T cells

2. Appropriately planned medical nutrition therapy is advantageous in individuals with cancer to specifically help mitigate extensive _____.

   a. anabolism
   b. catabolism
   c. depression
   d. inflammation

3. Which one of the following foods would a client who is having difficulty eating because of mucositis most likely tolerate?

   a. Cheese and crackers
   b. Chips and salsa
   c. Flavored yogurt
   d. Hot chili with beans

4. A disproportionate gaining of fat mass common to ART treatment is known as _____.

   a. cellulite
   b. cellulitis
   c. hyperlipidemia
   d. lipodystrophy

5. Which of the following evidence-based strategies help prevent cancer development?

   a. Avoiding consumption of any alcoholic beverages
   b. Maintaining energy balance with a plant-based diet
   c. Focusing on energy-dense meals and snacks
   d. Using vitamin and mineral supplements to ensure adequate intake

Next-Generation NCLEX® Examination-style Case Study

See answers in Appendix A.

A 65-year-old male (Ht.: 6'0" Wt.: 130 lbs.) was diagnosed with tongue cancer 1 month ago. Weight history shows that his usual body weight is 117 lbs. He mentions that he has had a cold for 6 weeks and has not been able to eat much due to lack of appetite. Swallowing has become more difficult for him because his mouth feels dry. He complains that food sticks in his throat, and it is hard to swallow. Since starting chemotherapy, he has felt nauseated at mealtimes. He passes bowel movements about once per week. When asked about his usual diet, he says that the eats ¼ cup of oatmeal in the morning, 5 crackers with 1 oz. of lunch meat at lunch, and ¼ cup of soup with ½ of a piece of bread at dinner. He drinks 2 liters of water per day because his mouth feels so dry. When he has the energy, he tries to go on his normal daily walk.

1. From the list below, select all factors from the client's history that are concerning.
   a. BMI
   b. Diet history
   c. Xerostomia
   d. Dysphagia
   e. Constipation
   f. Fluid intake

2. From the list below, select the options that are *most likely* the cause of the client's recent weight change.

   a. Increased metabolism
   b. Inadequate oral intake
   c. Increased nutrient and energy needs
   d. Feeding difficulty
   e. Fluid overload
   f. Excessive physical activity

3. Match the most appropriate nursing response option (provided below) to each client question.

CLIENT QUESTIONS	APPROPRIATE NURSE'S RESPONSE FOR EACH CLIENT QUESTION
"How can I eat enough calories when I don't feel hungry?"	
"What are some things I can do to help with my dry mouth?"	
"Are there foods that I can eat that are easier to swallow?"	
"What can I do to reduce feelings of nausea at mealtime?"	
"Is there something I can do to resolve my constipation?"	

Nurse's Response Options

a. "Eating moist foods, drinking fluids, and adding seasonings can help."
b. "Consuming foods that are high in calorie but low in volume can optimize intake."
c. "Adding sauces, gravies, and eating moist, soft foods can help."
d. "Consume small, frequent meals with foods that are cold or room temperature."
e. "Increase fiber and fluid intake and try to be physically active."
f. "Consume small, frequent meals that are hot and contain spices."
g. "Increase fiber, decrease fluids, and be physically active."
h. "Consuming foods that are high in volume and low in calories can optimize intake."

4. Match each medical nutrition therapy guideline to the most appropriate recommendation option provided.

MEDICAL NUTRITION THERAPY	ANSWERS	RECOMMENDATION
Calorie needs (Sedentary)		a. Butter, cream, whole milk, peanut butter, protein drinks
Protein needs		b. Strawberries, blueberries, raspberries
Antioxidants		c. Celery, cucumbers, cauliflower
Calorie-dense foods		d. Low-fat milk, coffee, popcorn
		e. 960 to 1125 kcals/day
		f. 1125 to 1350 kcals/day
		g. 1350 to 1680 kcal/day
		h. 38 to 45 g/day
		i. 45 to 68 g/day
		j. 68 to 96 g/day

Additional Learning Resources

Please refer to this text's Evolve website for answers to the Case Study Questions:
http://evolve.elsevier.com/Williams/basic/.
References and **Further Reading and Resources** in the back of the book provide additional resources for enhancing knowledge.

References

CHAPTER 1

1. U.S. Department of Health and Human Services. *Healthy People 2030*. health.gov/healthypeople. Published 2020. [Accessed 18 February, 2021].

2. U.S. Department of Health and Human Services. *Midcourse review: Progress made toward targets for leading health indicators*. www.healthypeople.gov/2020/data-search/ midcourse-review/lhi. Published 2014. [Accessed 30 August 2018].

3. U.S. Department of Health and Human Services. *The secretary's advisory committee for 2030: Committee reports and meetings*. www.healthypeople.gov/2020/about-healthy-people/development-healthy-people-2030/committee-meetings. Published 2019. [Accessed 22 October 2019].

4. Kochanek KD, M. S., Xu, J., & Arias, E. (2019). *Deaths: Final data for 2017, National Vital Statistics Reports*. Hyattsville, MD: National Center for Health Statistics.

5. U.S. Department of Agriculture and Agricultural Research Service. (2018). *Nutrient intakes per 1000 kcal from food and beverages: Mean energy and mean nutrient amounts per 1000 kcal consumed per individual, by gender and age, What We Eat in America, NHANES 2015–2016*.

6. Shlisky, J., et al. (2017). Nutritional considerations for healthy aging and reduction in age-related chronic disease. *Advances in Nutrition, 8*(1), 17–26.

7. Sudfeld, C. R., et al. (2015). Malnutrition and its determinants are associated with suboptimal cognitive, communication, and motor development in Tanzanian children. *Journal of Nutrition, 145*(12), 2705–2714.

8. Allard, J. P., et al. (2016). Decline in nutritional status is associated with prolonged length of stay in hospitalized patients admitted for 7 days or more: A prospective cohort study. *Clinical Nutrition, 35*(1), 144–152.

9. Kang, M. C., et al. (2018). Prevalence of malnutrition in hospitalized patients: A multicenter cross-sectional study. *Journal of Korean Medical Science, 33*(2), e10.

10. Allard, J. P., et al. (2016). Malnutrition at hospital admission-contributors and effect on length of stay: A prospective cohort study from the Canadian malnutrition task force. *JPEN Journal of Parenteral and Enteral Nutrition, 40*(4), 487–497.

11. Food and Nutrition Board and Institute of Medicine. (1997). *Dietary reference intakes for calcium, phosphorus, magnesium, vitamin D, and fluoride*. Washington, DC: National Academies Press.

12. Food and Nutrition Board and Institute of Medicine. (1998). *Dietary reference intakes for thiamin, riboflavin, niacin, vitamin B6, folate, vitamin B12, pantothenic acid, biotin, and choline*. Washington, DC: National Academies Press.

13. Food and Nutrition Board and Institute of Medicine. (2000). *Dietary reference intakes for vitamin C, vitamin E, selenium, and carotenoids*. Washington, DC: National Academies Press.

14. Food and Nutrition Board and Institute of Medicine. (2001). *Dietary reference intakes for vitamin A, vitamin K, arsenic, boron, chromium, copper, iodine, iron, manganese, molybdenum, nickel, silicon, vanadium, and zinc*. Washington, DC: National Academies Press.

15. Food and Nutrition Board and Institute of Medicine. (2002). *Dietary reference intakes for energy, carbohydrate, fiber, fat, fatty acids, cholesterol, protein, and amino acids*. Washington, DC: National Academies Press.

16. Food and Nutrition Board and Institute of Medicine. (2005). *Dietary reference intakes for water, potassium, sodium, chloride, and sulfate*. Washington, DC: National Academies Press.

17. Stallings, V. A., et al. (2019). The National Academies collection: Reports funded by National Institutes of Health. In *Dietary reference intakes for sodium and potassium*. Washington, DC: National Academies Press (U.S.), National Academy of Sciences.

18. U.S. Department of Agriculture. *USDA's MyPlate*. www.choosemyplate.gov. [Accessed 10 October 2018].

19. U.S. Department of Agriculture and U.S. Department of Health and Human Services. (December 2020). *Dietary Guidelines for Americans, 2020-2025* (9th ed.). Available at. www.dietaryguidelines.gov.

CHAPTER 2

1. Papanikolaou, Y., & Fulgoni, V. L. (2017). Certain grain foods can be meaningful contributors to nutrient density in the diets of U.S. children and adolescents: Data from the National Health and Nutrition Examination Survey, 2009–2012. *Nutrients, 9*(2).

2. Papanikolaou, Y., & Fulgoni, V. L. (2017). Grain foods are contributors of nutrient density for American adults and help close nutrient recommendation gaps: Data from the National Health and Nutrition Examination Survey, 2009–2012. *Nutrients, 9*(8).

3. Zong, G., et al. (2016). Whole grain intake and mortality from all causes, cardiovascular disease, and cancer: A meta-analysis of prospective cohort studies. *Circulation, 133*(24), 2370–2380.

4. U.S. Department of Health and Human Services. *Healthy People 2030*. health.gov/healthypeople. Published 2020. [Accessed 5 September, 2020].

5. U.S. Department of Agriculture and U.S. Department of Health and Human Services. (December 2020). *Dietary Guidelines for Americans, 2020-2025* (9th ed.). Available at: www.dietaryguidelines.gov.

6. U.S. Department of Agriculture and Agricultural Research Service. (2018). *Nutrient intakes from food and beverages: Mean amounts consumed per individual, by gender and age, What We Eat in America, NHANES 2015–2016*.

7. U.S. Department of Agriculture and Economic Research Service. *Caloric sweeteners: Per capita availability adjusted for loss*. www.ers.usda.gov/data-products/food-availability-per-capita-data-system/. Published 2017.

8. Food and Nutrition Board and Institute of Medicine. (2002). *Dietary reference intakes for energy, carbohydrate, fiber, fat, fatty acids, cholesterol, protein, and amino acids*. Washington, DC: National Academies Press.

9. Dahl, W. J., & Stewart, M. L. (2015). Position of the Academy of Nutrition and Dietetics: Health implications of dietary fiber. *Journal of the Academy of Nutrition and Dietetics, 115*(11), 1861–1870.

10. Ye, E. Q., et al. (2012). Greater whole-grain intake is associated with lower risk of type 2 diabetes, cardiovascular disease, and weight gain. *Journal of Nutrition, 142*(7), 1304–1313.

11. Veronese, N., et al. (2018). Dietary fiber and health outcomes: An umbrella review of systematic reviews and meta-analyses. *American Journal of Clinical Nutrition, 107*(3), 436–444.

12. Hollaender, P. L., Ross, A. B., & Kristensen, M. (2015). Whole-grain and blood lipid changes in apparently healthy adults: A systematic review and meta-analysis of randomized controlled studies. *Journal of Nutrition, 102*(3), 556–572.

13. Ho, H. V., et al. (2016). The effect of oat beta-glucan on LDL-cholesterol, non-HDL-cholesterol and apob for CVD risk reduction: A systematic review and meta-analysis of randomised-controlled trials. *British Journal of Nutrition, 116*(8), 1369–1382.

14. McRorie, J. W., Jr., & McKeown, N. M. (2017). Understanding the physics of functional fibers in the gastrointestinal tract: An evidence-based approach to resolving enduring misconceptions about insoluble and soluble fiber. *Journal of the Academy of Nutrition and Dietetics, 117*(2), 251–264.

15. Pilar, B., et al. (2017). Protective role of flaxseed oil and flaxseed lignan secoisolariciresinol diglucoside against oxidative stress in rats with metabolic syndrome. *Journal of Food Science, 82*(12), 3029–3036.

16. Damsgaard, C. T., et al. (2017). Whole-grain intake, reflected by dietary records and biomarkers, is inversely associated with circulating insulin and other cardiometabolic markers in 8- to 11-year-old children. *Journal of Nutrition, 147*(5), 816–824.

17. Li, X., et al. (2016). Short- and long-term effects of wholegrain oat intake on weight management and glucolipid metabolism in overweight type-2 diabetics: A randomized control led trial. *Nutrients, 8*(9).

18. Kirwan, J. P., et al. (2016). A whole-grain diet reduces cardiovascular risk factors in overweight and obese adults: A randomized controlled trial. *Journal of Nutrition, 146*(11), 2244–2251.

19. Moore, L. V., & Thompson, F. E. (2015). Adults meeting fruit and vegetable intake recommendations—United States, 2013. *MMWR Morbidity and Mortality Weekly Report, 64*(26), 709–713.

20. Albertson, A. M., et al. (2016). Whole grain consumption trends and associations with body weight measures in the United States: Results from the cross sectional National Health and Nutrition Examination Survey 2001–2012. *Nutrition Journal, 15*, 8.

21. U.S. Food and Drug Administration. *Additional information about high-intensity sweeteners permitted for use in food in the United States.* www.fda.gov/Food/IngredientsPackagingLabeling/FoodAdditivesIngredients/ucm397725.htm. Published 2018. [Accessed 30 September 2018].

22. National Institutes of Health and U.S. *Department of health and human services. Lactose intolerance.* ghr.nlm.nih.gov/condition/lactose-intolerance#statistics. Published 2018. [Accessed 22 September 2018].

23. U.S. Department of Agriculture. *USDA's MyPlate.* www.choosemyplate.gov.

CHAPTER 3

1. Food and Nutrition Board and Institute of Medicine. (2002). *Dietary reference intakes for energy, carbohydrate, fiber, fat, fatty acids, cholesterol, protein, and amino acids.* Washington, DC: National Academies Press.

2. de Souza, R. J., et al. (2015). Intake of saturated and trans unsaturated fatty acids and risk of all cause mortality, cardiovascular disease, and type 2 diabetes: Systematic review and meta-analysis of observational studies. *British Medical Journal, 351*, h3978.

3. Guasch-Ferre, M., et al. (2015). Dietary fat intake and risk of cardiovascular disease and all-cause mortality in a population at high risk of cardiovascular disease. *American Journal of Clinical Nutrition, 102*(6), 1563–1573.

4. Hooper, L., & Mann, J. (2016). Observational studies are compatible with an association between saturated and trans fats and cardiovascular disease. *Evidence Based Medicine, 21*(1), 37.

5. Food and Drug Administration. (2018). Final determination regarding partially hydrogenated oils. notification; declaratory order; extension of compliance date. *Federal Register, 83*(98), 23358–23359.

6. U.S. Department of Agriculture. *USDA's MyPlate.* www.choosemyplate.gov.

7. U.S. Department of Health and Human Services. *Healthy People 2020.* Published 2010. Updated 2019.

8. U.S. Department of Agriculture and U.S. Department of Health and Human Services. (December 2020). *Dietary Guidelines for Americans, 2020-2025* (9th ed.). Available at: www.dietaryguidelines.gov.

9. Xu, Z., McClure, S. T., & Appel, L. J. (2018). Dietary cholesterol intake and sources among U.S adults: Results from National Health and Nutrition Examination Surveys (NHANES), 2001–2014. *Nutrients, 10*(6).

10. Grundy, S. M. (2016). Does dietary cholesterol matter? *Current Atherosclerosis Reports, 18*(11), 68.

11. Baigent, C., et al. (2010). Efficacy and safety of more intensive lowering of ldl cholesterol: A meta-analysis of data from 170,000 participants in 26 randomised trials. *Lancet, 376*(9753), 1670–1681.

12. Ference, B. A., et al. (2012). Effect of long-term exposure to lower low-density lipoprotein cholesterol beginning early in life on the risk of coronary heart disease: A Mendelian randomization analysis. *Journal of the American College of Cardiology, 60*(25), 2631–2639.

13. United States Department of Agriculture and Agricultural Research Service. *USDA Food Composition Databases.* ndb.nal.usda.gov. Published 2018. [Accessed 15 May 2019].

14. U.S. Department of Agriculture and Center for Nutrition Policy and Promotion. Nutrient Content of the U.S. Food Supply. www.fns.usda.gov/resource/nutrient-content-us-food-supply-reports. Published 2014. [Accessed 15 May 2019].

15. Micha, R., et al. (2017). Association between dietary factors and mortality from heart disease, stroke, and type 2 diabetes in the United States. *Journal of the American Medical Association, 317*(9), 912–924.

16. Schwingshackl, L., et al. (2017). Food groups and risk of all-cause mortality: A systematic review and meta-analysis of prospective studies. *American Journal of Clinical Nutrition, 105*(6), 1462–1473.

17. Schwingshackl, L., et al. (2017). Food groups and risk of type 2 diabetes mellitus: A systematic review and meta-analysis of prospective studies. *European Journal of Epidemiology, 32*(5), 363–375.

18. Bernstein, A. M., et al. (2010). Major dietary protein sources and risk of coronary heart disease in women. *Circulation, 122*(9), 876–883.

19. Yu, E., Malik, V. S., & Hu, F. B. (2018). Cardiovascular disease prevention by diet modification: JACC health promotion series. *Journal of the American College of Cardiology, 72*(8), 914–926.

20. Petersen, K. S., et al. (2017). Healthy dietary patterns for preventing cardiometabolic disease: The role of plant-based foods and animal products. *Current Developments in Nutrition, 1*(12).

21. U.S. Food and Drug Administration. (2018). *Authorized health claims that meet the Significant Scientific Agreement (SSA) standard.* Silver Spring, MD: U.S. Department of Health and Human Services.

22. U.S. Department of Agriculture and Agricultural Research Service. (2018). *Nutrient intakes from food and beverages: Mean amounts consumed per individual, by gender and age, What We Eat in America, NHANES 2015–2016.*

23. Piche, M. E., et al. (2018). Overview of epidemiology and contribution of obesity and body fat distribution to cardiovascular disease: An update. *Progress in Cardiovascular Diseases, 61*(2), 103–113.

24. Global BMI Mortality Collaboration, et al. (2016). Body-mass index and all-cause mortality: Individual-participant-data meta-analysis of 239 prospective studies in four continents. *Lancet, 388*(10046), 776–786.

25. Aune, D., et al. (2016). BMI and all cause mortality: Systematic review and non-linear dose-response meta-analysis of 230 cohort studies with 3.74 million deaths among 30.3 million participants. *British Medical Journal, 353*, i2156.

26. Hamley, S. (2017). The effect of replacing saturated fat with mostly n-6 polyunsaturated fat on coronary heart disease: A meta-analysis of randomised controlled trials. *Nutrition Journal, 16*(1), 30.

27. Ramsden, C. E., et al. (2010). N-6 fatty acid-specific and mixed polyunsaturate dietary interventions have different effects on CHD risk: A meta-analysis of randomised controlled trials. *British Journal of Nutrition, 104*(11), 1586–1600.

28. Hooper, L., et al. (2018). Omega-6 fats for the primary and secondary prevention of cardiovascular disease. *Cochrane Database of Systematic Reviews, 7*, Cd011094.

29. Mozaffarian, D., & Wu, J. H. (2011). Omega-3 fatty acids and cardiovascular disease: Effects on risk factors, molecular pathways, and clinical events. *Journal of the American College of Cardiology, 58*(20), 2047–2067.

30. Abdelhamid, A. S., et al. (2018). Omega-3 fatty acids for the primary and secondary prevention of cardiovascular disease. *Cochrane Database of Systematic Reviews, 7*, Cd003177.

31. Sacks, F. M., et al. (2017). Dietary fats and cardiovascular disease: A presidential advisory from the American Heart Association. *Circulation, 136*(3), e1–e23.

32. Mozaffarian, D., Aro, A., & Willett, W. C. (2009). Health effects of trans-fatty acids: Experimental and observational evidence. *European Journal of Clinical Nutrition, 63*(Suppl. 2), S5–S21.

33. Centers for Disease Control and Prevention. (2016). Quickstats: Prevalence of abnormal cholesterol levels among young persons aged 6-19 years, by sex and weight status—National Health and Nutrition Examination Survey, United States, 2011–2014. *MMWR Morbidity and Mortality Weekly Report, 65*(24), 637.

CHAPTER 4

1. Food and Nutrition Board and Institute of Medicine. (2002). *Dietary reference intakes for energy, carbohydrate, fiber, fat, fatty acids, cholesterol, protein, and amino acids*. Washington, DC: National Academies Press.

2. Melina, V., Craig, W., & Levin, S. (2016). Position of the Academy of Nutrition and Dietetics: Vegetarian diets. *Journal of the Academy of Nutrition and Dietetics, 116*(12), 1970–1980.

3. Stahler, C. *How often do Americans eat vegetarian meals? And how many adults in the U.S. are vegetarian?* www.vrg.org/nutshell/Polls/2016_adults_veg.htm. Published 2016. [Accessed 17 May 2019].

4. Dinu, M., et al. (2017). Vegetarian, vegan diets and multiple health outcomes: A systematic review with meta-analysis of observational studies. *Critical Reviews in Food Science and Nutrition, 57*(17), 3640–3649.

5. Barnard, N. D., Levin, S. M., & Yokoyama, Y. (2015). A systematic review and meta-analysis of changes in body weight in clinical trials of vegetarian diets. *Journal of the Academy of Nutrition and Dietetics, 115*(6), 954–969.

6. Kahleova, H., & Pelikanova, T. (2015). Vegetarian diets in the prevention and treatment of type 2 diabetes. *Journal of the American College of Nutrition, 34*(5), 448–458.

7. Orlich, M. J., et al. (2015). Vegetarian dietary patterns and the risk of colorectal cancers. *JAMA Internal Medicine, 175*(5), 767–776.

8. Appleby, P. N., & Key, T. J. (2016). The long-term health of vegetarians and vegans. *Proceedings of the Nutrition Society, 75*(3), 287–293.

9. Turney, B. W., et al. (2014). Diet and risk of kidney stones in the Oxford cohort of the European Prospective Investigation into Cancer and Nutrition (EPIC). *European Journal of Epidemiology, 29*(5), 363–369.

10. Sabate, J., & Wien, W. (2015). A perspective on vegetarian dietary patterns and risk of metabolic syndrome. *British Journal of Nutrition, 113*(Suppl. 2), S136–S143.

11. Wang, F., et al. (2015). Effects of vegetarian diets on blood lipids: A systematic review and meta-analysis of randomized controlled trials. *Journal of the American Heart Association, 4*(10), e002408.

12. Satija, A., & Hu, F. B. (2018). Plant-based diets and cardiovascular health. *Trends in Cardiovascular Medicine, 28*(7), 437–441.

13. Clarys, P., et al. (2014). Comparison of nutritional quality of the vegan, vegetarian, semi-vegetarian, pesco-vegetarian and omnivorous diet. *Nutrients, 6*(3), 1318–1332.

14. Yokoyama, Y., et al. (2014). Vegetarian diets and blood pressure: A meta-analysis. *JAMA Internal Medicine, 174*(4), 577–587.

15. Chiu, Y. F., et al. (2015). Cross-sectional and longitudinal comparisons of metabolic profiles between vegetarian and non-vegetarian subjects: A matched cohort study. *British Journal of Nutrition, 114*(8), 1313–1320.

16. Tonstad, S., et al. (2013). Vegetarian diets and incidence of diabetes in the Adventist Health Study-2. *Nutrition Metabolism and Cardiovascular Diseases, 23*(4), 292–299.

17. Lee, Y., & Park, K. (2017). Adherence to a vegetarian diet and diabetes risk: A systematic review and meta-analysis of observational studies. *Nutrients, 9*(6).

18. Wallace, T. C., Reider, C., & Fulgoni, 3rd V. L., (2013). Calcium and vitamin D disparities are related to gender, age, race, household income level, and weight classification but not vegetarian status in the United States: Analysis of the NHANES 2001–2008 data set. *Journal of the American College of Nutrition, 32*(5), 321–330.

19. Hoffer, L. J. (2016). Human protein and amino acid requirements. *Journal of Parenteral and Enteral Nutrition, 40*(4), 460–474.

20. Food and Agriculture Organization of the United Nations (2013). Dietary protein quality evaluation in human nutrition. Report of an FAO Expert Consultation. *FAO Food & Nutrition Paper, 92*, 1–66.

21. Mathai, J. K., Liu, Y., & Stein, H. H. (2017). Values for digestible indispensable amino acid scores (DIAAS) for some dairy and plant proteins may better describe protein quality than values calculated using the concept for protein digestibility-corrected amino acid scores (PDCAAS). *British Journal of Nutrition, 117*(4), 490–499.

22. Rafii, M., et al. (2015). Dietary protein requirement of female adults >65 years determined by the indicator amino acid oxidation technique is higher than current recommendations. *Journal of Nutrition, 145*(1), 18–24.

23. Marinangeli, C. P. F., & House, J. D. (2017). Potential impact of the digestible indispensable amino acid score as a measure of protein quality on dietary regulations and health. *Nutrition Reviews, 75*(8), 658–667.

24. Crichton, M., et al. (2019). A systematic review, meta-analysis and meta-regression of the prevalence of protein-energy malnutrition: Associations with geographical region and sex. *Age and Ageing, 48*(1), 38–48.

25. Benjamin, O., & Lappin, S. L. (2018). Kwashiorkor. In *StatPearls*. Treasure Island, FL: StatPearls Publishing.

26. Asghari, G., et al. (2018). High dietary intake of branched-chain amino acids is associated with an increased risk of insulin resistance in adults. *Journal of Diabetes, 10*(5), 357–364.

27. Nie, C., et al. (2018). Branched chain amino acids: Beyond nutrition metabolism. *International Journal of Molecular Sciences, 19*(4).

28. Yoon, M. S. (2016). The emerging role of branched-chain amino acids in insulin resistance and metabolism. *Nutrients*, *8*(7).

29. U.S. Department of Agriculture and U.S. Department of Health and Human Services. (December 2020). *Dietary Guidelines for Americans, 2020-2025* (9th ed.). Available at: www.dietaryguidelines.gov.

30. U.S. Department of Agriculture. *USDA's MyPlate*. www.choosemyplate.gov.

CHAPTER 5

1. U.S. Department of Health and Human Services. *Phenylketonuria*. ghr.nlm.nih.gov/condition/phenylketonuria. Published 2018. [Accessed 17 May 2019].

2. Jurecki, E. R., et al. (2017). Adherence to clinic recommendations among patients with phenylketonuria in the United States. *Molecular Genetics and Metabolism*, *120*(3), 190–197.

3. Camp, K. M., et al. (2014). Phenylketonuria scientific review conference: State of the science and future research needs. *Molecular Genetics and Metabolism*, *112*(2), 87–122.

4. Strisciuglio, P., & Concolino, D. (2014). New strategies for the treatment of phenylketonuria (PKU). *Metabolites*, *4*(4), 1007–1017.

5. Manta-Vogli, P. D., et al. (2018). The phenylketonuria patient: A recent dietetic therapeutic approach. *Nutritional Neuroscience*, 1–12.

6. Sumaily, K. M., & Mujamammmi, A. H. (2017). Phenylketonuria: A new look at an old topic, advances in laboratory diagnosis, and therapeutic strategies. *International Journal of Health Sciences (Qassim)*, *11*(5), 63–70.

7. Thomas, J., et al. (2018). Pegvaliase for the treatment of phenylketonuria: Results of a long-term phase 3 clinical trial program (PRISM). *Molecular Genetics and Metabolism*, *124*(1), 27–38.

8. U.S. Department of Health and Human Services. *Galactosemia*. ghr.nlm.nih.gov/condition/galactosemia. Published 2018. [Accessed 17 May 2019].

9. Yuzyuk, T., et al. (2018). Biochemical changes and clinical outcomes in 34 patients with classic galactosemia. *Journal of Inherited Metabolic Disease*, *41*(2), 197–208.

10. Welling, L., et al. (2017). International clinical guideline for the management of classical galactosemia: Diagnosis, treatment, and follow-up. *Journal of Inherited Metabolic Disease*, *40*(2), 171–176.

11. U.S. Department of Health and Human Services. *Glycogen storage disease type I*. ghr.nlm.nih.gov/condition/glycogen-storage-disease-type-i. Published 2018. [Accessed 17 May 2019].

CHAPTER 6

1. U.S. Department of Agriculture. *USDA's MyPlate*. www.choosemyplate.gov.

2. U.S. Department of Agriculture and U.S. Department of Health and Human Services. (December 2020). *Dietary Guidelines for Americans, 2020-2025* (9th ed.). Available at: www.dietaryguidelines.gov.

3. Rangan, A. M., et al. (2016). Electronic dietary intake assessment (e-DIA): Relative validity of a mobile phone application to measure intake of food groups. *British Journal of Nutrition*, *115*(12), 2219–2226.

4. Pendergast, F. J., et al. (2017). Evaluation of a smartphone food diary application using objectively measured energy expenditure. *International Journal of Behavioral Nutrition and Physical Activity*, *14*(1), 30.

5. Boushey, C. J., et al. (2017). New mobile methods for dietary assessment: Review of image-assisted and image-based dietary assessment methods. *Proceedings of the Nutrition Society*, *76*(3), 283–294.

6. Food and Nutrition Board and Institute of Medicine. (2002). *Dietary reference intakes for energy, carbohydrate, fiber, fat, fatty acids, cholesterol, protein, and amino acids*. Washington, DC: National Academies Press.

7. Fullmer, S., et al. (2015). Evidence analysis library review of best practices for performing indirect calorimetry in healthy and non-critically ill individuals. *Journal of the Academy of Nutrition and Dietetics*, *115*(9), 1417–1446.e2.

8. Academy of Nutrition and Dietetics. (2018). Why and how is resting metabolic rate measured? And determination of energy needs in hospitalized patient. In *Nutrition Care Manual*. Chicago, IL: Academy of Nutrition and Dietetics.

9. Heymsfield, S. B., et al. (2019). The anatomy of resting energy expenditure: Body composition mechanisms. *European Journal of Clinical Nutrition*, *73*(2), 166–171.

10. Heymsfield, S. B., et al. (2018). Human energy expenditure: Advances in organ-tissue prediction models. *Obesity Reviews*, *19*(9), 1177–1188.

11. Geisler, C., et al. (2016). Age-dependent changes in resting energy expenditure (REE): Insights from detailed body composition analysis in normal and overweight healthy caucasians. *Nutrients*, *8*(6).

12. Muller, M. J., et al. (2013). Advances in the understanding of specific metabolic rates of major organs and tissues in humans. *Current Opinion in Clinical Nutrition and Metabolic Care*, *16*(5), 501–508.

13. Schoffelen, P. F. M., & Plasqui, G. (2018). Classical experiments in whole-body metabolism: Open-circuit respirometry-diluted flow chamber, hood, or facemask systems. *European Journal of Applied Physiology*, *118*(1), 33–49.

14. Hipskind, P., et al. (2011). Do handheld calorimeters have a role in assessment of nutrition needs in hospitalized patients? A systematic review of literature. *Nutrition in Clinical Practice*, *26*(4), 426–433.

15. Zhao, D., et al. (2014). A pocket-sized metabolic analyzer for assessment of resting energy expenditure. *Clinical Nutrition*, *33*(2), 341–347.

16. Woo, P., et al. (2017). Assessing resting energy expenditure in overweight and obese adolescents in a clinical setting: Validity of a handheld indirect calorimeter. *Pediatric Research*, *81*(1-1), 51–56.

17. Madden, A. M., Parker, L. J., & Amirabdollahian, F. (2013). Accuracy and preference of measuring resting energy expenditure using a handheld calorimeter in healthy adults. *Journal of Human Nutrition and Dietetics*, *26*(6), 587–595.

18. Anderson, E. J., et al. (2014). Comparison of energy assessment methods in overweight individuals. *Journal of the Academy of Nutrition and Dietetics*, *114*(2), 273–278.

19. Fares, S., et al. (2008). Measuring energy expenditure in community-dwelling older adults: Are portable methods valid and acceptable? *Journal of the American Dietetic Association*, *108*(3), 544–548.

20. Ringwald-Smith, K., et al. (2018). Comparison of resting energy expenditure assessment in pediatric oncology patients. *Nutrition in Clinical Practice*, *33*(2), 224–231.

21. Academy of Nutrition and Dietetics. (2018). How is resting metabolic rate best estimated in healthy people? In *Nutrition Care Manual*. Chicago, IL: Academy of Nutrition and Dietetics.

22. Schlein, K. M., & Coulter, S. P. (2014). Best practices for determining resting energy expenditure in critically ill adults. *Nutrition in Clinical Practice*, *29*(1), 44–55.

23. Ladd, A. K., et al. (2018). Preventing underfeeding and overfeeding: A clinician's guide to the acquisition and implementation of indirect calorimetry. *Nutrition in Clinical Practice*, *33*(2), 198–205.

24. Oshima, T., et al. (2017). Indirect calorimetry in nutritional therapy. A position paper by the ICALIC Study Group. *Clinical Nutrition*, *36*(3), 651–662.

25. Jotterand Chaparro, C., et al. (2017). Performance of predictive equations specifically developed to estimate resting energy expenditure in ventilated critically ill children. *The Journal of Pediatrics*, *184*, 220–226.e5.

26. Mifflin, M. D., et al. (1990). A new predictive equation for resting energy expenditure in healthy individuals. *American Journal of Clinical Nutrition, 51*(2), 241–247.

27. Butte, N. F., & King, J. C. (2005). Energy requirements during pregnancy and lactation. *Public Health Nutrition, 8*(7a), 1010–1027.

28. Arija, V., et al. (2018). Physical activity, cardiovascular health, quality of life and blood pressure control in hypertensive subjects: Randomized clinical trial. *Health and Quality of Life Outcomes, 16*(1), 184.

29. Wu, X. Y., et al. (2017). The influence of physical activity, sedentary behavior on health-related quality of life among the general population of children and adolescents: A systematic review. *PLoS One, 12*(11), e0187668.

30. Sanchez-Aguadero, N., et al. (2016). Diet and physical activity in people with intermediate cardiovascular risk and their relationship with the health-related quality of life: Results from the MARK study. *Health and Quality of Life Outcomes, 14*(1), 169.

31. Muros, J. J., et al. (2017). The association between healthy lifestyle behaviors and health-related quality of life among adolescents. *The Journal of Pediatrics (Rio J), 93*(4), 406–412.

32. Keys, A., Taylor, H. L., & Grande, F. (1973). Basal metabolism and age of adult man. *Metabolism, 22*(4), 579–587.

33. Henry, C. J. (2000). Mechanisms of changes in basal metabolism during ageing. *European Journal of Clinical Nutrition, 54*(Suppl. 3), S77–S791.

34. Schrack, J. A., et al. (2014). "IDEAL" aging is associated with lower resting metabolic rate: The Baltimore Longitudinal Study of Aging. *Journal of the American Geriatrics Society, 62*(4), 667–672.

35. Fabbri, E., et al. (2015). Energy metabolism and the burden of multimorbidity in older adults: Results from the BaltiMore Longitudinal Study of Aging. *The Journals of Gerontology Series A Biological Sciences and Medical Sciences, 70*(11), 1297–1303.

36. Nagel, A., et al. (2017). The impact of multimorbidity on resting metabolic rate in community-dwelling women over a ten-year period: A cross-sectional and longitudinal study. *The Journal of Nutrition, Health & Aging, 21*(7), 781–786.

37. Sowers, M., et al. (2007). Changes in body composition in women over six years at midlife: Ovarian and chronological aging. *The Journal of Clinical Endocrinology and Metabolism, 92*(3), 895–901.

38. Zaidi, M., et al. (2018). FSH, bone mass, body fat, and biological aging. *Endocrinology, 159*(10), 3503–3514.

CHAPTER 7

1. Mares, J. (2016). Lutein and zeaxanthin isomers in eye health and disease. *Annual Review of Nutrition, 36*, 571–602.

2. Bernstein, P. S., et al. (2016). Lutein, zeaxanthin, and meso-zeaxanthin: The basic and clinical science underlying carotenoid-based nutritional interventions against ocular disease. *Progress in Retinal and Eye Research, 50*, 34–66.

3. Wiseman, E. M., Bar-El Dadon, S., & Reifen, R. (2017). The vicious cycle of vitamin A deficiency: A review. *Critical Reviews in Food Science and Nutrition, 57*(17), 3703–3714.

4. Stevens, G. A., et al. (2015). Trends and mortality effects of vitamin A deficiency in children in 138 low-income and middle-income countries between 1991 and 2013: A pooled analysis of population-based surveys. *The Lancet Global Health, 3*(9), e528–e536.

5. Food and Nutrition Board and Institute of Medicine. (2001). *Dietary reference intakes for vitamin A, vitamin K, arsenic, boron, chromium, copper, iodine, iron, manganese, molybdenum, nickel, silicon, vanadium, and zinc*. Washington, DC: National Academies Press.

6. Moran, N. E., et al. (2018). Intrinsic and extrinsic factors impacting absorption, metabolism, and health effects of dietary carotenoids. *Advances in Nutrition, 9*(4), 465–492.

7. McCollum, E., et al. (1922). Studies on experimental rickets. XXI. An experimental demonstration of the existence of a vitamin which promotes calcium deposition. *Journal of Biological Chemistry, 53*, 293–312.

8. Cianferotti, L., et al. (2015). The clinical use of vitamin D metabolites and their potential developments: A position statement from the European Society for Clinical and Economic Aspects of Osteoporosis and Osteoarthritis (ESCEO) and the International Osteoporosis Foundation (IOF). *Endocrine, 50*(1), 12–26.

9. U.S. Department of Agriculture and Agricultural Research Service. (2018). *Nutrient intakes from food and beverages: Mean amounts consumed per individual, by gender and age, What We Eat in America, NHANES 2015–2016.*

10. Bendik, I., et al. (2014). Vitamin D: A critical and essential micronutrient for human health. *Frontiers in Physiology, 5*, 248.

11. Pfotenhauer, K. M., & Shubrook, J. H. (2017). Vitamin D deficiency, its role in health and disease, and current supplementation recommendations. *Journal of the American Osteopathic Association, 117*(5), 301–305.

12. Munns, C. F., et al. (2016). Global consensus recommendations on prevention and management of nutritional rickets. *The Journal of Clinical Endocrinology and Metabolism, 101*(2), 394–415.

13. Cashman, K. D., et al. (2017). Improved dietary guidelines for vitamin D: Application of Individual Participant Data (IPD)-level meta-regression analyses. *Nutrients, 9*(5).

14. Food and Nutrition Board and Institute of Medicine. (2011). *Dietary reference intakes for calcium and vitamin D*. Washington, DC: National Academies Press.

15. Evans, H. M., & Bishop, K. S. (1922). On the existence of a hitherto unrecognized dietary factor essential for reproduction. *Science, 56*(1458), 650–651.

16. Food and Nutrition Board and Institute of Medicine. (2000). *Dietary reference intakes for vitamin C, vitamin E, selenium, and carotenoids*. Washington, DC: National Academies Press.

17. Galli, F., et al. (2017). Vitamin E: Emerging aspects and new directions. *Free Radical Biology and Medicine, 102*, 16–36.

18. Traber, M. G. (2008). Vitamin E and K interactions—a 50-year-old problem. *Nutrition Reviews, 66*(11), 624–629.

19. Dam, H. (1935). The antihaemorrhagic vitamin of the chick. *The Biochemical Journal, 29*(6), 1273–1285.

20. Bollet, A. J. (1992). Politics and pellagra: The epidemic of pellagra in the U.S. in the early twentieth century. *Yale Journal of Biology and Medicine, 65*(3), 211–221.

21. Food and Nutrition Board and Institute of Medicine. (1988). *Dietary reference intakes for thiamin, riboflavin, niacin, vitamin B6, folate, vitamin B12, pantothenic acid, biotin, and choline*. Washington, DC: National Academies Press.

22. Marti-Carvajal, A. J., et al. (2017). Homocysteine-lowering interventions for preventing cardiovascular events. *Cochrane Database of Systematic Reviews, 8*, Cd006612.

23. Williams, J., et al. (2015). Updated estimates of neural tube defects prevented by mandatory folic acid fortification—United States, 1995–2011. *MMWR Morbidity and Mortality Weekly Report, 64*(1), 1–5.

24. Molloy, A. M., Pangilinan, F., & Brody, L. C. (2017). Genetic risk factors for folate-responsive neural tube defects. *Annual Review of Nutrition, 37*, 269–291.

25. Gong, R., et al. (2016). Effects of folic acid supplementation during different pregnancy periods and relationship with the other primary prevention measures to neural tube defects. *J Matern Fetal Neonatal Med, 29*(23), 3894–3901.

26. Buchman, A. L., et al. (2001). Choline deficiency causes reversible hepatic abnormalities in patients receiving parenteral nutrition: Proof of a human choline requirement: A placebo-controlled trial. *Journal of Parenteral and Enteral Nutrition, 25*(5), 260–268.

27. Biswas, S., & Giri, S. (2015). Importance of choline as essential nutrient and its role in prevention of various toxicities. *Prague Medical Report, 116*(1), 5–15.

28. Alissa, E. M., & Ferns, G. A. (2017). Dietary fruits and vegetables and cardiovascular diseases risk. *Critical Reviews in Food Science and Nutrition, 57*(9), 1950–1962.

29. Patel, H., et al. (2017). Plant-based nutrition: An essential component of cardiovascular disease prevention and management. *Current Cardiology Reports, 19*(10), 104.

30. Buil-Cosiales, P., et al. (2016). Association between dietary fibre intake and fruit, vegetable or whole-grain consumption and the risk of CVD: Results from the PREvencion con DIeta MEDiterrania (PREDIMED) trial. *British Journal of Nutrition, 116*(3), 534–546.

31. Aune, D., et al. (2017). Fruit and vegetable intake and the risk of cardiovascular disease, total cancer and all-cause mortality. A systematic review and dose-response meta-analysis of prospective studies. *International Journal of Epidemiology, 46*(3), 1029–1056.

32. U.S. Department of Agriculture. *USDA's MyPlate.* www.choosemyplate.gov.

33. Lee-Kwan, S. H., et al. (2017). Disparities in state-specific adult fruit and vegetable consumption - United States, 2015. *Morbidity and Mortality Weekly Report, 66*(45), 1241–1247.

34. Office of Dietary Supplements. *Mission statement.* ods.od.nih.gov/About/MissionOriginMandate.aspx. Published 2018. [Accessed 22 May 2019].

35. Kantor, E. D., et al. (2016). Trends in dietary supplement use among U.S. adults from 1999–2012. *Journal of the American Medical Association, 316*(14), 1464–1474.

36. Marra, M. V., & Bailey, R. L. (2018). Position of the Academy of Nutrition and Dietetics: Micronutrient supplementation. *Journal of the Academy of Nutrition and Dietetics, 118*(11), 2162–2173.

37. Melina, V., Craig, W., & Levin, S. (2016). Position of the Academy of Nutrition and Dietetics: Vegetarian diets. *Journal of the Academy of Nutrition and Dietetics, 116*(12), 1970–1980.

38. Karademirci, M., Kutlu, R., & Kilinc, I. (2018). Relationship between smoking and total antioxidant status, total oxidant status, oxidative stress index, vit C, vit E. *Clinical Respiratory Journal, 12*(6), 2006–2012.

39. Baineni, R., Gulati, R., & Delhi, C. K. (2017). Vitamin A toxicity presenting as bone pain. *Archives of Disease in Childhood, 102*(6), 556–558.

40. Hayman, R. M., & Dalziel, S. R. (2012). Acute vitamin A toxicity: A report of three paediatric cases. *Journal of Paediatrics and Child Health, 48*(3), E98–E100.

41. Cheruvattath, R., et al. (2006). Vitamin A toxicity: When one a day doesn't keep the doctor away. *Liver Transplantation, 12*(12), 1888–1891.

42. Garcia-Cortes, M., et al. (2016). Hepatotoxicity by dietary supplements: A tabular listing and clinical characteristics. *International Journal of Molecular Sciences, 17*(4), 537.

43. Brown, A. C. (2017). An overview of herb and dietary supplement efficacy, safety and government regulations in the United States with suggested improvements. Part 1 of 5 series. *Food and Chemical Toxicology, 107*(Pt A), 449–471.

44. Brown, A. C. (2017). Liver toxicity related to herbs and dietary supplements: Online table of case reports. Part 2 of 5 series. *Food and Chemical Toxicology, 107*(Pt A), 472–501.

45. Brown, A. C. (2017). Kidney toxicity related to herbs and dietary supplements: Online table of case reports. Part 3 of 5 series. *Food and Chemical Toxicology, 107*(Pt A), 502–519.

46. Brown, A. C. (2018). Heart toxicity related to herbs and dietary supplements: Online table of case reports. Part 4 of 5. *Journal of Dietary Supplements, 15*(4), 516–555.

47. Brown, A. C. (2018). Cancer related to herbs and dietary supplements: Online table of case reports. Part 5 of 5. *Journal of Dietary Supplements, 15*(4), 556–581.

48. Crowe, K. M., & Francis, C. (2013). Position of the Academy of Nutrition and Dietetics: Functional foods. *Journal of the Academy of Nutrition and Dietetics, 113*(8), 1096–1103.

CHAPTER 8

1. Adler, R. A. (2018). Update on osteoporosis in men. *Best Practice & Research Clinical Endocrinology & Metabolism, 32*(5), 759–772.

2. Alejandro, P., & Constantinescu, F. (2018). A review of osteoporosis in the older adult: An update. *Rheumatic Diseases Clinics of North America, 44*(3), 437–451.

3. Wright, N. C., et al. (2017). The impact of the new National Bone Health Alliance (NBHA) diagnostic criteria on the prevalence of osteoporosis in the USA. *Osteoporosis International, 28*(4), 1225–1232.

4. Williamson, S., et al. (2017). Costs of fragility hip fractures globally: A systematic review and meta-regression analysis. *Osteoporosis International, 28*(10), 2791–2800.

5. Cauley, J. A., et al. (2016). Risk factors for hip fracture in older men: The osteoporotic fractures in men study (MrOS). *Journal of Bone and Mineral Research, 31*(10), 1810–1819.

6. Cauley, J. A. (2017). Osteoporosis: Fracture epidemiology update 2016. *Current Opinion in Rheumatology, 29*(2), 150–156.

7. Modi, A., et al. (2017). Frequency of discontinuation of injectable osteoporosis therapies in U.S. patients over 2 years. *Osteoporosis International, 28*(4), 1355–1363.

8. Durden, E., et al. (2017). Two-year persistence and compliance with osteoporosis therapies among postmenopausal women in a commercially insured population in the United States. *Archives of Osteoporosis, 12*(1), 22.

9. U.S. Department of Agriculture and U.S. Department of Health and Human Services. (December 2020). *Dietary Guidelines for Americans, 2020-2025* (9th ed.). Available at: www.dietaryguidelines.gov.

10. Rizzoli, R. (2014). Nutritional aspects of bone health. *Best Practice & Research Clinical Endocrinology & Metabolism, 28*(6), 795–808.

11. Viljakainen, H. T. (2016). Factors influencing bone mass accrual: Focus on nutritional aspects. *Proceedings of the Nutrition Society, 75*(3), 415–419.

12. Kantor, E. D., et al. (2016). Trends in dietary supplement use among U.S. adults from 1999–2012. *Journal of the American Medical Association, 316*(14), 464–1474.

13. Pivnick, E. K., et al. (1995). Rickets secondary to phosphate depletion. A sequela of antacid use in infancy. *Clinical Pediatrics (Phila), 34*(2), 73–78.

14. Chines, A., & Pacifici, R. (1990). Antacid and sucralfate-induced hypophosphatemic osteomalacia: A case report and review of the literature. *Calcified Tissue International, 47*(5), 291–295.

15. Food and Nutrition Board and Institute of Medicine. (1997). *Dietary reference intakes for calcium, phosphorus, magnesium, vitamin D, and fluoride.* Washington, DC: National Academies Press.

16. Juraschek, S. P., et al. (2017). Effects of sodium reduction and the DASH diet in relation to baseline blood pressure. *Journal of the American College of Cardiology, 70*(23), 2841–2848.

17. Cook, N. R., Appel, L. J., & Whelton, P. K. (2016). Sodium intake and all-cause mortality over 20 years in the trials of hypertension prevention. *Journal of the American College of Cardiology, 68*(15), 1609–1617.

18. Rust, P., & Ekmekcioglu, C. (2017). Impact of salt intake on the pathogenesis and treatment of hypertension. *Advances in Experimental Medicine & Biology, 956*, 61–84.

19. Stallings, V. A., et al. (2019). *The National Academies Collection: Reports funded by National Institutes of Health, Dietary Reference Intakes for sodium and potassium.* Washington, DC: National Academies Press (U.S.), National Academy of Sciences.

20. U.S. Department of Agriculture and U.S. Department of Health and Human Services. (December 2020). *Dietary Guidelines for Americans, 2020-2025* (9th ed.). Available at: www.dietaryguidelines.gov.

21. Agus, Z. S. (2016). Mechanisms and causes of hypomagnesemia. *Current Opinion in Nephrology and Hypertension, 25*(4), 301–307.

22. Mawri, S., et al. (2017). Cardiac dysrhythmias and neurological dysregulation: Manifestations of profound hypomagnesemia. *Case Reports in Cardiology*, 6250312.

23. Food and Nutrition Board and Institute of Medicine. (2001). *Dietary reference intakes for vitamin A, vitamin K, arsenic, boron, chromium, copper, iodine, iron, manganese, molybdenum, nickel, silicon, vanadium, and zinc*. Washington, DC: National Academies Press.

24. Melina, V., Craig, W., & Levin, S. (2016). Position of the Academy of Nutrition and Dietetics: Vegetarian diets. *Journal of the Academy of Nutrition and Dietetics, 116*(12), 1970–1980.

25. Kassebaum, N. J., et al. (2014). A systematic analysis of global anemia burden from 1990 to 2010. *Blood, 123*(5), 615–624.

26. Global Burden of Disease Study 2013 Collaborators. (2015). Global, regional, and national incidence, prevalence, and years lived with disability for 301 acute and chronic diseases and injuries in 188 countries, 1990-2013: A systematic analysis for the global burden of disease study 2013. *Lancet, 386*(9995), 743–800.

27. World Health Organization. (2015). *The global prevalence of anaemia in 2011*. Geneva: World Health Organization.

28. Chang, T. P., & Rangan, C. (2011). Iron poisoning: A literature-based review of epidemiology, diagnosis, and management. *Pediatric Emergency Care, 27*(10), 978–985.

29. Crownover, B. K., & Covey, C. J. (2013). Hereditary hemochromatosis. *American Family Physician, 87*(3), 183–190.

30. Kawabata, H. (2018). The mechanisms of systemic iron homeostasis and etiology, diagnosis, and treatment of hereditary hemochromatosis. *International Journal of Hematology, 107*(1), 31–43.

31. U.S. Department of Agriculture and Agricultural Research Service. (2018). *Nutrient intakes per 1000 kcal from food and beverages: Mean energy and mean nutrient amounts per 1000 kcal consumed per individual, by gender and age, What We Eat in America, NHANES 2015–2016*.

32. Redman, K., et al. (2016). Iodine deficiency and the brain: Effects and mechanisms. *Critical Reviews in Food Science and Nutrition, 56*(16), 2695–2713.

33. Pearce, E. N., Andersson, M., & Zimmermann, M. B. (2013). Global iodine nutrition: Where do we stand in 2013? *Thyroid, 23*(5), 523–528.

34. Niwattisaiwong, S., Burman, K. D., & Li-Ng, M. (2017). Iodine deficiency: Clinical implications. *Cleveland Clinic Journal of Medicine, 84*(3), 236–244.

35. Hynes, K. L., et al. (2017). Reduced educational outcomes persist into adolescence following mild iodine deficiency in utero, despite adequacy in childhood: 15-year follow-up of the gestational iodine cohort investigating auditory processing speed and working memory. *Nutrients, 9*(12).

36. Markou, K. B., et al. (2008). Treating iodine deficiency: Long-term effects of iodine repletion on growth and pubertal development in school-age children. *Thyroid, 18*(4), 449–454.

37. Yakoob, M. Y., & Lo, C. W. (2017). Nutrition (micronutrients) in child growth and development: A systematic review on current evidence, recommendations and opportunities for further research. *Journal of Developmental and Behavioral Pediatrics, 38*(8), 665–679.

38. Zimmermann, M. B., & Boelaert, K. (2015). Iodine deficiency and thyroid disorders. *The Lancet Diabetes & Endocrinology, 3*(4), 286–295.

39. Dubbs, S. B., & Spangler, R. (2014). Hypothyroidism: Causes, killers, and life-saving treatments. *Emergency Medicine Clinics of North America, 32*(2), 303–317.

40. Wessels, I., Maywald, M., & Rink, L. (2017). Zinc as a gatekeeper of immune function. *Nutrients, 9*(12).

41. Bailey, R. L., West, K. P., Jr., & Black, R. E. (2015). The epidemiology of global micronutrient deficiencies. *Annals of Nutrition & Metabolism, 66*(Suppl. 2), 22–33.

42. Moghimi, M., et al. (2017). Maternal zinc deficiency and congenital anomalies in newborns. *Pediatrics International, 59*(4), 443–446.

43. Gammoh, N. Z., & Rink, L. (2017). Zinc in infection and inflammation. *Nutrients, 9*(6).

44. Food and Nutrition Board and Institute of Medicine. (2000). *Dietary reference intakes for vitamin C, vitamin E, selenium, and carotenoids*. Washington, DC: National Academies Press.

45. United States Department of Agriculture and Agricultural Research Service. *USDA Food Composition Databases*. ndb.nal.usda.gov. Published 2018. [Accessed 15 January 2019].

46. O'Connell, J., et al. (2016). Costs and savings associated with community water fluoridation in the United States. *Health Affairs (Millwood), 35*(12), 2224–2232.

47. Vairo, F. P. E., et al. (2019). A systematic review and evidence-based guideline for diagnosis and treatment of Menkes disease. *Molecular Genetics and Metabolism, 126*(1), 6–13.

48. Kathawala, M., & Hirschfield, G. M. (2017). Insights into the management of Wilson's disease. *Therapeutic Advances in Gastroenterology, 10*(11), 889–905.

49. Livingstone, C. (2018). Manganese provision in parenteral nutrition: An update. *Nutrition in Clinical Practice, 33*(3), 404–418.

50. European Food Safety Authority. (2014). Scientific opinion on dietary reference values for chromium. *The EFSA Journal, 12*, 38–45.

51. Vincent, J. B. (2017). New evidence against chromium as an essential trace element. *Journal of Nutrition, 147*(12), 2212–2219.

52. Cowan, A. E., et al. (2018). Dietary supplement use differs by socioeconomic and health-related characteristics among U.S. adults, NHANES 2011–2014. *Nutrients, 10*(8).

53. Food and Nutrition Board and Institute of Medicine. (2011). *Dietary reference intakes for calcium and vitamin D*. Washington, DC: National Academies Press.

CHAPTER 9

1. Cannon, W. B. (1932). *The wisdom of the body*. New York: W.W. Norton & Company.

2. Food and Nutrition Board and Institute of Medicine. (2005). *Dietary reference intakes for water, potassium, sodium, chloride, and sulfate*. Washington, DC: National Academies Press.

3. Thomas, D. T., Erdman, K. A., & Burke, L. M. (2016). Position of the Academy of Nutrition and Dietetics, Dietitians of Canada, and the American College of Sports Medicine: Nutrition and athletic performance. *Journal of the Academy of Nutrition and Dietetics, 116*(3), 501–528.

4. Zhang, Y., et al. (2015). Caffeine and diuresis during rest and exercise: A meta-analysis. *Journal of Science and Medicine in Sport, 18*(5), 569–574.

5. Seal, A. D., et al. (2017). Coffee with high but not low caffeine content augments fluid and electrolyte excretion at rest. *Frontiers in Nutrition, 4*, 40.

6. El-Sharkawy, A. M., Sahota, O., & Lobo, D. N. (2015). Acute and chronic effects of hydration status on health. *Nutrition Reviews, 2*(Suppl. 73), 97–109.

7. Liska, D., et al. (2019). Narrative review of hydration and selected health outcomes in the general population. *Nutrients, 11*(1).

8. Begg, D. P. (2017). Disturbances of thirst and fluid balance associated with aging. *Physiology & Behavior, 178*, 28–34.

9. Metheny, N. A., & Meert, K. L. (2018). Water intoxication and child abuse. *Journal of Emergency Nursing, 44*(1), 13–18.

10. Nagasawa, S., et al. (2014). Fatal water intoxication during olanzapine treatment: A case report. *Legal Medicine (Tokyo), 16*(2), 89–91.

11. Anil, S., et al. (2016). Xerostomia in geriatric patients: A burgeoning global concern. *Journal of Investigative and Clinical Dentistry, 7*(1), 5–12.

12. World Health Organization. *Diarrhoeal disease.* www.who.int/en/news-room/fact-sheets/detail/diarrhoeal-disease. Published 2019. [Accessed 17 May 2019].

CHAPTER 10

1. Simpson, J. W., Lawless, R. W., & Mitchell, A. C. (1975). Responsibility of the obstetrician to the fetus. II. Influence of prepregnancy weight and pregnancy weight gain on birthweight. *Obstetrics & Gynecology, 45*(5), 481–487.

2. Food and Nutrition Board and Institute of Medicine. (2011). *Dietary reference intakes for calcium and vitamin D.* Washington, DC: National Academies Press.

3. Food and Nutrition Board and Institute of Medicine. (1998). *Dietary reference intakes for thiamin, riboflavin, niacin, vitamin B6, folate, vitamin B12, pantothenic acid, biotin, and choline.* Washington, DC: National Academies Press.

4. Food and Nutrition Board and Institute of Medicine. (2000). *Dietary reference intakes for vitamin C, vitamin E, selenium, and carotenoids.* Washington, DC: National Academies Press.

5. Food and Nutrition Board and Institute of Medicine. (2001). *Dietary reference intakes for vitamin A, vitamin K, arsenic, boron, chromium, copper, iodine, iron, manganese, molybdenum, nickel, silicon, vanadium, and zinc.* Washington, DC: National Academies Press.

6. Food and Nutrition Board and Institute of Medicine. (2002). *Dietary reference intakes for energy, carbohydrate, fiber, fat, fatty acids, cholesterol, protein, and amino acids.* Washington, DC: National Academies Press.

7. Food and Nutrition Board and Institute of Medicine. (2004). *Dietary reference intakes for water, potassium, sodium, chloride, and sulfate.* Washington, DC: National Academies Press.

8. U.S. Department of Agriculture and U.S. Department of Health and Human Services. (December 2020). *Dietary Guidelines for Americans, 2020-2025* (9th ed.). Available at: www.dietaryguidelines.gov.

9. Kapral, N., et al. (2018). Associations between birthweight and overweight and obesity in school-age children. *Pediatric Obesity, 13*(6), 333–341.

10. Goldstein, R. F., et al. (2017). Association of gestational weight gain with maternal and infant outcomes: A systematic review and meta-analysis. *Journal of the American Medical Association, 317*(21), 2207–2225.

11. U.S. Department of Agriculture and Agricultural Research Service. (2018). *Nutrient intakes from food and beverages: Mean amounts consumed per individual, by gender and age, What We Eat in America, NHANES 2015–2016.*

12. Martínez-Galiano, J. M., et al. (2018). Maternal dietary consumption of legumes, vegetables and fruit during pregnancy, does it protect against small for gestational age? *BMC Pregnancy Childbirth, 18*(1), 486.

13. Amezcua-Prieto, C., et al. (2019). Types of carbohydrates intake during pregnancy and frequency of a small for gestational age newborn: A case-control study. *Nutrients, 11*(3).

14. Vannice, G., & Rasmussen, H. (2014). Position of the Academy of Nutrition and Dietetics: Dietary fatty acids for healthy adults. *Journal of the Academy of Nutrition and Dietetics, 114*(1), 136–153.

15. Zhang, Z., Fulgoni, V. L., Kris-Etherton, P. M., & Mitmesser, S. H. (2018). Dietary intakes of EPA and DHA omega-3 fatty acids among U.S. childbearing-age and pregnant women: An analysis of NHANES 2001–2014. *Nutrients, 10*(4).

16. Shulkin, M., et al. (2018). N-3 fatty acid supplementation in mothers, preterm infants, and term infants and childhood psychomotor and visual development: A systematic review and meta-analysis. *Journal of Nutrition, 148*(3), 409–418.

17. Mulder, K. A., Elango, R., & Innis, S. M. (2018). Fetal DHA inadequacy and the impact on child neurodevelopment: A follow-up of a randomised trial of maternal DHA supplementation in pregnancy. *British Journal of Nutrition, 119*(3), 271–279.

18. Calder, P. C. (2016). Docosahexaenoic acid. *Annals of Nutrition & Metabolism, 69*(Suppl. 1), 7–21.

19. Procter, S. B., & Campbell, C. G. (2014). Position of the Academy of Nutrition and Dietetics: Nutrition and lifestyle for a healthy pregnancy outcome. *Journal of the Academy of Nutrition and Dietetics, 114*(7), 1099–1103.

20. Rasmussen, K. M., & Yaktine, A. L. (Eds.). (2009). *Weight gain during pregnancy: Reexamining the guidelines.* Washington, DC: National Academies Press.

21. Siu, A. L., & U.S. Preventive Services Task Force. (2015). Screening for iron deficiency anemia and iron supplementation in pregnant women to improve maternal health and birth outcomes: U.S. preventive services task force recommendation statement. *Annals of Internal Medicine, 163*(7), 529–536.

22. Gupta, P. M., et al. (2017). Iron status of toddlers, nonpregnant females, and pregnant females in the United States. *American Journal of Clinical Nutrition, 106*(Suppl. 6), 1640S–1646S.

23. Blumberg, J. B., et al. (2017). Contribution of dietary supplements to nutritional adequacy by socioeconomic subgroups in adults of the United States. *Nutrients, 10*(1).

24. Toivonen, K. I., et al. (2018). Folic acid supplementation during the preconception period: A systematic review and meta-analysis. *Preventive Medicine, 114*, 1–17.

25. Kancherla, V., & Black, R. E. (2018). Historical perspective on folic acid and challenges in estimating global prevalence of neural tube defects. *Annals of the New York Academy, 1414*(1), 20–30.

26. Crider, K. S., et al. (2018). Modeling the impact of folic acid fortification and supplementation on red blood cell folate concentrations and predicted neural tube defect risk in the United States: Have we reached optimal prevention? *American Journal of Clinical Nutrition, 107*(6), 1027–1034.

27. Hollis, B. W., & Wagner, C. L. (2017). Vitamin D supplementation during pregnancy: Improvements in birth outcomes and complications through direct genomic alteration. *Molecular and Cellular Endocrinology, 453*, 113–130.

28. Wiedeman, A. M., et al. (2018). Dietary choline intake: Current state of knowledge across the life cycle. *Nutrients, 10*(10).

29. Wallace, T. C., et al. (2018). Choline: The underconsumed and underappreciated essential nutrient. *Nutrition Today, 53*(6), 240–253.

30. Matthews, A., et al. (2015). Interventions for nausea and vomiting in early pregnancy. *Cochrane Database of Systematic Reviews, 3*, CD007575.

31. Erick, M., Cox, J. T., & Mogensen, K. M. (2018). ACOG Practice Bulletin 189: Nausea and vomiting of pregnancy. *Obstetrics & Gynecology, 131*(5), 935.

32. McParlin, C., O'Donnell, A., Robson, S. C., et al. (2016). Treatments for HYPEREMESIS gravidarum and nausea and vomiting in pregnancy: A systematic review. *Journal of the American Medical Association, 316*(13), 1392–1401.

33. Austin, K., Wilson, K., & Saha, S. (2019). Hyperemesis gravidarum. *Nutrition in Clinical Practice, 34*(2), 226–241.

34. Centers for Disease Control and Prevention. *Pregnancy mortality surveillance system. Trends in pregnancy-related deaths 1987–2014.* www.cdc.gov/reproductivehealth/maternalinfanthealth/pregnancy-mortality-surveillance-system.htm. [Accessed 4 April 2019].

35. Hamilton, B. E., & Mathews, T. J. (2016). Continued declines in teen births in the United States, 2015. *NCHS Data Brief, 259*, 1–8.

36. Leftwich, H. K., & Alves, M. V. (2017). Adolescent pregnancy. *Pediatric Clinics of North America, 64*(2), 381–388.

37. Martin, J. A., et al. (2018). Births: Final data for 2016. *National Vital Statistics Reports, 1*, 67.

38. Pinheiro, R. L., Areia, A. L., Mota Pinto, A., & Donato, H. (2019). Advanced maternal age: Adverse outcomes of pregnancy, a meta-analysis. *Acta Médica Portuguesa, 32*(3), 219–226.

39. Class, Q. A., et al. (2017). Within-family analysis of interpregnancy interval and adverse birth outcomes. *Obstetrics & Gynecology, 130*(6), 1304–1311.

40. Leonard, S. A., Rasmussen, K. M., King, J. C., & Abrams, B. (2017). Trajectories of maternal weight from before pregnancy through postpartum and associations with childhood obesity. *American Journal of Clinical Nutrition, 106*(5), 1295–1301.

41. Popova, S., et al. (2017). Prevalence of alcohol consumption during pregnancy and fetal alcohol spectrum disorders among the general and aboriginal populations in Canada and the United States. *European Journal of Medical Genetics, 60*(1), 32–48.

42. Pregnancy Risk Assessment Monitoring System. (2018). *Prevalence of selected maternal and child health indicators for all PRAMS sites, Pregnancy Risk Assessment Monitoring System (PRAMS), 2012–2015.*

43. Shobeiri, F., & Jenabi, E. (2017). Smoking and placenta previa: A meta-analysis. *Journal of Maternal-Fetal and Neonatal Medicine, 30*(24), 2985–2990.

44. Dessì, A., Corona, L., Pintus, R., & Fanos, L. (2018). Exposure to tobacco smoke and low birth weight: From epidemiology to metabolomics. *Expert Rev Proteomics, 15*(8), 647–656.

45. Pereira, P. P., et al. (2017). Maternal active smoking during pregnancy and low birth weight in the Americas: A systematic review and meta-analysis. *Nicotine & Tobacco Research, 19*(5), 497–505.

46. Chatterton, Z., et al. (2017). In utero exposure to maternal smoking is associated with DNA methylation alterations and reduced neuronal content in the developing fetal brain. *Epigenetics & Chromatin, 10*, 4.

47. Ekblad, M., Lehtonen, L., Korkeila, J., & Gissler, M. (2017). Maternal smoking during pregnancy and the risk of psychiatric morbidity in singleton sibling pairs. *Nicotine & Tobacco Research, 19*, 597–604.

48. Friedmann, I., et al. (2017). Maternal and obstetrical predictors of sudden infant death syndrome (SIDS). *Journal of Maternal-Fetal and Neonatal Medicine, 30*(19), 2315–2323.

49. Kim, H. H., Monteiro, K., Larson, E., & Derisier, D. M. (2017). Effects of smoking and smoking cessation during pregnancy on adverse birth outcomes in Rhode Island, 2012–2014. *Rhode Island Medical Journal, 100*(6), 50–52.

50. Wouldes, T. A., & Lester, B. M. (2019). Stimulants: How big is the problem and what are the effects of prenatal exposure? *Seminars in Fetal and Neonatal Medicine, 24*(2), 155–160.

51. Grossman, M., & Berkwitt, A. (2019). Neonatal abstinence syndrome. *Seminars in Perinatology.* S0146-0005(19):30007-2.

52. Khiali, S., Gharekhani, A., & Entezari-Maleki, T. (2018). Isotretinoin: A review on the utilization pattern in pregnancy. *Advanced Pharmaceutical Bulletin, 8*(3), 377–382.

53. Wikoff, D., et al. (2017). Systematic review of the potential adverse effects of caffeine consumption in healthy adults, pregnant women, adolescents, and children. *Food and Chemical Toxicology, 109*(Pt 1), 585–648.

54. Miao, D., Young, S. L., & Golden, C. D. (2015). A meta-analysis of pica and micronutrient status. *American Journal of Human Biology, 27*(1), 84–93.

55. Leung, A. K. C., & Hon, K. L. (2019). Pica: A common condition that is commonly missed—an update review. *Current Pediatric Reviews, 15*(3), 164–169.

56. Roy, A., Fuentes-Afflick, E., Fernald, L. C. H., & Young, S. L. (2018). Pica is prevalent and strongly associated with iron deficiency among Hispanic pregnant women living in the United States. *Appetite, 120*, 163–170.

57. Beckert, R. H., et al. (2019). Maternal anemia and pregnancy outcomes: A population-based study. *Journal of Perinatology, 39*(7), 911–919.

58. Menon, K. C., et al. (2016). Effects of anemia at different stages of gestation on infant outcomes. *Nutrition, 32*(1), 61–65.

59. Dai, A. I., et al. (2015). Maternal iron deficiency anemia as a risk factor for the development of retinopathy of prematurity. *Pediatric Neurology, 53*, 146–150.

60. World Health Organization. (2015). *The global prevalence of anaemia in 2011.* Geneva: World Health Organization.

61. WHO guidelines approved by the Guidelines Review Committee. (2016). *Guideline: Daily iron supplementation in adult women and adolescent girls.* Geneva: World Health Organization.

62. WHO guidelines approved by the Guidelines Review Committee. (2012). *Guideline: Intermittent iron and folic acid supplementation in non-anaemic pregnant women.* Geneva: World Health Organization.

63. Lee, A. C., et al. (2017). Estimates of burden and consequences of infants born small for gestational age in low and middle income countries with INTERGROWTH-21(st) standard: Analysis of CHERG datasets. *British Medical Journal, 358*, j3677.

64. Fleiss, B., et al. (2019). Knowledge gaps and emerging research areas in intrauterine growth restriction-associated brain injury. *Frontiers in Endocrinology (Lausanne), 10*, 188.

65. Whelton, P. K., et al. (2018). 2017 ACC/AHA/AAPA/ABC/ACPM/AGS/APHA/ASH/ASPC/NMA/PCNA guideline for the prevention, detection, evaluation, and management of high blood pressure in adults: Executive summary: A report of the American College of Cardiology/American Heart Association task force on clinical practice guidelines. *Circulation, 138*(17).

66. Wilkerson, R. G., & Ogunbodede, A. C. (2019). Hypertensive disorders of pregnancy. *Emergency Medicine Clinics of North America, 37*(2), 301–316.

67. Magee, L. A., et al. (2014). Diagnosis, evaluation, and management of the hypertensive disorders of pregnancy: Executive summary. *Journal of Obstetrics and Gynaecology Canada, 36*(5), 416–441.

68. American Diabetes Association. (2019). *Classification and diagnosis of diabetes: Standards of medical care in diabetes. Diabetes Care, 42*(Suppl. 1), S13–s28.

69. Daly, B., et al. (2018). Increased risk of ischemic heart disease, hypertension, and type 2 diabetes in women with previous gestational diabetes mellitus, a target group in general practice for preventive interventions: A population-based cohort study. *PLoS Med, 15*(1), e1002488.

70. American Academy of Pediatrics Committee on Nutrition. (2012). Breastfeeding and the use of human milk. *Pediatrics, 129*(3), e827–e841.

71. Global Breastfeeding Collective. (2017). *Tracking breastfeeding policies and programmes. Global breastfeeding scorecard, 2017.* New York: United Nations Children Fund (UNICEF), World Health Organization.

72. Centers for Disease Control and Prevention, National Center for Chronic Disease Prevention and Health Promotion, Division of Nutrition, Physical Activity, and Obesity. (2020). Data, trend and maps. Available at: www.cdc.gov/nccdphp/dnpao/data-trends-maps/index.html. [Accessed 19 February 2021].

73. U.S. Department of Health and Human Services. *Healthy People 2030.* health.gov/healthypeople. Published 2020. [Accessed 18 February, 2021].

74. Schliep, K. C., et al. (2019). Factors in the hospital experience associated with postpartum breastfeeding success. *Breastfeeding Medicine, 14*(5), 334–341.

75. Biggs, K. V., et al. (2018). Formula milk supplementation on the postnatal ward: A cross-sectional analytical study. *Nutrients, 10*(5).

76. Preusting, I., et al. (2017). Obesity as a predictor of delayed lactogenesis II. *Journal of Human Lactation, 33*(4), 684–691.

77. Lind, J. N., Perrine, C. G., & Li, R. (2014). Relationship between use of labor pain medications and delayed onset of lactation. *Journal of Human Lactation, 30*(2), 167–173.

78. van Veldhuizen-Staas, C. G. (2007). Overabundant milk supply: An alternative way to intervene by full drainage and block feeding. *International Breastfeeding Journal, 2*, 11.

79. Sriraman, N. K., & Kellams, A. (2016). Breastfeeding: What are the barriers? Why women struggle to achieve their goals. *Journal of Women's Health (Larchmt), 25*(7), 714–722.

80. Coffman, L. (2019). The NP'S role in promoting and supporting breastfeeding. *Nurse Practitioner, 44*(3), 38–42.

81. Sayres, S., & Visentin, L. (2018). Breastfeeding: Uncovering barriers and offering solutions. *Current Opinion in Pediatrics, 30*(4), 591–596.

82. Horta, B. L., de Sousa, B. A., & de Mola, C. L. (2018). Breastfeeding and neurodevelopmental outcomes. *Current Opinion in Clinical Nutrition and Metabolic Care, 21*(3), 174–178.

83. Lessen, R., & Kavanagh, K. (2015). Position of the academy of nutrition and dietetics: Promoting and supporting breastfeeding. *Journal of the Academy of Nutrition and Dietetics, 115*(3), 444–449.

CHAPTER 11

1. Grummer-Strawn, L. M., et al. (2010). Use of World Health Organization and CDC growth charts for children aged 0-59 months in the United States. *MMWR Recommendations and Reports, 59*(RR-9), 1–15.

2. Food and Nutrition Board and Institute of Medicine. (2002). *Dietary reference intakes for energy, carbohydrate, fiber, fat, fatty acids, cholesterol, protein, and amino acids.* Washington, DC: National Academies Press.

3. Brennan, A. M., Murphy, B. P., & Kiely, M. E. (2016). Optimising preterm nutrition: Present and future. *Proceedings of the Nutrition Society, 75*(2), 154.

4. U.S. Department of Agriculture and Agricultural Research Service. (2018). *Nutrient intakes per 1000 kcal from food and beverages: Mean energy and mean nutrient amounts per 1000 kcal consumed per individual, by gender and age, What We Eat in America, NHANES 2015–2016.*

5. Sheppard, K. W., & Cheatham, C. L. (2018). Omega-6/Omega-3 fatty acid intake of children and older adults in the U.S.: Dietary intake in comparison to current dietary recommendations and the healthy eating index. *Lipids in Health and Disease, 17*(1), 43.

6. Thompson, M., et al. (2019). Omega-3 fatty acid intake by age, gender, and pregnancy status in the United States: National health and nutrition examination survey 2003–2014. *Nutrients, 11*(1).

7. Cardoso, C., Afonso, C., & Bandarra, N. M. (2018). Dietary DHA, bioaccessibility, and neurobehavioral development in children. *Critical Reviews in Food Science and Nutrition, 58*(15), 2617–2631.

8. Weaver, C. M., et al. (2016). The National Osteoporosis Foundation's position statement on peak bone mass development and lifestyle factors: A systematic review and implementation recommendations. *Osteoporosis International, 27*, 1281–1386.

9. Bailey, D. A., et al. (2000). Calcium accretion in girls and boys during puberty: A longitudinal analysis. *Journal of Bone and Mineral Research, 15*(11), 2245–2250.

10. van den Hooven, E. H., et al. (2015). Infant dietary patterns and bone mass in childhood: The generation R study. *Osteoporosis International, 26*, 1595–1604.

11. Bowman, S. A., et al. (2018). *Food patterns equivalents intakes by Americans: What We Eat in America, NHANES 2003–2004 and 2015–2016. Food surveys research group. Dietary data brief no. 20.*

12. U.S. Department of Agriculture and U.S. Department of Health and Human Services. (December 2020). *Dietary Guidelines for Americans, 2020-2025* (9th ed.). Available at: www.dietaryguidelines.gov.

13. Winzenberg, T., Shaw, K., Fryer, J., & Jones, G. (2006). Effects of calcium supplementation on bone density in healthy children: Meta-analysis of randomised controlled trials. *British Medical Journal, 333*, 775.

14. Georgieff, M. K., Ramel, S. E., & Cusick, S. E. (2018 Aug). Nutritional influences on brain development. *Acta Paediatrica, 107*(8), 1310–1321.

15. Food and Nutrition Board and Institute of Medicine. (2001). *Dietary reference intakes for vitamin A, vitamin K, arsenic, boron, chromium, copper, iodine, iron, manganese, molybdenum, nickel, silicon, vanadium, and zinc.* Washington, DC: National Academies Press.

16. Gupta, P. M., et al. (2017). Iron status of toddlers, nonpregnant females, and pregnant females in the United States. *American Journal of Clinical Nutrition, 106*(Suppl. 6), 1640S–1646S.

17. Brannon, P. M., Stover, P. J., & Taylor, C. L. (2017). Integrating themes, evidence gaps, and research needs identified by workshop on iron screening and supplementation in iron-replete pregnant women and young children. *American Journal of Clinical Nutrition, 106*(Suppl. 6), 1703S–1712S.

18. Jun, S., et al. (2018). Dietary supplement use among U.S. children by family income, food security level, and nutrition assistance program participation status in 2011–2014. *Nutrients, 10*(9).

19. American Academy of Pediatrics Committee on Nutrition. (2012). Breastfeeding and the use of human milk. *Pediatrics, 129*(3), e827–e841.

20. við Streym, S., et al. (2016). Vitamin D content in human breast milk: A 9-mo follow-up study. *American Journal of Clinical Nutrition, 103*(1), 107–114.

21. Wall, C. R., et al. (2016). Vitamin D activity of breast milk in women randomly assigned to vitamin D3 supplementation during pregnancy. *American Journal of Clinical Nutrition, 103*(2), 382–388.

22. March, K. M., et al. (2015). Maternal vitamin D$_3$ supplementation at 50 μg/d protects against low serum 25-hydroxyvitamin D in infants at 8 wk of age: A randomized controlled trial of 3 doses of vitamin D beginning in gestation and continued in lactation. *American Journal of Clinical Nutrition, 102*(2), 402–410.

23. Trend, S., et al. (2016). Levels of innate immune factors in preterm and term mothers' breast milk during the 1st month postpartum. *British Journal of Nutrition, 115*(7), 1178–1193.

24. Mimouni, F. B., Lubetzky, R., Yochpaz, S., & Mandel, D. (2017). Preterm human milk macronutrient and energy composition: A systematic review and meta-analysis. *Clinics in Perinatology, 44*(1), 165–172.

25. Ikonen, R., Paavilainen, E., & Kaunonen, M. (2015). Preterm infants' mothers' experiences with milk expression and breastfeeding: An integrative review. *Advances in Neonatal Care, 15*(6), 394–406.

26. Lessen, R., & Kavanagh, K. (2015). Position of the Academy of Nutrition and Dietetics: Promoting and supporting breastfeeding. *Journal of the Academy of Nutrition and Dietetics, 115*(3), 444–449.

27. Boué, G., et al. (2018). Public health risks and benefits associated with breast milk and infant formula consumption. *Critical Reviews in Food Science and Nutrition, 58*(1), 126–145.

28. Ellison, R. G., et al. (2017). Observations and conversations: Home preparation of infant formula among a sample of low-income mothers in the Southeastern U.S. *Journal of Nutrition Education and Behavior, 49*(7), 579–587.

29. American Academy of Pediatric Dentistry and American Academy of Pediatrics. (2016). Policy on early childhood caries (ECC): Classifications, consequences, and preventative strategies. Chicago: Oral health policies. *Pediatric Dentistry*, 38(6), 52–54.

30. Pluymen, L. P. M., et al. (2018). Early introduction of complementary foods and childhood overweight in breastfed and formula-fed infants in the Netherlands: The PIAMA birth cohort study. *European Journal of Nutrition*, 57(5), 1985–1993.

31. Heine, R. G. (2018). Food allergy prevention and treatment by targeted nutrition. *Annals of Nutrition & Metabolism*, 72(Suppl. 3), 33–45.

32. Moyer, V. A., & U.S. Preventive Services Task Force. (2014). Prevention of dental caries in children from birth through age 5 years: U.S. Preventive Services Task force recommendation statement. *Pediatrics*, 133(6), 1102–1111.

33. Vaughn, A. E., et al. (2016). Fundamental constructs in food parenting practices: A content map to guide future research. *Nutrition Reviews*, 74(2), 98–117.

34. Watts, A. W., et al. (2017). No time for family meals? Parenting practices associated with adolescent fruit and vegetable intake when family meals are not an option. *Journal of the Academy of Nutrition and Dietetics*, 117, 707–714.

35. Vaughn, A. E., Martin, C. L., & Ward, D. S. (2018). What matters most—what parents model or what parents eat? *Appetite*, 126, 102–107.

36. Verhage, C. L., Gillebaart, M., van der Veek, S. M. C., & Vereijken, C. M. J. L. (2018). The relation between family meals and health of infants and toddlers: A review. *Appetite*, 127, 97–109.

37. Jones, B. L. (2018). Making time for family meals: Parental influences, home eating environments, barriers and protective factors. *Physiology & Behavior*, 193(Pt B), 248–251.

38. Centers for Disease Control. *Screen time vs. Lean time infographic*. www.cdc.gov/nccdphp/dch/multimedia/infographics/getmoving.htm. [Accessed 14 April 2019].

39. Domingues-Montanari, S. (2017). Clinical and psychological effects of excessive screen time on children. *Journal of Paediatrics and Child Health*, 53(4), 333–338.

40. Nightingale, C. M., et al. (2017). Screen time is associated with adiposity and insulin resistance in children. *Archives of Disease in Childhood*, 102(7), 612–616.

41. Boyland, E. J., et al. (2016). Advertising as a cue to consume: A systematic review and meta–analysis of the effects of acute exposure to unhealthy food and nonalcoholic beverage advertising on intake in children and adults. *American Journal of Clinical Nutrition*, 103, 519–533.

42. Falbe, J., et al. (2014). Longitudinal relations of television, electronic games, and digital versatile discs with changes in diet in adolescents. *American Journal of Clinical Nutrition*, 100(4), 1173–1181.

43. American Academy of Pediatrics. (2013). Policy statement: Children, adolescents, and the media. *Pediatrics*, 132, 958–961.

44. American Academy of Pediatrics. (2016). Policy statement: Media use in school-aged children and adolescents. *Pediatrics*, 138(5).

45. Lopez, A., Cacoub, P., Macdougall, I. C., & Peyrin-Biroulet, L. (2016). Iron deficiency anaemia. *Lancet*, 387(10021), 907–916.

46. Hales, C. M., Carroll, M. D., Fryar, C. D., & Ogden, C. L. (2017). Prevalence of obesity among adults and youth: United States, 2015–2016. *NCHS Data Brief*, 288.

47. Gibson, L. Y., et al. (2017). The psychosocial burden of childhood overweight and obesity: Evidence for persisting difficulties in boys and girls. *European Journal of Pediatrics*, 176(7), 925–933.

48. Gurnani, M., Birken, C., & Hamilton, J. (2015). Childhood obesity: Causes, consequences, and management. *Pediatric Clinics of North America*, 62(4), 821–840.

49. U.S. Department of Health and Human Services. (2018). *Physical activity guidelines for Americans* (2nd ed.). Washington, DC: U.S. Department of Health and Human Services.

50. Li, W., et al. (2017). Association between obesity and puberty timing: A systematic review and meta-analysis. *International Journal of Environmental Research and Public Health*, 24(10), 14.

51. Luijken, J., van der Schouw, Y. T., Mensink, D., & Onland-Moret, N. C. (2017). Association between age at menarche and cardiovascular disease: A systematic review on risk and potential mechanisms. *Maturitas*, 104, 96–116.

52. Yee, A. Z., Lwin, M. O., & Ho, S. S. (2017). The influence of parental practices on child promotive and preventive food consumption behaviors: A systematic review and meta-analysis. *International Journal of Behavioral Nutrition and Physical Activity*, 14(1), 47.

CHAPTER 12

1. U.S. Department of Health and Human Services. *Healthy People 2030*. health.gov/healthypeople. Published 2020. [Accessed 28 April, 2021].

2. U.S. Census Bureau. (2018). *Projected age groups and sex composition of the population: Main projections series for the United States, 2017-2060*. Washington, DC: U.S. Government Printing Office.

3. Licher, S., et al. (2019). Lifetime risk and multimorbidity of non-communicable diseases and disease-free life expectancy in the general population: A population-based cohort study. *PLoS Med*, 16(2), e1002741.

4. Khan, S. S., et al. (2018). Association of body mass index with lifetime risk of cardiovascular disease and compression of morbidity. *JAMA Cardiology*, 3(4), 280–287.

5. U.S. Census Bureau. (2014). *Projected life expectancy at birth by sex, race, and hispanic origin for the United States: 2015 to 2060*. Washington, DC: U.S. Government Printing Office.

6. Singh, G. K., et al. (2017). Social determinants of health in the United States: Addressing major health inequality trends for the nation, 1935-2016. *The International Journal of Maternal and Child Health and AIDS*, 6(2), 139–164.

7. Davis, M. A., et al. (2017). Trends and disparities in the number of self-reported healthy older adults in the United States, 2000 to 2014. *JAMA Internal Medicine*, 177(11), 1683–1684.

8. Colman, I., et al. (2018). Depressive and anxious symptoms and 20-year mortality: Evidence from the stirling county study. *Depress Anxiety*, 35(7), 638–647.

9. Lasserre, A. M., et al. (2016). Clinical and course characteristics of depression and all-cause mortality: A prospective population-based study. *Journal of Affective Disorders*, 189, 17–24.

10. Borg, C., Hallberg, I. R., & Blomqvist, K. (2006). Life satisfaction among older people (65+) with reduced self-care capacity: The relationship to social, health and financial aspects. *Journal of Clinical Nursing*, 15(5), 607–618.

11. Hajek, A., Bock, J. O., & Konig, H. H. (2017). Psychosocial correlates of unintentional weight loss in the second half of life in the German general population. *PLoS One*, 12(10), e0185749.

12. McMinn, J., Steel, C., & Bowman, A. (2011). Investigation and management of unintentional weight loss in older adults. *British Medical Journal*, 342, d1732.

13. Gaddey, H. L., & Holder, K. (2014). Unintentional weight loss in older adults. *American Family Physician*, 89(9), 718–722.

14. Robertson, R. G., & Montagnini, M. (2004). Geriatric failure to thrive. *American Family Physician*, 70(2), 343–350.

15. Tan, M. E., et al. (2017). Employment status among the Singapore elderly and its correlates. *Psychogeriatrics*, 17(3), 155–163.

16. Lee, J., & Kim, M. H. (2017). The effect of employment transitions on physical health among the elderly in South Korea: A longitudinal analysis of the Korean retirement and income study. *Social Science & Medicine, 181*, 122–130.

17. Geisler, C., et al. (2016). Age-dependent changes in resting energy expenditure (REE): Insights from detailed body composition analysis in normal and overweight healthy Caucasians. *Nutrients, 8*(6).

18. Amdanee, N., et al. (2018). Age-associated changes of resting energy expenditure, body composition and fat distribution in Chinese Han Males. *Physiological Reports, 6*(23), e13940.

19. Yamada, M., et al. (2019). Synergistic effect of bodyweight resistance exercise and protein supplementation on skeletal muscle in sarcopenic or dynapenic older adults. *Geriatrics and Gerontology International*, 1–9.

20. Cruz-Jentoft, A. J., & Woo, J. (2019). Nutritional interventions to prevent and treat frailty. *Current Opinion in Clinical Nutrition and Metabolic Care*, 1–5.

21. Centers for Disease Control and Prevention, Division of Nutrition, Physical Activity and Obesity, National Center for Chronic Disease Prevention Health Promotion. (2018). *Adults need more physical activity*. Atlanta: U.S. Department of Health and Human Services.

22. U.S. Department of Health and Human Services. (2018). *Physical activity guidelines for Americans*. Washington, DC: U.S. Department of Health and Human Services.

23. Food and Nutrition Board and Institute of Medicine. (2002). *Dietary reference intakes for energy, carbohydrate, fiber, fat, fatty acids, cholesterol, protein, and amino acids*. Washington, DC: National Academies Press.

24. Hirani, V., et al. (2017). Longitudinal associations between body composition, sarcopenic obesity and outcomes of frailty, disability, institutionalisation and mortality in community-dwelling older men: The concord health and ageing in men project. *Age Ageing, 46*(3), 413–420.

25. Wannamethee, S. G., & Atkins, J. L. (2015). Muscle loss and obesity: The health implications of sarcopenia and sarcopenic obesity. *Proceedings of the Nutrition Society, 74*(4), 405–412.

26. U.S. Department of Agriculture and Agricultural Research Service. (2018). *Nutrient intakes from food and beverages: Mean amounts consumed per individual, by gender and age, What We Eat in America, NHANES 2015–2016*.

27. Deutz, N. E., et al. (2014). Protein intake and exercise for optimal muscle function with aging: Recommendations from the ESPEN expert group. *Clinical Nutrition, 33*(6), 929–936.

28. Franzke, B., et al. (2018). Dietary protein, muscle and physical function in the very old. *Nutrients, 10*(7).

29. Looker, A. C., et al. (2017). FRAX-based estimates of 10-year probability of hip and major osteoporotic fracture among adults aged 40 and over: United States, 2013 and 2014. *National Health Statistics Reports* (103), 1–16.

30. Food and Nutrition Board and Institute of Medicine. (1998). *Dietary reference intakes for thiamin, riboflavin, niacin, vitamin B6, folate, vitamin B12, pantothenic acid, biotin, and choline*. Washington, DC: National Academies Press.

31. Prentice, A. (2008). Vitamin D deficiency: A global perspective. *Nutrition Reviews, 66*(10 Suppl. 2), S153–S164.

32. Holick, M. F., & Chen, T. C. (2008). Vitamin D deficiency: A worldwide problem with health consequences. *American Journal of Clinical Nutrition, 87*(4), 1080s–1086s.

33. Norman, A. W., & Bouillon, R. (2010). Vitamin D nutritional policy needs a vision for the future. *Experimental Biology and Medicine, 235*(9), 1034–1045.

34. Manson, J. E., et al. (2016). Vitamin D deficiency—is there really a pandemic? *New England Journal of Medicine, 375*(19), 1817–1820.

35. Pfotenhauer, K. M., & Shubrook, J. H. (2017). Vitamin D deficiency, its role in health and disease, and current supplementation recommendations. *Journal of the American Osteopathic Association, 117*(5), 301–305.

36. LeFevre, M. L. (2015). Screening for vitamin D deficiency in adults: U.S. Preventive Services Task Force recommendation statement. *Annals of Internal Medicine, 162*(2), 133–140.

37. Food and Nutrition Board and Institute of Medicine. (2011). *Dietary reference intakes for calcium and vitamin D*. Washington, DC: National Academies Press.

38. Grossman, D. C., et al. (2018). Vitamin D, calcium, or combined supplementation for the primary prevention of fractures in community-dwelling adults: U.S. Preventive Services Task Force recommendation statement. *Journal of the American Medical Association, 319*(15), 1592–1599.

39. LeBlanc, E. S., et al. (2015). Screening for vitamin D deficiency: A systematic review for the U.S. Preventive Services Task Force. *Annals of Internal Medicine, 162*(2), 109–122.

40. Blumberg, J. B., et al. (2017). Contribution of dietary supplements to nutritional adequacy by socioeconomic subgroups in adults of the United States. *Nutrients, 10*(1).

41. Wallace, T. C., McBurney, M., & Fulgoni, V. L., 3rd. (2014). Multivitamin/mineral supplement contribution to micronutrient intakes in the United States, 2007-2010. *Journal of the American College of Nutrition, 33*(2), 94–102.

42. Donini, L. M., et al. (2016). Mini-nutritional assessment, malnutrition universal screening tool, and nutrition risk screening tool for the nutritional evaluation of older nursing home residents. *Journal of the American Medical Directors Association, 17*(10), 959. e11-e18.

43. Inoue, T., et al. (2019). Acute phase nutritional screening tool associated with functional outcomes of hip fracture patients: A longitudinal study to compare MNA-SF, MUST, NRS-2002 and GNRI. *Clinical Nutrition, 38*(1), 220–226.

44. Hoeksema, A. R., et al. (2018). Health and quality of life differ between community living older people with and without remaining teeth who recently received formal home care: A cross sectional study. *Clinical Oral Investigations, 22*(7), 2615–2622.

45. Wu, L. L., et al. (2018). Oral health indicators for risk of malnutrition in elders. *The Journal of Nutrition, Health & Aging, 22*(2), 254–261.

46. Begg, D. P. (2017). Disturbances of thirst and fluid balance associated with aging. *Physiology & Behavior, 178*, 28–34.

47. Koch, C. A., & Fulop, T. (2017). Clinical aspects of changes in water and sodium homeostasis in the elderly. *Reviews in Endocrine & Metabolic Disorders, 18*(1), 49–66.

48. Hales, C. M., et al. (2018). Trends in obesity and severe obesity prevalence in U.S. youth and adults by sex and age, 2007–2008 to 2015–2016. *Journal of the American Medical Association, 319*(16), 1723–1725.

49. Koolhaas, C. M., et al. (2018). Physical activity types and health-related quality of life among middle-aged and elderly adults: The Rotterdam study. *The Journal of Nutrition, Health & Aging, 22*(2), 246–253.

50. Cohen, A., Baker, J., & Ardern, C. I. (2016). Association between body mass index, physical activity, and health-related quality of life in Canadian adults. *Journal of Aging and Physical Activity, 24*(1), 32–38.

51. Liu, Z., et al. (2018). Effect of 24-month physical activity on cognitive frailty and the role of inflammation: The life randomized clinical trial. *BMC Medicine, 16*(1), 185.

52. U.S. Department of Agriculture and U.S. Department of Health and Human Services. (December 2020). *Dietary Guidelines for Americans, 2020-2025* (9th ed.). Available at: www.dietaryguidelines.gov.

53. Aguiar, E. J., et al. (2014). Efficacy of interventions that include diet, aerobic and resistance training components for type 2 diabetes prevention: A systematic review with meta-analysis. *International Journal of Behavioral Nutrition and Physical Activity, 11*, 2.

54. National Center for Chronic Disease Prevention and Health Promotion. *About chronic diseases*. www.cdc.gov/chronic disease/about/index.htm. Published 2019. [Accessed 24 March 2019].

55. National Center for Health Statistics. (2018). *Health, United States, 2017: With special feature on mortality*. Hyattsville, MD.

56. Administration for Community Living. (2019). *National survey of OAA participants, aging integrated database*. Department of Health and Human Services.

57. United States Department of Agriculture. (2018). *Trends in supplemental nutrition assistance program participation rates: Fiscal year 2010 to fiscal year 2016*. Food and Nutrition Service and Office of Policy Support. Washington, DC: United States Department of Agriculture.

58. Dorner, B., & Friedrich, E. K. (2018). Position of the Academy of Nutrition and Dietetics: Individualized nutrition approaches for older adults: Long-term care, post-acute care, and other settings. *Journal of the Academy of Nutrition and Dietetics, 118*(4), 724–735.

59. Keller, H. H., et al. (2017). Prevalence and determinants of poor food intake of residents living in long-term care. *Journal of the American Medical Directors Association, 18*(11), 941–947.

CHAPTER 13

1. U.S. Food and Drug Administration. (2004). *Food allergen labeling and consumer protection act of 2004*. Silver Spring, MD.

2. Cavaliere, A., De Marchi, E., & Banterle, A. (2017). Investigation on the role of consumer health orientation in the use of food labels. *Public Health, 147*, 119–127.

3. Miller, L. M., & Cassady, D. L. (2015). The effects of nutrition knowledge on food label use. A review of the literature. *Appetite, 92*, 207–216.

4. Haidar, A., et al. (2017). Self-reported use of nutrition labels to make food choices is associated with healthier dietary behaviours in adolescents. *Public Health Nutrition, 20*(13), 2329–2339.

5. Buyuktuncer, Z., et al. (2018). Promoting a healthy diet in young adults: The role of nutrition labeling. *Nutrients, 10*(10).

6. Christoph, M. J., et al. (2018). Nutrition facts panels: Who uses them, what do they use, and how does use relate to dietary intake? *Journal of the Academy of Nutrition and Dietetics, 118*(2), 217–228.

7. Jackey, B. A., Cotugna, N., & Orsega-Smith, E. (2017). Food label knowledge, usage and attitudes of older adults. *Journal of Nutrition in Gerontology and Geriatrics, 36*(1), 31–47.

8. Institute of Medicine (U.S.) Committee on the Nutrition Components of Food Labeling. (1990). *Nutrition labeling: Issues and directions for the 1990s*. Washington, DC: National Academies Press (U.S.).

9. Department of Health and Human Services. (2016). *Food labeling: REVISION of the nutrition and supplement facts labels*. U.S. Food and Drug Administration.

10. Gorski Findling, M. T., et al. (2018). Comparing five front-of-pack nutrition labels' influence on consumers' perceptions and purchase intentions. *Preventive Medicine, 106*, 114–121.

11. Egnell, M., et al. (2018). Objective understanding of Nutri-score front-of-package nutrition label according to individual characteristics of subjects: Comparisons with other format labels. *PLoS One, 13*(8), e0202095.

12. Egnell, M., et al. (2018). Objective understanding of front-of-package nutrition labels: An international comparative experimental study across 12 countries. *Nutrients, 10*(10).

13. Ducrot, P., et al. (2016). Impact of different front-of-pack nutrition labels on consumer purchasing intentions: A randomized controlled trial. *American Journal of Preventive Medicine, 50*(5), 627–636.

14. Fern, E. B., et al. (2015). The Nutrient Balance Concept: A new quality metric for composite meals and diets. *PLoS One, 10*(7), e0130491.

15. Lehmann, U., et al. (2017). Nutrient profiling for product reformulation: Public health impact and benefits for the consumer. *Proceedings of the Nutrition Society, 76*(3), 255–264.

16. Drewnowski, A. (2017). Uses of nutrient profiling to address public health needs: From regulation to reformulation. *Proceedings of the Nutrition Society, 76*(3), 220–229.

17. U.S. Department of Health and Human Services. (2013). *A food labeling guide: Guidance for industry*. College Park, MD: Center for Food Safety and Applied Nutrition, FDA.

18. U.S. Department of Agriculture. *National organic program*. www.ams.usda.gov/rules-regulations/organic. Published 2019. [Accessed 7 May 2019].

19. Brantsaeter, A. L., et al. (2017). Organic food in the diet: Exposure and health implications. *Annual Review of Public Health, 38*, 295–313.

20. Hurtado-Barroso, S., et al. (2019). Organic food and the impact on human health. *Critical Reviews in Food Science and Nutrition, 59*(4), 704–714.

21. Mie, A., et al. (2017). Human health implications of organic food and organic agriculture: A comprehensive review. *Environmental Health, 16*(1), 111.

22. U.S. Department of Agriculture and Economic Research Service. (2018). *Adoption of genetically engineered crops in the U.S.*. Washington, DC: National Agricultural Statistics Service, U.S. Department of Agriculture.

23. Edge, M. S., et al. (2018). 2015 evidence analysis library systematic review on advanced technology in food production. *Journal of the Academy of Nutrition and Dietetics, 118*(6), 1106–1127. e9.

24. U.S. Food and Drug Administration. *Food irradiation: What you need to know*. www.fda.gov/food/resourcesforyou/consumers/ucm261680.htm. Published 2018. [Accessed 22 April 2019].

25. Marder, E. P., et al. (2018). Preliminary incidence and trends of infections with pathogens transmitted commonly through food—foodborne diseases active surveillance network, 10 U.S. sites, 2006–2017. *Morbidity and Mortality Weekly Report, 67*(11), 324–328.

26. U.S. Department of Health and Human Services. *Healthy People 2030*. health.gov/healthypeople. Published 2020. [Accessed 28 April, 2021].

27. Dewey-Mattia, D., et al. (2018). Surveillance for foodborne disease outbreaks—United States, 2009–2015. *MMWR Surveillance Summaries, 67*(10), 1–11.

28. Centers for Disease Control and Prevention. (2018). *National salmonella surveillance annual report, 2016*. Atlanta: U.S. Department of Health and Human Services, CDC.

29. Centers for Disease Control and Prevention. (2018). *National shigella surveillance annual report, 2016*. Atlanta: U.S. Department of Health and Human Services, CDC.

30. Madjunkov, M., Chaudhry, S., & Ito, S. (2017). Listeriosis during pregnancy. *Archives of Gynecology and Obstetrics, 296*(2), 143–152.

31. Centers for Disease Control and Prevention. (2018). *National Shiga toxin-producing Escherichia coli (STEC) Surveillance Annual Report, 2016*. Atlanta: U.S. Department of Health and Human Services, CDC.

32. Jacobs Slifka, K. M., Newton, A. E., & Mahon, B. E. (2017). Vibrio alginolyticus infections in the USA, 1988–2012. *Epidemiology and Infection, 145*(7), 1491–1499.

33. Centers for Disease Control and Prevention. (2018). *Surveillance for foodborne disease outbreaks, United States, 2016, annual report*. Atlanta: U.S. Department of Health and Human Services, CDC.

34. Lanphear, B. P., et al. (2018). Low-level lead exposure and mortality in U.S. adults: A population-based cohort study. *Lancet Public Health, 3*(4), e177–e184.

35. Alvarez-Ortega, N., Caballero-Gallardo, K., & Olivero-Verbel, J. (2017). Low blood lead levels impair intellectual and hematological function in children from Cartagena, Caribbean coast of Colombia. *Journal of Trace Elements in Medicine & Biology, 44*, 233–240.

36. Wu, Y., et al. (2018). The relationship of children's intelligence quotient and blood lead and zinc levels: A meta-analysis and system review. *Biological Trace Element Research, 182*(2), 185–195.

37. Huang, S., et al. (2016). Childhood blood lead levels and symptoms of Attention Deficit Hyperactivity Disorder (ADHD): A cross-sectional study of Mexican children. *Environmental Health Perspectives, 124*(6), 868–874.

38. Barg, G., et al. (2018). Association of low lead levels with behavioral problems and executive function deficits in schoolers from Montevideo, Uruguay. *International Journal of Environmental Research and Public Health, 15*(12).

39. Gump, B. B., et al. (2017). Background lead and mercury exposures: Psychological and behavioral problems in children. *Environmental Research, 158*, 576–582.

40. O'Connor, D., et al. (2018). Lead-based paint remains a major public health concern: A critical review of global production, trade, use, exposure, health risk, and implications. *Environment International, 121*(Pt 1), 85–101.

41. Shen, Z., et al. (2018). Lead-based paint in children's toys sold on China's major online shopping platforms. *Environmental Pollution, 241*, 311–318.

42. Rocha, A., & Trujillo, K. A. (2019). Neurotoxicity of low-level lead exposure: History, mechanisms of action, and behavioral effects in humans and preclinical models. *Neurotoxicology, 73*, 58–80.

43. Reuben, A., et al. (2017). Association of childhood blood lead levels with cognitive function and socioeconomic status at age 38 years and with IQ change and socioeconomic mobility between childhood and adulthood. *Journal of the American Medical Association, 317*(12), 1244–1251.

44. Shah-Kulkarni, S., et al. (2016). Neurodevelopment in early childhood affected by prenatal lead exposure and iron intake. *Medicine (Baltimore), 95*(4), e2508.

45. Food and Agricultural Organization of the United Nations. (2018). *The state of food security and nutrition in the world 2018: Building climate resilience for food security and nutrition.* Rome, Italy: Food and Agricultural Organization of the United Nations.

46. Committee on World Food Security. (2017). *Global Strategic Framework for Food Security and Nutrition (GSF).* Rome, Italy: Food and Agriculture Organization of the United Nations.

47. Coleman-Jensen, A., et al. (2019). *Household food security in the United States in 2018, ERR-270.* U.S. Department of Agriculture, Economic Research Service.

48. United States Department of Agriculture. (2018). *Food and Nutrition Service Nutrition Program fact sheet; Commodity Supplemental Food Program.* Washington, DC: United States Department of Agriculture.

49. Food and Nutrition Services. (2019). *Supplemental Nutrition Assistance Program participation and costs.* Washington, DC: U.S. Department of Agriculture.

50. Food and Nutrition Services. (2019). *WIC program participation and costs.* Washington, DC: U.S. Department of Agriculture.

51. Food and Nutrition Services. (2019). *Monthly data–state level participation by category and program costs.* Washington, DC: U.S. Department of Agriculture.

52. U.S. Department of Agriculture. (2012). *Nutrition standards in the National School Lunch and School Breakfast Programs; final rule.* Washington, DC: Food and Nutrition Service, Federal Register.

53. Center for Nutrition Policy and Promotion. (2019). *USDA food plans: Cost of food at home at four levels U.S. average, February 2019.* Washington, DC: U.S. Food and Nutrition Service, U.S. Department of Agriculture.

CHAPTER 14

1. Emilien, C., & Hollis, J. H. (2017). A brief review of salient factors influencing adult eating behaviour. *Nutrition Research Reviews, 30*(2), 233–246.

2. Russell, C. G., & Russell, A. (2018). Biological and psychosocial processes in the development of children's appetitive traits: Insights from developmental theory and research. *Nutrients, 10*(6).

3. Tarragon, E., & Moreno, J. J. (2017). Role of endocannabinoids on sweet taste perception, food preference, and obesity-related disorders. *Chemical Senses, 43*(1), 3–16.

4. Garg, S., Nurgali, K., & Mishra, V. K. (2016). Food proteins as source of opioid peptides—a review. *Current Medicinal Chemistry, 23*(9), 893–910.

5. Ogle, A. D., et al. (2017). Influence of cartoon media characters on children's attention to and preference for food and beverage products. *Journal of the Academy of Nutrition and Dietetics, 117*(2), 265–270.e2.

6. Harris, J. L., & Kalnova, S. S. (2018). Food and beverage TV advertising to young children: Measuring exposure and potential impact. *Appetite, 123*, 49–55.

7. Coleman-Jensen, A., Rabbitt, M. P., Gregory, C. A., & Singh, A. (2018). *Household food security in the United States in 2017, ERR-256.* U.S. Department of Agriculture, Economic Research Service.

8. Fulgoni, V., III, & Drewnowski, A. (2019). An economic gap between the recommended healthy food patterns and existing diets of minority groups in the U.S. National Health and Nutrition Examination Survey 2013–14. *Frontiers in Nutrition, 6*, 37.

9. Berkowitz, S. A., et al. (2018). Food insecurity and health care expenditures in the United States, 2011-2013. *Health Services Research, 53*(3), 1600–1620.

10. Holben, D. H., & Marshall, M. B. (2017). Position of the Academy of Nutrition and Dietetics: Food insecurity in the United States. *Journal of the Academy of Nutrition and Dietetics, 117*(12), 1991–2002.

11. Wright, A., Smith, K. E., & Hellowell, M. (2017). Policy lessons from health taxes: A systematic review of empirical studies. *BMC Public Health, 17*(1), 583.

12. Setiloane, K. T. (2016). Beyond the melting pot and salad bowl views of cultural diversity: Advancing cultural diversity education of nutrition educators. *Journal of Nutrition Education and Behavior, 48*(9), 664–668.e1.

13. United States Census Bureau. (2017). *Profile America facts for features: CB17-FF.17.* Hispanic heritage month 2017. United States Department of Commerce Economics and Statistics Administration.

14. United States Census Bureau. (2018). *Profile America facts for features: CB18-FF.09 American Indian and Alaska native heritage month: November 2018.* United States Department of Commerce Economics and Statistics Administration.

15. Centers for Disease Control and Prevention. (2017). *National diabetes statistics report, 2017.* Atlanta: Centers for Disease Control and Prevention.

16. United States Census Bureau. *Quick facts United States.* www.census.gov/quickfacts/fact/table/US/RHI225217#RHI225217. Published 2019. [Accessed 18 June 2019].

17. Mintz, S. *The Gilder Lehrman Institute of American History. Facts about the slave trade and slavery.* www.gilderlehrman.org/content/historical-context-facts-about-slave-trade-and-slavery. Published 2019. [Accessed 18 June 2019].

18. Bhupathiraju, S. N., et al. (2018). Dietary patterns among Asian Indians living in the United States have distinct metabolomic profiles that are associated with cardiometabolic risk. *Journal of Nutrition, 148*(7), 1150–1159.

19. Dinu, M., et al. (2018). Mediterranean diet and multiple health outcomes: An umbrella review of meta-analyses of observational studies and randomised trials. *European Journal of Clinical Nutrition, 72*(1), 30–43.

20. United States Department of Labor Blog. *Women of working age*. www.dol.gov/wb/stats/NEWSTATS/latest/demographics.htm#wwcivilian. Published 2019. [Accessed 18 June 2019].

21. United States Department of Labor Blog. *12 stats about working women*. blog.dol.gov/2017/03/01/12-stats-about-working-women. Published 2019. [Accessed 18 June 2019].

22. Todd, J. E. (2017). Changes in consumption of food away from home and intakes of energy and other nutrients among U.S. working-age adults, 2005–2014. *Public Health Nutrition, 20*(18), 3238–3246.

23. Jones, B. L. (2018). Making time for family meals: Parental influences, home eating environments, barriers and protective factors. *Physiology & Behavior, 193*(Pt B), 248–251.

24. Kant, A. K. (2018). Eating patterns of U.S. adults: Meals, snacks, and time of eating. *Physiology & Behavior, 193*(Pt B), 270–278.

25. Kant, A. K., & Graubard, B. I. (2015). 40-year trends in meal and snack eating behaviors of American adults. *Journal of the Academy of Nutrition and Dietetics, 115*(1), 50–63.

26. Young, L. R., & Nestle, M. (2003). Expanding portion sizes in the U.S. marketplace: Implications for nutrition counseling. *Journal of the American Dietetic Association, 103*(2), 231–234.

27. McCrory, M. A., et al. (2019). Fast-food offerings in the United States in 1986, 1991, and 2016 show large increases in food variety, portion size, dietary energy, and selected micronutrients. *Journal of the Academy of Nutrition and Dietetics, 119*(6), 923–933.

28. Steenhuis, I., & Poelman, M. (2017). Portion size: Latest developments and interventions. *Current Obesity Reports, 6*(1), 10–17.

29. Zuraikat, F. M., et al. (2018). Comparing the portion size effect in women with and without extended training in portion control: A follow-up to the portion-control strategies trial. *Appetite, 123*, 334–342.

30. Stern, D., Ng, S. W., & Popkin, B. M. (2016). The nutrient content of U.S. household food purchases by store type. *American Journal of Preventive Medicine, 50*(2), 180–190.

CHAPTER 15

1. Hales, C. M., et al. (2018). Trends in obesity and severe obesity prevalence in us youth and adults by sex and age, 2007–2008 to 2015–2016. *Journal of the American Medical Association, 319*(16), 1723–1725.

2. National Center for Health Statistics. (2018). *Prevalence of overweight, obesity, and severe obesity among adults aged 20 and over: United States, 1960–1962 through 2015–2016*. Hyattsville, MD: U.S. Government Printing Office.

3. Loos, R. J. F., & Janssens, A. (2017). Predicting polygenic obesity using genetic information. *Cell Metabolism, 25*(3), 535–543.

4. Rost, S., et al. (2018). New indexes of body fat distribution and sex-specific risk of total and cause-specific mortality: A prospective cohort study. *BMC Public Health, 18*(1), 427.

5. Teigen, L. M., et al. (2017). The use of technology for estimating body composition: Strengths and weaknesses of common modalities in a clinical setting. *Nutrition in Clinical Practice, 32*(1), 20–29.

6. Haverkort, E. B., et al. (2015). Bioelectrical impedance analysis to estimate body composition in surgical and oncological patients: A systematic review. *European Journal of Clinical Nutrition, 69*(1), 3–13.

7. Mundi, M. S., Patel, J. J., & Martindale, R. (2019). Body composition technology: Implications for the ICU. *Nutrition in Clinical Practice, 34*(1), 48–58.

8. Bosy-Westphal, A., et al. (2017). Quantification of whole-body and segmental skeletal muscle mass using phase-sensitive 8-electrode medical bioelectrical impedance devices. *European Journal of Clinical Nutrition, 71*(9), 1061–1067.

9. Lowry, D. W., & Tomiyama, A. J. (2015). Air displacement plethysmography versus dual-energy x-ray absorptiometry in underweight, normal-weight, and overweight/obese individuals. *PLoS One, 10*(1), e0115086.

10. Delisle Nystrom, C., et al. (2018). The paediatric option for BodPod to assess body composition in preschool children: What fat-free mass density values should be used? *British Journal of Nutrition, 120*(7), 797–802.

11. Heymsfield, S. B., et al. (2016). Why are there race/ethnic differences in adult body mass index-adiposity relationships? A quantitative critical review. *Obesity Reviews, 17*(3), 262–275.

12. Santoro, A., et al. (2018). A cross-sectional analysis of body composition among healthy elderly from the European NU-AGE study: Sex and country specific features. *Frontiers in Physiology, 9*, 1693.

13. The Global BMI Mortality Collaboration. (2016). Body-mass index and all-cause mortality: Individual-participant-data meta-analysis of 239 prospective studies in four continents. *Lancet, 388*(10046), 776–786.

14. Baskaran, C., Misra, M., & Klibanski, A. (2017). Effects of anorexia nervosa on the endocrine system. *Pediatr Endocrinol Rev, 14*(3), 302–311.

15. Grigsby, M. R., et al. (2019). Low body mass index is associated with higher odds of COPD and lower lung function in low- and middle-income countries. *Journal of Chronic Obstructive Pulmonary Disease, 16*, 1–8.

16. Hruby, A., & Hu, F. B. (2015). The epidemiology of obesity: A big picture. *Pharmacoeconomics, 33*(7), 673–689.

17. Global Burden of Disease 2015 Obesity Collaborators. (2017). Health effects of overweight and obesity in 195 countries over 25 years. *New England Journal of Medicine, 377*(1), 13–27.

18. Bischoff, S. C., et al. (2017). Towards a multidisciplinary approach to understand and manage obesity and related diseases. *Clinical Nutrition, 36*(4), 917–938.

19. Beaulac, J., & Sandre, D. (2017). Critical review of bariatric surgery, medically supervised diets, and behavioural interventions for weight management in adults. *Perspectives in Public Health, 137*(3), 162–172.

20. Carter, S., Clifton, P. M., & Keogh, J. B. (2018). Effect of intermittent compared with continuous energy restricted diet on glycemic control in patients with type 2 diabetes: A randomized noninferiority trial. *JAMA Network Open, 1*(3), e180756.

21. Chin, S. H., Kahathuduwa, C. N., & Binks, M. (2016). Physical activity and obesity: What we know and what we need to know. *Obesity Reviews, 17*(12), 1226–1244.

22. Zhang, Y., et al. (1994). Positional cloning of the mouse obese gene and its human homologue. *Nature, 372*(6505), 425–432.

23. Cui, H., Lopez, M., & Rahmouni, K. (2017). The cellular and molecular bases of leptin and ghrelin resistance in obesity. *Nature Reviews Endocrinology, 13*(6), 338–351.

24. Farooqi, I. S., & O'Rahilly, S. (2014). 20 years of leptin: Human disorders of leptin action. *Journal of Endocrinology, 223*(1), T63–T70.

25. Wabitsch, M., et al. (2015). Biologically inactive leptin and early-onset extreme obesity. *New England Journal of Medicine, 372*(1), 48–54.

26. Ozsu, E., Ceylaner, S., & Onay, H. (2017). Early-onset severe obesity due to complete deletion of the leptin gene in a boy. *Journal of Pediatric Endocrinology & Metabolism, 30*(11), 1227–1230.

27. Lv, Y., et al. (2018). Ghrelin, a gastrointestinal hormone, regulates energy balance and lipid metabolism. *Bioscience Reports, 38*(5).

28. Thaker, V. V. (2017). Genetic and epigenetic causes of obesity. *Pediatricians Adolescent Medicine State of the Art Reviews, 28*(2), 379–405.

29. Lin, X., et al. (2017). Developmental pathways to adiposity begin before birth and are influenced by genotype, prenatal environment and epigenome. *BMC Medicine, 15*(1), 50.

30. van Dijk, S. J., et al. (2015). Recent developments on the role of epigenetics in obesity and metabolic disease. *Clinical Epigenetics, 7*, 66.

31. Vogelezang, S., et al. (2015). Adult adiposity susceptibility loci, early growth and general and abdominal fatness in childhood. The generation R study. *International Journal of Obesity (Lond), 39*, 1001–1009.

32. Ogata, B. N., & Hayes, D. (2014). Position of the Academy of Nutrition and Dietetics: Nutrition guidance for healthy children ages 2 to 11 years. *Journal of the Academy of Nutrition and Dietetics, 114*(8), 1257–1276.

33. Calonne, J., et al. (2019). Reduced skeletal muscle protein turnover and thyroid hormone metabolism in adaptive thermogenesis that facilitates body fat recovery during weight regain. *Frontiers in Endocrinology (Lausanne), 10*, 119.

34. Sachdev, M., et al. (2002). Effect of fenfluramine-derivative diet pills on cardiac valves: A meta-analysis of observational studies. *American Heart Journal, 144*(6), 1065–1073.

35. Rosa-Goncalves, P., & Majerowicz, D. (2019). Pharmacotherapy of obesity: Limits and perspectives. *American Journal of Cardiovascular Drugs, 19*(4), 349–364.

36. Raynor, H. A., & Champagne, C. M. (2016). Position of the Academy of Nutrition and Dietetics: Interventions for the treatment of overweight and obesity in adults. *Journal of the Academy of Nutrition and Dietetics, 116*(1), 129–147.

37. Fox, W., et al. (2019). Long-term micronutrient surveillance after gastric bypass surgery in an integrated healthcare system. *Surgery for Obesity and Related Diseases, 15*(3), 389–395.

38. Jensen, M. D., et al. (2014). 2013 AHA/ACC/TOS guideline for the management of overweight and obesity in adults: A report of the American College of Cardiology/American Heart Association Task Force on Practice Guidelines and The Obesity Society. *Circulation, 129*(25 Suppl. 2), S102–S138.

39. Yannakoulia, M., et al. (2019). Dietary modifications for weight loss and weight loss maintenance. *Metabolism, 92*, 153–162.

40. U.S. Department of Agriculture and U.S. Department of Health and Human Services. (December 2020). *Dietary Guidelines for Americans, 2020-2025* (9th ed.). Available at: www.dietaryguidelines.gov.

41. Academy of Nutrition and Dietetics. (2019). *Nutrition Care Manual*. Chicago, IL: Academy of Nutrition and Dietetics.

42. Kask, J., et al. (2016). Mortality in women with anorexia nervosa: The role of comorbid psychiatric disorders. *Psychosomatic Medicine, 78*(8), 910–919.

43. Kask, J., et al. (2017). Anorexia nervosa in males: Excess mortality and psychiatric co-morbidity in 609 Swedish inpatients. *Psychological Medicine, 47*(8), 1489–1499.

44. Lavender, J. M., Brown, T. A., & Murray, S. B. (2017). Men, muscles, and eating disorders: An overview of traditional and muscularity-oriented disordered eating. *Current Psychiatry Reports, 19*(6), 32.

45. Stice, E., et al. (2017). Risk factors that predict future onset of each DSM-5 eating disorder: Predictive specificity in high-risk adolescent females. *Journal of Abnormal Psychology, 126*(1), 38–51.

46. Racine, S. E., et al. (2017). Eating disorder-specific risk factors moderate the relationship between negative urgency and binge eating: A behavioral genetic investigation. *Journal of Abnormal Psychology, 126*(5), 481–494.

47. Smith, K. E., et al. (2018). A systematic review of reviews of neurocognitive functioning in eating disorders: The state-of-the-literature and future directions. *International Journal of Eating Disorders, 51*(8), 798–821.

48. Chojnacki, C., et al. (2016). Serotonin and melatonin secretion in postmenopausal women with eating disorders. *Endokrynologia Polska, 67*(3), 299–304.

49. Afifi, T. O., et al. (2017). Child maltreatment and eating disorders among men and women in adulthood: Results from a nationally representative United States sample. *International Journal of Eating Disorders, 50*(11), 1281–1296.

50. Udo, T., & Grilo, C. M. (2018). Prevalence and correlates of DSM-5-defined eating disorders in a nationally representative sample of U.S. adults. *Biological Psychiatry, 84*(5), 345–354.

51. Erzegovesi, S., & Bellodi, L. (2016). Eating disorders. *CNS Spectrums, 21*(4), 304–309.

52. Rowe, E. (2017). Early detection of eating disorders in general practice. *Australian Family Physician, 46*(11), 833–838.

53. Castillo, M., & Weiselberg, E. (2017). Bulimia nervosa/purging disorder. *Current Problems in Pediatric and Adolescent Health Care, 47*(4), 85–94.

54. Udo, T., & Grilo, C. M. (2019). Psychiatric and medical correlates of DSM-5 eating disorders in a nationally representative sample of adults in the United States. *International Journal of Eating Disorders, 52*(1), 42–50.

55. Hilbert, A. (2019). Binge-eating disorder. *The Psychiatric Clinics of North America, 42*(1), 33–43.

CHAPTER 16

1. Clarke, T. C., Norris, T., & Schiller, J. S. (2017). *Early release of selected estimates based on data from January–June 2017 National Health Interview Survey*. National Center for Health Statistics.

2. U.S. Department of Health and Human Services. *Healthy People 2030.* health.gov/healthypeople. Published 2020. [Accessed 18 February, 2021].

3. U.S. Department of Health and Human Services. (2018). *Physical activity guidelines for Americans* (2nd ed.). Washington, DC: U.S. Department of Health and Human Services.

4. Riebe, D., et al. (2015). Updating ACSM's recommendations for exercise preparticipation health screening. *Medicine & Science in Sports & Exercise, 47*(11), 2473–2479.

5. Gordon, B., Chen, S., & Durstine, J. L. (2014). The effects of exercise training on the traditional lipid profile and beyond. *Current Sports Medicine Reports, 13*(4), 253–259.

6. Mann, S., Beedie, C., & Jimenez, A. (2014). Differential effects of aerobic exercise, resistance training and combined exercise modalities on cholesterol and the lipid profile: Review, synthesis and recommendations. *Sports Medicine, 44*(2), 211–221.

7. Benjamin, E. J., et al. (2018). Heart disease and stroke statistics-2018 update: A report from the American Heart Association. *Circulation, 137*(12), e67–e492.

8. Wasfy, M. M., & Baggish, A. L. (2016). Exercise dose in clinical practice. *Circulation, 133*(23), 2297–2313.

9. Whelton, P. K., et al. (2018). 2017 ACC/AHA/AAPA/ABC/ACPM/AGS/APHA/ASH/ASPC/NMA/PCNA guideline for the prevention, detection, evaluation, and management of high blood pressure in adults: A report of the American College of Cardiology/American Heart Association Task Force on clinical practice guidelines. *Journal of the American College of Cardiology, 71*(19), e127–e248.

10. Colberg, S. R., et al. (2016). Physical activity/exercise and diabetes: A position statement of the American Diabetes Association. *Diabetes Care, 39*(11), 2065–2079.

11. Hansen, D., et al. (2018). Exercise prescription in patients with different combinations of cardiovascular disease risk factors: A consensus statement from the EXPERT Working Group. *Sports Medicine, 48*(8), 1781–1797.

12. Mikkelsen, K., et al. (2017). Exercise and mental health. *Maturitas, 106*, 48–56.

13. American College of Sports Medicine. (2009). American College of Sports Medicine position stand. Progression models in resistance training for healthy adults. *Medicine & Science in Sports & Exercise, 41*(3), 687–708.

14. Schuna, J. M., Jr., Johnson, W. D., & Tudor-Locke, C. (2013). Adult self-reported and objectively monitored physical activity and sedentary behavior: NHANES 2005–2006. *International Journal of Behavioral Nutrition and Physical Activity, 10*, 126.

15. Patterson, R., et al. (2018). Sedentary behaviour and risk of all-cause, cardiovascular and cancer mortality, and incident type 2 diabetes: A systematic review and dose response meta-analysis. *European Journal of Epidemiology, 33*(9), 811–829.

16. Horowitz, J. F., & Klein, S. (2000). Lipid metabolism during endurance exercise. *American Journal of Clinical Nutrition, 72*(Suppl. 2), 558S–563S.

17. Thomas, D. T., Erdman, K. A., & Burke, L. M. (2016). Position of the Academy of Nutrition and Dietetics, Dietitians of Canada, and the American College of Sports Medicine: Nutrition and athletic performance. *Journal of the Academy of Nutrition and Dietetics, 116*(3), 501–528.

18. Mountjoy, M., et al. (2018). International Olympic Committee (IOC) consensus statement on relative energy deficiency in sport (RED-S): 2018 update. *International Journal of Sport Nutrition and Exercise Metabolism, 28*(4), 316–331.

19. Close, G. L., et al. (2019). Nutrition for the prevention and treatment of injuries in track and field athletes. *International Journal of Sport Nutrition and Exercise Metabolism*, 1–26.

20. McDermott, B. P., et al. (2017). National Athletic Trainers' Association position statement: Fluid replacement for the physically active. *Journal of Athletic Training, 52*(9), 877–895.

21. Burke, L. M., et al. (2011). Carbohydrates for training and competition. *Journal of Sports Science, 29*(Suppl. 1), S17–S27.

22. Jager, R., et al. (2017). International Society of Sports Nutrition position stand: Protein and exercise. *Journal of Sports Science, 14*, 20.

23. U.S. Department of Agriculture and Agricultural Research Service. (2016). *Nutrient intakes from food and beverages: Mean amounts consumed per individual, by gender and age, What We Eat in America, NHANES 2013–2014.*

24. Ormsbee, M. J., Bach, C. W., & Baur, D. A. (2014). Pre-exercise nutrition: The role of macronutrients, modified starches and supplements on metabolism and endurance performance. *Nutrients, 6*(5), 1782–1808.

25. Burke, L. M., et al. (2018). Toward a common understanding of diet-exercise strategies to manipulate fuel availability for training and competition preparation in endurance sport. *International Journal of Sport Nutrition and Exercise Metabolism, 28*(5), 451–463.

26. Phillips, S. M. (2014). A brief review of critical processes in exercise-induced muscular hypertrophy. *Sports Medicine, 44*(Suppl. 1), S71–S77.

27. Kanayama, G., & Pope, H. G., Jr. (2018). History and epidemiology of anabolic androgens in athletes and non-athletes. *Molecular and Cellular Endocrinology, 464*, 4–13.

CHAPTER 17

1. Herdman, T., & Kamitsuru, S. (2018). *NANDA International, nursing diagnoses: Definitions and classification 2018–2020* (11th ed.). New York: Thieme Publishers.

2. Swan, W. I., et al. (2017). Nutrition care process and model update: Toward realizing people-centered care and outcomes management. *Journal of the Academy of Nutrition and Dietetics, 117*(12), 2003–2014.

3. Murakami, K., & Livingstone, M. B. (2016). Prevalence and characteristics of misreporting of energy intake in U.S. children and adolescents: National Health and Nutrition Examination Survey (NHANES) 2003–2012. *British Journal of Nutrition, 115*(2), 294–304.

4. Murakami, K., & Livingstone, M. B. (2015). Prevalence and characteristics of misreporting of energy intake in U.S. adults: NHANES 2003–2012. *British Journal of Nutrition, 114*(8), 1294–1303.

5. Tyrovolas, S., et al. (2016). Weight perception, satisfaction, control, and low energy dietary reporting in the U.S. adult population: Results from the National Health and Nutrition Examination Survey 2007–2012. *Journal of the Academy of Nutrition and Dietetics, 116*(4), 579–589.

6. Garriguet, D. (2018). Accounting for misreporting when comparing energy intake across time in Canada. *Health Reports, 29*(5), 3–12.

7. Leech, R. M., et al. (2018). The role of energy intake and energy misreporting in the associations between eating patterns and adiposity. *European Journal of Clinical Nutrition, 72*(1), 142–147.

8. Shaw, P. A., et al. (2019). Calibration of activity-related energy expenditure in the Hispanic Community Health Study/Study of Latinos (HCHS/SOL). *Journal of Science and Medicine in Sport, 22*(3), 300–306.

9. Matthews, C. E., et al. (2018). Measurement of active and sedentary behavior in context of large epidemiologic studies. *Medicine & Science in Sports & Exercise, 50*(2), 266–276.

10. Sardinha, L. B., & Judice, P. B. (2017). Usefulness of motion sensors to estimate energy expenditure in children and adults: A narrative review of studies using DLW. *European Journal of Clinical Nutrition, 71*(3), 331–339.

11. Correa, J. B., et al. (2016). Evaluation of the ability of three physical activity monitors to predict weight change and estimate energy expenditure. *Applied Physiology Nutrition and Metabolism, 41*(7), 758–766.

12. Jeran, S., Steinbrecher, A., & Pischon, T. (2016). Prediction of activity-related energy expenditure using accelerometer-derived physical activity under free-living conditions: A systematic review. *International Journal of Obesity (Lond), 40*(8), 1187–1197.

13. Mogensen, K. M., et al. (2019). Academy of Nutrition and Dietetics/American Society for Parenteral and Enteral Nutrition consensus malnutrition characteristics: Usability and association with outcomes. *Nutrition in Clinical Practice, 34*(5), 657–665.

14. Garvey, W. T., et al. (2016). American Association of Clinical Endocrinologists and American College of Endocrinology comprehensive clinical practice guidelines for medical care of patients with obesity executive summary. *Endocrine Practice, 22*(7), 842–884. (Complete guidelines available at www.aace.com/publications/guidelines).

15. Park, Y. M., et al. (2017). The association between metabolic health, obesity phenotype and the risk of breast cancer. *International Journal of Cancer, 140*(12), 2657–2666.

16. Eckel, N., et al. (2015). Characterization of metabolically unhealthy normal-weight individuals: Risk factors and their associations with type 2 diabetes. *Metabolism, 64*(8), 862–871.

17. Tunstall-Pedoe, H., et al. (2017). Twenty-year predictors of peripheral arterial disease compared with coronary heart disease in the Scottish Heart Health Extended Cohort (SHHEC). *Journal of the American Heart Association, 6*(9).

18. Kazempour-Ardebili, S., et al. (2017). Metabolic mediators of the impact of general and central adiposity measures on cardiovascular disease and mortality risks in older adults: Tehran Lipid and Glucose Study. *Geriatrics and Gerontology International, 17*(11), 2017–2024.

19. Sobiczewski, W., et al. (2015). Superiority of waist circumference and body mass index in cardiovascular risk assessment in hypertensive patients with coronary heart disease. *Blood Press, 24*(2), 90–95.

20. Song, X., et al. (2015). Cardiovascular and all-cause mortality in relation to various anthropometric measures of obesity in Europeans. *Nutrition Metabolism and Cardiovascular Diseases, 25*(3), 295–304.

21. Bell, C. L., Lee, A. S., & Tamura, B. K. (2015). Malnutrition in the nursing home. *Current Opinion in Clinical Nutrition and Metabolic Care, 18*(1), 17–23.

22. Li, I. C., Kuo, H. T., & Lin, Y. C. (2013). The mediating effects of depressive symptoms on nutritional status of older adults in long-term care facilities. *The Journal of Nutrition, Health & Aging, 17*(7), 633–636.

23. van Nie-Visser, N. C., et al. (2014). Which characteristics of nursing home residents influence differences in malnutrition prevalence? An international comparison of the Netherlands, Germany and Austria. *British Journal of Nutrition, 111*(6), 1129–1136.

24. Little, M. O. (2018). Updates in nutrition and polypharmacy. *Current Opinion in Clinical Nutrition and Metabolic Care, 21*(1), 4–9.

25. Peter, S., et al. (2017). Public health relevance of drug-nutrition interactions. *European Journal of Nutrition, 56*(Suppl. 2), 23–36.

26. Mohn, E. S., et al. (2018). Evidence of drug-nutrient interactions with chronic use of commonly prescribed medications: An update. *Pharmaceutics, 10*(1).

27. National Center for Health Statistics. (2018). *Health, United States, 2017: With special feature on mortality.* Hyattsville, MD.

28. Boullata, J. I., & Hudson, L. M. (2012). Drug-nutrient interactions: A broad view with implications for practice. *Journal of the Academy of Nutrition and Dietetics, 112*(4), 506–517.

29. Paine, M. F., et al. (2006). A furanocoumarin-free grapefruit juice establishes furanocoumarins as the mediators of the grapefruit juice-felodipine interaction. *American Journal of Clinical Nutrition, 83*(5), 1097–1105.

30. Choi, J. G., et al. (2016). A comprehensive review of recent studies on herb-drug interaction: A focus on pharmacodynamic interaction. *The Journal of Alternative and Complementary Medicine, 22*(4), 262–279.

31. Chrubasik-Hausmann, S., Vlachojannis, J., & McLachlan, A. J. (2019). Understanding drug interactions with St John's wort (*Hypericum perforatum*): Impact of hyperforin content. *The Journal of Pharmacy and Pharmacology, 71*(1), 129–138.

32. Asher, G. N., Corbett, A. H., & Hawke, R. L. (2017). Common herbal dietary supplement-drug interactions. *American Family Physician, 96*(2), 101–107.

33. Soleymani, S., et al. (2017). Clinical risks of St John's wort (*Hypericum perforatum*) co-administration. *Expert Opinion on Drug Metabolism & Toxicology, 13*(10), 1047–1062.

34. Russo, E., et al. (2014). *Hypericum perforatum:* Pharmacokinetic, mechanism of action, tolerability, and clinical drug-drug interactions. *Phytotherapy Research, 28*(5), 643–655.

35. Agbabiaka, T. B., et al. (2017). Concurrent use of prescription drugs and herbal medicinal products in older adults: A systematic review. *Drugs Aging, 34*(12), 891–905.

CHAPTER 18

1. Walsh, T., et al. (2019). Fluoride toothpastes of different concentrations for preventing dental caries. *Cochrane Database of Systematic Reviews, 3*, Cd007868.

2. National Center for Health Statistics. (2018). *Health, United States, 2017: With special feature on mortality.* Hyattsville, MD.

3. Kossioni, A. E. (2018). The association of poor oral health parameters with malnutrition in older adults: A review considering the potential implications for cognitive impairment. *Nutrients, 10*(11).

4. Zelig, R., et al. (2019). Associations between dental occlusion and nutritional status in community-dwelling older adults (P01-017-19). *Current Developments in Nutrition, 3*(Suppl. 1).

5. Watson, S., et al. (2019). The impact of dental status on perceived ability to eat certain foods and nutrient intakes in older adults: Cross-sectional analysis of the UK National Diet and Nutrition Survey 2008–2014. *International Journal of Behavioral Nutrition and Physical Activity, 16*(1), 43.

6. Dye, B. A., Weatherspoon, D. J., & Lopez Mitnik, G. (2019). Tooth loss among older adults according to poverty status in the United States from 1999 through 2004 and 2009 through 2014. *The Journal of the American Dental Association, 150*(1), 9–23. e3.

7. Nawaz, S., & Tulunay-Ugur, O. E. (2018). Dysphagia in the older patient. *Otolaryngologic Clinics of North America, 51*(4), 769–777.

8. Patel, D. A., et al. (2018). Economic and survival burden of dysphagia among inpatients in the United States. *Diseases of the Esophagus, 31*(1), 1–7.

9. Tagliaferri, S., et al. (2019). The risk of dysphagia is associated with malnutrition and poor functional outcomes in a large population of outpatient older individuals. *Clinical Nutrition, 38*(6), 2684–2689.

10. Beck, A. M., et al. (2018). Systematic review and evidence based recommendations on texture modified foods and thickened liquids for adults (above 17 years) with oropharyngeal dysphagia—an updated clinical guideline. *Clinical Nutrition, 37*(6 Pt A), 1980–1991.

11. O'Keeffe, S. T. (2018). Use of modified diets to prevent aspiration in oropharyngeal dysphagia: Is current practice justified? *BMC Geriatrics, 18*(1), 167.

12. Kaneoka, A., et al. (2017). A systematic review and meta-analysis of pneumonia associated with thin liquid vs. thickened liquid intake in patients who aspirate. *Clinical Rehabilitation, 31*(8), 1116–1125.

13. Chen, J., & Brady, P. (2019). Gastroesophageal reflux disease: Pathophysiology, diagnosis, and treatment. *Gastroenterology Nursing, 42*(1), 20–28.

14. Academy of Nutrition and Dietetics. (2019). *Nutrition Care Manual.* Chicago, IL: Academy of Nutrition and Dietetics.

15. de Bortoli, N., et al. (2016). Voluntary and controlled weight loss can reduce symptoms and proton pump inhibitor use and dosage in patients with gastroesophageal reflux disease: A comparative study. *Diseases of the Esophagus, 29*(2), 197–204.

16. Park, S. K., et al. (2017). Weight loss and waist reduction is associated with improvement in gastroesophageal disease reflux symptoms: A longitudinal study of 15,295 subjects undergoing health checkups. *Neuro-Gastroenterology and Motility, 29*(5).

17. Kroch, D. A., & Madanick, R. D. (2017). Medical treatment of gastroesophageal reflux disease. *World Journal of Surgery, 41*(7), 1678–1684.

18. Oor, J. E., et al. (2017). Seventeen-year outcome of a randomized clinical trial comparing laparoscopic and conventional nissen fundoplication: A plea for patient counseling and clarification. *Annals of Surgery, 266*(1), 23–28.

19. Hooi, J. K. Y., et al. (2017). Global prevalence of *Helicobacter pylori* infection: Systematic review and meta-analysis. *Gastroenterology, 153*(2), 420–429.

20. Leow, A. H., et al. (2016). Time trends in upper gastrointestinal diseases and *Helicobacter pylori* infection in a multiracial Asian population—a 20-year experience over three time periods. *Alimentary Pharmacology & Therapeutics, 43*(7), 831–837.

21. Malmi, H., et al. (2014). Incidence and complications of peptic ulcer disease requiring hospitalisation have markedly decreased in Finland. *Alimentary Pharmacology & Therapeutics, 39*(5), 496–506.

22. Lanas, A., & Chan, F. K. L. (2017). Peptic ulcer disease. *Lancet, 390*(10094), 613–624.

23. Levenstein, S., et al. (2015). Psychological stress increases risk for peptic ulcer, regardless of *Helicobacter pylori* infection or use of nonsteroidal anti-inflammatory drugs. *Clinical Gastroenterology and Hepatology*, 13(3), 498–506.e1.

24. Levenstein, S., et al. (2017). Mental vulnerability, *Helicobacter pylori*, and incidence of hospital-diagnosed peptic ulcer over 28 years in a population-based cohort. *Scandinavian Journal of Gastroenterology*, 52(9), 954–961.

25. Deding, U., et al. (2016). Perceived stress as a risk factor for peptic ulcers: A register-based cohort study. *BMC Gastroenterology*, 16(1), 140.

26. Panduro, A., et al. (2017). Genes, emotions and gut microbiota: The next frontier for the gastroenterologist. *World Journal of Gastroenterology*, 23(17), 3030–3042.

27. Kim, N., et al. (2018). Mind-altering with the gut: Modulation of the gut-brain axis with probiotics. *Journal of Microbiology*, 56(3), 172–182.

28. Proctor, C., et al. (2017). Diet, gut microbiota and cognition. *Metabolic Brain Disease*, 32(1), 1–17.

29. Kim, Y. K., & Shin, C. (2018). The microbiota-gut-brain axis in neuropsychiatric disorders: Pathophysiological mechanisms and novel treatments. *Current Neuropharmacology*, 16(5), 559–573.

30. Bruce-Keller, A. J., Salbaum, J. M., & Berthoud, H. R. (2018). Harnessing gut microbes for mental health: Getting from here to there. *Biological Psychiatry*, 83(3), 214–223.

31. Strandwitz, P. (2018). Neurotransmitter modulation by the gut microbiota. *Brain Research*, 1693(Pt B), 128–133.

32. Min, J. Y., & Min, K. B. (2018). Cumulative exposure to nighttime environmental noise and the incidence of peptic ulcer. *Environment International*, 121(Pt 2), 1172–1178.

33. Konturek, P. C., Brzozowski, T., & Konturek, S. J. (2011). Stress and the gut: Pathophysiology, clinical consequences, diagnostic approach and treatment options. *Journal of Physiology & Pharmacology*, 62(6), 591–599.

34. Kempenich, J. W., & Sirinek, K. R. (2018). Acid peptic disease. *The Surgical Clinics of North America*, 98(5), 933–944.

35. Satoh, K., et al. (2016). Evidence-based clinical practice guidelines for peptic ulcer disease 2015. *Journal of Gastroenterology*, 51(3), 177–194.

36. Perez, S., et al. (2017). Redox signaling in the gastrointestinal tract. *Free Radical Biology and Medicine*, 104, 75–103.

37. Farzaei, M. H., Abdollahi, M., & Rahimi, R. (2015). Role of dietary polyphenols in the management of peptic ulcer. *World Journal of Gastroenterology*, 21(21), 6499–6517.

38. Shanahan, E. R., et al. (2018). Influence of cigarette smoking on the human duodenal mucosa-associated microbiota. *Microbiome*, 6(1), 150.

39. Li, L. F., et al. (2014). Cigarette smoking and gastrointestinal diseases: The causal relationship and underlying molecular mechanisms (review). *International Journal of Molecular Medicine*, 34(2), 372–380.

40. National Institute of Health. *Cystic fibrosis*. ghr.nlm.nih.gov/condition/cystic-fibrosis. Published 2019. [Accessed 25 June 2019].

41. Kelsey, R., et al. (2019). Cystic fibrosis-related diabetes: Pathophysiology and therapeutic challenges. *Clinical Medicine Insights: Endocrinology and Diabetes*, 12, 1179551419851770.

42. Turck, D., et al. (2016). ESPEN-ESPGHAN-ECFS guidelines on nutrition care for infants, children, and adults with cystic fibrosis. *Clinical Nutrition*, 35(3), 557–577.

43. Lima, C. A., et al. (2017). Bone mineral density and inflammatory bowel disease severity. *Brazilian Journal of Medical and Biological Research*, 50(12), e6374.

44. Weisshof, R., & Chermesh, I. (2015). Micronutrient deficiencies in inflammatory bowel disease. *Current Opinion in Clinical Nutrition and Metabolic Care*, 18(6), 576–581.

45. Portela, F., et al. (2016). Anaemia in patients with inflammatory bowel disease—a nationwide cross-sectional study. *Digestion*, 93(3), 214–220.

46. van der Sloot, K. W. J., et al. (2017). Inflammatory bowel diseases: Review of known environmental protective and risk factors involved. *Inflammatory Bowel Diseases*, 23(9), 1499–1509.

47. Gungor, D., et al. (2019). Infant milk-feeding practices and diagnosed celiac disease and inflammatory bowel disease in offspring: A systematic review. *American Journal of Clinical Nutrition*, 109(Suppl. 7), 838s–851s.

48. Castro, F., & de Souza, H. S. P. (2019). Dietary composition and effects in inflammatory bowel disease. *Nutrients*, 11(6).

49. Nishida, A., et al. (2018). Gut microbiota in the pathogenesis of inflammatory bowel disease. *Clinical Journal of Gastroenterology*, 11(1), 1–10.

50. Ng, S. C., et al. (2018). Worldwide incidence and prevalence of inflammatory bowel disease in the 21st century: A systematic review of population-based studies. *Lancet*, 390(10114), 2769–2778.

51. Ruemmele, F. M., et al. (2014). Consensus guidelines of ECCO/ESPGHAN on the medical management of pediatric Crohn's disease. *The Journal of Crohn's and Colitis*, 8(10), 1179–1207.

52. Leung, A. K. C., et al. (2019). Travelers' diarrhea: A clinical review. *Recent Patents on Inflammation & Allergy Drug Discovery*.

53. GBD 2017 Causes of Death Collaborators. (2018). Global, regional, and national age-sex-specific mortality for 282 causes of death in 195 countries and territories, 1980–2017: A systematic analysis for the Global Burden of Disease Study 2017. *Lancet*, 392(10159), 1736–1788.

54. Peery, A. F., et al. (2019). Burden and cost of gastrointestinal, liver, and pancreatic diseases in the United States: Update 2018. *Gastroenterology*, 156(1), 254–272.e11.

55. Schafmayer, C., et al. (2019). Genome-wide association analysis of diverticular disease points towards neuromuscular, connective tissue and epithelial pathomechanisms. *Gut*, 68(5), 854–865.

56. Maguire, L. H., et al. (2018). Genome-wide association analyses identify 39 new susceptibility loci for diverticular disease. *Nature Genetics*, 50(10), 1359–1365.

57. Tursi, A. (2019). Current and evolving concepts on the pathogenesis of diverticular disease. *Journal of Gastrointestinal and Liver Diseases*, 28, 225–235.

58. Sperber, A. D., et al. (2017). The global prevalence of IBS in adults remains elusive due to the heterogeneity of studies: A Rome Foundation working team literature review. *Gut*, 66(6), 1075–1082.

59. Quigley, E. M., et al. (2016). World Gastroenterology Organisation Global guidelines irritable bowel syndrome: A global perspective update September 2015. *Journal of Clinical Gastroenterology*, 50(9), 704–713.

60. Simren, M., Palsson, O. S., & Whitehead, W. E. (2017). Update on Rome IV Criteria for colorectal disorders: Implications for clinical practice. *Current Gastroenterology Reports*, 19(4), 15.

61. Holtmann, G. J., Ford, A. C., & Talley, N. J. (2016). Pathophysiology of irritable bowel syndrome. *Lancet Gastroenterol Hepatol*, 1(2), 133–146.

62. Wald, A. (2016). Constipation: Advances in diagnosis and treatment. *Journal of the American Medical Association*, 315(2), 185–191.

63. Sicherer, S. H., et al. (2017). Critical issues in food allergy: A National Academies consensus report. *Pediatrics*, 140(2).

64. Dunlop, J. H., & Keet, C. A. (2018). Epidemiology of food allergy. *Immunology and Allergy Clinics of North America*, 38(1), 13–25.

65. National Academies of Sciences, Engineering, and Medicine. (2017). *Finding a path to safety in food allergy: Assessment of the global burden, causes, prevention, management, and public policy*. Washington, DC: National Academies Press.

66. Stukus, D. R., et al. (2016). Use of food allergy panels by pediatric care providers compared with allergists. *Pediatrics, 138*(6).

67. Gupta, R. S., et al. (2010). Food allergy knowledge, attitudes, and beliefs of primary care physicians. *Pediatrics, 125*(1), 126–132.

68. Muraro, A., et al. (2014). EAACI food allergy and anaphylaxis guidelines: Diagnosis and management of food allergy. *Allergy, 69*(8), 1008–1025.

69. Lessen, R., & Kavanagh, K. (2015). Position of the Academy of Nutrition and Dietetics: Promoting and supporting breastfeeding. *Journal of the Academy of Nutrition and Dietetics, 115*(3), 444–449.

70. Leonard, M. M., et al. (2017). Celiac disease and nonceliac gluten sensitivity: A review. *Journal of the American Medical Association, 318*(7), 647–656.

71. Choung, R. S., et al. (2015). Trends and racial/ethnic disparities in gluten-sensitive problems in the United States: Findings from the National Health and Nutrition Examination Surveys from 1988 to 2012. *American Journal of Gastroenterology, 110*(3), 455–461.

72. Leonard, M. M., et al. (2015). Genetics and celiac disease: The importance of screening. *Expert Review of Gastroenterology & Hepatology, 9*(2), 209–215.

73. Husby, S., Murray, J. A., & Katzka, D. A. (2019). AGA clinical practice update on diagnosis and monitoring of celiac disease-changing utility of serology and histologic measures: Expert review. *Gastroenterology, 156*(4), 885–889.

74. Dennis, M., Lee, A. R., & McCarthy, T. (2019). Nutritional considerations of the gluten-free diet. *Gastroenterology Clinics of North America, 48*(1), 53–72.

75. Ibis, C., et al. (2017). Factors affecting liver regeneration in living donors after hepatectomy. *Medical Science Monitor, 23,* 5986–5993.

76. Tsang, L. L., et al. (2016). Impact of graft type in living donor liver transplantation: Remnant liver regeneration and outcome in donors. *Transplantation Proceedings, 48*(4), 1015–1017.

77. Neuman, M. G., et al. (2016). Non-alcoholic steatohepatitis: Clinical and translational research. *Journal of Pharmacy and Pharmaceutical Sciences, 19*(1), 8–24.

78. Neuman, M. G., et al. (2017). Alcohol, microbiome, life style influence alcohol and non-alcoholic organ damage. *Experimental and Molecular Pathology, 102*(1), 162–180.

79. Valenti, L., et al. (2016). Nonalcoholic fatty liver disease: Cause or consequence of type 2 diabetes? *Liver International, 36*(11), 1563–1579.

80. Bemeur, C., & Butterworth, R. F. (2015). Reprint of: Nutrition in the management of cirrhosis and its neurological complications. *Journal of Clinical and Experimental Hepatology, 5*(Suppl. 1), S131–S140.

81. Chiu, E., et al. (2019). Malnutrition impacts health-related quality of life in cirrhosis: A cross-sectional study. *Nutrition in Clinical Practice.*

82. Weber, S. N., et al. (2019). Genetics of gallstone disease revisited: Updated inventory of human lithogenic genes. *Current Opinion in Gastroenterology, 35*(2), 82–87.

83. Di Ciaula, A., et al. (2017). The role of diet in the pathogenesis of cholesterol gallstones. *Current Medicinal Chemistry, 24,* 1–17.

84. Rebholz, C., Krawczyk, M., & Lammert, F. (2018). Genetics of gallstone disease. *European Journal of Clinical Investigation, 48*(7), e12935.

85. Talseth, A., et al. (2016). Risk factors for requiring cholecystectomy for gallstone disease in a prospective population-based cohort study. *British Journal of Surgery, 103*(10), 1350–1357.

86. Khoo, A. K., et al. (2014). Cholecystectomy in English children: Evidence of an epidemic (1997-2012). *Journal of Pediatric Surgery, 49*(2), 284–248;discussion 288.

87. Murphy, P. B., et al. (2016). The increasing incidence of gallbladder disease in children: A 20 year perspective. *Journal of Pediatric Surgery, 51*(5), 748–752.

88. Walker, S. K., et al. (2013). Etiology and incidence of pediatric gallbladder disease. *Surgery, 154*(4), 927–931; discussion 931-933.

89. Greer, D., et al. (2018). Is 14 the new 40: Trends in gallstone disease and cholecystectomy in Australian children. *Pediatric Surgery International, 34*(8), 845–849.

90. Chilimuri, S., et al. (2017). Symptomatic gallstones in the young: Changing trends of the gallstone disease-related hospitalization in the state of New York: 1996–2010. *Journal of Clinical Medicine Research, 9*(2), 117–123.

91. Mayerle, J., et al. (2019). Genetics, cell biology, and pathophysiology of pancreatitis. *Gastroenterology, 156*(7), 1951–1968.e1.

92. Crockett, S. D., et al. (2018). American Gastroenterological Association Institute guideline on initial management of acute pancreatitis. *Gastroenterology, 154*(4), 1096–1101.

CHAPTER 19

1. National Center for Health Statistics. (2018). *Health, United States, 2017: With special feature on mortality.* Hyattsville, MD.

2. Wilson, P. W. F., et al. (2019). Systematic review for the 2018 AHA/ACC/AACVPR/AAPA/ABC/ACPM/ADA/AGS/APHA/ASPC/NLA/PCNA guideline on the management of blood cholesterol: A report of the American College of Cardiology/American Heart Association Task Force on clinical practice guidelines. *Circulation, 139*(25), e1144–e1161.

3. Jellinger, P. S., et al. (2017). American Association of Clinical Endocrinologists and American College of Endocrinology guidelines for management of dyslipidemia and prevention of cardiovascular disease. *Endocrine Practice, 23*(Suppl. 2), 1–87.

4. Grundy, S. M., et al. (2019). 2018 AHA/ACC/AACVPR/AAPA/ABC/ACPM/ADA/AGS/APHA/ASPC/NLA/PCNA guideline on the management of blood cholesterol: A report of the American College of Cardiology/American Heart Association Task Force on clinical practice guidelines. *Journal of the American College of Cardiology, 73*(24), e285–e350.

5. Nassef, Y., et al. (2019). Association between aerobic exercise and high-density lipoprotein cholesterol levels across various ranges of body mass index and waist-hip ratio and the modulating role of the hepatic lipase rs1800588 variant. *Genes (Basel), 10*(6).

6. Arnett, D. K., et al. (2019). 2019 ACC/AHA guideline on the primary prevention of cardiovascular disease. *Circulation,* Cir0000000000000678.

7. Micha, R., et al. (2017). Association between dietary factors and mortality from heart disease, stroke, and type 2 diabetes in the United States. *Journal of the American Medical Association, 317*(9), 912–924.

8. Benjamin, E. J., et al. (2018). Heart disease and stroke statistics-2018 update: A report from the American Heart Association. *Circulation, 137*(12), e67–e492.

9. Gac, P., et al. (2017). Exposure to cigarette smoke and the morphology of atherosclerotic plaques in the extracranial arteries assessed by computed tomography angiography in patients with essential hypertension. *Cardiovasc Toxicol, 17*(1), 67–78.

10. Mokdad, A. H., et al. (2018). The state of U.S. health, 1990–2016: Burden of diseases, injuries, and risk factors among U.S. states. *Journal of the American Medical Association, 319*(14), 1444–1472.

11. Academy of Nutrition and Dietetics. (2019). *Nutrition Care Manual.* Chicago, IL: Academy of Nutrition and Dietetics.

12. Dinu, M., et al. (2018). Mediterranean diet and multiple health outcomes: An umbrella review of meta-analyses of observational studies and randomised trials. *European Journal of Clinical Nutrition, 72*(1), 30–43.

13. Panagiotakos, D. B., et al. (2009). Mediterranean diet and inflammatory response in myocardial infarction survivors. *International Journal of Epidemiology, 38*(3), 856–866.

14. Schwingshackl, L., & Hoffmann, G. (2014). Mediterranean dietary pattern, inflammation and endothelial function: A systematic review and meta-analysis of intervention trials. *Nutrition Metabolism and Cardiovascular Diseases, 24*(9), 929–939.

15. Stallings, V. A., et al. (2019). The National Academies Collection: Reports funded by National Institutes of Health. *Dietary reference intakes for sodium and potassium.* Washington, DC: National Academies Press (U.S.), National Academy of Sciences.

16. U.S. Department of Agriculture and Agricultural Research Service. (2018). *Nutrient intakes from food and beverages: Mean amounts consumed per individual, by gender and age, What We Eat in America, NHANES 2015–2016.*

17. Whelton, P. K., et al. (2018). 2017 ACC/AHA/AAPA/ABC/ACPM/AGS/APHA/ASH/ASPC/NMA/PCNA guideline for the prevention, detection, evaluation, and management of high blood pressure in adults: A report of the American College of Cardiology/American Heart Association Task Force on clinical practice guidelines. *Hypertension, 71*(6), e13–e115.

18. Miliku, K., et al. (2016). Associations of maternal and paternal blood pressure patterns and hypertensive disorders during pregnancy with childhood blood pressure. *Journal of the American Heart Association, 5*(10).

19. Urbina, E. M., et al. (2019). Relation of blood pressure in childhood to self-reported hypertension in adulthood. *Hypertension, 73*(6), 1224–1230.

20. Susic, D., & Varagic, J. (2017). Obesity: A perspective from hypertension. *The Medical Clinics of North America, 101*(1), 139–157.

21. Seravalle, G., & Grassi, G. (2017). Obesity and hypertension. *Pharmacological Research, 122*, 1–7.

22. Appel, L. J., et al. (1997). A clinical trial of the effects of dietary patterns on blood pressure. DASH Collaborative Research Group. *New England Journal of Medicine, 336*(16), 1117–1124.

23. Chiavaroli, L., et al. (2019). DASH dietary pattern and cardiometabolic outcomes: An umbrella review of systematic reviews and meta-analyses. *Nutrients, 11*(2).

24. Siervo, M., et al. (2015). Effects of the Dietary Approach to Stop Hypertension (DASH) diet on cardiovascular risk factors: A systematic review and meta-analysis. *British Journal of Nutrition, 113*(1), 1–15.

25. Juraschek, S. P., et al. (2017). Effects of sodium reduction and the DASH diet in relation to baseline blood pressure. *Journal of the American College of Cardiology, 70*(23), 2841–2848.

26. Graudal, N. A., Hubeck-Graudal, T., & Jurgens, G. (2017). Effects of low sodium diet versus high sodium diet on blood pressure, renin, aldosterone, catecholamines, cholesterol, and triglyceride. *Cochrane Database of Systematic Reviews, 4*, Cd004022.

27. Yang, G. H., et al. (2018). Effects of a low salt diet on isolated systolic hypertension: A community-based population study. *Medicine (Baltimore), 97*(14), e0342.

28. Pimenta, E., et al. (2009). Effects of dietary sodium reduction on blood pressure in subjects with resistant hypertension: Results from a randomized trial. *Hypertension, 54*(3), 475–481.

29. Overwyk, K. J., et al. (2019). Trends in blood pressure and usual dietary sodium intake among children and adolescents, National Health and Nutrition Examination Survey 2003 to 2016. *Hypertension, 74*(2), 260–266.

30. Newberry, S. J., et al. (2018). AHRQ comparative effectiveness reviews. In *Sodium and potassium intake: Effects on chronic disease outcomes and risks.* Rockville, MD: Agency for Healthcare Research and Quality (U.S.).

31. Luzardo, L., Noboa, O., & Boggia, J. (2015). Mechanisms of salt-sensitive hypertension. *Current Hypertension Reviews, 11*(1), 14–21.

32. Armando, I., Villar, V. A., & Jose, P. A. (2015). Genomics and pharmacogenomics of salt-sensitive hypertension. *Current Hypertension Reviews, 11*(1), 49–56.

33. Pilic, L., Pedlar, C. R., & Mavrommatis, Y. (2016). Salt-sensitive hypertension: Mechanisms and effects of dietary and other lifestyle factors. *Nutrition Reviews, 74*(10), 645–658.

34. U.S. Department of Agriculture and U.S. Department of Health and Human Services. (December 2020). *Dietary Guidelines for Americans, 2020-2025* (9th ed.). Available at: www.dietaryguidelines.gov.

35. Aburto, N. J., et al. (2013). Effect of increased potassium intake on cardiovascular risk factors and disease: Systematic review and meta-analyses. *British Medical Journal, 346*, f1378.

36. Yang, Y., et al. (2017). Association of husband smoking with wife's hypertension status in over 5 million Chinese females aged 20 to 49 years. *Journal of the American Heart Association, 6*(3).

37. Liu, M. Y., et al. (2017). Association between psychosocial stress and hypertension: A systematic review and meta-analysis. *Neurological Research, 39*(6), 573–580.

38. Blom, K., et al. (2014). Hypertension analysis of stress reduction using mindfulness meditation and yoga: Results from the harmony randomized controlled trial. *American Journal of Hypertension, 27*(1), 122–129.

39. Nagele, E., et al. (2014). Clinical effectiveness of stress-reduction techniques in patients with hypertension: Systematic review and meta-analysis. *Journal of Hypertension, 32*(10), 1936–1944; discussion 1944.

40. Kit, B. K., et al. (2015). Prevalence of and trends in dyslipidemia and blood pressure among U.S. children and adolescents, 1999–2012. *JAMA Pediatrics, 169*(3), 272–279.

41. Perak, A. M., et al. (2019). Trends in levels of lipids and apolipoprotein B in U.S. youths aged 6 to 19 years, 1999-2016. *Journal of the American Medical Association, 321*(19), 1895–1905.

42. Interator, H., et al. (2017). Distinct lipoprotein curves in normal weight, overweight, and obese children and adolescents. *Journal of Pediatric Gastroenterology and Nutrition, 65*(6), 673–680.

CHAPTER 20

1. Centers for Disease Control and Prevention. (2017). *National diabetes statistics report: Estimates of diabetes and its burden in the United States, 2017.* Atlanta: U.S. Department of Health and Human Services.

2. American Diabetes Association. (2019). Standards of medical care in diabetes–2019: Classification and diagnosis of diabetes. *Diabetes Care, 42*(Suppl. 1), S13–S28.

3. Skyler, J. S., et al. (2017). Differentiation of diabetes by pathophysiology, natural history, and prognosis. *Diabetes, 66*, 241–255.

4. Mayer-Davis, E. J., et al. (2017). Incidence trends of type 1 and type 2 diabetes among youth, 2002–2012. *The New England Journal of Medicine, 376*, 1419–1429.

5. Casegrande, S. S., et al. (2018). Prevalence of gestation diabetes and subsequent type 2 diabetes among U.S. women. *Diabetes Research and Clinical Practice, 141*, 200–208.

6. ACOG Practice Bulletin No. 190. (2018). Gestational diabetes mellitus. *Obstetrics & Gynecology, 131*, e49–e64.

7. American Diabetes Association. (2019). Standards of medical care in diabetes–2019: Management of diabetes in pregnancy. *Diabetes Care, 42*(Suppl. 1), S165–S172.

8. Butalia, S., et al. (2017). Short- and long-term outcomes of metformin compared with insulin alone in pregnancy: A systematic review and meta-analysis. *Diabetic Medicine, 34*(1), 27–36.

9. Song, R., et al. (2017). Comparison of glyburide and insulin in the management of gestational diabetes: A meta-analysis. *PLoS One, 12*, e0182488.

10. Aroda, V. R., et al. (2015). Diabetes Prevention Program Research Group. The effect of lifestyle intervention and metformin on preventing or delaying diabetes among women with and without gestational diabetes: The Diabetes Prevention Program Outcomes Study 10-year follow-up. *The Journal of Clinical Endocrinology and Metabolism, 100*(4), 1646–1653.

11. Knowler, W. C., et al. (2002). Reduction in incidence of type diabetes with lifestyle intervention or metformin. *New England Journal of Medicine, 346*(6), 393–403.

12. Diabetes Prevention Program Research Group., et al. (2009). 10-year follow-up of diabetes incidence and weight loss in the Diabetes Prevention Program Outcomes Study. *Lancet, 374*, 1677–1686.

13. Diabetes Prevention Program Research Group. (2015). Long-term effects of lifestyle intervention or metformin on diabetes development and microvascular complications over 15-year follow up. *The Lancet Diabetes & Endocrinology, 3*. 886-875.

14. Bird, S. R., et al. (2017). Update on the effects of physical activity on insulin sensitivity in humans. *BMJ Open Sport and Exercise Medicine, 2*(1), e000143.

15. Liu, Y., et al. (2019). Resistance exercise intensity is correlated with attenuation of HbA1c and insulin in patients with type 2 diabetes: A systematic review and meta-analysis. *International Journal of Environmental Research and Public Health, 16*(1), 140.

16. Rockette-Wagner, B., et al. (2017). Activity and sedentary time 10 years after a successful lifestyle intervention: The Diabetes Prevention Program. *American Journal of Preventive Medicine, 52*(3), 292–299.

17. Wilding, J. P. (2014). The role of the kidneys in glucose homeostasis in type 2 diabetes: Clinical implications and therapeutic significance through sodium glucose co-transporter 2 inhibitors. *Metabolism, 63*(10), 1228–1237.

18. Centers for Disease Control and Prevention. *Watch out for diabetic retinopathy.* www.cdc.gov/features/diabetic-retinopathy/. Published 2018. [Accessed 24 May 2019].

19. American Diabetes Association. (2019). Standards of medical care in diabetes–2019: Microvasular complications and foot care. *Diabetes Care, 42*(Suppl. 1), S124–S138.

20. Gubitosi-Klug, R. A., et al. (2016). Effects of prior intensive insulin therapy and risk factors on patient-reported visual function outcomes in the DCCT/EDIC. *JAMA Ophthalmology, 134*(2), 137–145.

21. Herman, W. H., et al. (2018). What are the clinical, quality-of-life, and cost consequences of 30 years of excellent vs. poor glycemic control in type 1 diabetes? *Journal of Diabetes and Its Complications, 32*(10), 911–915.

22. Ruospo, M., et al. (2017). Glucose targets for preventing diabetic kidney disease and its progression. *Cochrane Database of Systematic Reviews, 6*, CD010137.

23. Tiftikcioglu, B. I., et al. (2016). Autonomic neuropathy and endothelial dysfunction in patients with impaired glucose tolerance or type 2 diabetes mellitus. *Medicine (Baltimore), 95*(14), e3340.

24. Zilliox, L. A., et al. (2015). Clinical neuropathy scales in neuropathy associated with impaired glucose tolerance. *Journal of Diabetes and Its Complications, 29*(3), 372–377.

25. Pop-Busui, R., et al. (2016). Diabetic neuropathy: A position statement by the American Diabetes Association. *Diabetes Care, 40*(1), 136–154.

26. American Diabetes Association. (2019). Standards of medical care in diabetes–2019: Cardiovascular disease and risk management. *Diabetes Care, 42*(Suppl. 1), S103–S123.

27. Huo, X., et al. (2016). Risk of non-fatal cardiovascular diseases in early-onset versus late-onset type 2 diabetes in china: A cross-sectional study. *The Lancet Diabetes & Endocrinology, 4*(2), 115–124.

28. Danese, E., et al. (2015). Advantages and pitfalls of fructosamine and glycated albumin in the diagnosis and treatment of diabetes. *Journal of Diabetes Science and Technology, 9*(2), 169–175.

29. McGovern, A., et al. (2018). Comparison of medication adherence and persistence in type 2 diabetes: A systematic review and meta-analysis. *Diabetes Obesity & Metabolism, 20*(4), 1040–1043.

30. American Diabetes Association. (2019). Standards of medical care in diabetes–2019: Lifestyle management. *Diabetes Care, 42*(Suppl. 1), S46–S60.

31. Davies., et al. (2018). Management of hyperglycemia in type 2 diabetes, 2018. A consensus report by the American Diabetes Association (ADA) and the European Association for the Study of Diabetes (EASD). *Diabetes Care, 41*(12), 2669–2701.

32. Powers., et al. (2015). Diabetes self-management education and support in type 2 diabetes: A joint position statement of the American Diabetes Association, the American Association of Diabetes Educators, and the Academy of Nutrition and Dietetics. *Diabetes Care, 38*(7), 1372–1382.

33. Beck, J., et al. (2017). National standards for diabetes self-management education and support. *Diabetes Care, 40*(10), 1409–1419.

34. American Association of Diabetes Educators. *AADE7 self-care behaviors.* www.diabeteseducator.org/living-with-diabetes/aade7-self-care-behaviors. Published 2019. [Accessed 9 May 2019].

35. Franz, M. J., et al. (2017). Academy of Nutrition and Dietetics nutrition practice guideline for type 1 and type 2 diabetes in adults: Systematic review of evidence for medical nutrition therapy effectiveness and recommendations for integration into the nutrition care process. *Journal of the Academy of Nutrition and Dietetics, 117*(10), 1637–1658.

36. Evert, A. B., et al. (2019). Nutrition therapy for adults with diabetes or prediabetes: A consensus report. *Diabetes Care, 42*(5), 731–754.

37. Franz, M. J., et al. (2015). Lifestyle weight-loss intervention outcomes in overweight and obese adults with type 2 diabetes: A systematic review and meta-analysis of randomized clinical trials. *Journal of the Academy of Nutrition and Dietetics, 115*(9), 1447–1463.

38. Lean, M. E., et al. (2018). Primary care-led weight management for remission of type 2 diabetes (DiRECT). *Lancet, 391*(10120), 541–551.

39. MacLeod, J., et al. (2017). Academy of Nutrition and Dietetics nutrition practice guideline for type 1 and type 2 diabetes in adults; nutrition intervention evidence reviews and recommendations. *Journal of the Academy of Nutrition and Dietetics, 117*(10), 1637–1658.

40. Food and Nutrition Board and Institute of Medicine. (2002). *Dietary reference intakes for energy, carbohydrate, fiber, fat, fatty acids, cholesterol, protein, and amino acids.* Washington, DC: National Academies Press.

41. Johnson, R. K., et al. American Heart Association Nutrition Committee of the Council of Lifestyle and Cardiometabolic Health; Council on the Cardiovascular and Stroke Nursing; Council on the Clinical Cardiology; Council on Quality of Care and Outcomes Research, Stroke Council. (2018). Low-calorie sweetened beverages and cardiometabolic health: A science advisory from the American heart association. *Circulation, 138*(9), e126–e140.

42. Riddell, M., et al. (2017). Exercise management in type 1 diabetes: A consensus statement. *The Lancet Diabetes & Endocrinology*, 5(5), 377–390.

43. Snorgaard, O., et al. (2017). Systematic review and meta-analysis of dietary carbohydrate restriction in patients with type 2 diabetes. *BMJ Open Diabetes Research & Care*, 5(1), e000354.

44. van Zuuren, E. J., et al. (2018). Effects of low-carbohydrate compared with low-fat-diet interventions on metabolic control in people with type 2 diabetes: A systematic review including GRADE assessments. *American Journal of Clinical Nutrition*, 108(2), 330–331.

45. Sainsbury, E., et al. (2018). Effect of dietary carbohydrate restriction on glycemic control in adults with diabetes: A systematic review and meta-analysis. *Diabetes Research and Clinical Practice*, 139, 239–252.

46. American Diabetes Association. (2019). Standards of medical care in diabetes–2019: Glycemic targets. *Diabetes Care*, 42(Suppl. 1), S61–70.

47. American Diabetes Association. (2019). Standards of medical care in diabetes–2019: Comprehensive medical evaluation and assessment of comorbidities. *Diabetes Care*, 42(Suppl. 1), S34–S45.

CHAPTER 21

1. U.S. Renal Data System. (2018). *2018 Annual Data Report: Epidemiology of Kidney Disease in the United States*. Bethesda, MD: National Institutes of Health, National Institute of Diabetes and Digestive and Kidney Diseases.

2. Centers for Disease Control and Prevention, National Center for Health Statistics. *National health and nutrition examination survey questionnaire*. wwwn.cdc.gov/nchs/nhanes/continuousnhanes/overview.aspx?BeginYear=2015. Published 2015–2016. [Accessed 22 April 2019].

3. Kidney Disease: Improving Global Outcomes (KDIGO) CKD Work Group. (2013). KDIGO 2012 clinical practice guideline for the evaluation and management of chronic kidney disease. *Kidney International Supplements*, 3, 1–150.

4. Vart, P., et al. (2015). Mediators of the association between low socioeconomic status and chronic kidney disease in the United States. *American Journal of Epidemiology*, 181(6), 385–396.

5. Academy of Nutrition and Dietetics. (2019). *Nutrition Care Manual*. Chicago, IL: Academy of Nutrition and Dietetics.

6. Pavkov, M. E., Harding, J. L., & Burrows, N. R. (2018). Trends in hospitalizations for acute kidney injury– United States, 2000–2014. *Morbidity and Mortality Weekly Report*, 67, 289–293.

7. Moore, P. K., et al. (2018). Management of acute kidney injury: Core curriculum. *American Journal of Kidney Diseases*, 72(1), 136–148.

8. Zeng, X., et al. (2014). Incidence, outcomes, and comparisons across definitions of AKI in hospitalized individuals. *Clinical Journal of the American Society of Nephrology*, 9, 12–20.

9. Chawla, L. S., et al. (2017). Acute kidney disease and renal recovery: Consensus report of the Acute Disease Quality Initiative (ADQI) 16 workgroup. *Nature Reviews Nephrology*, 13, 241–257.

10. Basile, D. P., et al. (2016). Progression after AKI: Understanding maladaptive repair processes to predict and identify therapeutic treatments. *Journal of the American Society of Nephrology*, 27, 687–697.

11. Kidney Disease: Improving Global Outcomes (KDIGO) Anemia Work Group. (2012). KDIGO clinical practice guideline for anemia in chronic kidney disease. *Kidney International Supplements*, 2, 279–335.

12. Kidney Disease: Improving Global Outcomes (KDIGO) Blood Pressure Work Group. (2012). KDIGO clinical practice guideline for the management of blood pressure in chronic kidney disease. *Kidney International Supplements*, 2, 337–414.

13. Sung, W. L., et al. (2019). Dietary protein intake, protein energy wasting, and the progression of chronic kidney disease: Analysis from the KNOW-CKD study. *Nutrients*, 8(1), 11. pii:E121.

14. Koppe, L., Fouque, D., & Kalantar-Zadeh, K. (2019). Kidney cachexia or protein-energy wasting in chronic kidney disease: Facts and numbers. *The Journal of Cachexia Sarcopenia and Muscle*, 10(3), 479–484.

15. Sum, S. S., et al. (2017). Comparison of subjective global assessment and protein energy wasting score to nutrition evaluations conducted by registered dietitian nutritionists in identifying protein energy wasting risk in maintenance hemodialysis patients. *Journal of Renal Nutrition*, 27(5), 325–332.

16. Garg, A. X., et al. (2017). Patients receiving frequent hemodialysis have better health related quality of life compared to patients receiving conventional hemodialysis. *Kidney International*, 91(3), 746–754.

17. Lodebo, B. T., Shah, A., & Kopple, J. D. (2018). Is it important to prevent and treat protein-energy wasting in chronic kidney disease and chronic dialysis patients? *Journal of Renal Nutrition*, 28(6), 369–379.

18. Toyoda, K., et al. (2019). Effect of progression in malnutrition and inflammatory conditions on the adverse events and mortality in patients on maintenance hemodialysis. *Blood Purification*, 47(Suppl. 2), 3–11.

19. Zha, Y., & Qian, Q. (2017). Protein nutrition and malnutrition in CKD and ESRD. *Nutrients*, 9(3), 208.

20. Naderi, N., et al. (2018). Obesity paradox in advanced kidney disease: From bedside to the bench. *Progress in Cardiovascular Diseases*, 61, 168–181.

21. Kalantar-Zadeh, K., et al. (2017). The obesity paradox in kidney disease: How to reconcile it with obesity management. *Kidney International Reports*, 2, 271–281.

22. Held, P. J., McCormick, F., Ojo, J., & Roberts, J. P. (2016). A cost-benefit analysis of government compensation of kidney donors. *American Journal of Transplantation*, 16, 877–885.

23. Brown, R. O., & Compher, C. (2010). ASPEN clinical guidelines: Nutrition support in adult acute and chronic renal failure. *Journal of Parenteral and Enteral Nutrition*, 34(4), 366–377.

24. Chronic Kidney Disease-Mineral and Bone Disorder Work Group. (2017). Kidney Disease: Improving Global Outcomes (KDIGO). 2017 clinical practice guideline update for the diagnosis, evaluation, prevention, and treatment of chronic kidney disease-mineral and bone disorder (CKD-MBD). *Kidney International Supplements*, 7, 1–59.

25. Chen, Z., Prosperi, M., & Bird, V. Y. (2018). Prevalence of kidney stones in the USA: The National Health and Nutrition Evaluation Survey. *Journal of Clinical Urology*, 12(4), 296–302.

26. Assadi, F., & Moghtaderi, M. (2017). Preventative kidney stones: Continue medical education. *International Journal of Preventive Medicine*, 8, 67.

27. Khan, S. R., et al. (2017). Kidney stones. *Nature Reviews Disease Primers*, 2, 16008.

28. Antonelli J, Maalour N. Nephrolithiasis. *BMJ Best Practice*. bestpractice.bmj.com/topics/en-us/225. Published September 2018. [Accessed 20 May, 2019].

29. Ferraro, P. M., Curhan, G. C., Gambro, G., & Taylor, E. N. (2016). Total, dietary, and supplemental vitamin C intake and risk of incident kidney stones. *American Journal of Kidney Diseases*, 67(3), 400–407.

30. Jiang, K., et al. (2019). Ascorbic acid supplements and kidney stones incidence among men and women: A systematic review and meta-analysis. *The Journal of Urology*, 16(2), 115–120.

31. Jung, H., et al. (2017). Urolithiasis evaluation, dietary factors and medical management: An update of the 2014 SIU-ICUD international consultation on stone disease. *World Journal of Urology*, 35(9), 1331–1340.

32. Morgan, M. S. C., & Pearle, M. S. (2016). Medical management of renal stones. *British Medical Journal*, 352, i52.

33. Trinchieri, A., & Montanari, E. (2017). Prevalence of renal uric acid stones in the adult. *Urolithiasis*, 45, 553–562.

34. Ferraro, P. M., Mandel, E. I., & Curhan, G. C. (2016). Dietary protein and potassium, diet-dependent net acid load, and risk of incident kidney stones. *Clinical Journal of the American Society of Nephrology*, 11(10), 1834–1844.

35. Ferraro, P. M., Taylor, E. N., Gambro, G., & Curhan, G. C. (2017). Dietary and lifestyle risk factors associated with incident kidney stones in men and women. *The Journal Of Urology*, 198(4), 858–863.

36. Krieger, N. S., et al. (2016). Effect of potassium citrate on calcium phosphate stones in a model of hypercalciuria. *Journal of the American Society of Nephrology*, 25(12), 3001–3008.

37. Andreassen, K. H., Pedersen, K. V., Osther, S. S., et al. (2016). How should patients with cystine stone disease be evaluated and treated in the twenty-first century? *Urolithiasis*, 44, 65–76.

CHAPTER 22

1. Hiura, G., Lebwohl, B., & Seres, D. S. (2020). Malnutrition diagnosis in critically ill patients using 2012 Academy of Nutrition and Dietetics/American Society for Parenteral and Enteral Nutrition standardized diagnostic characteristics is associated with longer hospital and intensive care unit length of stay and increased in-hospital mortality. *Journal of Parenteral and Enteral Nutrition*, 44(2), 256–264.

2. Ihle, C., et al. (2017). Malnutrition-an underestimated factor in the inpatient treatment of traumatology and orthopedic patients: A prospective evaluation of 1055 patients. *Injury*, 48(3), 628–636.

3. Curtis, L. J., et al. (2017). Costs of hospital malnutrition. *Clinical Nutrition*, 36(5), 1391–1396.

4. Zhang, H., et al. (2017). Impact of nutrition support on clinical outcome and cost-effectiveness analysis in patients at nutritional risk: A prospective cohort study with propensity score matching. *Nutrition*, 37, 53–59.

5. Puvanesarajah, V., et al. (2017). Poor nutrition status and lumbar spine fusion surgery in the elderly: Readmissions, complications, and mortality. *Spine (Phila Pa 1976)*, 42(13), 979–983.

6. Moran Lopez, J. M., et al. (2017). Benefits of early specialized nutritional support in malnourished patients. *Medical Clinics (Barc)*, 148(7), 303–307.

7. Cano-Torres, E. A., et al. (2017). Impact of nutritional intervention on length of hospital stay and mortality among hospitalized patients with malnutrition: A clinical randomized controlled trial. *Journal of the American College of Nutrition*, 36(4), 235–239.

8. Wischmeyer, P. E., et al. (2017). A randomized trial of supplemental parenteral nutrition in underweight and overweight critically ill patients: The TOP-UP pilot trial. *Critical Care*, 21(1), 142.

9. White, J. V., et al. (2012). Consensus statement: Academy of Nutrition and Dietetics and American Society for Parenteral and Enteral Nutrition: Characteristics recommended for the identification and documentation of adult malnutrition (undernutrition). *Journal of Parenteral and Enteral Nutrition*, 36(3), 275–283.

10. Coss-Bu, J. A., et al. (2017). Protein requirements of the critically ill pediatric patient. *Nutrition in Clinical Practice*, 32(1S), 128S–141S.

11. Genaro Pde, S., et al. (2015). Dietary protein intake in elderly women: Association with muscle and bone mass. *Nutrition in Clinical Practice*, 30(2), 283–289.

12. Horosz, B., Nawrocka, K., & Malec-Milewska, M. (2016). Anaesthetic perioperative management according to the ERAS protocol. *Anaesthesiology Intensive Therapy*, 48(1), 49–54.

13. Yeh, D. D., et al. (2017). Implementation of an aggressive enteral nutrition protocol and the effect on clinical outcomes. *Nutrition in Clinical Practice*, 32(2), 175–181.

14. Elliott, J. A., et al. (2017). Sarcopenia: Prevalence, and impact on operative and oncologic outcomes in the multimodal management of locally advanced esophageal cancer. *Annals of Surgery*, 266(5), 822–830.

15. Myles, P. S., et al. (2017). Contemporary approaches to perioperative IV fluid therapy. *World Journal of Surgery*, 41(10), 2457–2463.

16. Badeaux, J. E., & Martin, J. B. (2018). Emerging adjunctive approach for the treatment of sepsis: Vitamin C and thiamine. *Critical Care Nursing Clinics of North America*, 30(3), 343–351.

17. Marik, P. E., et al. (2017). Hydrocortisone, vitamin C, and thiamine for the treatment of severe sepsis and septic shock: A retrospective before-after study. *Chest*, 151(6), 1229–1238.

18. Sadeghpour, A., et al. (2015). Impact of vitamin C supplementation on post-cardiac surgery ICU and hospital length of stay. *Anesthesiology and Pain Medicine*, 5(1), e25337.

19. Rodrigo, R., et al. (2013). A randomized controlled trial to prevent post-operative atrial fibrillation by antioxidant reinforcement. *Journal of the American College of Cardiology*, 62(16), 1457–1465.

20. Petersen, F., et al. (2017). The effects of polyunsaturated fatty acids and antioxidant vitamins on atrial oxidative stress, nitrotyrosine residues, and connexins following extracorporeal circulation in patients undergoing cardiac surgery. *Molecular and Cellular Biochemistry*, 433(1-2), 27–40.

21. Cereda, E., et al. (2015). A nutritional formula enriched with arginine, zinc, and antioxidants for the healing of pressure ulcers: A randomized trial. *Annals of Internal Medicine*, 162(3), 167–174.

22. Rech, M., et al. (2014). Heavy metal in the intensive care unit: A review of current literature on trace element supplementation in critically ill patients. *Nutrition in Clinical Practice*, 29(1), 78–89.

23. Mertens, K., et al. (2015). Low zinc and selenium concentrations in sepsis are associated with oxidative damage and inflammation. *British Journal of Anaesthesia*, 114(6), 990–999.

24. Stefanowicz, F., et al. (2014). Assessment of plasma and red cell trace element concentrations, disease severity, and outcome in patients with critical illness. *Journal of Critical Care*, 29(2), 214–218.

25. Lee, Y. H., et al. (2019). Serum concentrations of trace elements zinc, copper, selenium, and manganese in critically ill patients. *Biological Trace Element Research*, 188(2), 316–325.

26. Bonetti, L., et al. (2017). Prevalence of malnutrition among older people in medical and surgical wards in hospital and quality of nutritional care: A multicenter, cross-sectional study. *Journal of Clinical Nursing*, 26(23-24), 5082–5092.

27. Martos-Benitez, F. D., et al. (2018). Program of gastrointestinal rehabilitation and early postoperative enteral nutrition: A prospective study. *Updates in Surgery*, 70(1), 105–112.

28. Boullata, J. I., et al. (2017). ASPEN safe practices for enteral nutrition therapy. *Journal of Parenteral and Enteral Nutrition*, 41(1), 15–103.

29. McClanahan, D., et al. (2019). Pilot study of the effect of plant-based enteral nutrition on the gut microbiota in chronically ill tube-fed children. *Journal of Parenteral and Enteral Nutrition*, 43(7), 899–911.

30. Bobo, E. (2016). Reemergence of blenderized tube feedings: Exploring the evidence. *Nutrition in Clinical Practice*, 31(6), 730–735.

31. Savino, P. (2017). Knowledge of constituent ingredients in enteral nutrition formulas can make a difference in patient response to enteral feeding. *Nutrition in Clinical Practice*, 0884533617724759.

32. Academy of Nutrition and Dietetics. (2019). *Nutrition Care Manual*. Chicago, IL: Academy of Nutrition and Dietetics.

33. Ichimaru, S. (2018). Methods of enteral nutrition administration in critically ill patients: Continuous, cyclic, intermittent, and bolus feeding. *Nutrition in Clinical Practice, 33*(6), 790–795.

34. McClave, S. A., et al. (2016). Guidelines for the provision and assessment of nutrition support therapy in the adult critically ill patient. *Journal of Parenteral and Enteral Nutrition, 40*(2), 159–211.

35. Alberda, C., et al. (2017). Nutrition care in patients with head and neck or esophageal cancer: The patient perspective. *Nutrition in Clinical Practice, 32*(5), 664–674.

36. Laurenius, A., et al. (2017). Dumping symptoms is triggered by fat as well as carbohydrates in patients operated with Roux-en-Y gastric bypass. *Surgery for Obesity and Related Diseases, 13*(7), 1159–1164.

37. Frame-Peterson, L. A., et al. (2017). Nutrient deficiencies are common prior to bariatric surgery. *Nutrition in Clinical Practice, 32*(4), 463–469.

38. Sherf Dagan, S., et al. (2017). Nutritional recommendations for adult bariatric surgery patients: Clinical practice. *Advances in Nutrition, 8*(2), 382–394.

39. American Burn Association. *Burn incidence and treatment in the United States*. ameriburn.org/who-we-are/media/burn-incidence-fact-sheet/. Published 2016. [Accessed 15 May 2019].

40. Clark, A., et al. (2017). Nutrition and metabolism in burn patients. *Burns Trauma, 5*(1), 11.

CHAPTER 23

1. National Center for Health Statistics. (2019). *Health, United States, 2018*. Hyattsville, MD.

2. Sapienza, C., & Issa, J. P. (2016). Diet, nutrition, and cancer epigenetics. *Annual Review of Nutrition, 36*, 665–681.

3. International Agency for Research on Cancer. (2018). *Red meat and processed meat: IARC monographs on the evaluation of carcinogenic risks to humans* (Vol. 114). Lyon, France: International Agency for Research on Cancer, World Health Organization.

4. Chiavarini, M., et al. (2017). Dietary intake of meat cooking-related mutagens (HCAs) and risk of colorectal adenoma and cancer: A systematic review and meta-analysis. *Nutrients, 9*(5).

5. Nagle, C. M., et al. (2015). Cancers in Australia in 2010 attributable to the consumption of red and processed meat. *The Australian and New Zealand Journal of Public Health, 39*(5), 429–433.

6. Zhang, F. F., et al. (2019). Preventable cancer burden associated with poor diet in the United States. *JNCI Cancer Spectrum, 3*(2), pkz034.

7. Nagle, C. M., et al. (2015). Cancers in Australia in 2010 attributable to inadequate consumption of fruit, non-starchy vegetables and dietary fibre. *The Australian and New Zealand Journal of Public Health, 39*(5), 422–428.

8. Wu, S., et al. (2019). Fruit and vegetable intake is inversely associated with cancer risk in Mexican-Americans. *Nutrition and Cancer, 71*(8), 1254–1262.

9. Islami, F., et al. (2018). Proportion and number of cancer cases and deaths attributable to potentially modifiable risk factors in the United States. *CA Cancer Journal for Clinicians, 68*(1), 31–54.

10. Whiteman, D. C., & Wilson, L. F. (2016). The fractions of cancer attributable to modifiable factors: A global review. *Cancer Epidemiol, 44*, 203–221.

11. Brown, K. F., et al. (2018). The fraction of cancer attributable to modifiable risk factors in England, Wales, Scotland, Northern Ireland, and the United Kingdom in 2015. *British Journal of Cancer, 118*(8), 1130–1141.

12. World Cancer Research Fund/American Institute for Cancer Research, Diet, Nutrition, Physical Activity and Cancer: a Global Perspective. *Continuous Update Project Expert Report*. dietandcancerreport.org. Published 2018.

13. American Cancer Society. (2019). *Cancer prevention & early detection facts & figures 2019–2020*. Atlanta: American Cancer Society.

14. Vashi, P. G., et al. (2013). The relationship between baseline nutritional status with subsequent parenteral nutrition and clinical outcomes in cancer patients undergoing hyperthermic intraperitoneal chemotherapy. *Nutrition Journal, 12*, 118.

15. Reece, L., et al. (2019). Preoperative nutrition status and postoperative outcomes in patients undergoing cytoreductive surgery and hyperthermic intraperitoneal chemotherapy. *Annals of Surgical Oncology, 26*(8), 2622–2630.

16. Cardi, M., et al. (2019). Prognostic factors influencing infectious complications after cytoreductive surgery and HIPEC: Results from a tertiary referral center. *Gastroenterol Res Pract*, 2824073.

17. Vagnildhaug, O. M., et al. (2018). A cross-sectional study examining the prevalence of cachexia and areas of unmet need in patients with cancer. *Support Care Cancer, 26*(6), 1871–1880.

18. Arends, J., et al. (2017). ESPEN expert group recommendations for action against cancer-related malnutrition. *Clinical Nutrition, 36*(5), 1187–1196.

19. Arthur, S. T., et al. (2014). One-year prevalence, comorbidities and cost of cachexia-related inpatient admissions in the USA. *Drugs Context, 3*, 212265.

20. von Haehling, S., Anker, M. S., & Anker, S. D. (2016). Prevalence and clinical impact of cachexia in chronic illness in Europe, USA, and Japan: Facts and numbers update 2016. *The Journal of Cachexia Sarcopenia and Muscle, 7*(5), 507–509.

21. Aoyagi, T., et al. (2015). Cancer cachexia, mechanism and treatment. *World Journal of Gastrointestinal Oncology, 7*(4), 17–29.

22. Anderson, L. J., Albrecht, E. D., & Garcia, J. M. (2017). Update on management of cancer-related cachexia. *Current Oncology Reports, 19*(1), 3.

23. Mattox, T. W. (2017). Cancer cachexia: Cause, diagnosis, and treatment. *Nutrition in Clinical Practice, 32*(5), 599–606.

24. Thompson, K. L., et al. (2017). Oncology evidence-based nutrition practice guideline for adults. *Journal of the Academy of Nutrition and Dietetics, 117*(2), 297–310.e47.

25. Academy of Nutrition and Dietetics. (2019). *Nutrition Care Manual*. Chicago, IL: Academy of Nutrition and Dietetics.

26. Arends, J., et al. (2017). ESPEN guidelines on nutrition in cancer patients. *Clinical Nutrition, 36*(1), 11–48.

27. Purcell, S. A., et al. (2016). Key determinants of energy expenditure in cancer and implications for clinical practice. *European Journal of Clinical Nutrition, 70*(11), 1230–1238.

28. U.S. Food and Drug Administration. *Authorized health claims that meet the Significant Scientific Agreement (SSA) standard*. www.fda.gov/food/food-labeling-nutrition/authorized-health-claims-meet-significant-scientific-agreement-ssa-standard. Published 2018. [Accessed 17 August 2019].

29. Lohse, T., et al. (2016). Adherence to the cancer prevention recommendations of the World Cancer Research Fund/American Institute for Cancer Research and mortality: A census-linked cohort. *American Journal of Clinical Nutrition, 104*(3), 678–685.

30. Turati, F., et al. (2017). Adherence to the World Cancer Research Fund/American Institute for Cancer Research recommendations and colorectal cancer risk. *European Journal of Cancer, 85*, 86–94.

31. Vergnaud, A. C., et al. (2013). Adherence to the World Cancer Research Fund/American Institute for Cancer Research guidelines and risk of death in Europe: Results from the European Prospective Investigation into Nutrition and Cancer cohort study 1,4. *American Journal of Clinical Nutrition, 97*(5), 1107–1120.

32. Jankovic, N., et al. (2017). Adherence to the WCRF/AICR dietary recommendations for cancer prevention and risk of cancer in elderly from Europe and the United States: A meta-analysis within the CHANCES Project. *Cancer Epidemiol Biomarkers Prev, 26*(1), 136–144.

33. Kabat, G. C., et al. (2015). Adherence to cancer prevention guidelines and cancer incidence, cancer mortality, and total mortality: A prospective cohort study. *American Journal of Clinical Nutrition, 101*(3), 558–569.

34. U.S. Department of Health and Human Services. *Healthy People 2030.* health.gov/healthypeople. Published 2020. [Accessed 18 February, 2021].

35. Neuhouser, M. L., et al. (2015). Overweight, obesity, and postmenopausal invasive breast cancer risk: A secondary analysis of the Women's Health Initiative randomized clinical trials. *JAMA Oncology, 1*(5), 611–621.

36. World Cancer Research Fund/American Institute for Cancer Research. *Diet, Nutrition, Physical Activity and Cancer: a Global Perspective.* Continuous Update Project Expert Report. dietandcancerreport.org. Published 2018.

37. Iyengar, N. M., et al. (2019). Association of body fat and risk of breast cancer in postmenopausal women with normal body mass index: A secondary analysis of a randomized clinical trial and observational study. *JAMA Oncology, 5*(2), 155–163.

38. Dandamudi, A., et al. (2018). Dietary patterns and breast cancer risk: A systematic review. *Anticancer Research, 38*(6), 3209–3222.

39. Harris, H. R., Bergkvist, L., & Wolk, A. (2016). Adherence to the World Cancer Research Fund/American Institute for Cancer Research recommendations and breast cancer risk. *International Journal of Cancer, 138*(11), 2657–2664.

40. Bertuccio, P., et al. (2013). Dietary patterns and gastric cancer risk: A systematic review and meta-analysis. *Annals of Oncology, 24*(6), 1450–1458.

41. Fang, X., et al. (2015). Landscape of dietary factors associated with risk of gastric cancer: A systematic review and dose-response meta-analysis of prospective cohort studies. *European Journal of Cance, 51*(18), 2820–2832.

42. Centers for Disease Control and Prevention. *Cancer.* www.cdc.gov/cancer/. Published 2019. [Accessed 18 August 2019].

43. Luo, Q., & Asher, G. N. (2017). Complementary and alternative medicine use at a comprehensive cancer center. *Integrative Cancer Therapies, 16*(1), 104–109.

44. Judson, P. L., et al. (2017). Complementary and alternative medicine use in individuals presenting for care at a comprehensive cancer center. *Integrative Cancer Therapies, 16*(1), 96–103.

45. Greenlee, H., et al. (2016). Association between complementary and alternative medicine use and breast cancer chemotherapy initiation: The Breast Cancer Quality of Care (BQUAL) study. *JAMA Oncology, 2*(9), 1170–1176.

46. Wortmann, J. K., et al. (2016). Use of complementary and alternative medicine by patients with cancer: A cross-sectional study at different points of cancer care. *Medical Oncology, 33*(7), 78.

47. Sullivan, A., Gilbar, P., & Curtain, C. (2015). Complementary and alternative medicine use in cancer patients in rural Australia. *Integrative Cancer Therapies, 14*(4), 350–358.

48. Centers for Disease Control and Prevention. (2019). Estimated HIV incidence and prevalence in the United States, 2010–2016. *HIV Surveillance Suppl Report, 24*(1). Available at: www.cdc.gov/hiv/library/reports/hiv-surveillance.html.

49. Zhu, T., et al. (1998). An African HIV-1 sequence from 1959 and implications for the origin of the epidemic. *Nature, 391*(6667), 594–597.

50. UNAIDS. *Fact sheet—global aids update 2019.* www.unaids.org/sites/default/files/media_asset/UNAIDS_FactSheet_en.pdf. Published 2019. [Accessed 18 August 2019].

51. Centers for Disease Control and Prevention (2014). Revised surveillance case definition for HIV infection—United States, 2014. *MMWR Recommendations and Reports, 63*(Rr-03), 1–10.

52. Owens, D. K., et al. (2019). Screening for HIV infection: U.S. Preventive Services Task Force recommendation statement. *Journal of the American Medical Association, 321*(23), 2326–2336.

53. U.S. Department of Health and Human Services. *AIDSinfo: Drugs.* aidsinfo.nih.gov/drugs. Published 2019. [Accessed 18 August 2019].

54. U.S. Food and Drug Administration. *Vaccine product approval process.* www.fda.gov/vaccines-blood-biologics/development-approval-process-cber/vaccine-product-approval-process. Published 2018. [Accessed 18 August 2019].

55. Chou, R., et al. (2019). Preexposure prophylaxis for the prevention of HIV infection: Evidence report and systematic review for the U.S. Preventive Services Task Force. *Journal of the American Medical Association, 321*(22), 2214–2230.

56. Owens, D. K., et al. (2019). Preexposure prophylaxis for the prevention of HIV infection: U.S. Preventive Services Task Force recommendation statement. *Journal of the American Medical Association, 321*(22), 2203–2213.

57. Maluccio, J. A., et al. (2015). Improving health-related quality of life among people living with HIV: Results from an impact evaluation of a food assistance program in Uganda. *PLoS One, 10*(8), e0135879.

58. Derose, K. P., et al. (2018). Developing pilot interventions to address food insecurity and nutritional needs of people living with HIV in Latin America and the Caribbean: An interinstitutional approach using formative research. *Food and Nutrition Bulletin, 39*(4), 549–563.

59. Aberman, N. L., et al. (2014). Food security and nutrition interventions in response to the AIDS epidemic: Assessing global action and evidence. *AIDS and Behavior, 18*(Suppl. 5), S554–S565.

60. Bandera, A., et al. (2018). Altered gut microbiome composition in HIV infection: Causes, effects and potential intervention. *Current Opinion in HIV and AIDS, 13*(1), 73–80.

61. Pinto-Cardoso, S., Klatt, N. R., & Reyes-Teran, G. (2018). Impact of antiretroviral drugs on the microbiome: Unknown answers to important questions. *Current Opinion in HIV and AIDS, 13*(1), 53–60.

62. d'Ettorre, G., et al. (2017). Probiotic supplementation promotes a reduction in T-cell activation, an increase in Th17 frequencies, and a recovery of intestinal epithelium integrity and mitochondrial morphology in ART-treated HIV-1-positive patients. *Immunity Inflammation and Disease, 5*(3), 244–260.

63. Willig, A., Wright, L., & Galvin, T. A. (2018). Practice paper of the Academy of Nutrition and Dietetics: Nutrition intervention and human immunodeficiency virus infection. *Journal of the Academy of Nutrition and Dietetics, 118*(3), 486–498.

64. Vassimon, H. S., et al. (2012). Hypermetabolism and altered substrate oxidation in HIV-infected patients with lipodystrophy. *Nutrition, 28*(9), 912–916.

65. Bouatou, Y., et al. (2018). Lipodystrophy increases the risk of CKD development in HIV-positive patients in Switzerland: The LIPOKID study. *Kidney International Reports, 3*(5), 1089–1099.

66. Kingery, J. R., et al. (2016). Short-term and long-term cardiovascular risk, metabolic syndrome and HIV in Tanzania. *Heart, 102*(15), 1200–1205.

67. Benjamin, L. A., et al. (2016). HIV, antiretroviral treatment, hypertension, and stroke in Malawian adults: A case-control study. *Neurology, 86*(4), 324–333.

68. Pinto, D. S. M., & da Silva, M. (2018). Cardiovascular disease in the setting of human immunodeficiency virus infection. *Current Cardiology Reviews, 14*(1), 25–41.

69. Bhagwat, P., et al. (2018). Changes in waist circumference in HIV-infected individuals initiating a raltegravir or protease inhibitor regimen: Effects of sex and race. *Open Forum Infectious Diseases, 5*(11), ofy201.

Further Reading and Resources

CHAPTER 1

The following organizations are key sources of up-to-date information and research regarding nutrition. Each site has a unique focus and may be helpful for keeping abreast of current topics.

- Academy of Nutrition and Dietetics. www.eatright.org
- American Society for Nutrition. www.nutrition.org
- Dietary Guidelines for Americans. www.health.gov/dietaryguidelines
- Food and Agriculture Organization of the United Nations. www.fao.org
- Healthy People 2020. www.healthypeople.gov
- Society for Nutrition Education and Behavior. www.sneb.org
- USDA Choose MyPlate. www.choosemyplate.gov
- World Health Organization. www.who.int

CHAPTER 2

The following organizations are valuable resources for nutrition and health-related information, particularly regarding carbohydrates.

- USDA Choose MyPlate. www.choosemyplate.gov
- Women's Health (U.S. Department of Health and Human Services): Healthy Eating. www.womenshealth.gov/healthy-eating
- Food and Nutrition Information Center (USDA): Carbohydrate Information. www.nal.usda.gov/fnic/carbohydrates
- Whole Grains Council. https://wholegrainscouncil.org/
- Harvard's site for *The Nutrition Source* on Carbohydrates: www.hsph.harvard.edu/nutritionsource/carbohydrates/

CHAPTER 3

- Lipids in Health and Disease. www.lipidworld.com
  - An online journal of peer-reviewed articles about all aspects of lipids that is open access and free to the public
- Mayo Clinic. www.mayoclinic.com
  - A site search for "dietary fat" results in several informative articles
- USDA FoodData Central. https://fdc.nal.usda.gov/
  - A useful website for finding the nutrient content of the foods that you most enjoy, including their dietary fat content
- U.S. Food and Drug Administration. www.fda.gov
  - A site search for "trans fat" results in several informative articles regarding the current regulations on the use of partially hydrogenated oils in the food supply

CHAPTER 4

The following organizations are good sources of information about vegetarian diets.

- Food and Nutrition Information Center. www.nal.usda.gov/fnic
- Medline Plus: Vegetarian Diets. medlineplus.gov/vegetariandiet.html
- North American Vegetarian Society. navs-online.org/
- Vegetarian Nutrition Dietetic Practice Group. vndpg.org/ and veganhealth.org/
- The Vegetarian Resource Group. www.vrg.org
- Vegan Health. veganhealth.org/

CHAPTER 5

The following organizations provide up-to-date research and reliable information about matters of the GI tract and metabolism.

- The American College of Gastroenterology. www.gi.org
- The American Gastroenterological Association. www.gastro.org
- The American Journal of Gastroenterology. www.nature.com/ajg
- Metabolism. www.metabolism.com
- Nutrition & Metabolism. www.nutritionandmetabolism.biomedcentral.com

CHAPTER 6

The following websites provide methods for predicting total energy needs and for evaluating energy expenditure.

- Adult energy needs and healthy eating calculator. Search "energy needs" at www.bcm.edu
- Mayo Clinic. Search "burn calories" at www.mayoclinic.com
- USDA Choose MyPlate Daily Food Plans and Worksheets. www.choosemyplate.gov/MyPlatePlan
- National Institute of Health. Search "balance food and activity" at www.nhlbi.nih.gov

CHAPTER 7

For more information about the role of folic acid with regard to neural tube defects, see the following websites:

- Centers for Disease Control and Prevention: Spina Bifida. www.cdc.gov/ncbddd/spinabifida
- Spina Bifida Association. http://spinabifidaassociation.org

The following organizations and articles provide current information and guidelines regarding dietary recommendations for nutrient consumption and reliable information on dietary supplements:

- Centers for Disease Control and Prevention. Search "fruit and vegetable intake" and "vitamin intake". www.cdc.gov
- Center for Science in the Public Interest. cspinet.org
- National Science Foundation. Search "dietary supplements". www.nsf.org
- National Institutes of Health: Office of Dietary Supplements. ods.od.nih.gov
- The National Center for Complementary and Integrative Medicine. https://nccih.nih.gov
- U.S. Department of Defense: Operation Supplement Safety. www.opss.org/
- U.S. Food and Drug Administration: Dietary Supplements. www.fda.gov/Food/DietarySupplements

CHAPTER 8

The following websites are good sources for information about certain minerals in diets and their role in general health. You can also go to the National Heart, Lung, and Blood Institute website to learn about the relationship between several minerals (sodium, potassium, magnesium, and calcium) and hypertension. Examine the American Dental Association Oral Health Topics for more information about the protective role of fluoride in dental hygiene.

- American Dental Association. www.ada.org
- National Digestive Diseases Information Clearinghouse, hemochromatosis.www.niddk.nih.gov/health-information/liver-disease/hemochromatosis
- National Heart, Lung, and Blood Institute. www.nhlbi.nih.gov/health-topics/dash-eating-plan
- National Osteoporosis Foundation. www.nof.org

CHAPTER 9

The following organizations provide up-to-date recommendations regarding water and electrolyte balance in addition to a plethora of other health information.

- American College of Sports Medicine. Search "fluid requirements" at www.acsm.org
- Mayo Clinic. See "Nutrition and Healthy Eating" at www.mayoclinic.org/healthy-lifestyle

CHAPTER 10

Each of the following organizations has an earnest interest in the health care of pregnant women and their children. For information about a variety of topics involving pregnancy and lactation, explore their websites.

- American Academy of Pediatrics. www.aap.org
- Birth Defect Research for Children, Inc. www.birthdefects.org
- Canadian Paediatric Society. www.cps.ca
- La Leche League International, Inc. www.llli.org
- March of Dimes Birth Defects Foundation. www.marchofdimes.org
- U.S. Department of Agriculture WIC Program. www.fns.usda.gov/wic

CHAPTER 11

These websites are excellent resources for childhood nutrition information. One of the most important parts of working with parents and children on feeding and health issues is to have access to up-to-date information and ideas. Explore these sites to discover current topics that address the health and nutrition issues that face youth today.

- Ellyn Satter Institute for family feeding advice: www.ellynsatterinstitute.org
- Food and Nutrition Service. School Meals. Search "child nutrition program" at www.fns.usda.gov
- KidsHealth. www.kidshealth.org
- USDA Choose MyPlate tools for kids (6 to 11 years old). www.choosemyplate.gov/children
- National Center for Education in Maternal and Child Health. www.ncemch.org
- World Health Organization child growth standards. www.who.int/childgrowth/en/

CHAPTER 12

These organizations are excellent sources of information about nutrition, health, and community services for the elderly.

- Administration for Community Living. https://acl.gov/
- American Geriatrics Society. www.americangeriatrics.org
- Argentum (formerly known as Assisted Living Federation of America). www.argentum.org
- Centers for Disease Control and Prevention: Chronic Disease Prevention and Health Promotion. www.cdc.gov/chronicdisease/index.htm
- Centers for Medicare & Medicaid Services. www.cms.gov
- The Gerontological Society of America. www.geron.org
- LeadingAge. www.leadingage.org
- National Council on Aging. www.ncoa.org
- National Institute on Aging. www.nia.nih.gov
- National Osteoporosis Foundation. www.nof.org
- U.S. Department of Agriculture: Extension Services. nifa.usda.gov/extension
- U.S. Department of Agriculture: Commodity Supplemental Food Program. www.fns.usda.gov/csfp
- U.S. Department of Agriculture: Senior Farmers' Market Nutrition Program. www.fns.usda.gov/sfmnp
- U.S. Department of Agriculture: Supplemental Nutrition Assistance Program (SNAP). www.fns.usda.gov/snap

CHAPTER 13

Explore these websites for current information and regulations regarding food safety, food-borne illness, and food labeling standards.

- Centers for Disease Control and Prevention: Food-borne illness in the United States. www.cdc.gov/foodborneburden
- Food and Agriculture Organization of the United Nations: Economic and Social Development Department: www.fao.org/economic

- Food Value Analysis Tool: www.rti.org/impact/food-value-analysis-tool
This site provides data on the nutritional value and cost of food
- U.S. Department of Agriculture: Agricultural Marketing Service, The National Organic Program. www.ams.usda.gov/about-ams/programs-offices/national-organic-program
- U.S. Department of Agriculture: Food and Nutrition Services: Nutrition Assistance Programs. www.fns.usda.gov
- U.S. Food and Drug Administration: Ingredients, Packaging, and Labeling. www.fda.gov/food/food-ingredients-packaging
- U.S. Department of Agriculture: Food Safety Education. www.fsis.usda.gov/wps/portal/fsis/topics/food-safety-education

CHAPTER 14

- Association for the Study of Food and Society. www.food-culture.org
- Centers for Disease Control and Prevention: Minority Health. www.cdc.gov/minorityhealth
- Food and Agricultural Organization of the United Nations. www.fao.org/home/en/
- Society for the Anthropology of Food. https://foodanthro.com

CHAPTER 15

- Academy of Nutrition and Dietetics: Health and Wellness. www.eatright.org/health#wellness
- Academy of Nutrition and Dietetics. Search "staying away from fad diets" at www.eatright.org
- Centers for Disease Control and Prevention: Healthy Weight. www.cdc.gov/healthyweight/index.html
- Intuitive Eating. www.intuitiveeating.org
- Nutrition.gov: Weight Management. www.nutrition.gov/weight-management
- See the most recent health reports from the Office of the Surgeon General. Search "weight management" or "obesity" at www.hhs.gov/surgeongeneral

CHAPTER 16

Review the following websites for information, guidelines, research, and suggestions regarding exercise and physical fitness.
- American College of Sports Medicine. www.acsm.org
- Sports, Cardiovascular, and Wellness Nutrition. www.scandpg.org
- Nancy Clark's Sports Nutrition Guidebook. www.nancyclarkrd.com
- National Coalition for Promoting Physical Activity. www.ncppa.org
- National Institutes of Health: Office of Dietary Supplements. ods.od.nih.gov
- See the most recent physical fitness reports from the Office of the Surgeon General. Search "physical fitness" or "exercise" at www.hhs.gov/surgeongeneral

CHAPTER 17

- Academy of Nutrition and Dietetics. Search "nutrition care process" at www.eatrightpro.org
- American Society for Parenteral and Enteral Nutrition. www.nutritioncare.org
This association provides education, publications, conferences, and resources about clinical nutrition therapy for health care professionals. The association consists of physicians, dietitians, nurses, pharmacists, scientists, and other allied health care professionals.
- NANDA International. Search "diagnosis development" at www.nanda.org

CHAPTER 18

These organizations provide support for individuals who are affected by disorders of the gastrointestinal tract. Health care providers should be familiar with these organizations and their websites to refer patients to organizations that can continue to give them support, understanding, and up-to-date information about their diseases.
- American Academy of Allergy, Asthma, & Immunology. www.aaaai.org
- Asthma and Allergy Foundation of America. www.aafa.org
- Beyond Celiac. www.beyondceliac.org
- Celiac Disease Foundation. celiac.org
- Celiac Support Association. www.csaceliacs.org
- Crohn's and Colitis Foundation of America. www.crohnscolitisfoundation.org
- Cystic Fibrosis Foundation. www.cff.org
- Cystic Fibrosis. www.cysticfibrosis.com
- Dysphagia Research Society. dysphagiaresearch.site-ym.com
- International Foundation for Functional Gastrointestinal Disorders. www.iffgd.org
- National Institute of Diabetes and Digestive and Kidney Disease. See "digestive diseases" at www.niddk.nih.gov
- United Ostomy Associations of America. www.ostomy.org

CHAPTER 19

These organizations are valuable sources of information regarding the most current recommendations for healthy lifestyles to prevent and treat heart disease. The websites also provide educational materials for both health care professionals and the public.
- American Heart Association. www.heart.org
- Centers for Disease Control and Prevention: Heart disease prevention: What you can do. www.cdc.gov/HeartDisease/prevention.htm
- National Heart, Lung, and Blood Institute: Assessing cardiovascular risk: www.nhlbi.nih.gov/health-topics/assessing-cardiovascular-risk
- National Heart, Lung, and Blood Institute. Search "heart and vascular resources" at www.nhlbi.nih.gov

CHAPTER 20

The organizations listed below provide the most current information about the evaluation, treatment, and prevention of diabetes. These websites are excellent resources for both health care professionals and patients.

- Association of Diabetes Care and Education Specialists. www.diabeteseducator.org
- American Diabetes Association. www.diabetes.org
- Juvenile Diabetes Research Foundation International. www.jdrf.org
- National Institute of Diabetes and Digestive and Kidney Diseases. www.niddk.nih.gov

CHAPTER 21

These websites provide additional information about various forms of kidney disease. Several national organizations provide free education and support for health care providers, patients, and family members. Dietary restrictions for patients with kidney disease can sometimes be overwhelming. To understand such diets fully, continuous follow-up and feedback are needed.

- American Urological Association. www.urology health.org
- End Stage Renal Disease National Coordinating Center. esrdncc.org
- National Institute of Diabetes and Digestive and Kidney Diseases. www.niddk.nih.gov
- National Kidney Disease Education Program. http://nkdep.nih.gov

- National Kidney Foundation. www.kidney.org, a site search for "Understanding kidney disease and treatment options" will provide the viewer with an excellent series of short videos on kidney function, disease, and treatment modalities.

CHAPTER 22

- American Burn Association. ameriburn.org
- American Society for Parenteral and Enteral Nutrition. www.nutritioncare.org
- Burn Foundation. www.burnfoundation.org
- Critical Care Nutrition. www.criticalcarenutrition.com

CHAPTER 23

- AIDS information, education, and action. www.aids.org
- *AIDS*, the official journal of the International AIDS Society. journals.lww.com/aidsonline
- American Cancer Society. www.cancer.org
- Centers for Disease Control and Prevention: Cancer prevention and control. www.cdc.gov/cancer
- Centers for Disease Control and Prevention: National Center for HIV/AIDS, Viral Hepatitis, STD, and TB Prevention. www.cdc.gov/nchhstp
- HIV.gov. www.hiv.gov
- Joint United Nations Program on HIV/AIDS. www.unaids.org
- National Cancer Institute. www.cancer.gov
- The National Institute of Allergy and Infectious Diseases. HIV/AIDS. www.niaid.nih.gov/diseases-conditions/hivaids

Glossary

1α-hydroxylase the enzyme in the kidneys that catalyzes the hydroxylation reaction of 25-hydroxycholecalciferol (i.e., calcidiol) to calcitriol, which is the active form of vitamin D; 1α-hydroxylase activity is increased by parathyroid hormone when blood calcium levels are low.

A

abdominal thrusts (previously referred to as the *Heimlich maneuver*) a first-aid maneuver that is used to relieve a person who is choking from the blockage of the breathing passageway by a swallowed foreign object or food particle; to perform the maneuver, when standing behind the choking person, clasp the victim around the waist, place one fist just under the sternum (i.e., the breastbone), grasp the fist with the other hand, and then make a quick, hard, thrusting movement inward and upward to dislodge the object.

absorption (in terms of digestion and metabolism) the process by which nutrients are taken into the cells that line the gastrointestinal tract.

acculturation the process of an individual or group of people adopting the behaviors and lifestyle habits of a new culture.

acetone a major ketone compound that results from fat breakdown for energy in individuals with uncontrolled diabetes; persons with diabetes periodically take urinary acetone tests to monitor the status of ketone production.

achalasia a disorder of the esophagus in which the muscles of the tube fail to relax, thereby inhibiting normal swallowing.

acidic or alkaline diets diets based on the theory that diets high in acidic foods (e.g., animal protein, caffeine, simple sugars) will disrupt the body's normal pH balance, which is slightly alkaline.

acidosis a blood pH of less than 7.35; *respiratory acidosis* is caused by an accumulation of carbon dioxide (an acid); *metabolic acidosis* may be caused by a variety of conditions that result in the excess accumulation of acids in the body or by a significant loss of bicarbonate (a base).

adaptive thermogenesis an adjustment to heat production in response to changing environmental influences (e.g., external temperature, diet).

adipocytes fat cells.

adipose fat stored in the cells of adipose (fatty) tissue.

adipose tissue the storage site for excess fat.

aerobic capacity a state in which oxygen is required to proceed; milliliters of oxygen consumed per kilogram of body weight per minute as influenced by body composition.

albuminuria higher-than-normal levels of albumin in the urine; the health care team uses as a clinical tool to diagnosis and monitor kidney disease.

aldosterone a hormone of the adrenal glands that acts on the distal nephron tubule to stimulate the reabsorption of sodium in an ion exchange with potassium; the aldosterone mechanism is essentially a sodium-conserving mechanism, but it also indirectly conserves water, because water absorption follows sodium resorption.

aldosteronoma the excess secretion of aldosterone from the adrenal cortex; symptoms and complications include sodium retention, potassium wasting, alkalosis, weakness, paralysis, polyuria, polydipsia, hypertension, and cardiac arrhythmias.

alkaline diet diets that are low in animal protein and high in fruits and vegetables.

alkalosis a blood pH of more than 7.45; *respiratory alkalosis* is caused by hyperventilation and an excess loss of carbon dioxide; *metabolic alkalosis* is seen with extensive vomiting in which a significant amount of hydrochloric acid is lost and bicarbonate (a base) is secreted.

allergens food proteins that elicit an immune system response or an allergic reaction; symptoms may include itching, swelling, hives, diarrhea, and difficulty breathing as well as anaphylaxis in the worst cases.

allergy a state of hypersensitivity to particular substances in the environment that works on body tissues to produce problems in the functioning of the affected tissues; the agent involved (i.e., the allergen) may be a certain food that is eaten or a substance (e.g., pollen) that is inhaled or touched.

alpha-linolenic acid an essential fatty acid with 18 carbon atoms and 3 double bonds. The first double bond is located at the third carbon from the omega end, making it an omega-3 fatty acid. Found in soybean, canola, and flaxseed oil.

amenorrheic the absence of a menstrual period in a woman of reproductive age.

amino acids the nitrogen-bearing compounds that form the structural units of protein; after digestion, amino acids are available for the synthesis of required proteins.

aminopeptidase a specific protein-splitting enzyme secreted by glands in the walls of the small intestine that breaks off the nitrogen-containing amino end (i.e., NH_2) of the peptide chain, thereby producing smaller-chain peptides and free amino acids.

anabolism the metabolic process of building large substances from smaller parts; the opposite of catabolism.

anaerobic without oxygen; anaerobic microorganisms can live and grow in an oxygen-free environment.

anaphylactic shock a severe and sometimes fatal allergic reaction that results from exposure to a protein that the body perceives as foreign and that elicits a systemic response that involves multiple organs.

anemia a condition that is characterized by a decreased number of circulating red blood cells, decreased hemoglobin level, or both.

anencephaly the congenital absence of the brain that results from the incomplete closure of the upper end of the neural tube.

angina pectoris a spasmodic, choking chest pain caused by a lack of oxygen to the heart; this is a symptom of a heart attack, and it also may be caused by severe effort or excitement.

angiotensin I inactive peptide hormone that is the precursor to angiotensin II.

angiotensin-converting enzyme (ACE) the enzyme found on the capillary walls within the lungs that converts angiotensin I to angiotensin II. ACE is also present to a lesser extent in the endothelial cells and the epithelial cells within the kidneys.

angiotensin II an active hormone that constricts blood vessels and stimulates the release of aldosterone. Both actions lead to an increase in blood pressure.

angiotensinogen an inactive enzyme produced by the liver that circulates within the blood at all times. Angiotensinogen is activated by renin to become angiotensin I.

anorexia nervosa an extreme psychophysiologic aversion to food that results in life-threatening weight loss; a psychiatric eating disorder that results from a morbid fear of fatness in which a person's distorted body image is reflected as fat when the body is malnourished and extremely thin as a result of self-starvation.

anthropometric the physical measurements of the human body that are used for health assessment, including height, weight, skin fold thickness, and circumference (i.e., of the head, hip, waist, wrist, and mid-arm muscle).

anthropometric measurements the physical measurements of the human body that are used for health assessment, including height, weight, skin fold thickness, and circumference (i.e., of the head, hip, waist, wrist, and mid-arm muscle).

antibodies any of numerous protein molecules produced by β cells as a primary immune defense for attaching to specific related antigens.

antidiuretic hormone a hormone of the pituitary gland that acts on the distal nephron tubule to conserve water by reabsorption; also called *vasopressin.*

antigen any foreign or non-self–substance (e.g., toxins, viruses, bacteria, foreign proteins) that triggers the production of antibodies that are specifically designed to counteract their activity.

antioxidant a molecule that prevents the oxidation of cellular structures by free radicals.

anuria the absence of urine production; anuria indicates kidney failure.

appetite-regulating network a hormonally controlled system of appetite stimulation and suppression.

arteriole the smallest branch of an artery that connects with the capillaries.

ascites the accumulation of serous fluid (i.e., blood and lymph serum) in the abdominal cavity.

ascorbic acid the chemical name for vitamin C; the vitamin was named after its ability to cure scurvy.

assimilation the process in which a minority ethnic group or culture acquires the values, beliefs, and behaviors of a dominant ethnic or cultural group.

atherosclerosis the underlying pathology of coronary heart disease; a common form of arteriosclerosis that is characterized by the formation of fatty streaks that contain cholesterol and that develop into hardened plaques in the inner lining of major blood vessels such as the coronary arteries.

atonic without normal muscle tone.

atopy patch test a diagnostic test that is used to assess for allergic reactions on the skin.

atrophy tissue wasting.

auscultation listening to the sounds of the gastrointestinal tract with a stethoscope.

azotemia an excess of urea and other nitrogenous substances in the blood.

B

baby bottle tooth decay also known as *early childhood caries (ECC),* the decay of the baby teeth as a result of inappropriate feeding practices such as putting an infant to bed with a bottle; also called *nursing bottle caries, bottle mouth,* and *bottle caries.*

Barrett's esophagus complication of severe gastroesophageal reflux disease in which the squamous cell epithelium of the esophagus changes to resemble the tissue lining the small intestine; increases the risk of esophageal adenocarcinoma.

basal energy expenditure (BEE) the amount of energy (in kcal) needed by the body for the maintenance of life when a person is at complete digestive, physical, mental, thermal, and emotional rest (i.e., 10 to 12 hours after eating and 12 to 18 hours after physical activity); measured immediately upon waking. Also referred to as *basal metabolic rate (BMR).*

beriberi a disease of the peripheral nerves that is caused by a deficiency of thiamin (vitamin B_1) and is characterized by pain (neuritis) and paralysis of legs and arms, cardiovascular changes, and edema.

bile an emulsifying agent produced by the liver and transported to the gallbladder for concentration and storage; it is released into the duodenum in response to the hormone cholecystokinin to facilitate enzymatic fat digestion by acting as an emulsifier.

binge eating disorder a psychiatric eating disorder that is characterized by the occurrence of binge-eating episodes at least twice a week for a 6-month period.

bioavailability the extent to which a nutrient is available for use by the body.

biologic age age of the body relative to physiologic and maturity developmental standards.

Bitot's spots white or gray conjunctival lesions developing on the cornea because of vitamin A deficiency.

blood urea nitrogen a test of nephron function that measures the ability to filter urea nitrogen, which is a product of protein metabolism, from the blood.

body composition the relative sizes of the four body compartments that make up the total body: lean body mass (muscle mass), fat, water, and bone.

body dysmorphic disorder an obsession with a perceived defect of the body.

body mass index (BMI) the body weight in kilograms divided by the square of the height in meters (kg/m^2); this measurement correlates with body fatness and the health risks associated with obesity.

bolus feeding a volume of feeding administered by a syringe over a short period of time (usually 10 to 15 minutes) that is given in several feedings per day.

Bowman's capsule the membrane at the head of each nephron; this capsule was named for the English physician Sir William Bowman, who in 1843 first established the basis of plasma filtration and consequent urine secretion in the relationship of the blood-filled glomeruli and the filtration across the enveloping membrane.

branched-chain amino acids amino acids with branched side chains; three of the essential amino acids are branched-chain amino acids: leucine, isoleucine, and valine.

exclusively breastfed feeding the infant only breast milk with no supplemental liquids or solid foods, other than necessary medications or nutrient supplements when needed.

brush border the cells that are located on the microvilli within the lining of the intestinal tract; the microvilli are tiny hair-like projections that protrude from the mucosal cells and help to increase the surface area for the digestion and absorption of nutrients.

bulimia nervosa a psychiatric eating disorder related to a person's fear of fatness, in which cycles of gorging on large quantities of food are followed by compensatory mechanisms (e.g., self-induced vomiting, the use of diuretics and laxatives) to maintain a "normal" body weight.

C

cachexia a specific profound syndrome that is characterized by wasting, reduced food intake, and systemic inflammation.

Cajun a group of people with an enduring tradition whose French-Catholic ancestors established permanent communities in the southern Louisiana coastal waterways after being expelled from Acadia (now Nova Scotia, Canada) by the reigning English during the late 18th century; they developed a unique food pattern from a blend of native French influence and the Creole cooking that was found in the new land.

calcitriol the activated hormone form of vitamin D.

calorie a measure of heat; the energy necessary to do work is measured as the amount of heat produced by the body's work; the energy value of a food is expressed as the number of kilocalories that a specified portion of the food will yield when it is oxidized in the body.

carboxypeptidase a specific protein-splitting enzyme secreted as the inactive zymogen procarboxypeptidase by the pancreas; after it has been activated by trypsin, it acts in the small intestine to break off the acid (i.e., carboxyl) end of the peptide chain, thereby producing smaller-chain peptides and free amino acids.

carcinogenesis the transformation of normal cells into cancer cells.

carotene a group name for three red and yellow pigments (α-, β-, and γ-carotene) that are found in plant foods; β-carotene is most important to human nutrition because the body can convert it to vitamin A, thus making it a primary source of the vitamin.

carotenoids organic pigments that are found in plants; known to have functions such as scavenging free radicals, reducing the risk of certain types of cancer, and helping to prevent age-related eye diseases; more than 600 carotenoids have been identified, with β-carotene being the most well known.

catabolism the metabolic process of breaking down large substances to yield smaller building blocks.

catalyst a substance that increases the rate at which a specific chemical reaction proceeds but is not itself consumed during the reaction.

cellulitis the diffuse inflammation of soft or connective tissues from injury, bruises, or pressure sores that leads to infection; poor care may result in ulceration and abscess or gangrene.

cerebrovascular accident a stroke; a stroke is caused by arteriosclerosis within the blood vessels of the brain that cuts off oxygen supply to the affected portion of brain tissue, thereby paralyzing the actions that are controlled by the affected area.

chelator a ligand that binds to a metal to form a metal complex.

cholecalciferol the chemical name for vitamin D_3 in its inactive form; it is often shortened to *calciferol*.

cholecystectomy the removal of the gallbladder.

cholecystitis acute gallbladder inflammation.

cholecystokinin (CCK) hormone secreted from the mucosal epithelium of the small intestine in response to the presence of fat and certain amino acids in chyme. CCK inhibits gastric motility, increases the release of pancreatic enzymes, and stimulates the gallbladder to secrete bile into the small intestine.

cholelithiasis gallstones.

cholesterol a fat-related compound called a sterol that is synthesized only in animal tissues; a normal constituent of bile and a principal constituent of gallstones; in the body, cholesterol is primarily synthesized in the liver; in the diet, cholesterol is found in animal food sources.

chronic dieting syndrome a cyclic pattern of weight loss by dieting followed by rapid weight gain; this abnormal psychophysiologic food pattern becomes chronic, changing a person's natural body metabolism and relative body composition to the abnormal state of a metabolically obese person of normal weight.

chronic disease risk reduction (CDRR) a new category within the Dietary Reference Intakes that identifies the level of intake for which there is sufficient evidence to characterize a reduced risk for chronic disease. Sodium is the first nutrient to have an established CDRR.

chronic kidney disease-mineral and bone disorder (CKD-MBD) a clinical syndrome that develops as a systemic disorder of mineral and bone metabolism in patients with chronic kidney disease; results from abnormalities of calcium, phosphorus, parathyroid hormone, or vitamin D metabolism; causes abnormalities in bone turnover, mineralization, volume, linear growth, strength, and soft-tissue calcification.

chronologic age amount of time a person has lived.

chylomicron a lipoprotein formed in the intestinal cell that is composed of triglycerides, cholesterol, phospholipids, and protein; chylomicrons allow for the absorption of fat into the lymphatic circulatory system before entering the blood circulation.

chyme the semifluid food mass in the gastrointestinal tract that is present after gastric digestion.

chymotrypsin a protein-splitting enzyme secreted as the inactive zymogen chymotrypsinogen by the pancreas; after it has been activated by trypsin, it acts in the small intestine to continue breaking down proteins into shorter-chain polypeptides and dipeptides.

clinically severe or significant obesity a BMI of 40 kg/m^2 or more or a BMI of 35 to 39 kg/m^2 with at least one obesity-related disorder; also referred to as *extreme obesity* and *morbid obesity*.

cobalamin the chemical name for vitamin B_{12}; this vitamin is found mainly in animal protein food sources; it is closely related to amino acid metabolism and the formation of the heme portion of hemoglobin; the absence of hydrochloric acid and intrinsic factor leads to pernicious anemia and degenerative effects on the nervous system.

colloidal osmotic pressure (COP) the fluid pressure that is produced by protein molecules in the plasma and the cell; because proteins are large molecules, they do not pass through the separating membranes of the capillary walls; thus, they remain in their respective compartments and exert a constant osmotic pull that protects vital plasma and cell fluid volumes in these areas.

colostrum fluid secreted by the mammary glands for the first few days after birth, preceding the mature breast milk. Colostrum contains up to 20% protein, including a large amount of lactalbumin, minerals, and immunoglobulins that represent the antibodies found in maternal blood. It has less lactose and fat than mature milk.

complex carbohydrates large complex molecules of carbohydrates composed of many sugar units (polysaccharides); the complex forms of dietary carbohydrates are starch and dietary fiber.

conditionally indispensable amino acids the six amino acids that are normally considered dispensable amino acids because the body can make them; however, under certain circumstances (e.g., illness), the body cannot make them in high enough quantities, and they become indispensable (cannot do without) in the diet.

congenital obesity the excessive accumulation and storage of fat in the body that is present during infancy and/or childhood and is considered monogenetic.

congestive heart failure a chronic condition of gradually weakening heart muscle; the muscle is unable to pump normal blood through the heart-lung circulation, which results in the congestion of fluids in the lungs.

continuous feeding an enteral feeding schedule with which the formula is infused via a pump continuously over a 24-hour period.

continuous renal replacement therapy (CRRT) a method of blood purification that is used continuously (i.e., 24 h/day) for critically ill patients in intensive care settings. There are several forms of CRRT that vary according to the vascular access route, presence or absence of dialysate, type of semipermeable membrane used, and the mechanism of solute removal.

coronary heart disease the overall medical problem that results from the underlying disease of atherosclerosis in the coronary arteries, which serve the heart muscle with blood, oxygen, and nutrients.

crawfish boil traditional Louisiana Cajun festive meal. Typically includes crawfish, crab, shrimp, small ears of corn, new potatoes, onions, garlic and seasonings such as cayenne pepper, hot sauce, salt, lemons, and bay leaf. Smoked sausage links are occasionally added. All ingredients are added to a large pot and boiled. The contents are then spread out on newspaper-covered tables for everyone to eat from directly.

creatinine a nitrogen-carrying product of normal tissue protein breakdown; it is excreted in the urine; serum creatinine levels are an indicator of renal function.

Cushing's syndrome the excess secretion of glucocorticoids from the adrenal cortex; symptoms and complications include protein loss, obesity, fatigue, osteoporosis, edema, excess hair growth, diabetes, and skin discoloration.

D

deamination the removal of the nitrogen containing part (amino group) from an amino acid.

dehiscence a splitting open; the separation of the layers of a surgical wound that may be partial, superficial, or complete and that involves total disruption and resuturing.

dextrins intermediate starch breakdown products.

diabetes distress psychologic reaction to the intense emotional burden and negative impact of daily concerns when managing the serious and complex lifelong disease of diabetes.

diabetic ketoacidosis (DKA) also known as *ketoacidosis*, the excess production of ketones; a form of metabolic acidosis that occurs with unmanaged diabetes or starvation from burning body fat for energy fuel; a continuing uncontrolled state can result in coma and death.

dialysate the cleansing solution used in dialysis; contains dextrose and other chemicals similar to those in the body.

dialysis the process of separating crystalloids (i.e., crystal-forming substances) and colloids (i.e., glue-like substances) in solution by the difference in their rates of diffusion through a semipermeable membrane; crystalloids (e.g., blood glucose, other simple metabolites) pass through readily, and colloids (e.g., plasma proteins) pass through slowly or not at all. Dialysis is the process of removing waste and excess fluid from the blood when one's kidneys are not functioning.

Dietary Reference Intakes (DRIs) reference values for the nutrient intake needs of healthy individuals for each sex and age group.

dietetics the management of the diet and the use of food; the science concerned with nutrition planning, medical nutrition therapy, and the preparation of foods.

digestion the process by which food is broken down in the gastrointestinal tract to release nutrients in forms that the body can absorb.

dipeptidase the final enzyme in the protein-splitting system that releases free amino acids from dipeptide bonds.

dispensable amino acids the amino acids that the body can synthesize from other amino acids that are supplied through the diet and thus do not have to be consumed on a daily basis.

diuresis the increased excretion of urine.

diuretic any substance that induces urination and subsequent fluid loss.

diverticula small protruding pouches, or herniations, in the colonic mucosa through the muscular layer.

diverticulitis the inflammation of pockets of tissue (i.e., diverticula) in the lining of the mucous membrane of the colon.

doubly labeled water method gold standard for measuring energy expenditure. Participants ingest water labeled with a known concentration of isotopes of hydrogen and oxygen. Technicians measure the elimination of the isotopes to predict the energy expenditure and metabolic rate.

dual-energy x-ray absorptiometry radiography that makes use of two beams (i.e., dual) that measure bone density and body composition.

dumping syndrome condition in which there is a quick emptying of the stomach of a hyperosmolar content into the small intestine, causing fluid to shift into the intestinal lumen from the intravascular compartment.

dynamic equilibrium the process of maintaining balance (i.e., equilibrium) through constant change or motion by energy or action (i.e., dynamic).

dysbiosis imbalance of the intestinal microbiome.

dyslipidemia abnormal lipid profile (high total cholesterol, low-density lipoprotein cholesterol, or triglycerides; and/or low high-density lipoprotein cholesterol).

dysphagia difficulty swallowing.

E

early-onset obesity a genetically associated obesity that occurs during early childhood.

other specified feeding or eating disorder subthreshold disordered eating that is not consistent with the diagnostic criteria for bulimia nervosa or anorexia nervosa.

edema an unusual accumulation of fluid in the interstitial compartments (i.e., the small structural spaces between tissue parts) of the body.

estimated glomerular filtration rate (eGFR) equation used to measure kidney function.

element a single type of atom; a total of 118 elements have been identified, of which 94 occur naturally on Earth; elements cannot be broken down into smaller substances.

elemental formula a nutrition support formula that is composed of simple elemental nutrient components that require no further digestive breakdown and are thus readily absorbed; these formulas include protein as free amino acids and carbohydrate as the simple sugar glucose.

emulsifier an agent that breaks down large fat globules into smaller, uniformly distributed particles; the action is chiefly accomplished in the intestine by bile acids, which lower the surface tension of the fat particles, thereby breaking the fat into many smaller droplets and facilitating contact with the fat-digesting enzymes.

energy-yielding nutrients nutrients that break down to yield energy within the body, including carbohydrates, fat, protein.

enriched a word that is used to describe foods to which vitamins and minerals have been added back to a food after a refining process that caused a loss of some nutrients; for example, iron may be lost during the refining process of a grain, so the final product will be enriched with additional iron.

enteral a mode of feeding that makes use of the gastrointestinal tract through oral or tube feeding.

enterokinase an enzyme produced and secreted in the duodenum in response to food entering the small intestine; it activates trypsinogen to its active form of trypsin.

enzymes the proteins produced in the body that digest or change nutrients in specific chemical reactions without being changed themselves during the process, thus their action is that of a catalyst; digestive enzymes in gastrointestinal secretions act on food substances to break them down into simpler compounds. An enzyme usually is named after the substance (i.e., substrate) on which it acts, with the common word ending of -*ase*; for example, sucrase is the specific enzyme for sucrose, which it breaks down into glucose and fructose.

ergocalciferol the chemical name for vitamin D_2 in its inactive form; it is produced by some organisms (not humans) upon ultraviolet irradiation from the precursor ergosterol.

ergogenic the tendency to increase work output; various substances that increase work or exercise capacity and output.

erythropoietin hormone that stimulates the production of red blood cells in the bone marrow.

esophageal varices the pathologic dilation of the blood vessels within the wall of the esophagus as a result of liver cirrhosis; these vessels can continue to expand to the point of rupturing.

esophagitis inflammation of the esophagus.

essential (or primary) hypertension an inherent form of high blood pressure with no specific identifiable cause; it is considered to be familial.

essential nutrients nutrients a person must obtain from food because the body cannot make them for itself in sufficient quantity to meet physiologic needs.

estrogen hormones sex hormone produced primarily by the ovaries.

euglycemia normal blood glucose level.

euvolemia normal blood volume.

exogenous originating from outside the body.

expanded-criteria donors any donor who is older than 60 years old who has met the criteria for brain-death or a donor who is older than 50 years old with two of the following conditions: history of hypertension, a terminal serum creatinine level of at least 1.5 mg/dL, or death from a cerebrovascular accident.

extrusion reflex the normal infant reflex to protrude the tongue outward when it is touched.

exudate various materials such as cells, cellular debris, and fluids that have escaped from the blood vessels and that are deposited in or on the surface tissues, usually as a result of inflammation; the protein content of exudate is high.

F

familial hypercholesterolemia a genetic disorder that results in elevated blood cholesterol levels despite lifestyle modifications; this condition is caused by absent or nonfunctional low-density lipoprotein receptors, and it requires drug therapy for treatment.

familial hypertriglyceridemia a genetic disorder that results in elevated blood triglyceride levels despite lifestyle modifications; it requires drug therapy for treatment.

fatty acids the major structural components of fats.

ferritin the storage form of iron.

fetal alcohol spectrum disorders (FASD) a group of physical and mental birth defects that are found in infants who are born to mothers who used alcohol during pregnancy; the physical and mental disabilities vary in severity; there is no cure.

fetal alcohol syndrome (FAS) a combination of physical and mental birth defects that are found in infants who are born to mothers who used alcohol during pregnancy; this is the most severe of the fetal alcohol spectrum disorders; there is no cure.

filé powder a substance that is made from ground sassafras leaves; it seasons and thickens the dish into which it is added.

fistulas from the Latin word for "pipe," an abnormal opening or passageway within the body or to the outside.

fluorosis an excess intake of fluoride that causes the yellowing of teeth, white spots on the teeth, and the pitting or mottling of tooth enamel.

food insecurity limited or uncertain availability of nutritionally adequate and safe foods or limited or uncertain ability to acquire acceptable foods in socially acceptable ways.

food jag brief sprees or binges of eating one particular food.

food neophobia the fear of new food.

fundoplication a surgery that is used to treat gastroesophageal reflux disease; the upper portion of the stomach (i.e., the fundus) is wrapped around the esophagus and sewn into place so that the esophagus passes through the muscle of the stomach; this strengthens the esophageal sphincter to prevent acid reflux.

G

galactosemia an autosomal recessive genetic disorder in which the liver does not produce the enzyme that is needed to metabolize galactose.

gastric inhibitory peptide (GIP) a hormone secreted from the enterocytes of the duodenum and jejunum in response to the presence of glucose and fat. GIP stimulates insulin secretion from the pancreas and inhibits gastric motility.

gastrin a hormone that helps with gastric motility, that stimulates the secretion of gastric acid by the parietal cells of the stomach, and that stimulates the chief cells to secrete pepsinogen.

gastroscopy an examination of the upper intestinal tract with a flexible tube with a small camera on the end; the tube is approximately 9 mm in diameter, and it takes color pictures as well as biopsy samples, if necessary.

glomerular filtration rate (GFR) the volume of fluid that is filtered from the renal glomerular capillaries into Bowman's capsule per unit of time; this term is used clinically as a measure of kidney function.

glomerulus the first section of the nephron; a cluster of capillary loops that are cupped in the nephron head that serves as an initial filter.

glucagon a hormone secreted by the α cells of the pancreatic islets of Langerhans in response to hypoglycemia; it has an effect opposite to that of insulin in that it raises the blood glucose concentration and thus is used as a quick-acting antidote for a low blood glucose reaction; it also counteracts the overnight fast during sleep by breaking down liver glycogen to keep blood glucose levels normal and to maintain an adequate energy supply for normal nerve and brain function.

glucagonoma a very rare neuroendocrine tumor found in the α cells of the pancreas that leads to an overproduction of glucagon; may be characterized by diabetes, weight loss, high levels of glucagon, and hypoaminoacidemia.

gluconeogenesis the formation of glucose from noncarbohydrate substances such as amino acids.

GLUT4 an insulin-regulated protein that is responsible for glucose transport into cells.

glycemic control management of blood glucose levels within individualized targets.

glycemic index a ranking of foods relative to the increase above fasting in the blood glucose level more than 2 hours after the ingestion of a constant amount of that food divided by the response to a reference food.

glycerides the chemical group name for fats; fats are formed from a glycerol base with one, two, or three fatty acids attached to make monoglycerides, diglycerides, and triglycerides, respectively; glycerides are the principal constituents of adipose tissue, and they are found in animal and vegetable fats and oils.

glycogen a polysaccharide; a complex carbohydrate that is the main storage form of carbohydrates found in animal tissue that is composed of many glucose units linked together; stored primarily in the liver and to a lesser extent in muscle tissue.

glycogenesis the anabolic process of creating stored glycogen from glucose.

glycolipid a lipid with a carbohydrate attached.

goiter an enlarged thyroid gland that is usually caused by a lack of iodine to produce the thyroid hormone thyroxine.

gut microbiota microorganisms found in the gastrointestinal tract.

gynecomastia the excessive development of the male mammary glands, frequently as a result of increased estrogen levels.

H

Hamwi method a formula for estimating the ideal body weight on the basis of sex and height.

health a state of optimal physical, mental, and social well-being; relative freedom from disease or disability.

healthy eating index a measure of diet quality used to assess how well a food plan aligns with key recommendations of the *Dietary Guidelines for Americans*.

health promotion the active engagement in behaviors or programs that advance positive well-being.

hematuria the abnormal presence of blood in the urine.

hemochromatosis genetic disease resulting in iron overload.

hemoglobin a conjugated protein in red blood cells that is composed of a compact, rounded mass of polypeptide chains that forms globin (the protein portion) and that is attached to an iron-containing red pigment called *heme*; carries oxygen in the blood to cells.

hemolytic uremic syndrome a condition that results most often from infection with *Escherichia coli* and that presents with a destruction of red blood cells (i.e., hemolysis) and kidney failure.

hepatic encephalopathy a condition in which toxins in the blood lead to alterations in brain homeostasis as a result of liver disease; this results in apathy, confusion, inappropriate behavior, altered consciousness, and eventually coma.

hepatitis the inflammation of the liver cells; symptoms of acute hepatitis include flu-like symptoms, muscle and joint aches, fever, nausea, vomiting, diarrhea, headache, dark urine, and yellowing of the eyes and skin; symptoms of chronic hepatitis include jaundice, abdominal swelling and sensitivity, low-grade fever, and ascites.

hepatocyte cells of the liver.

homeostasis the state of relative dynamic equilibrium within the body's internal environment; a balance that is achieved through the operation of various interrelated physiologic mechanisms.

human milk fortifiers powder or liquid mixed with breast milk to increase the concentration of calories and protein in the milk for premature and low birth weight infants who need more kcal/mL than provided in breast milk.

hydrophilic water loving.

hydrophobic water fearing.

hydrostatic pressure the force exerted by a fluid pushing against a surface.

hydroxyapatite $(Ca_{10}[PO_4]6[OH]_2)$ the major mineral component of normal bone and teeth; provides structure and rigidity to bone; primary storage site of calcium and phosphorus in the body.

hypercalcemia a serum calcium level that is above normal.

hypercholesterolemia high cholesterol levels in the blood.

hyperemesis gravidarum a condition that involves prolonged and severe vomiting in pregnant women, with a loss of more than 5% of body weight and the presence of ketonuria, electrolyte disturbances, and dehydration.

hyperglycemia an elevated blood glucose level.

hyperhomocysteinemia the presence of high levels of homocysteine in the blood; associated with cardiovascular disease.

hyperkalemia a serum potassium level that is above normal.

hyperlipidemia high lipid levels in the blood.

hypernatremia a serum sodium level that is above normal.

hyperoxaluria excess oxalates in the urine.

hyperphosphatemia a serum phosphorus level that is above normal.

hypertension chronically elevated blood pressure; systolic blood pressure is consistently 130 mm Hg or more or diastolic blood pressure is consistently 85 mm Hg or more.

hypertriglyceridemia high levels of triglycerides in the blood.

hypocalcemia a serum calcium level that is below normal.

hypogeusia impaired taste.

hypoglycemia a low blood glucose level; a serious condition in diabetes management that requires immediate fast-acting glucose intake to increase blood glucose to safe levels.

hypokalemia a serum potassium level that is below normal.

hypomagnesemia a serum magnesium level that is below normal.

hyponatremia a serum sodium level that is below normal.

hypophosphatemia a serum phosphorus level that is below normal.

hyposmia impaired ability to smell.

hypotension low blood pressure.

hypovolemia low blood volume.

I

idiopathic of unknown cause.

ileum the third, and final, portion of the small intestine.

immunocompetence the ability or capacity to develop an immune response (i.e., antibody production or cell-mediated immunity) after exposure to an antigen.

indispensable amino acids the nine amino acids that must be obtained from the diet because the body does not make adequate amounts to support body needs.

insulin a hormone produced by the β cell in the pancreas, attaches to insulin receptors on cell membranes, and allows the absorption of glucose into the cell.

insulin secretagogues an oral medication that stimulates the β cells to secrete insulin to help lower overall blood glucose levels. Side effects are increased risk of hypoglycemia and weight gain.

intrauterine growth restriction (IUGR) a condition that occurs when a fetus weighs less than 10% of predicted weight for gestational age.

K

keratomalacia drying and clouding of the cornea because of vitamin A deficiency.

ketoacidosis the excess production of ketones; a form of metabolic acidosis that occurs with uncontrolled diabetes or starvation from burning body fat for energy fuel; a continuing uncontrolled state can result in coma and death.

ketogenesis a metabolic pathway that produces ketones bodies as an alternative source of energy for the body; manifests when carbohydrate stores are significantly reduced and the body breaks down fatty acids that are converted into acetone, acetoacetate, and β-hydroxybutyrate.

ketones the chemical name for a class of organic compounds that includes three keto acid bases that occur as intermediate products of fat metabolism.

ketosis the accumulation of ketones, which are intermediate products of fat metabolism, in the blood.

kilocalorie the general term *calorie* refers to a unit of heat measure, and it is used alone to designate the small calorie; the calorie that is used in nutrition science and the study of metabolism is the large Calorie or kilocalorie, which avoids the use of large numbers in calculations; a kilocalorie, which is composed of 1000 calories, is the measure of heat that is necessary to raise the temperature of 1000 g (1 L) of water by 1° C.

kinesiotherapist a health care professional who treats the effects of disease, injury, and congenital disorders through the application of scientifically based exercise principles that have been adapted to enhance the strength, endurance, and mobility of individuals with functional limitations or for those patients who require extended physical conditioning.

L

lactated Ringer's solution a sterile solution of calcium chloride, potassium chloride, sodium chloride, and sodium lactate in water that is given to replenish fluid and electrolytes; this solution was developed by the English physiologist Sidney Ringer (1835-1910).

lactation specialist health care professionals with specialized knowledge and clinical expertise in breastfeeding and human lactation. Also known as a *lactation consultant*.

large for gestational age (LGA) infant is larger than a sex- and gestational age–matched infant. Birth weight is above the 90th percentile.

life expectancy the number of years that a person of a given age may expect to live; this is affected by environment, lifestyle, sex, and race.

linoleic acid an essential fatty acid that consists of 18 carbon atoms and 2 double bonds. The first double bond is located at the sixth carbon from the omega end, making it an omega-6 fatty acid. Found in vegetable oils.

lipectomy the surgical removal of subcutaneous fat by suction through a tube that is inserted into a surface incision or by the removal of larger amounts of subcutaneous fat through a major surgical incision.

lipids the chemical group name for organic substances of a fatty nature; the lipids include fats, oils, waxes, and other fat-related compounds such as cholesterol.

lipiduria lipid droplets found in the urine that are composed mostly of cholesterol esters.

lipogenesis the anabolic process of forming fat.

lipoproteins chemical complexes of fat and protein that serve as the major carriers of lipids in the plasma; they vary in density according to the size of the fat load being carried (i.e., the lower the density, the higher the fat load); the combination package with water-soluble protein makes possible the transport of non–water-soluble fatty substances in the water-based blood circulation.

lobectomy surgical removal of a lobe of an organ.

M

macrosomia excessive fetal growth that results in an abnormally large infant.

major minerals the group of minerals that are required by the body in amounts of more than 100 mg/day.

masculinization a condition marked by the attainment of male characteristics (e.g., facial hair) either physiologically as part of male maturation or pathologically by either sex.

mechanical soft diet a meal plan that consists of foods that have been chopped, blended, ground, or prepared with extra fluid to make chewing and swallowing easier.

medical nutrition therapy a specific nutrition service and procedure that is used to treat an illness, injury, or condition; it involves an in-depth nutrition assessment of the patient, nutrition diagnosis, nutrition intervention (which may include diet therapy, counseling, and the use of specialized nutrition supplements), and nutrition monitoring and evaluation.

megacolon abnormally enlarged colon.

melatonin the hormone responsible for regulating body rhythms.

menopause the end of a woman's menstrual activity and capacity to bear children.

metabolic syndrome a combination of disorders that, when they occur together, increases the risk of cardiovascular disease and diabetes; it is also known as *syndrome X* and *insulin resistance syndrome*.

metabolism the sum of all chemical changes that take place in the body by which it maintains itself and produces energy for its functioning; products of the various reactions are called *metabolites*.

metastasis the spread to other tissue.

micelles packages of free fatty acids, monoglycerides, and bile salts; the hydrophobic fat particles are found in the middle of the package, whereas the hydrophilic part faces outward and allows for the absorption of fat into intestinal mucosal cells.

microalbuminuria low but abnormal levels of albumin in the urine.

microbiome microorganisms living in a specific environment.

microvilli extremely small, hair-like projections that cover all of the villi on the surface of the small intestine and that greatly increase the total absorbing surface area; they are visible through an electron microscope.

mucosal folds the large, visible folds of the mucous lining of the small intestine that increase the absorbing surface area.

mucositis an inflammation of the tissues around the mouth or other orifices of the body.

mutation a permanent transmissible change in a gene.

myocardial infarction (MI) a heart attack; a myocardial infarction is caused by the failure of the heart muscle to maintain normal blood circulation as a result of the blockage of the coronary arteries with fatty cholesterol plaques that cut off the delivery of oxygen to the affected part of the heart muscle.

MyPlate a visual pattern of the current basic five food groups—grains, vegetables, fruits, dairy, and protein—arranged on a plate to indicate proportionate amounts of daily food choices.

N

negative energy balance more total energy is expended than consumed.

neoplasm any new or abnormal cellular growth, specifically one that is uncontrolled and aggressive.

nephrolithiasis the formation of a kidney stone.

nephron the functional unit of the kidney that filters and reabsorbs essential blood constituents, secretes hydrogen ions as needed to maintain the acid-base balance, reabsorbs water, and forms and excretes a concentrated urine for the elimination of wastes.

nephrosis degenerative lesions of the renal tubules of the nephrons and especially of the thin basement membrane of the glomerulus that helps to support the capillary loops; marked by edema, albuminuria, and a decreased serum albumin level.

nephrotoxic toxic to the kidney.

niacin the chemical name for vitamin B_3; this vitamin was discovered in relation to the deficiency disease pellagra; it is important as a coenzyme factor in many cell reactions related to energy and protein metabolism.

nonessential nutrient a nutrient that can be manufactured in the body by means of other nutrients. Thus, it is not essential to consume regularly in the diet.

non–energy-yielding nutrients nutrients that do not break down to yield energy within the body, including vitamins, minerals, and water.

nursing diagnosis clinical judgment about individual, family, or community experiences/responses to actual or potential health problems/life processes. Nursing diagnoses provide the basis for selection of nursing interventions to achieve outcomes for which the nurse has accountability.

nursing process the means by which nurses deliver care to patients; it includes the following steps: assessment, diagnosis, planning, implementation, and evaluation.

nutrition the sum of the processes involved with the intake of nutrients as well as assimilating and using them to maintain body tissue and provide energy; a foundation for life and health.

nutrition care process model a systematic approach to providing high-quality individualized nutrition care. The model consists of the following steps: assessment, diagnosis, intervention, and monitoring and evaluation.

nutrition integrity a level of performance that ensures all foods and beverages available in schools are consistent with the *Dietary Guidelines for Americans,* and, when combined with nutrition education, physical activity, and a healthful school environment; contributes to enhanced learning and development of lifelong, healthful eating habits.

nutrition science the body of science, developed through controlled research, that relates to the processes involved in nutrition internationally, clinically, and in the community.

O

oliguria the secretion of small amounts of urine in relation to fluid intake (i.e., 0.5 mL/kg per hour or less).

"One-Step" A method for diagnosing diabetes using a 75-g oral glucose tolerance test. The patient's fasting plasma glucose level is measured, then the patient drinks a solution with 75 g of glucose; plasma glucose level is measured again at 1 hour and 2 hour postconsumption. Diagnostic criteria are based on the levels of plasma glucose at each measurement.

organic farming the use of farming methods that employ natural means of pest control and that meet the standards set by the National Organic Program of the U.S. Department of Agriculture; organic foods are grown or produced without the use of synthetic pesticides or fertilizers, sewage sludge, genetically modified organisms, or ionizing radiation.

osmosis the passage of a solvent (e.g., water) through a membrane that separates solutions of different concentrations and that tends to equalize the concentration pressures of the solutions on either side of the membrane.

osmotic pressure hydrostatic pressure across a semipermeable membrane that is necessary to maintain the normal movement of fluid between the capillaries and the surrounding tissue.

osteoblast cells that are responsible for the mineralization and formation of bone.

osteodystrophy an alteration of bone morphology found in patients with chronic kidney disease.

osteomalacia soft bones typically caused from a vitamin D or calcium deficiency.

osteopenia a condition that involves a low bone mass and an increased risk for fracture.

osteoporosis an abnormal thinning of the bone that produces a porous, fragile, lattice-like bone tissue of enlarged spaces that are prone to fracture or deformity.

outbreak of food-borne illness the occurrence of two or more similar illnesses resulting from ingestion of a common food.

oxytocin hormone released from the posterior pituitary gland that stimulates breast milk let-down.

P

pancreatic amylase a major starch-splitting enzyme that is secreted by the pancreas and that acts in the small intestine.

pancreatic lipase a major fat-splitting enzyme produced by the pancreas and secreted into the small intestine to digest fat.

pandemic a widespread epidemic distributed throughout a region, a continent, or the world.

pantothenic acid a B-complex vitamin that is found widely distributed in nature and that occurs throughout the body tissues; it is an essential constituent of the body's main activating agent, coenzyme A.

parasite an organism that lives in or on an organism of another species, known as the *host*, from whom all nourishment is obtained.

parenteral a mode of nourishment that does not make use of the gastrointestinal tract but that instead provides nutrition support via the intravenous delivery of nutrient solutions.

parotid glands the largest of the three pairs of salivary glands; the parotid glands lie, one on each side, above the angle of the jaw and below and in front of the ear; they continually secrete saliva, which passes along the duct of the gland and into the mouth through an opening in the inner cheek that is level with the second upper molar tooth.

pellagra the deficiency disease caused by a lack of dietary niacin and an inadequate amount of protein that contains the amino acid tryptophan, which is a precursor of niacin; pellagra is characterized by skin lesions that are aggravated by sunlight as well as by gastrointestinal, mucosal, neurologic, and mental symptoms.

pepsin the main gastric enzyme specific to proteins; it begins breaking large protein molecules into shorter-chain polypeptides; gastric hydrochloric acid is necessary for its activation.

peritoneal cavity a serous membrane that lines the abdominal and pelvic walls and the undersurface of the diaphragm to form a sac that encloses the body's vital visceral organs.

peritoneal dialysis is a form of dialysis in which the waste/excess fluid is filtered using the individual's peritoneal membrane. There are three basic steps: (1) fill the peritoneal membrane with dialysate, (2) allow the dialysate to dwell, (3) drain the dialysate, which now contains waste and excess fluid.

pernicious anemia a form of megaloblastic anemia resulting from vitamin B_{12} deficiency. Sometimes caused by insufficient or non-functioning gastric parietal cells that produce intrinsic factor; without intrinsic factor, vitamin B_{12} cannot be absorbed.

pharynx the muscular membranous passage that extends from the mouth to the posterior nasal passages, the larynx, and the esophagus.

pheochromocytoma a tumor of the adrenal medulla or the sympathetic nervous system in which the affected cells secrete excess epinephrine or norepinephrine and cause headache, hypertension, and nausea.

phospholipids class of lipids that are structural to the lipid bilayer of cell membranes. Composed of a glycerol backbone with two fatty acids and a phosphate group.

photosynthesis the process by which plants that contain chlorophyll are able to manufacture carbohydrates by combining carbon dioxide and water; sunlight is used as energy, and chlorophyll is a catalyst.

phylloquinone a fat-soluble vitamin of the K group that is found primarily in green plants.

plaque thick wax-like coating forming inside artery walls; primarily composed of cholesterol, fatty substances, cellular debris, calcium, and fibrin.

plasma protein any of a number of protein substances that are carried in the circulating blood; a major one is *albumin,* which maintains the fluid volume of the blood through colloidal osmotic pressure.

polarity the interaction between the positively charged end of one molecule and the negative end of another (or the same) molecule.

polydipsia excessive thirst and drinking.

polymeric formula a nutrition support formula that is composed of complete protein, polysaccharides, and fat as medium-chain fatty acids.

polypharmacy the use of multiple medications by the same patient.

polyuria excessive urination.

portal an entrance or gateway; for example, the portal blood circulation designates the entry of blood vessels from the intestines into the liver; it carries nutrients for liver metabolism, and it then drains into the body's main systemic circulation to deliver metabolic products to body cells.

portal hypertension high blood pressure in the portal vein.

postprandial after eating; normally 1 to 2 hours after a meal.

prebiotic nondigestible foods that promote the growth of beneficial microorganisms within the gut.

pregnancy-induced hypertension the development of hypertension during pregnancy after the 20th week of gestation. Also referred to as *hypertensive disorders of pregnancy.*

primary deficiency deficiency of a nutrient because of inadequate dietary intake. Different from secondary causes where the deficiency is due to malabsorption or other bioavailability hindrances.

probiotic a food that contains live microbials, which are thought to benefit the consumer by improving intestinal microbial balance (e.g., lactobacilli in yogurt).

proenzyme an inactive precursor (i.e., a forerunner substance from which another substance is made) that is converted to the active enzyme by the action of an acid, another enzyme, or other means.

prohormone a precursor substance that the body converts to a hormone; for example, a cholesterol compound in the skin is first irradiated by sunlight and then converted through successive enzyme actions in the liver and kidney into the active vitamin D hormone, which then regulates calcium absorption and bone development.

prolactin hormone released from the anterior pituitary gland that stimulates breast milk production.

proteinuria an abnormal excess of serum proteins (e.g., albumin) in the urine.

pulmonary edema an accumulation of fluid in the lung tissues.

pyridoxine the chemical name of vitamin B_6; in its activated phosphate form (i.e., B_2PO_4), pyridoxine functions as an important coenzyme factor in many reactions in cell metabolism that are related to amino acids, glucose, and fatty acids.

R

Ramadan the ninth month of the Muslim year, which is a period of daily fasting from sunrise to sunset.

Recommended Dietary Allowances (RDAs) the average daily dietary intake level that is sufficient to meet the nutrient requirement of nearly all healthy individuals in a group.

refeeding syndrome a potentially fatal condition that occurs when severely malnourished individuals are fed high-carbohydrate diets too aggressively; a sudden shift in electrolytes and fluid retention and a drastic drop in serum phosphorus, potassium, and magnesium levels cause a series of complications that involve several organs.

registered dietitian nutritionist (RDN) a professional dietitian accredited with an academic degree from an undergraduate or graduate study program who has passed required registration examinations administered by the Commission on Dietetic Registration (CDR). The RDN and RD (registered dietitian) credentials are legally protected titles that may only be used by authorized practitioners. The term *nutritionist* alone is not a legally protected or licensed title in most states. See www.eatright.org for more details.

renin an enzyme released from the kidney in the presence of hypovolemia; it converts angiotensinogen to angiotensin I.

rennin the milk-curdling enzyme of the gastric juice of human infants and young animals (e.g., calves); rennin should not be confused with renin, which is an important enzyme produced by the kidneys that plays a vital role in the activation of angiotensin.

residue any undigested or unabsorbed food remaining in the colon after digestion has taken place; includes fiber and substances that stimulate contractions of the GI tract.

resistant hypertension the presence of high blood pressure despite treatment with three antihypertensive medications.

resorption the destruction, loss, or dissolution of a tissue or a part of a tissue by biochemical activity (e.g., the loss of bone, the loss of tooth dentin).

resting energy expenditure (REE) the amount of energy (in kcal) needed by the body for the maintenance of life at rest over a 24-hour period; this is often used interchangeably with the term *basal energy expenditure*, but in actuality it is slightly higher because the protocol for measurement does not put the person at complete rest. Also referred to as *resting metabolic rate (RMR)*.

retinol the chemical name of vitamin A; the name is derived from the vitamin's visual functions related to the retina of the eye, which is the back inner lining of the eyeball that catches the light refractions of the lens to form images that are interpreted by the optic nerve and the brain and that makes the necessary light-dark adaptations.

riboflavin the chemical name for vitamin B_2; it has a role as a coenzyme factor in many cell reactions related to energy and protein metabolism.

rickets a disease of childhood that is characterized by the softening of the bones from an inadequate intake of vitamin D and insufficient exposure to sunlight; it is also associated with impaired calcium and phosphorus metabolism.

rooting reflex reflex that occurs when an infant's cheek is stroked or touched. The infant will turn toward the stimuli and make sucking (or rooting) motions in an effort to nurse.

S

saccharide the chemical name for sugar molecules; may occur as single molecules in monosaccharides (glucose, fructose, galactose), two molecules in disaccharides (sucrose, lactose, maltose), or multiple molecules in polysaccharides (starch, dietary fiber, glycogen).

salivary amylase a starch-splitting enzyme that is secreted by the salivary glands in the mouth and that is commonly called *ptyalin* (from the Greek word *ptyalon*, meaning "spittle").

sarcopenia loss of lean tissue mass associated with aging.

saturated the state of being filled; the state of fatty acid components being filled in all their available carbon bonds with hydrogen, thus making the fat harder and more solid at room temperature; such solid food fats are generally from animal sources.

school breakfast and lunch programs federally assisted meal programs that operate in public and nonprofit private schools and residential child-care institutions; these programs provide nutritionally balanced, low-cost, or free meals to children each school day.

scleroderma hardening and tightening of the skin and connective tissue.

screen time time spent in front of any electronic screen—television, computer, phone, DVD players, portable gaming devices, etc.

scurvy a hemorrhagic disease caused by a lack of vitamin C that is characterized by diffuse tissue bleeding, painful limbs and joints, thickened bones, and skin discoloration from bleeding; bones fracture easily, wounds do not heal, gums swell and tend to bleed, and the teeth loosen.

secondary hypertension an elevated blood pressure for which the cause can be identified and which is a symptom or side effect of another primary condition.

secretin a hormone that stimulates gastric and pancreatic secretions. Secretin stimulates the secretion of pepsinogen from the chief cells of the stomach. In response to a low pH in the duodenum, secretin stimulates the pancreatic release of bicarbonate to increase the pH to an alkaline environment.

senescence the process or condition of growing old.

sepsis a life-threatening immune response to a bacterial infection.

short-bowel syndrome malabsorption disorder caused by a lack of functional small intestine.

simple carbohydrates sugars with a simple structure of one or two single-sugar (saccharide) units; a monosaccharide is composed of one sugar unit, and a disaccharide is composed of two sugar units.

small for gestational age (SGA) infant is smaller than a sex- and gestational age–matched infant. Birth weight is below the 10th percentile.

sorbitol a sugar alcohol that is often used as a nutritive sugar substitute; it is named for where it was discovered in nature, in ripe berries of the *Sorbus aucuparia* tree; it also occurs naturally in small quantities in various other berries, cherries, plums, and pears.

speech-language pathologist a specialist in the assessment, diagnosis, treatment, and prevention of speech, language, cognitive communication, voice, swallowing, fluency, and other related disorders.

spina bifida a congenital defect in the embryonic fetal closing of the neural tube to form a portion of the lower spine, which leaves the spine unclosed and the spinal cord open to various degrees of exposure and damage.

state land grant universities an institution of higher education that has been designated by the state to receive unique federal support as a result of the Morrill Acts of 1862 and 1890.

steatorrhea fatty diarrhea; excessive amount of fat in the feces, which is often caused by malabsorption diseases.

steatosis accumulation of fat in the liver cells.

stillbirth the death of a fetus after the 20th week of pregnancy.

stoma the opening that is established in the abdominal wall that connects with the ileum or the colon for the elimination of intestinal waste after the surgical removal of nonfunctional portions of the intestines.

sugar alcohols nutritive sweeteners that provide 2 to 3 kcal/g; examples include sorbitol, mannitol, and xylitol; these are produced in food-industry laboratories for use as sweeteners in candies, chewing gum, beverages, and other foods.

supersaturation (pertaining to urine) excess concentration of solutes.

T

team-based care approach a multidisciplinary group of health care professionals working collaboratively.

teratogen a substance or factor resulting in birth defects or miscarriage of an embryo or fetus.

teratogenic causing a birth defect.

intensive lifestyle intervention an intensive lifestyle intervention that is focused on appropriate weight, diet, physical activity, and other controllable risk factors to reduce cholesterol levels and to prevent other complications of heart disease.

thermic effect of food an increase in energy expenditure caused by the activities of digestion, absorption, transport, and metabolism of ingested food; a meal that consists of a usual mixture of carbohydrates, protein, and fat increases the energy expenditure equivalent to approximately 10% of the food's energy content (e.g., a 300-kcal piece of pizza would elicit an energy expenditure of 30 kcal to digest the food).

thiamin the chemical name of vitamin B_1; this vitamin was discovered in relation to the classic deficiency disease beriberi, and it is important in body metabolism as a coenzyme factor in many cell reactions related to energy metabolism.

thyroid-stimulating hormone (TSH) hormone released from the anterior pituitary gland that regulates the activity of the thyroid gland; also known as *thyrotropin*.

thyrotropin-releasing hormone (TRH) a hormone produced by the hypothalamus that stimulates the release of thyroid-stimulating hormone by the pituitary.

thyroxine (T_4) an iodine-dependent thyroid prohormone; the active hormone form is T_3; it is the major controller of basal metabolic rate.

tocopherol the chemical name for vitamin E, which was named by early investigators because their initial work with rats indicated a reproductive function (Greek translation, "child bearing"); in people, vitamin E functions as a strong antioxidant that preserves structural membranes such as cell membranes.

trace minerals the group of elements that are required by the body in amounts of less than 100 mg/day.

transferrin a protein that binds and transports iron through the blood.

transport (in terms of nutrition and metabolism) the movement of nutrients through the circulatory system from one area of the body to another.

triglycerides the chemical name for fats in the body or in food; three fatty acids attached to a glycerol base.

trypsin a protein-splitting enzyme secreted as the inactive proenzyme trypsinogen by the pancreas and that is activated by enterokinase (or the presence of active trypsin); works in the small intestine to reduce proteins to shorter-chain polypeptides and dipeptides.

"Two-Step" A method for diagnosing diabetes using a two-step method of oral glucose tolerance test in a nonfasting patient. Step 1: The patient drinks a 50-g glucose solution and plasma glucose is measured at 1 hour postconsumption. If the patient's plasma glucose level is ≥140 g/dL, then the patient must return for Step 2, which is a fasting 100-g glucose tolerance test.

U

ultrasonography an ultrasound-based diagnostic imaging technique that is used to visualize the muscles and internal organs; also referred to as *sonography*.

unintentional weight loss weight loss of ≥5% of body weight over a 1- to 6-month period that is not intentional.

urea the chief nitrogen-carrying product of dietary protein metabolism; urea appears in the blood, lymph, and urine.

V

vacuole a small space or cavity that is formed in the protoplasm of the cell.

vagotomy the cutting of the vagus nerve, which supplies a major stimulus for gastric secretions.

vasculitis the inflammation of the walls of blood vessels.

vasopressin a hormone of the pituitary gland that acts on the distal nephron tubule to conserve water by reabsorption; also known as *antidiuretic hormone*.

villi small protrusions from the surface of a membrane; finger-like projections that cover the mucosal surfaces of the small intestine and that further increase the absorbing surface area; they are visible through a regular microscope.

VO_2max the maximal uptake volume of oxygen during exercise; this is used to measure the intensity and duration of exercise that a person can perform.

W

waist circumference the measurement of the waist at its narrowest point width-wise, just above the navel; waist circumference is a rough measurement of abdominal fat and a predictor of risk factors for cardiovascular disease; this risk factor increases with a waist measurement of more than 40 inches in men and of more than 35 inches in women.

weaning the process of gradually acclimating a young child to food other than the mother's milk or a breast milk substitute as the child's natural need to suckle wanes.

Wilson's disease an autosomal recessive genetic disorder in which copper accumulates in tissue and causes damage to organs.

X

xerophthalmia progressive ocular disease, frequently caused by vitamin A deficiency, beginning with severe dryness of the cornea and conjunctiva.

xerostomia the condition of dry mouth that results from a lack of saliva; saliva production can be hindered by certain diseases (e.g., diabetes, Parkinson's disease) and by some prescription and over-the-counter medications.

Z

zymogen an inactive enzyme precursor.

Answers to Chapter Review Questions

CHAPTER 1

Chapter Review Questions

1. a
2. a
3. b
4. d
5. a

Next-Generation NCLEX® Examination-style Case Study Answers

1. a, c, d, e

   Rationale: Signs of poor nutrition come in many different forms such as prolonged injury, frequent illness, and fatigue. We can also see poor nutrition in the physical appearance of hair, skin, and eyes. Behaviors such as restricting certain foods and eliminating whole food groups puts individuals at greater risk of poor nutrition since they are no longer getting nutrients from those foods. Consuming large amounts of fruits and vegetables provides many nutrients and contributes to good nutrition, provided the individual consumes adequate calories. Small, frequent meals are encouraged in clients with small appetites so that they can eat more food during the day. It would not necessarily lead to poor nutrition.

2. By eliminating most grains from her food intake, her diet may not provide adequate <u>B vitamins</u>. This could cause her to feel fatigued, as these nutrients have a role in <u>energy metabolisms</u>.

   Rationale: Grains are a rich source of many B vitamins. B vitamins do not provide calories themselves. However, they are necessary for the proper functioning of coenzymes that facilitate energy producing chemical reactions. Having a restricted diet can cause fatigue for many different reasons; inadequate B vitamin intake may be one of them.

3. c, d

   Rationale: Dietary Reference Intakes include the RDAs, EARs, AIs, and ULs. These are used for specific populations based as sex and age. Nutrient needs for an individual would be determined by using the RDA because it gives values that meet needs for ~97.5% of the specified population. When there is not enough data available to establish an RDA, then we use the AIs to estimate nutrient needs. Conversely, since the EAR only meets the needs for about 50% of the population, it would be more appropriate to use in group populations containing more than one person. The *Dietary Guidelines for Americans*, MyPlate, and Daily Values are not part of the DRI's, and give an overview of healthy eating patterns as opposed to specific nutrient recommendations.

4. a, b

   Rationale: MyPlate and the *Dietary Guidelines for Americans* outline basic nutrition behaviors that facilitate healthy eating patterns. Other resources such as DRI's are more specific to exact amounts of nutrients, as opposed to healthy meal patterns. *Healthy People 2030* provides goals that the nation wants the population to strive for but does not outline healthy eating patterns.

5.

OPTIONS	CARBOHYDRATES	PROTEIN	FAT
45–78 g			X
225–325 g	X		
50–175 g		X	
900–1300 g			
200–700 g			
400–700 g			

   Rationale: AMDR's are as follows: 45% to 65% for carbohydrates, 10% to 35% for protein, and 20% to 35% for fat. Once the calories are found, grams can be found by using the g/kcal for each macronutrient. The options provided fall into a range for each macronutrient.

6.

DIETARY CHANGES	EFFECTIVE	INEFFECTIVE
Makes ½ of her grains whole grains	X	
Makes ¼ of her plate fruits and vegetables		X
Drinks whole milk		X
Replaced sweet tea with water	X	
Eats meals on a bigger plate		X
Eats at the table to limit distractions	X	
Chooses canned vegetables with sodium		X

   Rationale: MyPlate has simple guidelines such as making ½ of all grains whole grains, filling ½ of the plate with fruits and vegetables, choosing low fat diary, replacing sugary beverages with water, choosing low sodium foods, using smaller dishes to reduce portions, and eating mindfully without distractions. View Figure 1.4 for more examples.

CHAPTER 2

Chapter Review Questions

1. a
2. c
3. b
4. d
5. b

Next-Generation NCLEX® Examination-style Unfolding Case Study Answers

1. Breakfast: sweetened cheerios (2 c.), skim milk (1 ¼ c.), banana (1 medium), black coffee (8 oz)
Lunch: turkey sandwich (2 pieces of white bread, 3 oz turkey, tomato, lettuce); pretzels (1 c.); carrots (1/2 c.); sweet tea (16 oz)
Dinner: chicken breast (4 oz), mashed potatoes with butter (3/4 c.), green beans (1/2 c.), dinner roll, soda

   Rationale: Carbohydrates increase blood glucose and sources include grains, dairy, fruits, and vegetables.

2. According to dietary guidelines, the client is within the total percent of calories from carbohydrate and needs to increase the total grams of fiber in his diet to meet recommendations.

   Rationale: The DRI's recommend consuming 45%-65% of calories from carbohydrates and 38 grams of fiber per day for males.

3. After analyzing the client's diet, the nurse identifies high intake of refined carbohydrates containing simple sugars most likely contribute to high blood glucose levels.

   Rationale: Refined carbohydrates have undergone processing that may remove fiber and other nutrients. Therefore refined carbohydrates contain less polysaccharides and are absorbed more rapidly by the body. This can cause a more rapid increase in blood glucose.

4.

FOOD ITEM	INDICATED	CONTRAINDICATED	IRRELEVANT
Dinner roll	X		
Chicken breast	X		
Soda		X	
Cheerios	X		
Pretzels	X		
Skim milk	X		
Mashed potatoes with butter		X	
Banana	X		
Black coffee			X

   Rationale: Simple sugars are foods containing mono- and disaccharides such as refined grains, corn syrup, fruit, honey, and dairy. These saccharides are rapidly digested and absorbed by the body. Complex sugars are foods containing polysaccharides such as whole grains, legumes, and vegetables. These foods are digested and absorbed at slower rates by the body than simple sugars.

5. Upon hearing these symptoms, the nurse educates the client that large amounts of fiber may be causing gastrointestinal discomfort, but it also may have contributed to his cholesterol levels due to its ability to form gels and absorb bile salts.

   Rationale: Consuming too much fiber can cause symptoms such as bloating, gas, and constipation. Soluble fiber can form gels and bind bile salts, which are released into the gastrointestinal tract during digestion in response to the presence of dietary fat. This allows bile salts to be excreted with the dietary fiber and can lower cholesterol levels in the blood.

6.

ASSESSMENT FINDING	EFFECTIVE	INEFFECTIVE	UNRELATED
Blood glucose 87 mg/dl	X		
Total cholesterol 195 mg/dl	X		
Client reports reduced bowel movements		X	
Client describes stomach pains throughout the day		X	
Client walks one mile daily	X		
Client's clothes have been fitting them better	X		
Client reports less acne on his skin			X

   Rationale: Consuming a well-balanced diet higher in fiber and complex carbohydrates can result in more manageable blood glucose levels, reduced cholesterol, increased energy, and weight loss. Whole grains, fruits, and vegetables found in a balanced diet are nutrient-dense and contain fiber and water. This helps to improve satiety and reduce total calorie intake, which may help them feel more energized and lose weight. However, too much fiber without adequate fluids or suddenly increasing fiber intake in large amounts may cause people to feel stomach pain, bloated, and constipated.

Next-Generation NCLEX® Examination-style Case Study Answers

1. a, d, e

   Rationale: The client's dietary recall indicates that she lacks carbohydrate rich foods such as fruits, whole grains, and legumes. She consumes foods high in protein and fat such as dairy, eggs, and meat. Eliminating food groups increases risk of nutrient deficiencies.

2. The client may not be maintaining euglycemia. Failing to refuel glycogen stores can cause fatigue and muscle catabolism.

   Rationale: The client's low carbohydrate intake is causing her to feel fatigue. Euglycemia describes normal glucose levels in the blood and is maintained when adequate carbohydrates are ingested. Inadequate carbohydrate intake fails to replenish glycogen stores found in the muscle and liver. Muscle glycogen is responsible for fueling muscles during exercise, while liver glycogen plays a role in blood glucose regulation. When the glycogen is depleted, the person will begin to feel fatigued. If glycogen is unavailable for use, the body will resort to breaking down lean body tissue for energy, which is an inefficient source of fuel.

3. e

Rationale: The AMDR for carbohydrates is 45% to 65% of total calories. Based on the client's needs of 2400 calories per day, she would need ~1080 calories to 1560 kcals. per day from carbohydrates. Since carbohydrates provide 4 calories per gram, she would need ~270 grams to 390 grams of carbohydrate per day.

4. c, e

Rationale: Carbohydrates provide energy to the body that is needed for physical activity. Foods such as oatmeal, toast, and fruit provide necessary carbohydrates. While cinnamon rolls provide carbohydrates, it wouldn't be considered the best option with all of the added sugar. Balanced meals containing carbohydrates are important to consume before participating in physical activity to provide necessary energy. However, meals with large amounts of sugar such as cinnamon roll with icing contain large amounts of added sugar and may have a negative impact on health and performance.

5.

ASSESSMENT FINDING	EFFECTIVE	INEFFECTIVE
Feels energized throughout the day	X	
Completes her workouts with less breaks	X	
Fears foods such as pasta and rice		X
Feels satisfied after meals	X	
Has irregular bowel movements		X
Consumes 200 g of carbohydrate/day		X

Rationale: Consuming carbohydrates will give the client energy throughout the day and during her workouts. Carbohydrate foods such as grains are also a good source of fiber that can help her feel more satisfied after eating. Fearing foods such as pasta and rice is not an effective outcome of establishing normal and balanced eating patterns. Consuming 200 grams of carbohydrates is under her recommendations of 270 g to 390 g of carbohydrate. Having irregular bowel movements may indicate that she is not meeting her daily fiber needs, or that the sudden increase in fiber without adequate fluids resulted in constipation.

CHAPTER 3

Chapter Review Questions

1. a
2. b
3. b
4. b
5. c

Next-Generation NCLEX® Examination-style Case Study Answers

1. b, c, f

Rationale: Saturated fats are commonly found in animal products such as meat and dairy and contribute to higher

cholesterol levels. Unsaturated fats are commonly found in plant foods such as olive oil and nuts and contribute to lower cholesterol levels. Omega-3 fatty acids have a positive impact on reducing cholesterol levels and can be found in fish and other types of seafood. The client's diet reflects high intakes of saturated fat and low intakes of unsaturated fats and omega 3 fatty acids.

2. The client has a high intake of saturated fat, which can raise cholesterol levels. These fats are generally solid at room temperature.

Rationale: Saturated fats are solid at room temperature and contribute to higher cholesterol levels. Unsaturated fats are liquid at room temperature and contribute to lower cholesterol levels. Monounsaturated and polyunsaturated fats are both types of unsaturated fat. Both essential fatty acids are polyunsaturated fats.

3. The client's symptoms of dry skin and blurred vision may be a result of his diet and medication. Questran binds to bile and inhibits reabsorption in the colon. This increases the use of cholesterol circulating in the bloodstream (to create more bile in the liver) but can also reduce absorption of fat-soluble vitamin.

Rationale: The client is showing signs of fat-soluble vitamin deficiency. This may be due to the medication he was placed on. Questran binds to bile and inhibits it from being reabsorbed in the colon. Instead, the Questran-bile complex is excreted in the feces. This allows the body to utilize more cholesterol from the blood stream, thereby lowering blood cholesterol levels. However, reduced bile reabsorption can also reduce the amount of fat-soluble vitamins absorbed and could lead to deficiencies.

4. a, b, e, f

Rationale: For this client, it is important to educate him on the different types of fats and their impact on the body so that he is aware of the better food choices. Since he is showing signs of fat-soluble vitamin deficiency, it would help to educate him about foods high in vitamins A, D, E, and K so that he can integrate them into his diet. Educating the client on dietary guidelines regarding dietary fat and the MyPlate guidelines will also help him structure his diet appropriately to create a healthy eating pattern. The ketogenic diet is a high-fat diet and would not be appropriate with this client. It would also not be necessary to avoid all types of fats, as fats contribute many functions to the body.

5.

OPTIONS	FAT	SATURATED FAT
450-788		
25		X
32		
50-88	X	
38		
225		

Rationale: The DRI's recommend consuming 20% to 35% of calories from fat and less than 10% of calories from saturated fat. Since fat contains 9 kcal/g, we can use this fuel factor to calculate the total grams per day.

6.

DIETARY CHANGES	EFFECTIVE	INEFFECTIVE
Consumes 35% kcals from saturated fat		X
Chooses fat-free milk and dairy	X	
Chooses lean cuts of chicken over red meats	X	
Uses butter instead of olive oil		X
Increases fruit and vegetable intake	X	
Consumes foods from all food groups	X	

Rationale: The *Dietary Guidelines for Americans* suggests consuming <10% of calories from saturated fat, choosing fat free milk and dairy, choosing lean meats, choosing unsaturated fats over saturated fats, and following a healthy diet pattern from all food groups.

CHAPTER 4

Chapter Review Questions

1. d
2. b
3. c

4. a
5. b

Next-Generation NCLEX® Examination-style Case Study Answers

1. a, c, d, f

Rationale: A vegan diet can be healthy throughout all life stages if followed correctly. However, it does eliminate certain types of foods, which may make it challenging for a picky eater to meet all of his needs. Plant-based foods contain inadequate amounts of all indispensable amino acids that cannot be produced by our body. Without careful planning, there is a high chance of not consuming enough protein or having an imbalance of amino acids.

2. From this client's diet recall, it does not appear that they are combining an appropriate array of different plant-based foods to ensure his intake of complementary proteins. This practice is important because most vegan-friendly foods on their own are deficient in one or more of the nine indispensable amino acids.

Rationale: Plant-based food sources contain incomplete proteins that do not contain all nine indispensable amino acids. These amino acid are not produced by our body and must be consumed in our diet. Animal sources contain complete proteins that contain all nine indispensable amino acids. However, plant-based foods with different amino acid profiles can be combined to meet all dietary protein needs.

3. The client may be in a state of catabolism since he is not getting all of the needed amino acids. He can combine different plant foods with different amino acid profiles to help achieve a positive nitrogen balance and encourage growth.

Rationale: When a person does not consume enough calories or protein, they go into a state of catabolism. Catabolism is when the muscle is broken down and the amino acids are used as building blocks or broken down into energy. This would put the client in a negative nitrogen balance, meaning that the body is excreting more nitrogen than it keeps.

4. a, b, e

Rationale: Plant sources contain various levels of different amino acids. Different plant foods with different amino acids can be combined to form a complete protein. Increasing calories and plant protein foods can increase the total amount of amino acids available for use. Whey protein is a product of milk and would not be appropriate for a vegan client. Consuming more soy products and soy protein would be helpful because soy is the only plant protein that is considered a complete protein.

5. b, c, e

Rationale: The following food combinations are often used to form complementary amino acids and complete proteins: Grains and peas, beans, or lentils; legumes and seeds; grains and dairy. Grains are low in threonine and high methionine while legumes and dairy are high in threonine and low in methionine. However, any combination with dairy would not be appropriate for this client who is following a vegan diet.

CHAPTER 5

Chapter Review Questions

1. c
2. a
3. b

4. a
5. c

Next-Generation NCLEX® Examination-style Case Study Answers

1. c

Rationale: The client experiences gastrointestinal signs of lactose intolerance after eating dairy foods such as milk, cheese, and ice cream. Clients with lactose intolerance are unable to digest the disaccharide found in dairy products. Instead, the bacteria in the large intestine ferment the disaccharide. This creates gas which can cause abdominal cramps, gas, and bloating. Having unabsorbed disaccharides in the lumen also increases the osmolality of the gastrointestinal contents, causing water to move into the lumen. This change in osmolality can also cause abdominal cramps and diarrhea. Fatigue and headaches are not necessarily associated with lactose intolerance but could be a result dehydration after experiencing frequent diarrhea and low blood glucose from skipping meals.

2. The client is not producing adequate amounts of the intestinal enzyme lactase, allowing lactose to move into the colon instead of undergoing digestion and absorption.

Rationale: Lactase is the enzyme associated with lactose intolerance. It is used to break down the disaccharide lactose into glucose and galactose. Without lactase, lactose moves through the small intestine and enters the colon undigested and unabsorbed. Lactose is then fermented by bacteria in the colon causing symptoms such as gas, bloating, and abdominal cramps.

3. a, b, c, f

Rationale: People experiencing lactose intolerance should limit or avoid dairy products. They can consume lactose-free products or products that add the enzyme lactase to break down the lactose. They may be able to identify an amount of diary that they are able to tolerate without symptoms through a systematic process of documenting foods and symptoms. The goal is to alleviate symptoms entirely. Fat-free dairy products do not necessarily contain less lactose. Lactose is the disaccharide found in milk. Removing the fat does not alter the presence of lactose.

4.

FOODS	EFFECTIVE	INEFFECTIVE
Lactaid milk	X	
Almond milk	X	
Eggs	X	
Cheese		X
Cow's milk		X
Yogurt		X
Soy milk	X	

Rationale: Dairy products such as cow's milk, cheese, and yogurt contain lactose. Plant-based milk products, such as soy and almond milk, do not contain lactose and are safe for consumption. Lactaid milk is milk that contains the lactase enzyme so it will not cause symptoms in the client. Eggs are not a dairy product, and therefore do not contain lactose.

CHAPTER 6

Chapter Review Questions

1. d
2. c
3. b
4. b
5. c

Next-Generation NCLEX® Examination-style Unfolding Case Study Answers

1. Breakfast: Cinnamon roll, apple juice, yogurt

   Lunch: Grilled chicken wrap (w/lettuce, tomato, spinach), potato chips, sweet tea, almonds
   Dinner: Chicken fried steak, baked potato, butter (with potato), asparagus, cookies

   Rationale: Calorie-dense foods contain large amounts of calories compared to overall volume. Nutrient-dense foods contain large amounts of nutrients compared to overall volume. It is possible for a food to be both calorie- and nutrient-dense.

2. The client is most likely feeling low-energy due to the depletion of glycogen stores throughout the night after long periods of fasting for 12-48 hours. These stores are responsible for maintaining blood glucose levels during sleep.

   Rationale: During periods of fasting, the body relies on glycogen stored in the body to provide energy and maintain blood glucose levels in attempt to maintain lean body mass.

3. a, c, d, g, h

   Rationale: There are multiple factors that can slow a person's BMR such as reduced lean body mass, fasting, hormonal imbalances, and reduced physical activity.

4. You determined that the client's hypothyroidism leads to reduced production of thyroxine, which slows metabolism. This would require the client have a larger calorie deficit to facilitate weight loss.

   Rationale: Hypothyroidism is a condition in which there is inadequate production of thyroxine in the body. Hypothyroidism can reduce the BMR; thus increasing the calorie-deficit required for weight loss.

5. Considering this client's new exercise regimen, the nurse found the client's BEE (kcal/kg/hr) and TEE (kcal/day) to be 1570 kcals/day and 2187 kcals/day respectively.

   Rationale: Basal energy expenditure can be found using the formula 1 kcal x kg body weight x 24 hours with women needing 0.9 kcal/kg body weight and men needing 1 kcal/kg of body weight. Total energy expenditure can be found using an activity factor of a certain activity and multiplying it by weight in pounds by the fraction of hour spent performing the activity.

6. a, b, c, e, g, h

   Rationale: Weight loss requires a negative energy balance. Choosing nutrient-dense foods, such as fruits and vegetables, over energy-dense foods allows a person to consume all of their micronutrients while not over-consuming total kcals. Increasing energy expenditure, through physical activity and exercise, helps to create a negative energy balance without having to cut kcal intake through food drastically or rapidly.

Next-Generation NCLEX® Examination-style Case Study Answers

1. b, c, f, g, h

   Rationale: Adults require less energy to sustain life in advanced years. This is related to many different factors such as loss of lean body mass and reduced levels of physical activity. Other hormonal factors such a menopause can lower the amount of energy required in older females.

2. The client is most likely consuming more energy than she is expending; this creates a positive energy balance, causing her to gain weight.

   Rationale: The client's weight gain suggests that she is in a positive energy balance, meaning that she is consuming more energy than she is expending. If the client's total energy expenditure is reduced due to aging, limited exercise, and menopause, but she is consuming the same number of calories, it would cause her to gain weight.

3.

INTERVENTION	EFFECTIVE	INEFFECTIVE
Reduce physical activity		X
Increase nutrient-dense foods	X	
Reduce calorie-dense food	X	
Skip meals		X
Build muscle mass through regular physical activity	X	
Create a positive energy balance		X
Create a negative energy balance	X	

Rationale: To reduce her calorie intake, the client would benefit from eating nutrient-dense foods that are low in calories, and limited calorie-dense foods that are high in calories. She would also benefit from building muscle through exercise because muscle mass helps maintain energy balance as a high-energy utilizing tissue. These behaviors combined would create a negative energy balance, helping her lose weight. We want to avoid any restrictive eating behaviors such as skipping meals because we want to create a healthy relationship with food and aging adults have high nutrient needs that may be hard to reach.

4. c

Rationale: The Mifflin St. Jeor equation with an activity factor can be used to find a person's total energy expenditure needs. This client is sedentary so her activity factor should be (10 x 95 kg + 6.25 x 163 cm – 5 x 70 y.o. – 161) x 1.0 = 1459 kcals/day.

CHAPTER 7

Chapter Review Questions

1. b   4. d
2. a   5. d
3. a

Next-Generation NCLEX® Examination-style Case Study Answers

1. a, b, d, f, g

Rationale: The client is on Warfarin because of her previous history with deep vein thrombosis. Any history or assessment related to changes in bleeding such as nose bleeds and bruises should require a follow up. Health care providers should continue to follow-up on clients taking any medication such as Warfarin and antibiotics to evaluate compliance and potential interactions. Likewise, health care providers should follow-up on diet history to evaluate for drug-nutrient interactions and nutrient deficiencies. Other assessment findings that are within normal ranges usually do not require follow-up.

2. The client's anticoagulant medication counteracts the function of vitamin K, which is to help form blood clots.

Rationale: Warfarin is an anticoagulant that thins the blood and prevents blood clotting. A common nutrient interaction with Warfarin is vitamin K. Vitamin K's function is to clot blood, therefore it is important to monitor the effects of these two components to ensure that they are in balance and working properly.

3. The gut contains bacteria that synthesize vitamin K. The client's recent use of antibiotics most likely eliminated this source of vitamin K and may have enhanced the function of Warfarin, causing the blood to be less viscous.

Rationale: Healthy gut bacteria synthesize vitamin K. However, antibiotics remove the bacteria in the gut; thus, reducing vitamin K production. This can have an impact on the vitamin K levels in the body and can enhance the blood thinning qualities of Warfarin.

4.

RECOMMENDATIONS	EFFECTIVE	INEFFECTIVE
Stop taking Warfarin		X
Avoid taking antibiotics again in the future		X
Consume consistent amounts of vitamin K daily	X	
Avoid as much vitamin K as possible		X
Take vitamin and mineral supplements consistently	X	

Rationale: Current recommendations for clients taking Warfarin or antibiotics are similar. It is safe to take these medications with vitamin K-rich foods; thus, there is no reason to avoid vitamin K-rich foods or the medications. Instead, clients should consume consistent amounts of food containing vitamin K so that the levels in their body remain consistent. This makes it easier to dose the medication and get the same effects repeatedly. Clients on anticoagulant medication should not take supplemental forms of vitamin K. Vitamin K intake through food should remain consistent daily. It is not beneficial to avoid vitamin K-rich food groups, because foods that are high in vitamin K also provide other essential nutrients.

5. b, c, e

Rationale: It is important to be aware of what foods are rich sources of vitamin K so that the client is aware of how much she is consuming. Common food sources of vitamin K include leafy green vegetables such as spinach, collard greens, and kale. Most meats, dairy, and beans do not contain much vitamin K.

6.

OUTCOMES	EFFECTIVE	INEFFECTIVE
Client states that her blood clots a lot quicker	X	
She is not sure how much vitamin K she eats daily		X
She continues to have bruising on arms and legs		X
Her nose bleeds have discontinued	X	
She feels more energetic	X	
She can identify foods with vitamin K and includes them in her diet	X	

Rationale: The client is more aware of what types of foods contain vitamin K and includes them in her diet. She feels more energetic, her coagulation time has returned to normal, and her frequent nose bleeds have stopped. These are all signs that her blood clotting function has returned to normal and that her vitamin K levels are again balanced with her anticoagulation medication. However, because she is not sure how much vitamin K she eats from day to day, it is hard to know if she is being consistent. This may explain why there are still bruises on her arms and legs. More education and self-monitoring would need to take place to get more control on the client's diet and symptoms.

CHAPTER 8

Chapter Review Questions

1. a
2. c
3. b
4. d
5. a

Next-Generation NCLEX® Examination-style Case Study Answers

1. a, b, c, f, g

Rationale: Older adults, especially females, are more at risk for osteoporosis. Other diseases, such as hyperthyroidism, can also contribute to calcium resorption from the bones. This can make bones weak and brittle. Failure to perform resistance exercise that puts stress on the bone can also increase risk of osteoporosis. Poor nutrient intake can reduce the amount of nutrients the client is getting, such as calcium and vitamin D, which contribute to bone strength, but also may contribute to low body weight. Having a small frame size increases the risk of developing osteoporosis. Although family history and alcohol use can both be contributing risk factors, this client does not have osteoporosis in her family history, and her alcohol use is limited.

2. a, c, d

Rationale: The client's dietary recall consists of small portion sizes and a relatively small amount of total food. This results in a diet that is low in calories and makes it difficult for the client to get all the nutrients that she needs. She consumes adequate fruits throughout the day but needs to improve her vegetable intake. She does not consume many foods that are high in calcium such as dairy. Spinach contains calcium, but it also contains oxalate acid (also found in tea), which inhibits absorption. The client's diet is low in phosphorous and iron-rich foods.

3. In addition to the client's diet, her poorly controlled hyperparathyroidism causes calcium from the bones to be resorbed, making them weak and brittle.

Rationale: The client has hyperthyroidism but forgets to take her medication. Too much parathyroid hormone results in calcium resorption from the bone and into the bloodstream to balance serum calcium levels. Without intervention, this hormonal imbalance can leave bones weak and brittle.

4.

INTERVENTION	EFFECTIVE	INEFFECTIVE
Consume dairy products	X	
Consume fortified foods with calcium	X	
Consume plant products with minimal oxalate acid	X	
Consume plant products with oxalate acid		X
Take a vitamin D supplement	X	
Increase low intensity exercise		X
Participating in resistance exercise	X	
Consistently take thyroid medication	X	

Rationale: Interventions to improve bone strength and density include a balanced diet, resistance exercise, and medication management. Foods high in calcium and vitamin D should be encouraged. The best source of calcium is dairy, but many plant-based foods also contain meaningful sources of calcium, depending on the amount of oxalate acid that they contain. Oxalate acid inhibits calcium absorption. Foods such as bok choy, collard greens, and calcium-fortified soy products have higher bioavailability than foods such as spinach and broccoli. Supplementing calcium and vitamin D can be helpful if the client's diet is inadequate. Resistance exercise that places stress on the bones is the most helpful way to increase bone density compared to other forms of exercise, and medications should be taken properly to avoid any nutrient imbalances.

5. a, c, d, e, g, i

Rationale: To increase her calcium levels, the health care team should encourage her to consume dairy or calcium-fortified dairy substitutes such as milk, cheese, and yogurt. Fish that contain bones (e.g., canned sardines) are also a good source of calcium, along with calcium-fortified soy products and juices. Plant foods that do not contain oxalate acid (e.g., bok choy) are a good source of calcium, because they have higher bioavailability than other plant foods, such as spinach.

CHAPTER 9

Chapter Review Questions

1. c
2. d
3. a
4. b
5. a

Next-Generation NCLEX® Examination-style Case Study Answers

1. a, c, d, e

Rationale: Medications such as diuretics and some antidepressants such as amitriptyline increase fluid losses and are a nutritional concern. The client lost weight after working out, which suggests that fluid was lost. Losing more than 1% to 2% of body weight increases the risk for dehydration. The client also stated that she does not eat or drink many fluids before the race, which is also a concern. Her age and exercise intensity are not concerning.

2. Diuretics and antidepressants increase the fluid needs of the client, and failure to consume enough fluids during exercise will mostly lead to dehydration.

Rationale: Diuretics and antidepressants increase fluid loss and require that the individual consume additional liquids to maintain hydration status and avoid dehydration. Exercise also increases total fluid needs to maintain hydration.

3.

CLIENT QUESTIONS	APPROPRIATE NURSE'S RESPONSE FOR EACH CLIENT QUESTION
"Where else in my diet can I get fluids?"	e
"If I don't use the bathroom as much, I probably don't lose as much water. Is that true?"	f
"Can I still exercise if I am taking diuretics and antidepressants?"	g
"How often should I drink water?"	d
"How much water should I drink two hours before exercise?"	a
"How much water should I drink after exercise?"	b
"Should I worry about dehydration if I lose a small amount of weight after a workout?"	c

Rationale: People can get fluids in their diet from liquids as well as foods that are high in water content. Fluids are lost through the kidneys, skin, lungs, and feces. We should consume fluids throughout the day and particularly around the time of physical activity. Individuals should consume 5 to 10 ml/kg of fluid 2 hours before exercise and should consume 20 to 24 oz of water for every pound of body weight lost during exercise. Weight loss during exercise is normal, because the body will lose fluids through sweat and respiration. However, individuals should aim to lose no more than 1% to 2% of body weight. Physical activity is safe for individuals taking diuretics and antidepressants. These medications do require larger amounts of fluid to maintain hydration.

4.

HEALTH TEACHING	INDICATED	CONTRAIN-DICATED	NONESSEN-TIAL
Drink 5 to 10 ml/kg of fluid 2 hours before working out and 20 to 24 ml per oz of body weight lost post workout.	X		
Utilize sports drinks with glucose and electrolytes if exercising for <60 minutes.			X
Consume energy drinks that contain taurine, guarana, and gingko biloba during exercise.		X	

HEALTH TEACHING	INDICATED	CONTRAIN-DICATED	NONESSEN-TIAL
Consume sports drinks with at least 500% of the RDA of most, if not all, vitamins and minerals.		X	
Sports drinks may be beneficial if exercise is 90 minutes or more.	X		
Drink 3 to 4 liters of water in 30 minutes during physical activity.			X

Rationale: It is important to prioritize hydration before and after workouts. Water is appropriate for most workouts, but sports drinks are beneficial for any activity that lasts for more than 60 to 90 minutes. The electrolytes in sports drinks allow the individual to retain more fluid and stay hydrated. Energy drinks are available on the market, but not a lot of research has been done regarding their effectiveness during exercise. Thus, they may not be safe. Sports drinks with megadoses of vitamins and minerals make it easy for individuals to overdose on these nutrients. Consuming excessive water in a short amount of time without adequate electrolytes may lead to water intoxication. This can result in hyponatremia and may eventually lead to coma or death without intervention. Individuals should avoid large volumes of water alone for long bouts of physical activity.

5.

ASSESSMENT FINDING	EFFECTIVE	INEFFECTIVE	UNRELATED
Lost ≤1% of body weight after exercising	X		
Urinates frequently	X		
Urine is light yellow	X		
Skin is moist and buoyant	X		
Muscles are sore after working out		X	
Feels sharp pain in foot			X
Consumes water before and after race	X		
Does not consume electrolytes during exercise exceeding 60 minutes		X	

Rationale: Losing 1% of weight after working out suggests that they hydrated effectively before the workout. Frequent urination and urine that is a light-yellow color both indicated adequate hydration. Having moist skin with low turgor is a sign of hydration. However, more education may need to take place for proper understanding about the appropriate use of sports drinks in exercise lasting more than 60 minutes. Having sore muscles may be related to dehydration, as well as intense exercise. However, foot pain in this situation is unrelated to hydration and is most likely due to the stress of the exercise itself.

CHAPTER 10

Chapter Review Questions

1. a   4. b
2. a   5. c
3. c

Next-Generation NCLEX® Examination-style Case Study Answers

1. a, b, c

   Rationale: Many factors and behaviors can contribute to iron-deficiency anemia. There is an increase in blood volume during pregnancy, and this contributes to pregnant women having higher iron requirements. Physicians usually recommend iron supplementation throughout pregnancy as part of a prenatal nutrient complex. Following a vegetarian diet can increase the risk for iron deficiency. Although some plant foods (e.g., spinach) contain iron, they also contain other compounds, such as oxalate acid, that bind iron and inhibit its absorption. In addition, taking iron supplements with meals allows for binding components located in food to bind to the iron and inhibit absorption. Prenatal supplements are important during pregnancy and should not be avoided in the case of iron-deficiency anemia. Iron in supplemental form is just as effective as the natural form. Last, dietary guidelines recommend that people consume a balance of plant and animal sources.

2. Although there are plant sources of iron in the client's diet, the bioavailability of iron is lower when compared to animal sources. Taking supplements with food can also lead to potential drug-nutrient interactions within the client.

   Rationale: Plant sources that contain iron also contain compounds, such as phytic acid and oxalic acid, that bind to iron and inhibit absorption. Absorption can also be limited when taking supplements with food that have similar binders.

3. The client consumes high-fiber foods containing phytic acid, which can bind to minerals, such as iron. This can make the minerals unavailable for absorption.

   Rationale: Phytic acid is a compound found in high-fiber, whole-grain foods that bind nutrients and inhibit absorption.

4.

METHODS	EFFECTIVE	INEFFECTIVE
Consume more plant proteins		X
Consume enriched grains	X	
Consume more animal proteins	X	
Take iron supplements with small amounts of food.	X	
Take iron supplements with calcium supplements		X
Take supplements with foods low in phytic acid	X	

Rationale: Enriched grains are grains that have nutrients, such as iron, added to them and can help increase iron intake. Consuming animal proteins that have greater bioavailability also help to increase intake as opposed to plant proteins that have lower bioavailability. Taking iron supplements on an empty stomach allows for higher levels of absorption because of lower chances of compounds, such as phytic acid, interfering with absorption. Calcium supplements can inhibit iron absorption, so they should be taken separately.

5. a, c, d, e

   Rationale: Iron-enriched foods are commonly breakfast cereal, pasta, bread, rice, and other grain products. Orange juice is fortified but mainly with vitamin D and calcium and not iron. However, vitamin C in orange juice does increase iron absorption. Spinach and ground beef contain iron, but they are not fortified.

CHAPTER 11

Chapter Review Questions

1. d   4. b
2. b   5. c
3. b

Next-Generation NCLEX® Examination-style Case Study Answers

1. a, b, e, f, g

   Rationale: It is important to follow up on the infant's growth because he was born at a low birthweight. His weight was disproportionally small for his gestational age because it was below the 10th percentile, but his length and head circumference were within the normal range. The American Academy of Pediatrics and the Academy of Nutrition and Dietetics recommend avoiding cow's milk until the infant turns 1 year old. Foods, such as scrambled eggs, that contain common food allergens should not be used as the first solid foods for infants. Although diarrhea can occur in infants, frequent and prolonged diarrhea should be followed up to determine potential underlying medical conditions. The feeding positions and supplement use were appropriate for this client.

2. Cow's milk is insufficient in <u>calories</u> and <u>essential fatty acids</u>, which maight hinder normal growth in the infant.

Rationale: Cow's milk is insufficient in calories and essential fatty acids, specifically linoleic acid, which can contribute to poor growth. Infants have immature digestive systems at birth that might not be able to handle the composition of cow's milk, which could explain the diarrhea and fussiness and contribute to poor growth.

3.

CLIENT QUESTIONS	APPROPRIATE NURSE'S RESPONSE FOR EACH CLIENT QUESTION
"How long should infants be breastfed?"	e
"What do I use to feed my 7-month-old infant if I don't want to breastfeed?	a
"Can I feed my 7-month-old infant water and juice?"	d
"When can infants drink cow's milk?"	c

Rationale: Infants should be breastfed for at least the first 6 months until solid foods are introduced. If the infant is not receiving breast milk, then the parents can use an iron-fortified breast milk substitute. Water and juice are appropriate for infants older than 6 months. Parents should not provide infants with cow's milk until the end of the first year of life.

4. c, f, g

Rationale: When first introducing solid foods to infants, parents should avoid common allergen-containing foods, such as citrus juice, nuts, eggs, and wheat. Better options would include soft fruits, vegetables, yogurt, and other soft foods. Allergen-containing foods can be introduced after a few solid foods are well tolerated.

5.

ASSESSMENT FINDING	EFFECTIVE	INEFFECTIVE
Infant is happy and cries less	X	
Normal bowel movements 1-2 times per day	X	
Weight increased 2 percentiles	X	
Parents feed infant peanuts and hotdogs		X
Infant is getting iron-fortified breast milk substitute if the mother is not breastfeeding	X	
Parents leave infant with a bottle of juice propped into the infant's mouth to feed		X

Rationale: The mother started to feed the infant iron-fortified breast milk substitute, which helped regulate the infant's bowel movements, mood, and growth. Peanuts and hot dogs are hard-to-swallow foods that should be avoided until the child is older. Propping bottles in the baby's mouth allows the juice to pool and can cause tooth decay and other complications. Parents need more education on those topics.

CHAPTER 12

Chapter Review Questions

1. b
2. d
3. b
4. c
5. c

Next-Generation NCLEX® Examination-style Case Study Answers

1. a, f

Rationale: The client is taking 5 different medications, known as polypharmacy, which puts him at risk for nutrient-drug interactions. While in quarantine and experiencing safety concerns regarding the grocery store, he has limited access to food. His food preparation skills, swallowing ability, and appetite are all in good condition, and therefore those are not concerning. He does not have dyspnea.

2. a, b

Rationale: Because the client is taking multiple medications and his daughter is not currently available to assist in his care, it is important to educate him on potential drug-food and drug-nutrient interactions. It is also important to address his food access and the assistance programs for which he might be eligible. Meals on Wheels would be the best choice for him because he meets the criteria, he is unable to leave his house, and he will be isolated for an unknown amount of time. This program will provide him with meals delivered to his house and will provide him with some social support. SNAP, commodity supplemental food programs, and senior farmers market nutrition programs are all for people that fall under the poverty level. Because this client is financially stable, it would be unlikely for him to qualify for those programs, and some of them would still require that he leave his home.

3.

DRUG CLASS	APPROPRIATE RECOMMENDATION
Antihypertensives	c
Antihistamines	e
Antihyperlipidemic	b
Nonsteroidal anti-inflammatory drugs	d
Antidepressants	a

Rationale: There are recommendations for each drug class regarding what foods and vitamins to avoid or include to avoid potentially dangerous interactions. See the "Drug Nutrient Interaction: Medication Use in the Adult" box for more information.

CHAPTER 13

Chapter Review Questions

1. d
2. a
3. a
4. c
5. b

Next-Generation NCLEX® Examination-style Unfolding Case Study Answers

1. a, d, e, f, g, h

   Rationale: Signs of foodborne illness include illness 1-6 hours after ingestion of food, severe cramping, abdominal pain, nausea, vomiting, diarrhea, sweating, fever, headache, and prostration. If the cream puffs were properly stored, then they would not have caused food-borne illness, so eating multiple cream puffs would not matter. Age is not a contributing factor in the risk of developing food-borne illness.

2. The couple's food-borne illness was most likely caused by the ingestion of <u>bacteria</u>, <u>viruses</u>, or <u>parasites</u>.

   Rationale: Foodborne illness is caused by the ingestion of bacteria, viruses, and parasites.

3. The agent that most likely caused the couple's illness was <u>poisoning</u>, a form of food <u>staphylococcus</u>.

   Rationale: Staphylococcus can be found in custard or cream-filled bakery goods as well as other foods. This bacterium causes food poisoning in people who consume foods that are contaminated.

4. a, c, d, e

   Rationale: Procedures should be in place to keep food safe from production until the point of service. Workers should wash their hands and put on a new pair of gloves for each new task. When they are leaving the kitchen or food preparation area, they need to remove their aprons to ensure that they do not become contaminated. Ready-to-eat foods that are consumed without further cooking should be kept separate form time temperature regulated foods such as raw meats to avoid cross contamination. Food should be kept at appropriate temperatures during storage and preparation to ensure that bacteria cannot grow and reproduce to cause food-borne illnesses.

5.

ACTION	CORRECT	INCORRECT
Cool food to room temperature before storing		X
Refrigerate food within 2 hours of serving	X	
Reheat leftovers until warm		X
Storing leftovers in open containers		X
Disposing trash and garbage appropriately	X	
Refrigerate food after 2 hours of serving		X
Reheat leftovers to specific temperature depending on the food	X	

Rationale: Leftover food should be stored immediately and within 2 hours of sitting to avoid temperatures that encourage bacterial growth. Hot food should not be set to cool to room temperature before putting in the refrigerator as that allows bacteria to grow. Any leftovers should be reheated to the appropriate temperature depending on the food to ensure that pathogens are killed before consumption. Trash and leftovers should be discarded appropriately to reduce cross contamination and spoilage of foods.

6. a, b, f

   Rationale: The worker should have had a band aid and gloves on if he had a cut on his finger to maintain proper sanitization. If the truck broke down, proper procedures should have been executed to maintain appropriate temperatures of the food so that quality would maintain. If the temperatures were out of range for too long in the truck or on the serving table, then the food should have been discarded.

Next-Generation NCLEX® Examination-style Case Study Answers

1. a, b, d, f

   Rationale: This family is food insecure and unable to provide their baby with enough nutrients. The baby's anthropometric measurements indicate poor growth, and the constipation suggests inadequate fiber and fluids because she is receiving inadequate nutrition. Housing and feeding strategies are not currently an issue in this case.

2. The infant's <u>poor growth</u> and <u>constipation</u> suggests that she is not getting enough nutrients through her feedings.

   Rationale: The infant is likely not getting enough calories or nutrients through her feeding, as evidenced by her poor growth and constipation.

3. a, b

   Rationale: The family would likely qualify for WIC and SNAP based on their income and having an infant less than 5 years of age. However, because the child is only 1 year old, she would not be in school and therefore would not be able to receive food from the National School Lunch and Breakfast Program. They would not qualify for Meals on Wheels because they are able to prepare their own food and have access to food.

4.

HEALTH TEACHING	INDICATED	CONTRAINDICATED
Look for sales in newspapers and online.	X	
Make a list of food and supplies before going to the grocery store.	X	
Read food labels.	X	

HEALTH TEACHING	INDICATED	CONTRAINDICATED
Store dry food in closed containers in a dry place and cool food to appropriate temperatures.	X	
Cook food to appropriate temperatures and use separate cutting boards for ready-to-eat foods.	X	
Go down every aisle of the store.		X
Thaw raw chicken on the counter before cooking.		X

Rationale: Client education regarding techniques to save money and proper voucher use might be helpful. Skills, such as planning, making lists, reading labels, and controlling food waste, might be helpful for this family as well. Practices related to lack of planning, such as going down every aisle and buying random ingredients, are not helpful. Improperly storing leftovers will put the family at risk for foodborne illness and increase the likelihood of food waste.

5.

ASSESSMENT FINDING	EFFECTIVE	INEFFECTIVE	UNRELATED
Parents use WIC vouchers to buy fruits, vegetables, and whole grains.	X		
Infant's height and weight are at the 15th percentile and continue to increase.	X		
Infant continues to have bowel movements every other day.		X	
Parents are able to purchase enough food to meet their needs.	X		
Infant is a picky eater when it comes to solid foods.			X

Rationale: The intervention is effective when the family is using WIC vouchers appropriately to buy foods that are high in nutrients, such as fruits, vegetables, and whole grains. These vouchers not only provide more food for the mother and father but also provide more food to the infant, which can help the infant grow appropriately. This is noted by the increase in the infant's height and weight to the 15th percentile. The infant might need more fiber and fluids daily because her bowel movements indicate that she is still experiencing constipation. The infant being a picky eater concerning solid foods is unrelated to the nutrition intervention focused on food security and growth.

CHAPTER 14

Chapter Review Questions

1. d   4. c
2. a   5. c
3. d

Next-Generation NCLEX® Examination-style Case Study Answers

1. a, c, d

   Rationale: The client snacks frequently throughout the day and consumes large portion sizes. She also chooses high-calorie foods. She consumes fast food about once per week, which is not excessive. She lacks nutrient-dense foods, such as fruits, vegetables, whole grains, and low-fat dairy.

2. b, e, g

   Rationale: The client's food choices, such as frozen foods, packaged snack items, and soda, are generally high in sodium, saturated fat, and added sugar. Nutrients that she is probably not getting enough of include vitamin A, vitamin K, calcium, fiber, and potassium because these are all found in plant-based whole foods.

3. The client's snacking increases overall calorie intake, and consuming energy-dense snacks increases the risk for overweight and obesity. In addition, the client's increased consumption of sodium might contribute to hypertension.

   Rationale: Frequent snacking, especially if the snack is high in calories, contributes to the increasing incidence in overweight and obesity. High intakes of sodium found in most processed foods contribute to elevated blood pressure.

4. a, b, d, e

   Rationale: For this client, it would be helpful for her to identify healthier food choices than the processed foods she is currently consuming. She would benefit from increasing her fruit, vegetable, whole-grain, and low-fat dairy intake. Because she eats frequently throughout the day, reducing her snacking frequency will likely reduce her calorie intake and establish set mealtimes. Reducing her portion sizes will also reduce her calorie intake and might make room for other foods that are higher in nutrients. Finally, planning meals ahead of time can make it easier for her to think about her food choices before consuming convenient snack foods during the day. Following a strict diet will likely add more stress to the client's life and is not beneficial. We want her to develop a healthy relationship with food, which is why we would not recommend eliminating food groups, such as carbohydrates or fats. Avoiding whole food groups is restrictive and eliminates essential nutrients that are needed in the diet.

5.

HEALTH TEACHING	INDICATED	CONTRAINDICATED
Aim to consume a meal pattern including 3 meals and 2 snacks.	X	
Increase your fruit and vegetable intake by trying to eat a fruit and vegetable at each meal.	X	
Consuming low-fat dairy and whole-grain foods will provide more nutrients than processed foods.	X	
Identify individual serving sizes on food labels.	X	
Consume the serving sizes served at restaurants because they are likely appropriate.		X
Consume high amounts of fruit juices to increase fiber and nutrients.		X
Skip meals at work if you forgot to pack a lunch.		X

Rationale: Creating a healthy meal pattern, such as 3 meals and 2 snacks per day, might be beneficial to the client in reducing her calories and improving her food choices. Aiming to consume a fruit and vegetable at each meal will increase her nutrient intake and reduce her calories. Low-fat dairy and whole-grain products will also add nutrients and reduce calories. Reading serving sizes located on nutrition labels can help reduce portion sizes, and being aware of large portion sizes at restaurants is beneficial. Although fruit juices do contain nutrients, these juices should not be consumed in large amounts because they are often high in added sugars, similar to soda. Skipping meals leads to irregular glucose levels and can leave the client feeling hungry and unfocused.

6.

ASSESSMENT FINDING	EFFECTIVE	INEFFECTIVE
Blood pressure changed from 130/90 mm Hg to 120/80 mm Hg	X	
Client lost 5 lbs. in the last 2 weeks	X	
Client skips breakfast and lunch 2 days out of the week		X
Client snacks less during the day	X	
Client consumes fast food 3 times per week		X
Client consumes at least 2 servings of fruit and vegetables every day	X	

Rationale: A decrease in blood pressure and weight loss are indicators of positive changes in her diet and health. Consuming less snacks during the day and increasing fruit and vegetable intake is beneficial. However, skipping meals and eating fast food 3 times per week are still areas that can be improved with time and continued education.

CHAPTER 15

Chapter Review Questions

1. c
2. b
3. a
4. b
5. c

Next-Generation NCLEX® Examination-style Unfolding Case Study Answers

1. a

Rationale: Using the Mifflin-St. Jeor equation with the client's weight in kilograms, height in cm, and age in years can find the client's basal metabolic rate. Then applying a physical activity factor to the basal metabolic rate will result in the client's total energy expenditure for the day.

2. Comparing the client's estimated energy needs to her current energy needs, she is currently in positive energy balance. This will result in weight gain.

   Rationale: Having a caloric intake greater than an individual's needs puts them in a positive energy balance, meaning that that they are taking in more energy than they are expending. This results in weight gain.

3. c

   Rationale: A deficit of 3500 kcals results in 1 lb of fat loss. Therefore to lose 1 lb a week, there would need to be a deficit of 500 kcals per day. This approach to weight loss can be more sustainable for clients and easier to maintain compared to larger caloric deficits that may make them feel hungry, irritable, and less likely to follow through with their goals.

4.

PRACTICES	EFFECTIVE	INEFFECTIVE
Increase physical activity	X	
Increase caloric deficit >500 kcals/day		X
Follow healthy eating patterns consuming a variety of foods	X	
Eat in front of the TV		X
Increase sedentary behavior		X
Create moderate calorie deficit ≤500 kcals/day	X	
Consume calorie dense foods		X
Consume less calories then expended	X	
Increase exercise	X	

Rationale: There are many strategies to create a negative energy balance. Consuming nutrient dense foods that are lower calories can help people consume less calories throughout the day without experiencing feelings of hunger. Caloric deficits are important for weight loss, but drastic deficits greater than 500 kcals/day may not be sustainable or pleasant for the client. Another strategy that can help a person reach negative energy balance is adding exercise and physical activity to increase total energy expended. Behaviors that are sedentary or allow for mindless eating like eating in front of a TV should also be avoided to help control caloric intake.

5. Based on the client's concerns, she should consider <u>aerobic</u> exercise for longer periods to increase use of <u>fat</u> for fuel instead of lean body mass.

Rationale: Aerobic exercise consists of activities that are long enough to draw on the body's fat reserve for fuel. While there is oxygen, lean body tissue burns fat, making aerobic exercise the best activity for high lean body mass and low fatty tissue in the body.

6. a

Rationale: BMI is not enough on its own to give enough information regarding body composition, and body composition does not give enough information regarding fat distribution. Therefore a combination of BMI, body composition, and waist circumference is the best way to measure overall weight and fat loss if possible.

Next-Generation NCLEX® Examination-style Case Study Answers

1. a, b ,d, e, g, h

Rationale: The client's weight, combined with small portion sizes and low calorie intake, indicates nutrition risk. Amenorrhea can be caused by inadequate energy intake and low body weight. Injuries, such as stress fractures, are common in persons with restricted calorie intake or eating disorders. Personality traits, such as being a perfectionist, can put an individual at risk of eating disorders. Although the client does exercise frequently, these patterns are not deemed to be excessive but can be harmful when paired with inadequate energy intake. She still socializes with her friends, and her overall food choices are healthy. However, she is not eating enough and does not have a healthy relationship with food.

2. c

Rationale: Anorexia nervosa is an extreme psychophysiological aversion to food that results in life-threatening weight loss. It is a psychiatric eating disorder that results from a morbid fear of fatness, in which a person's distorted body image is reflected as fat when the body is malnourished and extremely thin as a result of self-starvation. The client's avoidance of food and actions that suggest fear of weight gain suggest that she is struggling with anorexia nervosa.

3.

HEALTH PROFESSIONAL	NECESSARY	UNNECESSARY
Physician	X	
Physical trainer		X
Health coach		X
Registered dietitian nutritionist	X	
Psychologist	X	
Chiropractor		X
Nutritionist		X

Rationale: It is suggested that an individual struggling with an eating disorder work with an interdisciplinary team involving a physician, registered dietitian nutritionist, and psychologist. Other professions might be helpful but are not seen as necessary and could even be harmful if they are not qualified to work with a patient with such a complicated disorder.

4.

HEALTH TEACHING	INDICATED	CONTRAINDICATED
Consume a diet rich in energy and nutrients to establish a healthy weight.	X	
Consume foods, such as eggs, lean meat, legumes, and soy, to rebuild tissues.	X	
Focus on specifically eating foods that you have been avoiding.		X
Focus on drinking liquid supplements like Ensure so that you don't have to think about eating.		X
Choose foods, such as pasta, rice, and cereal, to provide quick digesting energy.	X	
You should eat a diet high in fat to provide essential fatty acids and boost calorie intake.		X
Focus on eating a variety of foods and be sure to include your favorite foods.	X	
You should avoid any foods that are high in saturated fat and added sugar like chips and cookies.		X
You should restrict carbohydrates, such as rice, bread, and pasta.		X

Rationale: It is recommended that clients with eating disorders try to get back to a healthy weight, establish healthy relationships with food, manage their physical and psychological health, and maintain social relationships. To get back to a healthy weight, a diet rich in energy and nutrients composed of a variety of foods is emphasized. High-protein foods are encouraged to rebuild body tissues and muscles. Carbohydrate foods are needed to supply quick digesting energy for the body. Consuming favorite foods can help to increase overall food intake and develop a healthy relationship with food. Slowly including foods that bring fear and anxiety without focusing solely on those foods is the best approach. Supplement drinks, such as Ensure, can help clients meet their calorie and protein needs, but the use of them should not be abused or used in place of food. We want clients to develop healthy eating habits and establish healthy eating relationships. A moderate-fat diet is recommended to encourage tolerance of higher volumes. Restricting and avoiding any type of food is discouraged.

5.

ASSESSMENT FINDING	EFFECTIVE	INEFFECTIVE
Gained 5 lbs. after 2 weeks of treatment	X	
Consumes 3 meals per day	X	
Consumes a variety of fruits and vegetables	X	
Feels distress after consuming large meals		X
Weighs herself twice per day		X
Purges after consuming dessert-like foods		X
Avoids foods, such as sour cream, oil, avocado, and cheese		X
Goes to the gym twice per day, 7 times per week		X
Started journaling her emotions in a notebook	X	
Eats meals with family and friends	X	

Rationale: The client is gaining weight and developing healthier meal patterns with a variety of nutrients. She is recognizing her feelings and emotions by journaling. Eating with family and friends can provide the support system that is needed to encourage healthy eating. However, if she is still feeling distress after consuming meals, avoids foods, purges through vomiting or exercise, and excessively weighs herself, these are signs that she might be relapsing and might need further education and treatment.

CHAPTER 16

Chapter Review Questions

1. c   4. c
2. b   5. d
3. b

Next-Generation NCLEX® Examination-style Case Study Answers

1. **b, c, d, g**

Rationale: Experiencing fatigue, exhaustion, injury, or infection might indicate that the athlete's nutrition regimen is inadequate. His exercise frequency is not abnormal as he consumes 3 meals and 3 snacks per day. He is getting 7 to 8 hours of sleep, which is the recommended amount.

2. The client's dietary intake indicates inadequate carbohydrate intake, which is the preferred source of energy during the athlete's endurance exercise.

Rationale: The athlete's dietary recall contains few foods that are good sources of complex carbohydrates, such as bread, rice, and pasta. Carbohydrates are important during endurance exercise because they are the main source of energy and help to replete glycogen stores located in the muscle and liver.

3. A few days before the triathlon, this client would benefit from carbohydrate loading to ensure maximal glycogen stores.

Rationale: Because carbohydrates replete glycogen stores, carbohydrate loading is often used in endurance athletes to ensure that these stores are filled to maximal capacity before competition. This practice increases the total duration of exercise the athlete can perform before experiencing fatigue.

4.

HEALTH TEACHING	INDICATED	CONTRAINDICATED
Consume carbohydrate foods 2 to 4 hours before exercise.	X	
Consume foods containing high amounts of fat, fiber, and protein 1 to 4 hours before exercise.		X
Consume carbohydrate during exercise lasting longer than 1 hour.	X	
Avoid consuming carbohydrate foods after exercise.		X
Consume foods with fat, protein, and fiber during exercise.		X

Rationale: Two to 4 hours before exercising, athletes should aim to consume carbohydrate-rich foods (e.g., pasta, bread, rice) that are low in fat and fiber and moderate in protein. These nutrients digest at a slower rate and cause discomfort if they are still in the stomach during exercise. During exercise, carbohydrate consumption is only necessary if exercise is longer than 1 hour. Carbohydrates consumed during exercise should be simple (e.g., sports drinks, chews, fruit) and contain little fat, protein, and fiber. After exercise, carbohydrates should be consumed as soon as possible (no later than 2 hours) to maximize glycogen repletion.

5.

ASSESSMENT FINDING	EFFECTIVE	INEFFECTIVE
Consumes cereal with non-fat milk 3 hours before exercise.	X	
Consumes sports drinks during training that lasts 45 minutes.		X
Consumes fruit chews during exercise lasting 2 hours.	X	
Consumes chicken and broccoli 2.5 hours after exercise.		X
Able to complete his workouts with fewer breaks.	X	

Rationale: Two to 4 hours before exercising, athletes should aim to consume carbohydrate-rich foods (e.g., pasta, bread, rice) that are low in fat and fiber and moderate in protein because these nutrients digest at a slower rate and cause discomfort if they are still in the stomach during exercise. During exercise, carbohydrates are only necessary if exercise is longer than 1 hour. These carbohydrates should be simple (e.g., sports drinks, chews, fruit) and contain little fat, protein, and fiber. After exercise, carbohydrates should be consumed as soon as possible (no later than 2 hours) to maximize glycogen repletion.

CHAPTER 17

Chapter Review Questions

1. a
2. c
3. c
4. a
5. b

Next-Generation NCLEX® Examination-style Unfolding Case Study Answers

1. The registered dietitian nutritionist (RDN) determines that the client's symptoms are most likely caused by surpassing the <u>tolerable upper intake level</u>, causing vitamin <u>toxicity</u>.

   Rationale: Tolerable upper level intake is the highest level of intake that will not result in adverse health effects. Therefore consuming nutrients above the UL puts the individual at risk for toxicity and adverse health effects.

2. e

   Rationale: The nutrition focused physical findings of the client are consistent with vitamin A toxicity. Refer to Table 17.2.

3. The client's vitamin <u>toxicity</u> is related to her liver damage because the liver is the main site of vitamin <u>storage and metabolism</u>.

   Rationale: The liver is the main site for vitamin activation, storage, and metabolism. Therefore high levels of vitamins put extra stress and work on the liver, resulting to liver damage. Vitamin A toxicity is particularly hepatotoxic.

4.

ITEM	SAFE	CONTRAINDICATED
Broccoli	X	
Alcohol		X
Sweet potato	X	
Multivitamins		X
Vitamin A supplements		X
Carrots	X	
Antioxidant supplements		X

Rationale: Although it is not necessary to suggest that all foods containing vitamin A should be avoided, supplements may lead to toxicity with the medication and alcohol should be avoided with the medication to avoid further liver damage.

5. c, d, f

   Rationale: Women that are planning to become pregnant should not take Accutane. Concerning her other conditions, it would benefit the client to speak to the doctor regarding what she should do and to discuss further drug-nutrient interactions. Because she is already experiencing signs of vitamin A toxicity, she should not be taking any other dietary supplements that contain vitamin A.

6. d, e

   Rationale: Liver enzymes such as ALT and AST are helpful to determine liver function. High levels of these enzymes suggest that the liver is damaged, and these enzymes are leaking into the blood.

Next-Generation NCLEX® Examination-style Case Study Answers

1. b, c, d, e

   Rationale: During the assessment period, it is important to follow-up on any symptoms that the client might be having, as well as obtain more information regarding medications, supplements, and diet history. Anthropometric measurements are important to assess. His BMI is 22.6 kg/m^2 and is not concerning.

2. b

   Rationale: Because the client has trouble remembering past events and information, the best method to collect dietary information from him would be a multiple-day food record. This is the only method that does not require memory. DEXA and BOD POD are not methods used to collect dietary intake information. We use DEXA and BOD POD to collect anthropometric data, such as body composition.

3.

INTERVENTIONS	INDICATED	CONTRAINDICATED
Plan out dietary supplement use around mealtimes.	X	
Educate the client on the effects and use of his supplements.	X	
Educate the client on proper dosing and timing of his supplements.	X	
Avoid coordinating with other health care professionals, if possible.		X
Educate the client with a 1-day strict meal plan that will avoid any drug-nutrient interactions.		X
Schedule meals and intake before considering the client's lifestyle.		X

Rationale: In cases of food-drug interactions, it is important to plan when the client should take his supplements in relation to his meals. Educating the client on the function of his dietary supplement and how it might interact with other supplements is also important. Coordinating with other health care professionals, such as pharmacists and physicians, might be helpful during this process, and therefore they should also be referred to, if needed. It is important to work with the client to learn more about his overall lifestyle and different foods that he likes to eat so that he can properly manage his medications at home by himself. Planning a strict 1-day meal plan might help the client or that day, but he might not know what to do on days that he eats other foods.

CHAPTER 18

Chapter Review Questions

1. b   4. d
2. b   5. a
3. c

Next-Generation NCLEX® Examination-style Unfolding Case Study Answers

Cystic Fibrosis case study

1. a, b, c, f

Rationale: Individuals with cystic fibrosis have increased energy needs due to the increased work of breathing, as well as their reduced ability to digest and absorb foods. Thick mucus often hinders the pancreas' ability to secrete digestive enzymes such as amylase, protease, and lipase, therefore reducing their ability to digest and absorb nutrients. Fat is a macronutrient of specific concern, and fat-soluble vitamins should be monitored in clients to avoid deficiencies. These clients may struggle to meet such increased needs whether it is inadequate intake or poor absorption, both of which increase their risk for malnutrition.

2.

ASSESSMENT DATA	ASSOCIATED CAUSE ANSWERS
Increased calorie needs	d
Undigested stool	b
Inadequate calorie intake	c
Underweight	a

Rationale: Individuals with cystic fibrosis are often underweight due to inadequate calorie intake. They also have increased needs due to increased work from breathing difficulty. Although breathing difficulties may contribute to the patient tiring easily while eating, not meeting her energy needs can also contribute to the patient's feelings of having low energy. Undigested stool is a sign of maldigestion and malabsorption, which is related to pancreatic insufficiency.

3. Although the client has increased her nutrient intake, she may not be gaining weight due to <u>pancreatic</u> insufficiency. She would most likely benefit from <u>enzyme</u> replacement therapy.

Rationale: Pancreatic enzyme replacement therapy is an effective strategy to help the body digest and absorb food if the pancreas is not producing enough digestive enzymes due to cystic fibrosis. These are usually taken as capsules before meals.

4. a, c, d, f

Rationale: Whereas all vitamins should be monitored in clients with cystic fibrosis, fat soluble vitamins (e.g., vitamins A, D, E, and K) should be of most concern as these patient's struggle to absorb adequate amounts of fat, which is needed for optimal fat-soluble vitamin absorption.

5.

STRATEGIES	EFFECTIVE	INEFFECTIVE
3 meals with 2-3 snacks per day	X	
High fat foods	X	
Restrict foods high in fat		X
Restrict foods high in sodium		X
Encourage a variety of foods from each food group	X	
Utilize oral supplements if needed	X	
Discourage use of calorie dense foods		X

Rationale: The main nutrition goal for individuals with cystic fibrosis is to meet their nutrient needs. Therefore we want to avoid restricting certain foods that may help them increase their calorie intake. Foods high in fat and foods high in sodium should be encouraged to help clients meet their calorie needs and balance their electrolytes from excess salt lost in sweat. A variety of foods is encouraged to ensure that the patient is getting a variety of vitamins and minerals, and small, frequent meals should be encouraged to increase total energy intake. Small meals also help avoid overly tiring the patient while eating.

6.

ASSESSMENT	EFFECTIVE	INEFFECTIVE	UNRELATED
BMI increased to 18.9	X		
Regular bowel movements	X		
Fat present in stool		X	
Consumes at least 75% of meals	X		
Has difficulty breathing			X
Has increased nutrient needs			X

Rationale: The intervention would be considered effective if the patient's BMI increased into a healthy range indicating weight gain. Regular bowel movements indicate that digestion is improving, but fat in the stool still indicates malabsorption. The patient consuming most of her meals increases her chances of meeting her calorie needs. Having difficulty breathing and an increased nutrient need is unrelated to nutrition interventions and will likely always be a consequence of her condition.

Hepatitis case study

1. **a, c, d**

   Rationale: Main signs and symptoms related to hepatitis include anorexia, jaundice, and malnutrition. The client is experiencing lack of appetite, yellowing of the skin, and has nausea, vomiting, and diarrhea. The combination of loss of fluids and nutrients with reduced food intake puts the client at risk of malnutrition. This would not result in constipation, fistulas, or dysphagia.

2. The client most likely has hepatitis A, which is a viral infection related to contaminated food or water.

   Rationale: Hepatitis A is a viral infection that can be transmitted via the fecal-oral route. This most likely occurs from contaminated food and water. The client stated that he was drinking from a water source where they also did laundry, bathing, etc. This is most likely a contaminated water source.

3. The client's lack of appetite puts him at risk for malnutrition. It is important for him to consume adequate amounts of energy and protein to encourage liver regeneration.

   Rationale: Inadequate intake and lack of appetite increases the client's risk of malnutrition. Hepatitis causes inflammation and damage to the liver, requiring higher calorie and protein needs to regenerate the tissue. If not enough calories, carbohydrates, or protein is consumed, then the body will have to resort to using protein for energy and the liver will not regenerate properly.

4. **b, e, f, g, h**

   Rationale: Clients with hepatitis need to rest and meet their energy needs. Dietary restrictions are usually avoided to encourage adequate food intake. High protein intake is needed to facilitate liver regeneration and adequate calories and carbohydrates are needed to avoid use of protein for fuel. Fat intake should not be over 30% of TEE to reduce stress put on the liver and to avoid or reduce severity of steatorrhea. The client may need to restrict sodium (e.g., <2000 mg) to reduce fluid retention.

5.

MACRONUTRIENTS	ANSWER
Carbohydrates	b
Protein	f
Fat	e

   Rationale: Medical nutrition therapy recommendations for macronutrients include protein 1-1.2 g/kg of body weight per day; 50% of calories from carbohydrate (4 kcal/g); and <30% of calories from fat (9 kcal/g). These recommendations can be used with the client's calorie needs to give specific macronutrient recommendations in grams/day.

6.

ASSESSMENT	EFFECTIVE	INEFFECTIVE
Increased appetite	X	
Weight loss		X
Slight yellowing of the skin		X
Increased calorie intake	X	
Solid bowel movements	X	
No feelings of nausea	X	
Body temperature 98.6°F	X	

   Rationale: The client's increased dietary intake is an improvement that shows that interventions were effective. However, weight loss shows that interventions may not be as effective, or he still may not be meeting all his needs. His normal bowel movements illustrate resolution of diarrhea and his normal body temperature is a good sign that he is progressing. Slight yellowing of the skin is an improvement, but also is a sign that the liver has not completely healed yet, so the intervention has not been 100% effective yet.

Next-Generation NCLEX® Examination-style Case Study Answers

1. **a, d, e ,f,**

   Rationale: The client is obese and does not get the recommended amounts of exercise. He also works a lot, which could add to his stress levels. Several aspects of his diet could be improved. Some beneficial changes include incorporating more fruits and vegetables and reducing foods high in fat, sodium, and sugar. He is not on any medications, and his dietary supplements are not of concern in this case.

2. The client's nutrition assessment indicates that his weight places him in the obese category. His diet is high in fat and sodium.

   Rationale: The client's height and weight data place his BMI of 33 kg/m² in the obese category. His dietary recall indicates that his food choices are high in fat and sodium.

3. **b**

   Rationale: Gastroesophageal reflux disease (GERD) occurs when regurgitated stomach acid enters the lower part of the esophagus. This can cause irritation and erosion of the mucosal lining. Clients with GERD often feel heartburn or pain in their chest after eating and might notice frequent belching or regurgitation of stomach contents. The client displays many risk factors of this condition, including being obese, consuming large meals that are high in fat, and drinking alcohol.

4.

CLIENT QUESTIONS	APPROPRIATE NURSE'S RESPONSE FOR EACH CLIENT QUESTION
"Are there medications that I can take to help my condition?"	c
"Can I still drink alcohol?"	e
"Should I lose weight?"	b
"How much physical activity should I be getting?"	g

Rationale: Lifestyle factors, such as diet, weight loss, and physical activity, can help manage this condition. Losing weight can reduce the pressure on the abdomen and reduce the amount of stomach acid that goes into the esophagus. Alcohol can further irritate the mucosa of the esophagus, and therefore it is recommended that alcohol is avoided or limited. Physical activity recommendations are to participate in at least 30 minutes of physical activity on most days of the week. If these changes are still not helping, there are medications that can help reduce symptoms, such as antacids and proton pump inhibitors. Antacids help reduce the acidity of stomach acid, and proton pump inhibitors help reduce the production of stomach acid.

5.

HEALTH TEACHING	INDICATED	CONTRAINDICATED
Consume meals in an upright position.	X	
After eating, it might help to lie down while your food is digesting.		X
Wear tight clothing, especially after consuming meals.		X
Consume small frequent meals instead of large meals.	X	
Drink large amounts of fluids with meals.		X
Avoid irritants, such as alcohol, caffeine, chocolate, carbonated beverages, tomatoes, and spicy foods.	X	
Consume foods that are lower in fat and high in fiber.	X	

Rationale: The client should sit in an upright position while eating and avoid laying down after mealtimes. This reduces the risk for stomach acid entering the esophagus. Clients with GERD should avoid tight clothing, especially after mealtimes, because it might increase abdominal pressure and increase the chances of reflux. Small frequent meals are recommended over large meals to reduce the amount of food and stomach acid in the stomach at once. Similarly, clients with GERD should sip liquids with meals and consume most liquids between meals to control the total volume in the stomach after eating. Clients might benefit from avoiding known irritants, such as alcohol, caffeine, chocolate, carbonated beverages, tomatoes, and spicy foods. Foods that are lower in fat and higher in fiber are encouraged.

6.

ASSESSMENT FINDING	EFFECTIVE	INEFFECTIVE
Lost 8 lbs. in 1 month	X	
Consumes fruits and vegetables throughout the day	X	
Replaced alcoholic beverages with soda		X
Has less chest pain after consuming meals	X	
Skips breakfast to lower calorie intake		X

Rationale: Weight loss is an effective means of reducing the risk and occurrence of GERD. Improving the diet by increasing fruits and vegetable intake, eating regular meals, and avoiding irritants such as alcohol are all effective methods of reducing the risk for GERD. Replacing alcohol intake with soda is contraindicated as soda contains carbonation. Suffering from less frequent chest pain following meals indicates his symptoms of GERD are improving.

CHAPTER 19

Chapter Review Questions

1. a
2. a
3. a
4. a
5. b

Next-Generation NCLEX® Examination-style Unfolding Case Study Answers

1. a, c, d, e, f, g, i, l

   Rationale: Risk factors for coronary heart disease include advanced age, genetics, heredity, elevated blood cholesterol, poor diet quality, physical inactivity, smoking, and comorbidities such as hypertension and being overweight.

2.

FACTORS	ANSWERS
Increasing age	b
Elevated blood cholesterol	c
Poor diet quality	a
Physical inactivity	e
Smoking	d
Hypertension/obesity	f

Rationale: Atherosclerosis is a progressive disease and worsens as an individual ages unless lifestyle changes are made. Elevated cholesterol levels facilitate plaque formation, as cholesterol is the main component of plaque. A poor-quality diet, including high sodium and saturated fat intake, contributes to plaque formation. Smoking is related to vasoconstriction and elevated blood pressure levels, which encourage plaque formation. Sedentary lifestyles, as well as other comorbidities such as hypertension and obesity, can increase the severity of atherosclerosis.

3. Excess consumption of <u>saturated</u> fat can lead to <u>atherosclerosis</u>, where plaque causes narrowing of the arteries. This plaque is mostly composed of <u>cholesterol</u>.

Rationale: Saturated fat increases the risk for plaque formation more so than unsaturated fat intake. Plaque is primarily composed of cholesterol, and dietary sources of saturated fat have higher cholesterol levels.

4. **a, c, e**

Rationale: The patient's diet was changed to allow ≤25% of calories from fat with an emphasis on unsaturated fat rather than saturated fat. This is because saturated fat contributes more to plaque formation and high blood cholesterol levels compared to unsaturated fat. Unsaturated fat can help to reduce cholesterol levels and inflammation.

5.

INTERVENTIONS	EFFECTIVE	INEFFECTIVE
Follow the Mediterranean Diet eating pattern	X	
Follow the Dietary Approach to Stop Hypertension eating pattern	X	
Follow a ketogenic diet		X
Limit sodium to 2400 mg per day		X
Consume fish twice per week	X	
Increase intake of refined grains		X
Increase fruit and vegetable intake	X	
Weight gain		X
Increase physical activity	X	

Rationale: Effective lifestyle changes include adopting diet patterns such as the Mediterranean diet and the DASH diet. These diets are generally higher in fruits, vegetables, unsaturated fats, and fish, while also lower in sodium and saturated fats. It is suggested that individuals consume fish two times per week and regularly participate in physical activity.

6. **a, b, c**

Rationale: Assessment measures such as BMI, blood pressure, cholesterol levels, triglyceride levels, and waist circumference are all important measures to assess the risk for cardiovascular disease. If these lab values are decreasing or within normal ranges, one can assume that the intervention is improving the patient's condition.

Next-Generation NCLEX® Examination-style Case Study Answers

1. The client's reduced renal blood flow can cause her adrenal glands to secrete <u>aldosterone</u>. This can cause retention of <u>water</u> and <u>sodium</u>, which is most likely contributing to her edema.

Rationale: Congestive heart failure results in reduced blood flow that reaches the kidneys. Normally, low renal blood flow indicates hypovolemia. The body's natural response to low blood flow is to increase the volume of blood in the body through the vasopressin and renin-angiotensin-aldosterone systems. However, in the case of congestive heart failure, the low renal blood flow does not indicate hypovolemia. Because the kidneys continue to increase blood volume, the blood becomes more dilute, and edema ensues.

2. **a, b, c, d, h**

Rationale: Diet recommendations for congestive heart failure include restricting fluid and sodium to normalize fluid balance. Diuretics can help to manage fluid retention, but the health care team should monitor potassium levels and supplement, if indicated. Supplements, such as folate, vitamin B_{12}, and magnesium, might be indicated in clients with congestive heart failure. Lastly, congestive heart failure can cause shortness of breath and make eating a challenge. The medical nutrition therapy guidelines for clients that feel exhausted during mealtime is to consume soft foods that do not require as much energy for physical digestion. Small frequent meals can also help these clients consume more total calories throughout the day.

3.

HEALTH TEACHING	INDICATED	CONTRAINDICATED
Use herbs to season foods.	X	
Avoid salty processed foods, such as chips, pickles, olives, and ham.	X	
Supplement thiamine and potassium if taking a diuretic.	X	
You do not have to limit alcohol consumption.		X
Limit meals to 2 or 3 per day if having difficulty eating enough calories.		X

Rationale: To restrict sodium, clients can use sodium-free herbs and spices during cooking. Clients should avoid salty processed foods and supplement thiamine and potassium, which might be lost with frequent diuretic use. Clients should avoid or limit alcohol to 1 drink per day. Small frequent meals, such as 5 to 6 meals per day, might be helpful for these clients to consume all their calorie needs.

4.

ASSESSMENT FINDING	EFFECTIVE	INEFFECTIVE
Reduced edema in the lower extremities	X	
Consumes 2300 mg of sodium per day		X
Limits fluid to 2 L per day	X	
Eats foods, such as mashed potatoes, applesauce, and pureed peas, when eating is difficult	X	
Has low potassium levels		X
Seasons chicken with sodium-free spices, such as pepper and garlic powder	X	

Rationale: Resolving edema is a sign that fluid balance is returning and that the intervention is working. The client is following the guidelines to limit fluid to 2 L per day, but he is consuming 2300 mg of sodium, which is over the recommended intake of 2000 mg per day. He is consuming soft foods and using sodium-free herbs and spices, such as pepper and garlic powder, to season foods. However, his low potassium levels indicate that he needs to supplement potassium to return those levels to normal.

CHAPTER 20

Chapter Review Questions

1. b
2. b
3. a
4. c
5. c

Next-Generation NCLEX® Examination-style Unfolding Case Study Answers

1. b, d, e, f

   Rationale: Having a regular schedule regarding meals and physical activity is important for people who are using exogenous insulin. They must plan accordingly to predict accurate amounts of insulin related to the amount of carbohydrates ingested and the length/intensity of physical activity. Carbohydrate intake increases blood glucose levels and physical activity reduces blood glucose levels. Inappropriately matching the insulin dose to that which is needed before a meal or exercise can result in abnormal blood glucose levels. Thus an effective insulin regimen will account for these factors. Stress can also elevate blood glucose levels and is something that the client must account for.

2. Irregularities in the client's diet and physical activity can result in hyperglycemia (i.e., high levels of glucose in the blood) and hypoglycemia (i.e., low levels of glucose in the blood).

   Rationale: Hyperglycemia means elevated blood glucose levels, while *hypoglycemia* means low blood glucose levels. Blood glucose increases with carbohydrate intake and decreases with physical activity Keeping a consistent schedule allows the individual to have a better idea of how much insulin to administer or how much food to consume to adequately control their blood glucose levels.

3. b, c

   Rationale: Administering too much insulin before a meal can lead to hypoglycemia, just as inadequate carbohydrate intake before or after exercise can lead to hypoglycemia.

4.

INTERVENTION	EFFECTIVE	INEFFECTIVE
Administer more insulin		X
Exercise		X
Consume rapid acting carbohydrates	X	
Consume a mixture of rapid and slow acting carbohydrates with protein	X	
Consume protein		X
Consume fat		X

Rationale: During a case of hypoglycemia, the best thing for an individual to do is consume a rapid acting carbohydrate source. This is a carbohydrate composed of simple sugars that digest and absorb quickly into the blood. Although it is true that slow acting carbohydrates (such as complex carbohydrates) can also raise blood glucose, they do not absorb as fast and would not be the best option for immediate treatment.

5. d, e

   Rationale: Simple carbohydrates containing monosaccharides and/or disaccharides are rapidly absorbed into the bloodstream to raise blood glucose levels. Examples of these foods include fruit, candy, fruit juices, etc.

6. b, e, f

   Rationale: Hypoglycemia is defined as blood glucose below 70 mg/dL. Therefore we would expect this individual's blood glucose to be between 70 and 100 mg/dL after consuming small amounts of rapid carbohydrate during a hypoglycemic episode. However, after eating, his blood glucose may be slightly higher than 100 mg/dL depending on how much carbohydrate he consumed. He would need to check his levels shortly after consumption.

Next-Generation NCLEX® Examination-style Case Study Answers

1. a, b, c, d, f

   Rationale: Risk factors related to type 2 diabetes include having a BMI of 25 kg/m² or greater, sedentary behavior, hypertension, history of cardiovascular disease or stroke, low HDL cholesterol levels, and high triglyceride levels. Refer to Box 20.1 in the textbook. The client has all these risk factors, except his HDL and LDL cholesterol levels are within normal ranges.

2. The client is experiencing polydipsia (increased thirst) and polyuria (increased urination). This is the body's attempt to remove excess glucose in the blood caused by insulin resistance.

   Rationale: Polydipsia (increased thirst) and polyuria (increased urination) are symptoms of type 2 diabetes. When there are high levels of glucose in the blood caused by insulin resistance, the body tries to regulate these levels by increasing fluid intake and increasing excretion through urinary output.

3. b, c, g

   Rationale: The medical nutrition therapy for type 2 diabetes includes weight loss, healthy eating, and physical activity to reduce insulin resistance. If this approach does not work, other interventions can be implemented, such as metformin.

4.

ASSESSMENT FINDING	EFFECTIVE	INEFFECTIVE
Client weighs 250 lbs. after 1 month	X	
Blood pressure: 120/85 mm Hg	X	
Triglycerides: 145 mmol/L	X	
Participates in 150 minutes of moderate intensity physical activity per week	X	

Continued

ASSESSMENT FINDING	EFFECTIVE	INEFFECTIVE
Avoids eating dinner with family and friends at restaurants		X
Replaced soda with diet soda	X	

Rationale: Weight loss greater than or equal to 5% of body weight is significant enough to improve insulin resistance. Reduced blood pressure, reduced triglyceride levels, and increased physical activity are all signs that the intervention is effective. Replacing soda with diet soda is an appropriate option for clients with diabetes because they consume non-nutritive sweeteners that do not influence blood sugar levels. However, avoiding food gatherings with family and friends is not effective and suggests an unhealthy relationship with food and/or insecurity in making food choices. The client should feel empowered to make healthy food choices in a variety of environments and still enjoy his social life.

CHAPTER 21

Chapter Review Questions

1. a
2. c
3. a
4. c
5. b

Next-Generation NCLEX® Examination-style Unfolding Case Study Answers

1. b, c, e, f, h

   Rationale: The kidneys work to filter particles and compounds in the blood to maintain electrolyte balance, acid-base balance, and fluid balance. The patient has protein and blood in the urine, high levels of urea and creatinine in the blood, and low glomerular filtration rate. Each of these clinical symptoms indicate kidney function decline.

2. The nurse recognizes that the patient's <u>electrolyte</u> imbalance is causing <u>edema</u>. The health care team needs to account for this when analyzing the patient's <u>weight</u>.

   Rationale: Decline in kidney function may lead to hyponatremia, hypervolemia, and hypoalbuminemia, which can lead to edema in the lower extremities. When a patient has signs of edema, it is important to note that their weight may not be accurate due to the increased fluid retention. Nurses may be able to find a patient's dry weight that excludes any potential fluid retention.

3. An increasing loss of <u>nephron</u> function requires external modifications to regulate <u>chemical</u> imbalances. This ensures that the body is in <u>homeostasis</u>.

   Rationale: A nephron is the basic functional unit of the kidney. It regulates chemical imbalances related to proteins, acids and bases, and electrolytes to ensure that the body is in a state of homeostasis. Damaged nephrons are unable to maintain these balances within the body. Thus patients must regulate levels of these compounds through external modifications such as nutrition and medication interventions.

4.

INTERVENTION	INDICATED	CONTRAINDICATED
Maintain lean body mass with adequate protein intake	X	
Restrict carbohydrates and fat		X
Restrict sodium intake to reduce fluid retention	X	
Restrict potassium	X	
Restrict phosphorous	X	
Encourage high intakes of calcium		X
Supplement vitamins A and E		X
Supplement vitamins D and K		X
Provide adequate fluid to meet patient's individualized needs	X	

Rationale: Patients with CKD may illustrate signs of malnutrition such as decreased appetite, edema, and unintended weight loss. For these patients, protein intake is important to ensure that they maintain lean body mass and do not lose further weight. Carbohydrates and fat intake should be adequate to ensure that the patient is meeting his or her calorie needs to avoid protein catabolism for energy. Sodium restrictions may need to be put into place to treat hypernatremia and hypervolemia., but fluid should still be provided to meet the individual's needs. Electrolytes such as K, P, and Ca can be elevated in patient's blood due to the kidney's decreased ability to filter and excrete these minerals appropriately. Because of this, these minerals are usually restricted, but it is highly individualized depending on the patient's lab values. Supplementing vitamins A and E are discouraged because a buildup of these vitamins can cause toxicity. Patients should also avoid vitamins D and K due to the kidney's inability to convert vitamin D to its active form, and the effect that excess vitamin K can have on blood clotting.

5. a, c, d, e

   Rationale: The patient is still losing weight and is deficient in many nutrients. His feelings of nausea, fatigue, and mouth pain suggest that he may not be eating enough calories, protein, or nutrients. Because of this, medical nutrition therapy guidelines suggest the use of soft foods that have a modified texture and foods high in protein. The patient should still avoid other foods that are high in minerals such as sodium, potassium, and phosphorous. Scrambled eggs are high in protein and soft in texture. Applesauce and cauliflower rice are texture modified and contain low amounts of sodium, potassium, and phosphorous. Baked salmon is a good option because it is easy to chew, moist, and provides adequate protein. The patient should avoid, or limit, foods in this list that are high in sodium, such as canned foods. However, "no sodium" and "low sodium" canned goods may be appropriate choices for these patients. Whole-wheat toast is dry and would likely cause this patient pain with his mouth sores. Whole grains also tend to be high in potassium and phosphorous. Thus MNK guidelines recommend white bread and refined grains for patients with CKD.

6. a, d, e, g

Rationale: When assessing patients with CKD, it is important to monitor their weight, electrolytes, minerals, and protein levels regularly. Weight and lean body mass are also important to assess to determine adequate intake and nutrition status. Health care providers use glomerular filtration rate to categorize different stages of CKD. Therefore increased GFR suggests that the patient's condition is improving rather than declining.

Next-Generation NCLEX® Examination-style Case Study Answers

1. b, c, e, g

Rationale: The client's height and weight, phosphorous intake, and glucose levels are within normal ranges. However, vitamin C intake exceeds the DRI, which increases the risk of kidney stones and could be a contributing factor. Her low calcium and fluid intake might have contributed to the kidney stone development. These factors would require a follow-up to ensure appropriate changes for treatment and future prevention. Clients with kidney stones are at greater risk of hypertension, and hypertension itself can also lead to stone formation, so it would be beneficial to get her blood pressure to normal levels.

2. After a dietary recall was collected from the client, the dietitian identified large amounts of foods high in oxalate, such as spinach and collard greens, which can increase the risk of kidney stone development.

Rationale: Foods high in oxalate are leafy greens, legumes beets, potatoes, bran products, cocoa, tea, and some nuts. Foods such as grains and animal proteins are generally low in oxalate. Large intake of oxalate can increase the risk of kidney stone development in some people.

3. a, d, e, g, h

Rationale: To resolve and prevent further development of kidney stones, the client should aim to maintain her current healthy weight. Protein restrictions are not necessary for clients with kidney stones, and limiting protein too much can increase the risk of stones. Instead, consuming the recommended 0.8 to 1 g/kg of protein per day is ideal. Reducing calcium intake is contraindicated, and the client should consume enough calcium to meet the DRI. Phosphorous intake should not exceed the DRI. Sodium and oxalate intake should be reduced because high intake of these compounds contributes to stone development in susceptible individuals. Lastly, the client should increase her fluid intake to 2 to 3 L/day to reduce the risk for stone formation.

4.

ASSESSMENT FINDING	EFFECTIVE	INEFFECTIVE
Client carries water bottle throughout the day to consume 2-3 L of fluid per day.	X	
Blood pressure: 119/79 mm Hg	X	
Client focuses on consuming more fruits and vegetables, such as oranges, grapefruits, and berries.	X	
Increased consumption of lean meats from animal sources.		X
Client consumes low-sodium dairy foods.	X	
Client reduces vitamin C supplementation to 60 mg of vitamin C per day.	X	
Client has resolution of hematuria.	X	

Rationale: For clients with kidney stones, increased fluid needs of 2 to 3 L/day is helpful to avoid formation of kidney stones. A reduction in blood pressure is a good sign that the body's stress response is normalizing. Focusing on fruits and vegetables that are high in citrate, such as oranges, grapefruits, and berries, is helpful to prevent crystallization of settled contents. Consuming low-sodium dairy foods is beneficial to meet calcium and vitamin D needs while also limiting sodium intake. The client decreasing her vitamin C supplementation below the UL of 2000 milligrams is recommended for kidney stone prevention. Consuming large amounts of protein from animal sources increases the risk of stone development and is not recommended. A resolution of hematuria (blood in the urine) is a good sign that the client's condition is improving.

CHAPTER 22

Chapter Review Questions

1. d
2. a
3. a
4. c
5. a

Next-Generation NCLEX® Examination-style Unfolding Case Study Answers

1. c, f, g, h, i, j

Rationale: A total gastrectomy involves the removal of the entire stomach. The stomach is one of the key organs involved in digesting foods, making food ready for absorption. With the removal of the stomach, patients are at risk of maldigestion, malabsorption, and malnutrition. Removing the stomach shortens the length of the gastrointestinal tract, which can also increase the speed of which food moves through the body. If food moves through the body at a faster rate, there is less time for digestion and absorption of the food. The procedure does not have an impact on the amount of bile or pancreatic enzymes secreted. It also does not affect the pancreas' ability to secrete insulin. Gastric surgery puts patients at risk of infection due to the surgical procedure, and they may experience physical complications such as fistulas and obstructions.

2. **c, e, f**

Rationale: After a gastrectomy, the medical nutrition guidelines recommend that patients consume small frequent meals to limit the amount of food going through the digestive tract at one time. This can improve digestion and absorption rates and slow the total transit time. Easily digestible foods are encouraged to put less stress on the gastrointestinal tract and to reduce complications related to obstructions and strictures that form from fibrous foods. Bland foods should be encouraged rather than foods that have large amounts of seasonings and spices, as these can irritate the GI tract. High quality protein foods are important to facilitate tissue healing and preserve lean body mass during the healing process.

3. The patient is most likely experiencing dumping syndrome. This can occur after consuming a meal with a large amount of readily absorbable carbohydrates that rapidly enter the small intestine.

Rationale: Dumping syndrome commonly occurs when large sections of the GI tract, such as the stomach, have been removed. This allows food to rapidly move into the small intestine. Readily absorbable carbohydrates (e.g., disaccharides and monosaccharides) are of specific concern because they rapidly form a concentrated food mass that pull water from the GI tract into the lumen. This attempt to maintain proper osmolality pulls water from the vascular system and causes symptoms of shock such as increased heart rate, weakness, sweating, dizziness, cramping, etc.

4.

INTERVENTION	INDICATED	CONTRAINDICATED
Consuming carbohydrates with a low glycemic index	X	
Drinking adequate fluids with meals		X
Eating meals slowly	X	
Reducing dietary fat	X	
Participating in physical activity shortly after eating		X
Laying down for 15-30 minutes after meals	X	

Rationale: Consuming carbohydrates with a lower glycemic index are used in dumping syndrome to reduce the osmolality in the GI tract. Eating slowly and avoiding fluid with meals can reduce the total volume of food going through the GI tract at one time. Patient's with dumping syndrome may illustrate signs of malabsorption as well. Because of this, they should avoid large amounts of dietary fat, which could otherwise lead to steatorrhea. After eating, patients may find it helpful to recline for 15-30 minutes to slow the transit time of food through the body. Physical activity increases the transit time

and should be avoided after meals in patients with dumping syndrome.

5. **b**

Rationale: Patients with dumping syndrome should avoid foods that contain simple sugars such as sweetened yogurts, baked goods, canned fruit, jellies, and sugar sweetened beverages. Liquids and soups eaten with solid foods should also be avoided. Breads, meats, unsweetened yogurt, fruits, and vegetables are encouraged.

6.

ASSESSMENT	EFFECTIVE	INEFFECTIVE
Weight has not returned to normal		X
Muscle mass has improved	X	
Less discomfort after meals	X	
Diarrhea		X
Displays feelings of fear towards foods		X
Avoids protein foods		X
Avoids carbohydrates with high GI index	X	
Consumes liquids with foods		X

Rationale: There are many signs that the intervention was not effective (e.g., the patient's weight has not returned to normal). This is probably because he displays feelings of fear towards foods, which may be why he is avoiding protein foods. He also consumes liquids with meals and is having diarrhea. This is a clear sign that the patient may need additional education to emphasize the importance of protein foods and to talk about other diet changes that he may not have understood. These changes may include avoiding liquids with meals to reduce the risk for diarrhea. However, it is good that he does have some improved muscle mass that may have come with increasing overall intake.

Next-Generation NCLEX® Examination-style Case Study Answers

1. **a, b, c, d**

Rationale: The patient has lost 5% of his body weight in 1 month, which is a sign of malnutrition. Height in the 8th percentile is a sign of stunted growth. His bowel resections and ulcerative colitis put him at risk for malabsorption, specifically because the ilium was removed. These procedures can negatively affect nutrient absorption. His overall caloric intake is very low. His history stated that he does not show signs of dysphagia and is able to eat food by mouth.

2. The patient's bowel resection might have resulted in short bowel syndrome. The patient's weight history indicates that this might have caused compromised digestion and absorption, resulting in impaired growth.

Rationale: Bowel resections can result in short bowel syndrome. Loss of the ileum can reduce the body's ability to digest food and absorb nutrients.

3. The patient's weight loss and oral intake indicate that he might not be getting enough calories and protein orally.

Rationale: Calories and protein are crucial for a child's growth, and when their oral intake is low, they are likely not meeting their needs. Although his calcium and vitamin D intake from food might be low, he takes a multivitamin that provides those nutrients. There is not enough information to determine his fluid or cholesterol intake.

4. **a, d**

Rationale: The patient still has a predominantly functioning digestive tract, and therefore it is best to use enteral nutrition to maintain the integrity and function of the gut. PPN and CPN are not necessary unless the patient is unable to tolerate EN feeds. Oral intake would also be encouraged because food is always the first approach if safe and able. There is no indication that he should be NPO.

5.

INTERVENTION	INDICATED	CONTRAINDICATED
Nasogastric tube	X	
Gastrointestinal tube		X
Standard formula		X
Elemental formula	X	
Continuous feeds	X	
Bolus feeds		X

Rationale: A nasogastric tube would be the first approach compared with a gastrointestinal tube. Nasogastric tubes are more comfortable to place and used for shorter periods until they can transition back to a regular diet. If the patient was unable to consume food for an extended period, then a gastrointestinal tube might be necessary. This patient is already having issues digesting and absorbing food, and therefore it is best that he is started on an elemental formula compared with a standard formula. Continuous feeds are suggested for individuals who have not been fed enterally before. Once the patient becomes more stable and tolerant of feeds, bolus feedings might be appropriate.

6.

ASSESSMENT FINDING	EFFECTIVE	INEFFECTIVE
Patient gained 200 g in the last 48 hours.	X	
Patient experienced vomiting.		X
Patient's chart shows 1 stool output over the last 46 hours.		X
Abdomen is distended.		X
Patient received 50% of recommended feeds.		X
Patient is taking a multivitamin.	X	
Small snacks are eaten throughout the day.	X	

Rationale: The patient is gaining weight, which might be a good sign that he is receiving proper nutrition. However, he is vomiting, is not producing adequate output, and has a distended abdomen. These are signs of intolerance. It would be appropriate to review the formula and feeding rate to adjust as needed. The patient is only receiving 50% of his recommended feeds, which means that he might not be

meeting his nutrient and energy needs. He is taking a multivitamin and eating small snacks throughout the day, which is good for maintaining the behavior of eating and helping to achieve his calorie needs.

CHAPTER 23

Chapter Review Questions

1. d
2. b
3. c
4. d
5. b

Next-Generation NCLEX® Examination-style Case Study Answers

1. **a, b, c, d, e**

Rationale: The client has lost 10% of his weight in 2 months, which is a sign of severe malnutrition. His diet history indicates that he is not consuming adequate energy or protein. His dry mouth and difficulty swallowing are concerns that may inhibit sufficient intake. Passing only one bowel movement per week is a sign of constipation and may be related to his lack of food intake. His fluid intake is normal and should be encouraged to help his dry mouth.

2. **a, b, c, d**

Rationale: Cancer and cancer treatment increase the client's metabolism and energy needs. When the client is not eating enough due to feeding difficulty or lack of appetite, weight loss can occur. He is not fluid-overloaded, because there are no signs of edema or excessive output, and his physical activity is reasonable.

3.

CLIENT QUESTIONS	APPROPRIATE NURSE'S RESPONSE FOR EACH CLIENT QUESTION
"How can I eat enough calories when I don't feel hungry?"	b
"What are some things I can do to help with my dry mouth?"	a
"Are there foods that I can eat that are easier to swallow?"	c
"What can I do to reduce feelings of nausea at mealtime?"	d
"Is there something I can do to resolve my constipation?"	e

Rationale: For hypermetabolic clients, it is essential to encourage the consumption of high-calorie foods that are low in volume. This helps the client get the most calories when their intake may not be adequate. With xerostomia, moist foods, seasonings, and fluids can facilitate saliva production and hydrate the mouth. Adding sauces, gravies, and soft, wet foods can help foods become more comfortable to swallow. If a client feels nausea around mealtimes, it is best to consume small, frequent meals containing cold or room-temperature foods. Constipated clients should be encouraged to increase their fiber, fluids, and physical activity to help stool move through the digestive tract.

4.

MEDICAL NUTRITION THERAPY	ANSWERS
Calorie needs (Sedentary)	f
Protein needs	i
Antioxidants	b
Calorie-dense foods	a

Rationale: Clients with cancer have calorie needs of about 25 to 30 kcal/kg, which would mean that this client's needs are ~1125 to 1350 kcals/day. Protein needs for clients with cancer are 1 to 1.5 g/kg, putting his needs at 45 to 68 gm/day. Antioxidants help reduce damage caused by oxidative stress and can be found in strawberries, blueberries, and raspberries. Lastly, calorie-dense foods can help improve the client's intake, so adding butter, cream, whole milk, and peanut butter to foods can add necessary calories and protein. Consuming protein drinks, when appropriate, can also help improve intake.

Dietary Reference Intake (DRI)

Dietary Reference Intakes (DRIs): Recommended Dietary Allowances and Adequate Intakes, Vitamins
Food and Nutrition Board, Institute of Medicine, National Academies

Life Stage Group	Vitamin A (mcg/d)a	Vitamin C (mg/d)	Vitamin D (IU/d)b,c	Vitamin E (mg/d)d	Vitamin K (mcg/d)	Thiamin (mg/d)	Riboflavin (mg/d)	Niacin (mg/d)e	Vitamin B6 (mg/d)	Folate (mcg/d)f	Vitamin B12 (mcg/d)	Pantothenic Acid (mg/d)	Biotin (mcg/d)	Choline (mg/d)g
Infants														
Birth–6mo	400*	40*	400	4*	2.0*	0.2*	0.3*	2*	0.1*	65*	0.4*	1.7*	5*	125*
6–12mo	500*	50*	400	5*	2.5*	0.3*	0.4*	4*	0.3*	80*	0.5*	1.8*	6*	150*
Children														
1–3yr	300	15	600	6	30*	0.5	0.5	6	0.5	150	0.9	2*	8*	200*
4–8yr	400	25	600	7	55*	0.6	0.6	8	0.6	200	1.2	3*	12*	250*
Males														
9–13yr	600	45	600	11	60*	0.9	0.9	12	1.0	300	1.8	4*	20*	375*
14–18yr	900	75	600	15	75*	1.2	1.3	16	1.3	400	2.4	5*	25*	550*
19–30yr	900	90	600	15	120*	1.2	1.3	16	1.3	400	2.4	5*	30*	550*
31–50yr	900	90	600	15	120*	1.2	1.3	16	1.3	400	2.4	5*	30*	550*
51–70yr	900	90	600	15	120*	1.2	1.3	16	1.7	400	2.4h	5*	30*	550*
>70yr	900	90	800	15	120*	1.2	1.3	16	1.7	400	2.4h	5*	30*	550*
Females														
9–13yr	600	45	600	11	60*	0.9	0.9	12	1.0	300	1.8	4*	20*	375*
14–18yr	700	65	600	15	75*	1.0	1.0	14	1.2	400i	2.4	5*	25*	400*
19–30yr	700	75	600	15	90*	1.1	1.1	14	1.3	400i	2.4	5*	30*	425*
31–50yr	700	75	600	15	90*	1.1	1.1	14	1.3	400i	2.4	5*	30*	425*
51–70yr	700	75	600	15	90*	1.1	1.1	14	1.5	400	2.4h	5*	30*	425*
>70yr	700	75	800	15	90*	1.1	1.1	14	1.5	400	2.4h	5*	30*	425*
Pregnancy														
14–18yr	750	80	600	15	75*	1.4	1.4	18	1.9	600i	2.6	6*	30*	450*
19–30yr	770	85	600	15	90*	1.4	1.4	18	1.9	600i	2.6	6*	30*	450*
31–50yr	770	85	600	15	90*	1.4	1.4	18	1.9	600i	2.6	6*	30*	450*
Lactation														
14–18yr	1200	115	600	19	75*	1.4	1.6	17	2.0	500	2.8	7*	35*	550*
19–30yr	1300	120	600	19	90*	1.4	1.6	17	2.0	500	2.8	7*	35*	550*
31–50yr	1300	120	600	19	90*	1.4	1.6	17	2.0	500	2.8	7*	35*	550*

Sources: Dietary Reference Intakes for Calcium, Phosphorus, Magnesium, Vitamin D, and Fluoride (1997); Dietary Reference Intakes for Thiamin, Riboflavin, Niacin, Vitamin B6, Folate, Vitamin B12, Pantothenic Acid, Biotin, and Choline (1998); Dietary Reference Intakes for Vitamin C, Vitamin E, Selenium, and Carotenoids (2000); Dietary Reference Intakes for Vitamin A, Vitamin K, Arsenic, Boron, Chromium, Copper, Iodine, Iron, Manganese, Molybdenum, Nickel, Silicon, Vanadium, and Zinc (2001); Dietary Reference Intakes for Water, Potassium, Sodium, Chloride, and Sulfate (2005); and Dietary Reference Intakes for Calcium and Vitamin D (2011). You may access these reports via www.nap.edu.

Note: This table (taken from the DRI reports, see www.nap.edu) presents Recommended Dietary Allowances (RDAs) in **boldface** type and Adequate Intakes (AIs) in lightface type followed by an asterisk (*). An RDA is the average daily dietary intake level; sufficient to meet the nutrient requirements of nearly all (97%–98%) healthy individuals in a group. It is calculated from an Estimated Average Requirement (EAR). If sufficient scientific evidence is not available to establish an EAR, and thus calculate an RDA, an AI is usually developed. For healthy breastfed infants, an AI is the mean intake. The AI for other life stage and sex groups is believed to cover the needs of all healthy individuals in the groups, but lack of data or uncertainty in the data prevent being able to specify with confidence of the percentage of individuals covered by this intake.

a As retinol activity equivalents (RAEs). 1 RAE = 1 mcg of retinol, 12 mcg of β-carotene, 24 mcg of α-carotene, or 24 mcg of β-cryptoxanthin. The RAE for dietary provitamin A carotenoids is twofold greater than retinol equivalents (REs), whereas the RAE for preformed vitamin A is the same as the RE for vitamin A.

b As cholecalciferol. 1 mcg of cholecalciferol = 40 IU of vitamin D.

c Under the assumption of minimal sunlight.

d As α-tocopherol. α-Tocopherol includes RRR-α-tocopherol, the only form of α-tocopherol that occurs naturally in foods, and the 2R-stereoisomeric forms of α-tocopherol (RRR-, RSR-, RRS-, and RSS-α-tocopherol) that occur in fortified foods and supplements. It does not include the 2S-stereoisomeric forms of α-tocopherol (SRR-, SSR-, SRS-, and SSS-α-tocopherol), also found in fortified foods and supplements.

e As niacin equivalents (NEs). 1 mg of niacin = 60 mg of tryptophan; 0–6 months = preformed niacin (not NE).

f As dietary folate equivalents (DFEs). 1 DFE = 1 mcg of food folate = 0.6 mcg of folic acid from fortified food or as a supplement consumed with food = 0.5 mcg of a supplement taken on an empty stomach.

g Although AIs have been established for choline, there are few data to assess whether a dietary supply of choline is needed at all stages of the life cycle, and it may be that the choline requirement can be met by endogenous synthesis at some of these stages.

h Because 10% to 30% of older people may malabsorb food-bound B12, it is advisable for those older than 50 years to meet their RDA mainly by consuming foods fortified with B12 or a supplement containing B12.

i In view of evidence linking folate intake with neural tube defects in the fetus, it is recommended that all women capable of becoming pregnant consume 400 mcg from supplements or fortified foods in addition to intake of food folate from a varied diet.

It is assumed that women will continue consuming 400 mcg from supplements or fortified food until their pregnancy is confirmed and they enter prenatal care, which ordinarily occurs after the end of the periconceptional period—the critical time for formation of the neural tube.

Dietary Reference Intakes (DRIs): Recommended Dietary Allowances and Adequate Intakes, Minerals
Food and Nutrition Board, Institute of Medicine, National Academies

Life Stage Group	Calcium (mg/d)	Chromium (mcg/d)	Copper (mcg/d)	Fluoride (mg/d)	Iodine (mcg/d)	Iron (mg/d)	Magnesium (mg/d)	Manganese (mg/d)	Molybdenum (mcg/d)	Phosphorus (mg/d)	Selenium (mcg/d)	Zinc (mg/d)	Potassium (mg/d)	Sodium (mg/d)	Chloride (g/d)
Infants															
Birth–6 mo	200*	0.2*	200*	0.01*	110*	0.27*	30*	0.003*	2*	100*	15*	2*	400*	110*	0.18*
6–12 mo	260*	5.5*	220*	0.5*	130*	11	75*	0.6*	3*	275*	20*	3	860*	370*	0.57*
Children															
1–3 yr	700	11*	340	0.7*	90	7	80	1.2*	17	460	20	3	2000*	800*	1.5*
4–8 yr	1000	15*	440	1*	90	10	130	1.5*	22	500	30	5	2300*	1000*	1.9*
Males															
9–13 yr	1300	25*	700	2*	120	8	240	1.9*	34	1250	40	8	2500*	1200*	2.3*
14–18 yr	1300	35*	890	3*	150	11	410	2.2*	43	1250	55	11	3000*	1500*	2.3*
19–30 yr	1000	35*	900	4*	150	8	400	2.3*	45	700	55	11	3400*	1500*	2.3*
31–50 yr	1000	35*	900	4*	150	8	420	2.3*	45	700	55	11	3400*	1500*	2.3*
51–70 yr	1000	30*	900	4*	150	8	420	2.3*	45	700	55	11	3400*	1500*	2.0*
>70 yr	1200	30*	900	4*	150	8	420	2.3*	45	700	55	11	3400*	1500*	1.8*
Females															
9–13 yr	1300	21*	700	2*	120	8	240	1.6*	34	1250	40	8	2300*	1200*	2.3*
14–18 yr	1300	24*	890	3*	150	15	360	1.6*	43	1250	55	9	2300*	1500*	2.3*
19–30 yr	1000	25*	900	3*	150	18	310	1.8*	45	700	55	8	2600*	1500*	2.3*
31–50 yr	1000	25*	900	3*	150	18	320	1.8*	45	700	55	8	2600*	1500*	2.3*
51–70 yr	1200	20*	900	3*	150	8	320	1.8*	45	700	55	8	2600*	1500*	2.0*
>70 yr	1200	20*	900	3*	150	8	320	1.8*	45	700	55	8	2600*	1500*	1.8*
Pregnancy															
14–18 yr	1300	29*	1000	3*	220	27	400	2.0*	50	1250	60	12	2600*	1500*	2.3*
19–30 yr	1000	30*	1000	3*	220	27	350	2.0*	50	700	60	11	2900*	1500*	2.3*
31–50 yr	1000	30*	1000	3*	220	27	360	2.0*	50	700	60	11	2900*	1500*	2.3*
Lactation															
14–18 yr	1300	44*	1300	3*	290	10	360	2.6*	50	1250	70	13	2500*	1500*	2.3*
19–30 yr	1000	45*	1300	3*	290	9	310	2.6*	50	700	70	12	2800*	1500*	2.3*
31–50 yr	1000	45*	1300	3*	290	9	320	2.6*	50	700	70	12	2800*	1500*	2.3*

Sources: Dietary Reference Intakes for Calcium, Phosphorus, Magnesium, Vitamin D, and Fluoride (1997); Dietary Reference Intakes for Thiamin, Riboflavin, Niacin, Vitamin B₆, Folate, Vitamin B₁₂, Pantothenic Acid, Biotin, and Choline (1998); Dietary Reference Intakes for Vitamin C, Vitamin E, Selenium, and Carotenoids (2000); Dietary Reference Intakes for Vitamin A, Vitamin K, Arsenic, Boron, Chromium, Copper, Iodine, Iron, Manganese, Molybdenum, Nickel, Silicon, Vanadium, and Zinc (2001); Dietary Reference Intakes for Water, Potassium, Sodium, Chloride, and Sulfate (2005); Dietary Reference Intakes for Calcium and Vitamin D (2011); and Dietary Reference Intakes for Sodium and Potassium (2019). You may access these reports via www.nap.edu.

Note: This table (taken from the DRI reports, see www.nap.edu) presents Recommended Dietary Allowances (RDAs) in **boldface type** and Adequate Intakes (AIs) in lightface type followed by an asterisk (*). An RDA is the average daily dietary intake level; sufficient to meet the nutrient requirements of nearly all (97%–98%) healthy individuals in a group. It is calculated from an Estimated Average Requirement (EAR). If sufficient scientific evidence is not available to establish an EAR, and thus calculate an RDA, an AI is usually developed. For healthy breastfed infants, an AI is the mean intake. The AI for other life stage and sex groups is believed to cover the needs of all healthy individuals in the groups, but lack of data or uncertainty in the data prevent being able to specify with confidence of the percentage of individuals covered by this intake.

Dietary Reference Intake of Energy From Birth to 18 Years of Age Per Day
Food and Nutrition Board, Institute of Medicine, National Academies

	Age	Estimated Energy Requirement
Infants	0 to 3 months	$(89 \times \text{Weight [kg]} - 100) + 175\,\text{kcal}$
	4 to 6 months	$(89 \times \text{Weight [kg]} - 100) + 56\,\text{kcal}$
	7 to 12 months	$(89 \times \text{Weight [kg]} - 100) + 22\,\text{kcal}$
	13 to 36 months	$(89 \times \text{Weight [kg]} - 100) + 20\,\text{kcal}$
Boys	3 to 8 years	$88.5 - (61.9 \times \text{Age [yr]}) + \text{PA} \times (26.7 \times \text{Weight [kg]} + 903 \times \text{Height [m]}) + 20\,\text{kcal}$
	9 to 18 years	$88.5 - (61.9 \times \text{Age [yr]}) + \text{PA} \times (26.7 \times \text{Weight [kg]} + 903 \times \text{Height [m]}) + 25\,\text{kcal}$
Girls	3 to 8 years	$135.3 - (30.8 \times \text{Age [yr]}) + \text{PA} \times (10.0 \times \text{Weight [kg]} + 934 \times \text{Height [m]}) + 20\,\text{kcal}$
	9 to 18 years	$135.3 - (30.8 \times \text{Age [yr]}) + \text{PA} \times (10.0 \times \text{Weight [kg]} + 934 \times \text{Height [m]}) + 25\,\text{kcal}$

PA, Physical activity level. Data from Food and Nutrition Board. (2002). *Dietary Reference Intakes for energy, carbohydrate, fiber, fat, fatty acids, cholesterol, protein, and amino acids (macronutrients)*. Institute of Medicine. Washington, DC: National Academies Press.

Dietary Reference Intakes (DRIs): Recommended Dietary Allowances and Adequate Intakes, Total Water, Fiber, Essential Fatty Acids, and Protein
Food and Nutrition Board, Institute of Medicine, National Academies

Life Stage Group	Total Water[a] (L/d)	Total Fiber (g/d)	Linoleic Acid (g/d)	α-Linolenic Acid (g/d)	Protein[b] (g/d)
Infants					
Birth–6 mo	0.7*	ND	4.4*	0.5*	9.1*
6–12 mo	0.8*	ND	4.6*	0.5*	**11.0**
Children					
1–3 yr	1.3*	19*	7*	0.7*	**13**
4–8 yr	1.7*	25*	10*	0.9*	**19**
Males					
9–13 yr	2.4*	31*	12*	1.2*	**34**
14–18 yr	3.3*	38*	16*	1.6*	**52**
19–30 yr	3.7*	38*	17*	1.6*	**56**
31–50 yr	3.7*	38*	17*	1.6*	**56**
51–70 yr	3.7*	30*	14*	1.6*	**56**
>70 yr	3.7*	30*	14*	1.6*	**56**
Females					
9–13 yr	2.1*	26*	10*	1.0*	**34**
14–18 yr	2.3*	26*	11*	1.1*	**46**
19–30 yr	2.7*	25*	12*	1.1*	**46**
31–50 yr	2.7*	25*	12*	1.1*	**46**
51–70 yr	2.7*	21*	11*	1.1*	**46**
>70 yr	2.7*	21*	11*	1.1*	**46**
Pregnancy					
14–18 yr	3.0*	28*	13*	1.4*	**71**
19–30 yr	3.0*	28*	13*	1.4*	**71**
31–50 yr	3.0*	28*	13*	1.4*	**71**
Lactation					
14–18 yr	3.8*	29*	13*	1.3*	**71**
19–30 yr	3.8*	29*	13*	1.3*	**71**
31–50 yr	3.8*	29*	13*	1.3*	**71**

Source: Dietary Reference Intakes for Energy, Carbohydrate, Fiber, Fat, Fatty Acids, Cholesterol, Protein, and Amino Acids (2002/2005) and Dietary Reference Intakes for Water, Potassium, Sodium, Chloride, and Sulfate (2005). The reports may be accessed via www.nap.edu.

NOTE: This table (taken from the DRI reports, see www.nap.edu) presents Recommended Dietary Allowances (RDA) in **boldface type** and Adequate Intakes (AIs) in ordinary type followed by an asterisk (*). An RDA is the average daily dietary intake level; sufficient to meet the nutrient requirements of nearly all (97%–98%) healthy individuals in a group. It is calculated from an Estimated Average Requirement (EAR).

If sufficient scientific evidence is not available to establish an EAR, and thus calculate an RDA, an AI is usually developed. For healthy breastfed infants, an AI is the mean intake. The AI for other life stage and sex groups is believed to cover the needs of all healthy individuals in the groups, but lack of data or uncertainty in the data prevents being able to specify with confidence the percentage of individuals covered by this intake.

[a]Total water includes all water contained in food, beverages, and drinking water.

[b]Based on grams of protein per kilogram of body weight for the reference body weight (e.g., for adults 0.8 g/kg body weight for the reference body weight).

Dietary Reference Intakes (DRIs): Acceptable Macronutrient Distribution Ranges
Food and Nutrition Board, Institute of Medicine, National Academies

Macronutrient	RANGE (PERCENT OF TOTAL ENERGY)		
	Children, 1–3 yr	Children, 4–18 yr	Adults
Fat	30–40	25–35	20–35
n-6 polyunsaturated fatty acids[a] (linoleic acid)	5–10	5–10	5–10
n-3 polyunsaturated fatty acids[a] (α-linolenic acid)	0.6–1.2	0.6–1.2	0.6–1.2
Carbohydrate	45–65	45–65	45–65
Protein	5–20	10–30	10–35
Dietary Elements to Limit	**Recommendation**		
Dietary cholesterol	As low as possible while consuming a nutritionally adequate diet		
Trans fatty acids	As low as possible while consuming a nutritionally adequate diet		
Saturated fatty acids	As low as possible while consuming a nutritionally adequate diet		
Added sugars[b]	Limit to no more than 25% of total energy		

[a]Approximately 10% of the total can come from longer-chain n-3 or n-6 fatty acids.
[b]Not a recommended intake. A daily intake of added sugars that individuals should aim for to achieve a healthful diet was not set.
Source: Dietary Reference Intakes for Energy, Carbohydrate, Fiber, Fat, Fatty Acids, Cholesterol, Protein, and Amino Acids (2002/2005). You may access the report via www.nap.edu.

Dietary Reference Intakes (DRIs): Tolerable Upper Intake Levels, Vitamins
Food and Nutrition Board, Institute of Medicine, National Academies

Life Stage Group	Vitamin A (mcg/d)[a]	Vitamin C (mg/d)	Vitamin D (IU/d)	Vitamin E (mg/d)[b,c]	Niacin (mg/d)[c]	Vitamin B₆ (mg/d)	Folate (mcg/d)[c]	Choline (g/d)	Carotenoids[d]
Infants									
Birth–6 mo	600	ND	1000	ND	ND	ND	ND	ND	ND
6–12 mo	600	ND	1500	ND	ND	ND	ND	ND	ND
Children									
1–3 yr	600	400	2500	200	10	30	300	1.0	ND
4–8 yr	900	650	3000	300	15	40	400	1.0	ND
Males									
9–13 yr	1700	1200	4000	600	20	60	600	2.0	ND
14–18 yr	2800	1800	4000	800	30	80	800	3.0	ND
19–30 yr	3000	2000	4000	1000	35	100	1000	3.5	ND
31–50 yr	3000	2000	4000	1000	35	100	1000	3.5	ND
51–70 yr	3000	2000	4000	1000	35	100	1000	3.5	ND
>70 yr	3000	2000	4000	1000	35	100	1000	3.5	ND
Females									
9–13 yr	1700	1200	4000	600	20	60	600	2.0	ND
14–18 yr	2800	1800	4000	800	30	80	800	3.0	ND
19–30 yr	3000	2000	4000	1000	35	100	1000	3.5	ND
31–50 yr	3000	2000	4000	1000	35	100	1000	3.5	ND
51–70 yr	3000	2000	4000	1000	35	100	1000	3.5	ND
>70 yr	3000	2000	4000	1000	35	100	1000	3.5	ND
Pregnancy									
14–18 yr	2800	1800	4000	800	30	80	800	3.0	ND
19–30 yr	3000	2000	4000	1000	35	100	1000	3.5	ND
31–50 yr	3000	2000	4000	1000	35	100	1000	3.5	ND
Lactation									
14–18 yr	2800	1800	4000	800	30	80	800	3.0	ND
19–30 yr	3000	2000	4000	1000	35	100	1000	3.5	ND
31–50 yr	3000	2000	4000	1000	35	100	1000	3.5	ND

Note: A Tolerable Upper Intake Level (UL) is the highest level of daily nutrient intake that is likely to pose no risk of adverse health effects to almost all individuals in the general population. Unless otherwise specified, the UL represents total intake from food, water, and supplements. Because of a lack of suitable data, ULs could not be established for vitamin K, thiamin, riboflavin, vitamin B₁₂, pantothenic acid, biotin, and carotenoids. In the absence of a UL, extra caution may be warranted in consuming levels above recommended intakes. Members of the general population should be advised not to routinely exceed the UL. The UL is not meant to apply to individuals who are treated with the nutrient under medical supervision or to individuals with predisposing conditions that modify their sensitivity to the nutrient.
[a]As preformed vitamin A only.
[b]As α-tocopherol; applies to any form of supplemental α-tocopherol.
[c]The ULs for vitamin E, niacin, and folate apply to synthetic forms obtained from supplements, fortified foods, or a combination of the two.
[d]β-Carotene supplements are advised only to serve as a provitamin A source for individuals at risk of vitamin A deficiency.
ND = Not determinable because of lack of data of adverse effects in this age group and concern with regard to lack of ability to handle excess amounts. Source of intake should be from food only to prevent high levels of intake.
Sources: Dietary Reference Intakes for Calcium, Phosphorus, Magnesium, Vitamin D, and Fluoride (1997); Dietary Reference Intakes for Thiamin, Riboflavin, Niacin, Vitamin B₆, Folate, Vitamin B₁₂, Pantothenic Acid, Biotin, and Choline (1998); Dietary Reference Intakes for Vitamin C, Vitamin E, Selenium, and Carotenoids (2000); Dietary Reference Intakes for Vitamin A, Vitamin K, Arsenic, Boron, Chromium, Copper, Iodine, Iron, Manganese, Molybdenum, Nickel, Silicon, Vanadium, and Zinc (2001); and Dietary Reference Intakes for Calcium and Vitamin D (2011). You may access these reports via www.nap.edu.

Dietary Reference Intakes (DRIs): Tolerable Upper Intake Levels, Minerals
Food and Nutrition Board, Institute of Medicine, National Academies

Life Stage Group	Arsenic[a]	Boron (mg/d)	Calcium (mg/d)	Copper (mcg/d)	Fluoride (mg/d)	Iodine (mcg/d)	Iron (mg/d)	Magnesium (mg/d)[b]	Manganese (mg/d)
Infants									
Birth–6 mo	ND	ND	1000	ND	0.7	ND	40	ND	ND
6–12 mo	ND	ND	1500	ND	0.9	ND	40	ND	ND
Children									
1–3 yr	ND	3	2500	1000	1.3	200	40	65	2
4–8 yr	ND	6	2500	3000	2.2	300	40	110	3
Males									
9–13 yr	ND	11	3000	5000	10	600	40	350	6
14–18 yr	ND	17	3000	8000	10	900	45	350	9
19–30 yr	ND	20	2500	10000	10	1100	45	350	11
31–50 yr	ND	20	2500	10000	10	1100	45	350	11
51–70 yr	ND	20	2000	10000	10	1100	45	350	11
>70 yr	ND	20	2000	10000	10	1100	45	350	11
Females									
9–13 yr	ND	11	3000	5000	10	600	40	350	6
14–18 yr	ND	17	3000	8000	10	900	45	350	9
19–30 yr	ND	20	2500	10000	10	1100	45	350	11
31–50 yr	ND	20	2500	10000	10	1100	45	350	11
51–70 yr	ND	20	2000	10000	10	1100	45	350	11
>70 yr	ND	20	2000	10000	10	1100	45	350	11
Pregnancy									
14–18 yr	ND	17	3000	8000	10	900	45	350	9
19–30 yr	ND	20	2500	10000	10	1100	45	350	11
31–50 yr	ND	20	2500	10000	10	1100	45	350	11
Lactation									
14–18 yr	ND	17	3000	8000	10	900	45	350	9
19–30 yr	ND	20	2500	10000	10	1100	45	350	11
31–50 yr	ND	20	2500	10000	10	1100	45	350	11

Sources: Dietary Reference Intakes for Calcium, Phosphorus, Magnesium, Vitamin D, and Fluoride (1997); Dietary Reference Intakes for Thiamin, Riboflavin, Niacin, Vitamin B_6, Folate, Vitamin B_{12}, Pantothenic Acid, Biotin, and Choline (1998); Dietary Reference Intakes for Vitamin C, Vitamin E, Selenium, and Carotenoids (2000); Dietary Reference Intakes for Vitamin A, Vitamin K, Arsenic, Boron, Chromium, Copper, Iodine, Iron, Manganese, Molybdenum, Nickel, Silicon, Vanadium, and Zinc (2001); Dietary Reference Intakes for Calcium and Vitamin D (2011); and Dietary Reference Intakes for Sodium and Potassium (2019). You may access these reports via www.nap.edu.

NOTE: A Tolerable Upper Intake Level (UL) is the highest level of daily nutrient intake that is likely to pose no risk of adverse health effects to almost all individuals in the general population. Unless otherwise specified, the UL represents total intake from food, water, and supplements. Because of a lack of suitable data, ULs could not be established for all minerals. In the absence of a UL, extra caution may be warranted in consuming levels above recommended intakes. Members of the general population should be advised not to routinely exceed the UL. The UL is not meant to apply to individuals who are treated with the nutrient under medical supervision or to individuals with predisposing conditions that modify their sensitivity to the nutrient.

[a] Although the UL was not determined for arsenic, there is no justification for adding arsenic to food or supplements.

[b] The ULs for magnesium represent intake from a pharmacologic agent only and do not include intake from food and water.

[c] Although silicon has not been shown to cause adverse effects in humans, there is no justification for adding silicon to supplements.

[d] Although vanadium in food has not been shown to cause adverse effects in humans, there is no justification for adding vanadium to food, and vanadium supplements should be used with caution. The UL is based on adverse effects in laboratory animals, and these data could be used to set a UL for adults but not children and adolescents.

[e] There are no ULs established for sodium. However, there are Chronic Disease Risk Reduction Intake levels specific for each sex and age group, as follows: children 1–3 yr, reduce intakes if above 1200 mg/d; children 4–8 yr, reduce intakes if above 1500 mg/d; males and females, 9–13 yr, reduce intakes if above 1800 mg/d; males and females (including pregnant or lactating women), 14+ years, reduce intakes if above 2300 mg/d.

ND = Not determinable because of lack of data of adverse effects in this age group and concern with regard to lack of ability to handle excess amounts. Source of intake should be from food only to prevent high levels of intake.

Molybdenum (mcg/d)	Nickel (mg/d)	Phosphorus (g/d)	Selenium (mcg/d)	Silicon[c]	Vanadium (mg/d)[d]	Zinc (mg/d)	Sodium[e] (g/d)	Chloride (g/d)
ND	ND	ND	45	ND	ND	4	ND	ND
ND	ND	ND	60	ND	ND	5	ND	ND
300	0.2	3	90	ND	ND	7	ND[e]	2.3
600	0.3	3	150	ND	ND	12	ND[e]	2.9
1100	0.6	4	280	ND	ND	23	ND[e]	3.4
1700	1.0	4	400	ND	ND	34	ND[e]	3.6
2000	1.0	4	400	ND	1.8	40	ND[e]	3.6
2000	1.0	4	400	ND	1.8	40	ND[e]	3.6
2000	1.0	4	400	ND	1.8	40	ND[e]	3.6
2000	1.0	3	400	ND	1.8	40	ND[e]	3.6
1100	0.6	4	280	ND	ND	23	ND[e]	3.4
1700	1.0	4	400	ND	ND	34	ND[e]	3.6
2000	1.0	4	400	ND	1.8	40	ND[e]	3.6
2000	1.0	4	400	ND	1.8	40	ND[e]	3.6
2000	1.0	4	400	ND	1.8	40	ND[e]	3.6
2000	1.0	3	400	ND	1.8	40	ND[e]	3.6
1700	1.0	3.5	400	ND	ND	34	ND[e]	3.6
2000	1.0	3.5	400	ND	ND	40	ND[e]	3.6
2000	1.0	3.5	400	ND	ND	40	ND[e]	3.6
1700	1.0	4	400	ND	ND	34	ND[e]	3.6
2000	1.0	4	400	ND	ND	40	ND[e]	3.6
2000	1.0	4	400	ND	ND	40	ND[e]	3.6

Sodium and Potassium Content of Foods, 100 g, Edible Portion

FOOD AND DESCRIPTION	SODIUM (mg)	POTASSIUM (mg)
Bread, Grain, Cereal, and Pasta		
Biscuits, plain or buttermilk, frozen, baked	942	224
Biscuits, mixed grain, refrigerated dough	670	456
Bran cereal	356	661
Bran flakes, wheat cereal	590	564
Bran, raisin and bran flake cereal	356	661
Bread crumbs, dry, grated, plain	732	196
Bread, stuffing, dry mix, prepared	479	67
Breads		
Cracked wheat	538	177
French or Vienna, enriched	602	117
Italian, enriched	618	124
Raisin	347	227
Rye	603	166
White enriched, made with nonfat dry milk	336	111
Whole-wheat, commercially prepared	455	254
Bulgur, cooked	5	68
Corn grits, white, enriched, cooked without salt	2	27
Corn products used mainly as ready-to-eat breakfast cereals		
Corn flakes, sweetened	463	73
Corn flakes, unsweetened	571	107
Corn, puffs	267	—
Bread, cornbread, dry mix, prepared with 2% milk, 80% margarine, and eggs	599	133
Cornmeal, yellow, degermed, enriched, dry form	7	142
Crackers		
Butter (e.g., Ritz)	882	119
Graham, plain	659	177
Saltines	1133	100
Sandwich type, peanut butter filling	801	215
Farina, cereal, enriched, cooked with water and salt	126	23
Macaroni, unenriched, cooked without salt	1	44
Muffins		
Blueberry	417	83
Corn, commercially prepared	385	69
English, wheat	353	186
Noodles, egg, enriched, cooked	5	38
Oats, cereal, regular and quick, unenriched, cooked with water, without salt	4	70
Pancakes, plain, dry mix, complete, prepared	628	175
Popcorn, popped		
Plain, air-popped	8	329
Oil and salt added	764	240
Pretzels. hard, plain, salted	1240	223
Rice, cooked, unsalted		
Brown	4	61
White, long-grain, regular, enriched	1	35
Wild	3	101

FOOD AND DESCRIPTION	SODIUM (mg)	POTASSIUM (mg)
Rice, puffed, fortified, ready-to-eat cereal	3	113
Rolls and buns, commercial, commercially prepared		
Hard rolls, enriched	544	108
Plain (pan rolls), enriched	467	139
Sweet rolls	253	149
Rye wafers, plain	557	495
Spaghetti, enriched, cooked, without salt	1	44
Tapioca, dry	1	11
Waffles, frozen, plain, heated	467	144
Zwieback	227	305
Fruit and Fruit Juice		
Apple juice, canned or bottled, unsweetened	4	101
Apple, raw, with skin	1	107
Applesauce, canned, sweetened, without salt	2	75
Apricot nectar, canned	8	67
Apricot		
Canned, syrup pack, light	4	138
Dried, sulfured, uncooked	10	1162
Raw	1	259
Avocado, raw, all commercial varieties	7	485
Banana, raw	1	358
Blackberries		
Canned, syrup pack, heavy	3	99
Raw	1	162
Blueberries		
Frozen, unsweetened	1	54
Raw	1	77
Boysenberries, frozen, unsweetened	1	139
Cherries		
Canned		
Sour, red, solids and liquid, water pack	7	98
Sweet, solids and liquid, water pack, light	1	131
Frozen, not thawed, sweetened	2	130
Raw, sweet	0	222
Cranberries		
Juice cocktail, bottled	2	14
Raw	2	80
Sauce, sweetened, canned	5	28
Dates, deglet noor	2	656
Figs, raw	1	232
Fruit, cocktail, canned, solids and liquid, juice pack	4	95
Gooseberries, canned, solids and liquid, syrup pack, light	2	77
Grapefruit		
Canned, juice, sweetened	2	162
Raw, pulp, pink, red, white, all varieties	0	135
Grapes, raw, red or green	2	191
Grape juice, canned or bottled, unsweetened	5	104
Guava, whole, raw, common	2	417
Lemon juice, raw	1	103
Lime juice, raw	2	117
Loganberries, frozen	1	145
Melons, cantaloupe, raw	16	267
Nectarine, raw	0	201
Olives, pickled, canned or bottled		
Green	1556	42
Ripe, jumbo super-colossal	735	9
Orange, raw, all commercial varieties	0	181
Orange juice		
Canned, unsweetened	4	184
Frozen concentrate, unsweetened, diluted with three parts water, by volume	4	158
Raw, all commercial varieties	1	200

Continued

FOOD AND DESCRIPTION	SODIUM (mg)	POTASSIUM (mg)
Peach		
Canned, solids and liquid, water pack	3	99
Frozen, sliced, sweetened	6	124
Raw	0	190
Pear		
Canned, solids and liquid, water pack, light	2	53
Raw	1	116
Pineapple		
Frozen chunks, sweetened, not thawed	2	100
Raw, all varieties	1	109
Plum		
Canned, purple, solids and liquid, juice pack	1	154
Raw	0	157
Prunes, dried, uncooked	2	732
Raisins, dark, seedless	26	744
Raspberries		
Frozen, red, sweetened, not thawed	1	114
Raw	1	151
Strawberries		
Frozen, sweetened, sliced	3	98
Raw	1	153
Tangerine, (mandarin oranges), raw	2	166
Watermelon, raw	1	112
Vegetables and Vegetable Juices		
Asparagus		
Canned, canned, no salt added, solids and liquids	26	172
Cooked, boiled, drained	14	224
Frozen, cooked, boiled, drained, without salt	3	172
Beet greens, cooked, boiled, drained, without salt	241	909
Broccoli		
Cooked, boiled, drained, without salt	41	293
Frozen, chopped, cooked, boiled, drained, with salt	260	142
Brussels sprouts, frozen, cooked, boiled, drained, without salt	21	317
Cabbage		
Chinese (pak-choi), cooked, boiled, drained, without salt	34	371
Cooked, boiled, drained, without salt	8	196
Raw	18	170
Red, raw	27	243
Carrots		
Cooked, boiled, drained, without salt	58	235
Raw	69	320
Cauliflower		
Cooked, boiled, drained, without salt	15	142
Raw	30	299
Celery		
Cooked, boiled, drained, without salt	91	284
Raw	80	260
Chard, Swiss, cooked, boiled, drained, without salt	179	549
Chicory, witloof (also called *French* or *Belgian endive*), raw	2	211
Collards, cooked, boiled, drained, without salt	15	117
Corn, sweet yellow		
Canned, cream style, regular pack	261	134
Canned, whole kernel, drained solids	205	132
Cooked, boiled, drained, without salt	1	218
Frozen, kernels cut off cob, cooked, boiled, drained, without salt	1	233
Cress, garden, raw	14	606
Cucumbers, with peel, raw	2	147
Eggplant, cooked, boiled, drained, without salt	1	123
Endive, raw	22	314
Garlic, raw	17	401
Ginger root, raw	13	415
Kale, cooked, boiled, drained, without salt	16	144

FOOD AND DESCRIPTION	SODIUM (mg)	POTASSIUM (mg)
Lettuce		
Arugula, raw	27	369
Butterhead varieties such as Boston and bibb, raw	5	238
Crisphead varieties such as iceberg, raw	10	144
Mushrooms		
Canned, drained solids	425	129
White, raw	5	318
Mustard greens, cooked, boiled, drained, without salt	9	162
Okra		
Cooked, boiled, drained, without salt	6	135
Raw	7	299
Onions		
Raw	4	146
Spring or scallions (including tops and bulb), raw	16	276
Parsnips, cooked, boiled, drained, without salt	10	367
Peppers		
Hot, chili, red, raw	9	322
Sweet, green, raw	3	175
Pickles, cucumber, dill	809	117
Potatoes		
Sweet, boiled, in skin, flesh, without salt	4	379
Sweet, canned, mashed	75	210
White, cooked, boiled in skin, without salt	4	379
White, dehydrated, mashed, flakes, prepared without milk	164	164
Pumpkin		
Canned	241	206
Cooked, boiled, drained, without salt	1	230
Radishes, raw	39	233
Rhubarb, frozen, cooked with sugar	1	96
Rutabagas, cooked, boiled, drained, without salt	5	216
Sauerkraut, canned, solids and liquid	661	170
Spinach		
Canned, regular pack, drained solids	322	346
Cooked, boiled, drained, without salt	70	466
Frozen, chopped, cooked, boiled, drained, without salt	97	302
Squash		
Summer, all varieties, cooked, boiled, drained, without salt	1	192
Winter, acorn, cooked, baked, without salt	4	437
Winter, spaghetti, cooked, baked, drained, without salt	18	117
Tomato juice, canned or bottled, with salt	253	217
Tomato puree, canned		
With salt added	202	439
Without salt added	28	439
Tomatoes, ripe		
Red, canned, solids and liquid, packed in juice	115	191
Red, raw, year round average	5	237
Turnips, cooked, boiled, drained, without salt	16	177
Turnip greens, cooked, boiled, drained, without salt	29	203
Watercress, raw	41	330
Nuts, Seeds, Peas, and Legumes		
Almonds		
Dry roasted with salt added	234	713
Dry roasted without salt	4	363
Beans, mature seeds		
Red, cooked, boiled, without salt	2	403
White, canned	340	454
White, cooked, boiled, without salt	2	463
Beans, lima, immature seeds		
Canned, solids and liquids	252	285
Cooked, boiled, drained, without salt	17	570
Frozen, cooked, boiled, drained, without salt	69	304

Continued

FOOD AND DESCRIPTION	SODIUM (mg)	POTASSIUM (mg)
Beans, mung, sprouted seeds, cooked, boiled, with salt	238	266
Beans, snap		
Green, canned, regular pack, solids and liquids	192	92
Green, cooked, boiled, drained, without salt	1	146
Green, frozen, cooked, boiled, drained, without salt	1	159
Green, raw	6	211
Yellow, canned, regular pack, solids and liquids		
Yellow, frozen, cooked, boiled, drained, without salt	9	126
Yellow or wax, cooked, boiled, drained, without salt	3	299
Brazil nuts, dried, unblanched	3	659
Cashews, dry roasted, without salt	16	565
Coconut meat, raw	20	356
Cowpeas, including black-eyed peas		
Common, mature seeds, canned, plain	293	172
Immature seeds, cooked, boiled, drained, without salt	4	418
Macadamia nuts, raw	5	368
Peanut butter made with salt	426	558
Peanuts		
Dry roasted without salt	6	634
Oil roasted with salt	320	726
Peas, green		
Cooked, boiled, drained, without salt	3	271
Frozen, cooked, boiled, drained, with salt	323	110
Raw	5	244
Peas and carrots, frozen, cooked, boiled, drained, with salt	304	158
Pecans	0	410
Sunflower seeds, dry-roasted, without salt	3	850
Walnuts		
Black, dried	2	523
Persian or English	2	441
Dairy and Dairy Substitutes		
Buttermilk, liquid, whole	105	135
Cheeses		
Natural cheeses		
Cheddar	653	76
Cottage (large or small curd)	315	104
Cream	314	132
Parmesan, shredded	1696	97
Swiss	187	72
Pasteurized processed cheese, American	1671	132
Pasteurized processed cheese spread, American	1625	242
Cream, liquid, light, coffee or table	72	136
Cream substitutes, powered	124	669
Milk, cow		
Canned, evaporated	106	303
Dry, whole	371	1330
Liquid (pasteurized and raw)		
Skim	52	166
Whole, 3.7% fat	43	132
Yogurt, plain, whole milk	46	155
Beef, Lamb, Pork, and Meat Products		
Beef		
Cured, corned beef, canned	897	136
Hamburger, regular ground, cooked	85	353
Liver, cooked, pan-fried	77	351
Rib eye steak, trimmed to ⅛ th inch fat, grilled	59	296
Round, top round, trimmed to ⅛ th inch fat, braised	45	319
Lamb		
Ground, cooked, broiled	81	339
New Zealand, neck chops, cooked, braised	91	276

FOOD AND DESCRIPTION	SODIUM (mg)	POTASSIUM (mg)
Pork		
Bacon		
Canadian, cooked, pan-fried	993	999
Cured, cooked, baked	2193	539
Ham, cured, whole, roasted	1327	316
Loin chops, cooked, broiled	55	344
Salt pork, cured, raw	2684	66
Sausage, cold cuts, and luncheon meats		
Bologna, beef and pork	960	315
Frankfurters, meat, heated	1013	141
Luncheon meat, pork with ham, minced, canned, includes Spam	1411	409
Pork sausage, links/patty, cooked, pan-fried	814	342
Veal, loin, cooked, braised	80	280
Poultry		
Chicken		
Broilers or fryers, dark meat, including skin, cooked, roasted	87	220
Broilers or fryers, light meat, including skin, cooked, roasted	75	227
Broilers or fryers, leg, including skin, battered, cooked, fried,	279	189
Gizzard, chicken, all classes, cooked, simmered	56	179
Duck, domesticated, meat only, cooked, roasted	65	252
Eggs, chicken		
Whole, cooked, scrambled	145	132
Whites, fresh, raw	166	163
Yolks, fresh, raw	48	109
Goose, domesticated, meat only, cooked, roasted	76	388
Turkey		
Whole, light meat, including skin, cooked, roasted	101	248
Whole, light and dark meat, including skin, cooked, roasted	116	242
Fish and Seafood		
Bass, striped, cooked, dry heat	88	328
Bluefish, cooked, dry heat	77	477
Carp, cooked, dry heat	63	427
Catfish, wild, cooked, dry heat	50	419
Caviar, black and red, granular	1500	181
Clams, mixed species		
Canned, drained solids	112	628
Cooked, breaded and fried	364	326
Raw	601	46
Cod, Pacific, cooked	134	372
Crab		
Alaska king, cooked, moist heat	1072	262
Blue, cooked, moist heat	395	259
Croaker, Atlantic, cooked, breaded and fried	348	340
Flat fish (flounder and sole species), cooked, dry heat	363	197
Haddock, cooked, dry heat	261	351
Halibut, Atlantic and Pacific, cooked, dry heat	82	528
Herring, Pacific, cooked, dry heat	95	542
Lobster		
Northern, cooked, moist heat	486	230
Spiny, mixed species, cooked, moist heat	227	208
Mussels, blue, cooked, moist heat	369	268
Ocean perch, Atlantic, cooked, dry heat	347	226
Oysters		
Eastern, wild, cooked, moist heat	166	139
Eastern, wild, raw	85	156
Perch, mixed species, cooked, dry heat	79	344
Pike, walleye, cooked, dry heat	65	499

Continued

FOOD AND DESCRIPTION	SODIUM (mg)	POTASSIUM (mg)
Rockfish, Pacific, mixed species, cooked, dry heat	89	467
Roe, mixed species, raw	91	221
Salmon		
Chinook, smoked	672	175
Coho, wild, cooked, moist heat	53	455
Sockeye, cooked, dry heat	92	436
Sardines		
Atlantic, canned in oil, drained solids	307	397
Pacific, canned in tomato sauce, drained solids	414	341
Scallops, bay and sea, cooked, steamed	667	314
Sea bass, mixed species, cooked, dry heat	87	328
Sturgeon, mixed species, cooked, dry heat	69	364
Tuna		
Light, canned in oil, drained solids	416	207
Light, canned in water, drained solids	247	179
Yellowfin, cooked, dry heat	54	527
Fats and Oils		
Butter		
Salted	643	24
Unsalted	11	24
Margarine, regular, soybean	943	42
Oils (canola, coconut, olive)	0	0
Dressings, Sauces, Gravy, and Seasonings		
Bouillon, beef, powder, dry	26000	446
Horseradish, prepared	420	246
Mayonnaise, regular	635	20
Mustard, prepared, yellow	1104	152
Salad dressings, commercial		
Bleu or Roquefort cheese, regular	642	88
Caesar, regular	1209	29
French, regular	661	108
Italian, regular	993	84
Thousand Island	962	107
Soy sauce, made from soy and wheat, regular	5493	435
Tartar sauce, regular	667	68
Tomato catsup, regular	907	281
Vinegar, cider	5	73
Sweets, Sweetened Beverages, Desserts		
Cakes, commercially prepared		
Angel food	749	93
Boston cream pie	254	39
Cheesecake	438	90
Coffeecake, crème-filled with chocolate frosting	323	78
Gingerbread	327	439
Snack cake, crème-filled, chocolate with frosting	332	176
White, prepared without frosting	327	95
Candy		
Caramels	245	214
Chocolate, sweet	6	2901
Chocolate fudge	45	134
Gum drops, starch jelly pieces	44	5
Hard	38	5
Marshmallows	80	5
Peanut bars	156	407
Chocolate		
Drink, liquid, milk and soy based	63	245
Hot cocoa mix	850	0
Syrup, fudge type	346	284
Unsweetened squares	24	830

FOOD AND DESCRIPTION	SODIUM (mg)	POTASSIUM (mg)
Coconut cream (liquid expressed from grated coconut meat)	4	325
Cookies		
Butter, commercially prepared	282	111
Chocolate chip, refrigerated dough, baked	232	200
Fortune	31	41
Gingersnaps	555	346
Molasses	459	346
Oatmeal with raisins	322	230
Peanut butter, commercially prepared	336	107
Vanilla wafer, lower fat	388	97
Cream puffs, éclair, with custard or cream filling	265	68
Custard, egg, baked	61	148
Doughnuts, cake type, plain, sugared or glazed	402	102
Honey	4	52
Ice cream		
Chocolate	76	249
Vanilla	80	199
Ice cream cone, cake or wafer-type	256	112
Jams and preserves	32	77
Molasses	37	1464
Pie crust, made with enriched flour, baked	467	114
Pies, baked, pie crust made with unenriched flour		
Apple	201	65
Cherry	246	81
Pecan	275	99
Pumpkin	239	167
Pudding mixes and puddings made from mixes		
Banana, prepared with 2% milk	296	131
Tapioca	120	131
Vanilla, prepared with whole milk	286	128
Sugar		
Cane	58	63
Brown	28	133
Tea, black, sweetened	3	14
Mixed Dishes, Fast Food, Soups		
Beans and frankfurters, canned, prepared with equal volume water	437	191
Beef potpie, commercial, frozen, prepared	365	115
Beef stew, canned entrée	388	163
Biscuit and sausage, fast food	814	153
Burrito		
Bean and cheese, frozen entrée	351	210
Beef and bean, frozen entrée	587	221
Fast food, with beans, cheese, and beef	451	204
Cheeseburger, fast food, double, large patty, with condiments, lettuce, and tomato	405	202
Chicken potpie, commercial, frozen, prepared	393	110
Chicken sandwich, fast food, grilled, with bacon, tomato, lettuce, cheese, and mayonnaise	630	226
Chili, no beans, canned entrée	411	185
Chili con carne with beans, canned entrée	449	264
Croissant, fast food, with egg, cheese, and ham	711	179
Fish sandwich, fast food, with tartar sauce and cheese	434	220
Lasagna with meat and sauce, frozen entrée, prepared	347	184
Macaroni and cheese, boxed, prepared	460	80
Nachos, fast food, with cheese	313	362
Pizza		
Fast food pizza chain, sausage topping, thick crust	637	190
Frozen, cheese topping, regular crust, cooked	447	152
Ravioli, cheese and tomato sauce, frozen	280	233
Rice bowl with chicken, frozen entrée, prepared (includes fried, teriyaki, and sweet and sour varieties)	333	123

Continued

FOOD AND DESCRIPTION	SODIUM (mg)	POTASSIUM (mg)
Soups, commercial, canned		
Beef broth, bouillon, and consommé, prepared with an equal volume of water	264	64
Chicken noodle, prepared with an equal volume of water	335	24
Tomato, prepared with an equal volume of water	186	275
Vegetable beef, prepared with an equal volume of water	349	69
Spaghetti, with meatballs in tomato sauce, canned	280	217
Submarine sandwich, fast food, with cold cuts, lettuce, and tomato on white bread	575	282
Taco		
Fast food, with beef, cheese, and lettuce, hard shell	397	209
Fast food, with chicken, cheese, and lettuce, soft shell	613	217
Turkey and gravy, frozen entrée	554	61

Source: United States Department of Agriculture and Agricultural Research Service (2019). *USDA Food Composition Databases*. Retrieved August 31, 2019, from https://ndb.nal.usda.gov.

Index

Note: Page numbers followed by "f" indicate figures "t" indicate tables and "b" indicate boxes.